MODERN PERSPECTIVES IN PSYCHIATRY
Edited by John G. Howells

3

MODERN PERSPECTIVES IN INTERNATIONAL CHILD PSYCHIATRY

MODERN PERSPECTIVES IN PSYCHIATRY
Edited by John G. Howells

1. Modern Perspectives in Child Psychiatry (2nd ed. 1967)
2. Modern Perspectives in World Psychiatry (1968), Introduced by Lord Adrian, O.M.
3. Modern Perspectives in International Child Psychiatry (1969), Introduced by Leo Kanner, M.D.

IN PREPARATION

4. Modern Perspectives in Adolescent Psychiatry
5. Modern Perspectives in Psycho-Obstetrics

MODERN PERSPECTIVES IN INTERNATIONAL CHILD PSYCHIATRY

Edited by
JOHN G. HOWELLS
M.D., D.P.M.

Director, The Institute of Family Psychiatry
Ipswich and East Suffolk Hospital
England

Introduced by
LEO KANNER
M.D.

OLIVER & BOYD · EDINBURGH

OLIVER AND BOYD LTD

Tweeddale Court
Edinburgh 1

First Published 1969

© 1969, Oliver & Boyd Ltd

05 001819 1

Printed in Great Britain by
T. & A. Constable Ltd., Hopetoun Street, Edinburgh

EDITOR'S FOREWORD

Each volume in 'Modern Perspectives in Psychiatry' aims to bring the facts from the growing points in a particular field of psychiatry to the clinician at as early a stage as possible. Thus, a single volume in this Series is not a textbook; a psychiatric textbook has the double disadvantage of rapidly becoming out of date and of restricting to one, or at best to a few, authors the coverage of a field as large as psychiatry. However, the eventual scope of the volumes in the whole Series is such as to constitute a complete international system in the theory and practice of psychiatry.

Contributions likely to be significant in the development of international psychiatry are selected from all over the world. It is hoped that the Series will be a factor in effecting integration of world psychiatry and that it will supply a forum for the expression of creative opinion wherever it may arise.

The present volume has benefited from the contributions of authorities from Canada, France, Germany, Israel, Italy, Japan, Sweden, the United Kingdom, the Union of Soviet Socialist Republics and the United States of America. Each chapter is written by an acknowledged expert, often the leading authority in his field. He was entrusted with the task of selecting, appraising and explaining his special subject for the benefit of colleagues who may be less well acquainted with it. Each chapter is not an exhaustive review of the literature on the subject, but contains what the contributor regards as relevant to clinical practice in that field. The volume will be valuable to the psychiatrist in training. The place of the Series as an indispensable reference source is assured by the appearance of a cumulative index in each volume.

Volumes in 'Modern Perspectives in Psychiatry' are complementary. Readers of this volume will find interest in the already published volume 1, *Modern Perspectives in Child Psychiatry*. That volume gave special attention to the scientific basis of child psychiatry, while the present volume gives the same attention to psychopathology; both books, in addition, have contributions in clinical psychiatry. Together, they make an unrivalled source book of child psychiatry.

Volume 2, *Modern Perspectives in World Psychiatry*, also contains material relevant to child psychiatry. This volume is to be followed by *Modern Perspectives in Psycho-Obstetrics* and *Modern Perspectives in Adolescent Psychiatry*; both are of special interest to the child psychiatrist.

The list of contents of the volumes already published will be found at the back of this volume.

The Editor has pleasure again in acknowledging the thoughtful, careful, inexhaustible effort of his editorial assistant, Mrs Maria-Livia Osborn. The valuable cumulative indices are also her work.

Grateful acknowledgement is also made to the following publishers and editors of journals, and to the authors concerned, for kind permission to reproduce the material mentioned: Dr Leo Kanner's introduction is based on his Maudsley Lecture reprinted from the *Journal of Mental Science*, 1959, **105**, 581; *Rivista Sperimentale di Freniatria*, 1908, **32**, for the paper by Professor de Sanctis; *Journal of Nervous and Mental Diseases*, 1954, **119**, for the paper by Theordor Heller; *Nervous Child*, 1943, **2**, for the paper by Dr Kanner; The Prado Museum, Madrid, Ch. V, Fig. 1; Barnard's Studios, Ltd., Ch. V. Fig. 2; Methuen, London, and N. Tinbergen, Ch. V, Fig. 3 (from *Social Behaviour in Animals*); Andre Deutsch, and L. Williams, Ch. V, Fig. 4 (from *Man and Monkey*); Churchill, London, and R. W. B. Ellis, Ch. V, Fig. 5 (from *Child Health and Development*, 1966); Paul Popper Ltd. Ch. V, Fig. 6; Bodleian Library, Oxford, Ch. V, Fig. 8; N.S.P.C.C. Ch. IX, Figs. 1 and 2.

CONTENTS

EDITOR'S FOREWORD v

INTRODUCTION, Trends in Child Psychiatry, *Leo Kanner* 1

* * *

Part One

PSYCHOPATHOLOGY

I THE CHILD'S HAZARDS *IN UTERO* . . *D. H. STOTT*
    1. The Folklore 19
    2. The Zoological Breakthrough 20
        Virus Infections 20
        Other Infections 23
    3. Emotional Stress 27
    4. Mental Retardation 37
    5. Infantile Ill-health 39
    6. Malformation 41
    7. Behaviour-disturbance 42
    8. Cleft Lip and Palate 45
    9. Mongolism 47
  10. Drugs as Teratogens 50
  11. Research Perspectives 53

II GENESIS OF BEHAVIOUR DISORDERS . *STELLA CHESS*
    1. Theories of Child Development 61
    2. Problems of Retrospective Investigation ... 62
    3. Selectivity of Child's Responses to Pathogenic Influence ... 65
    4. Anterospective Longitudinal Studies of Child Development ... 66
    5. Temperamental Individuality 68
    6. Temperamental Clusters 69
    7. Temperament-environment Interaction ... 70
    8. Selectivity of Stress 70
    9. Temperament in Brain-damaged Children ... 74
  10. Parental Effectiveness 75
  11. Temperament in Mentally Retarded Children ... 76
  12. Child Care Practices 77
  13. Role of Anxiety 77
  14. Summary 78

CONTENTS

III MOTHER-INFANT RELATIONS AT BIRTH . . . . . PETER H. WOLFF

1. INTRODUCTION 80
    Related Studies 81
2. THE OBSERVATIONS 84
    The Mother's Concerns Before Labour 85
    The Events During Labour and Delivery 86
    The First Interaction After Birth 88
    The Evolution of the Interaction 89
    The Return Home 93
    The Infant's Contribution to the Interaction 93
    Summary and Conclusions 95

IV MOTHER-CHILD RELATIONSHIP   MYRIAM DAVID & GENEVIEVE APPELL

1. INTRODUCTION 98
2. MOTHER-CHILD INTERACTION 99
3. CASE STUDIES 100
    Molly A 100
    Bob B 102
    Louise C 103
    Lewis D 104
    Frank E 105
4. DISCUSSION OF INTERACTION AT AGE ONE 106
    Interaction per se 106
    Content of Interaction 108
5. INTERACTION AND RELATIONSHIP 111
    Quantity of Interaction in Relation to Space 111
    Form of Interaction in Relation to Closeness/Distance in Relationship 112
    Situation, and Modes of Interaction in Relation to Maturity Level 113
    Tonality of Interaction and in Relation to Intensity and Quality of Investment 113
    Areas of Interaction and Emotional Content of Relationship 113
    Evolution of the Pattern of Interaction 114
6. EMOTIONAL CONTENT OF INTERACTION: ITS IMPACT ON THE CHILD'S DEVELOPMENT 115
7. SUMMARY 120

V FATHERING . . . . . . JOHN G. HOWELLS

1. INTRODUCTION 125
2. THE ANIMAL KINGDOM 127
    Diverse Parental Care 128
    Care by Father 130
    Care of the Young in other Anthropoids 131
    Summary 132
3. ANTHROPOLOGY 133
    The Family 133
    Parenting 136
    Fathering 136
    Summary 138
4. FATHERING IN CONTEMPORARY SOCIETY 138
    National Practices 139

The Absence of Father	140
Father and Child Development	141
The Role of Father	142
Father Participation	143
Summary	144
5. FATHERING AND PSYCHIATRY	144
Neuroses	144
Delinquency	145
Sex Role Identity	146
Treatment	146
Psychosis	146
Clinical Practice	147
Summary	148
6. CONCLUSION	148

VI THE CHILD'S NEEDS FOR HIS EMOTIONAL HEALTH . . . . S. A. SZUREK

1. INTRODUCTION	157
2. THE NEEDS OF THE NEWBORN	158
The First Smile	161
Developmental Deviations	161
3. REMAINDER OF THE FIRST YEAR OF LIFE	162
Sucking	163
Elimination	164
Emotional Needs after the Fourth Month	164
4. THE VIEWS OF SPITZ	168
Coma in the Newborn	170
Three Months Colic	171
Infantile Eczema	171
Rocking	172
Fecal Play and Coprophagia	173
The Hyperthermic Child	174
Emotional Deficiency Diseases	174
Appendix by *W. G. Cobliner*	176
5. THE NEEDS OF THE TODDLER AND THE YOUNG CHILD	177
Tendency to Regression	179
Sexual Interests and Sensuality	179
Aggressive Assertiveness	182
The Beginnings of a Sense of Self	185
Deviations in Development	187
Development of Character Traits	189
Learning to Love	191
6. THE NEEDS OF THE CHILD FROM SIX TO TWELVE—LATENCY	192
The Latency Child's Need for Continued Firm Parental Guidance	195
7. SUMMARY	198

VII DEVELOPMENTS IN PSYCHOANALYTIC THEORY AS APPLIED TO CHILDREN . S. LEBOVICI

1. INTRODUCTION	200
2. OBJECT RELATIONS IN CHILDREN	201
Early Precursors of the Object: the Smile	204
Recognition of the Object and Anxiety at Eight Months	206
The Origins and Beginnings of Semantic Communication	207

CONTENTS

    3. CHILD FANTASIES   210
    4. RECENT PSYCHOANALYTICAL STUDIES OF CHILD DEVELOPMENT   215
    5. CONCLUSION   218

VIII SOME RECENT DEVELOPMENTS IN CHILD PSYCHOANALYSIS AT THE HAMPSTEAD CLINIC . . . *JOSEPH SANDLER & JACK NOVICK*

    1. HISTORICAL DEVELOPMENT   221
    2. THE CLINIC   223
        Clinical Services   223
        Preventive and Educational Services   224
        Research Projects and Study Groups   225
        Community Education   229
    3. REVIEW OF CLINIC PUBLICATIONS   230
        General Studies of Normal and Abnormal Development   230
        Specific Studies of Abnormal Development   236
        Studies from the Hampstead Index   245

IX SEPARATION AND DEPRIVATION   *JOHN G. HOWELLS*

    1. INTRODUCTION   254
        Contemporary Child Care   255
    2. A DIRECT INVESTIGATION ON SEPARATION   258
        General   258
        Incidence of Separation   258
        The Effects of Separation Experiences   267
        Causes of Separation   273
        Care of the Child during Separations   276
        Summary of Whole Investigation   278
    3. ADDITIONAL STUDIES ON SEPARATION   279
    4. PARENT–CHILD SEPARATION AS A THERAPEUTIC PROCEDURE   284
        Family Psychiatry   285
        Vector Therapy   286
        Therapeutic Uses of Separation   287
    5. CONCLUSION   289

X CULTURE AND CHILD REARING   . *MARVIN K. OPLER*

    1. INTRODUCTION   292
    2. NEO-FREUDIAN INFLUENCES   297
    3. CULTURAL FACTORS   304
    4. SUMMARY   317

XI CHILD REARING IN THE KIBBUTZ .   . *LOUIS MILLER*

    The Kibbutz Community   321
    The Kibbutz Family   322
    Collective Child Care and Education   323
    The Child and the Metapelet   324
    The Child and his Peer Group   326
    The Child and his Parents   330
    The Child and the Kibbutz Community   331
    'Familistic' Trends on the Kibbutz   332
    Theory of Kibbutz Education   334
    The Adolescent on the Kibbutz   336
    The Study of the Kibbutz-reared Child   339

CONTENTS

XII PARENTAL ATTITUDE AND FAMILY DYNAMICS ON CHILDRENS' PROBLEMS IN JAPAN . . . KIYOSHI MAKITA & KEIGO OKONOGI
  1. INTRODUCTION — 347
  2. GENERAL CONSIDERATION ON THE PARENTAL ATTITUDE AND ITS RESPONSE — 348
  3. DETERMINANTS OF PARENTAL ATTITUDE IN JAPAN — 350
     Over Protection — 351
     Rejection — 354
     Perfectionism — 355
  4. DETERMINANTS OF FAMILY DYNAMICS IN JAPAN — 356
     Method of the Study — 357
     Partial Results of the Family Study — 361
     The Pre-War Autocratic Family Pattern — 362
     The Post-War Modernized Family — 365
  5. SUMMARY — 368

PART TWO

CLINICAL

XIII TRENDS IN THE INVESTIGATION OF CLINICAL PROBLEMS IN CHILD PSYCHIATRY . G. K. USHAKOV
  1. HISTORICAL INTRODUCTION — 375
  2. PSYCHIATRIC RESEARCH BY COMPARISON-BY-AGE-GROUP METHOD — 378
     As Applied to Psychosis — 378
     As Applied to Neurosis — 379
  3. COMPARISON-BY-AGE-GROUP METHOD OF SYMPTOMS AND SYNDROMES — 380
  4. PROBLEMS IN THE ANALYSIS OF CLINICAL SYNDROMES — 382
  5. INVESTIGATION OF THE PROCESSES OF COMPENSATION AND CORRECTION OF DISORDERS — 385
  6. MAIN METHODS OF CLINICAL INVESTIGATION — 387

XIV THE DEVELOPMENT OF ELECTROCEREBRAL ACTIVITY IN CHILDREN . . . W. GREY WALTER
  1. INTRODUCTION — 391
     Problems Encountered in Obtaining EEGs in Young Children — 391
     Interpretation of Intrinsic Rhythms — 392
     Application of Telemetry — 393
     Abnormalities in the EEG — 393
     Origin and Functions of Intrinsic Rhythms — 395
     Techniques for Detecting Evoked Responses — 396
     Features of Evoked Responses — 397
     Contingent Negative Variation — 399
     Origin and Functions of the CNV — 401

CONTENTS

2. Evoked Responses and CNV in Children — 402
   Subject Material — 402
   Clinical and EEG Features — 402
   Autonomic Variables — 403
3. Cerebral Responsiveness in Normal Children — 404
4. Cerebral Responsiveness in Disturbed Children — 407
5. Recent Developments — 408
6. Cerebral Responsiveness in Organic Disorders — 410
   Recovery from Encephalitis — 411
7. Relation between Electrocerebral and Psychosocial Development — 413

XV SLEEP DISTURBANCES IN CHILDREN . . . . . MELITTA SPERLING

1. Introduction — 418
2. General Remarks — 419
3. Sleep Disturbances in Infancy — 420
   The Oral Phase of Development of the Child During the First Year of Life — 420
4. The Role of the Mother-child Relationship in the Genesis of Infantile Sleep Disturbance and the Role of Infantile Sleep Disturbance in the Etiology of Severe Emotional Disturbance in Childhood — 423
5. Sleep Disturbances During the Anal Phase of Development between Ages One to Three — 426
   Management — 427
6. Sleep Disturbances During the Oedipal Phase between Three and Five Years — 428
7. Sleepwalking (Somnambulism) and Allied Phenomena and their Relation to Neurotic Insomnia — 430
   Typical Fears Associated with the Sleep Disturbances of the Oedipal Phase and Some Remarks on Management — 436
8. Pavor Nocturnus — 440
   Nocturnal Psychosomatic Symptoms, Enuresis and Soiling — 450
   Sleep Phobias, Sleep Rituals, Habitual Waking up — 451

XVI PICA   REGINALD S. LOURIE & FRANCIS K. MILLICAN

1. Introduction — 455
2. Psychiatric Study — 456
3. Children's Hospital Research Study of Children with Pica — 456
   Subjects and Methods — 456
4. Illustrative Cases — 457
   Family A — 457
   Family B — 459
   Family C — 461
5. Results of the Research and Implications — 462
   Constitutional Factors — 462
   Environmental Factors — 462
   Nutritional Factors — 464
   Psychodynamic Factors — 464
   Psychopathology Accompanying Pica — 465
   Relationship of Pica to Addiction — 467

CONTENTS xiii

6. OUTPATIENT TREATMENT OF PICA 467
   Medical Evaluation 467
7. PREVENTIVE MEASURES 469

XVII PEPTIC ULCERS IN CHILDREN . *THOMAS P. MILLAR*
1. INTRODUCTION 471
2. INCIDENCE 471
3. DIAGNOSIS 472
4. PSYCHOPATHOLOGY: CLINICAL REPORTS 472
5. THEORETICAL MODELS 474
6. GASTRIC FUNCTION AND PEPTIC ULCER 475
7. CLINICAL OBSERVATIONS 476
   Presenting Problems 476
   Adjustment Problems 476
   Family History 477
   Developmental History 478
   The Child 479
   Recapitulation 481
8. DYNAMIC FORMULATION 481
   Intolerance for Delay 482
   Egocentricity 483
   Omnipotence and Autonomy 483
   Impaired Self-Esteem 484
   Peptic Ulcers in Children: a Tentative Formulation 485
9. TREATMENT CONSIDERATIONS 486
   The Acute Phase 487
   Promoting the Adaptive Maturity of the Child 488
10. CONCLUSION 492

XVIII THE MANAGEMENT OF ULCERATIVE COLITIS
       IN CHILDHOOD . *DANE G. PRUGH & KENT JORDAN*
1. INTRODUCTION 494
2. EPIDEMIOLOGIC ASPECTS 495
3. PATHOLOGY OF THE BOWEL 495
4. SOMATIC CLINICAL PICTURE 495
5. PSYCHOSOCIAL OBSERVATIONS 496
6. PSYCHOPHYSIOLOGIC INTERRELATIONSHIPS 498
7. MULTIPLE ETIOLOGIC CONSIDERATIONS 499
8. MANAGEMENT AND THERAPY 500
   Medical Aspects 501
   Surgical Aspects 506
   Formal Psychotherapeutic Aspects 510
   Specific Therapeutic Considerations 515
   Other Psychotherapeutic Approaches 520
   A Comprehensive Approach to Treatment 521
9. PREVENTION 524
10. SUMMARY 524

XIX PSYCHOGENIC RETARDATION . *ANDREW CROWCROFT*
1. INTRODUCTION 531
2. SEVERE SUBNORMALITY 532
3. WASTAGE OF ABILITY 533

CONTENTS

4. Cultural Deprivation		534
Maternal Deprivation		536
5. Language, Learning and Culture		537
6. Family Studies		538
7. Individual Studies		540
8. Ego Theories—the Vulnerability Factor		541
9. Conclusion		544

XX DEVELOPMENT AND BREAKDOWN OF SPEECH . . . . *MOYRA WILLIAMS*

1. Introduction	547
2. Development of Speech in Normal Children	549
Pre-linguistic Utterances	549
Early Linguistic Utterances	550
3. Development of Speech in the Deaf and Hard of Hearing	554
4. Development of Speech in Subnormal Children	555
5. Development of Speech in Psychotic Children	557
6. Development of Speech in Aphasic Children	559
Comparison between the Aquisition of Speech by Children and Adults	560
7. The Breakdown of Language Associated with Cerebral Lesions	560
8. The Breakdown of Language in Senile Dementia	563
9. The Breakdown of Speech in Schizophrenics	564

XXI DYSFUNCTIONS OF PARENTING: THE BATTERED CHILD, THE NEGLECTED CHILD, THE EXPLOITED CHILD . . . *RICHARD GALDSTON*

1. Introduction	571
2. The Battered Child	572
Definition	572
Description	572
Parents	573
3. The Neglected Child	575
Definition	575
Description	575
Parents	577
4. The Exploited Child	579
Definition	579
Description	580
Parents	582
5. Summary	584

XXII THREE HISTORIC PAPERS 589

1. On some Varieties of Dementia Præcox, *Sante de Sanctis*	590
Introductory Note by the Editor	590
Introduction	590
Premonitory Signs	605
Conclusion	605
2. About Dementia Infantilis, *Theodor Heller*	610
Introductory Remarks by the Translator	610

3. AUTISTIC DISTURBANCES OF AFFECTIVE CONTACT, *Leo Kanner* 617
   Discussion 639
   Comment 646

XXIII THE NATURE OF CHILDHOOD PSYCHOSIS . . . . . *LAURETTA BENDER*
1. DEFINITION 649
2. HISTORICAL NOTES 651
3. REVIEW: CHILDHOOD PSYCHOSIS, UNITED STATES, TO 1956 653
   Introduction 653
   Childhood Schizophrenia: Lauretta Bender and Associates 653
   Paul Schilder's Contributions 655
   Leo Kanner's Syndrome: Early Infantile Autism 656
   Margaret Mahler's Symbiotic Psychosis 658
   Children with Atypical Development: Beata Rank and Co-workers 658
   Emotional Deprivation 659
   Ego Psychology and Psychoanalysis 660
4. MODERN PERSPECTIVES IN CHILDHOOD PSYCHOSIS, 1956–66 661
   Organic Factors Emphasized in the United States 661
   Recent United States Books on Childhood Psychosis 662
   New York Contributions: Lauretta Bender and Associates 667
   Autonomic Nervous System and Childhood Psychosis 669
   Schizophrenic Infants: Barbara Fish 669
   Biochemical Studies: Siva Sankar 670
   Psychological Studies 671
   Language of Schizophrenic Children 671
   Summary of United States Studies: Paul Hoch 672
   British Studies in Child Psychosis 672
   Childhood Psychoses in Western Europe 674
   Childhood Psychoses in Eastern Europe 675
   Childhood Psychoses in Japan 675
   Israel 676
   India 678

XXIV THERAPEUTIC MANAGEMENT OF SCHIZOPHRENIC CHILDREN . . . . . *WILLIAM GOLDFARB*
1. INTRODUCTION 685
2. CORRECTIVE SOCIALIZATION 688
   Diagnosis of Childhood Schizophrenia 688
   Adaptive Deficiencies of Schizophrenic Children 689
   Causal Factors 691
   Treatment Objectives 692
   The Therapeutic Environment 692
   Professional Coordination 695
   Chemotherapy 696
   Milieu Therapy 698
   Individual Therapy 698
   Family Treatment 701
3. COMMUNITY PLANNING 703
   Preferred Size of Treatment Unit 703
   Duration of Treatment 703
   Variety of Services 703

CONTENTS

XXV ACUTE ORGANIC PSYCHOSES OF CHILDHOOD . . . . . *G. BOLLEA*
1. INTRODUCTION 706
2. AETIOLOGY 709
   Introduction 709
   Cerebral Causes 710
   Extra-cerebral Causes 712
   Physical Agents 715
3. SYMPTOMATOLOGY 716
   Disorders of Consciousness 718
   Disorders of Ego Awareness 725
   Psychosensory Disorders 726
   Thought Disorders 727
   Affective Disorders 728
   Psycho-motor Disorders 729
   Behaviour Disorders 730
4. CONCLUSION 731

XXVI THE CHILD AT SCHOOL . . *JOHN C. GLIDEWELL*
1. THE PSYCHO-SOCIAL CONTEXT OF LIFE AT SCHOOL 733
   The Development of Classroom Social Structure 733
   The Components of Social Structure in the Classroom 734
   Dimensions of Social Structure in the Classroom 735
   Teacher Power and Its Use 735
   Stress at School 736
   Summary 738
2. MANIFESTATIONS OF DISTRESS AT SCHOOL 739
   The Search for Syndromes 739
   Identification of Emotional Problems 740
   Prevalence and Incidence 741
3. ANTECEDENTS OF DISTRESS AT SCHOOL 743
   Constitution and Temperament 743
   Intellectual Resources 744
   Family Dynamics 745
   Socio-cultural Background 746
   Community Contra-cultures 748
4. PREVENTION OF BEHAVIOUR PROBLEMS AT SCHOOL 749
   General 749
   Parent Education 749
   Teacher Training 751
   Preschool Check-up 753
   Mental Health Consultation in Schools 753
   System Intervention in Schools 754
5. CLINICAL SERVICES IN THE SCHOOL 754
   General 754
   Referral and Relief 755
   Social Class Mediation 755
   The Educational Institution and the Health Institution 756
6. SUMMARY 756

XXVII RESIDENTIAL CARE OF CHILDREN . . *SVEN AHNSJÖ*
1. INTRODUCTION 764
   Institutions and their Development 764
   Institutions: a Necessary Evil 765
   Fundamental Requirements for Child-care Institutions 765

2. Institutional Care on Social Indications	767
3. Institutional Care for Physically Handicapped Children and Adolescents	768
Institutions for the Blind	769
Institutions for the Deaf	769
Institutions for the Children and Adolescents with Motor Disorders	769
4. Institutional Care for Mentally Ill Children and Adolescents	770
Child and Youth Psychiatric Hospital Departments	770
Treatment Homes Connected with Child and Youth Psychiatric Departments	771
Institutions for Psychotic Children and Adolescents (Mental Hospitals)	773
Mental Nursing-homes for Children and Adolescents	774
Institutional Care and Schools for the Intellectually Retarded	774
Institutions for Care (Nursing-homes)	775
Schools for the Mentally Retarded	776
5. Institutional Care for Children with Epileptic Symptoms	777
6. Residential Care of Juvenile Delinquents	778
School Homes	779
Vocational Schools	780
Spare-time Activity	781
Special Detention Departments	781
Aftercare	782
7. The Future Development of Institutional Care	782

XXVIII THE STRATEGY OF FOLLOW-UP STUDIES, WITH SPECIAL REFERENCE TO CHILDREN . *LEE N. ROBINS & PATRICIA L. O'NEAL*

1. Uses for the Follow-up Study	785
Natural Histories and the Evaluation of Therapy	785
Can Follow-up Studies Reveal Causes?	786
2. Issues in the Overall Design of Follow-up Studies	787
The Study Population	787
Prospective or *post facto* Follow-ups?	792
Records, Interviews or Both?	795
Adults or Children as Index Cases?	796
3. Tactics for Solving Problems Inherent in Follow-up Studies	797
The Inequality of Time Intervals	797
Criteria for Inclusion of Subjects	799
Methods of Locating Subjects to Maximize Recovery Rates	799
Maximizing Cooperation	801
Avoiding Contamination of Intake and Follow-up Data	802
Author Index	805
Subject Index	835
Contents of *Modern Perspectives in Child Psychiatry*	879
Contents of *Modern Perspectives in World Psychiatry*	880

INTRODUCTION

TRENDS IN CHILD PSYCHIATRY

Leo Kanner
M.D.
Baltimore, Maryland, U.S.A.

Introduction

In the light of present-day usage, it sounds incredible that the term child psychiatry itself had not acquired formal citizenship in the realm of professional or any other parlance until a little less than three decades ago. In the early 1930s, Tramer introduced it in its German form, *Kinderpsychiatrie*, as part of the name of the journal which he founded and which he has so capably edited throughout the years. In 1935, I chose *Child Psychiatry* as the title of my textbook. In 1937, at the initiative of Heuyer, an international congress in Paris, called together under the heading of *Psychiatrie infantile*, voted, not without opposition, to give legitimate status to the term. In 1938, finally, Schröder could proclaim that this name 'has apparently become conventional in most civilized countries'.

In a way, these baptismal quandaries and their comparatively recent resolution tell the story—a story which goes beyond a mere exercise in semantic niceties—of the origins of a branch of science which has become a respectable ingredient of our contemporary cultural milieu. I venture to say that child psychiatry and the name by which it goes today have arrived on the scene at approximately the same time. I am ready to defend the thesis that prior to the 1920s there was no body of knowledge or of clinical practice integrated enough to merit being set aside as an organized specialty.

Child psychiatry is the result of the convergence of a number of interests which for about half a century have existed alongside each other, with only sporadically and tenuously maintained areas of mutual contact. So long as these interests remained separated and confined to narrowly delimited spheres of activity, they each no doubt afforded highly significant insights which then, however, were applicable solely or principally within the constricted range in which the observations had been made. It was not until they could be brought together in one place that the edifice of child psychiatry could be erected as a comfortable dwelling unit with interconnecting rooms where a family of scientists could indulge in a fruitfully collaborative exchange of ideas and cognitions. Child psychiatry, in brief, is a fusion of what used to be a collection of more or less loosely scattered segments.

With your indulgence, I should like to have some of these segments pass in parade before you. It would seem reasonable to let psychiatry take the lead.

The Contribution of Psychiatry

In the second half of the nineteenth century, several texts were published on 'psychic disorders', 'mental diseases', or 'insanity' of children. Behavioural deviations interested Emminghaus (1887), Moreau de Tours (1888), Ireland (1898), and Manheimer (1899) chiefly as they seemed to fit diagnoses in accordance with classifications devised for adults. There was a tendency toward fatalism which saw in the reported disorders the irreversible results of heredity, degeneracy, excessive masturbation, overwork, or religious preoccupation. These texts, nevertheless, offered a wealth of illustrative case material, no matter how sketchily some of it was presented in the form of anecdotal snapshots.

But let it not be said that the psychiatrists of that era were satisfied to be merely the mechanical recorders of observed or quoted instances. In the refreshing vigour of expanded curiosities, we sometimes, paying half-hearted homage to the psychiatric leaders of the past—and not too remote a past at that—are inclined to dismiss their formulations as obsolete relics, of consequence only to the medical historian. Those men certainly did pay attention to, and did try to find explanations for, psychotic manifestations in childhood, the very existence of which was questioned or even denied by many in the early part of this century. No more fitting example can be offered than that of Henry Maudsley. In his *Physiology and Pathology of Mind*, published in 1867, Maudsley included a 34-page chapter on 'Insanity of Early Life'. In it, he not only attempted to correlate symptomatology with the patient's developmental status at the time of onset but also suggested an elaborate seven-point classification of the infantile psychoses. Anyone superciliously critical of either the terminology or the intrinsic cohesion of the grouping may well be reminded that the classification of the childhood psychoses is to this day a matter of controversial floundering.

Maudsley, as you know, rewrote his book a number of times. I cannot refrain from reproducing the introductory paragraph of the chapter on children in the revision of 1880. He began:

'How unnatural! is an exclamation of pained surprise which some of the more striking instances of insanity in young children are apt to provoke. However, to call a thing unnatural is not to take it out of the domain of natural law, notwithstanding that when it has been so designated it is sometimes thought that no more needs to be said. Anomalies, when rightly studied, yield rare instruction; they witness and attract attention to the operation of hidden laws or of known laws under new and unknown conditions; and so set the enquirer on new and fruitful paths of research. For this reason it will not be amiss to occupy a separate chapter with a consideration of the abnormal phenomena of mental derangement in children.'

The 'abnormal phenomena of mental derangement' continued for some time to be the almost exclusive interest which academic psychiatry had for children. This type of preoccupation found its culmination in the second edition of Ziehen's treatise on the mental diseases (*Geisteskrankheiten*) of childhood which appeared as late as in 1925. Unparalleled as a reference book and as an exhaustive bibliographic guide, it started out with this categorical statement: 'For childhood the same division of psychoses is recommended as for the later ages, namely (*a*) psychoses *with* intellectual defect and (*b*) psychoses *without* intellectual defect.' Ziehen's book was, indeed, on the whole an almost literal translation of adult psychiatry into terms of how much of it one might find in children. The author must have proceeded in about the following manner: 'My readers are, of course, familiar with paranoia, melancholia, hebephrenia, stupor, hysteria, etc., in adults; now let us see how frequently these things are seen in children and how similarly or dissimilarly they manifest themselves.' Abnormalities of the cortical structure and constitutional predisposition were considered as the dominant aetiological factors.

An avowed emphasis on an organic and genetic background prevailed also in Sancte de Sanctis' *Neuropsichiatria infantile*, published in the same year as Ziehen's book. De Sanctis, scorning the modern direction toward 'clinical individualism', complained that 'the study of individual differences causes some to lose the aspect of group characteristics' and that 'the investigation of intimate psychodynamics distracts the view of others from the inevitable play of its nervous or, more generally, vital partner'. He went to the other extreme of losing sight of personality because of his strict adherence to somatic and localizing preoccupations.

The Contribution of Studies on Mental Deficiency

This summary completes the psychiatric vanguard of the procession of segments, covering the efforts over a period of about eight decades, partly before and some time after the initial publication of Kraepelin's monumental work. Another segment is represented by the occupation with the problems of mental deficiency. During a long period of stagnation, interrupted only by Paracelsus' discovery of the connection between endemic goitre and intellectual stunting, the feebleminded were regarded as a homogeneous group. The seemingly solid wall believed to be made up of identical material was dented slightly by Langdon Down's description in 1866 of what he first called Kalmuck idiocy and later came to be spoken of as mongolism. From then onwards, ever new entities were singled out and studied separately. Contributions came from various sources. We owe the knowledge of amaurotic family idiocy to the British ophthalmologist-surgeon Tay and the American neurologist Sachs; of dementia infantilis to the Austrian educator Heller; of phenylketonuria to the Norwegian veterinarian Fölling. A compact unit emerged which had its own experts, facilities, journals, and congresses. It sequestered itself from the rest of the concerns about child development and child behaviour to the extent that, at least on the North American continent, only a negligible fraction of the medical members of the American Association on Mental Deficiency have found it necessary to affiliate themselves with the American Psychiatric or Orthopsychiatric Association. Exciting things have happened within this unit, especially in the past three decades, owing to advances made in neuropathology, endocrinology, biophysics, biochemistry, psychology, and education.

The Contribution of Education

As the parade of segments marches past, education is next in line. After compulsory school attendance had become an established institution, the educators became increasingly concerned about problems of learning and conduct among their pupils. Psychiatrists, for the most part, kept themselves aloof and thereby forced the teaching profession to look for its own solutions. The movement began in France and was pursued there with remarkable vigour. In Central Europe, a group, under the banner of what was termed *Heilpädagogik* (remedial education), undertook, under the leadership of Heller, Hanselmann, Isserlin, and Busemann, to make itself responsible for as much amelioration as was possible in the educational setting. Much was accomplished in this enforced isolation. The second edition of Hanselmann's *Einführung in die Heilpädagogik* (1933) showed a breadth of experience which might well arouse the envy of many a psychiatrist. The labours of these educators resulted in Europe and in America in organized practical arrangements for the special education of the intellectually, sensorily, neuro-orthopaedically, and neurotically handicapped children.

The Contribution of Criminology

A delegation from criminology is next in the procession. In the 1890s a number of civic-spirited men and women found the then existing retaliatory attitude toward young offenders objectionable and detrimental to their development. They exerted all the political influence they could muster. As a result, South Australia in 1895, Illinois and Colorado in 1899 passed statutes establishing juvenile courts in which delinquent children were to be handled separately and differently from adult violators of the law. Since then, juvenile courts have become an established institution. The presiding officers are mostly jurists, assisted often by a staff of social workers, paediatricians, and psychiatrists. In the case of the more severe offenders, re-education and rehabilitation, with or without the aid of psychotherapy, are channelled through special units known as reformatories, correctional or training schools. The names of William Healy, August Aichhorn, Sheldon and Eleanor Gluck are intimately connected with the study of juvenile delinquents.

The Contribution of Psychology

The procession continues. Psychology joins the ranks. Around the turn of the century, psychologists shifted their emphasis from armchair contemplations to actual attention to real people. Alfred Binet is usually and, I believe, correctly hailed as the great innovator. No longer speculating about the attributes of an abstract soul, he let live children come unto him and, initially for the benefit of French school authorities, inaugurated an era of concrete study and the measured comparison of individuals with regard to certain areas of functioning. There came, after a few earlier examples set by Preyer in Germany, Sully in England, and Compayré in France, a spurt of stage-by-stage examinations and recordings of the gradual emergence of motor, perceptual, conceptual, linguistic, and social behaviour. Diaries, interrogations, and a variety of test batteries combined to get together a set of data which, as developmental psychology, has made invaluable contributions. Much information has come—to name but a few —from the work of the Bühlers, William Stern, David Katz, E. Claparède, Jean Piaget, and Kurt Lewin. Following this trend, Arnold Gesell and his co-workers were able to set up a normative scale of infantile development, beginning within a few weeks after birth.

The Contribution of Psycho-analysis

The next marcher in the parade, psychoanalysis, passes by with éclat and fanfare. The awe-inspiring genius of one man created a fascinating system which has had a powerful influence on Western civilization. Freud, on the basis of anthologies of neurotic adults, more or less directly elicited reminiscences, published his theory of infantile sexuality in 1905, three years before he saw any one child professionally. He gave special heed to a set of lawfully progressing centrifugal forces centred around a broadened concept of libido and assumed to govern the development of children's personalities. Freud's profound wisdom and honesty is evident in every one of the 24 pages of the second of the Three Contributions to the Theory of Sex, entitled *Infantile Sexuality*. In this short space, there are not fewer than 55 passages in which the remarks are qualified by 'probably', 'perhaps', 'apparently', 'I believe', 'it is possible', 'as it were', 'so to say', 'may well be', 'it might be supposed', 'it may be assumed', 'we may gain the impression', etc. This collection of probabilities, possibilities, assumptions, beliefs, opinions, conjectures, impressions, and analogies, not as yet validated by dispassionate scrutiny, was somehow transformed into certainties and decreed truths and formed the foundation of an all-embracing credo enveloping all aetiology and therapy. This insistence by many, though by no means all, of Freud's followers has threatened to make of psychoanalysis an orthodox all-or-none proposition of the kind which Adolf Meyer liked to characterize as 'exclusive salvationism'. On the other hand, the excellent accomplishments of Anna Freud are witness to the fact that, with a less dogmatic and more flexible application, psychoanalysis can make significant contributions to the observation and treatment of children.

The Contribution of Child Guidance Clinics

The column of paraders which next appears on the scene is made up by the child guidance clinics which were inaugurated in the early 1920s. The seeds for their growth were implanted toward the end of the first decade of this century when Clifford Beers, with the encouragement of Adolf Meyer, John Dewey, Stanley Hall, and others, founded the National Committee for Mental Hygiene. Prevention of insanity and delinquency was the key word. The idea of setting up insanity and delinquency as targets to shoot at with the arrows of preventive efforts was laudable enough, to be sure. But it implied an orientation which started out with a vision of calamity, looked upon young nonconformists as wayward youths to be snatched in time from the gates of asylums and prisons, and indulged in the practice of throwing inkwells at devils painted on the wall. Actual work with children taught the workers that proper mental hygiene is not primarily an exercise in trying to prove alarmists wrong, that emotionally upset children deserve treatment of what bothers them because it bothers them *now*, and that the greatest benefit can be derived from dealing effectively with what Douglas Thom aptly referred to as 'the everyday problems of the everyday child'. Under Thom's leadership, the Boston Habit Clinic opened its doors in 1921. In 1922, 'demonstration child guidance clinics' were established in several cities with the aid of the Commonwealth Fund. They were called so because they were meant to demonstrate their usefulness to the communities in which they were set up. By the end of the decade, there were about 500 such clinics on the North American Continent alone. In 1930, the governments of more than 50 countries sent delegates to the first International Congress of Mental Hygiene, which was held in Washington, D.C.

The greatest contribution made by these clinics to the understanding of children's behaviour was the departure from the almost universal tendency to look for explanations one-sidedly in an individual's inherent, genetically, constitutionally, and endopathologically determined, centrifugal propensities for disturbing deviations. The focus of enquiry was broadened, beyond the curiosity about that which goes on *within* a child as he reaches out into his environment, to include the external, centripetal forces which do things *to* him and thereby help to shape his feelings and resulting demeanour. Thus ensued a searching investigation of interpersonal relationships at home and in school as motivating factors. Children's behaviour began to be correlated with parents' and teachers' attitudes, which were taken into account as part of the therapeutic strategy. The newly created concept of attitude therapy made it possible to help parents and teachers to examine, discuss, and modify those of their emotional problems which were found to be detrimental to individual children. Simultaneously, through what was called relationship and release therapy, the children themselves were given an opportunity to bring their conflicts to the surface and deal with them in a manner more comfortable and serviceable than theretofore.

The child guidance clinics, aware of the psychological and sociological implications of their job, set up the so-called clinical team of psychiatrist, psychologist, and social worker. This novel and wholesome arrangement, however, was from the beginning allowed to be frozen into a rigid system which came to regard itself as a complete, self-contained unit. Much was made of this 'interdisciplinary' collaboration which closed the door to all but three disciplines, and much time, meditation, and printer's ink were spent on trying to figure out and delineate the exact role of each member of what, because of the exhibited air of sacred solemnity, I have sometimes facetiously dubbed 'the Holy Trinity'. There being no perfection in human enterprise, the great benefit derived from making certain types of children's behaviour problems a matter of community concern had in its wake a consciously cultivated estrangement from medicine and an exclusion of all those other types of handicaps which did not fit the clinic's self-imposed limitations. Saying this does not in any way imply a detraction of the historical importance of the work of those clinics. The insights gained from the study of parent-child, sibling-sibling, teacher-pupil, and therapist-patient relationships formed a truly indispensable addition to the sum total of information gathered by the other segments which we have met in the procession.

The parade has come to an end. Psychiatry, the study of mental deficiency, education, criminology, psychology, psychoanalysis, and child guidance have each displayed before you their particular areas of interest, enquiry, and helpfulness. Few of them had more than a nodding acquaintance with one another. I must hasten to add that in every one of those pursuits there were men whose vision went beyond the circumscribed scope of the specific segment. But it was not until 32 years ago that one man, without identifying himself with any one of the segments, managed to blend all of them into a single discipline which viewed the child as the core of psychiatric endeavour—not selectively the psychotic, feebleminded, educationally maladjusted, delinquent, or parentally mismanaged child but every child who needed psychiatric investigation and amelioration.

August Homburger

Such is the nature of public acclaim that the spectacular takes precedence over calm, diligent, unobtrusively persistent labour. It is perhaps because of this that the present generation has lost sight of the merits of him who should be honoured as the first all-round, comprehensive child psychiatrist. August Homburger was commissioned in 1917 by his chief, Franz Nissl, to establish a psychiatric outpatient department at the University of Heidelberg. He began to centre his interest more and more on the problems of children. It is amazing how much creative work and organizational activity he was able to pack into the 13 years between 1917 and 1930, the time of his death at the age of 57 years. He stepped out of the monastic seclusion of the psychiatric department of his university and got the community at large to participate in the concerns for mental hygiene. He worked in close collaboration with courts, schools, and social agencies. He introduced a series of university lectures on psychotherapy. Mayer-Gross, in his moving obituary, has pointed out how much courage it must have taken to do this 'at a time when neither official psychiatry nor official internal medicine paid the slightest attention to the significance and effects of psychogenic factors'. In 1926, Homburger published his *Lectures on the Psychopathology of Childhood*. His broad orientation could not abide by the therapeutically sterile and aetiologically one-sided categorizing of Ziehen and de Sanctis. His background had given him a mastery of neurology, which served admirably in his work with children, but at the same time made him aware of the fact that cerebral anomalies alone could not account for social, attitudinal and other factors in his young patients' experiences. He set out, with a critical eye and with remarkable fairness, to round up and present to his readers the sum and substance brought together by the various segments as well as the existing theories and hypotheses. Prophetically foreseeing his role as a pacemaker, he wrote in the preface to his book: 'The psychopathology of childhood will—of this I am firmly convinced—experience much deepening and enrichment in the years to come. Whatever I may have to say in these chapters bears the nature of transitoriness and is still anchored in tradition.' His modesty apparently did not allow him to admit to himself fully that, with all due respect for precedent and while putting up a warehouse of accumulated knowledge and thought, he himself was the originator of a new tradition—that of an inclusive concept of the psychopathology of childhood or child psychiatry.

Paediatrics

It was toward the end of 1930, the year of Homburger's death, the year of the first International Congress of Mental Hygiene, the year of the White House Conference on Child Health and Protection, that Adolf Meyer, Edwards A. Park, Stewart Paton, and Ludwig Kast of the Josiah Macy, Jr., Foundation engaged me for an excursion into territory until then neglected by psychiatrists. The preliminary task assigned to me was to consist of 'an investigation of the rank and file of patients in the paediatric clinics for the formulation of psychiatric problems, the mastery of which should be made accessible to the paediatrician to serve him as the psychopathological principles in dealing with children'.

You have undoubtedly noticed, and possibly been puzzled by, the fact that paediatrics, contrary to logically justified expectation, was conspicuously absent from the procession which has passed before you. Lest the inference be drawn therefrom that the medical child specialists were indifferent about issues involving their patients' intellectual, emotional, and social functioning, it is well to remember that as far back as in 1889 Jacobi, one of the pioneers of American paediatrics, spoke of the desirability of making use of psychiatric knowledge in his specialty. But as no help was offered from psychiatric quarters, a few paediatricians went forth to explore the field for themselves. Rachford's *Neurotic Disorders in Childhood* (New York, 1905), Guthrie's *Functional Nervous Disorders in Childhood* (London, 1907), and Czerny's *Der Artzt als Erzieher des Kindes* (Berlin, 1908) were outstanding efforts in this direction. This essentially homegrown crop was kept from withering by a few members of the paediatric specialty. It is not generally known, for example, that the more recent detailed studies by Goldfarb, Spitz, and Bowlby of the effects of early psychological deprivation were preceded by pertinent observations on the part of two paediatricians. In 1915, Chapin, in an article entitled *Are Institutions for Infants Necessary?* advocated the boarding out of infants so that they might receive individual care and affection. In 1942, just one year before Goldfarb's first report, Bakwin's classical paper, *Loneliness in Infants,* painted a 'fairly well defined' clinical picture of the hospitalized infant whose personal needs are neglected aside from the exclusive attention to his somatic illness. Nor should one overlook the fact that in 1919, before the advent of the child guidance clinics, Hector Charles Cameron, physician in charge of the children's department of Guy's Hospital, gave evidence of much sympathetic understanding of emotional features and parent-child relationship in a charming, often reprinted book, *The Nervous Child*, and later in a chapter contained in the 1929 edition of Garrod, Batten and Thursfield's textbook of paediatrics.

But these insights were sporadic and not at all the common property of the paediatric profession, even though its practititioners, often prodded by the demands of sophisticated parents, became increasingly eager to receive assistance from psychiatry. What did they find? The child guidance clinics, as they came along, ignored them completely; the 'team' gave them the cold shoulder. Perusal of the literature resulted in bewilderment. Veeder, shortly before he became editor of the *Journal of Pediatrics*, had this to say at the White House Conference in 1930: 'I have a very definite feeling that the psychiatrist and psychologist have contributed somewhat to the paediatric attitude of suspicion, or scepticism. The psychiatrist above all other people with whom I come into close contact has a penchant for obfuscating his thought with a most perplexing, and I feel unnecessarily complicated verbiage.'

Such was the situation when, in November 1930, I set foot at the Harriet Lane Home, the children's division of the Johns Hopkins University School of Medicine, as the first pseudopodium stretching out into paediatrics from the psychiatric amoeba. A cautious attempt by von Pirquet in 1911 to have a psychiatric observation station, headed by E. Lazar, at the University Children's Hospital in Vienna was not even locally too successful because at that time child psychiatry and paediatric concern with it were both still in the stage of embryonic incipiency.

Very soon after the assumption of my duties, an anonymous donor, to whom I shall be forever grateful, left on my desk the reprint of an article, just off the press, entitled *The Menace of Psychiatry*. Its author was Joseph Brennemann, an eminent paediatrician known for his long experience and sound judgment, a man whose word had a great resonance among his colleagues. Brennemann declared unequivocally: 'There is not only a menace of psychiatry, but it is already seriously in our midst.' He castigated the blatant overpopularization and oversentimentalization of child psychology, the overevaluation of certain standardized tests, and the conflicting claims of some of the speculative, aggressively vociferous, and overbearingly dogmatic 'schools'. Thus Brennemann's blast presented a healthy challenge, the call for a sweeping house-cleaning which deserved to be at least as welcome to psychiatrists as to the paediatric group which he addressed. For here was sound criticism of features which were not so much a menace *of* psychiatry as they were a menace *to* psychiatry.

Brennemann's warning enhanced my already firm resolution to avoid these and many other pitfalls. Coming from a pluricultural and plurilingual background, having emancipated myself from the theological and political absolutism fed me in my youth, falling easily into step with Meyer's practised advocacy of a scientifically objective, self-scrutinizing, pluralistic and relativistic attitude, I found it impossible to limit myself to any of the segments which have passed before you in the procession. Besides, the setting itself made any such restricted alignment impractical. The children who came to the wards and outpatient department just did not sort themselves in accordance with anybody's preoccupations. They were brought in because they were feverish, coughed, had rashes, lost weight, had fractured a bone, were jaundiced, convulsed, held their breath, stuttered, wet the bed, stole, did poorly in their studies. They came with these and many other complaints. Here, then, was an unprecedented opportunity, offered in no other setting, to study children and their manifold problems in an environment from which no patient was ever kept away for any reason and in which the watchfully and hopefully waiting paediatricians were trying to assess the services rendered by psychiatry and its invited representative. For paediatricians are, as all medical men and all other scientists everywhere should well be, governed by the desire for factual demonstrations, for the careful perception of reality which hesitates to accept even the most beautifully constructed hypotheses unquestionably at their face value.

Synthesis

This psychiatric-paediatric alliance in the daily work with individual children made it possible to utilize all the previously recorded observations and discoveries and to introduce the sum total as the discipline of child psychiatry as a medical concern with psychological, educational, social, and cultural ramifications; as a legitimate science within the framework of medical practice, teaching, and research; as a child-centred enterprise engaged in the diagnosis, treatment, and prevention of developmental and behavioural deviations with and without organic involvements. That this trend toward synthesis has more recently spread over the entire field of psychiatry, has been made clear by the publication in 1957 of a volume edited skilfully by H. D. Kruse and entitled *Integrating the Approaches to Mental Disease*. Starting with the deplored awareness of what was referred to as insular grouping, fragmentation, segmentation, and provincialism, an attempt was made by 48 men, including Hargreaves, Rees, Richter, and Slater, to get together on fundamentals and outline areas of acceptance by all and of non-acceptance by some. It is rather pleasing to know that child psychiatry, under the influence of Adolf Meyer, has gone a long way in striving for this aim over a period of nearly 30 years.

This is not to say that, even though the ranks have been closing, there is complete uniformity of opinion and method. As a matter of fact, I am not sure that such uniformity is a condition to be coveted before that day in the distant future when all the aetiological, diagnostic, remedial, and prophylactic facts will lie palpably in the palms of our hands. On the contrary, some of us have found it necessary to speak out against a recurrent tendency to impose an inflexible system of thought and action on all patients, regardless of the nature of their difficulties. This tendency seems to have persisted, in one form or another, since the time of Maudsley who, asserting that 'whosoever distinguishes well teaches well', felt called upon to militate against uniform procedure. He wrote that for adequate strategy 'it would be necessary to have a full and exact knowledge of the construction of the individual mind as well as of the proper remedy: to know the particular character, the special fault of it, the kind of disorder to which the fault was prone to lead, and the exact conditions of life which would be the fit remedy; for different pursuits might wisely be used as so many remedies for different defects of character'.

These words, written in 1895, have a peculiarly familiar ring if one considers the still existing controversies about the need for diagnostic accuracy and for investigative as well as therapeutic methodology. The issue, highlighted so well by Maudsley half a century ago and still alive in our midst, is essentially this:

There are those whose medical training has kept in the foreground of their responsibility the obligation to view each patient as—if I may use Meyer's term—a unique experiment of nature. It is the physician's duty to devise and refine means of investigation that would help him to become cognizant of this uniqueness as an indispensable preparation for the regime best adapted to the requirements of the individual. In so doing, whether he be an ophthalmologist, a cardiologist, an orthopaedist, or an adult or child psychiatrist, he notices that there are certain combinations of features which, though never completely identical, are similar enough to justify the recognition of specific diagnostic categories. This, after all, has been Kraepelin's great accomplishment, that he perceived, described, and studied these similarities and thus brought order into the hitherto unorganized welter of mental diseases. This search for diagnostic clarity is still going on in the wide area of child psychiatry, with the added awareness that, within each sufficiently defined category, the imperative consideration of genetic, physical, intellectual, situational, and experiential differences presents a fascinating invitation to deal with each child as an exceptional, unduplicated specimen.

This, however, is not a universally established tradition among child psychiatrists. There are those who, rightly dissatisfied with what sometimes, I believe erroneously, has been identified as the only concern of medicine, are inclined to turn their backs to organ pathology, description, and classification. Intrigued, as everybody should be, by the relatively new emphasis on psychodynamics, there has been a tendency to elevate intrapsychic and interpersonal factors to the rank of sole determinants of behaviour, or at least as the sole determinants worthy of psychiatric attention. Certain theories have been put forth and certain methods of enquiry and treatment have been laid down which are transmitted from teacher to learner as ultimate, catechistic truths. In the process, theory and method have gained ascendancy over the patient, to whom they are applied with little curiosity about his microcosmic uniqueness. If the standard concepts and rules are not suited to his specific problem, then they are either tried out on him for a time anyway or he is sent home unaided. Under these circumstances, with medicine pushed aside, it is not surprising that the door has been opened wide to lay people, with or without a preliminary medical diploma, who have qualified as adept repeaters of the catechism.

Infantile Psychoses

A concrete example may serve as an illustration of the manner in which the two groups have approached the problem of diagnosis. During the past two decades, there has been a revival of interest in the infantile psychoses. There has been, especially in the United States, an unprecedented wealth of publications on childhood schizophrenia. In them, two more or less antithetical trends are clearly discernible: one which tries to single out specific, circumscribed, carefully defined syndromes on the basis of precise semeiology, and one which tends to dilute the concept of schizophrenia, with not too much regard for the intricacies of differentiation not only between those syndromes themselves but also between them and conditions of innate mental deficiency. It is true, of course, that, as instances of spontaneous or therapeutically induced improvement have demonstrated, average or better than average original endowment can be dammed up by the psychotic process. It is also true that, as Weygandt pointed out in his monograph written for Aschaffenburg's *Handbuch* in 1915, idiotic and imbecile children can present oddities of behaviour reminiscent of schizophrenic phenomena. There is no denying that overlapping symptomatology creates problems in trying to distinguish between different illnesses which have a number of features in common. But the problem is definitely not solved by the decree that the sharing of symptoms makes the conditions identical or that because of the partial resemblance a differentiation is unnecessary.

Nevertheless, on the assumption that lack of adequate mother-child relationship underlies *all* arrest or fragmentation of personality structure at different stages of development, Beata Rank advocated the sweeping notion of the 'atypical child'. She declared that, in using this term, she referred to 'more severe disturbances in early development which have been variously described as Heller's disease, childhood psychosis, childhood schizophrenia, autism, or mental deficiency'. Similarly, Szurek, announcing the consensus of his co-workers at the Langley-Porter Clinic in San Francisco, made this statement: 'We are beginning to consider it clinically (that is, prognostically) fruitless, or even unnecessary, to draw any sharp dividing lines between a condition that one could call psychoneurotic and another that one could call psychosis, autism, atypical development, or schizophrenia.' This is a return to pre-Kraepelinian looseness which throws all the laboriously assembled and refined diagnostic criteria to the winds as irrelevant impediments on the road to treatment. Treatment, under these circumstances, has become a more or less stereotyped method applied to all comers and dispensed as hours of psychotherapy. The therapeutic cart is put before the diagnostic horse and it seems that sometimes the horse is left out altogether.

Psychotherapy

It is perhaps not out of place if, at this juncture, I beg of you to let me dwell briefly on the role of psychotherapy in child psychiatry. Let me begin with an expression of unreserved admiration for the methods which have been introduced in order to help children to reveal their feelings to themselves and to the therapist. Play, drawing, clay modelling, thematic apperception tests, and other projective tools have proved of inestimable value. Having said this, I wish to add that psychotherapy, no matter how essential it is in the overall remedial strategy, is but a part of the therapist's responsibility. While it aims at an adjustment from within outward, there is ample room for help extended from without inward. I think you will agree with me that, while our professional literature abounds in detailed accounts of excellent observations and more or less realistic interpretations of happenings during therapeutic interviews, the intrinsic goal of psychiatric treatment has never been defined clearly and unequivocally. Is it the purpose to learn and teach specific methods or, as some say, techniques to be employed indiscriminately in every instance, unmindful of the uniqueness of the problems which confront us? I shall never forget the young man just out of training who on a visit to our clinic was stunned by the absence of a sand box and running water in the treatment rooms; it was incomprehensible to him how there could be any child psychiatry without those two implements which, so he had been taught, were absolutely essential parts of the arrangement. Does not this smack too much of an attitude which fosters the rearing of a generation of therapeutic mechanics?

If I may venture a concise statement about the goal of psychiatric treatment, it is this: The sum total of efforts expended in order to help a patient to attain *his* optimal condition of comfort and smoothness of functioning. Such a formulation recognizes that, with the great variety of conditions encountered in the wide realm of child psychiatry, the attainable optimum differs with each individual's somatic, intellectual, and sociocultural propensities, all of which must therefore be investigated carefully before a plan for treatment is outlined. The plan may, depending on the findings, involve parent counselling, psychotherapy with the child, the correction of impaired vision, adequate classroom placement, the supply of sufficient food and clothes, and any other arrangements in keeping with the patient's specific needs. Patient-centred, individualized programmes with concrete aims differ essentially from less goal-defined, method-centred journeys into the unknown with the diffuse hope that somehow this will eventually produce a state of blissful 'normalcy' in the image of the therapist's conception of suburbanite propriety.

The children who come streaming to a large paediatric clinic and to its psychiatric station recruit themselves from mansions, middle-class homes, tenement houses, and shacks, from psychometrically intelligent and unintelligent families, from backgrounds of affectionate acceptance, agitated overprotection, perfectionistic disapproval, or overt hostility and neglect. They arrive with healthy bodies, minor physical ailments, and more severe congenital or acquired anomalies and diseases. They are brought with no complaints about their behaviour, with everyday problems from which I for sure was not, and possibly some of you were not, totally exempt, with varying degrees of developmentally determined intellectual shortcomings, with anxiety-laden neuroses, and occasionally with major psychotic disturbances. Not one of them deserves to be pushed aside or sent off because he does not fit the preordained requirements of a selectively dosed therapeutic procedure. No physician would, or should, be content with an attitude which makes the choice of patients depend on the method instead of making the choice of methods depend on the needs of the individual patient.

Conclusion

I realize that some of the trends of which I have spoken pertain to psychiatric work with adults as well as with children. I also realize that child psychiatry, being a newcomer among the medical sciences, still experiences enough uncertainty to warrant a great deal of experimentation. I grant that some of the restricted preoccupations with psychodynamic factors can be understood as an overreaction to the earlier disregard of these factors and to earlier satisfaction with the mere description of symptoms and with mere diagnostic labelling with little or no heed to the foundation and meaning of the patient's emotional involvement. But I believe that the time has come when all of us in the field should be willing to submit theories and methods to a sober evaluation of results. It is time for a bit of reality testing. It is time to examine the existing free-floating generalizations in relation to available data of observation and at the same time to build further generalizations on the basis of such data. With this in mind, I can find no more suitable quotation with which to conclude than the reiteration of a plea by Henry Maudsley, who said: 'Observation should begin with simple instances, ascent being made from them step by step through appropriate generalizations, and no particulars should be neglected.'

PART ONE

PSYCHOPATHOLOGY

I

THE CHILD'S HAZARDS *IN UTERO*

D. H. STOTT

*Professor and Head of the Department of Psychology
University of Guelph, Guelph, Ontario, Canada*

1
The Folklore

There has been an extensive folklore about prenatal influences. Its logic is akin to that of the magic of effigy-making: the content of the mother's thoughts was supposed to become impressed upon the soma of the foetus. If the mother developed a liking for strawberries during the pregnancy, the baby might have a strawberry-like birth mark. A mother once explained that her baby clung to her tightly on being carried upstairs because she had seen her mother fall on the stairs when she was pregnant. A baby's being born with the cord round its neck is attributed to the mother's having had an affair with a sailor. These are instances of the folklore of maternal impression which, very occasionally, one meets nowadays. But they have become rare collector's pieces like all ancient superstition and magic. The assurances of family doctors have effectively killed them. One can say that at present in Britain women have ceased to search in their pregnancies for the causes of their children's handicaps. The possible exception is that they tend to remember falling, mostly during the late pregnancy; but it is doubtful if they seriously attribute the handicap to such.

Nevertheless the folklore has had an unfortunate delayed effect. In the course of its eradication a counter-myth arose—that nothing that happened during the pregnancy could affect the child, that nature completely protected the foetus. Scientifically it became taboo to relate the events of the pregnancy with the condition of the child. Anyone who entertained such an idea was contaminating science with superstition. The implication of the counter-myth was that whereas at every other stage of its growth the living organism is affected for better or for worse by its environment, this did not hold of the period of gestation, although this is the time of its most rapid growth, when it would need an abundant supply of food and oxygen. These nine months were treated as if they were an unbiological phase of completely predetermined development, for which no counterpart existed in nature. Even today genetic and environmental (postnatal) influences are often juxtaposed as if they were clear alternatives. In studies of the effects of mother-child separation seldom is any enquiry made about pregnancy and birth history. The same factors are ignored or dismissed in twin-studies.

2

The Zoological Breakthrough

Meanwhile in experimental zoology—at a safe distance from taunts about maternal impression—findings were beginning to accumulate about the sensitivity of the embryo to adverse environment.

In the early years of the twentieth century it had been observed that malformations could be produced in fishes and amphibians by subjecting the eggs to an unfavourable environment (Stockard[73]). Perhaps because these findings did not find an echo in the genetic interests of the time they were not developed as they should have been. However, Landauer[45, 46] devoted many years of fundamental work to the study of adverse factors on embryonic development in the domestic fowl. It was only in 1935 that malformations were produced experimentally in a mammal; Hale[33] showed that the offspring of sows deprived of vitamin A tended to show eye defects and other malformations. Analogous results were obtained by Warkany and Nelson[89] and many other workers in respect of a number of animals and domestic birds.

Virus Infection

Gregg's[32] discovery of the tendency to malformation following prenatal rubella came opportunely to demonstrate that the human foetus was not invulnerable, as previously thought, to environmental influence. Because, however, the earlier confirmatory studies were retrospective, no reliable data were obtained as to the number of mothers who had had rubella during the pregnancy without harm to the infant.

Carefully planned prospective studies showed that the risk was less than anticipated. In a summary of 11 such, including their own, made by Greenberg and his associates[31], only 12 per cent of the children were malformed and 7·2 per cent were still born after the mothers had had rubella during the first trimester. In Sweden Lundström[48] was able to carry out a large study following a rubella epidemic by arranging for 1,067 mothers to be questioned in maternity wards soon after delivery or at the time of spontaneous abortion. When the infection had occurred during the first four months the total casualty rate, including foetal death, malformation and prematurity, was 16·6 per cent compared with 7·2 per cent among the controls; but it reached over 25 per cent for the second-month infections (some 14 per cent for death and/or malformation only). In a prospective study by Bradford Hill et al.[10] in Britain four malformed children and one stillbirth were found among 18 births following first-trimester rubella. But in a French study by Lamy and Seror[10], quoted by the above, the proportion of malformed infants was as high as 22 out of 40 (55 per cent), with five abortions.

The most comprehensive prospective study of the effects of rubella during pregnancy is that by Manson[51] in Britain. She confirmed that the proportion of the resulting children who were adversely affected was smaller than anticipated. Among the 578 cases, 6·8 per cent had major malformations compared with 2·3 per cent in the control-group. When the infection occurred during the first 12 weeks the incidence of malformation was 15·8 per cent, with 4·2 per cent in the 12- to 16-week cases. The percentage incidence of other birth casualty following infection in the first 12 weeks was found to be as follows:

	Abortions	Stillbirth	Death before 2 years
Rubella	5·0	4·5	6·9
Control	2·4	2·4	2·4

The total reproductive casualty for this early stage of infection—covering abortion, stillbirth, death under two years, malformation and deafness—amounted to 25·8 per cent. There were also a very few additional cases in which mental backwardness or heart murmur were the only symptoms.

Bradford Hill and his colleagues consider that the differences in incidence reported are greater than can be explained by chance or by differences in the methods of investigation; they suggest that the effect of rubella may vary regionally or from time to time. It is possible, for example, that it may have a facilitating effect after the manner of the noxious agents found in experiments upon animals. In this case the incidence of casualty would be higher in those ethnic groups more genetically liable to the malformations in question, or in social groups heavily exposed to influences producing genetic anomaly.

It is still not finally established to what extent other virus diseases can damage the foetus. Coffey and Jessop[17], anticipating the arrival of the virus of Asian influenza in Dublin in the course of the epidemic of 1957, designed a prospective study of those women who were infected during pregnancy. Among their children 2·4 times as many were malformed as in an uninfected control-group, the difference being significant at a risk of less than 1 in 50. This result points to some connection between maternal influenza in pregnancy and malformation, but it adds to the mystery of the etiological process: of the 663 infected mothers there were born in fact only 24 (3·6 per cent) malformed children. Such a low proportion suggests that the influenza plays a marginal role in a complicated series of events.

Acheson[1] pointed out that the women attending the three Dublin hospitals, from which the cases were taken, were an underprivileged group and suggested that, 'it is not the infecting agent itself, but the systematic disturbance of a severe infection in a woman who is already sorely taxed in supporting her pregnancy, which is the factor that damages the foetus'. Ingalls and his colleagues[40] have put forward a hypothesis of cumulative maternal factors in mongolism. This may well be true of other malformations in which environmental factors are suspected of being in part responsible.

The evidence of other studies of influenza as a possible teratogen would seem, when examined closely, to give some support to the above findings. Pleydell[61] made a small prospective study, finding three malformed children born to mothers who had Asian influenza during their pregnancies (7 per cent compared with 1·35 per cent among 1,040 controls). Among the 163 cases of the virus A prime infection which Manson and her co-workers studied along with their rubella survey there was only a slightly higher incidence of major defect (3·7 per cent compared with 2·3 per cent in the controls), and the infections in question occurred between the 13th and 27th weeks. There was a higher infant death-rate when the influenza occurred during the second trimester, 5 of the 97 live-born children dying under two years as against an expectation of 2 to 3. As the authors state, the above hardly constitutes evidence of a risk to the child following influenza in pregnancy but it equally does not rule out this risk.

Two other studies of the effects of Asian influenza during pregnancy have reported negative results, but neither was on a large enough scale to detect the marginal type of difference reported by Coffey and Jessop, and some methodological criticisms may be made of both of them. Walker and McKee[88] found 13 anomalies, amounting to a rate of 33 per 1,000, but it was not ascertained whether in fact the women had had influenza, it being merely recorded that since the epidemic was prevalent during September-November 1957, their exposure to infection would have occurred during the first and second trimesters. Of those reckoned to have been exposed only 53 per cent could report having had the disease. What was even more disconcerting was that of 101 consecutive cases tested in the maternity hospital all showed positive antibodies. This rendered a control-group out of the question, so the authors were forced to fall back, by way of comparison, upon an incidence of malformation of 42 per 1,000 obtained at another time by different workers in a different population. Such a procedure is open to several methodological objections: apart from probable variations in method of examination between one physician and another, the incidence of malformation is known to vary as between ethnic groups and social classes. The second study suggesting a negative relationship between Asian influenza and malformation was that of Wilson *et al.*[96]. They carried out titre counts for Asian influenza on 126 women at the end of the second trimester of pregnancy, 75 reacting positively and 51 negatively. It was remarkable that these reactions bore no relation to influenza as diagnosed by the women's doctors, 18 of the 40 doctors' cases having a negative antibody count. Only four malformations were found, and it is formally true, as the authors state, that no significant teratogenic effect was demonstrated. But two of the four anomalies were cases of anencephaly born to mothers with positive titres and who moreover reported nose and throat infections during the first trimester. The other two anomalies were born to mothers with negative titres. One was a cleft palate, but since a sibling had the same defect the malformation was probably of a genetic type. The other was a generalized hypotonia, and hardly a malformation in the accepted sense. The upshot is that neither of the above studies can be regarded as detracting from the findings of Coffey and Jessop. However, one gets the impression that whatever the influence of this and other virus diseases apart from rubella may be, it is relatively slight and is possibly contingent upon what other unfavourable factors are present. Almost certainly the American populations within which the negative findings were made would have enjoyed vastly better social amenities than did the Dublin women who were the subject of the positive findings.

As regards the remaining virus infections, the evidence is that if they have any effect on the foetus it is even more marginal than that of influenza. Along with their rubella study Manson and her co-workers followed the outcome of 103 cases of measles in pregnancy, and found a suggestively higher incidence both of infant deaths, namely 6 among the 35 infants born after first trimester infection, whereas one only would have been expected, and of malformations, amounting to 7 per cent compared with 2 per cent in the controls but with the infections spread over all the trimesters. They concluded cautiously that it is possible that maternal measles will harm the child, but that the evidence is not strong.

Other infections

The evidence concerning poliomyelitis has been well summarized by Flamm[27]. Many studies show that pregnant women are more prone to the infection, or at least to show it clinically, and that this holds even when pregnant and non-pregnant women of the same age-groups are compared. As regards the effects upon the embryo, Flamm brought together the results of 50 studies of poliomyelitis in the first trimester, covering 323 cases; these showed no abnormal incidence of true malformation. He quotes Anderson *et al.*[4] as arriving at a similar result in their study of 75 cases during the Minnesota epidemic of 1946. On the other hand, Flamm quotes 30 reported cases in which there was clear evidence of polio virus passing the placental barrier and infecting the foetus, and 23 further cases in which this probably happened. The sequelae consisted of damage to the central nervous system similar to that caused by postnatal poliomyelitis. This disease can consequently be a cause of brain damage, but in a different way from rubella in that the injury takes the form not of maldevelopment but of destruction of already formed tissue.

The protozoon responsible for toxoplasmosis can also be transmitted to the foetus, in which it can produce neural lesion. The symptoms in the child of such prenatal infection are characteristic—hydrocephalus, cerebral calcification, chorio-retinitis, respiratory disease, strabismus, epilepsy and above all damage to the central nervous system. However, the picture is similar to that arising from other forms of brain damage, and in only a small proportion of the cases is a particular symptom such as hydrocephaly or chorio-retinitis found to be due to congenital toxoplasmosis. Diagnosis depends upon the ascertainment of antibodies in the mother and child in a density commensurate with the age of the child. It would appear that most instances of prenatal infection result in the death of the foetus or neonate. Unfortunately, however, so little work has been carried out on toxoplasmosis in Britain, or indeed anywhere from an epidemiological angle, that it is impossible to estimate the amount of brain damage in surviving children which may be attributed thereto. To judge by the work of Thalhammer[83], it may possibly be found to be the cause of many times more mental subnormality than all the virus diseases together. From a sample of brain-damaged children he excluded all those with congenital malformation evidently originating in the organogenetic phase and all those who, by the clinical symptoms, were obviously cases of congenital toxoplasmosis. Of the 288 remaining cases he found that 17 per cent reacted positively to the Sabin-Feldman dye test during their first year, compared with none at all in a sample of mentally unimpaired children of similar age drawn from the same population. Moreover he showed that for the higher age-groups the excess of positive-reactors among the brain-damaged remained fairly constant (Fig. 1). In effect, if both groups were equally exposed to postnatal infection, the excess would be expected to narrow somewhat, as seen in the diagram, since there would always be a smaller proportion in the brain-damaged group still to be infected. Thalhammer's sample was taken in Vienna, where a fairly high proportion of the population were found to carry antibodies (42 per cent). In Sheffield (England) the proportion has been found to be only 19 per cent, and in colder regions less still, so that elsewhere fewer than 17 per cent of the hitherto unaccountable cases of brain damage may be attributable to toxoplasmosis. It is not certain however that the techniques used were comparable, and systematic surveys need to be undertaken.

Thalhammer's sample of brain-damaged children was taken from admissions to a children's hospital, and so his results are not contradicted by those of Burkinshaw, Kirman and Sorsby[13] obtained from a hospital for mental defectives. They concluded that toxoplasmosis is not an important cause of the latter; but among institutionalized patients there would be a great preponderance of low-grade cases, and Thalhammer points out that the degree of brain damage in his positive cases was not generally of the severest type. Moreover, he excluded cases of probable other etiology, while the above authors included all the patients in their hospital, including mongols, within their survey. There is in effect some internal evidence that toxoplasmosis was causative in a certain number of their cases. The three most frequent types of abnormality—epilepsy, hemiplegia, and strabismus —which together made up half the total of 48 defects observed in the positive cases, are mentioned by Thalhammer as typical sequelae of toxoplasmosis. The authors discount the high proportion of positive-reactors among their population by the suggestion that toxoplasma infection would

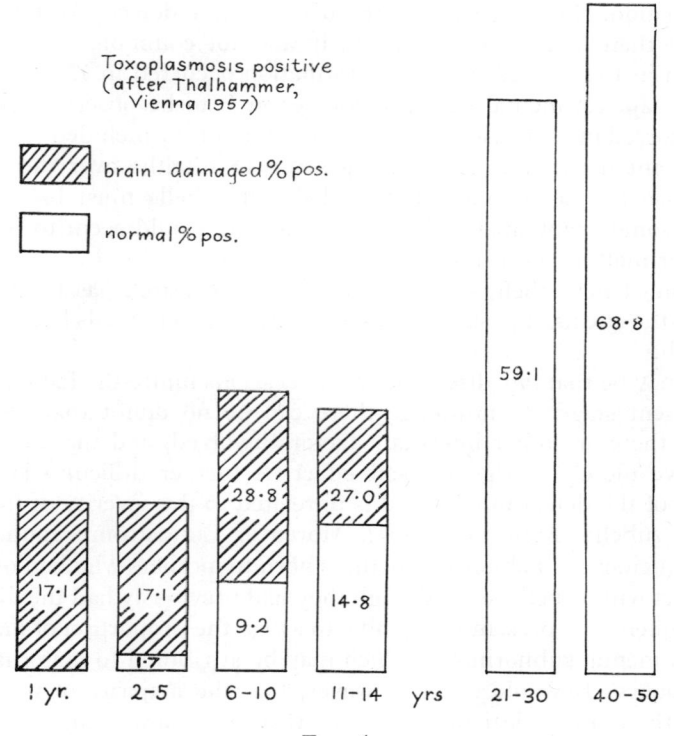

FIG. 1.

spread equally rapidly within an institution as in the community. This however is contradicted by their finding of only two (3½ per cent) toxoplasmosis-positive mongols.

Very recently Robertson[64] has shown a significant association between toxoplasmosis and stillbirth. In a small town in which an undue number of the latter had occurred over successive years an exhaustive enquiry was made into all possible causes, but the only significant difference found was in the incidence of toxoplasma infection shown by titre counts. Of the 19 mothers of the stillborns 13 had counts greater than 1/32. Only four of a similar number of mothers of live-born healthy children in a nearby town reacted positively by this criterion, and for one of these the count was so high as to point to postnatal infection. The counts of the stillborn group were of an order to be expected if the women had been infected during their pregnancies, and the longer the interval that had elapsed since the stillbirth the higher the median titre was found to be. Robertson estimated that 10 of the 19 stillbirths could have been due to toxoplasmosis.

It is, in summary, extremely difficult to sum up the total effects of infectious diseases during pregnancy. As Manson and her co-workers point out, maternal rubella is not, owing to its rarity, a significant cause even of malformation. This is even more so of mental defect. Although more frequent than in the control-group, it was not common. Whereas, with infection in the first 12 weeks, malformation occurred in 15·8 per cent of the pregnancies, mental defect serious enough to be observed in infancy only occurred in four cases, or 2 per cent. The survey included the majority of pregnant married women during some 18 months over the whole of Britain, so that as a cause of mental defect rubella must be negligible. Barring some unanticipated discovery the same would seem to be true of the other malformation-producing virus diseases.

It must nevertheless be emphasized that research has been directed towards the effects of particular illnesses rather than towards heterogeneous ill-health.

It may be that *any* disease may on occasions injure the foetus. Even at our present stage of knowledge there can be no doubt that, even with rubella, there are other important factors involved, and that an infection may have merely a triggering-off effect. A further difficulty is that the severity of the defect in the child is unrelated to the severity of the symptoms of rubella (Manson *et al.*[51]). Moreover Lundström[48] found an increased incidence of abnormal foetuses born to mothers who had only been in contact with rubella, even though they had previously had the disease. It is consequently at present impossible to assess the proportion of malformation and mental subnormality which may be attributed to maternal illness in pregnancy. It would seem, however, that the majority of pregnancies leading thereto are clear of disease, so that, as is now recognized, only a small proportion of reproductive casualty can be explained by such.

On the other hand Pleydell[61], working from another angle, that of the local distribution of anencephaly, adduced some suggestive evidence that 'there is a much greater association between maternal infection and congenital abnormalities than is at present accepted'. Not only was anencephaly some four times more common in the industrial than in the rural areas of the county he studied, but cases tended to occur in the same few streets on the same days or nearly so. Within these concentrations anencephaly tended to be associated with other malformations. It must also be borne in mind that the great majority of malformations cannot be attributed to any cause, and it is very seldom that the factors responsible for congenital brain damage can be diagnosed.

There is a mounting volume of indirect evidence which points to the vulnerability of the foetus to unfavourable intrauterine environment. Several malformations show a higher incidence among first-borns on the one hand, and among fourth and later children on the other, or alternatively with very young and elderly mothers. The outstanding example, mongolism, is too well known to need more than mention. Similar findings are reported for malformations of the central nervous system (Record and McKeown[62]), and for hare-lip and cleft palate (MacMahon and McKeown[50]). Klebanov[41] found that of 1,430 children born to Jewish women released from German concentration camps 58 were malformed. This is only four to five times the normal rate, but it is significant that 12 of this number were mongols, a rate of 1 in 35 compared with 1 in about 650 as found in the European populations. The majority of the mothers of the 'mongols' were under 30, so that high maternal age could not have accounted for the high incidence.

The incidence of reproductive casualty has been found to vary with social conditions. Anderson, Baird and Thomson[5] found that in the four principal Scottish cities the anencephaly rate varied inversely with the amenities of living, and was also consistently higher in the industrial than in the rural counties. Edwards[25], also in Scotland, showed it to be about four times higher in the Registrar-General's social class V (unskilled labourers) than in the highest social class. In the United States Pasamanick and Knobloch[59] and in Britain Drillien and Richmond[23], and Drillien[21] have shown that premature birth is associated with low social class. Stewart[71] reported similarly both of prematurity and perinatal death.

Perhaps the most surprising of these environmental indications are those which relate to season of conception. Pasamanick, Dinitz and Knobloch[60], analysing the seasonal variations in births by groups of States of the U.S.A., found that a spring decrease was most marked in those in which the summers were uncomfortably hot. They had earlier reported (Knobloch and Pasamanick[43]) a preponderance of mentally deficient children born during the winter months, contrary to the general tendency for the number of births in lower-class families to fall off during these months. Other studies indicating the vulnerability of the gestational period are reviewed below owing to their possible relevance to emotional factors, and indeed it may be such rather than infections which produce the correlation with changes in environment. Nevertheless the reasons for these correlations are not yet established, and it may be that unsuspected infections are responsible.

3

Emotional Stress

The etiological possibility remaining to be explored is that of emotional or 'psychological' stress during pregnancy. The old duality between mind and body, while persisting as an ingrained habit of mind going back in European philosophy at least as far as Plato, does not fit what is known of the bodily changes following the arousal of emotion. The most modern point of view has been succinctly stated by Stafford Clark[69]: 'As doctors we have long known that sudden shock can produce sudden and sometimes catastrophic physical and mental responses. We have begun to see that, in a comparable way, the long-continued battle with stress and tension which it is the lot of so many of us to fight is not a battle in which it is always very profitable to distinguish between hard knocks and hard feelings; nor are the scars borne separately on body or upon mind.'

The possibility that mental stresses may damage the foetus is strengthened by parallel findings in experiments with animals. Thompson and Sontag[84] subjected 12 female rats to the continuous ringing of an electric bell, this being repeated twice daily between the 5th and 18th days of pregnancy to the point where the animals broke down in seizures. Of the offspring 24 were chosen, and these were switched randomly with other litters to equalize postnatal environment. At maze learning they were found to be significantly slower than the controls. One might say that the ringing of the bell either 'got on the nerves' of the pregnant rats, or played on fear reactions to such an extent that, with the disintegration of behaviour, a gross physical side-effect ensued. It could thus be argued that although the behaviour disturbance was psychogenic the insult to the foetuses was somatic. This reservation would not apply to the subsequent experiment of Thompson[85], in which he exposed pregnant rats to anxiety without somatic stress. Five female rats were trained, prior to mating, to expect an electric shock at the sound of a buzzer, and to escape by opening a door. After mating they were placed three times daily for the duration of the pregnancy in the shock compartment and given the buzzer signal without the shock being applied, but with the escape door fastened. The 30 offspring and 30 controls were switched systematically between the experimental and control mothers in order to equalize a possible postnatal effect from the former upon their offspring. The differences in the performances of the two groups of young rats in tests of 'emotionality' were striking and statistically significant. The experimental group at the ages of 30 to 40 days was more sluggish, moving about some 36 per cent less, taking twice as long in leaving their cage when it was open and nearly three times as long to reach food when hungry. At 130 to 140 days the behavioural differences were still significant, but somewhat less. Thompson drew the reasonable conclusion that stress in the form of anxiety applied to female rats during pregnancy produced a disturbed emotionality in the offspring. It is noteworthy that this took the same form—that of an apparent lack of confidence and enterprise—as reported by the present writer below in respect of children whose mothers had had a disturbed pregnancy.

Several experiments demonstrate that exposure of animals to unfavourable psychological relationships, in this sense, have somatic sequelae. Barnett and his co-workers (Barnett[8], Barnett et al.[9]) found that in male wild rats attack by another male of the same species can produce well-marked endocrine disturbance (adrenal-cortical depletion, followed by hypertrophy) and even death, although the animal attacked suffered no physical injury. Bruce[11] noted from an accident of laboratory routine that mice mated with their stud male, with whom they were familiar, often reverted to a non-pregnant state if put shortly afterwards with strange males. Systematic experiment showed that when the latter were of a different strain this occurred in up to 80 per cent of the cases. There could have been no physical interference because the females were kept caged separately from the strange males, and could only see, smell and hear them. No similar failure of pregnancy occurred following contact with the stud male or with other females, the few cases of infertility then being associated with pseudopregnancy and not with the early abortion or resorbtion which must have followed proximity to the strange males. In both these studies the objective physical change was the result of a state of affairs outside the animal's body, that is to say, owing to its being aware of what was presumably an unfavourable or unpleasant 'personal' relationship. Bruce[12] subsequently isolated the smell of the strange male as the effective agent producing pregnancy failure, since this occurred merely by letting the female smell nesting material with which the males had previously been in contact.

A striking rise in the malformation rate was noted in a number of centres in Germany during the hardships of the early post-war period, which the investigators attributed to a combination of the nutritional deficiencies and psychological stresses arising from destruction of living accommodation, food shortages, refugeeism, etc. In effect, the rate began to rise from the *beginning* of the war, before nutritional deficiencies would have arisen. At the Leipzig Maternity Hospital the mean for 1940-45 showed an increase over that for 1936-39 of 49 per cent, which was significant at less than 1 in a 1,000 ($\chi^2 = 13\cdot7$) (Aresin and Sommer)[6]. From the results of a large survey by Eichmann and Gesenius[26] covering 36 Berlin and 19 other hospitals it can be seen (Fig. 2) that the increase for the region they covered began with the seizure of power by Hitler in January 1933. For the seven years up to then the rate was 1·25 per cent, for the seven years thereafter it was 2·38 per cent. During the war years (1940-45) there was a further increase to 2·58 per cent, and a startling one, to 6·5 per cent, for the 1946-50, which were years of great hardship. The above authors, and investigators in other centres, showed that the war and post-war increases were confined almost entirely to malformations of the central nervous system. Nowak[58] emphasized that this could not be a side-effect of higher maternal age, since it was the mothers in the 22 to 35 age-group who were most affected. The only obvious difference between life in the pre- and post-Hitler periods, and between the pre-war years and those of the early war years, would be in greater psychological stress to certain sections of the community—fear of the Storm troopers, racial victimization, mobilization and the general anxieties and disturbance associated with war. It is of interest that there are historical references to an increase in malformations during the Thirty Years and Napoleonic Wars, and after the siege of Paris in 1870-71 (Gesenius[29]).

For Britain no general survey of trends in malformation has been published. Logan[47] showed that the mortality of infants under one year owing to congenital malformation was distinctly higher for the years 1940-

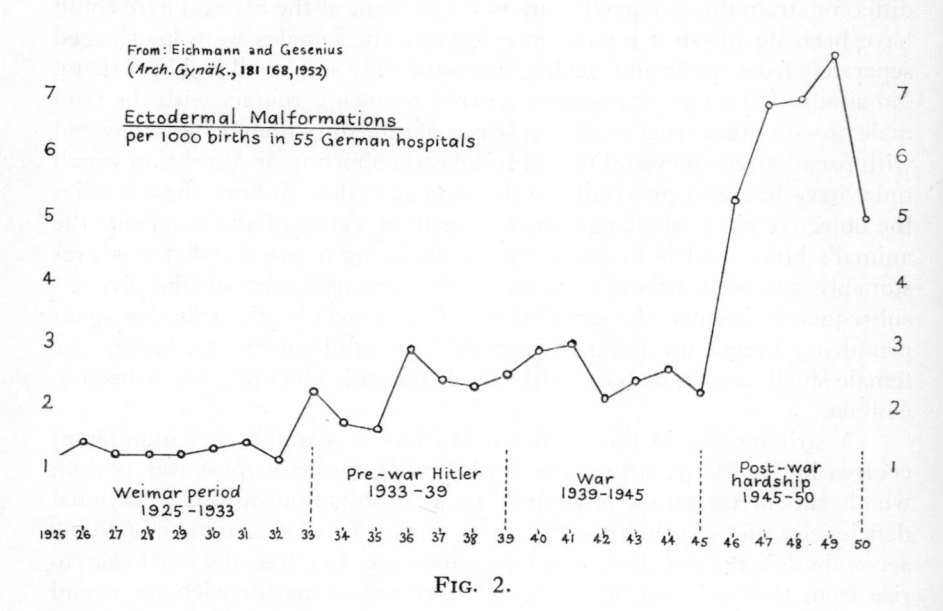

From: Eichmann and Gesenius
(*Arch. Gynäk.*, 181 168, 1952)

Ectodermal Malformations
per 1000 births in 55 German hospitals

Weimar period 1925-1933
Pre-war Hitler 1933-39
War 1939-1945
Post-war hardship 1945-50

FIG. 2.

1942 than at any time since 1931, but fell steadily from 1943 onwards. Not having the evidence from Germany available, he concluded that the incidence of malformation could not have altered, so that the wartime rise of death therefrom must have been due to a temporary disorganization of antenatal and obstetric services. It is fortunate, however, that the reports of the Registrar-General for England and Wales, from whom Logan took his data, also include the totals of children by sexes dying from malformation during the first four weeks of life. In Fig. 3 these are reduced to rates per 1,000 live births. It is seen that for both sexes they remain fairly stable for the years 1932-39, but reach a peak during the years 1940-43. For the remaining war years they return to the pre-war level, but then fall abruptly to a new level representative of the post-war years. For several reasons these trends cannot in the main be accounted for by variations in the quality of medical care. Malformations proving lethal within four weeks would include a greater proportion which would have been so anyway, compared with those causing death within the first year. They would also have included a higher proportion of anencephaly, which occurs three times more frequently among females (Stevenson et al.)[70]. It is therefore significant that the wartime rise—comparing the average rates for 1932-39 and 1940-43—is practically twice as high for females as for males (14·3 per cent and 7·5 per cent respectively). Moreover, the close parallelism of the annual fluctuations for the two sexes taken over the whole period up to 1957 could hardly be accounted for by annual changes in the quality of medical care. It is more reasonable to assume, with the German data in mind, that the wartime rise was due to greater prenatal stress. Garry and

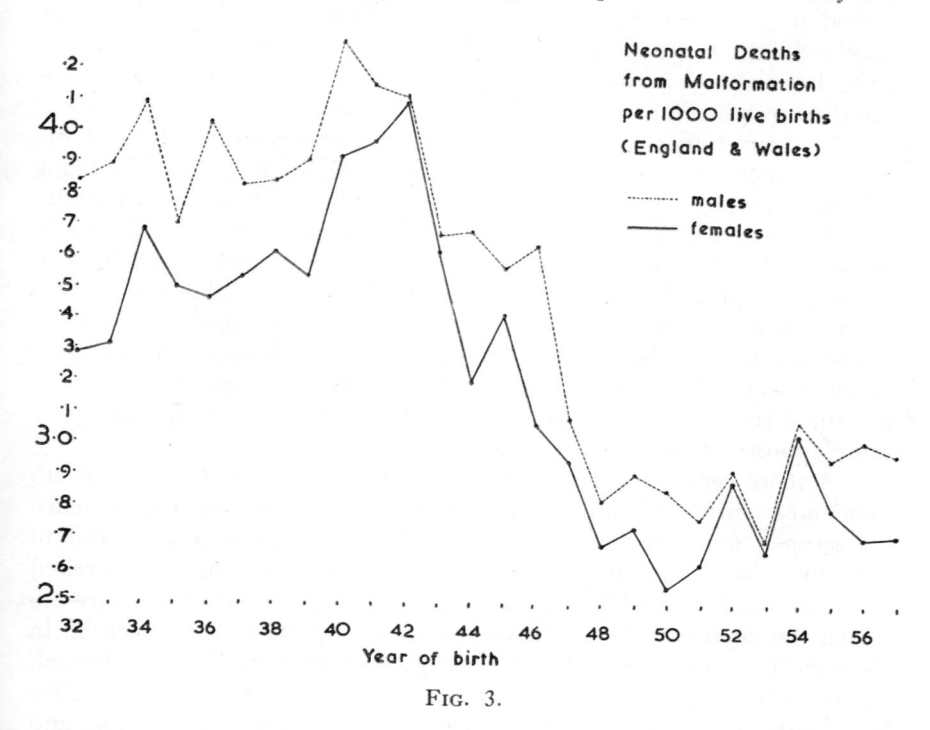

Neonatal Deaths from Malformation per 1000 live births (England & Wales)

.... males
——— females

FIG. 3.

Wood[28] found that as a result of the efficient rationing system and of high earning power consequent upon full employment, 'the general standard of nutrition, especially of pregnant and nursing mothers, was raised above the level of the pre-war years'. Fewer wartime infants died in infancy, and the average weight of babies up to 1 year of age rose. Poorer nutrition during pregnancy can thus be ruled out as the reason for the rise in the number of deaths from malformation. The only feasible alternative is the undoubted high incidence of anxieties and fears (no epidemic having occurred at this period).

The epidemiological studies of malformations of the central nervous system made at Birmingham are also compatible with the above hypothesis. Record and McKeown found that the rates for anencephaly and spina bifida followed the same pattern as that for deaths from malformation over

England and Wales given above. They began to rise sharply in Birmingham during 1938-39, the time of Britain's entry into the war, reaching a peak during 1940-43, and falling thereafter by stages to below the pre-war level. The investigators themselves write that 'We have no explanation for these secular variations, but are satisfied that they are not associated to any considerable extent with fluctuations in the parity composition of the general population of births'. It will however be noted that besides the anxieties attendant upon wartime conditions the peak coincided with the period of the most intense bombing. The same authors show that in Scotland, where there was very little bombing, there was no significant peak, but only the post-war fall coincident with the improvement in the standard of life compared with the pre-war period.

In their studies of the epidemiology of anencephaly McKeown and Record[54] report consistent seasonal variations, the highest incidence being related to conception during May to August and the lowest during October to February. But this seasonal variation was almost entirely confined to first-borns. If it was purely 'biological', associated with first births in general, no *seasonal* trend would be expected. If on the other hand it had been caused by a seasonal infectious disease or by climatic conditions it would surely have been found irrespective of birth-rank. In seeking a factor which operates more strongly among first-borns conceived during the summer months one is tempted to reflect that this season may offer more opportunities for premarital conception.

A more recent study by Edwards[25] of the trend of anencephaly in Scotland confirms this apparently anomalous tendency, that 'the influence of season is more marked on first births'. His attempts to relate this to notifiable diseases and temperatures during the previous summers proved unsuccessful. He found that despite improvements in social conditions—to which the anencephaly rate is very sensitive—there had been no fall in Scotland between 1939 and 1956. But the apparent stability, he showed, disguised two opposing trends. During the years 1939-43 the incidence for later births was consistently high, reaching an all-high peak in 1942, and during these years it was higher than for first births. That for first births became markedly greater in 1944 and 1945, and except for two years, when the two rates were about equal, it has remained greater. The high total incidence for 1951-54 was due entirely to a great excess for first births. There would thus appear to be two distinct social influences, the one reducing the incidence for later births, which one may assume was the general betterment of social conditions, the other some factor affecting specifically first births. The suggestion that this might reflect a change in the sexual habits of younger adults, with a resultant increase in extra-marital conception, gains some support from the Report of the Chief Medical Officer for England and Wales[14]. He points to the alarming rise in the annual number of new cases of gonorrhoea in recent years, especially among both males and females aged 18 to 19 years.

The evidence provided by the above studies as to the relevance of mental stress in pregnancy is inferential, the feasibility of this hypothesis resting upon the lack of obvious alternative interpretations of the data. Scattered in the literature are a number of case-reports relating malformation or mental defect to psychological stress. MacGillivray[49] has mentioned as a possible etiological factor in a case of hypertelorism the shock sustained by a woman about three months pregnant when a child standing beside her was killed by an automobile. Klotz[42] reported two cases which strongly suggested psychological causation, one involving shock following the news of the wounding of the husband immediately prior to conception, which was followed by anencephalic birth; the second of a woman who, having had to flee for political reasons in early pregnancy, gave birth to a mentally defective child. In both cases the mothers had a clear heredity, were organically healthy and had been subjected to no dietary deficiency. The geneticist Grebe[30] mentions four cases of acrocephalosyndactyly, two of which followed psychological stresses produced by bombing and refugeeism. He also reports a case of monozygotic twins of whom one only was an anencephalic; the mother had been thrown downstairs in an air-raid at the second week of pregnancy. In a case referred to the present writer the mother reported that, at the end of the sixth month of pregnancy, 'My husband was in Switzerland. I lived in my parents' house in Germany. As it was a Jewish home the Nazis came in on the 8th of November, 1938, destroyed the furniture and locked my mother and myself in the bathroom. It was a great shock. Afterwards I had very strong movements.' The male child which resulted from this pregnancy was a mental defective without speech, but in accordance with the stage of pregnancy of the shock was of completely normal physical appearance. The strong foetal movements recall Sontag's finding of such when the mother suffers emotional disturbance.

It is sometimes pointed out that if mental stress is a significant factor this would be revealed in a larger number of malformed children among the illegitimate. Murphy[57] found that this was not the case in his extensive study. There are, however, several considerations which may explain this result. Illegitimacy is a legal rather than a biological concept, and many children deemed such are in fact the product of stable unions (e.g. where one of the marriage partners cannot be released from a former marriage, or where the marriage ceremony would have been inconvenient or thought not worth while). The greatest incidence of illegitimate birth occurs in very young mothers. In a published psychiatric study of the illegitimate pregnancies of nine girls of under 16 years of age, who were not abnormally deviant either mentally or emotionally from their contemporaries, Anderson et al.[2] found less emotional distress than expected. In two cases the girls' condition had to be pointed out to them by others. In none of the nine was there severe depression or panic leading to attempted abortion, and 'mixed feelings of fear, anxiety and guilt gradually yielded to single-minded concentration on getting the child born'. In the whole group eventually investigated of 60 such cases, 'the actual fact of extramarital pregnancy caused the majority of them very little distress, and after the pregnancy came to be accepted, the child was in very many instances . . . looked forward to' (Anderson)[3]. It may be surmised that the young woman would often be counting on marrying the putative father, and even in some cases envisaging pregnancy as a device for bringing about marriage. In others the pregnancy may have been unconsciously welcomed, as the counterpart of delinquency in a youth, as a means for example of working off hostility or resentment against a parent.

It must often happen that the very young mother-to-be deceives herself as to her condition until the organogenetic phase is past. Anxiety about the eventual marriage would also tend to come to a head during the later pregnancy, so that the effects upon the child are more likely to be such as can result from stress in mid- and late pregnancy.

In effect, since the illegitimate offspring of stable cohabitations are thereby excluded, premarital conception may be more associated with emotional stress than illegitimate birth. A greater incidence of prematurity and of perinatal death among extramaritally conceived children has indeed emerged from studies of which this was not the main subject of enquiry. Studying the effects of employment during pregnancy Stewart[71] found that in a group of extramaritally conceived children (48 illegitimate and 162 legitimate premaritally conceived) prematurity was over twice and perinatal death nearly three times as frequent as among the postmaritally conceived. In a further paper Stewart, et al.[72] reported a significantly greater proportion of foetal deaths among the premaritally conceived. This could not have been a side-effect of first parity, for the proportion of foetal deaths in that group was only slightly above expectation.

Clokie[16] found that first babies born within a year of marriage ran a 50 per cent above normal risk of prematurity, while the percentage of illegitimacy among prematures was 7·4 compared with 4·4 among all births for Northamptonshire as a whole.

This consensus of findings as to the disadvantages of extramarital conception is of course open to different interpretations. Drillien and Richmond[23] discount the general assumption of the greater biological risk involved in very young motherhood, pointing out that beside the preponderance of underweight babies born to women under 20 there is also a greater proportion of babies of over 7½ lb (namely 60 per cent, compared with 40 per cent in mothers of 20 to 24 years, and less than 18 per cent in primiparae over 35 years). They conclude that 'from a biological point of view the youngest mothers are most successful in their pregnancies'. The bi-modal distribution of birthweight in children of very young mothers in effect fits a hypothesis of high biological efficiency coupled with some occasional reason for impairment which is associated with young motherhood. The reason suggested by the above authors is that in the case of some extramaritally conceived children premature labour may have been induced by attempted abortion. How many very young mothers would be sophisticated enough to attempt such is an open question. On the other hand an element of anxiety and distress would be present in many if not most cases, and this may have set up hormonal reactions unfavourable to foetal development. It is moreover relevant that the incidence of congenital defect has been found to be some seven times greater among premature babies (Douglas and Blomfield)[20]. This suggests that the prematurity is in many cases a concomitant of multiple impairments, which could hardly originate from mechanical intervention at a late stage of pregnancy. In so far as these congenital defects could be classed as damage rather than true malformation they may in part be accounted for by lack of antenatal care in view of the tendency of some types of mother, notably those subject to preoccupations and stress (which see below), to come to clinics later in pregnancy. Nevertheless the factor probably most specific to extramarital conception is mental stress, and so there is a case for investigating the association between congenital defect and this hitherto neglected factor.

There have been only a few studies which have taken account of mental stress, but they raise important methodological considerations that justify their discussion in some detail. Record[63] reported shortly upon a retrospective study of the incidence of certain disturbances of pregnancy as obtained from the mothers. He did not say under what conditions the latter were interviewed, so that it is not known whether the interviews were of a type to elicit reasonably complete information. It is hard to believe that 742 mothers of normal controls would report not a single fall or other accident during the pregnancy and that only two mothers would report emotional shock. In a study by the present writer (Stott)[77] 344 mothers of normal controls reported 22 (6·4 per cent) shocks and severe falls (ordinary falls being left out of account), as opposed to 19·8 per cent among the 849 defectives. In Record's survey there must have been considerable under-reporting by mothers of both normal and malformed children. Nevertheless the emotional shocks which did come to light were consistently higher for all the categories of malformation (averaging 2·2 per cent compared with 0·3 per cent for the controls, $P = <0.0001$), and the same applied to the falls (4·3 per cent compared with 0·0 per cent). Although, as Record suggests, the preponderance of these shock-factors in the malformed group may well have been due to the mothers' attempts to account for the defect—a central methodological consideration discussed below—the fact remains that there were more reported in the malformed group, so that the hypothesis of mental stress is not disproved. Record is inclined to discount this factor from internal evidence, pointing out, first, that pyloric stenosis—one of the malformations included—is dependent, at least in part, on factors in the postnatal environment. But liability to non-epidemic diseases, including pyloric stenosis and others of the digestive system, seem by the evidence of the study reported subsequently to be related to pregnancy stresses in which mental stresses predominated. The same counter-objections could be made against Record's reference to two other malformations, patent ductus arteriosus and congenital dislocation of the hip, which he mentions as being in some cases related to conditions of birth. There is moreover the evidence of Sontag[67, 68] that emotional stress in the mother can produce hyperactivity in the foetus which may entail foetal injury or abnormal presentation. There are grounds, then, for suggesting that Record may have been unduly cautious in interpreting his data. As a further reason for not attaching causal significance to the above statistical relationships between emotional shock and all the types of malformation taken together, he considers it unlikely that any one disorder of pregnancy could cause them all. But to produce a statistical association it would only be necessary for a significant number of types of malformation to be produced by emotional shock. The experimental production of malformation in animals shows that the particular form taken depends more upon genetic dispositions than upon type of insult, and the sequelae of rubella undoubtedly vary with stage of gestation.

The second statistical study taking account of prenatal emotional factors (McDonald)[53] had the initial advantage of being a prospective one, but it serves to illustrate that this method also has its pitfalls. Over 3,000 women were interviewed during the fourth or fifth month of pregnancy concerning the events of the first 12 weeks. The incidences of spontaneous abortion, perinatal death and major or minor defects were subsequently noted. Although McDonald claims that the sample, being a straight run of women booking in at an antenatal clinic, was unbiased, this method of selection in itself must have resulted in a considerable degree of bias. She herself admits that the low abortion rate among those women conceiving extramaritally (2·9 per cent compared with 7·1 per cent for 'postmaritals') was due to the tendency of 'extramaritals' to report to the clinic later in the pregnancy, and hence many earlier abortions were missed. But the similarly low figure of 2·7 per cent for perinatal death among extramaritally conceived children suggests the operation of some more subtle selective factor. As quoted above, Stewart found perinatal death to be nearly three times more frequent among the extramaritally conceived, with a risk of chance of less than 1 in a 1,000. That McDonald found almost exactly the reverse—$2\frac{1}{2}$ times more among the postmarital—could be interpreted to mean that such 'extramaritals' as did report in early pregnancy were a highly self-selected sample, namely those whose circumstances were very favourable to a successful pregnancy. One might hazard a guess that they tended to be those for whom the fact of pregnancy was not the subject of alarm.

McDonald found only a slightly higher incidence of malformation among the extramaritals. But if shock and anxiety can result in malformation, and if it was those extramaritally conceiving women experiencing most mental stress who stayed away, then this would produce an understating of the incidence of malformation among the extramaritally conceived infants.

One may also ask whether there was not a tendency for mothers experiencing anxiety or shock in high degree for any reason to stay away. This might easily have been the case where the mental stress was so acute as to have brought on illness or depression, or where it was of a preoccupying nature such as the illness of husband or child. In assessing the degree of selection it is noteworthy that among the women who could not be traced subsequent to interview, there was a much higher amount on the one hand of marked anxiety and emotional shock (30 per cent compared with 13½ per cent among those who produced normal infants) and on the other of attempted abortion (18 per cent compared to 5·4 per cent). It would thus appear that the women suffering mental stresses tended to exclude themselves from McDonald's sample.

Apart from the patent bias of the sample, the manner in which the expectant mothers were interviewed virtually invalidated the study on methodological grounds. It was, to say the least, somewhat insensitive to confront a woman immediately after a physical examination, itself associated with some anxiety as to whether the pregnancy was normal, with questions as to whether her husband was the father of the child and whether she had attempted an abortion. McDonald furthermore admitted in her paper that there was a lack of privacy, and (in answer to a question after her paper read to the Royal Society of Medicine in London) that they were conducted in hurried and uncomfortable conditions. It can be well understood that women who had probably been kept waiting some time for their examination, as Douglas[19] shows happens in these circumstances, would not be in the mood to answer questions. Even if they did not feel insulted by the imputations of the questions many of them would be preoccupied with getting home, so that they would not be in a condition to remember, or would have answered as shortly as possible, that is to say, negatively. Moreover the two questions about mental stress were put in very general terms, of the nature of: 'Did you have any marked anxiety?' and 'Did you have any emotional shock?' rather than taking the form of enquiries about actual events such as, 'Were any of your children ill?', 'Did anyone die whom you were fond of?' It is sometimes not realized that just as precise techniques are required for obtaining data through interviews as are required in the conduct of a physical examination.

4

Mental Retardation

As the basis for an exploratory study, without formulated hypotheses, of the causes of mental retardation the present writer obtained exhaustive case-histories of two groups of children (Scott[75]). The first was of 40 mental defectives, of IQ less than 50, selected from a junior training centre as being of normal physical appearance (some malformations being subsequently found among them). The second, a mentally subnormal group of 65 with an

IQ range of 50 to 80, was drawn from special schools. In view of the rubella finding, and since the object of the study was to cast further afield for possible causes of retardation, detailed pregnancy-histories were taken, in which not only maternal illnesses but all the circumstances of the mothers' family lives were recorded. A series of control-groups of mentally normal children were obtained, the parents of whom, in order to get large numbers, were interviewed for the most part in groups and helped to complete a questionnaire concerning the same pregnancy and early-life factors as for the retarded. For one of the control-groups—that consisting of the siblings of the latter—the interviews were conducted by exactly the same procedure as for the survey group of retarded. In the course of this study a great preponderance both of adverse pregnancy factors and of non-epidemic early illness became apparent among the retarded, to such an extent that the writer formulated the hypothesis that there were two major, prenatal and a postnatal, etiological classes. In the course of the analysis of the data, however, a close relationship emerged between the adverse pregnancy-factors and non-epidemic disease below the age of 3 years.

The adverse pregnancy-factors taken into account were, in the first place, maternal illnesses, from which however colds and mild bronchitis were excluded. In the small category of mental illness were included only what a psychiatrist would term anxiety-state, with obsessional sobbing, hysteria, fainting, etc., and other objective evidence of mental breakdown such as the removal of the mother on that account to hospital. The category of mental or emotional stress was most difficult to define. All what were at the time common and ordinary anxieties and fears, such as uncertainties over the husband's employment, his absence in the Forces during the war, dissatisfaction over living accommodation, living in a bombed area, were excluded. On the other hand, accommodation problems involving bad human relationships or threat of eviction were rated as stressful. The same applied to severe illness of the husband or of a son or daughter, news that the husband was a war casualty, and bombing incidents involving the house or such as were otherwise particularly frightening to the mother. Marital disagreements were rated as stressful only if they reached the point of violence, mental cruelty from an unbalanced husband, or desertion or infidelity of the husband during the pregnancy. The criterion, in sum, was that the pregnant woman had suffered acute mental distress arising from circumstances which threatened to bring calamity to her life or actually did so. Purely physical shock hardly occurred in this sample apart from involvement in bombing incidents; falls and slight accidents were ignored.

Nevertheless, because there were no previous studies available to provide criteria of the level of severity of stress which might affect the offspring, it was often difficult to decide whether a particular stress should be included. For this reason the stressful pregnancies were divided in those which clearly met the above criterion, and those which were on the borderline.[1] These are referred to subsequently as P and $P?$.

INFANTILE ILL-HEALTH

In Table 1 it is seen that P is between $2\frac{1}{2}$ and 3 times as great for the retarded group and $P+P?$ over twice as great.

TABLE 1

	P No. of cases	%	$P+P?$ No. of cases	%
Retarded samples (102)	49	48·0	67	65·7
Controls (450)	80	17·8	135	30·0

The significance of the above results requires no statistical corroboration. It can be noted however that as between the retarded and their 91 siblings—for whom interview-methods were exactly similar—it gave a χ^2 of 26·35 with $P<0·001$.

5

Infantile Ill-health

The above finding was open to the methodological objection that the mothers of the retarded children might be more prone to think back into their pregnancies in order to discover some reason for their children's mental deficiency or mental subnormality. In effect, as will be shown subsequently from Drillien's investigation of this possibility, mothers seldom make any connection between the events of their pregnancies and the condition of their children. Nevertheless, a means of overcoming this element of uncertainty was at hand in the relationship between the pregnancy-stresses and infantile ill-health: it could not be supposed that mothers of mentally defective or subnormal children would have attributed only infantile ill-health to pregnancy factors or would have held these to be the cause of the mental retardation only when their children happened in addition to have some ill health in infancy. Hence a relationship between pregnancy stress and infantile ill-health could not feasibly be due to maternal bias. Table 2 shows this relationship for 102 out of the 105 (for one the pregnancy and for two the early-life histories were unobtainable).

Where the mother reported physical or mental stress during the pregnancy which met the above criteria, 75·5 per cent of the infants suffered fairly serious ill-health at some time or other during their first three years. This applied to only 28·5 per cent of the infants following a clear pregnancy. The borderline group occupied an intermediate position with 44·5 per cent. When the latter are included with the definite stresses $\chi^2 = 13·86$; when with clear pregnancies 17·75. In either case the relationship between stressful pregnancy and infantile ill-health is highly significant statistically ($P<0.001$).

This result was not a reflection of a social-class factor, since the proportions of stressful pregnancy in the cases from adequate- and inadequate-standard homes were almost identical (65 and 67·5 per cent). Moreover the relationship between stressful pregnancy and infantile early illness was found to be just as close in the cases from adequate-standard homes as in the sample as a whole.

TABLE 2

Non-epidemic illness 0·3 yr	Pregnancy stress			Total
	Definite	Borderline	None	
Reported	37	8	10	55
Not reported	12	10	25	47
	49	18	35	102

A possible explanation of this relationship is that the ill-health and vicissitudes to which the mothers were subjected reduced them to such a state of depression or debility that they neglected their children. Such neglect would occur, however, only in cases of mental breakdown in women of very unstable personality. And among the 59 rated as stable the proportion of those in whom a stressful pregnancy resulted in an unhealthy infant was 70 per cent, rather higher than for the sample as a whole, and the relationship remained significant.

The relationship between stressful pregnancy and infantile ill-health extended to the control children, as shown in Table 3.

TABLE 3

	Serious ill-health in infancy	Healthy infancy	Total
Definite or borderline pregnancy stress	45 (33%)	90 (67%)	135
Clear pregnancy	36 (11%)	279 (89%)	315
	81	369	450

It is seen that among a fairly representative sample of children only one-third of those born following a stressful pregnancy are affected in their health up to the age of three years. This is not a sufficiently high proportion to attract attention in general medical practice; even if the doctor suspected any connection between pregnancy events and infantile ill-health, he would dismiss it because two out of three children born following a stressful pregnancy would be healthy. Nevertheless the reality of the tendency is brought out by the statistic that only 11 per cent of the children born following a stress-free pregnancy suffered infantile ill-health.

Broken down by sexes an even more striking picture emerges. It is known that boys are more prone to childhood illnesses than girls. This is reflected in the controls, in that—taking the purely non-backward groups numbering 359—21·1 per cent of the boys but only 9·1 per cent of the girls had serious illness below the age of three. Table 4 shows the relationship of the latter to stressful pregnancy for each sex.

TABLE 4

| | Serious ill-health in infancy || Healthy infancy ||
	Boys	Girls	Boys	Girls
Definite or borderline pregnancy stress	20 (35·7%)*	11 (20·8%)	36	46
Clear pregnancy	21 (15·2%)	4 (3·6%)	117	108

* Percentages affected within each pregnancy-category.

It is remarkable that among the 112 girls born following a clear pregnancy, only four met the criterion for serious non-epidemic illness under three years. Of these the sole illness of three was enteritis, which might well have been the result of high exposure to infection and could be classed as epidemic. The fourth girl developed eczema at 18 months. Thus, among the girls early ill-health was almost entirely the sequel of stressful pregnancy. That among the boys about half the cases of unhealthy infancy were not associated with pregnancy-stress suggests either that among males the genetic determinants of such are more potent, or that their ill-health was related to pregnancy-stresses insufficiently severe to meet the criteria used in the study. There may thus be different triggering-off points for impairment in each sex.

6

Malformation

Among the 105 children of the retarded sample 15 congenital malformations were identified; among the 450 controls there were 9 if naevi are included. Of the total of 24 only 6 were unrelated to classified pregnancy stress, and of these 4 were slight or vestigial such as might have been due to a heterozygous gene. The relationship between stressful pregnancy and congenital malformation for the retarded and controls combined gave a χ^2 of 15·84 ($P<0.001$). All the stresses occurred within, or included the first trimester. Of the 18 pregnancies in question, 11 were affected by purely mental stresses, 3 combined mental and physical, and 4 consisted of maternal illness only.

7

Behaviour-disturbance

It is a matter of clinical observation that non-mongol mentally retarded children show a high incidence of disturbed behaviour. The social adjustment of the retarded sample, as rated in the Bristol Social Adjustment Guides (Stott and Sykes[81], Stott[76]), was much inferior to that of a sample of primary school children drawn from the same locality which had served as controls for another study. Of the retarded, 45·2 per cent showed noticeable timidity compared with 28·5 of these controls; for other forms of disturbed behaviour the proportions were respectively 31·4 and 20·1 per cent. Since the timidity (the syndrome of Unforthcomingness in the Bristol Guides) represented the most clear-cut form of temperamental impairment, and was so much more prevalent among the retarded, a test was made of its relationship to pregnancy stress. Within the retarded group of 102 this was significant at a χ^2 of 10·17, giving P approaching 0·001. The relationship of timidity to early ill-health was one of pure chance ($\chi^2 = 0.14$). This ruled out the possibility that the timidity could have been the result of the ill-health or the concomitant hospitalization,* but raised the question of why there should be a complete lack of relationship between two dependent variables each of which was fairly closely related to the same independent variable. Further analysis of the data revealed a higher incidence of specifically late pregnancy stress, or much aggravated stress, among the behaviourally disturbed; conversely, among the disturbed children those with a history of predominantly late-pregnancy stresses had significantly less early illness ($\chi^2 = 6.95$ $P<0.01$) (Stott[78]). There was no relationship between type of impairment and type of pregnancy-stress; however, the type of impairment seemed to be related to stage of pregnancy, but further work needs to be done with prospective or immediately retrospective data before this suggestion can be confirmed.

The upshot of this study was that four major types of impairment—mental retardation, ill-health, malformation and personality-defect—were

---

* Relatively few (25·4 per cent) of the unforthcoming retarded children had been hospitalized in infancy compared with the stable retarded (34·3 per cent) or of the otherwise disturbed retarded (33·3 per cent). Among them personality defect seemed quite unrelated to separation from the mother, although this occurred in some cases for long periods (Stott)[74]

found to follow a stressful pregnancy. In view of the genetic factor which has been established in all common childhood illness by twin-studies (Marshall, Hutchinson and Honisett[52]), it may also be concluded that the effect of pregnancy-stress depends in part upon the genetic constitution of the child. Consequently no one sort of impairment results inevitably from stress, even at a given stage, and it has been seen that in mentally normal children only about one-third suffer early ill-health following a stressful pregnancy. In this respect the chances of impairment are of the same order as for prenatal rubella.

A vulnerability to postnatal stresses conferred by complications of pregnancy and delivery was demonstrated in Drillien's[21] follow-up study of prematurely born children. The pregnancy-stresses included such conditions as toxaemia (other than mild), threatened abortion, antepartum haemorrhage and chronic diseases such as essential hypertension, cardiac conditions and diabetes. Mental stresses were not taken into account, but to judge from the foregoing study would have been associated with the first group of diseases. Using the Bristol Social Adjustment Guides she found a quite marked excess of behaviour-disturbance at 7 years, in both the premature and mature-born groups, when there was a history of complications of pregnancy and/or delivery. Her results are summarized in Table 5, which gives the means for indications of behaviour disturbance.

TABLE 5

($+$ = present, $-$ = absent)

	Severe family stress		t	P
	$-$	$+$		
(a) Birth weight 4·8 lb and under (132 cases)				
Complications of pregnancy $-$	6·4	13·1	3·209	<0·01
and/or delivery $+$	10·5	20·0	5·941	<0·001
t	2·045	1·466		
p	<0·05	not sig.		
(b) Birth weight 5·9 lb and over (165 cases)				
Complications of pregnancy $-$	4·9	7·5	4·722	<0·001
and/or delivery $+$	8·2	15·6	1·712	not sig.
t	7·029	4·313		
p	<0·001	<0·001		

(Drillien)[21]

A clear picture emerges of a congenital disadvantage arising from prematurity and complications of pregnancy and/or delivery when it comes to resisting the disturbing effects of family stresses. Those comparisons which do not reach significance seem not to do so only because of insufficient numbers, since the trend is no less marked in them. For example the prematurely born children with a history of pregnancy/birth complications who were also subjected to severe familial stress gained a mean BSAG score of 20·0, which is the criterion for maladjustment.

McKerracher[55] made a study of boys aged 13 years using the same criteria of pregnancy-stress and illness as Stott. He found that physical, emotional and mixed pregnancy-stresses were all significantly related to behaviour-disturbance between 5 and 12 years, this being three times more frequent for all types of stress together than in the controls. However this was not reflected in the teachers' assessments when the group was aged 13 years, which he interprets as 'a strong tendency to overcome initial setbacks'. However, only one-third of the cases with a history of stressful pregnancy gained entry to a senior secondary (more academic) school compared with two-thirds of the controls.

The relationship between pregnancy-stress and personality-defect was demonstrated in a small but carefully conducted study by Scott[65]. She carried out observations upon 30 4-year-old children in a Nursery School, assessing the effectiveness-motivation of each child. The concept underlying this variable, proposed by White[95] and Stott[79] is the extent to which a child attempts to deal in a progressively more advanced or complicated manner with the objects at its disposal, tries different tasks, likes to create spectacular effects, is eager to find out things for himself, will attempt to establish dominance or at least equality vis-à-vis other children, and generally establishes a relationship of personal effectiveness with his environment. It is the opposite of the attitude of unforthcomingness mentioned earlier. The 30 children were awarded total scores according to the 'effectiveness' of their behaviour in 20 categories. They were then divided at the median to give Effective and Ineffective groups of 15 each. The mothers were then interviewed and the results recorded on an experimental edition of the Systematic Interview Guides (Stott[80]). The number of stress-factors during their pregnancies reported by the mothers was 10 for the Effective and 28 for the Ineffective, giving means of 0·66 and 1·86, which was significant at nearly the 0·02 level. Those reported for the Ineffective group tended to be more severe. By Stott's criteria of definite and borderline stress, and giving 2 points for the former and 1 for the latter, the pregnancy-stress score of the Effective group came to 12, compared with 45 for the Ineffective. None of the children was obviously retarded, and indeed represented all the 4-year-olds in a particular community Day-Nursery (Kindergarten). Thus the mothers had no reason for regarding them as abnormal, and those of the Ineffective could hardly have had any incentive to account for a handicap by searching in their pregnancies. This study may thus be taken as confirming the earlier finding of a relationship between stressful pregnancy and unforthcomingness (effectiveness-deficit).

Its importance lies in suggesting prenatal factors as a determinant of personality differences in a normal population.

8

Cleft Lip and Palate

The part played by pregnancy-stresses in the etiology of cleft lip and palate has been well brought out by Drillien, Ingram and Wilkinson[22]. Of the 172 children born with the malformations in South-East Scotland and Fife during the years 1953-61 they were able to obtain comprehensive life-history data of 169. To these were added 21 of the 29 stillbirths or neonatal deaths with the same malformation born within this period. They were matched by a control group of 124 maturely born children without cleft palate.

By utilizing the observation that this malformation sometimes recurs in families and is sometimes found in isolation they were able to divide the cleft lip/palate group into subgroups of primarily genetic and non-genetic etiology. In the one, the malformation may appear spontaneously or to the accompaniment of minimal stress; in the other, such genetic factor as there may be is only activated by adverse conditions of gestation. The subgroups were termed the family-history positive (primarily genetic) consisting of 64 cases, and the family-history negative of 105 cases.

Significant differences in maternal reproductive history were found between the two subgroups. The mothers of the history-negative cases had lost relatively more children of other conceptions from abortion, stillbirth or neonatal death and had more liveborn with congenital defects. The same applied to the small group whose children were stillborn or died neonatally. On the other hand there was no difference in the above respects between the history-positive subgroup and the control group.

The incidence of pregnancy stresses for the two subgroups and the controls is given in Table 6. Threatened abortion and hyperemesis (persistent nausea and vomiting throughout the day for three months or more) showed a high incidence among the cleft lip/palate cases irrespective of family-history. The authors suggest that the threatened abortions were secondary to the primary developmental defect, by which they presumably imply some natural tendency towards disposal of malformed embryos. For the similar incidence of hyperemesis among the history-positive they have no explanation except the possibility that mothers tended to exaggerate the degree of sickness when the outcome of the pregnancy was a malformed child. In general mothers have a clear memory of the incidence of sickness in each of their pregnancies, and it is hard to appreciate what motivation there could be for exaggeration of the order shown, since mothers tend to accept malformations fatalistically and without guilt. One is tempted to ask whether the hyperemesis was also a reaction caused by the presence of an abnormal embryo.

Among the remaining stresses a fairly consistent picture emerges of similarity between the history-positive and the controls, but of excess among the history-negative and stillborn/neonatal death subgroups. As the authors point out, there can be no reason why the mothers of the history-negative cases should be more prone to report pregnancy-stresses than those of the history-positive. Consequently this feature of the experimental design provided a neat test of the credibility of mothers' accounts of their pregnancies. If there had been any significant tendency to over-report

TABLE 6

Per cent incidence of pregnancy-stresses

	Cleft lip/palate FH+ve	Cleft lip/palate FH−ve	Stillborn neonat. d.	Controls
Early pregnancy				
Threatened abortion	8·2	8·6	7·4	0·8
Hyperemesis	9·8	8·6	14·8	0·0
Chronic diseases (ess. hypertension, cardiac, serious anaemia, respiratory, thyroid)	9·8	16·2	11·1	7·3
Accidents (1st trim.)	1·6	6·7	5·0	?
Infections (1st trim.)	6·6	1·9	10·0	?
Emotional stress (1st trim.)	9·8	16·2	35·0	9·0
Emotional stress (2nd and 3rd trim.)	9·8	8·6	20·0	3·0

conditions when the child was malformed, one would have thought that this would have produced an excess of stresses among the history-positive relative to the controls.

The emotional stresses taken account of were experiences likely to cause severe emotional disturbances to a normally stable woman. Those mentioned are marital discord resulting in separation or divorce, death after distressing illness of a near relative, or prolonged anxiety requiring medical treatment. The authors rightly considered it unlikely that such experiences could be fabricated, especially as many were open to independent verification. The greater incidence of such stresses among the history-negative subgroup compared with the controls did not reach statistical significance, but that among the stillborn/neonatal-death group did so at a χ^2 of 10·039 and a P approaching the 0·001 level. The higher incidence of emotional stresses in the history-negative subgroup is given further credibility in that it does not apply to the second and third trimesters.

9
Mongolism

The discovery of a chromosomal anomaly in mongolism, important and well-established as it is, has had the unfortunate effect that this has come to be regarded as *the* cause of this condition. Since the nondisjunction must almost certainly occur at or prior to conception, the possibility that the events of pregnancy may also play some part has been dismissed. It has been overlooked that a not inconsiderable proportion of embryos never proceed to term, and that those expelled or resorbed tend to be malformed. Hertig[38] found that of 36 human embryos examined upon hysterectomy 13 (36 per cent) were abnormal. Since the above proportion is many times in excess of the incidence of malformed children actually born it would seem to follow that the abnormal embryos are, in the normal course of events, weeded out by some natural process. It will be recalled that in their cleft lip/palate study summarized above Drillien and her co-workers were led to regard the equal incidence of threatened abortion and hyperemesis among the history-positive and history-negative cases as secondary to the existence of the malformation, which must be taken to mean that the anomaly tends to activate some expelling mechanism. What this may be can only be surmised, but it is feasible that it produces antigens against which the maternal body normally reacts. The degree to which the latter rejects or tolerates abnormal embryos would seem to depend upon hormonal balance. Woollam and Millen[97] reduced the incidence of harelip in mice by administrating thyroxine, but since litter-size was also reduced thereby one may suppose that this hormone facilitates the destruction of abnormal embryos. Conversely, Woollam and his co-workers[98] were able to increase the number of malformed eyes in the offspring of irradiated rats by means of large doses of vitamins; litter-size was correspondingly increased, so that the effect was presumably to induce greater tolerance of malformed embryos. To this must be added the finding of Tough *et al.*[86] that ordinary X-ray treatment produces large numbers of abnormal cells containing extra chromosomes, all of which however are reduced to the normal level within five days. The production of a mongol child may consequently depend not only on an initial chromosomal anomaly but also upon a failure of the maternal body to react in a way that would have resulted in its destruction.

The present writer made an enquiry of parents by questionnaire through the (English) National Society for Mentally Handicapped Children regarding shocks sustained in each month of pregnancy. The questionnaire used enquired about incidents and circumstances of a factual nature, such as exposure to personal danger, horrifying experience, fears for the safety or health of husband or child, death of near relative or close friend, infidelity of husband, and physical traumata such as injury from road accidents, burns or physical violence. The mothers' reports were assessed on an overall criterion of degree of stress by an experienced psychiatric social worker who was unaware of the hypothesis or of the differential effects of stage of pregnancy. For mongol defectives under 21 years of age 739 forms were received. The controls consisted of 400 non-mongol defectives, in respect of whom questionnaires were received and treated in exactly the same manner. At the time they were completed (1957-58) very few people knew about the organogenetic phase of gestation, and this was true even of a large number of general medical practitioners. Consequently any difference in the timing of pregnancy stresses as between the mongol and non-mongol groups could hardly be attributed to bias in maternal reporting. Moreover, since both the mongols and the controls suffered from an approximately

TABLE 7

Percentage Distribution by trimester of stressful experiences and of minor accidents

	Trimester		
	First	Second	Third
Stressful experience:			
Mongols (276)	48·1	31·5	20·5
Non-mongols (113)	29·5	37·4	33·2
Light accidents and falls:			
Mongols (144)	21·3	44·8	33·8
Non-mongols (67)	21·3	48·8	29·8

equal degree of mental deficiency (the Society in question consisting almost exclusively of parents of children who had been excluded from schooling as ineducable) there could have been no incentive for the mothers of one group to emphasize certain pregnancy events more than another.

A markedly higher incidence of stressful experiences was reported for the mongol-pregnancies during the second and third months. An internal check on the possibility, despite the precautions taken in the design of the experiment, of a maternal-bias effect was provided by a similar analysis by month of light accidents and ordinary falls. In Table 7 these are grouped by trimester, and the incidence of major stressful experience portrayed by months in Fig. 4.

It is seen that there is virtually no difference in the incidence of light accidents and falls as between the mongol and the non-mongol groups. Moreover the mothers tended to report more of them during the second and third trimesters. More severe physical traumata showed a similar distribution. Consequently it would appear that physical traumata of any type, without emotional stress, have no effect in facilitating mongol outcome.

In order to assess the specific effects of emotional stress those cases were chosen in which such experience occurred in a single month, without physical illness or trauma at any time during the pregnancy. When this was done the concentration of stress within the first trimester of the mongol-pregnancies is even more marked.

That emotionally stressful experiences should be so much more effective in facilitating mongol outcome (if in fact the relationship is a causal one) suggests that the physiological link is a hormonal one. It could

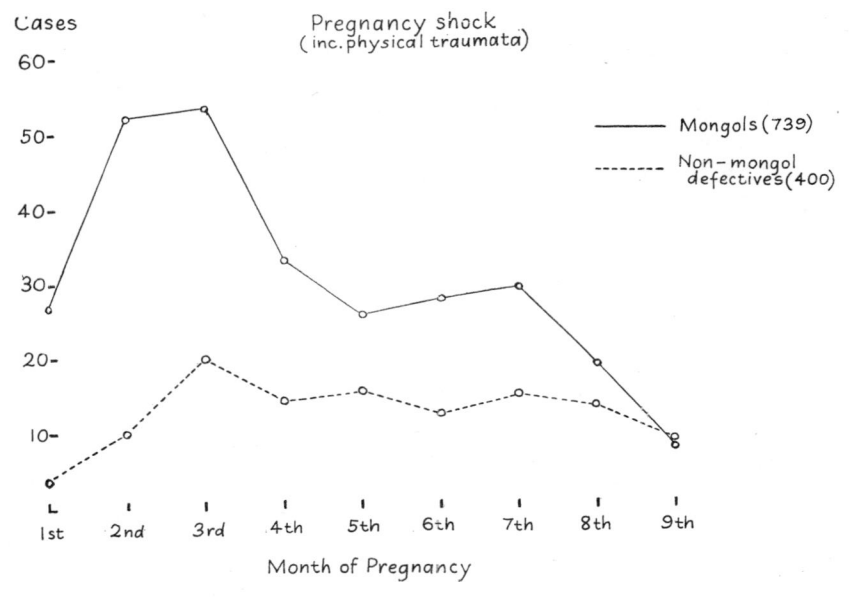

FIG. 4.

be argued that physical trauma, without distressing aftermath, is too short-lived to induce hormonal exhaustion or serious imbalance. In this case it could be predicted that short-lived emotional traumata would be less effective than those which were more lasting. The emotionally stressful experiences were accordingly divided into the 'ephemeral', such as a burglary or a fire incident, and the 'lasting' which initiated a period of distress, such as the onset of serious illness in a close relative, or the death of such. These lasting stresses showed a greater concentration in the first trimester compared with the ephemeral (χ^2 of 7·69 and $P<0·05$).

In sum, this study brought out a relationship between mongol birth and emotionally stressful experiences of some duration occurring in the second and third months of the pregnancy, which was significantly greater than chance. The design of the experiment—in comparing the pregnancy-histories of mongol with non-mongol defectives, and the independent assessment of the stresses—makes it difficult to dismiss this finding on methodological grounds, since it is inconceivable that the mothers could have attributed their having mongoloid children so selectively to lasting emotional stress at a given stage of pregnancy.

Drillien and Wilkinson[24] were able to repeat the above study by using a group of 227 mentally defective children, of whom one third were mongols. They did so in the expectation, as they stated, of a negative result in view of their findings from the cleft lip/palate study. They used the same criteria of stressful emotional experience as in the study by Stott. In the event their findings not only confirmed his but suggested a greater etiological significance for stressful experience. The latter were present during the first trimester in 35·7 per cent of the mongol pregnancies compared with 12·9 per cent of those in the non-mongol defective cases. This amounts to a relatively greater incidence for the mongols of 2·75 times compared with 2·17 times in Stott's study. The difference may be due to the fact that whereas he had obtained his data by questionnaire Drillien and Wilkinson did so by personal interviews conducted by an experienced caseworker, who had also played the same role in the cleft lip/palate study. It is not known whether she was able to obtain more candid accounts of the pregnancies, or whether the criteria for assessing emotional stress were somewhat broader.

Drillien and Wilkinson took the precaution, in order to assess the extent to which Stott's results were due to maternal bias, of asking the parents to what they attributed their children's mental deficiency. Three-quarters of those of mongol children could give no reason at all. Of the mothers reporting several stressful experiences two-thirds thought it unlikely that this could have anything to do with the defect. Rather more (37·5 per cent) who experienced such in the later pregnancy gave it as the reason. The general finding, however, was that the mothers did not think back to their pregnancies for an explanation of their child's mongolism.

10

Drugs as Teratogens

Little attention had been given to the possible teratogenic effects of drugs during pregnancy until the dramatic outbreak of *phocomelia* in Germany in 1960-61. This malformation consists in the absence or shortening of the limb bones and gross malformation of the hands and feet. Previously it had been very rare and usually affected only one limb. Several cases were observed in 1959; already by 1960 it had reached epidemic proportions; but nevertheless increased fourfold in the following year. Later in that year the enquiries of Lenz at Hamburg revealed that a large proportion of the mothers of the malformed children had taken Contergan, the West German trade name for thalidomide, during the pregnancy. Almost simultaneously McBride in Australia and Spiers in Scotland made the same discovery in relation to Distaval, the English marketed name of thalidomide. A subsequent careful investigation by Lenz showed that this drug produces the above malformation when taken in the second month of pregnancy.

In Germany thalidomide had been regarded as a harmless sleep-producer, and was initially sold without prescription, hence the large number of children who were affected, put by Taussig[82] probably at well over 4,000. In Britain the number has been estimated at 500. It was not possible to find out what proportion of the women who took the drug during the critical month had normal children. In Düsseldorf the children of one-half of the women who had taken it were malformed, but since the enquiry was necessarily retrospective the exact month in which it was taken could not be ascertained with certainty. It could therefore be that as a teratogen thalidomide is exceptional in that it is noxious in probably the great majority of cases and possibly—if taken at exactly the critical time—in all. It is also exceptional in tending to produce a characteristic type of malformation which is otherwise very rare. Such associated malformations as have been observed are chiefly of the head, face and heart. The affected children seem mentally normal. Thus thalidomide has some effect quite distinct from rubella, which causes a variety of defects and only in a small proportion of cases.

Hellmann et al.[37] found that the administration of thalidomide to mice delayed the rejection of skin-homografts. This prompted him[36] to make an ingenious suggestion about the mode of action of the drug in relation to malformation. He points out that in genetically heterogeneous animals the foetus is a homograft on the mother, and that if early spontaneous abortions, many of which are malformed, are homograft rejections, an immuno-suppressive drug might permit the malformed to reach term. He quotes the opinion of His[39] that the lymphocytes which he saw in aborted foetuses originated from the mother and served to destroy the foetus. (The immunological rejection of homografts is mainly due to the action of lymphocytes.) Hellmann cannot explain why normal foetuses remain unrejected, even though having an antigenic effect. One can only suppose, if his theory is correct, that the normal foetus is robust enough to resist the maternal antibodies. He argues that just as it is important for the survival of the individual that mutant, and particularly malignant, cells should normally be eliminated as antigens so the same process occurs at the multicellular level. 'The rejection of malformed foetuses could therefore be regarded as an active fundamental homeostatic mechanism essential for the survival of the species.' The relevance of this argument for the reconciliation of the chromosomal and early-pregnancy findings in mongolism needs no emphasis. Phocomelia, however, cannot be simply explained in this way for two reasons. The first is that the affected children show no chromosomal anomaly. The second is that, if the thalidomide merely acts as a suppressor of an antigenic mechanism, why its use was not followed by a number of different malformations. This, and the rarity of *phocomelia* apart from thalidomide, induced Hellmann to suggest that the latter has the double effect of directly causing the malformation and of suppressing the mechanism for the rejection of the abnormal embryo.

That the medical world was taken by surprise by the phocomelia outbreak and was long in recognizing its origin is an index both of how little is known of the effects of drugs taken during pregnancy, and of the lack of system in the recording of pregnancy-data. A large number of drugs are known to be teratogenic in animals and some—notably penicillin, streptomycin and tetracycline—have been found to produce malformations of the limbs (Millen)[56]. It is only fair to the firms which marketed thalidomide to mention that it had been found to have no effect on animals. This is but one example of the bewildering species-specific nature of teratogens, another example being that cortisone produces malformation in mice but not in rats.

A number of studies have shown that the prenatal administration of sedative drugs to rats affects the offspring. Harned *et al.*[35] found that an amount of sodium bromide sufficient only to produce a mild apathy in the gravid animal impaired the ability of the offspring at maze-learning. Hamilton[34] obtained the same result with rats on a three-table test, which demanded memory and a high type of learning, as also did Armitage[7] using sodium barbital and sodium pentobarbital. Werboff and Havlena[93] found that reserpine, chlorpromazine and meprobamate administered prenatally decreased activity and emotionality measured on the open-field test and reduced liability to seizure on exposure to a stressful audile stimulus. However, it was later found that only the meprobamate impaired maze-learning (Werboff and Kesner)[94]. All three produced significantly more neonatal deaths (Werboff and Dembicki)[90]. Other drugs—5HTP and BAS—significantly increased activity and emotionality, but none the less reduced the number born and the viability of the offspring, and the survivors were lighter in weight than the controls. There was also a greater susceptibility to audiogenic seizure, but not impairment in learning (Werboff *et al.*)[92]. It could be argued that since the activity-level of the offspring of the untreated rats would have evolved to the optimum level, the increase following the drugs would represent an impairment. In human beings hyperactivity and abnormal acceleration of maturation are recognized types of dysfunction, the former markedly associated with brain damage and the latter nearly always associated with sub-average mental development. The administration of alcohol to gravid rats was found by Vincent[87] to decrease emotionality in the offspring in small, and to increase it in large doses. Since both dosages reduced maze-learning ability, this would support the view that either higher or lower emotionality must be regarded as impairment. Dispensa and Hornbeck[18] found that thyroid hormone administered during pregnancy improved the maze-learning ability of the offspring whereas anterior pituitary hormone had no such effect. Subsequently Clendinnen and Eayrs[15] found that the latter, in the form of somatotrophin, produced hypertrophy of the neurons of the cerebral cortex, earlier maturation and enhanced higher-level behaviour. In studying the effects of the prenatal use of drugs in human beings acceleration and hyper-reactivity should be noted as well as retardation and unresponsiveness.

Very few results are available, apart from those for thalidomide, of the effects of the use of sedative drugs during human pregnancy. Kris[44] found that the children of 14 pregnant psychiatric patients who had received chlorpromazine showed no birth anomalies and were normal after four years. On the other hand Sobel[66] observed increased respiratory distress in the newborn, antepartum bleeding, prematurity and infant mortality following prenatal dosage with reserpine and chlorpromazine. Such contradictory results serve to emphasize the need for a systematic and comprehensive system for the recording of infantile conditions and behaviour and of concomitant pregnancy stresses, as advocated below in the discussion of research perspectives in the general area of prenatal influences. In a general review article Werboff and Gottlieb[91] recommend that, considering the present uncertain state of knowledge about the effects of drugs, 'practitioners must weigh the immediate benefits of administering a particular drug to a pregnant woman against the possible toxic or delayed behavioural effects of the drug on the offspring'.

11

Research Perspectives

It would have been gratifying, in this review of work on prenatal influences, to have been able to quote a large number of definitive studies. Only those relating to rubella and thalidomide can be regarded as 'proved' in the usual sense of the word. Such work as has been done has served to destroy the myth that the foetus is completely protected from outside influences. Indeed the evidence suggests that the foetus is peculiarly sensitive to its environment within the maternal host, and to stresses which affect the mother. At least the possiblity has been established that the major determinants of viability, physical growth and health, mental ability and personality, may be those which operate during gestation. It has now become mandatory to take cognizance of prenatal factors in any study of the etiology of differences in personality, intelligence or health. One may be forgiven for naïvely wondering, considering the vast potential importance of such knowledge for the human race, why it has not been given higher priority as a field of research. Even if the slenderest chance were shown to exist for exposing the cause, and leading to the prevention of a larger proportion of mental subnormalities and physical and mental ill-health—or the slightest possibility showed itself of our being able to improve the intelligence and health of the human race on a grand scale—surely it would be worthwhile to endow research institutes and attract the best scholars for work in this field. The reasons for its neglect lie in the sociology and psychology of contemporary research. All but a dedicated and culturally atypical few reject topics of research that will be unlikely to advance their careers. This means that the project must be of limited duration, the research design impeccable, the variables clearly defined and the topic fashionable. The field of prenatal influences offers none of these advantages. It demands years of painstaking work with variables that are difficult to define, within a field contaminated by superstition. The scientific climate is also unfavourable for risk-taking at the present time. The cry is for 'proof', although the very idea that anything can be proved is foreign to empirically won knowledge. Proof requires elimination of every other possible explanation, and this implies omniscience. Science has to limit itself to the establishment of regularities from which the probability of events can be inferred. To say that a postulate is 'not proved' does not justify the assumption that it is false or that it may safely be ignored. If the knowledge to be gained is potentially valuable, the necessary techniques must be developed. The rub is to find the workers who in the meantime are prepared to brave taunts of lack of rigour, and risk having little to show by way of formal results after years of patient trial.

The study of prenatal influences has been handicapped in addition by a particular confusion of thought in methodology. This has consisted in the demand for prospective studies as the only sort worthy of credence, and the consequent rejection of results from retrospective studies. It goes without saying that the prospective type of investigation makes for high reliability in the data, eliminates retrospective bias and carries conviction. But one must first know what kinds of data to collect, that is to say, what will probably be relevant and significant. Such knowledge can only be provided by preliminary retrospective studies. Failure to make these has in some cases (notably in child development, with the neglect of prenatal data) made a longer term prospective study a waste of time from its inception. The prospective rubella study by Manson and her co-workers, while well designed for what they set out to find, affords a good example of lost opportunities. No enquiry was made of other types of maternal stress, or other maternal variables, and so the mystery of why only a small proportion of the infants were affected even though the mothers had rubella in the first trimester remained unsolved. And no enquiry was made concerning the effects upon the child's temperament and behaviour of rubella contracted in the later trimesters.

Prospective studies have other disadvantages. Unless they can be carried through expeditiously the hypotheses which they were designed to test may be out of date before the results are obtained. With conditions such as mongolism, which occur once in several hundred births, the prospective study has to be on a vast scale if a sufficient number of cases are to be included. In such instances the only practicable means of obtaining a statistically significant result is by a retrospective study. It is a question of choosing a research design which maximizes the reliability of the data, while ensuring that such unreliability as remains works against the significance of the results. The cleft-palate study of Drillien, Ingram and Wilkinson[22], which compared the familial with the non-familial causes, is a good example of this technique. In assessing the validity of results the cardinal question is the probability of bias; a prospective investigation is a good, but not the sole, way of meeting this criterion.

The variable around which most difficulties have centred has been that of emotional stress. Paradoxically it is the one which has emerged as possibly the most significant in more than one study (in which the authors have none the less fought shy of it). In other studies it has been treated with appalling carelessness. Its proper handling is the first prerequisite to progress in our knowledge of prenatal influences. In effect it consists of two interrelated variables—the nature of the experience, and the stress tolerance of the individual mother. The second is the more difficult to evaluate, and probably it is best not to attempt to do more than to take into account a small number of objective indications such as a record of psychiatric treatment for 'nerves', symptoms of anxiety-state, etc. An alternative is—at the expense of a certain loss of statistical significance—to ignore this variable altogether and to concentrate upon an assessment of stressful events judged capable of causing emotional upset to the majority of women. Suggestions for standardizing such assessments are given in the Manual and Scoring Key to the Systematic Interview Guides (Stott[80]).

Severity of certain pregnancy illnesses such as toxaemia can be similarly assessed according to the treatment (1 point if treated at home without the mother being put to bed; 2 if put to bed and 3 if taken to the hospital). With other diseases, such as rubella, the severity of symptoms is no guide to the degree to which they affect the foetus, and their assessment will depend upon what is progressively discovered about their effects. Since there is reason for believing that the effects of diverse stresses are cumulative, it would make sense, in a study of the etiology of childhood conditions, to summate the ratings for all the types of stress incurred within a pregnancy.

The condition of the child can be quantified in a similar way, a rating from 1 to 3 being given for each disease according to its lethality or degree of handicap if left untreated. The mode of quantification of impairment—if any is required—is obviously something that must be decided by the objective of each investigation. The above method would be convenient, for example, in examining the role of prenatal stresses in various types of behavioural abnormality or criminalism. A general measure of multiple impairment in childhood would be useful both in assessing the noxiousness of prenatal factors. The number of ways in which the child may be affected presents a difficulty in determining the effects of, say, influenza or toxoplasmosis. It may be overcome by an over-all score for impairment.

The above mentioned Systematic Interview Guides represent only a first attempt at such quantification, which will have to be progressively modified with the progress of knowledge. One of the advantages of their use at the present time is in ensuring that, in the taking of a case-history from the mother, there is a record of the factors which are absent as well as those that are present. In the use of unsystematic case-records, however thoroughly they may be compiled, the lack of specific reference to a condition may mean either that it was absent or simply that the mother was not asked.

For this and many other reasons it is seldom possible to base a research upon administrative records. At the same time, the vast amount of case-material handled in antenatal and child welfare clinics would solve the difficulty of scale in prospective studies, if only the data could be systematized with a view to possible research use. In order to do this a standard interview schedule would be required (which also has the advantage for current clinical work that the essential facts can be found, and a general overview of the case made, in the space of a few minutes). For the study of prenatal influences, a detailed and systematic method of recording not only physical data but the events of the expectant mother's family life at intervals prior to delivery could easily be related by the research department of a local health authority to the outcome of the pregnancy and the conditions of the child in its early years. In sum, definitive progress in this field must depend upon large-scale investigations, best carried out by Institutes or administrative authorities whose future does not depend upon finding significant correlations within a given time.

REFERENCES

1. ACHESON, R. M., 1960. Maternal influenza and congenital deformities (Letter to the *Lancet*, i, 981).
2. ANDERSON, E. W., HAMILTON, M. W., and KEENA, J. C., 1957. Psychiatric, social and psychological aspects of illegitimate pregnancy in girls under sixteen years. *Psyschiatr. Neurolog.* **133**, 207-20.
3. ANDERSON, E. W., 1960. Personal communication.
4. ANDERSON, G. W., ANDERSON, G., SKAAR, A., and SANDLER, F., 1952. Poliomyelitis in pregnancy. *Amer. J. Hyg.*, **55**, 127-39.
5. ANDERSON, W. J. R., BAIRD, D., and THOMSON, A. M., 1958. Epidemiology of stillbirth and infant deaths due to congenital malformations. *Lancet*, i, 1304-06.
6. ARESIN, N., SOMMER, K. H., 1950. Missbildungen und Umweltfaktoren. *Zb. F. Gynäk.*, **72**, 1329-36.
7. ARMITAGE, S. G., 1952. The effect of barbiturates on the behaviour of rat offspring as measured on learning and reasoning situations. *J. Comp. Physiol. Psychol.*, **45**, 146.
8. BARNETT, S. A., 1958. Physiological effects of 'social stress' in wild rats. I. The adrenal cortex. *J. Psychosom. Res.*, **3**, 1-11.

REFERENCES

9. BARNETT, S. A., EATON, J. C., and MCCALLUM, H. M., 1960. Physiological effects of 'social stress' in wild rats. II. Liver glycogen and blood glucose. *J. Psychosom. Res.*, **4**, 251-60.
10. BRADFORD HILL, A., DOLL, R., GALLOWAY, T. McL., and HUGHES, J. P. W., 1958. Virus diseases in pregnancy and congenital defects. *Brit. J. prev. soc. Med.*, **12**, 1-7.
11. BRUCE, H. M., 1960a. A block to pregnancy in the mouse caused by the proximity of strange males. *J. Reprod. Fertil.*, **1**, 96-103.
12. BRUCE, H. M., 1960b. Further observations on the pregnancy block in mice caused by the proximity of strange males. *J. Reprod. Fertil.*, **3**, 310-11.
13. BURKINSHAW, J., KIRMAN, B. H., and SORSBY, A., 1953. Toxoplasmosis in relation to mental deficiency. *Brit. Med. J.*, i, 702-04.
14. *Chief Medical Officer for England and Wales, report 1959.* London, H.M.S.O.
15. CLENDINNEN, B. G., and EAYRS, J. T., 1961. The anatomical and physiological effects of prenatally administered somatotrophins on cerebral development in rats. *J. Endocrinal.*, **22**, 183.
16. CLOKIE, H., 1959. Premature babies born in Northamptonshire in 1952. *Med. Officer*, **101**, 119.
17. COFFEY, V. P., and JESSOP, W. J. E., 1959. Maternal influenza and congenital deformities. *Lancet*, ii, 935.
18. DISPENSA, J., and HORNBECK, R. T., 1941. Can intelligence be improved by prenatal endocrine therapy? *J. Psychol.*, **12**, 209.
19. DOUGLAS, J. W. B., 1948. *Maternity in Great Britain.* Oxford, Univ. Press.
20. DOUGLAS, J. W. B., and BLOMFIELD, J. M., 1958. *Children under five.* London, Allen and Unwin.
21. DRILLIEN, C. M., 1964. *The growth and development of the prematurely born infant.* Edinburgh, Livingstone.
22. DRILLIEN, C. M., INGRAM, T. T. S., and WILKINSON, E. M., 1966. *The causes and natural history of cleft lip and palate.* Edinburgh, Livingstone.
23. DRILLIEN, C. M., and RICHMOND, F., 1956. Prematurity in Edinburgh. *Archs Dis. Child.*, **31**, 390.
24. DRILLIEN, C. M., and WILKINSON, E. M., 1964. Emotional stress and mongoloid birth. *Devel. Med. Child. Neurol.*, **6**, 140-43.
25. EDWARDS, J. H., 1958. Congenital malformations of the central nervous system in Scotland. *Brit. J. prev. soc. Med.*, **12**, 115-30.
26. EICHMANN, E., and GESENIUS, H., 1952. Die Missgenburtenzunahme in Berlin und Umgebung in den Nachkriegsjahren. *Arch. Gynäk.*, **181**, 168-84.
27. FLAMM, H., 1959. *Die pränatalen Infektionen des Menschen.* Stuttgart, G. Thieme.
28. GARRY, R. C., and WOOD, H. O., 1946. Dietary requirements in human pregnancy and lactation. A review of recent work. *Nutr. Abstr.*, **15**, 591-621.
29. GESENIUS, H., 1951. Missgeburten im Wechsel der Jahrhunderte. *Berliner Med. Zeitschrift*, **2**, 359-62.
30. GREBE, H., 1955. Die Grundlagen menschlicher Missbildungen. *Naturwissenschaftliche Rundschau*, **5**, 189.
31. GREENBERG, M., PELLITERI, O., and BARTON, J., 1957. Frequency of defects in infants whose mothers had rubella during pregnancy. *J. Amer. med. Assn*, **165**, 675.
32. GREGG, N. McA., 1941. Congenital cataract following German measles in the mother. *Trans. ophthalm. Soc. Austral.*, **3**, 35.
33. HALE, F., 1935. Relation of vitamin A to anophthalmos in pigs. *Amer. J. Ophth.*, **18**, 1087-93.

34. HAMILTON, H. C., 1944. The effect of administration of sodium bromide to pregnant rats on the learning ability of the offspring. III. Three-table test. *J. Psychol.*, **18**, 183-95.
35. HARNED, B. K., HAMILTON, H. C., and BORRUS, J. C., 1940. The effect of bromide administered to pregnant rats on the learning ability of offspring. *Amer. J. Med. Sci.*, **200**, 846.
36. HELLMANN, K., 1966. Immunosuppression by thalidomide: implications for teratology. *Lancet*, i, 1136-37.
37. HELLMANN, K., DUKE, D. I., and TUCKER, D. F., 1965. Prolongation of skin homograft survival by thalidomide. *Brit. Med. J.*, ii, 687.
38. HERTIG, A. T., 1953. *Traumatic abortion and prenatal death of the embryo*. Proc. Cong. on prematurity and congenital malformations sponsored by the Society for the Aid of Crippled Children, New York.
39. HIS, W., 1891. *Int. Beitr. Wissen. Med.*, **1**, 177.
40. INGALLS, T. H., BABOTT, J., and PHILBROOK, R., 1957. The mothers of mongoloid babies: a retrospective appraisal of their health during pregnancy. *Amer. J. Obstet. Gynaec.*, **74**, S72-81.
41. KLEBANOV, D., 1948. Hunger und psychische Erregungen als Ovar und Keimschädigungen, *Geburtsh. u. Frauenheilk.*, **7-8**, 812.
42. KLOTZ, R., 1952. Das psychische Trauma in der Genese der Missgeburt. *Zentralblatt. F. Gynäk.*, **74**, 906.
43. KNOBLOCH, H., and PASAMANICK, B., 1958. Seasonal variation in the births of the mentally deficient. *Amer. J. Pub. Hlth*, **48**, 1201.
44. KRIS, E. B., 1962. Children born to mothers maintained on pharmacotherapy during pregnancy and postpartum. *Rec. Adv. Biol. Psychiat.*, **4**, 180.
45. LANDAUER, W., 1929. Experimental studies concerning the development of the chicken embryo. 1. The toxic action of lithium and magnesium salts. *Poultry Sci.* **8**, 301-12.
46. LANDAUER, W., 1932. The effects of irradiating eggs with ultra-violet light upon the development of chicken embryo. Experiments with Frizzle and Creeper fowl. *Storrs Agri. Exper. Station Bull.*, **179**.
47. LOGAN, W. P. D., 1951. Incidence of congenital malformation and their relation to virus infections during pregnancy. *Brit. med. J.*, ii, 641.
48. LUNDSTRÖM, R., 1952. Rubella during pregnancy. *Acta paediat. Stockh.*, **41**, S83-94.
49. MACGILLIVRAY, R. C., 1957. Hypertelorism with unusual associated anomalies. *Amer. J. Ment. Def.*, **62**, 288.
50. MACMAHON, T., and MCKEOWN, T., 1953. Incidence of hardship and cleft palate related to birth rank and maternal age. *Amer. J. Hum. Gen.*, **5**, 176.
51. MANSON, M. M., LOGAN, W. P. D., and LOY, R. M., 1960. *Rubella and other virus infections during pregnancy*. London, H.M.S.O.
52. MARSHALL, A. G., HUTCHINSON, E. O., and HONISETT, J., 1962. Heredity in common diseases: a retrospective study of twins in a hospital population. *Brit. med. J.*, ii, 1-6.
53. MCDONALD, A. D., 1958. Maternal health and congenital defect. *New England J. Med.*, **258**, 767-73.
54. MCKEOWN, T., and RECORD, R. G., 1951. Seasonal incidence of congenital malformation of the central nervous system. *Lancet*, i, 102.
55. MCKERRACHER, D. W., 1961. *Effects of physical and emotional pregnancy stress upon the development of children*. Ed. M. thesis, University of Glasgow.
56. MILLEN, J. W., 1962. Thalidomide and limb deformities. *Lancet*, ii, 599-600.
57. MURPHY, D. P., 1947. *Congenital malformation*. Philadelphia, Lippincott.
58. NOWAK, J., 1950. Häufigkeit der Missgeburten in den Nachkriegsjahren 1945-1949. *Zb. F. Gynäk.*, **72**, 1313-28.

59. PASAMANICK, B., and KNOBLOCH, H., 1957. Some early precursors of racial behavioral differences. *J. Nat. Med. Assn*, **49**, 372.
60. PASAMANICK, B., DINITZ, S., and KNOBLOCH, H., 1959. Geographic and seasonal variations on births. *Pub. Hlth Rep.*, **74**, 285.
61. PLEYDELL, M. J., 1960. Anencephaly and other congenital malformations. *Brit. med. J.*, i, 309-14.
62. RECORD, R. G., and MCKEOWN, T., 1950. Congenital malformation of the central nervous system. *Brit. J. Soc. Med.*, **4**, 217.
63. RECORD, R. G., 1958. Environmental influences in the aetiology of congenital malformations. *Proc. Roy. Doc. Med.*, **51**, 147.
64. ROBERTSON, J. S., 1960. Excessive perinatal mortality in a small town associated with evidence of toxoplasmosis. *Brit. med. J.*, ii, 91-96.
65. SCOTT, J. K., 1965. *Effectiveness behaviour and its relation to congenital factors in four year old children*. M.A. thesis, University of Glasgow.
66. SOBEL, D. E., 1960. Foetal damage due to ECT, insulin coma, chlorpromazine, or reserpine. *Arch. Gen. Psychiat.*, **2**, 606.
67. SONTAG, L. W., 1941. Significance of fetal environmental differences. *Amer. J. Obst. Gynec.*, **42**, 996-1003.
68. SONTAG, L. W., 1944. Differences in the modifiability of fetal behavior and physiology. *Psychosom. Med.*, **6**, 151-54.
69. STAFFORD-CLARK, D., 1959. The foundations of research in psychiatry. *Brit. med. J.*, ii, 1199.
70. STEVENSON, S. S., WORCESTER, J., and RICE, R. G., 1950. 677 congenitally malformed infants and associated gestational characteristics. *Pediatrics*, **6**, 37.
71. STEWART, A. M., 1955. A note on the obstetric effects of work during pregnancy. *Brit. J. prev. soc. Med.*, **9**, 159.
72. STEWART, A., WEBB, J. W., and HEWITT, D., 1955. Observations on 1,078 perinatal deaths. *Brit. J. prev. soc. Med.*, **9**, 57.
73. STOCKARD, C. R., 1910. The influence of alcohol and other anaesthetics on embryonic development. *Amer. J. Anat.*, **10**, 369.
74. STOTT, D. H., 1956. The effects of separation from the mother in early life. *Lancet*, i, 624-28.
75. STOTT, D. H., 1957. Physical and mental handicaps following a disturbed pregnancy. *Lancet*, i, 1006-12.
76. STOTT, D. H., 1958a. *The social adjustment of children*. London, Univ. Press. Manual to the Bristol Social Adjustment Guides.
77. STOTT, D. H., 1958b. Some psychosomatic aspects of casualty in reproduction. *J. Psychosomat. Res.*, **3**, 42.
78. STOTT, D. H., 1959. Evidence for prenatal impairment of temperament in mentally retarded children. *Vita Humana*, **2**, 125.
79. STOTT, D. H., 1961. Mongolism related to emotional shock in early pregnancy. *Vita Humana*, **4**, 57-76.
80. STOTT, D. H., 1967. *The systematic interview guides*. London, Univ. Press.
81. STOTT, D. H., and SYKES, E. G., 1956. *The Bristol social adjustment guides*. London, Univ. Press.
82. TAUSSIG, H. B., 1962. A study of the German outbreak of phocomelia. *J. Amer. med. Assn*, 1106-14.
83. THALHAMMER, O., 1957. *Die Toxoplasmose bei Mensch und Tier*. Vienna, W. Maudrich.
84. THOMPSON, W. R., and SONTAG, L. W., 1956. Behavioral effects in the offspring of rats subjected to audiogenic seizure during the gestational period. *J. comp. physiol. Psychol.*, **49**, 454-66.
85. THOMPSON, W. R., 1957. Influence of prenatal maternal anxiety on emotionality of young rats. *Science*, **125**, 698.

86. TOUGH, I. M., BUCKTON, K. E., BAIKIE, A. G., and COURT-BROWN, W. M., 1960. X-ray induced chromosome damage in man. *Lancet*, ii, 849-51.
87. VINCENT, N. M., 1958. The effect of prenatal alcohol upon motivation, emotionality and learning in the rat. *Amer. Psychol.*, **13**, 401.
88. WALKER, W. M., and MCKEE, A. F., 1959. Asian influenza in pregnancy. *Obstet. Gynec.*, **13**, 394-98.
89. WARKANY, J., and NELSON, R. C., 1940. Appearance of skeletal abnormalities in the offspring of rats reared on a deficient diet. *Science*, **92**, 383-84.
90. WERBOFF, J., and DEMBICKI, E. L., 1962. Toxic effects of tranquillizers administered to gravid rats. *J. Neuropsychiat.*, **4**, 87-91.
91. WERBOFF, J., and GOTTLIEB, J. S., 1963. Drugs in pregnancy: behavioral teratology. *Obstet. Gynec. Survey*, **18**, 420-23.
92. WERBOFF, J., GOTTLIEB, J. S., HAVLENA, J., and WORD, T. J., 1961. Behavioral effects of prenatal drug administration in the white rat. *Pediatrics*, **27**, 318-24.
93. WERBOFF, J., and HAVLENA, J., 1962. Postnatal behavioral effects of tranquilizers administered to the gravid rat. *Exper. Neurol.*, **6**, 263-69.
94. WERBOFF, J., and KESNER, R., 1963. Learning defects of offspring after administration of tranquillizing drugs to the mothers. *Nature, Lond.*, **197**, 106-07.
95. WHITE, R. W., 1959. Motivation reconsidered: the concept of competence. *Psychol. Rev.*, **66**, 297-333.
96. WILSON, M. G., HEINS, H. L., IMAGAWA, D. T., and ADAMS, J. M., 1959. Teratogenic effects of Asian flu. *J. Amer. med. Assn.* **171**, 638-41.
97. WOLLAM, D. H. M., and MILLEN, J. W., 1960. Influence of thyroxine on the incidence of harelip in the 'Strong A' line of mice. *Brit. med. J.*, i, 1253-64.
98. WOOLLAM, D. H. M., PRATT, C. W. M., and FOZZARD, J. A. F., 1957. Influence of vitamins upon some teratogenic effects of radiation. *Brit. med. J.*, i, 1219-21.

II

GENESIS OF BEHAVIOUR DISORDERS

STELLA CHESS
M.D.

Associate Professor of Psychiatry—New York University School of Medicine

Many studies and investigations carried out during the past few decades have yielded much suggestive data and a number of important insights into the circumstances which may contribute to the development of a behaviour disorder in a child. Hereditary and genetic factors, prenatal and perinatal brain damage, biochemical and neurophysiological disturbances, unfavourable parental attitudes and practices, intrafamilial conflict, conditions of social stress and deprivation and distortions of the learning processes involved in the child's socialization all have been incriminated as factors which can contribute to the production of disturbance in behavioural development.

1

Theories of Child Development

However, despite the accumulation of voluminous literature, there is as yet no body of evidence sufficient to provide solid support for any single theory about the genesis of behaviour problems in childhood. On the contrary, the fields of child development and child psychiatry currently are besieged by a number of differing theoretical formulations competing for acceptance, each of which has been used as a didactic framework within which an approach to the question of the origin of behaviour disorders has been made. Basically, current theories are interactionist. However, the relative weight given to constitution and environment varies in crucial ways. Traditional Freudian child psychiatry adheres strictly to the classical thesis of the primacy of hypothesized instinctual drive states and views behaviour disturbance as the outcome of conflicts between these drives seeking expression and satisfaction and repressing forces originating in the environment which seek to inhibit or contain them. A number of Freudian theoreticians have modified this classical approach in recent years to include the 'autonomous ego' as an additional prime determinant of behaviour and its disorders. The 'neo-Freudians' emphasize the importance of interpersonal relationships, socio-cultural factors or adaptational mechanisms in the genesis of disorders. Learning theory, deriving in varying degrees from the work of Pavlov, Skinner, Hull and others, is utilized either in combination with psychoanalytic concepts or alone to establish a developmental theory fundamentally antithetical to psychoanalysis wherein disturbances are viewed as conditioned maladaptive learned patterns based on conditioned reflex formation. Other researchers focus on the role of predetermined developmental sequences in the ontogeny of normal as well as disordered behaviour and cognition. Still other investigators consider prenatal and perinatal brain damage to be responsible not only for the obvious organic brain syndromes but also for a variety of behaviour disorders usually considered to be of functional origin. Finally, there is the now generally discredited constitutionalist position in which the emergence of behaviour disorder is viewed as a direct reflection of innate characteristics in the basic biological organization of the child.

Consideration of the reasons for the inconclusiveness of data obtained from these innumerable investigations into the origins of behaviour disorders in childhood involves two issues of critical importance. In the first place, none of these studies has provided enough data to validate its underlying theoretical formulations and thus deductions from these theories about the nature of individual child development remain assumptions rather than facts. Secondly, the vast majority of studies have offered as primary evidence information about the events and course of psychological development in early childhood obtained retrospectively from individuals suffering from behaviour disturbances or from the parents of such individuals. This method of studying the early developmental history of children recently has been shown to be unreliable on several accounts and significant distortions in parental recall and report have been revealed (Chess et al.[7]; Robbins[16]; Wenar[23]; Thomas et al.[21]).

2

Problems of Retrospective Investigation

Freud was the first to recognize the necessity for questioning the accuracy of recall in retrospective reports. As is well known, he discovered that his patients' reports of sexual seduction in their early childhood were frequently false. These episodes, which were recalled vividly and with convincing detail, in reality had not occurred. Freud concluded that these reports were memories of early childhood phantasies. He further assumed that the phantasies were as influential in the causation of disturbed psychological development as the actual events themselves would have been. Neither

Freud nor his followers appear to have given serious consideration to the possibility that the phantasies, too, might suffer from distortion of retrospective recall, and be either misplaced in regard to the time of actual occurrence, or altered from the actual original content of the childhood phantasy, or both.

Nevertheless, the assumption that retrospectively obtained personal histories of early childhood events, feelings and phantasies represented a valid body of evidence on which to base a theory of child development went virtually unchallenged until recently. However, as has been shown by Jerome D. Frank[9], not only the memories of patients, but even their free associations and dreams can be influenced by the theoretical bias of the psychotherapist. Thus, their use as accurate information about the past is greatly limited.

The validity of the other major source of retrospective data, namely, mothers' reports on the early development of their children, has also been subjected to investigation. Two studies of the accuracy of such parental recall derived from the New York Longitudinal Study of child development. One involved the recall by parents when the child was 3 years old of the facts of their child-rearing practices and the child's development during infancy (Robbins[16]). The other study considered the recall of the child's developmental course by parents of behaviourally disturbed children (Chess)[6]. In both studies, the accuracy of recall was tested by comparison with anterospective data on the children and parents gathered previously during the course of the longitudinal study.

In the first study, a number of inaccuracies of recall were found, especially about items dealing with the ages of weaning and toilet training, the occurrence of thumbsucking and whether the child was fed on schedule or demand. Although mothers generally recalled more accurately than fathers, significant discrepancies were found in the reports of the former. These findings, together with those of several other related studies in the literature, have been summarized recently by Wenar[23] with the conclusion that 'a good deal of past research has leaned heavily on the slenderest of reeds. It may well be that mothers' histories mislead more often than they illuminate and, as yet, we are in a poor position to know when they are doing one or the other.'

Besides the various idiosyncratic factors which may produce distortions of recall, it has been suggested that socio-cultural norms may influence the direction of the inaccuracies (Robbins[16]). The basis for this hypothesis is the fact that in several instances where inaccuracies of recall occurred there was a significant correlation between the direction of error and the recommendations of accepted experts in the child-care field. American middle-class mothers, particularly, tended to report practices that conformed to the recommendations of Spock[19] and others rather than their actual functioning when this was not correctly recalled.

Even greater degrees of unreliability were found, as had been expected, in the second study which tested the accuracy of recall of significant events by the parents of children with behaviour problems (Chess[6]). The staff child psychiatrist obtained a retrospective history of the child's early developmental course from the parents when the child first was brought for consultation about disturbances in behavioural functioning. Comparison of this report with information on the child's development collected longitudinally revealed significant distortions in 12 of the 33 cases studied. In many instances, the discrepancies were expected and explainable. Thus, parental defensiveness led to inability to recall pertinent past behaviour and to denial or minimization of the problem. And, just as inaccuracies in recall by parents of normally developing children reflected current popular recommendations about child care, similarly, distortions in timing reported by parents of children with behaviour problems showed the influence of currently popular theories about the causes for psychopathology such as sibling rivalry or failure of the mother to provide adequate feelings of security for the child. For example, incidents dealing with the initial signs of difficulty were reported first occurring after a new sibling was born or after the mother returned to work when, in fact, the anterospective records showed clearly that the episodes of malfunctioning preceded these events.

Distortions such as these, in which timing is shifted so that the sequence of events conforms to prevalent theories of causation, are of special importance because they indicate that a theory of child development which explains the origin of problem behaviour may generate 'evidence' to support itself once it gains wide acceptance. Awareness of the danger of such a self-fulfilling prophecy makes it imperative that retrospective behavioural data be scrutinized carefully, especially in cases where the recall could be influenced by a knowledge of the theory. Such a caution applies not only to parental recall but also to reports of their childhood given by adult patients undergoing examination or treatment.

Another interesting finding in this study was the lack of systematic relationship between the consistency and fluency of the parent's report at the time of clinical interview and the accuracy of the report when judged against the body of available anterospective data. Since the temptation is always to accept those responses that are precise, apparently factual and clearly pertinent to the questions asked, it should be noted that a number of the mothers who gave such responses outlined developmental histories grossly at variance with the anterospective data, while one of the consistently accurate reports of antecedent behaviour was given by a disorganized and circumstantial mother. No systematic relation existed between the character of the child's presenting problem and either the frequency or type of distortion in parental recall.

Retrospective investigation also may be inaccurate in ways which do not directly involve errors in parental recall but rather reflect the prejudgments of the psychiatrist or psychologist who already has knowledge of the existence of a specific problem. For instance, if a child is brought for psychiatric consultation with presenting problems that suggest marked neurotic tendencies, the professional gathering information on his earlier development (whether from the patient himself, the parents, or other sources) may give primary attention only to the data which appear to be influential in this regard. He may, for example, seek information on the causation of dependency, such as maternal overprotection. And, as a result, he may not explore with the same thoroughness equally significant facts in development which appear to him to be irrelevant or contradictory to the formation of the dependency trait. Because the investigator is aware of a problem in the child, he may automatically have in mind the issues he considers significant in determining the development of the disturbance and may focus selectively only on those items in the past history that support his formulation.

3

Selectivity of Child's Responses to Pathogenic Influences

A further question which requires anterospective longitudinal data for adequate exploration is the inability of any of the current theoretical concepts about the origins of behavioural disturbance to explain the fact that only some of the children subjected to the presumed pathogenic influences do in fact develop such disturbances. While it is true that the constitutionalist approach does offer an explanation in terms of inborn differences in the children, the evidence for such inborn differences turns out to be the fact of difference in development—a classic example of circular reasoning.

With all the other theoretical formulations, however, whether they emphasize prenatal and perinatal pathology, parental characteristics, other intrafamilial influences or extrafamilial environmental factors, it is possible to identify significant numbers of children who, though they are subjected to these influences, develop normally. In brief, the selective effectiveness of each particular influence or factor is not accounted for and current theories continue to be plagued by their inability to explain individual differences in the type of disturbance which may develop. Why does one child who is subjected to an oppressively domineering and rigid parent become a passive submissive individual while another who is subjected to the same influence develops a rebellious and aggressively negativistic character? Is the fact that one child with postencephalitic brain damage shows impulsivity and distractibility while another manifests primarily repetitive and stereotyped behaviour to be explained entirely on the basis of brain areas involved? Why does one conditioned maladaptive learning experience lead to a phobia and another to a compulsion? Why does socio-economic deprivation lead one individual to defeatism and inertia and another to intensive activity for achievement and success?

Beiser[1] has recently described the problem posed by these facts for the currently favoured thesis which emphasizes the decisive role of the parent by saying, 'there is not a direct quantitative relationship between pathology in a parent and pathology in a child . . . the helpless position of a child does not always make him the victim of the parent. This presents a great problem for the development of any pertinent generalizations concerning the influence of parents on children. It is to be hoped that ongoing longitudinal studies of very young children and their parents will contribute to some general principles.'

Freud himself recognized the limitations of theorizing retrospectively about the etiology of behavioural disorder when he said, 'so long as we trace the development (of a mental process) backwards, the connection appears continuous, and we feel we have gained an insight which is completely satisfactory or even exhaustive. But if we proceed the reverse way, if we start from the premises inferred from the analysis and try to follow these up to the final result, then we no longer get the impression of an inevitable sequence of events which could not have been otherwise determined. We notice at once that there might be another result, and that we might have been just as well able to understand and explain the latter.'[10] This aspect of the partial if not illusory nature of retrospective information offers a possible explanation of the failure of any past or current theory to explain these developmental differences between children and shows that attempts to reconstruct the sequences of forces involved in the evolution of individuality should not be made dependent on information obtained retrospectively.

4

Anterospective Longitudinal Studies of Child Development

All of these discussions which indicate the inadequacy of retrospective data as a basis for studying the genesis of behaviour disorders have led to an increasing awareness of the need for longitudinal developmental studies in which data can be gathered anterospectively. Although such longitudinal studies are time-consuming and present special problems of data collection and data analysis, they have the unique advantage of permitting the collection of information that is unaffected by errors of retrospective recall or by knowledge of the existence of a problem at each age-stage of a child's development.

Previous longitudinal studies at Berkeley (MacFarlane[14]), the Fels Institute (Kagan[12]), Yale (Kris[13]) and Topeka (Murphy[15]) have made important contributions to the understanding of the evolution of behaviour disorders. In these studies the possible significance of temperamental characteristics of the child in interaction with parental function has been indicated. A lack of correlation between the child's patterns of psychodynamic defenses and the occurrence of behavioural dysfunction has been found (Murphy)[15]. Symptoms typical of various age periods have been tabulated, their vicissitudes over time traced and correlations among different symptoms determined (MacFarlane[14]). However, each of these studies has been limited either by small sample size, which has not permitted generalization of the findings or, in the case of Berkeley where there was adequate sample size, by the absence of systematic psychiatric evaluation of the children, which has severely restricted the possibility of categorizing the behaviour disturbances and of making meaningful correlations with the longitudinal behavioural data.

In order for a longitudinal developmental study to give adequate consideration to the genesis of behaviour disorders in childhood, three basic conditions must be satisfied.

1. The study sample should be of sufficient size so that the number and variety of behaviour problems that develop are large enough to permit generalizations from the findings. Only a few children can be expected to show significant difficulties in development if the sample is small; the findings would then of necessity be restricted to individual case studies. In such instances, meaningful overall comparisons between the disturbed and nondisturbed children, and especially any analyses of specific types of disorder, will not be possible.

2. An *a priori* theoretical framework should not be imposed upon the collection or analysis of the data. Such an imposition makes it impossible to test the validity of the particular theory against the data and interferes with the exploration of alternative possibilities. For example, if a 3-year-old's slow participation in peer group activity is categorized *a priori* as an expression of anxiety, it is then not possible to utilize the characteristics of peer involvement to study the role of anxiety in the genesis of behaviour problems. Similarly, if it is assumed that a mother's attitude toward toileting necessarily determines her child's reaction to toilet training, then the toilet training experience can not be used to investigate the influences of the mother on the child's development. If the data collection and analysis are not insulated from theoretical formulations about the nature of psychological development, then the investigation will take on the qualities of a self-fulfilling prophecy.

3. Clinical psychiatric evaluation of each child presenting with a behaviour problem should be done independently of the other data collected in the ongoing longitudinal study. Only if these two bodies of data are obtained separately and independently will it be possible to use them effectively for various correlational analyses.

The New York Longitudinal Study has had available both a total sample of substantial size and independent clinical evaluation of each of the children with a behaviour problem. In addition, we were able to develop an economical method for the continual collection of valid and representative data. By means of a structured interview which focuses on gathering information on a descriptive, factual level, we have found that it is possible to use the parents as a rich source of meaningful, accurate, ongoing data on the child's behaviour. The parental reports have correlated closely with descriptions of behaviour obtained by independent, direct observation. They have also been broad and detailed enough to permit content analysis (Thomas[21]).

The data on the total sample include information gathered longitudinally and anterospectively at sequential age levels from early infancy onwards on the nature of each child's own individual characteristics of functioning at home, in school and in standard test situations; on parental attitudes and child care practices; on special environmental events and the child's reaction to them; and other pertinent neurological or physical information. In addition, a psychiatric evaluation by the staff child psychiatrist has been made of each child presenting symptoms. Wherever indicated, special neurological, perceptual or psychological testing also has been done. Clinical follow-up of each child with a problem has been carried out systematically.

The information on the 136 children in the study who have been and are continuing to be followed since March, 1956, has been culled from anterospective parental interviews, periods of direct observation in the homes of most of the children, detailed observation of each child's behaviour during standard play and psychological test situations, direct observation of the child's behaviour in school and teacher interviews.

It was our belief that since there is at present no adequate theoretical foundation on which to base a deductive approach to individual child development, a useful hypothetical framework could be constructed only from inductive analysis of anterospective data concerning the details of behavioural functioning in infancy and childhood. Collected longitudinally, such data also provides information on the evolution of adaptive response patterns and temperamental characteristics.

5

Temperamental Individuality

Many child psychiatrists and other researchers have made token acknowledgment of the fact that children differ. Our study has investigated *how* they differ and how the dynamics of such individuality influenced each child's psychological development. Inductive content analysis of the anterospective data on infant behaviour provided a description of the behavioural style of each child from two to three months onward. We have used the word 'temperament' to describe this primary reactive style and it is emphasized that this contains no inference as to genetic, somatologic, endocrine or environmental etiologies. Temperament applies only to the *how* of behaviour, not to the *what* or to the *why*, and neither permanence nor immutability is implicated in this concept.

The temperamental attributes of each child have been subsumed in nine categories: activity level, rhythmicity (regularity of biological functions), approach-withdrawal (positive or negative initial response to new stimulation be this a new person, activity or toy), adaptability (the ease with which behaviour can be changed in response to changed circumstances), positive or negative quality of mood (laughing or smiling as opposed to crying or fussing), intensity of mood (irrespective of its direction or quality), level of sensory threshold (the intensity of stimuli required to evoke a discernible response), distractibility, and finally a combination of attention span and persistence. Discrete descriptive behavioural items in each protocol were scored for each of the nine temperamental categories in accordance with the definitions used in the study, employing a three-point scale. Various techniques were employed to minimize halo effect and enhance internal validity and scorer reliability. The details of the scoring procedures and the statistical results have been reported elsewhere (Chess[4]; Thomas[22]). Using the totalled item scores, the initial temperamental style of each of the 136 children in the study was identified. When followed through the years, temperamental identity was found to be generally consistent. Although the behaviour content keeps changing as the child matures, the formal pattern of reactivity tends to remain constant.

6
Temperamental Clusters

Qualitative and quantitative factor analysis of the temperamental profiles revealed that certain categories tended to cluster together and this permitted the identification of groups of similarly reactive children. The largest such group was characteristically regular, easily adaptable to change, showed positive approaches to new stimuli and tended to have a preponderantly positive mood of mild to moderate intensity. We have called an individual in this group an 'easy child' and the fact that such a child quickly develops sleep and feeding schedules, takes to most new foods from the start, easily adapts to a new school and learns the rules quickly and accepts most frustrations with a minimum of fuss, fully justifies our appellation.

Contrasting behavioural reactivity was identified in a smaller group of children who exhibited irregularity, slow adaptability to change, predominantly negative responses to new stimuli and frequent negative mood of high intensity. The 'difficult child' in this group does not easily conform to feeding, bathing, dressing or sleeping schedules or routines. His initial exposure to strange faces, new activities or new places may produce loud protest or crying and frustration may precipitate a tantrum. It should be noted, however, that these children can and do function easily, consistently and energetically after they have adapted to the new.

One further temperamental cluster warrants description here and children in this group combine negative responses of mild intensity to a new stimulus, be it a person, place, school or food, with slow adaptability following repeated contact. 'Slow to warm up' seems an apt label for such children.

7
Temperament-Environment Interaction

No one temperamental characteristic or combination of such characteristics necessarily produced a behaviour problem or made the child immune to one. Behaviour problems, as well as the absence of behaviour problems, were found among children with very different characteristics. However, for each of the 39 children in whom a disturbance did develop, it was possible to define the etiological factors in the genesis and course of the problem in terms of the child's significant characteristics (temperament and other additional components such as brain damage or physical handicap) and his specific interactive process with influential features of the environment (parental functioning and extrafamilial circumstances such as school and peer group). It should be emphasized that behavioural normality as well as disturbance depends on this interaction between the child with his given temperament and characteristics and significant features of his developmental environment (Chess[5]; Thomas[20]).

8
Selectivity of Stress

An equally important additional finding has been that each of the children has a specific reaction to stress and that for each child a different situation or experience is stressful. Those environmental demands and expectations which are most stressful for a child can be correlated with his temperamental characteristics; that which may be pathogenic for one child and lead to symptom formation may not be so for another. This complex interplay of factors at the core of a child's behaviour problem can be refined into three fundamental considerations: (*i*) the child's characteristic temperamental pattern, (*ii*) the environmental demands which are most stressful for children with this type of behaviour style, and (*iii*) the parental and/or environmental approaches which intensify such stressful demands to the point of symptom formation in the child.

Those children with the temperamental cluster we categorized as 'difficult,' perhaps 10 per cent of the total sample, showed the greatest frequency of behaviour problem development. Yet there is no evidence that the parents of the difficult infants were essentially different as a group from other parents or that the difficulty of the child *per se* leads to the development of behaviour problems. Rather, it is the parent-child interaction that is crucial, for these difficult infants require unusually consistent, firm, patient and tolerant handling if they are to learn to adapt to new demands with a minimum of stress (Rutter[18]). The demands of socialization, in particular the need to alter spontaneous responses and patterns to conform to the rules of family, school or peer group, are typically stressful for these children. Inconsistent, impatient or punitive approaches to these children intensify the stress and may make effective behaviour change impossible. Such suboptimal handling often leads to negativism and behaviour problem development.

An example of how the temperament-environment interaction is dynamically involved in the genesis of behaviour problems in these difficult children is seen in a pair of children, a boy and a girl, both of whom were irregular, non-adaptable, highly reactive and negative in infancy. Adaptation to nursery school at age 4 was also a difficult and lengthy process for both of them.

These early close similarities between the children were not matched by comparable parental attitudes and practices. The girl's father gave the impression of disliking the child, was punitive and angry and spent little or no recreational time with her. Although the mother seemed quite concerned for the child and more understanding and permissive, she proved to be quite inconsistent. Only in terms of safety rules and choice of clothing were the parents firm and consistent with their daughter and themselves.

In contrast, the boy's parents were unusually consistent and tolerant. They took the child's lengthy adjustment periods in stride, waited out his negative moods without getting angry and were not embarrassed by his unexpected tantrums in public places. They were permissive, but at the same time set safety limits and consistently pointed out to him the need to recognize the interests of his peers.

By the time they were $5\frac{1}{2}$ years of age, these two initially similar children showed qualitative behavioural differences. The boy had adjusted to nursery school, was a constructive member of his class and functioned smoothly in the major areas of daily living. The girl, however, had developed a number of increasingly severe symptoms including explosive anger, negativism, fear of the dark, encopresis, thumbsucking, poor peer relationships and protective lying. Only in the two areas where parental functioning had been firm and consistent, safety rules and choice of clothing, was there no symptomatology or negativism.

She was given a psychiatric examination at age $5\frac{1}{2}$ and during the play interviews was co-operative and free of negativism. She expressed no awareness of problems verbally, in the selection of play objects, or in the content of play which was appropriate to age and sex. Denial was prominent throughout the session. A moderately severe neurotic behaviour disorder was diagnosed and direct psychotherapy was advised. This was carried through and at follow-up at 6 years, 3 months, the stealing and encopresis had ceased and limits were more readily accepted.

It should not be inferred from this history that the parents alone were responsible for the child's difficulties. This *'mal de mère'* (Chess[3]) approach to children's problems is prevalent but unjustified in many instances, including this case. With a child of a different temperament, the same parental handling might have led to no or minor behaviour disorder. A child who was more quickly adaptive might have developed compensatory positive peer ties or a constructive teacher relationship. A number of other alternative child reactions to such parents are possible, given differing child individuality.

Easy children usually adapt to the demands of socialization with little or no stress and, as a group, tend to develop fewer behaviour problems than the difficult infants. However, the very ease with which they adapt may be one of the factors underlying behaviour problem development, especially and particularly when there is a severe dissonance between the demands and expectations of the intra- and extrafamilial environments. During the first few years of life, the easy child adapts quickly to the standards and behaviour expectations of his parents. Stress and malfunctioning develop, however, when he moves into situations involving peer play groups and school whose standards and demands conflict sharply with what he has learned at home.

For example, the parents of one such easy child had a high regard for individuality of expression and disapproved of any of their child's attitudes or behaviour which they identified as stereotypical or unimaginative. They encouraged self-expression and discouraged conformity and attentiveness to rules impressed by others even though they were distressed by her ill manners and bossy disdain for the desires of others.

The child thus came to insist always on her own preferences and this led to an attrition of friends and increasing isolation from her peer group. Her difficulty in listening to and following directions led to very unsatisfactory progress in school.

Because of the child's mounting problems with peer group and school activities, the parents were advised to restructure their functioning with her. They were encouraged to place less emphasis on individuality and to teach her to respond to the needs of others and conform constructively in class and with her peers. The parents, due to their awareness of the child's social isolation and the potential seriousness of her educational problem, were able to carry out this plan consistently. Although they continued to place a high value on creativity as opposed to conformity, the parents gave the child a set of rules which thus reduced the dissonance between intra- and extrafamilial standards. At follow-up six months later, the child had adapted to the new rules, the conflict between standards within and without the home had become minimal, she had become a participating member of a peer group and had caught up to grade level in academic work.

It is of interest that although the severe dissonance between intra- and extrafamilial demands and expectations may produce stress and disturbance in other types of children, it appears that this factor is especially pathogenic for the easy children. Quite another specific situation is typically stressful for those youngsters who slowly adapt to new stimuli following mild negative initial responses, the 'slow to warm up children,' namely, insistence by parents or teachers upon immediate positive involvement with the new. To fulfil this demand is difficult or impossible for such a child. If there is recognition that the child's slow adaptation to new friends, a new school or a new academic subject is his normal temperamental style and if patient encouragement is offered, positive involvement in activities will gradually occur. However, if the child's slowness to warm up is interpreted as timidity or lack of interest and he is confronted with the impatience of others and pressure to adapt more quickly than he can, the child may react to this stress with an intensification of his withdrawal tendency. And, if this increased holding back in turn stimulates increased impatience and pressure by a parent or teacher, a destructive child-environment interactive process will be set in motion.

These slow to warm up children may labour under incorrect teacher judgments. In some instances, slow adaptation was attributed to underlying anxiety and, in other cases, slow initial mastery of new subjects was equated with inadequate intellectual capacity. When the longitudinal records of these children were studied and shown to document a slow to warm up temperamental style, we recommended that the children be given a longer period of contact with the new situation before the teacher's judgment was acted upon. This was carried out and subsequent successful mastery of the new demands clarified the fact that temperamental style, not psychopathology or poor intellectual capacity, was responsible for the initial difficulty.

The persistent and non-distractible child represents still another constellation of temperamental characteristics which results in a tendency to resist interference or attempts to divert him from an activity in which he is absorbed. Interruptions during the course of an ongoing activity in which the child is pleasurably engaged may be specifically stressful to a child with this type of temperamental individuality. And, if the adult interference is arbitrary and forceful, tension and frustration mount quickly and may reach explosive proportions.

Children with still other temperamental qualities can be identified and type-specific sources of stress similarly categorized, such as an unrealistic restriction on the motor activity of a highly active child or an insistence that a highly distractible child maintain a long, uninterrupted concentration on a particular task. Other studies in the field have further expanded our knowledge of the role the child's own temperament plays in the development of behavioural disturbance and its symptoms.

Ross[17], in a recent study of children who achieve poorly in school, has identified what he calls the 'unorganized child,' one whose particular disturbance results from the interaction of the temperamental qualities of high distractibility, low persistence and short attention span with a disorganized or overpermissive environment in which little has been expected of the child. He notes that children with the opposite temperamental qualities in an identical environment will not develop the syndrome because they need little outside encouragement to develop organized behaviour patterns while children with the same temperamental characteristics in a highly structured and demanding environment also will not develop the symptoms of the unorganized child.

The unorganized child tends to be restless, unable to meet school requirements unless he is strictly supervised and demanding of attention as a substitute for the satisfaction he cannot gain from accomplishment. Ross further suggests that specific manifestations of this syndrome will vary in relation to the other temperamental qualities of the child, especially his activity level and intensity of mood. Thus, 'a highly active unorganized child is likely to be a disturbing influence both at home and at school because of his inattentiveness and restlessness, and his tendency to chatter disruptively and to involve himself with trivia. If he is less active, his inattentiveness may take the form primarily of daydreaming. If his reactions are intense, the intensity may be manifested by tantrums when he is frustrated' (p. 112). It is of interest that the symptoms as well as the origin of the basic disturbance in development are both fundamentally related to the basic interaction we have found underlying the genesis of all problem behaviour.

9

Temperament in Brain-damaged Children

From the study of three children in the longitudinal study population who suffered brain damage, we culled additional evidence of the importance of temperament-environment interactions in the psychological development of children (Birch[2]). The behavioural sequelae of brain damage in childhood are most diverse and may range from no apparent behaviour disturbance or absence of behavioural disturbance but presence of mental subnormality to serious disorganizations of interpersonal, intellectual and social functioning which are phenomenologically indistinguishable from the major psychoses of childhood.

While recognition of the existence of a variety of behavioural patterns in children with brain damage is important, it is necessary to go further and to identify those factors in development which contribute to the emergence of the above-noted abnormal behaviour manifestations if they are to be understood. On one hand, the differences may stem from physiological sources and pertain to the type, size or locus of the lesion, the time of life at which the nervous system was damaged and the character of the pathologic process. On the other hand, interactions between the child's temperamental style and parental environmental influences may be responsible for the development of behaviour differences just as this dynamic interplay was seen to be crucial for non-brain-damaged children.

The three children with brain damage in the study population have been considered in terms of this second set of influences and the findings have been reported in detail. The question to which we addressed ourselves was why two of the children with brain damage were able to achieve positive social adaptation and environmental mastery whereas the third had increasingly poor environmental control, maladaptation and, eventually, severe psychopathology. This question was important because the degree of intellectual deficit attendant upon brain damage did not in itself account for the differences in developmental course. Two of the children, one who had a superior IQ and one who was mentally subnormal, both made effective adjustments, while the third child, whose level of general intellectual functioning was at the population average, developed several maladaptations.

10

Parental Effectiveness

The family of the child with superior intelligence was inconsistent with regard to permissiveness versus insistence on the fulfilment of rules. The increasing evidences of the child's superior intellectual ability were met with relief and applause, as this quality was highly prized by both parents. The parents of the child with mental subnormality tended toward permissiveness and followed few absolute rules in the handling of the youngster and his older normal sibs. Their growing awareness of his intellectual slowness was accompanied first by avoidance of recognition of the fact and then by appropriate educational placement but maintenance of his participation in the neighbourhood informal play groups in so far as he was tolerated. The parents of the child with average intelligence initially handled her in a manner which strongly resembled that of the first parents described; they were inconsistently permissive. As the child's disturbing behaviour became more prominent, the parental inconsistency also became more crucial.

We found that temperamental organization in conjunction with familial environment could explain the difference in development and predict the future course of functioning. The two children who were primarily regular in biological functioning, positive in mood, moderately active, mild in intensity, readily adaptive and had no significant lowering of response threshold had a relatively good behavioural outcome. The child who was irregular (arhythmic), negative in mood, highly active, intensely reactive, non-adaptive and had a low threshold had an increasingly disturbed behavioural course.

Again, this is not to assume or imply that temperament alone was responsible for the poor behavioural consequence since several of the other children in the study who had equally difficult temperamental characteristics had a good behavioural outcome, probably as a result of a favourable combination of parental-environmental circumstances. Rather, the findings imply that the course of behaviour development in brain-damaged children is determined by the complex interaction of parental functioning and general environmental demands with the child's given set of response tendencies.

Parents may modify their practices so that they are in accord with the child's personality type, but the resultant response of the child in the direction the parents desire depends to some extent again on the child's temperamental characteristics. Those who are adaptable, positive and rhythmic are most amenable and responsive to parental changes and the prognosis is good. Those who are non-adaptive, negative and arhythmic with a low response threshold and short attention span are much less likely to respond with modified behaviour to changes in parental procedures. Extraordinary parental patience and consistency coupled with a stable and well-structured environment may eventually result in affecting the desired developmental course with some of these children but, in most cases, the ineffectiveness of their efforts to direct the child's behaviour results in parental feelings of helplessness, frustration, anger and guilt. Unfortunately, these understandable reactions then further diminish the parents' effectiveness and not uncommonly there will be progressive worsening of the behaviour of parents and child, increasing familial disorganization and conflict and the eventual inability to retain the child within the family setting.

11

Temperament in Mentally Retarded Children

Mentally retarded children, as a group, repeatedly have been reported to have a higher proportion of behaviour disorders than do intellectually normal children. It is assumed that behaviour which, while chronological age inappropriate, is appropriate to mental age, is not to be included here in the count of behaviour problems of mentally retarded youngsters. The higher probability in this group that there will be brain damage with direct behavioural representation as well as excessive environmental stress explains much but probably not all of the behavioural pathology. The author is currently engaged in a study of the contribution temperamental individuality makes to the behaviour patterns of intellectually defective youngsters. The same temperamental clusters described above with regard to intellectually normal children are also to be found amongst retarded children. Benign parent-child interaction has resulted in socially acceptable children who apparently are competent to the fullest extent of their mental capacity. Where temperamental vulnerability has been matched by environmental stress, specific for the particular temperamental cluster, the data to date suggest that the negative potentials of other etiological factors are enhanced. Such children not only perform below mental age expectancy but also exhibit behavioural patterns which often cause families to limit their own social interactions to a severe degree. As a part of this study, a parent discussion is held after all the data on the child in question have been examined. In this guidance conference, the dimension of temperament is given equal consideration with other etiological factors which act as determinants of the child's behaviour and recommendations are made for optimum parental attitudes and management of the child. The productivity of this approach will be assessed at a follow-up after the lapse of several years.

12

Child Care Practices

Consideration of temperamental type specific vulnerabilities and strengths leads directly to the conclusion that child care practices must be individually determined in order that they may be optimal. Thus the responsibility lies with parents and their advisors to make themselves aware of the infant's reactive pattern and modify general child care rules to make them appropriate to the particular youngster. While this approach does indeed demand an examination of parental attitudes and practices when studying the origins of a behaviour disorder in a child, a sharp disagreement is to be expressed with the all too fashionable professional attitude which can be summed up as 'to know Johnny's mother is to understand his problem.' This way of thinking is a facile substitute for a study of all the complex factors which may have produced a disturbance in development. This unidirectional preoccupation with the pathogenic role of the mother has often restricted diagnostic procedures to studies of the mother's functioning and has also frequently limited treatment methods to changing maternal attitudes. By unjustly holding many mothers exclusively or primarily responsible for their children's problems, proponents of this *'mal de mère'* (Chess[3]) view have unnecessarily burdened them with deep feelings of guilt and inadequacy without delving sufficiently and appropriately into the true nature of parent-child interaction. Of necessity, this involves the influences of the child's individual characteristics on the parent as well as parental influences on the child.

13

Role of Anxiety

The findings of our study also do not support psychoanalytic theories of the genesis of behaviour problems in which primary emphasis is placed on the roles of anxiety, intrapsychic conflict and psychodynamic defences. We have found that when these phenomena do appear in the course of behaviour problem development they are secondary features which result from the stressful, maladaptive character of the unhealthy temperament-environment interaction. Lois Murphy and her colleagues in the Topeka Study[15] have similarly found that there is no definite primary relationship between the patterns of psychodynamic defences and the adjustment of pre-school children.

Past retrospective studies have encouraged an intrapsychic explanation for the origin of behaviour disorders because when a child finally presents an extensively elaborated psychological disturbance, anxiety and conflict obviously will be present. Nevertheless, anterospective data reveal that these phenomena appear secondarily and influence the subsequent course of the behaviour problem only by adding a new dimension to the dynamics of the child-environment interaction. It should be remembered, too, that if temperamental individuality is not given serious attention, certain reactive patterns such as those of the difficult or slow to warm up child easily may be misinterpreted as the result of anxiety or as defences against anxiety.

14

Summary

Our studies of the importance of temperamental characteristics in influencing the developmental course of brain-damaged children and children with and without behaviour problems emphasize the necessity to study the entire child—his temperamental characteristics, neurological status, intellectual capacities, and physical handicaps. Such studies reveal that the influence of the parents can be understood only by a simultaneous consideration of the child's temperament and the influence of temperament only by a simultaneous consideration of environmental influences. The interactional process is of basic importance in studying the genesis and etiology of behaviour disorders in childhood. For, to automatically assume that a child who does not partake fully in peer activities is anxious and insecure is to overlook the possibility that he may be a normal, slow to warm up child. Similarly, to classify peremptorily a 6-year-old who explodes with anger at his teacher's command as aggressive and oppositional may be to ignore the fact that he is a persistent child who will normally and characteristically show frustration when an activity in which he is deeply absorbed is abruptly interrupted. And, just as a deep-seated neurosis may cause a mother's guilt and anxiety, so, too, might her confusion and problems in dealing with a temperamentally difficult child. Each of these opposed possibilities must be considered or else questions of etiology, diagnosis and therapy are answered by rote without the necessary regard for the vital facts. It is only through serious investigation of the various aspects of parent and child individuality and their interaction with each other that fundamental knowledge of normal and particularly problem behaviour will be gathered.

REFERENCES

1. BEISER, H. R., 1964. Discrepancies in the symptomology of parents and children. *J. Am. Acad. Child Psychiat.*, **3**, 459.
2. BIRCH, H. G., THOMAS, A., and CHESS, S., 1964. Behavioral development in brain-damaged children. *Arch. gen. Psychiat.*, **11**, 596.
3. CHESS, S., 1964. Editorial: Mal de Mère. *Am. J. Orthopsychiat.*, **34**, 613.
4. CHESS, S., HERTZIG, M., BIRCH, H. G., and THOMAS, A., 1962. Methodology of a study of adaptive functions of the preschool child. *J. Amer. Acad. Child Psychiat.*, **1**, 236.
5. CHESS, S., THOMAS, A., and BIRCH, H. G., 1967. Behavior problems revisited: findings of an anterospective study. *J. Amer. Acad. Child Psychiat.* **6**, 321.
6. CHESS, S., THOMAS, A., and BIRCH, H. G., 1966. Distortions in developmental reporting made by parents of behaviorally disturbed children. *J. Amer. Acad. Child Psychiat.*, **5**, 226.
7. CHESS, S., THOMAS, A., BIRCH, H. G., and HERTZIG, M., 1960. Implications of a longitudinal study of child development for child psychiatry. *Amer. J. Psychiat.*, **117**, 434.
8. CHESS, S., THOMAS, A., RUTTER, M., and BIRCH, H. G., 1963. Interaction of temperament and environment in the production of behavior disturbance in children. *Am. J. Psychiat.*, **120**, 144.
9. FRANK, JEROME D., 1962. *Persuasion and healing.* Baltimore, J. Hopkins.
10. FREUD, S., 1950. *Collected papers.* London, Hogarth.
11. JONES, ERNEST, 1953. *Life and work of Sigmund Freud*, vol. 1. New York, Basic Books.
12. KAGAN, J., and MOSS, H. A., 1962. *Birth to maturity.* New York, John Wiley.
13. KRIS, M., 1957. The use of prediction in a longitudinal study. *Psy. Study Child*, **12**, 175.
14. MACFARLANE, J. W., ALLEN, L., and HONZIK, M. P., 1962. *Developmental study of the behavior problems of normal children between 24 months and 14 years.* Berkeley, Univ. Calif. Press.
15. MURPHY, L. B., and Associates, 1962. *The widening world of childhood.* New York, Basic Books.
16. ROBBINS, L. C., 1963. The accuracy of parental recall of aspects of child development and of child rearing practices. *J. abnorm. soc. Psychol.*, **66**, 261.
17. ROSS, D. C., 1966. Poor school achievement: a psychiatric study and classification. *Clin. Pediatrics*, **5**, 109.
18. RUTTER, M., BIRCH, H. G., THOMAS, A., and CHESS, S., 1964. Temperamental characteristics in infancy and the later development of behaviour disorders. *Brit. J. Psychiat.*, **110**, 651.
19. SPOCK, B., 1958. *Baby and child care.* New York, Cardinal Giant.
20. THOMAS, A., CHESS, S., and BIRCH, H. G., 1966. *A 10-year study of the development of behavior problems in childhood.* Presented to APA May 1966.
21. THOMAS, A., CHESS, S., BIRCH, H. G., and HERTZIG, M., 1960. A longitudinal study of primary reaction patterns in childhood. *Comprehensive Psychiat.*, **1**, 103.
22. THOMAS, A., CHESS, S., BIRCH, H. G., HERTZIG, M., and KORN, S., 1964. *Behavioural individuality in early childhood.* London, Univ. Press.
23. WENAR, C., 1963. The reliability of developmental histories. *Psychosom. Med.*, **25**, 505.

III

MOTHER-INFANT RELATIONS AT BIRTH*

Peter H. Wolff
M.D.

Assistant Professor, Psychiatry, Harvard Medical School, Boston, Massachusetts

1
Introduction

Technological societies tend to leave a mother no opportunity to establish any relation with her infant immediately after birth, and very little opportunity for a close relation during the lying-in period. Obstetrical and pediatric factors often conspire to obscure that natural sequence surrounding birth which is apparent in the less 'advanced' societies: Thus general anaesthesia may make it impossible for a mother to hear, see, or hold her new baby during the first twelve hours after delivery; the physical separation of mother and infant in hospital, except during feedings, not only limits the length of their contact, but restricts their interchanges to a few simple operations. Our information about the earliest mother-infant transactions is therefore limited to retrospective accounts, which may be grossly distorted by pre-delivery medication like scopolamine; to cross-correlational studies which while useful do not reveal the underlying psychological mechanisms of the earliest mother-infant transactions; to direct observations which, as I have pointed out, are limited in their scope; and to biographical accounts by a few unusual women who have kept diaries of their labour and delivery (e.g., Karmel[11]; Painter[16]). Had I therefore interpreted the limits of my assignment too closely, I would have had few established data to contribute to this volume.

---

* Work for this report was completed while the author was supported in full by a Career Development Award of the U.S.P.H.S.-N.I.M.H. (KMH-3461), and a research grant of the U.S.P.H.S. (MH-06034).

INTRODUCTION

If, on the other hand, I had interpreted the assignment more liberally to include events leading up to and following delivery, it would have been difficult to specify its limits, since a mother's relation to her new baby is influenced by experiences that occurred long before she has conceived, while the individuation of infant and mother that is necessary for any true reciprocal interaction is not achieved all at once with the expulsion of the foetus, but may require months or years. In this account I have confined my remarks to the events of labour and delivery and the first encounters of mother and infant, for the most part as these could be inferred from direct observation. An adequate discussion of post-partum depressions and other psychiatric conditions causally related to delivery, would require a detailed clinical exploration of the mothers' pre-morbid personalities; I have therefore left their consideration to other contributors.

Since present methods of investigation preclude any systematic study of the psychological interactions between mother and foetus, observational studies of infant behaviour and of the earliest mother-infant relation have usually taken the moment of birth as their point of departure. This pragmatic limitation has unfortunately led to a categorical distinction between the events before and the events after birth, and to a theoretical oversimplification which regards the events before delivery as pertaining to 'constitutional' or genetic factors, the events after delivery as pertaining to experience. The fact that a particular capacity cannot be observed at birth does not warrant the assumption that this capacity is 'learned' in the usual sense (as, for example, in the case of form-perception and language acquisition). Nor does our limited information about the pre-functional organization of human behaviour justify the assumption that heredity alone accounts for the infant's neuropsychological status at birth. The endless disputes between those subscribing to a 'nativists' or a 'learning theorists' formulation of early development are pertinent to this topic in so far as they touch on questions regarding the baby's inherent coordination with certain stimulus qualities in the mother, and on questions regarding the mother's inherent foreknowledge of infant care—in other words, her maternal instinct.

Related Studies

Working with non-human mammals, Schneirla and his collaborators, among others, have accumulated an impressive empirical literature to discredit the concept of a unitary maternal instinct that blindly directs all of a mother's care-taking functions (Rosenblatt et al.[22]; Schneirla et al.,[23]). For one after another of the 'instinctive' maternal acts, these investigators have demonstrated that it is not a pre-formed instinct, but the outcome of an intricate interplay of forces which includes hormonal factors, previous maternal experiences, experiences not directly related to the care of the young, search for relief from visceral pain (e.g., breast engorgement), etc.; and that under normal circumstances these various part-functions appear as the goal-directed sequence which we call maternal behaviour. Such studies have been successful in reducing the task traditionally assigned to the maternal instinct; yet they have not excluded the contribution of species-specific structures to the regulation of the earliest mother-infant relations. Evidence from the fields of cognition, perception, and language acquisition argues strongly for the presence of complex inborn structures, and even inborn thought structures in the human infant (Lenneberg[13], Klüver[12], Chomsky[4], Wolff[28].) Evidence from comparative psychology indicates that the species-specific structures implied by the concepts of *imprinting, fixed action pattern,* and *innate releaser mechanism* regulate a good deal of the parent-offspring transactions in non-human mammals and non-mammalian vertebrates (Thorpe[26]). Wherever animal behaviourists have sought to demonstrate that such co-ordinations are 'learned', they have simply questioned claims about the particular content of the inborn structures, without invalidating the essential point that one must postulate pre-functional or *a priori* psychological structures to account for the naïve organism's relation to his environment, and for his capacity to integrate experiences. Ethological 'mechanisms' must therefore be considered in all systematic discussions of human mother-infant relations, even though we are totally ignorant of the extent to which (if any) they are relevant. Bowlby's discussion of 'attachment behaviour' may be a beginning in this direction, but is by itself sufficient to account for the enormous plasticity and diversity of interacting sequences that guarantee the solidity of mother-infant relations at birth in the human species (Bowlby[3]).

As it was originally defined by Konrad Lorenz, imprinting refers to a form of rapid and irreversible learning which has been observed in selected species of vertebrates but rarely in mammals (Hediger[9]; Thorpe[26]). The looser concept of *critical period* defined in different ways by various authors, appears to have a much wider representation in mammals, and may in its most general form also be relevant for human learning. While the concept usually refers to a period in *early* ontogenesis when the organism rapidly assimilates articulated experiences, including the species-specific characteristics of the parent, it has also been defined to include a circumscribed period during which parents and offspring most readily establish a social bond. Fortunately, it is impossible to perform the crucial experiments on humans from which one could analyse the relative contributions of parent and offspring to the social bond defined under 'critical' period, so that we have no information about the relevance of the concept for the human species; or, if it is relevant, whether it applies to the infant's or the mother's heightened sensitivity to particular actions of the social partner.

Studies of the relation between adoptive parents and adopted children do not help materially, since long-lasting emotional factors above and beyond those of a critical period may be operative. The clinical observation of mothers of premature infants who have had no direct contact with their baby for up to two months, suggests that in the early months they may feel estranged. Again, however, extraneous factors like the infant's almost total isolation in the incubator, his precarious physical and neurological status, and the mother's residual concern about her infant's health may be at work, which present added obstacles to a mother's feeling of intimacy with her infant. Questions about a critical period of mother-infant attachment in the first week can therefore not be resolved directly by the study of premature infants with their mothers, even though the possibility cannot be discounted; and perhaps the effort should be made to maximize the periods of contact between mother and infant during the early post-partum period.

Aside from a consideration of inborn coordinations and critical periods, investigators have pointed to the effect which a mother's emotional condition may have on the baby's physical and psychological status before birth. Sontag has shown, for example, that a mother's emotional state can influence foetal motility, that foetal hyperactivity is related to hypermotility after birth, and consequently that a mother's emotional condition during pregnancy may affect the kind of baby she produces (Sontag[25]). Other studies have concluded that the mother's psychological state in pregnancy influences the course and length of her labour (Kann[10]; Grimm[8]; Scott[24]); and that the mother's emotional attitude (her acceptance or rejection of the expected child) is related to her adjustment to the infant once it arrives (Newton[14]; Zemlich and Watson[29]). Wherever such studies are based on questionnaire methods, their categories for classifying the data tend to be too gross for a meaningful assessment of either the mother's specific emotional condition or the baby's motoric response it engenders; it is therefore difficult to draw any conclusions from questionnaire studies about the mechanisms which determine a mother's ties to her infant before birth, or the quality of their relation after birth.

Psychoanalytic investigations concerning the symbolic significance of pregnancy, labour and delivery have indicated an intimate association between a woman's adjustment to menstruation, coitus, and marriage, her experiences in labour, and her feelings about her new baby. It has been suggested, for example, that the meaning of genital orgasm is functionally related to that of labour, as well as to the feelings a mother has for her infant; that sexual intercourse has many features in common with delivery; and that the new baby represents to the mother a recompense for her lack of a penis (Helene Deutsch[5]; Newton[14]). Using direct observations and detailed prospective and retrospective interviews, Dr. C. Gill, however, found no such correlation between pre-pregnancy sexual experiences and behaviour during labour (unpublished findings). By cross-correlational techniques, Dr. Newton has traced the inter-relations among the various aspects of a woman's sexual function, and has concluded that attitudes towards menstruation, coitus and feminine identity are related to maternal feelings, but that this relationship is by no means clear-cut (Newton[14]).

A detailed study now in progress by Dr. Bibring and her associates on the psychological processes of pregnancy and the earliest mother-child relationship may go a long way toward clarifying those questions which at present we can only ask; unfortunately the findings and conclusions are not yet published. In a preliminary report these authors have formally outlined the complexity of developmental shifts that must occur if a woman is to make the transition from wife to mother smoothly:

'... The special task that has to be solved by pregnancy and by becoming a mother lies within the sphere of distribution and shifts between the cathexis of self-representation and of object-representation.

'To say it in other words; any normal girl, though she may have intense wishes for a child, and though she might love the man who will be the father of this child, still must make a major developmental move in becoming a mother. This step takes place between her being a single, circumscribed, self-contained organism (though capable of intense closeness in her love relationship), to reproducing herself and her love object in a child who will from then on remain an object outside of herself. And yet a special relationship will be established to this child—different from any other earlier or later. It will persist in the form of a synthesis of her relationship to the child, representing a person in his own right, of her relationship to the child, representing her husband, and last, not least, of her relationship to the child, representing herself' (Bibring *et al.*[2], pp. 16-17).

These shifts in a woman's relationships to important persons in her life, and the fluidity in levels of developmental differentiation they imply, make late pregnancy and the early puerperium a period of primary interest for developmental and personality psychology.

2

The Observations

The material I will present does little to clarify these larger issues. Its scientific status is dubious, as these observations of the mother-infant relation were peripheral to my effort to obtain a detailed account of the obstetrical events and an accurate assessment of the infant's neurological status shortly after birth. The report is based on the observation of fourteen mothers, ten of them American primiparae and multiparae, four of them Japanese mothers from an urban community in Japan, whom I have included for comparative purposes since their behaviour during delivery differed markedly from that of the American mothers.

As part of a larger study on the development of affect expressions in young infants, I interviewed the parents of prospective subjects shortly before the mother's date of confinement, attended her delivery, observed her contacts with her infant in hospital, and observed the infant's development in the home for a one-, three- or six-month period. Although the material is purely descriptive and in many respects incomplete, I am presenting it on the assumption that one must begin somewhere, and that a phenomenal description of the events is essential before more elaborate hypotheses can be formulated and tested systematically.

The Mother's Concerns Before Labour

The baby's sex preoccupies almost all parents at some time during the course of the mother's pregnancy. While this concern may cover up a host of more significant unconscious doubts the parents have about themselves, the baby's sex also is an issue in its own right, and one which parents invariably discuss as they look forward to the arrival of their baby. It may appear in the signs and symptoms from which they infer that they will have either a girl or a boy; it may be apparent from the list of names they have selected; or from the clothes they have bought. Both the preferences and the reasons for it will vary from culture to culture, from couple to couple within a culture, and between husband and wife. A wife may wish for a boy to please her husband, or for a girl because she thinks girls are easier to take care of. A husband may hope for a boy to carry on his name or preserve his fortune, or he may wish for a girl to be a companion to his wife. In Dr Newton's study maternal women were more likely to hope for a girl, and women who resented their feminine identity preferred boys (Newton[14]). In my small sample no such relationships were apparent, and our study made no assessment of a woman's feminine or masculine identification. Yet such a simplistic categorization as masculine and feminine women seems insufficient to account for the many variations and combinations in character structure which can determine why a woman should want either a boy or a girl.

The significance of the issue is also reflected in the folklore by which members of a particular social group diagnose the infant's gender—the astrological, meteorological and personal circumstances at the time of conception, the size of the woman's abdomen, the amount of foetal activity, the mother's discomfort, the size of her mask of pregnancy, and in some instances the techniques the couple used to influence their baby's sex at the time of conception (Ploss and Bartels[19]). According to the economic requirements of the group, tradition may assign different values to sons and daughters, and this in turn will surely influence the parents' preference. Finally, one must consider that the issue may not always be the baby's *sex* but the need to form some concrete image of the baby which occupies the parents, and that this is difficult to do as long as the foetus remains an amorphous 'it'.

Although several fathers showed their disappointment and remained distant or indifferent to the baby for some time, a mother's unfulfilled wish did not seem to influence her relation to the infant adversely in home observations, even when her preference was definite and the couple had 'tried again' to balance an already large family by adding one child of the unrepresented sex. However, since my observations did not extend beyond the first six months of the baby's life, the absence of adverse responses to disappointment is inconclusive; long-term follow-up studies may very well show that frustrated pre-delivery expectations can influence how a mother will feel about her child when his or her sex-specific behaviour becomes more apparent.

Of equal importance, although perhaps not so openly expressed, are the parents' concerns about the baby's physical condition. In the past such worries found their expression in a folklore which listed the various dangers to a woman when she encountered a cripple, had a great emotional shock, saw a rabbit or a goat, or was looked on by someone possessed of the evil eye, while she was pregnant (Ploss and Bartels[19]). In Western societies technological advances have rationalized these fears so that a woman in the United States, for example, is more likely to worry about biological incompatibilities between herself and her husband, about infections during pregnancy, exposure to radiation, toxic drugs, and the like.

While there are, to my knowledge, no specific studies on this point, it seems likely from clinical reconstruction that every primigravida, and most multiparae, worry about the physical condition of their foetus at some time during pregnancy, and ruminate whether they have harmed it accidentally by their activity, their diet, or their emotional state. From the observations of a worried mother's first leisurely encounter with her baby (see below), it seems that she must carefully inspect all parts of her baby before she can firmly believe he is all right.

The four Japanese mothers observed in the home, and several other Japanese women who did not participate in the study, emphatically volunteered doubts about their ability to provide enough breast milk for their baby, and planned to supplement the breast milk with a formula. The four mothers in the study all resorted to supplementary feedings in the first month, although there was no indication they lacked breast milk. In contrast, no American mothers in the group who planned to nurse their babies had any doubt that they would be able to, and none of them supplemented nursing with bottle milk or formula until at least the end of the third month. My sample is far too small, however, even for tentative conclusions on this point, since American mothers who nurse, unlike the Japanese mothers, are likely to be a very select group.

The Events During Labour and Delivery

These then are some of the preoccupations with which an expectant mother enters hospital. As labour progresses and the strength of her uterine contractions increases, a woman is likely to go through a remarkable psychological transformation. From a self-sufficient, reserved individual, she may become compliant and ingenuous in her relation to the doctor and nurse; she will cling to anyone who is willing to hold her hand, beg for assistance like a small child, or become petulant in her demands for relief from pain and other discomforts. Although each mother has her own way of responding to active labour, provided she is awake and alert, the transformation is of a general type which usually can be described as an increased dependence on, and passivity in relation to, the adults around her, which exceeds in degree what is commonly observed in any adult who is hospitalized for other reasons. During labour a mother puts herself entirely in the hands of the doctor and nurses, and cooperates almost too eagerly with their instructions. Experienced nurses seem particularly sensitive to a mother's greater dependence, and will scold her benignly when she does the wrong thing, praise her excessively when she is 'doing well'. The psychological impact of delivery on those present seems to be so compelling that they all assist physically or psychologically in getting the baby out even when they have attended hundreds of deliveries before. If things go smoothly in the delivery room, a sensitive balance of interacting participants is achieved that is rarely observed under other circumstances.

In Japan this balance was dramatically illustrated several times by the changes in verbal interchange between patient and physician during labour. A reserved and dignified primigravida, for example, entered hospital during the early second stage of labour, retained her composure and addressed her doctor, nurses, and the observer in a respectful mode until the contractions became the primary focus of her attention. Then she switched to a different mode which is commonly used only by Japanese children when they address their parents or other adults, but under ordinary circumstances is inappropriate for conversations between adults. Her physician who until then had also spoken to her in the polite form, immediately responded to her appeal, and addressed her as a parent would speak to his child. While the form of his address was 'familiar', it had none of the condescension implicit to the words 'honey', 'mother', or 'sweetheart', with which obstetricians in this country sometimes address their patients. Throughout the second stage of labour, patient and doctor conversed in this way, the doctor giving encouragement, the patient drawing support from his reassurances. Once the baby was delivered, however, first the mother, and then the doctor, immediately reverted to a more formal address. These 'transformations' were paralleled by the nurses' sympathetic support of the mother during delivery, and their return to a more disinterested professional attitude as soon as the baby was born.

Another more experienced Japanese woman was equally reserved until the middle of the second phase of labour, but then clutched my thigh with each contraction, and implored me in the same childish language to help her with her pain. After delivery she also returned to polite speech without any signs of embarrassment.

Such a shift in the levels of relationship can also be observed in the behaviour of American mothers, but rarely as clearly in the verbal interchanges. Some women will call out to their mothers for help, or damn them for not being there to help, or plead with the doctor to 'put them out'. The relationship between physician and patient seems to be less intimate, the atmosphere in the delivery room more professional in the United States, and I have never observed the same sensitive response to a woman's specific needs of the moment as in Japan. Neither this nor the other comparisons to follow between Japanese and American cultural patterns of mother and infant care, however, are intended as an invidious judgment of the West; only an assessment which would take the entire cultural context into account could lead to valid conclusions concerning the advantages and disadvantages of either pattern of maternal and infant care.

Near the end of the second stage, the mother turns all her attention to her own body; her absorption in her inner processes is so complete that she resents gratuitous advice or questions which she considers to be irrelevant at that time; her face turns purple and the sweat stands out on her forehead as she strains with each contraction, and her threshold to external events seems to be markedly elevated (see Karmel[11]). Rarely does one observe a woman performing such hard physical work as during a natural labour, so that it is no wonder the successful completion of labour represents to a woman an enormous achievement. Its significance goes beyond the awareness of having delivered a baby, and refers specifically to the physical task that is now behind her, and that has restored her body to its former shape. A number of the mothers have, for example, felt their flat bellies immediately after delivery and commented with relief that they were back to their normal shape, or that they could see their feet again.

My account so far pertains to the usual sequence when labour and delivery go smoothly. The specific effect of a complicated delivery on the mother's subsequent relation to her child remains for the most part unknown. It seems unlikely that a painful or traumatic delivery, which nevertheless produces a viable and healthy infant, would influence a mother's feelings for her child permanently, unless predisposing psychological factors gave the obstetrical complications a special meaning. In clinical case histories one reads, for example, that a woman has blamed her child for having 'torn her apart', and therefore has always felt at odds with him; but more often than not the same history indicates that the woman in question would have found some other pretext to formulate her conflict if the delivery had gone smoothly. Dr H. Deutsch has called attention to the possibility that deliveries conducted under general anaesthesia can precipitate paranoid ideations; that a disturbed mother may wonder, for example, what was done to her or her baby while she was unconscious, and for years afterwards wonder whether the baby handed to her was really hers. In this small sample of mothers I have observed neither these pathological reactions, nor any approaching a true post-partum depression.

The First Interaction After Birth

With the expulsion of foetus, a woman's relation to her baby enters into a qualitatively new phase. Until she could hear and see her baby, she generally treated it as an organic part of herself even though she could feel it move and at times referred to it as an individual in its own right. After delivery the baby is clearly no longer physically a part of her; yet a mother continues to identify with the baby, and to identify it with herself so that we must distinguish the physical separation *per se* from the psychological individuation that follows from it. While a mother's lack of differentiation from her infant seems to be an essential dimension of her transactions with him in the early months, it would go poorly with the child's development if the mother did not accept her baby at the same time as an autonomous organization which she must allow to develop according to its own dictates, and to whose unique individual traits she must adapt. The first encounters between mother and infant in hospital thus represent in concrete terms the essential and inevitable contradictions which will characterize their developing interactions in the months to come; and with a formal analysis of their interchanges in the first week, the investigator can study some of the operations used by mother and infant to resolve this contradiction that remain constant over time.

Immediately after the foetus is delivered, and before the placenta has been expelled, a waking mother will turn her attention to the baby. Since the obstetrician often announces to her the sex of the baby while it is being delivered, one of her most pressing questions has been settled before she begins to ask. Next she usually asks about the baby's health, but the physician's reassurances on this score are usually far less acceptable to her than his diagnosis of the baby's sex. Although the birth cry is her concrete evidence that the baby is alive, she will not believe it until she has actually seen him move, heard him cry, or held him in her arms. When the geographical arrangements of the delivery room are such that a mother cannot see her baby, she anxiously listens for subsequent cries, sighing with relief after each cry and commenting, 'That's what I wanted to hear', or 'listen to him screech'. Several mothers whom I observed during two consecutive deliveries, both times wanted to know first how much the baby weighed before they asked either about the sex or the physical state; they, however, belonged to an American sub-culture where large babies and strong men are held in high esteem.

The mother's initial reaction to holding her baby or being at least allowed to inspect him, is obviously a moment of profound significance for her; an observer who is not too preoccupied with making detailed observations will recognize from the mother's silent tears, her look of awe, and the tenderness with which her arms reach out, that he is participating vicariously in one of woman's most intimate experiences, and at such a moment will find it difficult to intrude on her privacy.

The Evolution of the Interaction

All mothers delivered in hospital will rest for at least 12 to 18 hours before they see their infants again; and during their second encounter the first active interchanges between mother and infant become evident, especially in women who were not conscious immediately after delivery.

The range of mothers' reactions to their baby at this time will vary considerably, and is as much a function of their past experiences with babies as of their general style. Some women are definitely frightened to hold their baby, and hardly dare to touch it for fear that they will break it (see also Painter[16]). Some women 'confess' in subsequent months that they were shocked by the baby's ugly, wrinkled appearance, and had to pretend tender emotions for several days to suppress their indifference or repugnance. Since many more *inexperienced* mothers react to this encounter with fear than either multiparae or primiparae who have cared for other babies in the past, it seems unlikely that the irrational fears brought out by the baby reflect unconscious pathological conflicts, unless they are part of a more general and more ominous pathological configuration. Instead these are probably natural reactions of unfamiliarity, and the expressions of anxiety women feel when their capacity to function as mothers is challenged for the first time.

If comparative studies of non-human mammals are at all pertinent to human mother-infant couples, they emphasize the fallacy of postulating that the 'natural' mother knows exactly what to do; that the initial reactions of confusion and repulsion are part of the price woman has paid for becoming civilized; or that the more primitive a particular social group is, the more adequate will its mothers be. Primiparous chimpanzees may flee away from their new infant in a panic and make no effort to care for it (Elder and Yerkes[6]; Nissen and Yerkes[15]); cats are at first indifferent to their litters and do not actively seek out their kittens until the third day (Schneirla *et al.*[23]); many species of larger mammals (in zoos) are so helpless at first that the perinatal mortality among their firstborns is very high (Hediger[9]).

When an unpractised human mother is given her baby to feed for the first time, she may show the same helpless surrender that was apparent during labour and delivery; and again the presence of an older and experienced woman can be of great help to her at this critical moment. Although many urban Japanese women are now delivered in hospital rather than at home, this has not prevented grandmothers from visiting their daughters and being present at the first feeding. On several occasions, therefore, I had the opportunity in Japan to observe how much strength and support a mother can draw from her own mother at this critical time. One inexperienced mother, for example, refused the assistance of a nurse and struggled with an uncooperative baby for 15 minutes, but remained composed and stoic in her efforts to feed him until she saw her own mother approaching along the corridor. Then she shouted 'Mama', held out her arms in supplication, relaxed with relief, and surrendered herself into the grandmother's arms. For the next half hour the two women worked in complete harmony, together holding the baby, directing its mouth to the nipple, and squeezing the breast; for at least one feeding on each day of the remaining days in hospital, the grandmother came to help. By the time the mother went home she was efficient in her movements, competent in her care, and sensitive to the baby's changing needs; two weeks later she handled a minor medical crisis concerning the baby like a veteran.

A more helpless Japanese mother, whose own mother could not visit for geographical reasons, was in a panic when the nurse first brought her the baby to feed, clutched the nurse's hand and refused to let it go. The nurse responded sympathetically, helped her in adjusting the baby to the breast, and answered endless questions until the mother felt confident enough for that day to continue on her own. On subsequent days the nurse looked in frequently to see if she could help, and (to me) seemed extraordinarily tolerant of the mother's 'babyish' ways; but this mother also went home with a feeling of some assurance that she would be able to care for the baby on her own.

Similar reactions can be observed in American women, although I have not seen anything like the intimacy between mother and grandmother that we saw in the Japanese women; and I doubt that the American women in my sample would have tolerated such close physical contact with their mothers. They were not only more restrained in their behaviour, but valued their autonomy and independence from their mothers far too much to permit any interference with their handling of the baby. Whenever a grandmother volunteered to help at home, the mother either refused such assistance outright, or else "allowed" the grandmother to clean the house, but jealously took over the care of the baby herself. The nursing mothers in the group, moreover, seemed to know as much about breast feeding as the nurses who explained it to them, and resented any gratuitous advice.

After feeding her baby for the first time, a mother almost invariably turns to an inspection of his body and searches his face assiduously for family resemblances. All the women I have observed, both in the United States and Japan, have inspected the baby's hands with great care (before or) after the first feeding. Some did so with hesitation, as if they only dared to look at one (and then always the right) hand; others explored the whole body, including the hands, the feet, and the genitals, with confidence. From the observations it was not clear why the hands were so important, and why so many women were surprised that the hands were already well formed. More generally mothers were surprised that their babies could function at all (for example, that they could breathe), and that their grasp and rooting reflexes were intact; half playfully they tested the various reflexes repeatedly, as if to convince themselves that their baby was really 'operational'.

A mother's first conversations with her baby may also reveal something of her early maternal feeling when considered in a broader context. Some mothers in the group spoke only to the observer for the first several days, or to the nurse who brought the baby, and asked anxious questions, but they did not address the baby directly. The same mothers were clumsy about holding the baby, kept him at a physical distance during the feeding, were afraid they might touch the baby's 'soft spot' (i.e., anterior fontanelle), and moved with hesitation. It took some mothers three or four days to direct meaningful phrases to their baby; all of them, however, eventually did.

More experienced or 'competent' mothers immediately addressed their remarks to their baby, sympathized with his struggles in the cruel world, or laughed and discussed his future with him. These mothers also seemed to have a more immediate sense of their baby's needs, held him closely, and moved smoothly while shifting his position.

Such crude distinctions among mothers as I have drawn here are not intended as a classification to distinguish between 'good' and 'bad' mothers; nor should they imply that a mother's initial lack of intimacy with a new baby signifies anything about her subsequent relation to him. All one can conclude from these observations is that the quality of verbal and motor interchanges may discriminate between mothers who have, and those who have not, had previous experiences in handling babies; furthermore, that one does not have to assume a preformed maternal instinct as the necessary and sufficient condition for a satisfactory relation between mother and infant. It is impressive how quickly the inept, distant and helpless new mothers acquired competence and decisiveness in their movements, how soon they addressed their babies as individuals, both in speech and action. Although several of the inexperienced mothers in the group did not establish solid communication with their babies until the fourth week, the quality of their interaction at that time seemed to be excellent, and differed in no apparent way from that of mothers who had been self-assured or competent at the beginning. Similarly, some multiparous women with three or more children at home acted blasé about their new baby, and were not interested until the baby gave signs of recognizing them by smiling selectively to their faces or making 'eye-to-eye' contact (Wolff[27]).

A mother's initial conversations with her infant may be one convenient clue about her maternal feelings, but they are only one of many dimensions which reveal something about the *quality* of her initial relation to her infant. Probably of much greater significance, although harder to record, is the *quality* of the mother's movements as she approaches and holds the baby, as she puts him to breast, bathes and changes him, and plays with him. The critical information to be gotten from such observations is not *what* or even *how much* a mother does, but *how* she does it, and *when* in relation to the baby's organismic state or stage of development. At present we have no language to describe either the quality of the mother's movements or the transactional aspects of the mother-infant relation, in satisfactory categories. Yet an 'objective' quantitative assessment of total body-body contact, of spatial limb displacements, or even a precise count of how many interchanges were initiated by whom, will not suffice to describe the quality of the interchanges adequately. It is here that a viewpoint which equates quantification with mathematization in psychology is most apparently deficient (see, for example, Piaget[17]; Rapaport[21]).

The Return Home

The different reactions that mothers show as they prepare to take their baby home may reflect still other aspects of their early maternal feelings. Although many women at first looked forward to their confinement as a period of rest, many of them were already restless on the third day and asked to be discharged before the appointed time, claiming that they were needed at home, or that they could not put up with the inconvenient hospital routines; very few allowed themselves to enjoy the luxury of the full five days in hospital. Dr Escalona has noted that such an intolerance of passivity, when it is present, is already apparent during pregnancy; and that the psychological conflicts relating to activity and passivity that such intolerance implies, may backfire in the subsequent weeks when the mother feels drained by her infant's excessive demands[7]. In my home observations it was clear that those mothers who could indulge themselves while still in hospital or during the first weeks at home, also had more patience and tolerance of the infant's needs in later months than mothers who valiantly resumed all their pre-delivery activity at once and tried to put themselves entirely at their baby's disposal.

Japanese tradition recognizes a woman's need for time to recover her body integrity and to re-structure her self-image; it therefore dictates that a woman should remain inactive during the first month after giving birth. In traditional homes the young mother is relieved by her mother or mother-in-law, from doing certain tasks, lest she do irreparable damage to her body. Urban mothers have modified this tradition to fit their own circumstances, by hiring a midwife who makes daily visits to bathe the infant, offers advice, and chats with the mother on a variety of subjects, to which the mother listens attentively even though the answers are as familiar to her as to the midwife. A Western observer may be puzzled to see an experienced Japanese mother sitting respectfully on the sidelines while a midwife explains every step of the bath which the mother has done hundreds of times before. Yet such ritual support seems to respect a woman's special psychological state after delivery, and to guarantee that at least the psychological, even if not the physical, burdens of a new mother are made lighter.

In urban American families the grandmother still has the vestige of a similar function, and when a mother is not too resentful of intrusion she may allow her mother to help although, as I have mentioned, she will be very careful to protect her maternal prerogatives and leave only the care of the older children and the household chores to her mother.

The Infant's Contribution to the Interaction

By confining my remarks to the mother's behaviour, I have left out the baby's significant and positive contributions to their transactions. The omission, in which I indulged for convenience, also reflects a general deficiency in the literature, which has explored the mother's influence on the baby in some detail, but taken insufficient cognizance of the fact that the baby's activity influences a mother's activities with him as much as her past experience and tradition. The infant's skill in searching for and sucking on the nipple are a primary determinant in the formation of the satisfactory nursing couple. In my observations the first 'true' contact between the nursing mother and her infant was sometimes not established until the baby had taken at least one satisfactory feeding. Some mothers reported that they felt inadequate as long as their baby did not suck well; that the physician's efforts to reassure them by 'blaming' the baby did not help their self-esteem; and that only after an adequate feeding pattern had been established did they feel they were really mothers. By doing what he should, the baby seemed to give his mother confidence that what she did was right, and allowed her the freedom to explore and refine her methods of child care. At the same time he helped her to overcome the fears of inadequacy which, if they had persisted, might have impaired her subsequent efficiency. How important the baby's contribution in this respect can be, becomes clear when something goes wrong—when, for example, the baby is sleepy whenever he is brought to the mother for a feeding: he will nurse poorly, return to the nursery unsatisfied, and cry until he is given a supplementary bottle feeding in the nursery so that he is sleepy again at the next scheduled feeding. Under such conditions a mother will sooner or later give up nursing in desperation, not only because she has failed too many times, but because the combined effect of her increasing distress and the lack of stimulation to her breast tissue have made her physiologically incapable of nursing.

Feeding is only one of many instances where the infant's behaviour will directly influence a mother's emotional state and actions. Anxious mothers may worry about the baby's spontaneous jerks and hover over him, especially if they have been sensitized by any suspicion that something is physically wrong. Most mothers get nervous at one time or another about their baby's breathing during sleep; some mothers place the baby near them during the night for fear that he will choke; others cannot tolerate the constant anticipation of the next breath and put the baby out of earshot.

No matter how meaningless the infant's smile may be from a behaviourist's point of view, it delights the mother and elicits tender comments from her. The tonal quality of a baby's cry may be extremely irritating (as in brain-damaged but also some normal infants), or it may sound sweet and appealing to the mother. Not only the mother's way of hearing, but the particular acoustic properties of the cry, will affect her response to the baby's vocal distress.

From the beginning of their relationship, the baby's body posture and muscle tonus seem to have a profound effect on the mother's movements and way of holding him. Careful neurological examination of the neonate with adequate follow-up studies indicate that hyper- or hypo-tonicity may be related to minimal brain damage, which in turn may influence the mother-child relation adversely (Prechtl and Stemmer[20]). Even infants without neurological complications show considerable variation in muscle tonus; some babies are 'cuddly' at birth, others stiffen out as soon as they are held. The developmental histories reported by parents of psychologically disturbed children make frequent references to the fact that the deviant child 'never cuddled as a baby'. From such accounts it is not clear, however, whether the infants were 'stiff' from the very beginning, whether they were responding to something unique in the mother's way of holding them, or whether a congenital stiffness in the baby triggered an anxious response in the mother, which in turn alarmed the baby into a more rigid posture. When a child is 'stiff' at birth, a sensitive mother may interpret this as the baby's rejection of her, while a more confident mother may accept it as the baby's way. Another baby may become stiff in his mother's arms because of the way she holds him, but mould easily into someone else's arms. One mother may take this selective response to heart and force the issue by holding him as closely as possible; another may compromise and assume that the baby 'has a will of his own'. Whatever the specific content of the interchange, the infant's actions from the very beginning clearly influence the mother's response. Congenital differences in muscle tonus, motility, duration of alertness, vigour of sucking, frequency of smiling, and stability of sleep-waking cycle, certainly contribute as much to the mother-infant relation as the mother's individuality. Yet an exhaustive description of the baby's characteristics, no matter how objective and scientific, will be of little relevance to the study of mother-infant relations, unless the functional significance of each trait for a particular mother is taken into account.

Summary and Conclusions

A further discussion of the developing interactions between a unique baby and a unique mother would go beyond my assigned topic. From this limited inventory it should, however, be apparent that mother-infant relations at birth, short though they are, reveal in a condensed form many of the significant mother-child encounters that are distributed in more disconnected fashion at other times. In this respect, the rapid shift in levels of transaction during labour, delivery and the puerperium were most apparent to direct observation. What might have appeared as a pathological regression to an infantile position in another context was the general, and perhaps even the adaptive, prelude to a woman's nurturing relation to her new infant. The transactions between mother and obstetrician, and between mother and grandmother or other mature women, which prepared the mother to accept the baby on the one hand as a needful organism, on the other hand as an individual in his own right, were found to be complex and fluid. From the observation of primiparous women with their infants during the first week, and from a comparison of primiparous and multiparous women, it seemed clear that experience contributes significantly but not exclusively to the quality in which a mother handles her baby; studies on non-human mammalian parent-offspring relations were introduced to suggest that the concept of a maternal instinct need not be invoked in order to account for the stable relation of mother and infant, either among civilized or primitive mammals.

The limited description also made it clear that the early patterns of social interaction between mother and infant can be understood from a *developmental* point of view only after a descriptive language and conceptual framework are devised which treat the mother and infant as a system in its own right. I tried to indicate further why no causal analysis of mother and infant as functionally separate systems alone would clarify this crucial issue of human transactions.

Whether the relevant concepts can be imported from a mathematical theory of games (as, for example, Piaget[18] has suggested), or whether a 'general systems' theory (Bertalanffy[1]) can be modified and made sufficiently humble to aid in the study of parent-offspring pairs, are questions that seem worthy of further exploration. It is unlikely that questionnaires, correlational studies, or physiological measurement by themselves, will bring the relevant answers.

REFERENCES

1. BERTALANFFY, L. VON, 1952. *Problems of life*. New York, Wiley.
2. BIBRING, G. L., DWYER, T. F., HUNTINGTON, D. S., and VALENSTEIN, A. F., 1961. A study of the psychological processes in pregnancy and of the earliest mother-child relationships. I. Some propositions and comments. *Psychoanal. Study Child*, **16**, 9-24.
3. BOWLBY, J., 1958. The nature of the child's tie to his mother. *Int. J. Psychoanal.*, **39**, 350-73.
4. CHOMSKY, N., 1965. *Aspects of the theory of syntax*. Cambridge, Mass., M.I.T. Press.
5. DEUTSCH, H., 1944. *The psychology of women: a psychoanalytic interpretation*. New York, Grune and Stratton.
6. ELDER, E. H., and YERKES, R. M., 1936. Chimpanzee births in captivity: a typical case history and report of 16 births. *Proc. Roy. Soc., Ser. B.*, **120**, 409.
7. ESCALONA, S., 1949. The psychological relation of mother and child upon return from the hospital. *Conferences on infancy and childhood*. New York, Josiah Macy, Jr., Foundation.
8. GRIMM, E. R., 1961. Psychological tension in pregnancy: *Psychosom. Med.*, **23**, 520.
9. HEDIGER, H., 1955. *Psychology of animals in zoos and circuses*. New York, Criterion Books.
10. KANN, J., 1950. An exploratory study of the relationship of certain psychological variables to the degree of difficulty of birth. *Unpublished Ph.D. Dissertation*, Univ. of Pittsburgh.
11. KARMEL, M., 1959. *Thank You, Dr. Lamaze*. New York, Lippincott.
12. KLÜVER, H., 1962. Psychological specificity—does it exist? In *Macromolecular specificity and biological memory*. Ed. Schmitt, F. O. Cambridge, Mass., M.I.T. Press.

REFERENCES

13. LENNEBERG, E. H., 1960. Language, evolution, and purposive behavior. In *Culture in history: essays in honor of Paul Radin*. Ed. Diamond, S. New York, Columbia Univ. Press.
14. NEWTON, N., 1955. *Maternal emotions*. New York, Hoeber.
15. NISSEN, H. W., and YERKES, R. M., 1943. Reproduction in the chimpanzee: report of forty-nine births. *Anat. Rec.*, **86**, 567.
16. PAINTER, C., 1965. *Who made the lamb?* New York, New American Library (Signet).
17. PIAGET, J., 1950. *L'epistemologie genetique*, vol. I. Paris, Presses Universitaires.
18. PIAGET, J., 1956. The general problems of the psychobiological development of the child. In *Discussions on child development*, vol. IV. Eds. Tanner, J. M., and Inhelder, B. New York, Internat. Univ. Press.
19. PLOSS, H., and BARTELS, M., 1908. *Das Weib in der Natur und Völkerkunde*, vol. I. Leipzig, Th. Grieben.
20. PRECHTL, H. F. R., and STEMMER, Ch. J., 1962. The choreiform syndrome in children. *Developm. Med. Child Neurol.*, **4**, 119-27.
21. RAPAPORT, D., 1959. The structure of psychoanalytic theory: a systematizing attempt. In *Psychology: a study of a science*. Vol. 3. Ed. Koch, S. New York, McGraw-Hill.
22. ROSENBLATT, J. S., TURKEVITZ, G. T., and SCHNEIRLA, T. C., 1962. Development of sucking and related behavior in neonite kittens. In *Roots of Behavior*. Ed. Bliss, E. L. New York, Hoeber.
23. SCHNEIRLA, T. C., ROSENBLATT, J. S., and TOBACH, E., 1963. Maternal behavior in the cat. In *Maternal behavior in mammals*. Ed. Rheingold, H. L. New York, Wiley.
24. SCOTT, E. M., and THOMPSON, M., 1956. A psychological investigation of primigravidae—IV. Psychological factors in the clinical phenomenon of labour. *J. Obst. Gynec. Brit. Emp.*, **63**, 502.
25. SONTAG, L. W., 1944. Differences in modifiability of foetal behavior. *Psychosom. Med.*, **6**, 151.
26. THORPE, W. H., 1956. *Learning and instinct in animals*. Cambridge, Univ. Press.
27. WOLFF, P. H., 1963. The early development of smiling. In *Determinants of Infant Behaviour—II*. Ed. Foss, B. London, Methuen.
28. WOLFF, P. H., 1966. La théorie sensori-motrice de l'intelligence et la psychologie du développement général. In *Psychologie et Epistemologie Génétiques; Thèmes Piagètiens*. Paris, Dunod.
29. ZEMLICH, M. S., and WATSON, R. I., 1953. Maternal attitudes of acceptance and rejection during and after pregnancy. *Amer. J. Orthopsychiat.*, **23**, 520.

IV

MOTHER-CHILD RELATIONSHIP

MYRIAM DAVID

AND

GENEVIEVE APPELL

Paris, France

1

Introduction

From the dawn of history, all cultures have recognized the value of the mother to the child and of the child to the mother. Experienced at an emotional level by all human beings, this relationship has been studied by psychoanalysts, psychiatrists and psychologists, changing what was a credo into a more definite knowledge.

Psychoanalytic practice has shown how a maternal image is built into the adult psyche, carried over from an infantile experience, and how it remains active at an unconscious level in adult relationship adjustments. Nowadays most child psychiatrists agree that the child builds his personality through the relationship which develops between himself and his mother and father; disturbances in the child are often related to a disturbed mother-child relationship.

Although all psychologists agree that early childhood experiences are important for the development of the child, some disagreement remains as to what is the decisive factor. For the psychoanalytic school of thought it is the emotional tie between mother and child, whereas for behaviourists and advocates of learning theory it is the environmental stimuli, the mother being the usual, but not the only possible channel through which these stimuli reach the child.

In clinical work the concept of mother-child relationship remains vague, however widely used. Professional workers often speak of a good or of a poor relationship, but may imply many different things: by 'a poor relationship' meaning that the child is not wanted; or not loved; or that hate and frustration are prevalent; or that mother is careless and oblivious of the child's needs; or that she projects on the child her own needs, the child being a narcissistic object whose needs are not distinguished from her own; it may mean also that she is overprotective, indulging, or strict and rigid, etc. . . . At times all professional workers dealing with human beings seem to have a definite image of an ideal mother-child relationship, but this image differs greatly from one worker to another, and is never fully actualized.

A study of 1-year-old infants and their mothers has made it possible to distinguish different modes of mother-child interaction, and their impact on the child's behaviour and development. This study will be presented in order to illuminate the content of mother-child relationship. Previous communications by the authors[2, 19, 20, 21] will be found in the bibliography, which includes also references to relevant literature.

2

Mother-child Interaction

In the framework of a research on the effects of early and brief mother-child separation (in the three first months of life), and in an attempt to define and compare the maternal care the children received when returned to their homes, these infants were followed up until age $2\frac{1}{2}$.*

Twenty-five families have been regularly visited. Home visits lasted for an average of three hours. They were made daily for the first week of family reunion, and then once a week up to 6 months, then twice a month till 15 months, and once a month till $2\frac{1}{2}$-years-old.

During these home visits direct observations of child and mother were recorded, as well as interviews with the mother. The material included usual everyday routine, occasional play with the child, tests in his natural setting; there were also sessions at the office of the professional worker at 13 and 18 months, and at 2 and $2\frac{1}{2}$ years.

Every effort was made to minimize the intrusion which the research might represent to the family. The method of observing and the kind of relationship to be established with the parents, were carefully devised from this point of view.

The material thus collected has been analysed from the point of view of mother-child interaction at 12 months. Five cases will be used to illustrate the subject in the following pages.

Though limited to this age and to a restricted number of cases, this analysis has proved to be a fruitful way of looking at mother-child relationship.

* This investigation is part of a research programme sponsored by a grant from the Foundations' Fund for Research in Psychiatry, Yale University, New Haven.

3

Case Studies

Molly A

Family background. Mr and Mrs A belong to the working class. Father is a house painter, mother left school early and did not work before marriage. She does all the house work. The flat lacks space and comfort, but they are strongly tied to it by childhood memories.

Mrs A lived there, with three older brothers and her mother to whom she felt very close, her father having died when she was still a small girl. She was still a child during the war and was left alone with her mother when her brothers were called up. They seem to have loved each other dearly, with a mutual dependance, as Mrs A's mother was often sick and Mrs A cared for her until she died, leaving her 16-year-old daughter at a loss.

Mr A, abandoned in early childhood by his parents, was brought up by a neighbour and friend of Mrs A's mother. As a child he spent most of his time in playing with his future wife in her home. He shared her devotion to her mother, whom he admired and loved.

United by this common love they remained together and eventually married. Father deeply respects mother and her family, is protective towards her, which she enjoys. His tie to her is very much like the relationship he had with her mother and she seems to appreciate this; she is cheerful and warm in spite of frequent illness and is the leading central figure of the family.

Study of interaction. Molly and her mother are in constant interaction, which takes the form of long chains of response in which one partner answers the other, the latter responds in turn and so on. Interaction then can be schematized $A \rightarrow B \rightarrow A \rightarrow B \rightarrow A$ etc. . . . Arising from all the incidents of household routine and the child's spontaneous interests, these chains are as often initiated by one partner as by the other. The following is an illustration:

Molly, under a table, is playing peek-a-boo with the observer, and smiling at her. Mother says to observer: 'You see she is copying Susan', and, addressing Molly: →'Come along, let's go and fetch Susan'. →Molly forgets her game with the observer, promptly comes out of her hiding-place, responds to mother with happy sounds, takes mother's hand→and they both go towards the door; mother asks Molly to say 'bye-bye' to observer,→Molly ignores this but tries to open the door;→the mother, wishing to stop her doing this, picks her up,→Molly protests strongly;→ mother says 'Come along, it isn't time yet', and to distract her gives her Susan's doll;→Molly takes hold of the doll and speaks to it;→mother puts Molly down;→but Molly goes (clings?) back to mother and wants to be picked up;→mother says cheerfully 'always Mummy', and gives her another doll; →Molly smiles broadly at mother, and mother announces reluctantly 'I won't look at you any more'; →Molly seems content / and retires to play under table; →but mother looks down at her and says 'what are you doing there?' →Molly comes out and stands up, helping herself by holding mother's legs; she takes hold of mother's hand and pulls it. →Mother says 'what do you want?' →Molly pulls her towards Susan's doll (though the doll was at hand) →and mother seems happy to be pulled by Molly and to comply; she gives her the doll →and Molly takes hold of it and cuddles it, saying 'Te-Te Te', →so mother leaves her and goes to stir the fire in the next room, the kitchen. →Molly, however follows her towards the kitchen and sits in the doorway, →mother says 'I don't like you to be there' and comes back; →Molly rises to her feet and calls 'Mum, Mum, Mum', she holds doll against her heart, then holds it out to mother, going towards her making imitative noises; while doing this she falls, →mother says 'Boum', →Molly gets up and wants to be picked up; →mother does not respond, / and Molly proceeds to play with the closet door; →mother rushes to stop her, and says: 'At her age Susan was less demanding' while Molly →says 'Pa, papa' to which mother →answers 'Papa will come, so take care of your bottom', adding joyfully that she is scared of Daddy; // Molly goes back to fiddle with closet door; this time mother pays no attention, and then the interaction stops for a moment. Molly leaves the closet and quietly goes into parent's bedroom, while mother speaks of Sue; however a few instants later, Molly being out of sight→mother goes to see what Molly is doing in other room and a new chain of interaction is set off.

As this example shows, the ending of interaction is often delayed, either by Molly, or by mother, who regains her daughter's attention in subtle ways.

The tone of interaction is on the whole cheerful, noisy and boisterous, while the greatest variety of modes of interaction are intensely used by both parties.

Baby-care is achieved in a casual way, and brings no problems. Occurring in the midst of this ongoing interchange, the task to be done seems far less important than the pleasure of being together and interacting. Almost every action or sound made by Molly is an exciting event for mother, who turns it into an occasion of interaction.

Strong mutual need for togetherness creates a maximum avoidance of separation, and puts some limits to Molly's relations with other people. The obstacle comes not from Molly, whose fear is mitigated by great interest, but from mother, who gently interferes, always attracting her daughter's attention.

The intense pleasure derived from this proximity is the striking feature of this pair. Each one finds intense satisfaction in the other, and expresses it actively and openly.

Occasions of conflict exist, however, when mother teases Molly for the pleasure of giving in the next minute, which restores mutual gratification; or when mother resents her daughter's great possessiveness. Then interaction becomes limitative, on mother's part, with an angry Molly showing aggressiveness and indignation very much a reflection of her mother's anger. Such episodes are short, and finish with pleasurable reconciliation.

Bob B

Family background. Bob's parents live in a small, but charming flat near relatives. They enjoy a close and harmonious relationship, are both socially responsible members of their community, sharing common interests in the home and outside.

Father is an engineer, and little is known of his family background. Mother lost her father when she was five, and her mother died when she was 16. She always evokes warm memories about her mother, whom she describes as a person who gave a great deal to her children through her use of imagination. As a young girl Mrs B took responsibility for her mentally ill brother and the problems of a difficult sister.

Mrs B was trained as a nursery school teacher, then worked as a secretary, but gave this up after Bob's birth. She enjoys baby-care and housekeeping, but it is vital for her not to be confined to them. She is well organized, and does most of the housework, but manages to find time for social events and for helping those in need. It is of value and interest for father and mother to invest much of their free time in social and cultural activities, leaving Bob to the care of a neighbour and reciprocating the service more than generously and willingly.

Study of interaction. Interaction between Bob and his mother, also a very happy pair, is however in sharp contrast with that observed in Molly's case.

The chains of interaction are rare and brief; they are released mostly by Bob's reactions to separation, hurt and fear, or by the few restrictions which mother imposes.

Physical care is quick and efficient, but carried on without interchange, although mutual tolerance and empathy in ways of handling are obvious, mother being a quiet, clever, and firm leader and Bob a contented complier.

The characteristic interaction of this couple is mutual silent watching of each other, without interfering in each other's activity. This provides them both with quiet but intense pleasure, and is their way of sharing each other's interests.

Mother derives from this a fine knowledge of Bob's abilities, likes and dislikes, and by taking them into account she provides a rich and stimulating environment, of which he makes an active and cheerful use, pleasing her by his autonomy and his creative activity.

She constantly gives him opportunities to discover the outside world, the pleasure of relationships with others; these are of great value to her, and she lets him master situations and his own emotions unaided and at his own pace. She never imposes herself on him in these spheres. And he, under mother's eyes, makes brilliant use of such opportunities.

This pattern serves to maintain a skilful balance between closeness and distance and provides for most of the time great satisfaction to both.

However, Bob asks for more closeness than mother is ready to give. He cannot stand mother's remoteness when she happens to be absorbed in her own activity, and he reacts with acute distress to the short, but somewhat frequent separations he is exposed to. Mother cannot stand these demands, which make her feel angry and depressed. This is the only source of conflict, and at this age they have found no solution.

Louise C

Family background. Louise is the youngest of a family of three children. Her father is a qualified worker in an important firm, her mother plans to return to secretarial work, while the paternal grandmother, who lives with them shares the housework.

The whole family strives for a perfect household, upward social mobility and rising prosperity. Good organization, thrift, strict order, and extreme cleanliness, no time wasting, and restricted social life, is the rule for every one, and few events ever break this routine. The chief exponent is the stern paternal grandmother, it is approved by the hard-working father, and accepted without protest by the pretty, narcissistic mother.

The children are part of this bee-hive life and must fit into it by avoiding mess, noise, disorder, and any interference in the work to be done. Therefore they are not allowed to play together, and are left confined in small spaces with no toys or very few. All excitement is immediately quelled, while good manners and good habits are highly valued.

Physical health is also a preoccupation and seems to be the only sphere where a certain amount of self-indulgence is allowed.

Study of interaction. Among all the pairs observed, interaction between Louise and her mother is the least frequent and the poorest.

A few short chains are observed during physical care, apart from which Louise and mother are hardly ever together. Mother, absorbed in her housework, ignores Louise's discreet signals, and seems blind to her expressions of distress, fear or fatigue.

A few words, smiles and glances, occasional little smacks or caresses, brief babyish social games are the only modes of interaction to be observed between this undemonstrative couple.

The few chains of interaction to be seen occur only on mother's initiative, arising from the strict limitations she imposes upon Louise concerning touching, playing, moving around. All self-expression seemed to be shocking, while the children's achievements in any area have no interest for mother.

The one exception is toilet-training. From 12 months on, a strict routine is introduced. Severely scolded for accidents, gently congratulated for exerting control, Louise is trained amazingly quickly, to the greatest satisfaction of mother and grandmother.

On the whole Louise conforms to this limiting and empty world. However at times she resists and mother then gives in easily, rather laughingly, when the matter is unimportant. When she feels it is worth while to insist she is firm, but does not get angry if Louise protests; she ignores her crying, and then Louise gives in.

Looking after Louise is no burden for mother. It is even a pleasurable task, and since Louise is a beautiful, undemanding and compliant baby, she is proud and satisfied. Her feeling about Louise is one of pleasure, but although she tells the observer about this, she never shows it to the little girl by cuddling, or by gifts which might please her.

Lack of proximity in this couple is most striking, but both accept this mutual distance, which does not create any conflict.

Lewis D

Family background. Lewis is the second child of a working class family; his older brother, aged four, goes to school. Father is an unskilled worker, and though in stable and regular work, is anxious about unemployment. They live in an uncomfortable little flat.

Both parents have had unhappy childhoods and present disturbed personalities. The father appears to be anxious, with phobias and temper tantrums, and seems unable to make decisions and take responsibilities. The mother is depressed, and they both have poor relationships with relatives and neighbours. Their marital life is a failure. Daily family life is riddled with quarrels and frustrations for all members of the family.

Mrs D is deeply entangled in her past. The usual chores of life and many features of Lewis revive in her many miserable feelings linked to painful childhood memories: resentful feelings towards a father who abandoned her mentally ill mother in a psychiatric hospital, where she died; who left her as a young girl without letters nor visits in a tuberculosis hospital, while marrying a woman who had a girl of Mrs D's age, for whom he seems to care more than for his own daughter.

Her son, her husband and her father are often linked together as the cause of her misery, while at the same time, she shows tremendous anxiety, resulting from guilt, fear and resentment, about her mother's insanity.

Though often deeply depressed, she carries somewhere within her the feeling of a better self, which is somehow connected with her eldest son. And indeed, she is intelligent and sensitive, ambitious and successful in keeping up the standards of the family life, the house, the children and herself. Under suitable conditions she could develop a positive relationship of mutual consideration.

Study of interaction. Although mother's interaction with Lewis is average in total amount, it is very irregularly scattered over time.

Long periods of isolation, during which Lewis remains alone in a room or in the flat, are followed by long sequences of interaction. These are initiated for purposes of mothercraft, but she often makes a gesture arousing Lewis's hopes, and then ignores his disappointment when she turns away towards something else.

She also initiates long periods of physical contact, not always for mothercraft purposes. During such periods she becomes, at times, immersed in her inner thoughts and oblivious of the child who, sitting in her lap, tries again and again to get her attention. Then she suddenly seems to discover that he is there and for a brief moment gives herself up to a close enveloping physical contact, only to be absent again the following minute. After a long period of such alternation Lewis tries to free himself and leaves her alone.

However, he comes back after a while, and starts to follow her around, asking for attention that she is not ready to give. She then either ignores him, or angrily pushes him away, leaving him, in either case, unsatisfied and demanding.

The modes of interaction are compulsive and primitive, very different from other cases. Both mother and child seem to seek for physical symbiotic contact, but when this appears it never leads to long chains, since neither partner ever takes into account what the other is doing, but simply follow their own impulses.

Mother appears to be for Lewis a desirable and provocative object which always disappoints him. He is for mother a burden, a part of her personal unhappiness. She cannot see, hear, stimulate, consider what he spontaneously does. Nor can she give him pleasure, any more than she finds pleasure in him. However, her mothercraft is adequate; Lewis does not suffer physically and enjoys his freedom in this atmosphere of half-abandonment.

The general tone of interaction is one of deep frustration.

Frank E

Family background. Mr and Mrs E, a middle-class couple, live in a comfortable flat in a suburb close to Mr E's engineering work. The two children, Liliane ($2\frac{1}{2}$) and Frank (1) enjoy a large private balcony and the public garden.

Mother is devoted to her children and her household duties, for which she has some help. Reserved and somewhat shy, she keeps the neighbours at a distance. The only visitors are the two grandmothers, and occasionally an uncle or an aunt. To be good parents seems to be the main ambition shared by both parents.

Study of interaction. Interaction between Frank and his mother is average in amount, and takes variety of shapes and modes during mothercraft, which is accurate and enjoyable for both partners. However, beyond physical care, mother shows little interest in the boy's activities, nor does she respond much to his strong orientation towards her. She is mainly responsive to a slight motor disability in the child, who is clumsy, poorly coordinated, often falls down and is unable to get up or sit up again.

Thus motor activity at 1 year old appears to be the main occasion and mode of interaction. The child's disability acts as an anxiety-producing signal, inducing the mother to rush towards him, either to prevent him from falling or to pick him up, and also to test his walking again and again. This becomes the only way in which Frank can gain her attention, and he falls back on it when other means have failed. Interaction is then often loaded with anxiety, fatigue and sometimes anger in the mother, and with impulsivity, fear and frustration on the part of Frank, who in turn is felt by mother as a naughty demanding boy.

On the other hand, mother is much more responsive to Liliane, who is then felt to be 'sweet and weak'. Interaction with her is outstandingly richer in all its various aspects.

Frank and Liliane have little difficulty when alone. However quite often Mrs E., needing closeness with her daughter introduces Liliane into her own interaction with Frank, which is frustrating to him and gratifying for Liliane. For instance, she invites Liliane to help her to teach Frank walk, which he fears. He becomes upset, she scolds him and praises Liliane: she is a good girl and he a bad boy. Or mother puts him down and picks up Liliane, or leaves the room with Liliane, leaving Frank crying behind. The opposite situation is never seen.

4

Discussion of Interaction at Age One

Summaries of these five cases illustrate the great differences which exist between one mother-child pair and another.

These differences have been studied from the angle of mother-child interaction, which can be described in various ways:

Interaction per se.

This has a general configuration which can be defined along five main points: (*i*) quantity, (*ii*) beginning and end, (*iii*) form, (*iv*) mode, (*v*) tone.

Interaction in each mother-child pair differs from the others in each of these aspects. These characteristic differences are stable throughout the material. Thus each case has its own specific pattern, which can be precisely described, point by point.

1. *Quantity of interaction* is indeed so great in Molly's case as to be almost continuous during waking hours; it is scarce in Louise's case, irregular in Lewis's case, average in Frank's, with Bob coming somewhere between Molly and Frank.

2. *Beginning and end of interaction.* In many instances it is hard to say

who starts and ends an interaction. It may begin on the initiative of either mother or child from an inner wish. This wish in A however may appear in relation to his partner's behaviour (B) which acts as a releasing signal inducing A to start interaction, whether the signal is intended or not by the partner's at a conscious or unconscious level.

The children resemble each other in their ways of starting interaction, differing from one another only by their greater or lesser eagerness to begin. On the other hand, each mother responds to different behaviours in the child as releasors which stimulate her to initiate interaction. Thus Molly's mother seems to notice and enjoy all aspects of her little girl and makes them into opportunities for interaction; Bob's mother is more selective (preferring usually his constructive, imaginative activities and his powers of observation); Frank's mother is even more selective responding mainly to his walking and motor disability. For Louise and Lewis, interaction initiated by mother is rarely a response to anything coming from the child, but arises from an impulse of her own (Lewis's mother) or some plan of her own (Louise's mother).

At this age, the child seem always to respond to mother's-initiated interaction, turning it into a chain by his response (M→C→M); whereas all the mothers ignore a number of interactions started by the child (C→M). Even Molly's enthusiastic mother does not always respond to her girl; however she responds more often than she fails to do so, while Louise's mother shows the opposite pattern.

Mutual consent in initiating interaction varies also from one case to another: it is highest with Molly and her mother, whereas in Lewis's case consent on mother's part is at the lowest.

As to the ending of interaction, Louise is the only child who is always willing to accept it, whereas the other children show now and then some reluctance when their mother ends the interaction: this is infrequent in Molly's case, since mother is always ready to start again at the slightest sign from her daughter; coming next in the reluctance to stop interaction is Bob, who still shows some tolerance, with Frank and Lewis as the least amenable of the group.

On the other hand, only Molly's and Lewis's mother occasionally show some unwillingness to let the child break off the interaction: Molly's mother, however, easily finds a way to reopen it, since Molly is so responsive; at the other extreme Lewis's mother attempts to keep him on her lap when he wants to get off and this leads to a smothered fight.

3. *Form of interaction.* Interaction can take the form of *chains* (A→B →A→B→), but only in Molly's case were these chains endless like the one described.

Interaction can be *direct and simple* (A→B or B→A) when the partner does not reply. This occurs for instance when one partner is busy watching the other. All children can be seen watching their mothers, without any response from the mother. Bob's mother is the only one for whom watching her son is a predominant form and mode of interaction. Some mothers, like Louise's, do not seem to watch the child at all; some, like Molly's, cannot watch without interfering, and thus gives the interaction the form of a chain.

In Bob's case, direct simple visual interaction leads to a third form of interaction: *indirect interaction* through environment and objects (A→E; E→B): mother provides the child with a rich environment of people and objects, and a diversity of experiences which she knows he will enjoy, Bob indeed uses these on his own in a constructive, active, imaginative way and shows continual pleasure, which in turn stimulates mother's interest and watching.

4. *Modes of interaction.* Rich and manifold in Molly's case, all to be used: looking, talking, laughing at each other; kissing, petting; give and take; calling for attention and giving it in all sorts of ways; carrying, helping the child to walk, etc. . . . This is much more restricted in Bob's case, where *visual* attention is a highly predominant mode; so is *walking* in Frank's case, while *primitive modes* are used exclusively in Lewis's case, such as pinching, mouthing, and touching which are not seen at this age in Bob, Molly and Frank.

5. *The tone* of interaction can be defined by its intensity and quality. It is intense in Molly, Bob, Frank and Lewis, in contrast to the flatness in Louise's case. It is happy and predominantly pleasurable in Molly's and Bob's cases, in contrast to the highly predominant mutual dissatisfaction in Lewis's case; it is happy and boisterous in Molly; happy but quiet in Bob.

Content of interaction

It is fruitful also to observe in each case how this pattern of interaction is displayed in the current circumstances of day-to-day life.

The daily life and events are rather similar for these five children. They are all at the same level of development: in each child new capacities are appearing, new ways of being and acting due to their development, such as: moving about and walking; increased understanding, leading to a new sort of play with objects. Holding and manipulation have been mastered, and give way to putting things here and there, in and out, together and apart. The children begin to give such play symbolical meanings; they are starting to understand speech and to be able to make their wants understood.

They all have to cope with the same basic emotional problems; separation anxiety, fear of strangers, wishes to do things themselves while still wanting mother's participation; beginning awareness of the toilet-training procedures, of their own possibilities and wants which are sometimes in conflict with mother's demands, not only as regards toilet-training, but in respect of all habits, so-called good manners, etc. . . .

It is interesting to examine all these different aspects of behaviour from the angle of interaction, in the following situations:

(*i*) interdependency situations: i.e. situations such as feeding, toileting, carrying the child, having the child in the arms, on the lap;

(*ii*) activities of the child, such as: locomotor, manual activities and play; speech;

(*iii*) mother's activities not related to the child;

(*iv*) in relationships with others: father, siblings, strangers;

(*v*) situations of separation and others arousing frustration and/or anxiety.

(*a*) First of all, it is striking to find how, in one given area of behaviour, interaction can differ from one mother-child pair to another.

For instance, if one considers toilet-training, it is for Louise and her mother a preponderant occasion of interaction, the only one really invested with strong feelings, which gives to interaction a quality of unusual tension. At the opposite extreme, it is one of the few things which rarely produce interaction in Molly's case. Mother lets Molly go about in her wet pants; makes no attempt to train her; but laughs at her, telling her how she is dirty, jokingly threatens her with father's punishment. In Bob and Frank it leads to very different types of pleasurable interaction: mother keeps Bob very clean, Bob lends himself passively, but with obvious pleasure to mother's clever, silent, efficient manipulation. For Frank and his mother this, as well as all physical care, is an occasion of cheerful interchange. Whereas for Lewis, mother acts on sudden impulses to change diapers in a rough and frightening way which leads to screaming, and this in turn leads mother to give up.

Another good illustration of the differences in the pattern of mother-child interaction in a given area of behaviour is provided by the study of interaction in separation situations:

For Molly no such situations seem to exist, since mother never goes out of the flat without taking Molly along with her. Even in the flat, togetherness is constantly insured, and active avoidance of separation by both partners accounts for these endless chains of interaction, Molly on the one hand free to walk about, can follow mother wherever she goes; on the other hand Molly's disappearance next door, or even under the table brings her mother promptly in search.

We have seen how Bob's mother manages to maintain a certain amount of separation in the house by keeping him in areas which are limited, though wide and well furnished, not allowing him in the kitchen or the living-room. When his mother disappears into the next room, Bob reacts by watching her come and go, he listens and recognizes by the sounds if mother is putting on her coat to go out, he becomes apprehensive and starts to yell when she opens the door of the flat. Mother is upset by this screaming, but nevertheless is firmly determined not to give in; she leaves the screaming boy alone while she does a quick errand. These separation situations are always short since usually mother takes him with her on shopping expeditions. However she leaves him once a week with a cousin, whose children she takes care of at other times. Bob cries a bit when she leaves him, but not for long; on the other hand, he yells when she occasionally leaves him in the evening with an unknown baby-sitter: such situations are unknown to Molly.

Lewis's mother seldom takes her son with her when she goes out, leaving behind her for a long time a desperate Lewis, who is still upset when she comes back; at home the only occasions of interaction apart from interdependency situations, consist of Lewis following mother, and mother responding by pushing him away impatiently and putting him in a distant corner or in the next room. This sort of interaction is never seen in Bob's case; his mother manages situations in such a way that Bob is quite content to be at some distance with his wealth of possessions, as long as she is in sight.

For Louise, separation is so constant that it does not give rise to any interaction. Mother and grandmother sit in a room next door, where Louise cannot see them or hear them. She notices when mother comes in the room, and sometimes smiles at her, but mother seldom notices, and goes out without responding. Louise does not react when mother goes out nor does she mind, or even seem to notice, when mother is out of the flat for several hours, leaving Louise with her sister and grandmother.

For all the areas of behaviour and situations listed above, the differences from one mother-child pair to another are equally striking.

(b) It appears moreover that interaction is never evenly distributed throughout all these circumstances. Some areas of behaviour give rise to no interaction at all, whereas other areas of behaviour seem to be selected as important. The pattern of interaction for a given case has various shadings from one area to another.

For instance, for Louise, interaction is related only to physical care, and mother consistently stops all her attempts to interfere, touch things or move, while imposing upon her the procedures of toilet-training. For Lewis too, almost all interaction is found in interdependency situations, but for him physical care is followed by long and more or less satisfactory periods on mother's lap. For Frank, the interactions are somewhat evenly shared between physical care, which is pleasurable to him and his mother, and his locomotor activities which are tinged with anxiety and frustration for both.

For Molly and Bob the greater and richer part of interaction is found outside interdependency situations.

For Molly and her mother the avoidance of separation is one of the main source of interaction: it accounts for the endless chains and the constant active interference in each other's activities, both mother and child being unable to allow the other to get involved with anything or anybody else. Molly's clever motor activities, completely unlimited by mother, are also a source of cheerful interaction, the only occasions where mother does not interfere physically, but gives purely verbal encouragement; all other activities being turned into an occasion of interchange.

Whereas, for Bob, speech and motor activities are hardly ever an occasion of direct or indirect interaction, the pattern of quiet, pleasurable, visual and indirect interaction relates only to play and social activities.

Thus, through the systematic study of the various situations common to all mothers and children of this age group, one sees how each pair selects its own specific areas for mutual interaction, and that strong interacting emotional attitudes are attached to each area of interaction. These attitudes guide the interaction, and, as will be seen in the following section, are responsible for organizing it into its specific pattern. This raises the question of the connection between interaction and relationship.

5

Interaction and Relationship

Interaction is not relationship, but its observable counterpart. It is the means for expressing and translating into action the emotional content of relationships. Moreover, it serves as a regulating device for various aspects of the mother-child relationship which the study of interaction helps us to distinguish. Relationship can indeed be considered from angles which correspond point by point to those under which interaction has been described.

Quantity of interaction in relation to space

Out of the comparative study of these five cases emerges a strong impression that the mother invites, or allows the child to take more or less space in her life. By 'giving space' is meant giving time and taking the child along with her in the different sectors of her life.

The quantity of interaction reflects the amount of 'space' accessible to the child. He is not the only person to whom mother devotes space; there may be some spaces from which he is excluded, and he may share his space with others.

For instance Molly has plenty of space, she is allowed to occupy the total space along with her sister; at times she shares it also with father, to whom mother assigns a much smaller space. Louise has very little space, which she has to share with her brother and sister, while mother keeps a wider space for herself alone, and another space, somewhat distinct from these, for her husband. Bob has a large space, which he shares with father, who is always present in the background; but there are areas for father alone and for mother and father as a couple, from which Bob is excluded. Lewis's mother oscillates between allowing him to invade the total space,

I

and then excluding him; he seldom shares it with his brother, who enjoys a wider space, or with his father, whose space in mother's life seems to be distinct from the children's, but to have the same characteristics as Lewis's.

Expressed through the quantity of interaction, the 'space' is controlled by mother through the readiness or reluctance with which she decides to start and end interaction, or to respond to the child's approaches.

This control of the quantity of interaction is closely linked on one hand with the overall pleasure/frustration which mother and child exchange (which will be studied further), and on the other hand with the balance of their mutual need for closeness/distance, which will be examined now.

Form of interaction in relation to closeness/distance in relationship

Closeness versus distance is a second interesting aspect of relationship which is determined mostly by the form of interaction; the use of various combinations of forms insuring in each case a specific equilibrium between closeness and distance.

Mutual need for closeness in Molly's case is expressed and gratified through very long chains of interaction which are not seen in the other cases (A→B→A→B→A→B etc . . .). Whereas in Bob's case closeness and distance are simultaneously enjoyed through the double form of interaction so characteristic in this case: *simple direct visual* interaction; *indirect interaction* (A→E; E→B), while chains are short and surprisingly scarce. While in Louise's case simple direct interaction predominantly expresses and insures distance.

Lewis's often disappointed search for closeness, alternating with extreme distance is expressed on the one hand by long interdependency situations, when he is kept on his mother's lap, and they both try without success to obtain some pleasurable response from the other; on the other hand by short chains, where Lewis's pursuit of mother provokes her to push him away (L→M→L), to an extreme distance, with total lack of interaction, during which mother is absorbed by her own distress, while Lewis engages in hyperactive lonely play, which is rather sterile if not destructive.

This mutual need or search for a balance of closeness/ and distance is connected in each case with the mutual attitude towards separation, and affects the degree of the mother's interference in the child's activities, through which she creates more or less dependency or autonomy. This applies to all the children in whatever sector of life. For instance Bob, so self-sufficient in his play, in his relationships with children, even with strangers, is as dependent as Louise in respect of physical care, for which he takes as yet no initiative and lets himself be cleaned, fed, put here and there by mother with sheer delight.

Whereas Molly, who needs and enjoys so much attention in all her deeds and misdeeds, is much more independent than Bob in feeding, running around and moving about.

Situation, and modes of interaction in relation to maturity level

It is well known that the younger the infant, the greater the interaction for physical care, the intervals being mostly filled with sleep, whereas for the growing infant, these in between times become richer in interaction, while physical care takes less time and becomes more casual.

Lack of interaction apart from physical care shows the mother to be uninterested in the child's spontaneous activities which are left outside the relationship. In such a case the child exists for the mother only through the care she gives, his smiles and looks towards her, not through his capacity to be or do on his own.

We have seen that our five cases divide sharply in two categories: in one, Bob, Molly and Frank, in the other, Louise and Lewis; for these last two children interaction occurs mostly in interdependency.

In this respect, the interaction between Lewis and his mother is at an even more primitive level than that between Louise and her mother, such as occurs as a rule with infants only a few weeks old, at a symbiotic level in mother's arms or on her lap; whereas for Louise, it occurs in a face-to-face relationship during physical care, as it mostly does for infants during the second half of the first year.

The modes of interaction are revealing of this. For Lewis, holding and being held, clinging, petting, mouthing, pinching mother's arm and face are primitive modes, whereas for Louise and her mother the main mode is imitative games initiated by mother, mild exploratory touching by Louise, which mother tries to prevent; quite different also from the modes used by Bob, Molly, Frank and their mothers, where look, smile, touch, speech and mimics are used in a give-and-take mode, in which each partner is distinct from the other and collaborates actively.

Tonality of interaction in relation to intensity and quality of investment

The tonality of interaction conveys through mimicry, smiles, laughter, cries, gesture, facial and corporal expression, both the intensity and the nature of the feelings invested by each partner in the relationship.

The general tone of interaction gives an overall impression of the relationship, whether it be the predominant deep pleasure, as with Bob and Molly, frustration for Lewis, pleasure mitigated with anxiety in Frank's, flatness for Louise. It is probably one of the main means through which child and mother feel each other as good or bad objects.

To summarize, one sees how the quantity, form, modes and tonality of interaction express and regulate different important aspects of relationship: space, closeness-distance, maturity level, intensity and quality of invested feelings.

Areas of interaction and emotional content of relationship

The predominance of interaction in certain areas of behaviour, the feelings attached to them, as well as the attitudes displayed, indicate what and where are the areas of mutual pleasure, love and satisfaction, and those of mutual frustration and conflict. Moreover, in each case there appears to be a central core of the relationship. This emerged from the material and appears to be preponderant organizing force in interaction.

Molly and her mother have this intense pleasure in togetherness; violent but short storms about possessiveness, in which each strongly opposes the other, followed quickly by mutual consolation.

Bob and his mother have intense pleasure in side-by-side autonomous activity, with violent, open conflict about separation.

For Frank and his mother 'walking' is invested with the strong ambivalent feelings of both, and tied up with mother's feelings towards Frank as a boy, and as an intruder in her relationship with Liliane.

For Louise and her mother, there is neither pleasure nor conflict, except in the one area of toilet-training, where mutual obstinacy of mother and child leads to dramatic scolding by mother and crying by Louise, ending in success and pride on both sides.

Lewis and his mother have everlasting overwhelming mutual frustration in all areas of behaviour, whether feeding, sleeping, walking, cleanliness, activities, which goes together with constant searching on Lewis's part, a frequent rejection on mother's part.

In each case, this predominant trend permeates the whole interaction, using all the circumstances and all the means at its disposal, and thus creates a tight interdependency between all the manners in which interaction is displayed. This accounts not only for the consistency of the pattern of interaction throughout, but for its great degree of cohesion.

For instance in Molly's case the need for togetherness is responsible for the great amount of interaction, the avoidance of separation and the interference in each other's activities, all combining to shape interaction into these long chains, while using the greatest variety of modes. It is also responsible, as will be seen further on, for the stimulating ways in which interaction is displayed in speech and locomotor activities, favouring by this means both interchange and togetherness, while the ways in which interaction is displayed, in play activity and relationship with others, serve to prevent mother and child from getting involved elsewhere and otherwise, while the opposite pattern appears with Bob.

Thus it appears that interaction is more than an accurate reflection of relationship, it has important functions: it provides the basis on which emotional relationship can exert itself, express itself, regulate itself. One can also see how the consistency and cohesion of the pattern of interaction which exerts itself in all sectors of the child's life is a moulding force for his development.

Evolution of the pattern of interaction

In comparing those five children at an early age (4-5 months) and later ($2\frac{1}{2}$ years) it was striking to find the same main differences in the patterns of the mother-child pairs. It was noticed indeed that the overall percentage of interaction during waking periods and the form of interaction is not much modified during the two first years, a certain specificity of the individual pattern remaining constant throughout the developmental process.

However, in the realm of this consistency, there is room for evolutive changes brought about by the growth of the child. As has been said when discussing maturity level, new acquisitions provide new grounds for interaction, while some previous circumstances lose their interest and are abandoned, making way for new ones, to which interaction will be applied in the way which best serves the basic dominant attitude of the pair.

The tone may then change considerably, according to whether or not new acquisitions can be taken into the interaction and become a source of mutual pleasure.

As to the modes of interaction, in some mother-child pairs, these seem to develop with the growth of the child's equipment, as following a parallel maturational process (Molly, Frank). However in other cases it is not so. We have seen, for instance, that the modes of Lewis and his mother were the same at 1 year old as at 3 months. This seemed to bring about some discomfort and displeasure, possibly because it was out of step with the child's needs, as related to the rhythm of development.

Bob's mother, as we said, apart from physical care, used almost exclusively a visual mode of interaction. Though Bob liked to be cuddled in the nursery, his use of visual contact was also noted. At home, he seemed to accept the absence of cuddling, and was content with the visual mode of interaction provided by his mother. However, around 11 months old, he developed, as is usual, separation anxiety, together with a mild sleeping problem. It was only after some time that mother, intolerant of Bob's crying, eventually found that a long cuddle before bed time had a soothing effect on Bob, who then went readily to sleep. Cuddling appeared in this instance as a late compensatory mode of interaction, readily abandoned as soon as it was found unnecessary.

6

Emotional Content of Interaction: Its Impact on the Child's Development

Coming back to the mother-child couples, in their emotional attitudes towards various issues, five different outcomes may occur, each one has a determining effect on the behaviour by which it is brought about.

1. *Mutual pleasure has constructive effects at two levels:*

(*a*) Attitudes towards each other which are pleasurable to both mother and child seem to create in each the desire and the ability to promote situations and occasions to enjoy them. In such cases it is hard to say who is the responsible leader. We seem to be confronted with a resonance phenomenon: the pleasure of each corresponds to and reinforces the pleasure of the other, while inducing in both an eagerness and ability to create situations in which they can enjoy each other in such ways. We can see this between Molly and her mother in respect of 'togetherness'; between Bob and his mother in their mutual pleasure in side-by-side autonomous activities, with little direct interchange.

Each time this occurs, the child is found to have outstanding abilities in these areas of activity which are a dominant and pleasurable source of interaction.

For instance Molly is outstanding, and rank-ordered first, for loco-motor activities and speech, which are enjoyable for both mother and child and facilitate togetherness. Bob is unusual for his age in his constructive use of objects, and his play with other children; we have seen how mother encourages this, enjoying it as much as her son, while these activities insure a combination of closeness-distance which is pleasurable to both.

(b) Mutual pleasure also creates a mutual responsiveness which has a reinforcing effect: for instance all five children are oriented towards their mothers: watching, following, welcoming them. But the intensity of their orientation is at the level of mother's responses: lowest in Louise, greatest in Molly and Bob, though taking different forms. It is worth mentioning incidentally that the intensity of orientation of the child corresponds with a similar intensity in its intolerance of separation.

Moreover it appears that whenever this deep satisfaction in each other is an overall dominating trend, the child shows strength in his drives and develops early abilities for mastery and defence, either independently or using mother as a prop, a sort of extension of himself.

For instance, confronted with a stranger Bob controls the situation by watching the latter. His obvious interest in her, mitigated by fear, induces a cautious and progressive approach: prolonged and distant observation of her belongings, which he does not take when she offers them but only later when she leaves them on the table; sending his beloved toys in her direction, and so coming nearer and nearer; finally engaging in play with her, able to defend himself when she teases him without interrupting their game.

Molly's interest in the stranger is as great as Bob's, but she displays more overt fear and clings to mother as to a haven of safety. Only from this shelter does she dare to look at the stranger, then step by step, she leaves mother's lap while still touching her. Slowly she emerges further, always running back to mother as soon as the unknown creature moves or makes a tentative approach. Only after a long while does she feel secure enough to daringly provoke the stranger.

2. At the opposite extreme, some areas of behaviour remain in the shade, somewhat ignored by both mother and child. They do not become

a source of interaction, or hardly at all. The performance of the child is then low mean average.

For instance, neither Bob nor his mother are interested in locomotor activities. Mother does not comment on his new abilities or disabilities in respect of locomotion. She disregards this to the extent of not mentioning his first step. And Bob, so far ahead in play activities, is not interested; he can move around to get what he wants by necessity but not as a pleasure. Moreover, there is an advantage for both of them in Bob's relative immobility, since mother likes to carry him quickly from here to there at her convenience, and he enjoys it. So he is not stimulated to walk, and remains clumsy, which, far from annoying mother, makes her laugh; his clumsiness is no frustration for Bob, since he has at hand everything he needs to play with and to enjoy himself. It is the same with speech. Mother shares Bob's interest in sounds, and provides musical toys and games, and indeed Bob is highly auditory. But she is not interested in speech, she does not speak much herself nor does she answer to Bob's sounds by sounds, attempting to turn them into language, as Molly's mother does; Bob's interest remains at the same level, using sounds for play, but not for interchange with mother.

The same applies to Molly and her mother in respect of play activities: neither of them is much interested in constructive or imaginative play. Moreover, if Molly happens to show some interest, mother will divert her attention towards herself, so that play with objects is mainly converted into 'give-and-take' games, which favour interchange and togetherness but reinforce Molly's pleasure in possession, and does not stimulate the pleasure of doing tests, which show that she has only a low mean level.

Louise shows lack of pleasure, indifference in walking, moving, doing, together with poor performance; she is rank-ordered last in all these areas.

Here again it is hard to say whether the lack of mutual interest, by depriving the child of stimulation, promotes poor performance, or if the poor performance is responsible for the mutual lack of interest. But just as with mutual pleasure, what is obvious is the association of the three elements: lack of interest and responsiveness in both mother and child, and poor performance, each reinforcing the other two.

3. In some areas of behaviour mothers make firm demands or consistent impediments. Often they do this in such a matter-of-fact, noiseless, subtle way, that it could easily be overlooked. All the more since in all these instances the children comply in the same noiseless matter-of-fact way, without experiencing frustration, or at least without showing any sign of it, as if there were a mutual agreement to abandon certain types of behaviour or activity.

From one mother-child pair to another the areas of encouragement and discouragement differ.

For instance, Molly's mother, in contrast with her usual attitudes, decides very firmly when Molly must sleep: she knows it, and has a way of putting her to bed with a bottle, leaving her alone, with the door shut, insisting that no one must stay in the room; and Molly is never observed protesting, she goes to sleep as soon as the bottle is empty, without asking for any attention.

Mother was surprisingly successful in restricting Louise in subtle, but firm and consistent ways in all areas of behaviour, without Louise showing the slightest sign of frustration: she seemed quite content to stand and look with nothing to do, and no freedom to move about.

In similar ways Bob's mother made him respect the invisible barriers which prevented him from touching some of her belongings, from going in a forbidden room, from interfering in mother's business.

Indeed, the least frustrated children are Louise and Bob, whose mothers are always consistent in the limitations they impose.

In Louise, where these limitations were widespread, with no compensations of mutual pleasure, we found an inhibited child with a real lack of spirit.

Bob, whose restrictions were few, and counterbalanced by many areas of pleasurable stimulation, showed outstanding and increasing growing ability to conform, even in mother's absence, without suppressing the strength of his underlying wishes, which he displaced on to permitted or valued activities.

Thus one can see how consistent limitation leads to a consenting child, who inhibits his behaviour, whereas mutual pleasure leads to stimulation and reinforcement, with somewhere in between the no-man's-land of 'indifference', where abilities are left to grow uncultivated on fallow land.

4. There are instances in which mothers are intolerant towards certain features, or behaviours of the child, without being then able to stop the child, as these mothers did.

In such instances the mother's limitations or demands are occasional and inconsistent. They seem to have a reinforcing effect on the behaviour of the child.

For instance, this is striking with Molly's mother who sometimes allows her to touch or to take, then suddenly forbids her. This reinforces Molly's possessiveness and stubborn determination to get what she wants. In the same way, Lewis's mother seems to encourage him to pursue her by often pushing him away, while she also responds now and then by long interdependency situations, during which she lends herself to closeness of contact.

These inconsistent restrictions create a vicious circle of mutual frustration and opposition. In this respect Frank's, Molly's and Lewis's records are much richer in frustrations than those of the two other children.

However, Frank, and even more so Molly, are able to fight back to assert themselves, and oppose their mothers strongly.

While Lewis, the most frustrated of all five children, reacts to frustration by whining and hyperactivity, not by defying his mother, he cannot fight his brother either. His fragility, in contrast to the fighting strength of the two others, seems to be related to the deep mutual dissatisfaction and anxiety which in this case overflowed the relationship, as is seen in 5. below.

In Bob's case the consistency of limitations, as well as the multiple areas of mutual pleasure, leave no room for any opposition between Bob and his mother, who remains at large the undisputed master of the situation.

5. In other instances the child, either in general, or in some restricted area of behaviour, arouses deep dissatisfaction and/or anxiety in the mother.

In such instances, mothers are apt to blame the child, feeling him to be a heavy and tiresome burden, which arouses their hostility. Not only do they lose all ability to respond by offering an acceptable outlet, but their inadequate responses rub in the child's failures, and eventually produce inability; a vicious circle is thus created, about which they both express open anxiety and strong depressive feelings.

Even Bob's mother does not altogether avoid this, though in all other respects she is so gratified by her son. So clever in managing all the other aspects of their relationship to the greatest satisfaction of both, she is unable for a long time to cope with Bob's separation anxiety. Similarly Bob, usually so clever in avoiding frustration as well as in coping with stranger anxiety, is in this instance completely helpless, crying desperately, rocking, unable to sleep.

In Frank's case his mother's intolerance of his slight motor disability makes it into a major problem. By her way of meeting it in their interaction, she enhances his dysfunction.

As to Lewis's mother, who belittles all features and activities of her son: the counterpart is a child who is by far the most frequently frustrated in everyday life, who often looks miserable, sometimes excited, but never really contented, he also shows the lowest ability in organizing speech, locomotion, activity in meaningful and constructive ways, and little ability to develop personal means of coping with frustration and anxieties.

Such a study of the impact of mother-child relationship on the development of the child is far from being exhaustive. However it shows clearly how the child is deeply influenced by the mother-child relationship in all areas of his personality. Though mothers are not aware of it, each one of them makes consistent and significant conscious and unconscious choices as to what she selects in the child to stimulate, prevent, or distort according to whether his behaviour arouses in her pleasure, indifference, displeasure, anxiety.

By talking with each of the mothers, one gets a partial hypothetical understanding and knowledge of the motivations which arouse in each specific feelings towards her child as a whole, or towards specific trends, areas of behaviour, developmental features or emotional problems. Whether these are linked with the past history of each mother, her early parental relationship, her socio-cultural value system, or her present tie to her husband, her idiosyncratic sensitiveness corresponded to her own development of personality.

Be that as it may, from the emotions stirred in a mother by her child results her specific way to rule her relationship in all its aspects, space, closeness, maturity, intensity—quality and zones of investment, through the pattern of interaction.

It is true that the child brings into the interaction his own special gifts, his handicaps and perhaps his own spontaneous emotional trends. However they are braced through interaction with his mother, and out of this grows the child, his equipment and his ego strength; in this way also progressively built up his ability to relate to his mother. We have few means with which to explore the inner life of the child at this pre-verbal age, but Spitz has shown, through direct observation and an experimental approach, the genesis of mother-child relationship during the first year of life. Similar studies could lead to better understanding of the components and the shape of the internalized mother image during the following years, as affected by the two first years of mother-child interaction and relationship.

7

Summary

In conclusion, one sees how the study of interaction provides a more precise knowledge of mother-child relationship. It shows how in each mother-child couple some basic emotional attitudes pervade the relationship and are a key-note for interaction. Expressed and acted out all through the interaction they organize it in a pattern which can be described in terms of quantity, beginning and end, form, mode, tone and content, specific for each couple. Though consistent, far from giving rise to stereotyped behaviours, the pattern is displayed in a wide variety of ways.

It also appears that interaction is not only a means of expression and acting out of relationship but also through its various aspects (quantity, shape, mode, tone, content) is a regulating device through which all aspects of relationship are very finely controlled e.g. space, closeness, maturity level, intensity, quality and zones of emotional investment.

Moreover interaction between mother and child shows how, through his characteristics, impulses, and spontaneous behaviour, the child evokes strong feelings in his mother, leaving her either more sensitive or less so to different areas of behaviour and development (language games, motor activity, social interplay, separation situation, etc. . . .); how mother's emotional attitudes correspond with those of the child: it is precisely these emotional responses to one another which organize interaction into its pattern, giving it its specificity, cohesion and consistency. Displayed in various circumstances and in different areas of behaviour it acts as a main dynamic organizing force for the child's personality development.

REFERENCES

1. AINSWORTH, M., and BOWLBY, J., 1954. Research strategy in the study of mother-child separation. *Courrier*, **4**, 105-31.
2. AINSWORTH, M., and BOWLBY, J., 1962. The effects of maternal deprivation: A review of findings and controversy in the context of research strategy. *Public Health Papers*, No. 14. World Health Organization.
3. APPELL, G., and DAVID, M., 1965. A study of mother-child interaction at 13 months. In *Determinants of infant behaviour*, vol. 3. Ed. Foss, B. London, Methuen.
4. BALINT, M., 1948. Individual differences of behaviour in early infancy and an objective method for recording them. *J. Genet. Psychol.*, **73**.
5. BAYLEY, N., and SCHAEFER, E., 1960. Relationship between the socio-economical variables and the behaviour of mothers towards young children. *J. Genet. Psychol.* **96**, 61-67.
6. BENJAMIN, J., 1959. Prediction and psychopathological theory. In *Dynamic psychopathology in childhood*. Eds. Jessner, L., and Pavenstedt, E. Grune and Stratton, New York.
7. BENJAMIN, J., 1961. Some developmental observations relating to the Theory of Anxiety. *J. Am. Psychoanalyt. Assn*, **9**.
8. BERGMAN, P., and ESCALONA, S., 1949. Unusual sensitivities in very young children. *Psychoanalytic Study of the Child*, 3-4. New York, Intern. Univ. Press.
9. BERGMANN, T., in coll. FREUD, A., 1965. *Children in hospitals*. New York, Intern. Univ. Press.
10. BOLLAND, J., and SANDLER, J., 1965. Study of a psychoanalytic case material of a two-year-old child. *The Hampstead psychoanalytic index*. New York, Intern. Univ. Press.
11. BOWLBY, J, 1957. An ethological approach to research in child development. *Brit. J. Med. Psychol.*, **30**, 230-40.
12. BOWLBY, J., 1958. The nature of the child's tie to his mother. *Internat. J. Psychoanal.*, **39**, 350-73.
13. BOWLBY, J., 1960. Ethology and the development of object relations. *Internat. J. Psychoanal.*, **41**, 313-17.
14. BOWLBY, J., 1960. Separation anxiety. *Internat. J. Psychoanal.*, **41**, 89-113.
15. BOWLBY, J., 1960. Separation anxiety: A critical review of the literature. *J. Child Psychol. Psychiat.*, **1**, 251-69.
16. BRAZELTON, T. B., 1964. The early mother-infant adjustment. *Pediatrics*, **32**, 931-37.
17. BRODY, S., 1956. *Patterns of mothering*. New York, Intern. Univ. Press.
18. COLEMAN, R. W., KRIS, E., and PROVENCE, S., 1953. The study of variations of early parental attitudes. *Psychoanalytic study of the child*, **8**. New York, Intern. Univ. Press.

19. DAVID, M., and APPELL, G., 1961. A study of nursing care and nurse-infant interaction. In *Determinants of infant behaviour*. Ed. Foss, B. London, Methuen.
20. DAVID, M., and APPELL, G., 1961. Etude des Facteurs de carence affective dans une pouponnière. Paris. *La psychiatrie de l'enfant*, vol. 4. P.U.F.
21. DAVID, M., and APPELL, G., 1966. La relation mère-enfant. Paris. *La psychiatrie de l'enfant*, vol. 9.
22. DER HEYDT, V. VON, 1964. The role of the father in the early mental development. *Brit. J. Med. Psychol.*, **37**, 123-31.
23. ERIKSON, E. H., 1959. Growth and crisis of the healthy personality. *Psychological Issues*, **1**.
24. ESCALONA, S., LEITCH, M., et al., 1952. Early phases of personality development. *Monogr. Soc. Res. Child Development*, **17**, No. 1.
25. ESCALONA, S., LEITCH, M., et al., 1953, 1954. Emotional development in the first year of life. *Problems of infancy and childhood*. New York. Josiah Macy Jr. Foundation.
26. FOSS, B., Ed., 1959-65. *Determinants of infant behaviour*, vols. 1-3. Proceedings of a Tavistock Study Group on Mother-Infant Interaction. London, Methuen.
27. FREUD, A., 1950. L'importance de l'evolution de la psychologie psychanalytique de l'enfance. *International psychiatric congress*. Paris, Rapports Hermann et Cie.
28. FREUD, A., 1953. Some remarks on infant observation. *Psychoanalytic study of the child*, **8**, 19. New York, Intern. Univ. Press.
29. FREUD, A., 1958. Child observation and prediction of development. *Psychoanalytic study of the child*, **13**, 92. New York Intern. Univ. Press.
30. FREUD, A., and SPITZ, M., 1960. Discussion of Dr J. Bowlby's paper. *Psychoanalytic Study of the Child*, **15**. New York, Intern. Univ. Press.
31. GREENACRE, P., et al., 1961. *La theorie de la relation parent-enfant. Remarques complémentaires*. Special number, 22nd International Congress of Psychoanalysis, Edinburgh, 30th July-3rd August. Also, 1963, *Revue Française de Psychanalyse*, Paris, **27**, 483-527.
32. Groupe Lyonnaise d'Etudes Medicales et Psychologiques et Biologiques, 1963. Amour Maternel, Paris, Spes. Pg. 240.
33. HARLOW, H. F., 1958. The Nature of Love. *Am. Psychologist*, **13**, 673.
34. HARLOW, H. F., 1960. Primary affectional patterns in primates. *Am. J. Orthopsychiat.*, **30**, 676.
35. HARLOW, H. F., 1963. The maternal affectional system. In *Determinants of Infant Behaviour*. vol. II. Ed. Foss. B. London, Methuen.
36. HARLOW, H. F., and ZIMMERMAN, R., 1959. Affectional responses in the infant monkey. *Science*, **130**.
37. HARTMANN, H., and KRIS, E., 1945. The genetic approach in psychoanalysis. *Psychoanalytic Study of the Child*, **1**. New York, Intern. Univ. Press.
38. HARTMANN, H., KRIS, E., and LOEWENSTEIN, R. M., 1946. Comments on the formation of the psychic structure. *Psychoanalytic Study of the Child*, **2**, New York, Intern. Univ. Press.
39. HELLMANN, I., 1963. Analyse simultanée de la mère et de son enfant. *Revue Française de Psychanalyse*, **27**, 619-39.
40. LATIL, J., 1966. L'enfant et ses premières experiences familiales. *Pedagogie*, Paris, 342-50.
41. LEBOVICI, S., 1950. Notions nouvelles sur le developpement du nourrisson dans ses repercussions psychologiques ulterieures. *La Semaine des Hôpitaux*, **26**.
42. LEBOVICI, S., 1964. Quelques reflexions à propos de l'abord écologique en psychiatrie infantile. *Psychiatrie de l'Enfant*, **7**, 198-268.

REFERENCES

43. LEVY, D. M., 1958. Behavioural analysis. *Analysis of clinical observations of behaviour, as applied to mother-newborn relationship.* Springfield, Ill., Charles C. Thomas.
44. LEWIN, K. K., 1936. *Principles of topological psychology.* New York, McGraw-Hill.
45. LEZINE, I., 1956. Recherche sur la psychologie du premier âge. *Schweiz. Ztschr. F. Psych.*, **15**.
46. LEZINE, I., 1964. *Psychopedagogie du premier âge.* P.U.F., Coll. Le Psychologue.
47. MANDLER, G., 1963. Parent and child in the development of the Oedipus complex. *J. Ment. Dis.*, **136**, 226-35.
48. MOSS, A., 1965. Methodological issues in studying mother-infant interaction. *Am. J. Orthopsychiat.*, **35**, 482-86.
49. PUTNAM, M. C., RANK, B., PAVENSTEDT, E., ANDERSON, A. N., and RAWSON, I., 1948. Case study of atypical two-and-a-half-year-old. *Am. J. Orthopsychiat.*, **28**.
50. RACAMIER, P. C., SENS, C., and CARRETIER, L., 1961. La mère et l'enfant dans les psychosis du post-partum. *L'Evolution Psychiatrique*, **4**, 525-69.
51. RAPAPORT, D., 1960. Psychoanalysis as a developmental psychology. In *Perspectives in psychological theory.* Eds. Kaplan, B., and Wapner, S. New York, Intern. Univ. Press.
52. RHEINGOLD, H., 1958. A method for measuring maternal care. *Amer. Psychol.*, **13**, 319 (Abstract).
53. RHEINGOLD, H., and BAYLEY, N., 1959. The later effects of an experimental modification of mothering. *Child Development*, **30**, 363-72.
54. RHEINGOLD, H., 1960. The measurement of maternal care. *Soc. Res. Child Development*, **3**, 565-75.
55. RITVO, S., and SOLNIT, S. A., 1958. Influences of early mother-child interaction on identification processes. *Psychoanalytic Study of the Child*, **13**, New York, Internat. Univ. Press.
56. ROBERTSON, J., 1962. Mothering as an influence on early development. *Psychoanalytic Study of the Child*, **17**, New York, Internat. Univ. Press.
57. RUBINFINE, D. L., 1962. Maternal stimulation, psychic structure and early object relations, with special reference to aggression and denial. *Psychoanalytic Study of the Child*, **17**, New York, Intern. Univ. Press.
58. SANDLER, L., 1962. Issue in early mother-child interaction. *J. Child Psychiat.*, **1**.
59. SCHAEFER, S., 1960. Consistency of maternal behaviour from infancy to preadolescence. *J. Abnorm. Psychol.*, **61**, 1.
60. SCHAEFER, S., and BAYLEY, N., 1963. Maternal behaviour and their intercorrelation from infancy through adolescence. *Monogr. Soc. Res. Child Development*, **28**.
61. SCHUR, M., 1960. Discussion of Dr John Bowlby's Paper. *Psychoanalytic Study of the Child*, **15**. New York, Internat. Univ. Press.
62. SPITZ, R., 1954. Genèse des premières relations objectales. *Revue Française de Psychanalyse*, **18**, 479-575.
63. SPITZ, R., 1959. La cavité primitive. Trad. J. Mallet. *Revue Fraçnaise de Psychanalyse*, **23**.
64. SPITZ, R., 1962. Le non et le oui. *La genèse de la communication humaine*, A. M. Rocheblave-Spenle, Paris, Presses Univ. de France.
65. SPITZ, R., 1958. *La première année de l'enfant.* P.U.F.
66. SPITZ, R., 1960. Discussion of Dr John Bowlby's paper. *Psychoanalytic study of the child*, **15**. New York, Intern. Univ. Press.
67. SPITZ, R., 1964. Quelques prototypes précoces de défense du Moi. *Revue Française de Psychanalyse*, **28**, 185-215.

68. WINNICOTT, D., 1945. Primitive emotional development. *Internat. J. Psychoanal.*, **26**, 137-43.
69. WINNICOTT, D., 1953. Transitional objects and transitional phenomena. *Internat. J. Psychoanal.*, **34**, 1-9.
70. WINNICOTT, D., 1964. *The family and individual development*. London, Tavistock Publications.
71. YARROW, L. J., and GOODWIN, M. S., 1965. Some conceptual issues in the study of mother-infant interaction. *Am. J. Orthopsychiat.*, **35**, 473-81.

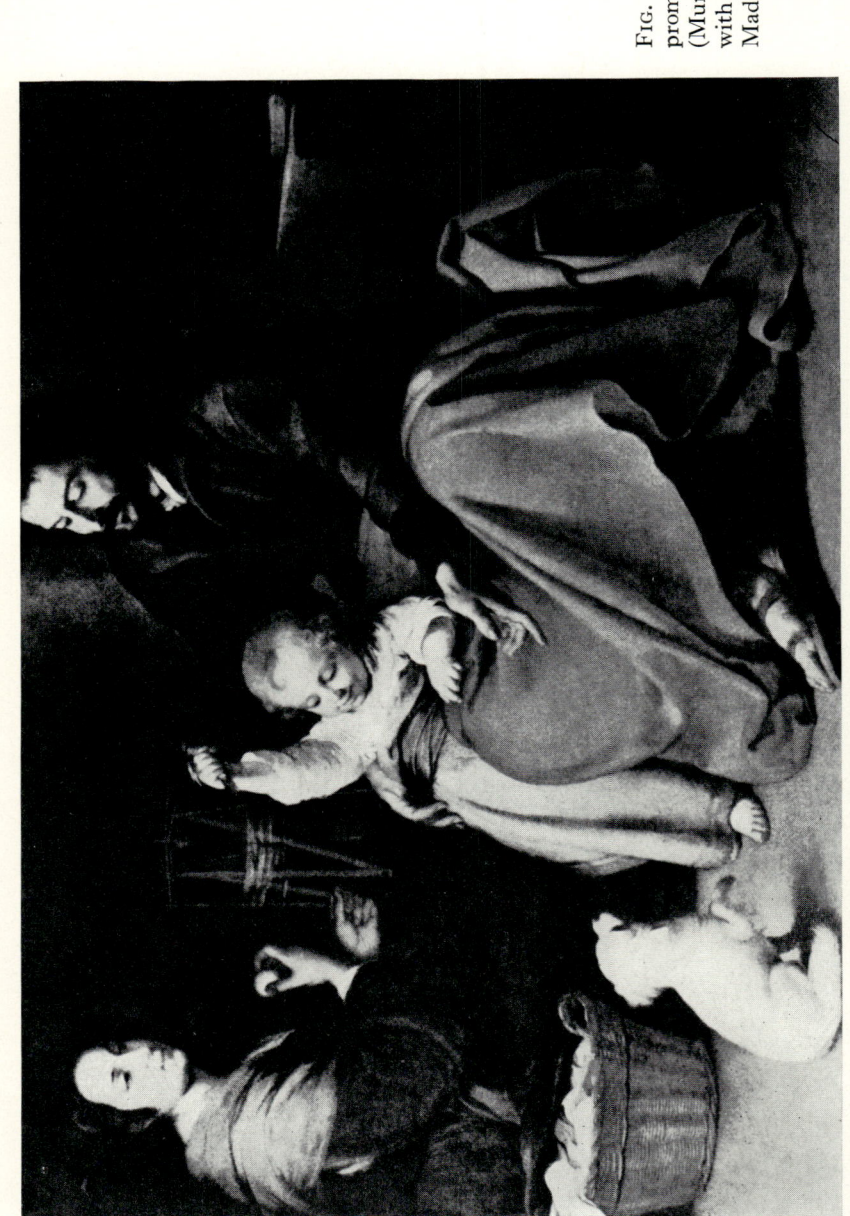

FIG. 1. Father given prominence in the family. (Murillo, the holy family with the little bird. Madrid, Prado.)

V

FATHERING

John G. Howells

*Director, The Institute of Family Psychiatry,
Ipswich and East Suffolk Hospital, Ipswich, England*

> I'll meet the raging of the skies,
> But not an angry father.
>
> (Thomas Campbell:
> *Lord Ullin's Daughter*)

1

Introduction

Fathering is an element in family life as distinct as mothering. Yet legal enactions, social policy, art forms, in western culture, although not in all cultures, neglect fathering in comparison to mothering. The neglect of fathering is at its greatest in contemporary child psychiatry and psychology.

Some psychoanalytical writers do not regard fathering as an element in family life as distinct as mothering. In this connection, Ackerman[2] states: 'I am inclined to believe that there is no separate fathering instinct'. Later in an admirable section on the 'Disturbances of fathering', the same writer gives such a definite place to father in family life that the reader might reasonably question his thesis. Proponents of this point of view regard any tender, kind, solicitous care of the infant by father as 'mothering'. This carries the implication that such behaviour by men is not masculine—yet is regarded as a virtue in the marriage relationship. The same view regards these qualities as borrowed from, or an imitation of, the mother and not intrinsic to the father.

Again, this viewpoint tends to emphasize the biological function of the mother in child care—that she alone bears and breast feeds the child. Furthermore, it is assumed that father is a latecomer to the child's life—only when the child begins to talk and be independent. All these views can be challenged.

The author asserts that fathering is an element in family life as significant as mothering. Fathering and mothering may have many components; most are probably in common, a few may be dissimilar. There are more likenesses in mothering and fathering than there are differences. Both are the product of an intimate emotional experience with their own parents of both sexes; they must absorb components from both. Both also have much in common with relatedness elsewhere—foster parenting, adoptive parenting, marital relatedness, grandparenting, etc. A child in his tender years requires this protective relatedness from any source—normally, it is given equally by father and mother, sometimes better by father or mother, and sometimes better by others. Each situation is unique.

Again, to emphasize mother's biological role in bearing the infant is to overlook the psychological climate of pregnancy and conception. The acceptance of father by mother may be the predominant factor in leading to the acceptance of a child from him, and uniquely from him. Thereafter the parents become a pair linked in a common endeavour, in which, however, only one of them can physically bear the yet unborn child. The father's thoughts, feelings and actions influence the mother's regard for her child and thus indirectly the child. Striking evidence of the father's involvement is seen in the couvade syndrome. The first child emerges into an already formed psychological group situation of father, mother and child. The group of a second child is a larger one consisting of four people. The child may be introduced to the group in any order—often he meets father first, if the mother is incapacitated. Thereafter, what he receives from each member of the group is dependent on their feelings for him, their capacity for relating, and the roles given them. This is infinitely variable and unique for each family. The one thing that a father cannot do for his child is to breast feed him—although there are isolated instances of the child being soothed at his father's nipples. In the contemporary bottle-feeding society, this is not the handicap that it might appear. All else his father can do directly for him. When not directly participating in his care, the father still influences his child through his intimate relationship with the mother; after all a father normally regards a child as a tangible evidence of his own union with the mother. The child is fortunate in the insurance of two parents, whereby one can compensate for the other. Father supports mother and child. Equally, mother supports father and child. The part played by a particular father, or a particular mother, is dependent on his own previous family, clan and social experiences.

The view that seeks to diminish the role of father leans on historical accounts that suggest, as did Briffault[18], that the role of mother is central and that of father unessential and secondary. In support of this thesis, it is even suggested that early man's ignorance of his role in impregnation led to his neglect of fatherhood. These views, too, are open to challenge. Westermarck[153] sees father as having had a significant place in the family from earliest times. It is difficult to see how man could fail to see the link

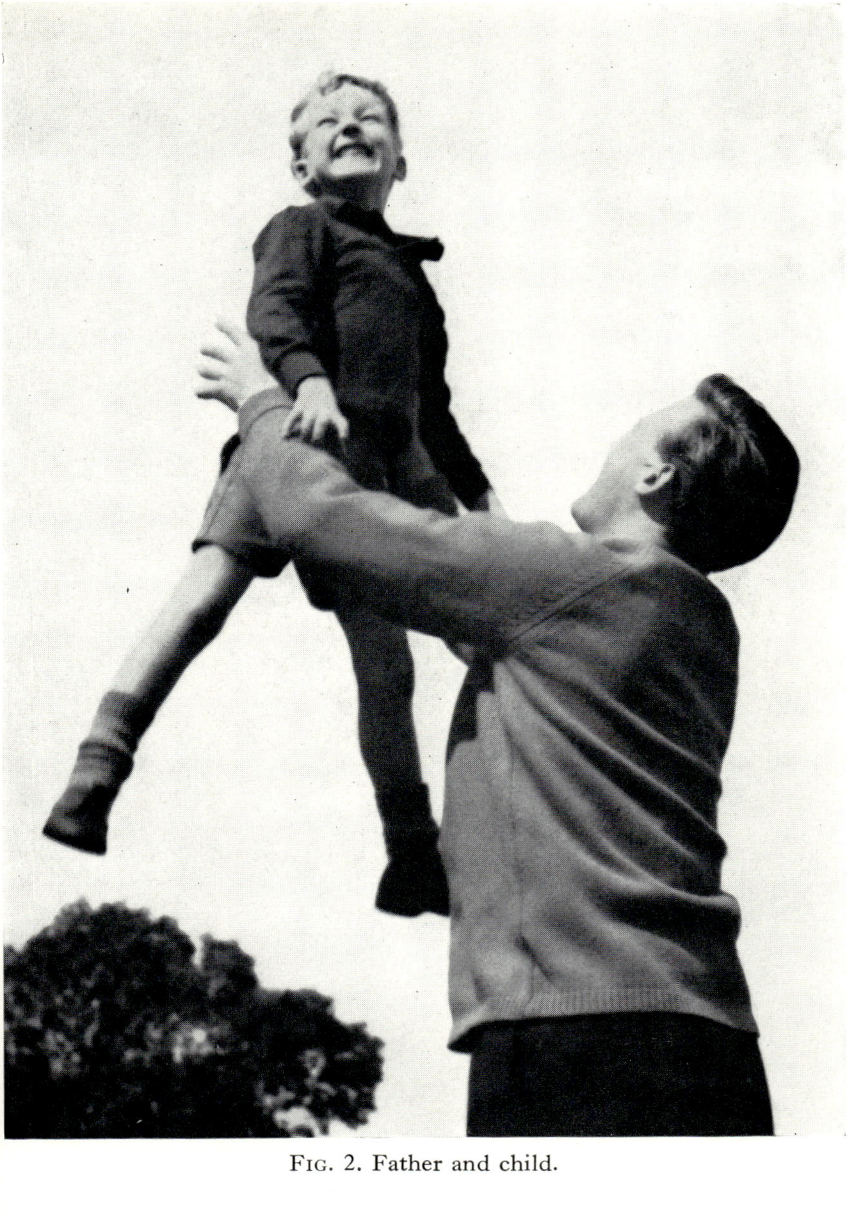

FIG. 2. Father and child.

between impregnation and conception, an event with such a direct causal link. When he fails to see it, there may be strong cultural pressures to believe otherwise—as revealed by Malinowski[93], amongst the Trobriands.

Fathering is an essential element of the family group, a group that receives increasing attention in psychiatry. Child psychiatry is moving away from the concept of a sick child with intra-psychic pathology in whose management the mother requires only guidance. It is increasingly accepted that the child is responding to a situation—usually within his family. When account is taken of the mother and child as a dyad, we arrive at child and mother psychiatry; when father is included to make a triad—child and parent psychiatry; when account is taken of siblings as well, child and family psychiatry emerges. In all these approaches the child is the focus of attention. But, in family psychiatry[63] the family is the unit and the focus of attention is on it as a whole. If the child is the referred member of a family, he is regarded as an index of a sick family, and it is this family that becomes the object of investigation and treatment; the restoration of health to the family restores the child's health and guarantees the child's future well-being.

This complex unit, the family, can be conceptualized[65] in five dimensions in the Past, Present and Future time sequence. These five dimensions are those of the Individual, of the Relationship, of the Group Dynamics, of the Material Circumstances and of the Family Community Interaction. The father-child relationship is one of the four most important relationships in the Dimension of the Relationships, these being: father-mother, mother-child, father-child, and child-child. It is essential to understand that each relationship is reciprocal, e.g. father-child and child-father. This chapter is concerned with one of these—fathering—the father-child relationship.

After a brief discussion of fathering in the animal kingdom and in anthropology, fathering will be evaluated as it stands in contemporary society. This will lead to an account of the place of fathering in contemporary child psychiatry. Without diminishing the role of the mother it is hoped that the role of the father will emerge as an essential component of family group life.

2

The Animal Kingdom

By selecting the appropriate facts from a mass of evidence, most points of view can be supported. Students of child nurture have not hesitated to seek support for their hypotheses from ethology—both in the study of animal life in the artificial conditions of the laboratory and in the wild. Again, it is mothering which is invariably the focus of study. Argument from analogy is always dangerous and never more so than here.

Studies of parental care in animals in the laboratory must be treated with great caution. So biased is present day opinion in favour of exclusive maternal care, that the bias is often imposed on the animals. Paternal and other forms of care are not feasible in the conditions set by the experiments. Rheingold[120] states in this connection: 'But among mammals care is given the young not only by the mother and father but often by other members of the group, males as well as females, juveniles as well as adults. Then, under the conditions of many of the studies reported here, all but the mother and her offspring were excluded'. Furthermore, in captivity, due to the artificial conditions, aberrations of behaviour appear in animals as in humans, e.g. in monkey colonies in laboratories there is more sex perversion, as rank order amongst the monkeys tends to disappear.

The variety and flexibility of nature can be seen in its methods of reproduction—division, budding, autogamy, conjugation, mutation, copulation and parthenogenesis. Nature will use what meets the requirements of the situation—in summer, green aphids reproduce by parthenogenesis, but male and females pair in the autumn. Some animals, e.g. snails, are hermaphrodite and either fertilize themselves or from one another.

Similarly, the main lesson to be found from the study of the care given to young animals is that nature is flexible. The need is to nurture the young so as to continue the species. Depending on the situation, nature will use a variety of means to achieve its purpose. As will be seen, parenting in many forms will be employed; paternal care will often be an ingredient in this, and sometimes it will be the only care. Most important to the young is not *who* offers the care, but that care is given. The intensity of care and quality of care varies with the species—nature meets the need by means appropriate to the situation with a broad concept of parenting and a flexible utilization of the means available. *Parenting* is more important than the parent.

Diverse Parental Care

To demonstrate the great variety of types of parental care in animals, examples will be given of some before concentrating on fathering in the animal kingdom.

1. *No care by parents*. The grayling butterflies, male and female, meet only to mate. The female lays her eggs on objects that will provide food for the caterpillars and thereafter leaves them. Many female fish lay their eggs and then give them no further care. Turtles, frogs and spiders behave similarly. In some species of shell fish and sea urchins, the male and female cells are discharged, meet by chance, and are given no parental care. The worm supplies the protection of a cocoon, but no care.

2. *Equal care by parents*. In the herring gull, the parents take turns in sitting on the eggs. The eggs are never left alone. After hatching, each

parent will feed the chicks by regurgitation and defend them against predators. In the Ringed Plover, male and female take turns in looking after the young from the first hatch and the eggs of the second hatch. Hobbies, unlike herring gulls, have a strict division of labour between male and female. The female, who is the larger of the two, stands guard over the young, while the male does the food hunting for the whole family. With foxes, the male at first feeds the female and the young; later both feed the young. Adelie and King penguins share the care of the young.

3. *Switching of roles.* In some animals it is possible for a switching of roles to take place. In kestrels, for instance, should the female die, the male will take on her task of feeding the young in addition to his own task of hunting for the food. Again, among partridges[81], the father spends most of his time on the look out, while the mother cares for the offspring and in moments of great danger conducts them to safety. But if the mother should die, the father takes over the task of protecting the young and finding food for them.

4. *Care mainly by the female.* In sheep there is exclusive care of the lambs by the ewe. In some varieties of Cichlid fish, the eggs are hatched and young cared for in the mouth of the female. In kestrels, the male hunts for food and the female protects the young and cares for them. Some female scorpions devour the male after copulation; therefore no male care is possible. Praying mantises also devour the male after copulation.

5. *Multiple mothering.* In a pride of lions, the young will be fed by the nearest lioness. Amongst elephants, in order to protect them from tigers, the young are placed between the mother and another female elephant, the 'Aunt', both of whom offer care.

6. *Care by the group.* Rowell[123] observed juvenile hamsters retrieving infant hamsters and Beniest-Noirot[10] reported the presence of several 'maternal' activities in virgin female, adult bachelor male, and immature mice.

7. *Foster parents.* The female cuckoo lays her eggs in the nest of another species and the young cuckoo is thereafter cared for by the foster parents. Both in scorpions and tarantulas the female will take the offspring of others and foster them—as noted originally by Fabre. In elephants, the tendency to foster is so well developed that the adult childless female elephants may adopt calves of others, or even human children; they may become greatly attached to a child who may be able to take great liberties with the huge foster parents (Sanderson[126]).

8. *Care by servants.* In the honey bee, the male fertilizes the queen, the queen lays the eggs; all other duties are performed by worker bees, infertile females. One of the functions of the worker is the care of the young —to be a nanny. Similar conditions are found in termites.

9. *Care in a crèche.* When the young Emperor penguins are of an age

when both parents have to search for food, they are cared for in a crèche. Adelie penguins also have these kindergartens.

10. *Care by Siblings*. In moth mites, the male offspring assist in the birth of the females and then immediately impregnate them—demonstrating sibling care and incest.

Care by Father

In the stickleback, the male selects the territory for his nest and builds it. He attracts the female and persuades her to spawn in his nest. The male may receive eggs from a number of females. Their work consists only in

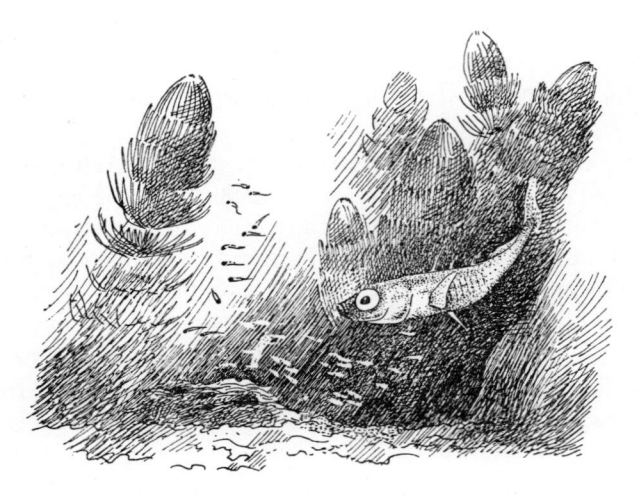

FIG. 3. The male stickleback fathering his young.
Reproduced by kind permission of the author and publishers from: Tinbergen, N., *Social Behaviour in Animals*. London: Methuen.

supplying the eggs and after that is completely over. Thereafter the male fertilizes the eggs, cares for them and brings up the young. Caring for the eggs includes guarding them and 'fanning' them by inducing a flow of current over them. The young are kept together in a swarm by the father, who is quick to chase and catch in his mouth the wandering young.

The males of some marine catfish and of other catfish found in the rivers of South America, carry the eggs in their mouths until they hatch. They do not eat at all during this period. The father's interest in his duties does not wane even after the young fish hatch, for he swims with them for a time and, when danger threatens, holds his mouth open so that the frightened youngsters can dash into it to safety.

In Emperor penguins, care is predominantly by the male as the young live in the male pouch while the female goes off in search of fish. The Phalarope bird[17] builds the nest, is courted by the female, and after the eggs are laid, takes over the entire responsibility of incubating them. In most ostrich-like birds, the males undertake the incubation of the eggs.

Darwin's frogs of Chile use the male vocal pouch as a nest where the young are incubated and emerge as young frogs. In the Midwife toad of south-west Europe, the male looks after the strings of eggs and, when these are ripe, hatches them in water. The female sea-horse lays her eggs in a pouch within the male, who thereafter has the care of the eggs and of the young.

Sometimes, the paternal care is selective; in wild cattle, the male calves, but not the female, are looked after by the herd bull. Nature may also offer substitute paternal care. The female hornbill, for instance, is imprisoned in a tree hole and fed by the male. Should this male die, another unattached male hornbill will take over the fathering.

Care of the Young in other Anthropoids

Especial attention must be given to the primate animals most closely related to man. As in man, diversity of methods of care is the striking finding and it may include care by males.

Infant care can be a group activity involving different age groups and both adult sexes. Russell's[125] commentary on hierarchies in Japanese monkey bands states that the females approve of male interest in infants and, when females with young are having their next babies, middle rank male leaders and middle rank sub-leaders may take charge of the 1 year olds. Baby sitting is a way of ingratiating themselves with the females. Hinde[59] reports on care by other females in a group of rhesus monkeys: 'It is thus clear that the attentions of 'aunts' may profoundly affect the environment of a young rhesus not only directly, but also by influencing the degree of permissiveness shown by the infant's own mother'.

The social unit for the protection and nourishment of the newborn langur does not include the adult male. Adult male langurs, Jay[72] states, are indifferent to a newborn and are seldom within 15 feet of one. The loudest squeals of a newborn do not draw the attention of an adult male and when an infant needs help, assistance is given by either the mother or another adult female. If an adult male accidentally frightens an infant, the mother instantly threatens, chases, and often slaps the male. Other adult females near the infant may join the mother and chase the male as far as 25 yards.

This is in contrast to the care in baboons when, as Devore[30] reports, the birth of a new infant absorbs the attention of the entire troop. From the moment the birth is discovered, the mother is continuously surrounded by the other baboons, who walk beside her and sit as close as possible when she rests. Juvenile and young adult male express only perfunctory interest in the infant, but older males frequently come and touch the infant. The degree of interest, Devore states, shown by adult males varies considerably. On several occasions the most dominant males carried young infants on their bellies, as long as 20 minutes in one instance. All the adult males of the troop are sensitive to the slightest distress cries of a young infant and will viciously attack any human who comes between an infant and the troop. Adult males, even young adult males, allow infants to crawl all over them with impunity. Jealous protection by the adult males continues unabated as the infants grow and the older infants and young juveniles increase their efforts to entice them into a play group. By the end of the 10th month the infant, who until now has depended largely upon its mother for both companionship and protection, looks to its peers for companionship and to the adult males for protection. In the description of the mother-infant relations in the baboon, Devore stresses that the relationship of the infant to the adult males is important at every stage of the infant's maturation.

From the two month observation of an infant female that had lost its mother, Devore illustrates how close a relationship can become between a female infant and an adult male. The other adult females are less tolerant than the males and thus it was natural that a very dominant male should protect the infant. The sick infant was the male's constant companion, grooming him through the day, walking in his shadow when the troop moved, and sleeping beside him in the trees at night. She even stayed beside him while he was in consort with an estrous female.

Devore goes on to mention additional examples of male care. Zuckerman[161] describes what appears to be a very similar relationship in the London Zoo colony between an infant and an adult male hamadryas baboon after the death of the infant's mother. Itani[70] has described in detail a routinized form of paternal care in Japanese macaques during the birth season. Devore concludes that the evidence from baboons and Japanese macaques suggests that social bonds between adult males and infants are very strong in these terrestrial species, in striking contrast to the weak bonds between infants and adult males in more arboreal species, for example, in langurs as mentioned earlier.

Perhaps the most striking example of exclusive male care is provided by the marmosets of South America[152]; the male takes the young to the female for suckling, but this is the only child care allowed to her.

It appears that in anthropoid primates many varieties of child care are found—whole group, joint male and female, exclusively female, multiple female, kindergarten and exclusively male.

Summary

This brief study of infant care demonstrates the variety of methods employed in the animal kingdom for the care of the young, methods that

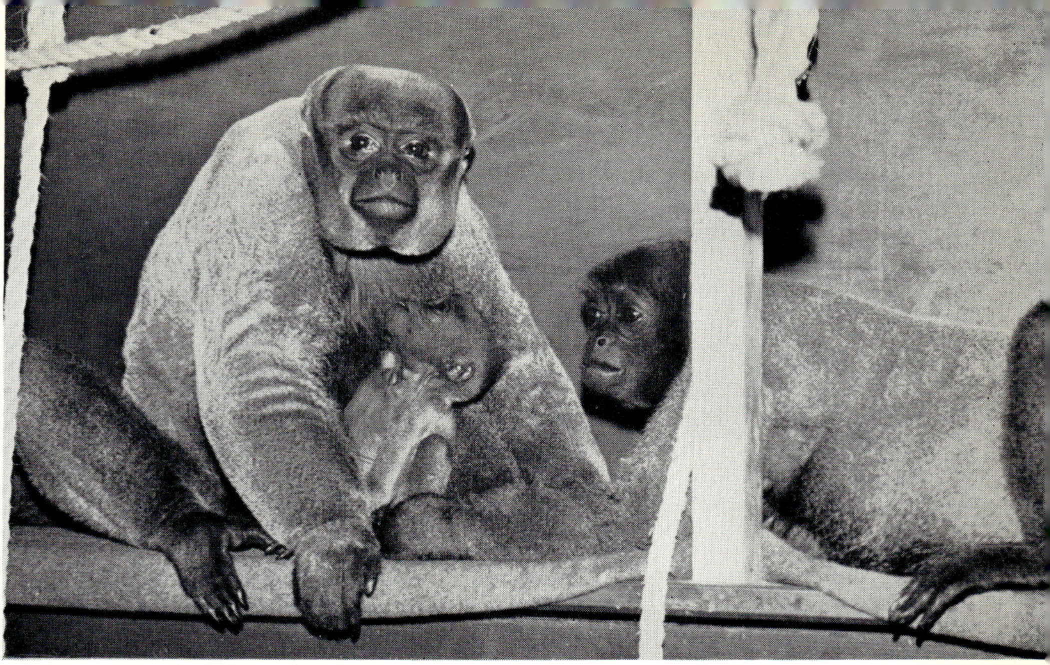

FIG. 4. Jojo, the dominant male, cuddles Charlie, his infant by Lulu.

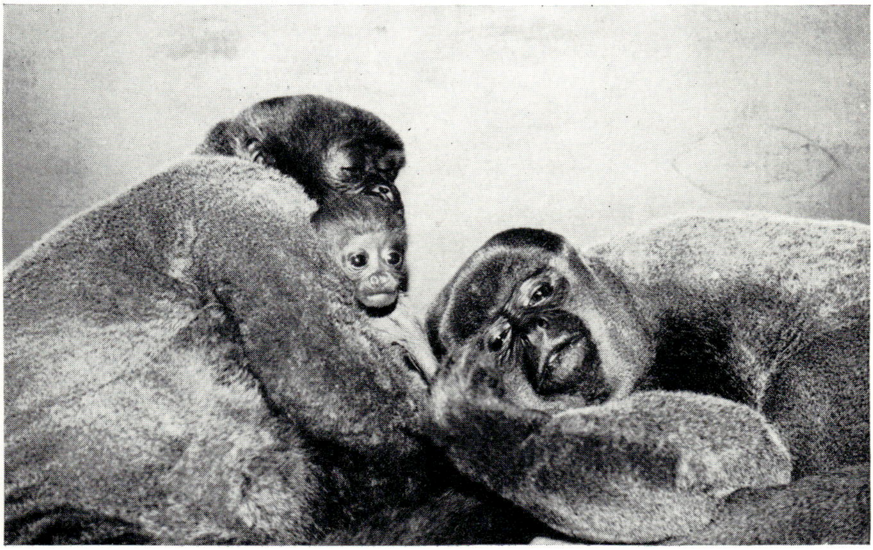

are repeated in human societies. That care is given, is more important than the method, or the individual employed.

Nature is flexible and takes the situation into account, replacing one method by another, if this is more efficacious in a new situation. In chimpanzees, as clan feeling is not well developed, the young must rely on a strong and sustained maternal interest; but in the socially inclined baboons maternal care can be less strong. A chimp, or a baboon infant in the situation of the other would be lost.

That there can be great variety within one order or even within one family of animals is also noted; hence the danger of generalizing within even one family. It may be that the capacity to adjust by replacing one method by another is greatest in the higher vertebrates and is put to its maximum use in homo sapiens.

It should be noted that fathering in the animal kingdom is an entity as well defined as mothering—if the term 'instinct' is employed it would apply as much to fathering as to mothering.

3

Anthropology

Each culture imagines that its way of child rearing and family life to be the best. An appraisal of history and of many cultures today shows how varied are family patterns and child care practices. As in the animal kingdom, nature is more concerned that the human child should have the required care, than she is about the way in which the care is given; over the latter, she displays variety and flexibility. Her main instrument for child nurture is a group, the family. Fathering, within the group, is not neglected.

The Family

The family, in some form, appears to be universal; at times, it may be diffuse and not easily identified as a unit. The *Oxford Dictionary*[130] offers the following definitions of the family: (*i*) 'The body of persons who live in one house or under one head, including parents, children, servants, etc.' (*ii*) 'The group consisting of parents and their children, whether living together or not; in wider sense, all those who are nearly connected by blood or affinity.' (*iii*) 'A person's children regarded collectively.' (*iv*) 'Those descended or claiming descent from a common ancestor.'

The first definition conforms most clearly to modern ideas of the 'nuclear family'. The nuclear family, sometimes termed the 'immediate family', or the 'elementary family', can be defined as a sub-system of the social system, consisting of two adults of different sexes who undertake a parenting role to one or more children. The 'family of orientation' is often used to designate the nuclear family in which a person has, or has had, the status of a child, and the term 'family of procreation' in which a person has, or has had, the status of a parent. When authority is based on a male as head of the family we speak of a patriarchy, and when on a female as a matriarchy.

The term 'extended family' is used to refer to any grouping, related by descent, marriage or adoption, which is broader than the nuclear family and which conforms most closely to the second definition of the Oxford Dictionary. 'Lateral' extension would embrace uncles, aunts, cousins, etc., while 'vertical' extensions would embrace two or more generations.

A family exists for a particular purpose in the social context in which it finds itself, and is shaped by this fact. The unit may be a small or large nuclear family, a nuclear family extended laterally or vertically or both, an extended family large enough to merit the term 'clan', or it may melt into a community that regards itself as the effective unit.

In psychiatry, concern should be with individuals who have emotional significance as a group. This, most commonly, is the family. But a blood tie is of secondary importance to an emotional tie, e.g. a servant given intimate care of the children may have more significance for them than the natural parents. Thus, in clinical practice, the concept of the family may have to be widened to take account of this.

Families in some form are universal. Attempts to prove the historical development of the family through various forms to the present highly regarded nuclear family have failed. The form of the family is its response to its social background. It shows many variations.

Murdock[104] states that of 192 societies studied, 47 (24 per cent) have normally a nuclear family, 92 (48 per cent) possess some form of extended family, and 53 (28 per cent) have polygamous, but not extended, families.

An extended family, sometimes termed a 'joint' family, consists of two or more nuclear families—the extension may be lateral, or, more commonly, vertical. Among the Hindus, for example, may be found an extended family consisting of kinsmen over three or four generations and their wives and offspring. It constitutes a perpetual corporation owning property generation after generation, and not dissolving after the death of every husband. When descent is dependent on the female side of the family, it is termed matrilineal, when on the male side, patrilineal. Under the patrilineal system, as with us, the children inherit the rank, property, and clan or phratry of the father and look to him as their chief protector and representative. But under the matrilineal system the difference is almost startling, for the children inherit the mother's phratry or clan, and have nothing to do with that of the father. The mother's brother is more important. For example: Malinowski[94] pointed out that the Trobriard Islanders did not recognize father, but vested disciplinary functions in a child's mother's brother. The male, the uncle, however, is still an important figure.

A polygamous family is dependent on plural marriage. There are two or more nuclear families having one married partner in common. In polygyny there is marriage of one man with more than one woman simultaneously. In sororal polygyny (wives are sisters) the family was more indulgent than in non-sororal polygyny[155]. Sisters exhibit less rivalry, are co-operative and often share the same home with the common husband. Polygyny may be due to economic factors, or as a means of ensuring an heir. By Koranic law a man may have four wives. The Mormons of Utah practised polygyny until 1890. In polyandry one woman is married simultaneously to more than one man. It is usually associated with matrilineal descent and matriarchy. When the co-husbands are brothers, it is known as Adelphic Polyandry. Sometimes the family is informal, the woman being visited by a succession of men and dwelling alone with her children. Hobhouse, Wheeler and Ginsberg[61] found monogamy in 66 societies, polygamy in 409 societies (polygyny in 378 and polyandry in 31).

Mead[97] gives two examples of extreme family variants. In Mentawei, off Sumatra, the male head of the family is so important that he cannot work. Thus he cannot marry until old enough to have a son to do the work. This situation is solved by the children being adopted at birth by their maternal grandmother, and by the young maternal uncles doing all the work and supporting the children. When a son is old enough to work, his father marries his mother, adopts the children and sets up house. Among the Nairs of Malabar, as the men object to having the women under the dominance of a man outside the family, the children are married very young and divorced the same day. The women live at home with their parents and have lovers. The man keeps all control of their sisters and their sisters' children.

Variants have their counterpart in modern society, close examination of which shows the diversity of family forms and that the nuclear family is not universal. Howells[67] found that in a random sample of families in an English town, approximately 70 per cent followed the pattern of a nuclear family, 20 per cent had an extended family pattern, and 10 per cent had an anomalous family structure. This last group contained a variety of unusual patterns. For example, mother and children alone; father and children alone; mother, grandmother and children; polygamy, etc. These modern variants are of great research interest and test many of the hypotheses concerning family functioning. Clinical practice tends to be based on an idealized concept of the family, an ideal often coming from personal prejudice, or personal experience of the worker, and usually conforming to the model of the nuclear family. Atypical family formations are not necessarily unhealthy. The real issue is not the structure of the family, but whether the needs of the family members are being met.

Families are resilient. The main functions of the family are so fundamental that however social circumstances change, means are found to carry them out. Young and Willmott[159] gave a fascinating account of the movement of families from a long-established community in East London, to a new estate on the outskirts of the city. Child rearing in London was dependent on an extended family system, which made the maternal grandmother the mother's principal aid in the care of the children—an extended family. Outside London the mother's principal aid became the previously neglected father—a tight nuclear family. In either event children received care. Family resilience is highly correlated with family emotional health; thus breakdown at acculturization may be an index of family ill-health rather than a product of change.

Parenting

Children are usually brought up within some form of family structure; but other methods are practised, for example, the communal or semi-communal upbringing of the Kibbutz[101]. In some extended families, where many women may be present, the word meaning 'mother' is used by the child to refer to other women around him as well. Thus it is as if the child were brought up by many mothers.

The child has a number of requirements and as long as they are met, the method employed to satisfy them can fit the social system. The methods are variable. Commonly the care is supplied within a nuclear family which supplies care by two adults—an insurance against the loss of one. Within the family, child care may be equally shared by the parents; mother care may be predominant; care may be by mother alone, for example, in old American Negro slave families, when the males might be sold; care may be by older children (Mead and MacGregor[99]); care by relations and friends (Leighton and Kluckholn[85]); care may be predominantly by fathers; care may be fathers alone; care may be provided outside the family—the child not differentiating between the women around him; or care may be offered by the whole community. Mead[96] suggests that the latter may be the best type of care; the child cannot usually select his parents, but under this system can choose those that meet his requirements best. Mead states '. . . cross-cultural studies suggest that adjustment is most facilitated if the child is cared for by many warm, friendly people'. The only life worth living in the ages of the Greek civilization was that of citizen service; the family possessed little interest and the son, when of age, left his father and mother. Plato replaced the private household by a single state-family.

Fathering

There is a distinction between the man who is socially and legally responsible for a woman's children, and the man who actually begat them. The legal father is the 'pater' and socially recognized guardian, and the biological father, the begetter, is the 'genitor'. A Dinka husband may depute a kinsman to sleep with his wife if, for some reason or another, he

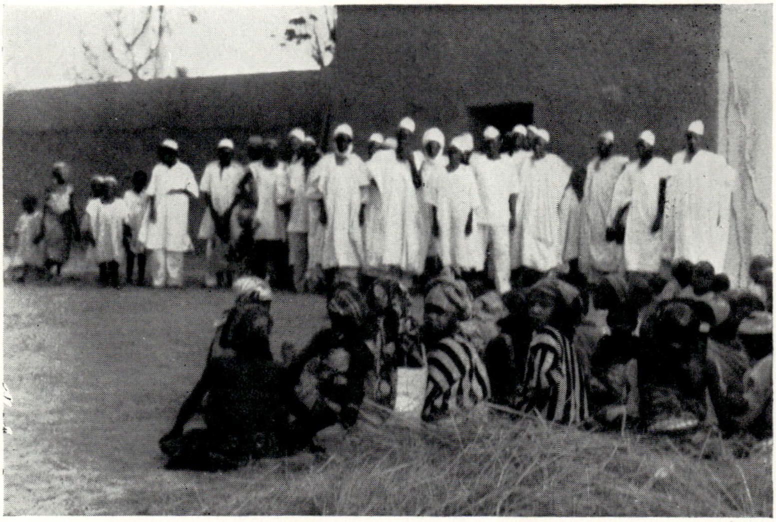

FIG. 5. Children and fathers at a children's clinic in Northern Nigeria. The mothers remain at home in purdah.

cannot fill the complete role of husband, provided always that he may claim the children. He is 'pater', his kinsman 'genitor'. Again, a widow may sometimes be allowed to choose her own lover, when it is clearly recognized that any children born of this union are the legal children of the man in whose name cattle were originally given for her in marriage. However, in modern Western society, pater and genitor are usually the same person.

A number of terms are employed in relation to father and his family: patrilocal (family lives where father lives); patrinomal (family takes father's name); patrilineal (descent is through father's line); patrimony (property inherited through father); patriarchy or pater familias (father is head of the family).

In the Roman family, the father was predominant. The father as head of the family (paterfamilias) possessed absolute authority (patria potestas) over the persons and goods of his wife, sons, unmarried daughters and slaves. Within the family, he was sole owner of property, sole priest and guardian of the family 'sacra', and sole judge. He had the right to put to death his wife and children and in his hands alone it lay to rear or 'expose' his new-born offspring. He saw personally to the training of his son.

Anthropological studies quote instances where care of children is often a primary activity of the father and sometimes predominantly that of the father.

Amongst the Arapesh, for instance, Mead[95] states that the father plays an equal part with the mother during pregnancy. The child is thought of as the product of father's semen and mother's blood. The child's conception is a joint endeavour, and during the early weeks of pregnancy following the cessation of menstruation the father 'works' to produce his child by strenuous sexual activity with his wife. His involvement with mother and infant after the child's birth is so close as to earn the phrase that he is 'in bed having a baby'. The child's strength is also thought to be dependent on the father, who is forbidden sexual intercourse until the child can walk and is then believed strong enough to withstand the parents' sexuality again. The care of children is regarded as the task of both men and women.

Again, on the island of Manus, in the Admiralty Islands, Mead[98], for instance, reports that the father is the dominant and the tender, loving parent. After the birth of her first child, the mother lives with her family. Then she returns to her husband's house and from the first he takes a fiercely possessive interest in the child, male or female. As soon as the child can stand, the father takes the child from the mother. She is set to work, while he spends all the time left free from his fishing with the child. The child is his constant companion and at night sleeps with him (the female child until she is 7 or 8 years old). The second born gives mother a child for a few months, but, at this time, the first born moves even closer to his father. The life of all the children is around the father, whether he be their natural or adoptive father. There is a strong personality resemblance between the adopted children and their adoptive father.

As often appertains in primitive societies, should the social work economy require father and sons to work together, then father may exert a great influence on the upbringing of sons, and mothers, conversely, on the upbringing of their daughters.

Anthropological studies challenge, too, an over-rigid definition of the qualities required in 'masculinity' and 'feminity'. Mead[95] quotes her experiences in New Guinea. The Arapesh ideal of a man is that he should be mild and responsive; the Arapesh ideal woman should be the same. The Mundugumer ideal is that of a violent aggressive male and female. The Tchambuli reverse what we commonly regard as masculine and feminine attitudes—their ideal woman is dominant, impersonal and managing, while the man is dependent, art loving and unmanaging.

Summary

Social anthropology, like ethology, illustrates the variability and flexibility of methods employed by nature in the upbringing of the human child. The family group is basic, but has many varieties, and within it parenting is supplied in a flexible manner by the utilization of mothering, of fathering and of care by others. Fathering is an important element in child care; occasionally it may be employed exclusively. 'Masculinity' and 'feminity' are again flexible elements, greatly dependent on the needs and dictates of the cultural situation.

4

Fathering in Contemporary Society

In civilized countries, the male and the father are frequently given a preeminent place—mother and children take his name, live where he lives, move when he moves and he may have privileged rights in that society. But, in most societies he is assumed to be secondary to the mother in the care of the children; child care is seen as matricentric. Indeed, parental care is often assumed to be mother care; deprivation of parenting is often assumed to be deprivation of mothering. Bowlby[15] in this context states in his review of maternal care and deprivation, that 'In the young child's eyes father plays second fiddle . . . but is of indirect value as an economic and emotional support of the mother'.

This is the impression given by sociological, psychological and psychiatric literature. The facts, however, may be different. The father may share parenting, often equally, sometimes predominantly, and sometimes subordinately. But few facts are available. Research largely ignores the father; in addition, he is less accessible than the mother. Eron *et al.*[36] emphasize the importance of a direct approach to fathers, rather than an approach through the mother which can be inaccurate in giving a picture of father's interaction with his children.

This neglect in the literature can be illustrated by taking Winnicott's[157] important book on the theory of emotional development; while the index refers to 50 insertions on the mother, it refers to only 3 on the father. Carmichael's Manual of Child Psychology[23] does not list father in the index. This neglect of the father is the subject of comment in Thompson's comprehensive and balanced volume on child psychology[139]. 'Fathers and siblings have been too long neglected as important influences on the child'— and again by Nash[107], English[35], Gilloran[48], and Hoffman[62].

In the main, the available literature deals with four aspects of fathering —the effect of father on child development, the role of father, the effects of father's absence on the child, and father's participation. Each will be briefly considered after a short review of the position in a number of countries.

National Practices

That child care is regarded as matricentric is almost universal in contemporary national literature about child rearing practices.

Nash[108] makes a thorough review of the position in the United States of America. He quotes Gorer[50], who epitomized American society as the 'Motherland' and regards father as vestigial. Kluckhohn[82], Nash states, takes up a similar position and believes that the American father has largely abdicated control of his children. This mother centredness is also emphasized by Rohrer and Edmondson[122], and Rubenstein and Levitt[124], while Ostrovsky[111] deplores the lack of father substitutes, as school teachers are predominantly female. Sunley[137], after reviewing 19th century American literature, states that the mother's role was paramount at that time also.

In Europe, again the literature emphasizes the major role of mother in child rearing. MacCalman[90] states in regard to the position in the United Kingdom: 'In many families the father has little influence on his baby'. Henriques[57] in the same volume analysed material from popular magazines and said that scarcely any magazines dealt with father's role.

Métraux[100] states in regard to the German literature: 'The central character in the child care literature is the mother'. Favez-Boutonier[38] gives second place to the paternal function in the first two years, but regards the complementary influence of father as important thereafter in child development patterns in France. Aubry[5], from the same country, is more definite in emphasizing the predominant role of the mother in child care in an otherwise strongly patriarchal society.

Makarenko[92] has had considerable influence on child rearing practices in the Soviet Union. His emphasis is different and interesting. His appeal is always to the 'parents' as a couple: 'Dear parents, above all you should remember the great importance of this business and your great responsibility for it.' Again: 'Punishment is a very difficult business that demands unerring tact and care on the part of the educator. Therefore, we recommend parents to avoid punishment as much as possible, and to try first of all to restore the proper routine. This, of course, takes a long time, but you must be patient and wait calmly for results'.

Makarenko stresses the value of co-operation between the parents in everything and the need to speak with an agreed voice—even in matters appertaining to small children:

'Parents should learn to give such orders at a very early stage, when the first child is 1½ to 2 years old. It is not difficult at all.'

When Makarenko refers to father and mother, he puts father first.

On rare occasions he makes a direct appeal to the father, never to mother:

'You are not only a citizen, however. You are also a Father. And you must do your parental job to the best of your ability. Herein lie the roots of your authority. First of all, you should know what your child's interests are, what he likes and dislikes, what he wants and does not want. You should know who his friends are, whom he plays with and what he plays at, what he reads and how he understands what he has read. When he goes to school it is your business to know what his attitude is to his school and his teachers, what difficulties he meets with, and how he behaves in the classroom. You should know all this always, from your child's earliest years.' Again: 'A child catches the slightest inflection in your tone; every turn of thought reaches him by invisible paths. You do not notice these things. And if you are rude at home, if you are boastful, or drunk, or, still worse, if you insult his mother, you do not have to think of upbringing any more—you are already bringing up your children, bringing them up badly, and no amount of good advice or methods can help you.'

The Absence of Father

Fathers are absent from the home at least as often as mother (Howells[68]). Great significance has been given to separation of a child from his mother but not to the break between father and child. When a child is separated from his family, any ill effects noted are frequently put down to the break with mother, although that with father co-exists.

Father's absence makes an Oedipus situation invalid, removes the possibility of a father to identify with, makes the children dependent on mother's idea of father, makes substitute fathering more of a necessity, also changes the family by its effects on the mother and produces problems of readjustment on father's return. Nevertheless the dire consequences sometimes predicted at the loss of the father do not necessarily come about; families have a capacity for adjustment. Absence of father may not confuse the child's sex role; the mother, for instance, as well as the father is anxious to impose a masculine role on her sons.

A number of studies concern themselves with the absent father.

Bach[6] studied the wartime phantasies of children with absent fathers and found that the children tended to 'feminize' their fathers, who became, in their phantasies, more affectionate and companionable. Sears et al.[128] again found less aggression in the phantasies of boys from homes with an absent father. The father's absence had little effect on girl's aggression. It was deducted that the father normally supplied social control. An extensive study by Stolz et al.[134] showed that the return of father from the war produced a severe stress situation for father and first born child. Winch[156] showed that the courtship behaviour of college students suffered if their fathers were absent. Stephens[133] found some evidence that boys of fatherless families are anxious about sex and more effeminate than when the families had fathers. Seplin[129] found that father's absence caused children to cling to their mothers and to precipitate emotional problems. Lynn and Sawrey[89] found that children with absent fathers had difficulties in peer adjustment. Other studies were conducted on father absent families by Freud and Burlingham[43], Hill[58], Tiller[142], Grønsetti[52], Bradburn[16], and Ancona et al.[3] Wynn[158] considers the problems arising in helping fatherless families.

Father and Child Development

Gardner[45] and Simpson[132] have shown that children of both sexes prefer their mother's presence to their father's when in personal-social difficulties. Children of both sexes would like to resemble the parent of the same sex, but rate the parent of the opposite sex rather higher in geniality and character—Gardner[45]. Kagan[78] found that children saw their mother as friendlier than father and father more punitive and dominant; older children, however, saw the same sex parent as more dominant. Burchinal[20] found that fathers were less accepting of children than were mothers. Harris and Tseng[54] found that children in general hold favourable opinions of their parents—rather more so of mother than of father—while girls show a sharp increase of positive attitudes towards father as they grow older.

Mueller[103] has shown that dominating fathers have an adverse effect on the adjustment of both boys and girls; a change in father's behaviour brings an improvement in his children. Aberle and Naegels[1] found that the fathers of middle-class homes have definite aspirations for their children and, in general, wish boys to be masculine and girls to be docile and marriageable. According to Gray[51] boys who see themselves as being like their father show the most favourable personal-social adjustment, while Lazowick[84] states that they are also less anxious. Levin and Sears[86] have studied the incorporation of paternal characteristics by the child. Eron et al.[36] found that father is an important model for aggression in children.

Dyer[31] showed that the father's job satisfaction is transferred to the child and affects the parents' aspirations for the child. Strong[136] showed that about 25 per cent of sons have interests similar to their father's interests. Remstad and Rothney[118] have also explored this area.

Elder[33] found that progressively orientated fathers reported more interaction with their children, while traditionally orientated fathers disciplined for a larger number of reasons though using a smaller variety of punishments.

Radke[116] in an extensive investigation found that there was an increase in father's responsibility for the discipline of young children. Even so, the children saw mother as the more influential in their lives; fathers tended to be more severe in punishment. Jackson[71], however, found mothers more coercive. Block[14] comments on the qualities of fathers—restrictive fathers are submissive, suggestible and inadequate, while permissive fathers are more self reliant and ascendant.

Mussen[105] shows that adolescent boys of high masculinity due to identification with father are better adjusted than those of low masculinity. Mussen and Distler[106] report that high masculinity boys have stronger emotional bonds with their fathers and these fathers take more interest in their sons' upbringing. Johnson[74] suggests that the girl development of sex-role orientation depends upon her identification with her father. Hjelholt[60] has emphasized the importance of father in superego development.

Josselyn[75] argues that fathers have biological roots and psychological satisfaction in the care of their children. Katy[80] has defended fathers' importance in child rearing.

The Role of Father

In infancy, Winnicott[157], quoting a view frequently held by psychoanalysts, gives reality to two people only—mother and infant: 'The original two body relationship is that of the infant and the mother or mother substitute, before any property of the mother has been sorted out and moulded into the idea of a father'. At another point he states: 'I leave out infant-father relationships in this context because I am referring to early phenomena, those that concern the infant's relationship to the mother, or *to the father as another mother*. The father at this early stage has not become significant as a male person' (my italics). It is difficult to see why *both* mother and father cannot be given identities, and not in terms of one another, but in terms of both being parents.

Tasch[138] has studied the role of the father in the family and considers it in relation to the greater freedom of the modern family. Fathers regarded themselves as having a primary role in relation to child care, enjoying direct participation with their offspring rather than being merely indirectly supportive through the mothers. Bernhardt[11] is optimistic about the improved role of the father in the family. Gardner[44] considered that fathers had ample time for fathering, but did not use their opportunities. Jackson[71]

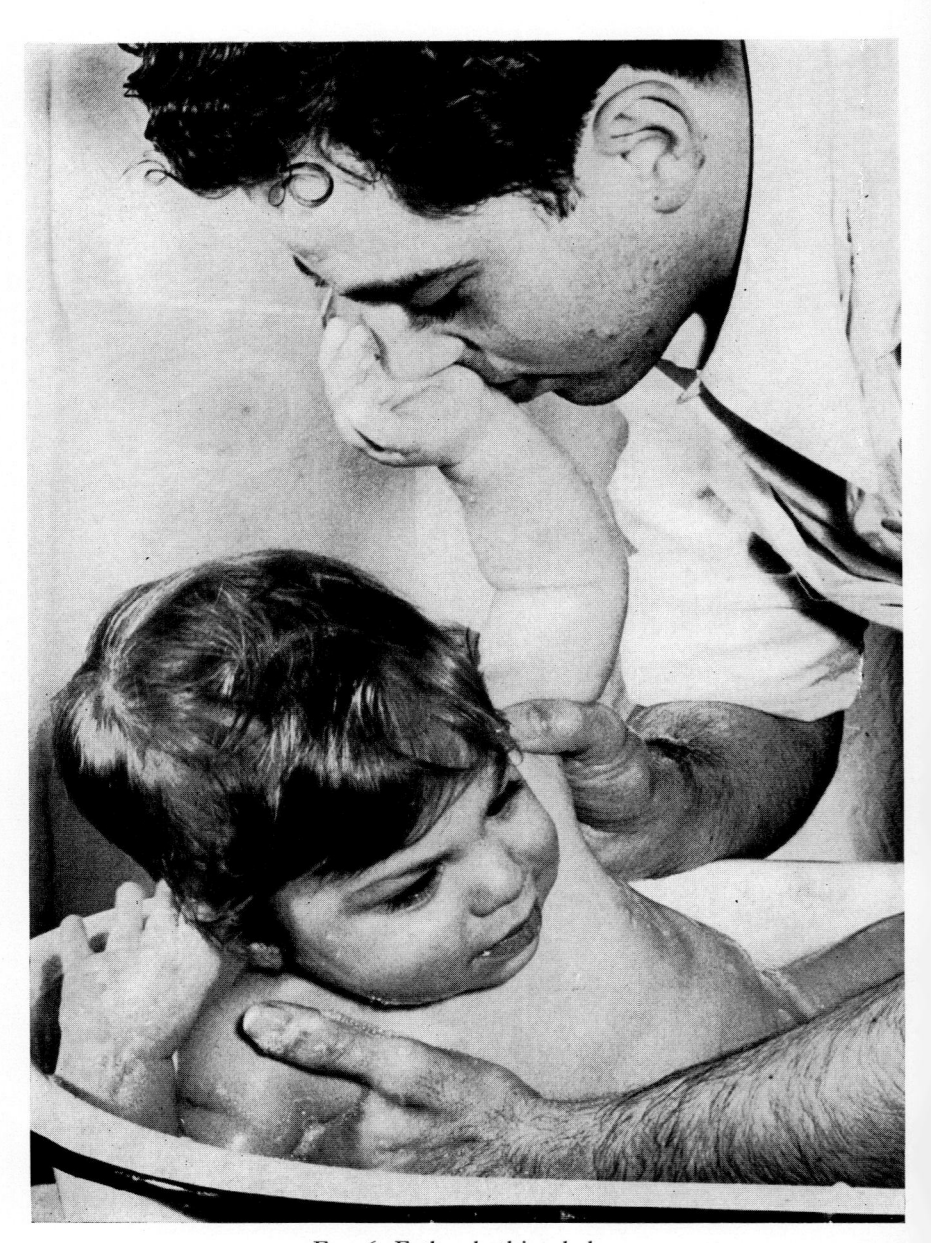

FIG. 6. Father bathing baby.

found that the stereotype of punitive male and passive female was not supported by the responses of parents using a projection technique. Sears, Maceroy and Levin[127] consider from their study that when the father is warmer than the mother, he is the most effective punisher; conversely should mother be warmer, her spanking is more effective. Birdwhistell[13] considers the stereotype of American father and its progress in a changing society.

Father Participation

The Newsons[109] found a high degree of participation by fathers in the lives of the children they observed. They found for example that 57 per cent of Social Class I and II (upper professional) fathers were highly participant, 61 per cent of Social Class III (white collar), 51 per cent of Social Class III (skilled manual), 55 per cent of Social Class IV and 36 per cent of Social Class V (unskilled).

Gavron[46] in a sample of middle-class parents, found 44 per cent of the fathers would do, and in fact did everything required for their children from playing with them to soothing them when they cried at night, from feeding them to changing their nappies. A further 21 per cent were rated very helpful by their wives, which meant they would do most things as a matter of course, but drew the line at one or two things, usually changing nappies. 31 per cent of the wives rated their husbands as interested but not helpful. Only 4 per cent of the wives in the entire sample rated their husbands as non-participant.

In working-class families Gavron found, as with the middle-class families, that the degree to which the father participated in the lives of his children was quite striking, and the degree of participation was even greater than among the middle-class families. 52 per cent of fathers were rated by their wives as doing anything and everything for their children as a matter of course. A further 27 per cent were prepared to do most things, drawing the line as did some middle-class fathers over changing nappies, and getting up at night. Of the remainder, 21 per cent, 12 per cent were considered 'interested but not helpful' and just over half to be uninvolved in their children's lives.

It is questionable whether fathering is a recent phenomenon; to a considerable extent it has always been active However, some writers have assumed a recent increase in fathering, and give a number of reasons for the change. It is argued that the small modern home brings the child closer to father; but the poorer classes have always lived in small houses. The absence of servants forces the father to help mother with the children; but most families have never had servants. That mother now tends to work, again forces father to help; but in many societies, women have always worked. The equality of the sexes, it is thought, may make the modern woman more independent of her husband, and thus able to demand help from him. Furthermore she sees her role in terms not too different from his; thus sharing of roles is more possible. Affluence in society calls for less hours of work, and father can participate more readily in family life. It should be noted that, in varying degrees at different times, these reasons have always applied in some societies.

Summary

Father is largely neglected in contemporary social literature on the family in most countries, and the available literature concentrates on a few aspects of fathering only. There is support for the idea that the absence of father may have an adverse effect on the family. This carries the implication that he means something when present. The literature suggests that he plays a part in child development, but authorities disagree about its nature. Some see father as secondary in the contemporary family, while others give him a more powerful role. Some direct studies suggest that his participation is greater than expected.

5

Fathering and Psychiatry

The literature of contemporary societies makes little reference to fathering. In psychiatry, the literature is at its most meagre, while that on mothering would have overflowed this volume. The neglect of the father is striking, and this fact has often hampered the use of procedures in child psychiatry. The available literature on fathering in child psychiatry will be briefly reviewed.

Neuroses

Freud gave a central place to the Oedipus situation in his schema for psychopathology, and father had an equal place in the family triad. Perhaps, its supposed operation later than in early childhood, allowed it to be inferred that the father was less important in these early years. But, in fact, the neglect was also extended to later years. The Oedipus situation with rivalry of father and son must exist, but so do many other combinations and permutations of interaction—in all age groups. Fenichel[39] regards the positive Oedipus complex as starting in the third year of life, reaching its climax at the fourth and fifth year. 'I love mother and hate father, because he takes mother for himself' is the positive complex. The negative Oedipus complex is when the boy's love for his father prevails and the mother is hated as a disturbing element in the relationship. The positive and negative complexes can sometimes exist together. Fenichel states the girl undergoes one more step of development than the boy—the transfer of attachment from mother to father between the ages of three and six. The girl in turn comes to hate her mother and to love father. Another central Freudian concept, the Superego, is dependent largely on the father. It is held that in the usual patriarchal family, identification is with the frustrating authority of father; in both sexes the fatherly superego is decisive although mother can make a contribution, and in girls may be a positive ego ideal.

Jung[77] regards father as one of the child's archetypes—there being unconscious predisposition towards a primitive mode of thought. The father archetype is in some ways the opposite of the mother archetype and signifies strength, authority, movement, activity and the creative breath. This father image is associated with storms, lightning, wars, raging animals and violent events. Jung wrote one paper on the father, 'The significance of the father in the destiny of the individual'[76]. However, generally in his writings he refers much more frequently to mother than to father. Von der Heyd[146] has enlarged on the Jungian view of fathering.

Father as a possible contributor to pathology has been the subject of comment by some authors. Cavallin[24] has commented on incestuous fathers. Petersen et al.[113] conclude that father's behaviour is as important as the mothers in causing maladjustment in children. Heinicke and Westheimer[56] comment on the child's reaction to father during separation and on reunion—during separation they manifested less affection to father and on reunion, developed a strong interest in the presents he brought. After reunion, they quickly resumed affectionate relations with him. In children with school phobia, fathers were said to be passive and dependent.[145]

The expectant father has come under observation, with particular attention to the couvade reaction (Trethowen[144]). He is now so frequently an attender in the labour ward that an advice leaflet[37] is available to him. His mental health is vulnerable during his wife's pregnancy as has been reported by Hartman and Nicolay[55] and others[19, 29, 42, 143, 150, 154, 160].

Father is implicated in psychosomatic disorders. In Jewish children with eating problems[88], fathers were said to be ineffectual and undependable. Subordination was also the feature of fathers of obese children[19]. A number of writers (Finch and Hess[40], Langford[83], Mohr et al.[102], Prugh[115], and Wenar et al.[151]) have felt that the fathers of children with ulcerative colitis are passive and withdrawn from the family.

Delinquency

Fathers have a bad reputation in relation to delinquency in their children. Andry[4] found that delinquent boys tended to get on less well with their parents, especially father, than non-delinquent boys. Logan and Goldberg[87] found a similar tendency. Defects in the fathers of delinquents have been reported by the Gluecks[49], Thrasher[140], Crane[28], Becker[8], and Ostrovsky[111]. Fathers absence in early childhood is linked to antisocial behaviour later—Siegman[131]. Similar views are expounded by Parsons[112];

Bacon, Child and Barry[7]; Cohen[27], and Chinn[26]. There is some disagreement to the above in the views of McCord et al.[91]

Sex Role Identity

As the general belief is held that mothers play a predominant part in child rearing, it was natural from this supposition to wonder what effect this might have on sex-role identity and even the etiology of homosexuality. The anxiety at times manifest in the literature almost mounts to neurotic proportions, and were the worst predictions fulfilled, the result would be so obvious as to make investigation unnecessary. It seems to have been overlooked that the person who needs man and cares for him most is the woman; she is thus very anxious to produce masculinity in her boys. Indeed, possibly the mother makes patriarchal society. An early writer on this theme of sex-role identity was Flügel[41]. Nash[108] brings the subject up to date in an excellent review that covers other aspects of fathering.

Treatment

The father in treatment has been the subject of some comment. Bell et al.[9] analyse fathers' resistance. His involvement in treatment is a matter discussed by Beron[12], Burgum[21], Richards[119], Rubenstein and Levitt[124], Walton[149], Strean[135], and Grunebaum and Strean[53]. Grunebaum[53] discusses the group psychotherapy of fathers. Mueller[103] refers to the fathers' influence on results.

Psychosis

In considering father in the etiology of adult schizophrenia, he is often linked with studies on the mother. Conclusions drawn from parent-schizophrenic studies are contradictory, as is illustrated by consideration of some of the studies. Ellison and Hamilton[34] found the mothers overprotective and the fathers over-aggressive. Johnston et al.[73] found physical assault of children by the parents. Wahl[147, 148] found the loss of a parent in childhood or adolescence. Reichard and Tillman[117] described overtly rejecting mothers and domineering fathers. The work of Tietze[141], Gerard and Siegel[47], and Kasanin et al.[79], supported the notion of dominant mothers and passive fathers. Caputo[22] investigated this last possibility and found that it required qualification; he found a hostile atmosphere in the homes of schizophrenics and that both parents contributed to it. Prout and White[114] compared the parents of schizophrenics and those of normal males, and found no significant differences between them. Rogler and Hollingshead[121] found that experiences in the childhood and adolescence of schizophrenic persons do not differ noticeably from those of people who are not afflicted by the illness.

Father alone in relation to schizophrenia has received less attention. The small amount of literature available is again contradictory—some described father as passive and ineffectual, others as harsh and domineering —as observed in a review by Cheek[25]. Parental factors, including paternal families, in the etiology of child psychoses have been the subject of reviews by Eisenberg[32], and O'Gorman[110], and again by Bender in this volume (Chapter XXIII). No mention will be made here of the family as an agent in the etiology of schizophrenia as the author has reviewed the subject elsewhere[66].

Clinical Practice

Pre-eminently, opinions have emphasized the importance of the child's intra-psychic emotional events. That these are fed by, and are continuous with, extra-personal emotional events has been given less prominence. The child was sick in himself, as if he had caught measles, and the unfortunate family, usually through the mother, needed guidance to help him. That he was an inseparable part of them, with a continuous emotional field, and only sick when they were sick was overlooked. When extrapsychic events came into prominence at all, it was the mother who was selected for attention.

Referral systems in child psychiatry have often been content to ignore father. Yet, by addressing the attendance request to both parents, he will often respond. Enquiries as to specially convenient times also help. Evening clinics will bring in the stragglers.

Individual psychiatry, including child psychiatry, is outmoded, (Howells[64]). Accepting the family as the sick unit throws light on the inseparability of all family members, including the father. If father is never a direct interactor with a child, he is still an integral part of the family's total emotional climate; in fact he is both.

Clinical investigations that exclude father cannot give a true picture of the family. Nor will mother's opinion on father's supposed actions be accurate, as Eron *et al.*[36] have shown. The contact must be direct. Never should the investigator deny himself the opportunity, through family group diagnosis[65], of seeing father's as well as mother's interactions with their children. Surprising matters come to light. The children may congregate around mother; but sometimes it will be father. The baby may never leave father's knee, or is handed to him for soothing when it becomes fractious. The family with all this pathology might have crashed—but it can be seen how in some instances father keeps it together. Conversely, his place as an augmentor of stress may emerge. Projective techniques such as the *Family Relations Indicator*[69] should be given to the father as often as to the mother if a true picture of the family dynamics is to emerge. The Indicator is planned to throw light on fathering as well as other family elements (see Fig. 7).

An assessment of the true family situation will lead to realistic therapy. Father as often as mother requires help as part of the sick family. He may be the family element of choice for individual therapy, or a participant in dyadic therapy, or in family group therapy. He, as much as any member of the family, may need his field of emotional forces to be repatterned by vector therapy[65].

Saddest of all, father's place as a compensating factor, as a benevolent influence, as a therapeutic agent is ignored. Elaborate measures outside the family may be made to compensate a child for deprivation of mothering,

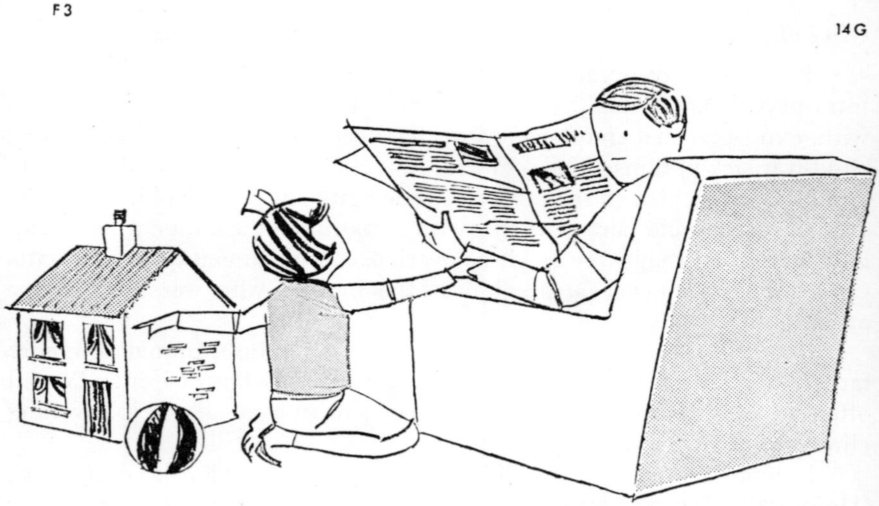

FIG. 7. Card from the Family Relations Indicator involving father-child relationships.

when a simple re-allocation of roles within the family may produce an equally satisfactory, or a better result. It was no ill chance that a child was given two parents, one was meant to compensate for the other.

Summary

Fathering has suffered gross neglect in both the theory and practice of child psychiatry.

6

Conclusion

A brief review of parenting in the animal kingdom displayed the variability and flexibility of nature. The crucial goal of care of the young is achieved by means appropriate to the situation of the young, with a broad concept of parenting, and a flexible utilization of the means available. Parenting is

FIG. 8. An Egyptian boy's letter to his father, in Greek, on papyrus, 2nd or 3rd century A.D. Part of it reads: 'It was a fine thing of you not to take me with you to town. If you won't take me with you to Alexandria I won't write you a letter or speak to you or greet you. ... Mother said to Archelus, "He upsets me. Take him away." ... So send for me, I implore you. If you don't, I won't eat, I won't drink; so there!'
Reproduced by kind permission of the Bodlein Library, Oxford.

more important than the parent. Parenting may be undertaken by male and female parents. At times mothering alone is employed. In certain other situations paternal care is the sole means utilized. In yet other situations there is no parenting by the natural parents. As an entity, or 'instinct', fathering is as well defined as mothering.

Social anthropology reveals the same variability and flexibility in the care of the young homo sapiens as in the animal kingdom. What is appropriate in a given situation is the means employed. The family group is paramount, and within it fathering has an important place; in a particular milieu there may even be exclusive care by the father.

The neglect of father in the literature on contemporary society is striking; in most of it, it is assumed that child care is matricentric. The small available literature is contradictory; research on such an important topic is small, often indirect and, in general, concerned with secondary issues. Some direct studies suggest that father participation is greater than expected. Research is rarely concerned with the nature of fathering. This issue requires further comment here.

Reasons for this neglect in the western world may be several. In the Christian religion a far more prominent place is given to Christ's mother, Mary, in His upbringing than is accorded to His father, Joseph. The Madonna and child are a frequent subject for the artist in the last 1900 years; Joseph and child are rarely depicted. Again, by tradition in the western world the man assumes the main role of breadwinner, while the woman has charge of home and children. This may help to explain how, where women traditionally work, the parenting is more likely to be a shared responsibility.

Just as bad mothering has a capacity to cause pathology in the child, so has bad fathering. That this is largely ignored in psychiatry is apparent from the brief review of its literature. The neglect seriously limits the practice of child psychiatry. The father is a significant element in the child's life from conception—he influences the child, for good or evil, directly, through the mother, and as a contributor to the family climate. The child's meaning to the father determines father's attitudes. Father may be a focus of stress to a child, to several children or to the whole family—but meaningful only in that particular family. Like the rest of the family, father may help to shape the symptomatology of the child faced with his stressful family situation. He may be a sick family element in need of therapy, he may conversely carry considerable potential as an ameliorating therapeutic force. Thus the father must be evaluated as an element in any clinical exploration of the family. Legal provisions have yet to give father a just place when guardianship of children is considered at divorce; the needs and rights of the unmarried father has had even less consideration. The neglect of father in any study of child care is a serious omission in the assessment of an important variable. Research should not only be directed to fathering, but also to the factors that have led to his neglect hitherto.

The reasons for the neglect of fathering in child psychiatry that may emerge from an investigation could include the following: the tendency for mothers to accompany children to clinics may lead to neglect of fathers and the assumption that the mother alone is involved in the child's problem. The fact that child psychiatrists are frequently women may introduce a bias by her empathy with the female parent. Again there is sometimes a tendency for attention to focus on the intra-psychic illness of the child patient, for which his parents are assumed to have no etiological significance, and his mother only was assumed to need guidance in the management of his illness as the operative parent. In the childhood of adults, and of child psychiatrists there may be more subtle factors that, in the western world, sets up a preoccupation with the mother—especially the idealization of the mother. For example, preoccupation with the problems of family life is greatest in those who have suffered adverse family experiences. Thus selection factors may bring less well-adjusted individuals into the field of child care, who would assume that their anomalous backgrounds are characteristic of family life generally. There may also be selection in terms of social class; child workers may come from backgrounds where servants, and thus less participation by father, were common.

To conclude, the means of child care are less important than the needs of child care. Parenting is more important than the parents. It is maintained here that in parenting, fathering is as distinct an entity as mothering. While pleading the acceptance of this truth, it must be understood that both are but two elements in the total family matrix. Neglect of this latter truth can also lead to serious limitation of the practice of child psychiatry.

REFERENCES

1. ABERLE, D. F., and NAEGELS, K. D., 1952. Middle-class father's occupational role and attitudes towards children. *Amer. J. Orthopsychiat.*, **22**, 366.
2. ACKERMAN, N. W., 1958. *The psychodynamics of family life*. New York, Basic Books.
3. ANCONA, L., CESA BIANTHI, M., and BOCQUET, F., 1963. Identification with father in the absence of the paternal model. *Arch. Psychol. Neurol. Psychiat.*, **24**, 539.
4. ANDRY, R. G., 1960. *Delinquency and parent pathology*. London, Methuen.
5. AUBRY, J., 1955. Comparative studies of French case-histories. In *Mental Health and Infant Development*, vol. 1. Ed. Soddy, K. London, Routledge and Kegan Paul.
6. BACH, G. R., 1960. Father-fantasies and father-typing in father-separated children. *Child Develpm.*, **17**, 63.
7. BACON, H. K., CHILD, I. L., and BARRY, H. A. A., 1963. Cross-cultural study of correlates of crime. *J. abnorm. soc. Psychol.*, **66**, 291.
8. BECKER, W. C., 1960. The relationship of factors in parental ratings of self and each other to the behaviour of kindergarten children. *J. consult. Psychol.*, **24**, 507.

REFERENCES

9. BELL, N., TRIESCHMAN, A., and VOGEL, E., 1961. A sociocultural analysis of the resistances of working-class fathers treated in a child psychiatric clinic. *Am. J. Orthopsychiat.*, **31**, 388.
10. BENIEST-NOIROT, E., 1958. Analyse du comportement dit maternal chez la souris. *Monographies Françaises de Psychologie*, I. Paris, Centre National de la Recherche Scientifique.
11. BERNHARDT, K. S., 1957. The father in the family. *Bull. Inst. Child Stud.*, **19**, 2.
12. BERON, L., 1944. Fathers as clients of a child guidance clinic. *Smith Coll. Stud. soc. Wk*, **14**, 351.
13. BIRDWHISTELL, R. L., 1957. Is there an ideal father? *Child Study*, **34**, 29.
14. BLOCK, J., 1955. Personality characteristics associated with father's attitudes towards child-rearing. *Child Develpm.*, **26**, 41.
15. BOWLBY, J., 1951. *Maternal care and mental health.* Geneva, W.H.O.
16. BRADBURN, N. M., 1963. Achievement and father dominance in Turkey. *J. abnorm. Soc. Psychol.*, **67**, 464.
17. BRELAND, O. P., 1948. *Animal facts and fallacies.* London, Faber and Faber.
18. BRIFFAULT, R., 1927. *The mothers.* New York, Macmillan.
19. BRUCH, H., 1947. Psychological aspects of obesity. *Psychiatry*, **10**, 373.
20. BURCHINAL, L. G., 1958. Mothers' and fathers' differences in the acceptance of children. *J. genet. Psychol.*, **92**, 103.
21. BURGUM, M., 1942. The father gets worse: a child guidance problem. *Am. J. Orthopsychiat.*, **12**, 474.
22. CAPUTO, D. V., 1963. The parents of the schizophrenic. *Family Process*, **2**, 339.
23. CARMICHAEL, L., 1954. *Manual of child psychology.* London, New York, John Wiley.
24. CAVALLIN, H., 1966. Incestuous fathers: a clinical report. *Am. J. Psychiat.*, **122**, 1132.
25. CHEEK, F. E., 1965. The father of the schizophrenic. *Archs gen. Psychiat.*, **13**, 336.
26. CHINN, W. L., 1938. A brief survey of nearly 1,000 juvenile delinquents. *Brit. J. educ. Psychol.*, **8**, 78.
27. COHEN, A. K., 1955. *Delinquent boys: the culture of the gang.* Glencoe, Ill., Free Press.
28. CRANE, A. R., 1951. A note on pre-adolescent gangs. *Aust. J. Psychol.*, **3**, 43.
29. CURTIS, J. L., 1955. A psychiatric study of 55 expectant fathers. *U.S. Armed Forces med. J.*, **6**, 937.
30. DEVORE, I., 1963. Mother-infant relations in free-ranging baboons. In *Maternal behaviour in mammals.* Ed. Rheingold, H. L. London, New York, John Wiley.
31. DYER, W. G., 1956. A comparison of families of high and low job satisfaction. *Marriage and Family Living*, **18**, 58.
32. EISENBERG, L., 1957. The fathers of autistic children. *Amer. J. Orthopsychiat.*, **27**, 715.
33. ELDER, R. A., 1949. Traditional and developmental conceptions of fatherhood. *Marriage and Family Living II*, **106**, 98-100.
34. ELLISON, E. A., and HAMILTON, D. M., 1949. Hospital treatment of dementia praecox. *Am J. Psychiat.*, **106**, 454.
35. ENGLISH, SPURGEON O., 1954. The psychological role of the father in the family. *Soc. Casework.*, **35**, 323.
36. ERON, L. D., BANTA, T. J., VALDER, L. O., and LAULICHT, J. H., 1961. Comparison of data obtained from mothers and fathers on child rearing practices and their relation to child aggression. *Child Develpm.*, **32**, 457.
37. *Expectant Fathers' Leaflet*, 1966. The National Childbirth Trust, London.

38. FAVEZ-BOUTONIER, J., 1955. Child Development patterns in France. In *Mental health and infant development*, vol. 1, Ed. Soddy, K. London, Routledge and Kegan Paul.
39. FENICHEL, O., 1945. *The psychoanalytic theory of neuroses*. New York, Norton.
40. FINCH, S. M., and HESS, J. H., 1962. Ulcerative colitis in children. *Am. J. Psychiat.*, **118**, 819.
41. FLUGEL, J. C., 1921. *The psychoanalytic study of the family*. London, Hogarth.
42. FREEMAN, T., 1951. Pregnancy as a precipitant of mental illness in men. *Brit. J. med. Psychol.*, **24**, 49.
43. FREUD, A., and BURLINGHAM, D., 1944. *Infants without families*. New York, Intern. Univ. Press.
44. GARDNER, L. P., 1943. A survey of the attitudes and activities of fathers. *J. genet. Psychol.*, **63**, 15.
45. GARDNER, L. P., 1947. An analysis of children's attitudes towards fathers. *J. genet. Psychol.*, **70**, 3.
46. GAVRON, H., 1966. *The captive wife: conflicts of housebound mothers*. London, Routledge and Kegan Paul.
47. GERARD, D. L., and SIEGEL, J., 1950. The family background of schizophrenia. *Psychiat. Q.*, **24**, 47.
48. GILLORAN, J. L., 1965. Family happiness: the father's angle. *J. Roy. Soc. M.* **4**, 211.
49. GLUECK, S., and GLUECK, E. T., 1950. *Unravelling juvenile delinquency*. New York, Commonwealth Fund.
50. GORER, G., 1948. *The American People: a study of national character*. New York, Norton.
51. GRAY, S. W., 1959. Perceived similarity to parents in adjustment. *Child Develpm.*, **30**, 91.
52. GRØNSETTI, E., 1957. The impact of father-absence in sailor families upon the personality structure and social adjustment of adult sailor sons. Part I. In *Studies of the family*, vol. 2, Ed. Anderson, N. Göttingen, Vandenhoek and Ruprecht.
53. GRUNEBAUM, H. V., and STREAN, H. S., 1964. Some consideration of the therapeutic neglect of fathers in child guidance. *J. Child Psychol. Psychiat.*, **5**, 241.
    GRUNEBAUM, H., 1962. Group psychotherapy of fathers. *Br. J. Med. Psychol.*, **35**, 147.
54. HARRIS, D. B., and TSENG, S. C., 1957. Children's attitudes toward peers and parents as revealed by sentence completions. *Child Develpm.*, **28**, 401.
55. HARTMAN, A. A., and NICOLAY, R. C., 1966. Sexually deviant behaviour in expectant fathers. *J. abnorm. Psychol.*, **71**, 232.
56. HEINICKE, C. M., and WESTHEIMER, I. J., 1965. *Brief Separations*. London, Longmans.
57. HENRIQUES, F., 1955. Popular magazines and the upbringing of children. In *Mental health and infant development*, vol. 1, Ed. Soddy, K. London, Routledge and Kegan Paul.
58. HILL, R., 1949. *Families under stress*. New York, Harper.
59. HINDE, R. A., 1965. Rhesus monkey aunts. In *Determinants of infant behaviour* III. Ed. Foss, B. M. London, Methuen.
60. HJELHOLT, G., 1958. The neglected parent. *Nord. Psykol.*, **10**, 179.
61. HOBHOUSE, WHEELER, and GINSBERG., 1900. Quoted by Bell, N. W., and Vogel E. F., (Eds.). In *The family*. Glencoe, Ill., Free Press.
62. HOFFMAN, L. W., 1961. *The father's role in the family*. Merrill Palmer Quart.

63. HOWELLS, J. G., 1963. *Family psychiatry*. Edinburgh, Oliver and Boyd.
64. HOWELLS, J. G., 1965. Child psychiatry as an aspect of family psychiatry. *Acta paedopsychiatrica*, **32**, 35.
65. HOWELLS, J. G., 1968. *Theory and practice of family psychiatry*. Edinburgh, Oliver and Boyd.
66. HOWELLS, J. G., 1968. Schizophrenia and family psychopathology. In *Modern perspectives in world psychiatry*. Ed. Howells, J. G. Edinburgh, Oliver and Boyd.
67. HOWELLS, J. G. Unpublished study.
68. HOWELLS, J. G., and LAYNG, J., 1955. Separation experiences and mental health. *Lancet*, ii, 285.
69. HOWELLS, J. G., and LICKORISH, J. R., 1967. Family relations indicator (2nd ed.). Edinburgh, Oliver and Boyd.
70. ITANI, J., 1962. Paternal care in the wild Japanese monkey, Macaca fuscata Fuscata. *Primates, J. Primatol.*, **2**, 61-93.
71. JACKSON, P. W., 1956. Verbal solutions to parent-child problems. *Child Develpm.*, **27**, 339.
72. JAY, PHYLLIS, 1963. Mother-infant relations in Langurs. In *Maternal behaviour in mammals*. Ed. Rheingold, H. L. New York and London, John Wiley.
73. JOHNSON, A. M., GRIFFIN, M. E., WATSON, J., and BECKETT, P. S., 1956. Studies in schizophrenia at Mayo Clinic. *Psychiatry*, **19**, 143.
74. JOHNSON, M. M., 1963. Sex-role learning in the nuclear family. *Child Develpm.*, **34**, 319.
75. JOSSELYN, I. M., 1956. Cultural forces, motherliness and fatherliness. *Amer. J. Orthopsychiat.*, **26**, 264.
76. JUNG, C. G., 1949. *The significance of the father in the destiny of the individual*. Zürich, Rascher.
77. JUNG, C. G., 1959. *The basic writings of Jung*. (edited by De Lasylo). New York, Modern Library.
78. KAGAN, J., 1956. The child's perception of the parent. *J. abnorm. soc. Psych.*, **53**, 257.
79. KASANIN, J., KNIGHT, E., and SAGE, P., 1934. The parent-child relationship in schizophrenia. *J. nerv. ment. Dis.*, **79**, 249.
80. KATY, R., 1957. The role of the father. *Mental hygiene*, **41**, 517.
81. KATZ, D., 1953. *Animals and men*. Harmondsworth, Pelican books. (First published in Germany 1937.)
82. KLUCKHOHN, C., 1949. *Mirror for man*. New York, McGraw-Hill.
83. LANGFORD, W. S., 1964. The psychological aspects of ulcerative colitis. *Clin. Proc. Children's Hosp., Wash.*, **20**, 89.
84. LAZOWICK, L. M., 1955. On the nature of identification. *J. abnorm. soc. Psychol.*, **51**, 175.
85. LEIGHTON, D., and KLUCKHOHN, C., 1947. *Children of the people*. Cambridge, Mass., Harvard Univ. Press.
86. LEVIN, H., and SEARS, R. R., 1956. Identification with parents as a determinant of doll-play aggression. *Child Develpm.*, **27**, 135.
87. LOGAN, R. F. L., and GOLDBERG, E. M., 1953. Rising eighteen in a London suburb. *Brit. J. Sociol.*, **4**, 323.
88. LURIE, O. R., 1941. Psychological factors associated with eating difficulties in children. *Am. J. Orthopsychiat.*, **11**, 452.
89. LYNN, D., and SAWREY, W. L., 1959. The effects of father-absence on Norwegian boys and girls. *J. abnorm. soc. Psychol.*, **59**, 258.
90. MACCALMAN, D. R., 1955. Background to child development patterns in the United Kingdom. In *Mental health and infant development*, vol. 1. Ed. Soddy, K. London, Routledge and Kegan Paul.

91. McCord, J., McCord, W., and Thurber, E., 1962. Some effects of paternal absence on male children. *J. abnorm. soc. Psychol.*, **64**, 361.
92. *Makarenko, His Life and Work*. Trans. from Russian by Issacs, B. Moscow, Foreign Languages Publishing House.
93. Malinowski, B., 1927. *The father in primitive psychology*. London, Routledge and Kegan Paul.
94. Malinowski, B., 1927. *Sex and parenting in savage societies*. London, Routledge and Kegan Paul.
95. Mead, M., 1935. *Sex and temperament in three primitive societies*. London, Routledge and Kegan Paul.
96. Mead, M., 1954. *Am. J. Orthopsychiat.*, **24**, 471.
97. Mead, M., 1955. In *Mental health and infant development*. Part 4. Ed. Soddy, K. London, Routledge and Kegan Paul.
98. Mead, M., 1962. *Growing up in New Guinea*. London, Penguin Books.
99. Mead, M., and MacGregor, F. M. C., 1951. *Growth and Culture*. New York.
100. Métraux, R., 1955. Parents and children: an analysis of contemporary German child-care and youth-guidance literature. In *Childhood in contemporary culture*. Eds. Mead, M., and Wolfenstein, M. Chicago, Univ. Press.
101. Miller, L., 1968. The significance of child rearing in the Kibbutz. Chapter VIII in this volume.
102. Mohr, G. J., Josselyn, I. M., Spurlock, J., and Barron, S. H., 1958. Studies in ulcerative colitis. *Amer. J. Psychiat.*, **114**, 1067.
103. Mueller, D. D., 1945. Paternal domination: Its influence on child guidance results. *Smith Coll. Stud. soc. Wk.*, **15**, 184.
104. Murdock, G. P., 1960. The universality of the nuclear family. In *The family*. Bell, N. W., and Vogel, E. F. Glencoe, Ill., Free Press.
105. Mussen, P., 1961. Some antecedents and consequences of masculine sex-typing in adolescent boys. *Psychol. Monogr.*, **75**, No. 2.
106. Mussen, P., and Distler, L., 1960. Child-rearing antecedents of masculine identification in kindergarten boys. *Child Develpm.*, **31**, 89.
107. Nash, J., 1952. Fathers and sons: A neglected aspect of child care. *Child Care*, **6**, 19.
108. Nash, J., 1965. The father in contemporary culture and current psychological literature. *Child Develpm.*, **36**, 261.
109. Newson, J., and Newson, E., 1963. *Infant care in an urban community*. London, Allen and Unwin.
110. O'Gorman, G., 1965. The psychoses of childhood. In *Modern perspectives in child psychiatry*, Ed. Howells, J. G. Edinburgh, Oliver and Boyd.
111. Ostrovsky, E. S., 1959. *Father to the child*. New York, G. P. Putnam.
112. Parsons, T., 1947. Certain sources and patterns of aggression in the social structure of the western world. *Psychiatry*, **10**, 172.
113. Petersen, D. R., Becker, W. C., Hellmer, L. A., Shoemaker, D. J., and Quay, H. C., 1959. Parental attitudes and child development. *Child Develpm.*, **30**, 119.
114. Prout, C. T., and White, M. A., 1950. A controlled study of personality relationships in mothers of schizophrenia male patients. *Am. J. Psychiat.*, **107**, 251.
115. Prugh, D. G., 1951. The role of emotional factors in ulcerative colitis in childhood. *Gastroenterol.*, **18**, 339.
116. Radke, M. J., 1946. The relation of parental authority to children's behaviour and attitudes. *Univ. Minn. Child Welf. Monogr.*, No. 22.
117. Reichard, S., and Tillman, C., 1950. Patterns of parent-child relationships in schizophrenia. *Psychiatry*, **13**, 247

REFERENCES

118. REMSTAD, R., and ROTHNEY, J. W. M., 1958. Occupational classification and research results. *Personnel Guid. J.*, **36**, 465.
119. RICHARDS, M. E., 1949. When to include the father in child guidance. *Smith Coll. Stud. soc. Wk*, **19**, 79.
120. RHEINGOLD, H. L., 1963. Introduction to *Maternal Behaviour in Mammals*, Ed. Rheingold, H. L. New York and London, John Wiley.
121. ROGLER, L. H., and HOLLINGSHEAD, A. B., 1965. *Trapped: Families and schizophrenia*. New York and London, John Wiley.
122. ROHRER, J. H., and EDMONDSON, M. S., 1960. *The eighth generation*. New York, Harper.
123. ROWELL, T. E., 1961. Maternal behaviour in non-maternal Golden Hamsters (*Mesocricetus auratus*). *Animal Behaviour*, **9**, 11.
124. RUBENSTEIN, B. O., and LEVITT, M., 1957. Some observations regarding the role of fathers in child psychotherapy. *Bull. Menninger Clin.*, **21**, 16.
125. RUSSELL, 1967. *The listener*, **77**, No. 1985.
126. SANDERSON, W. T., 1963. *The Dynasty of Abu*. London, Cassell.
127. SEARS, R. R., MACEROY, E. E., and LEVIN, H., 1957. *Patterns of child rearing*. New York, Peterson.
128. SEARS, R. R., PINTLER, M. H., and SEARS, P. S., 1946. Effect of father separation on preschool children's doll play aggression. *Child Develpm.*, **17**, 219.
129. SEPLIN, C. D., 1952. A study of the influence of the father's absence for military service. *Smith Coll. Stud. soc. Wk*, **22**, 123.
130. *Shorter Oxford English Dictionary*. 1933. 3rd ed. Oxford, Univ. Press.
131. SIEGMAN, A. W., 1966. Father absence during early childhood and anti-social behaviour. *J. abnorm. soc. Psychol.*, **71**, 71.
132. SIMPSON, M., 1935. Parent preferences of young children. *Teach. Coll. Contrib. Educ.*, No. 652.
133. STEPHENS, W. N., 1961. Judgements by social workers on boys and mothers in fatherless families. *J. genet. Psychol.*, **99**, 59.
134. STOLZ, L. M., et al., 1954. *Father relations of war-born children*. Stanford, Calif., Univ. Press.
135. STREAN, H. S., 1962. A means of involving father in family treatment. *Am. J. Orthopsychiat.*, **32**, 719.
136. STRONG, E. K., 1957. Interests of fathers and sons. *J. Appl. Psychol.*, **41**, 284.
137. SUNLEY, R., 1955. Early nineteenth century American literature on child-rearing. In *Childhood in contemporary cultures*. Eds. Mead, M., and Wolfenstein, M. Chicago, Univ. Press.
138. TASCH, R. J., 1952. The role of the father in the family. *J. exp. Educ.*, **20**, 319.
139. THOMPSON, G. G., 1962. *Child psychology*. Boston, Houghton Mifflin.
140. THRASHER, F. M., 1927. *The gang*. Chicago, Univ. Press.
141. TIETZE, T., 1949. A study of mothers of schizophrenic patients. *Psychiatry*, **12**, 55.
142. TILLER, P. O., 1958. Father absence and personality development of children in sailor families. *Nordisk Psykologi's Monogr. Ser.*, No. 9.
143. TOWNE, R. D., and AFTERMAN, J., 1955. Psychosis in males related to parenthood. *Bull. Menninger Clin.*, **19**, 19.
144. TRETHOWAN, W. H., and CONLON, M. F., 1965. The couvade syndrome. *Brit. J. Psychiat.*, **111**, 57.
145. VAN HOUTEN, J., 1948. Mother-child relationships in school phobia. *Smith Coll. Stud. soc. Wk*, **18**, 161.
146. VON DER HEYDT, VERA., 1964. The role of the father in early mental development. *Brit. J. med. Psychol.*, **37**, 123.
147. WAHL, C. W., 1954. Some antecedent factors in family histories of schizophrenics. *Am. J. Psychiat.*, **110**, 668.

148. WAHL, C. W., 1956. Some antecedent factors in the family histories of schizophrenics in the U.S. Navy. *Am. J. Psychiat.*, **113**, 201.
149. WALTON, E., 1940. The role of the father in treatment at a child guidance clinic. *Smith Coll. Stud. soc. Wk*, **11**, 155.
150. WEINER, A., and STEINHILBER, R., 1961. The post-partum psychoses. *J. Intern. Coll. Surgeons*, **36**, 490.
151. WENAR, C., HANDLON, M. W., and GARNER, A. M., 1962. *Origins of psychosomatic and emotional disturbances: A study of mother-child relationships*. New York, Paul B. Heober.
152. WENDT, H., 1965. *The sex life of the animals*. London, Arthur Baker.
153. WESTERMARCK, E. A., 1921. *History of human marriage*. New York, Macmillan.
154. WHITE, M. A., PROUT, C. T., FIXSEN, C., and FONDEUR, M., 1957. Obstetricians' role in post-partum mental illness. *J. Am. med. Assn*, **165**, 138.
155. WHITING, J. W. M., and CHILD, I., 1953. *Child training and personality*. Yale Univ. Press.
156. WINCH, R., 1950. Some data bearing on the oedipal hypothesis. *J. abnorm. soc. Psychol.*, **45**, 481.
157. WINNICOTT, D. W., 1965. *The maturational process and the facilitating environment*. London, Hogarth.
158. WYNN, M., 1964. *Fatherless families*. London, Michael Joseph.
159. YOUNG, M., and WILLMOTT, P., 1957. *Family and kinships in East London*. London, Macmillan.
160. ZILBOORG, G., 1931. Depressive reactions related to parenthood. *Am. J. Psychiat.*, **10**, 927.
161. ZUCKERMAN, S., 1931. *The social life of monkeys and apes*. London, Kegan Paul, Trench, Trubner.

VI

THE CHILD'S NEEDS FOR HIS EMOTIONAL HEALTH

S. A. Szurek
M.D.

Professor, Department of Psychiatry
University of California School of Medicine, San Francisco, California

Director, Children's Service,
Langley Porter Neuropsychiatric Institute, San Francisco, California

1

Introduction

The needs of a child that promote his emotional health, when satisfied, are intimately and inextricably related to the emotional health and well being of his parents or their surrogates. Their needs when satisfied increase the probability that his needs will be fulfilled as well.

For many obvious reasons it has been difficult in many discussions to maintain such a comprehensive attention upon the family as whole, upon each individual in it and their mutual influence upon each other. Even when a discussant makes every effort to describe accurately sequences of emotional processes in each person of the family and the reactions of others to them, it very frequently happens that his audience or readers misunderstand him. It seems to be extremely difficult for many people—also for obvious reasons—not to confuse a dispassionate description of the cycles and circles of cause and effect (becoming cause of the next effect) in emotional processes with either praise, admiration and exhortation to emulation, or on the other hand, with blame, condemnation, derogation or contempt. What is or what actually happens becomes what should, ought or must happen or what should not, ought not or must not happen. Moralistic and legalistic attitudes creep in. These pervasive attitudes becloud understanding and retard learning from experiments of nature how that which is integrative and fortunate can be repeated and that which is destructive and tragic can be reduced or avoided if possible.

Such misunderstandings have resulted in heated discussions in defence of children or on the other hand in defence of parents which have shed little light upon the life of the family. The present writer hopes at least not to contribute to this or to a similar holy war.

It is a truism that the child's needs change in kind or degree from one period of his life to another. This fact is used in this essay to give order to the discussion.

It is also a truism that the needs of the parents, of the family as a whole, also change. Such changes of their needs and the manner and degree of their satisfactions although closely relevant will only be indicated as necessary to complete the description.

Although very important, special and particular needs of the child and his parents arising from handicaps imposed by disease or injury will not be considered central to this discussion.

2

The Needs of the Newborn

'His second folly was that he (Frederick II, 1194-1250, Holy Roman Emperor) wanted to find out what kind of speech and what manner of speech children would have when they grew up, if they spoke to no one beforehand. So he bade foster mothers and nurses to suckle the children, to bathe and wash them, but in no way to prattle with them or to speak to them, for he wanted to learn whether they would speak the Hebrew language, which was the oldest, or Greek or Latin or Arabic, or perhaps the language of their parents, of whom they had been born. But he laboured in vain, because the children all died. For they could not live without petting and the joyful faces and loving words of their foster mothers. And so the songs called "swaddling songs", which a woman sings while she is rocking the cradle, to put a child to sleep, and without them a child sleeps badly and has no rest'. Salimbene*[5].

Many, if not most parents anticipate with eagerness the birth of their child as a fulfilment of their marriage and as a satisfaction of their deep individual and common wish to be fully a man and woman. They have thoughtfully prepared in every way for its coming with an effort to repeat, and if possible to improve, for their child, on their own life experience each with his own parents. The father, content with his own vocational skill and achievement, is proud and assured of his strength and of his persistence in work and of his capacity to provide for his wife and family. His sexual drive towards his wife, infused with deep and considerate tenderness, is usually satisfied and adds to his sense of power. His sense of competence is increased by his realistic assessment of what living needs are

* The writer is indebted to a colleague, John I. Langdell, M.D., for bringing to his attention this early experimentation in human development.

to be provided now and in the future. His child will be not only another evidence of his own maturity but a further stimulus to his own effort.

The mother, with a satisfactory experience and relation to her own mother and father, feels deeply fulfilled as a woman in her pregnancy and her mothering impulse after the child's birth. Her deep pride in her creative role sustains her in every effort to maintain her own health and strength from such current learning as she can find. Her love flows freely, eagerly and fully in sex and in daily experience towards her husband and her child.

They each respect each other's competence and each is warmed by loving exchanges with the other. The sex of the child, although perhaps differently tinged in each of their wishes, is relatively less important than the fact of this being their child. If it is their first child, they seek appropriate and wise advice from their parents or from professional medical sources about healthful daily practices for each phase of pregnancy and in preparation for its fruition in the mother's labour and delivery. They find mutual support in the practices which maintain or develop adequate nutrition, and strength of the mother for the process of birth whether it is to occur with or without anaesthesia.

Both father and mother experience from each of their own parents and family, individually and together, the fond eagerness for a grandchild and their helpful, affectionate acceptance as a couple, as a new family to become a part of the larger one. To become 'a part of the large family' may have different meanings in specific details in different cultures and subcultures. In each such culture, however, the integration into such a larger family connotes those matters of mutual consideration or obligation which is satisfying to the needs of self-regard of each person involved and their individual wishes.

Such a description—perhaps too idyllic for any given situation—is to be understood as needs for emotional health more or less adequately fulfilled especially for the expectant parents concerned. Each has chosen the other with a definitely positive balance in their feelings of pride and hopeful anticipation of complementary satisfaction in life with the other as an attractive mate and loving person.

Under such circumstances the pregnancy generally progresses smoothly with often even a greater than usual sense of well-being on the part of the expectant mother. This comes about from her continuing, or increasing physical fitness from appropriate exercise, diet and sufficient rest and from a deepening experience of satisfying mutuality with her husband during this period. Generally, too, the birth of the child at full term, although arduous, is satisfying to the mother and proceeds without seriously untoward events to either child or mother. In recent years in modern hospital confinements, the trend is to keep the newly born child at his mother's side. This is to continue those aspects of the prenatal symbiosis essential to his further development and the satisfaction of the maternal impulse and need to provide the care that his immaturity requires.

Fathers, too, have more opportunities in visits—than through the previous glass window of the nursery—to embark on the first part of their voyage of mutual adaptation.

In the situation where most of the aspects described are present, or more of them are more often present than not, the fortunate newly born infant enters a world where most of the needs of his further growth and development are very likely to be met. He has an individual mother. He has an informed mother eager to complete herself in the task of satisfying every need of his helplessness, she can understand and discover. Until her milk flows, she responds to his every cry with gentle stroking of his head, with cuddling, lowering his head, rocking and with soothing sounds. All this stimulates his respiration—so recently reversed as regards the direction of the movements of his diaphragm from what they were while he was still in the womb. His brain, most incompletely developed of all the organs and very rapidly growing, is hungry for oxygen. His shallow and rapid respirations are deepened by her response. His oxygen need is more satisfied, his cry subsides, and he sinks into his tense, semiconscious silence —until the need brings the next cry. His mother also protects him to the extent that she can against sudden loud sounds, against extremes of temperature, against preventable pain, undue pressure and overlong wetness. She protects him against sudden changes in his sense of equilibrium by shifting his position slowly.

When her milk begins to flow she makes sure he is able to suck. If he is one of the 40 per cent of newly born infants who appears unready, she helps him learn to suck by making sure the nipple is well in his mouth, and by rhythmically and gently moving his chin up and down so that his tongue and palate are stimulated. When this activity, the next one after breathing, is mastered by such practice and help and by the maturation of the neuromuscular complex of organs involved, he is more fully equipped to get and take those elements of the world he needs as nourishment and pleasurable exercise.

She notices that he sucks more than would be necessary for the amount of milk he takes into his stomach. He eagerly sucks in this way beyond his merely nutritional needs not only at her breast, but also on pacifier, sugared cloth and eventually his own fingers and thumb. In response to this enthusiastic sucking she unquestioningly, undisturbedly permits his impulse its full satisfaction at her own nipple or provides a substitute nipple. For she learns from these experiences that only when this impulse for pleasure sucking is fully gratiated does he slip back into what is his rest and sleep.

As these first days and weeks go by she is guided by *his* stirring and *his* crying as to when to provide him with opportunity to suck for his food and for his pleasurable exercise. She permits him gradually to establish his own rhythm about all this and intuitively—if not from modern professional advice—knows that the only reliable clock is that which expresses his organismic processes however varying and irregular the periods it indicates in these first weeks of life.

Thus it is that the neonate's three primary hungers[4] for adequate oxygen, especially for his brain, for sucking for food and for satisfaction, and for the pleasant sensory stimulation of fondling, caressing and singing during bathing, feeding and so on are satiated by the hunger of the mother to provide them. She maintains her own readiness for such responsiveness to his needs by adjusting her other work, her needs for adequate nutrition, exercise and rest with her husband's understanding help if necessary. She is then rewarded and satisfied in her mothering needs by the infant's steady growth in size and vigour, by a gradual steadying of his rhythm of need for such ministrations into more regular and predictable periods, and by the gradual general relaxation of the tenseness of his posture awake or asleep.

The First Smile

This relaxation is evident also in his facial muscles and expression. She observes a smile one day in about the fourth week, after some days of abortive mouthings and facial changes. She may attribute this as his response to the sight of her face, but since his sight develops more slowly (and even blind babies smile) this facial change is more likely to come in a moment when he is generally content, probably when he hears the affectionate tone of her voice. In any case her delighted reaction encourages him to repeat and practice his smile. It becomes a communicative signal between them which powerfully enhances their mutual pleasure and this, with all else good that happens to him, forms for him those rudiments of feeling which could be called trust.

Developmental Deviations

Pathological deviations in development during early infancy such as marasmus and the underlying etiological factors, although very important for more thorough understanding, cannot be here discussed for reasons of space. Instead of such a discussion the writer wishes to call the reader's attention to a very lucid discussion by Dr Rene Spitz[6] a careful student of this period of life.

Any extreme reaction in infancy to rather marked privation emphasizes the need of the child during the early weeks of his life for individual and consistent mothering love for both his physical and psychological growth. It points up, too, the probable reasons for the milder, or more severe but transient, disturbances in the absence of any identifiable diseases of infants who do not suffer the total loss of the presence in the home of a loving, nurturant mothering person. In these latter instances the maternal response to the cues given by the infant is likely to be partly interfered with, somewhat reduced in its full expression of adequacy and tenderness, and/or in the accuracy of its modulation to the actual need of the infant at a given moment or period of time. Such interferences to the maternal impulse may be any one of a great variety: from transient preoccupations to longer lasting internalized conflicts arising from untoward events in the mother's daily life and personal relations.

Such severe reactions also suggest that the rather severe maldevelopments called childhood psychosis may have their roots in troubled mother-infant experiences, even though not all clinical students of early childhood agree that any, or all of the psychotic disorders of early childhood are entirely experientially determined. Some of these clinicians consider that some hereditary factors, or still obscure disease of the child contribute to the genesis of the problem. Further close research already begun is needed to settle the question.

3

Remainder of First Year of Life

The needs of the infant between the first or second month of life and the end of the first year usually change rapidly with the progressive maturation of his body and their vital functions. It is predominantly a period—especially in the first four to five or six months—of biological rather than cultural emphasis. Nevertheless, these biological processes when, as most often is the case, are nurtured and supported by the parents (particularly the mother) are of profound importance for the full development of later mental functioning and emotional integration.

In most families this growth of the infant is generally smooth and the mother's nurturing care becomes so promptly adapted to each phase of child's growth that any problems in the mutual adaptation are hardly noticed. Sucking and breathing become gradually well and firmly established. This occurs in the first weeks in large part in response to the mother's prompt nursing at the breast or with bottle while holding the infant firmly and gently at every hunger cry. Such development occurs smoothly particularly if the mother strokes his head, holds him in her lap rocking him gently for a few minutes before feeding him for a full 20 to 30 minutes. Most mothers await the spontaneous waking of the baby and permit only a few minutes of crying as a breathing exercise before picking him up for feeding. Diapering is done by such a mother only after the feeding and after elimination occurs which happens only three to five times a day in the first one or two months, followed by a gradual reduction in their number. She is not concerned much by wetness in the intervals while the child sleeps after such feedings, nor by the number of, or the intervals between, such awakenings for food, for stimulation and at one of them for exercise and bath. The number of these awakenings gradually decrease in the third and fourth month as the child begins to sleep longer at night.

In short the average mother's observance of the rhythm of her baby's physiological processes in these first three months is rewarded by a progressive steadying of this rhythm with more predictably longer intervals between the awakenings at night, and between eliminations. She is rewarded, too, by not only the gain in weight, size of her infant but also by both a gradual increase in his alertness, greater activity while awake and by greater relaxation of his tense posture during sleep. He responds with an obvious sense of general well-being to his warm bath or an oil massage. He thrives upon such skin stimulation as well as upon his mother's gentle rocking, cuddling and upon his hearing her voice as she sings or speaks to him during feedings, at bath or during lengthening periods of wakefulness as his growth proceeds.

Sucking

The healthy mother is particularly attentive to the full satisfaction of infant's need for sucking not only for his nutritional needs but also for his pleasurable needs. It is obvious to her that early in this period the mouth is the first developed effector organ by means of which he has the most satisfying active contact with her breast, eventually with her as a person, as a representative of the world outside. She observes that the intensity and eagerness with which her baby sucks increases until about the fourth month. Thereafter it tends to diminish as the baby begins to vocalize, to bite and grasp with his hands. It diminishes, that is, if it has been fully and agreeably exercised up to this time.

Students of infancy like Ribble[4] have found that infants whose sucking needs and the other needs for the variety of gentle stimulation previously outlined, grow and mature in every way more promptly, with less tendency towards functional retrogressions and delays in growth. Such children are alert and responsive sooner. The smiling and vocalizing appears earlier, and eventually they develop speech better and earlier than others not so fully satisfied. Finger and thumb sucking in such children are also much less frequent, less persistent. Children who are rocked in the mother's arms or in cradles also are less likely to manifest less tendency to habitual self-rocking, self-rolling or head-banging.

These students of infancy also emphasize that such mothering provides the nutrition, the oxygen, the stimulation needed for the growth and maturation of the brain especially but also for all parts of the nervous system of the sensory and motor organs. This maturation of the nervous system is evident in the obvious progressive use of vision, greater strength and vigour of movement of the head, trunk, arms and legs, increasing span of attention to mother's approach, to the sound of her voice, to the sight of her face. It becomes evident in a general sense anticipatory excitement in movements, wriggling, arm waving eventually stretching or reaching towards her at feeding and play periods or at bath times. These are called by Ribble 'premental' behaviour. All the infant's inner hungers for food, oxygen and growing other needs for sensory experience and activity satisfactions are focused upon the mother. With her necessary help in this period of biological immaturity he obtains the necessities for his survival and growth quite insistently and 'selfishly'. The average mother hardly thinks of this as 'selfishness' but as biological need which coincides with her need to provide it so that his actual dependency can with further maturation progress to eager self-dependency. It never occurs to her to thwart her infant in any of these important respects of his needs. Experiencing such loving care forms the basis for the infant's ability to love well and to learn with sustained and eager curiosity.

Elimination

During these first three to six months elimination is another of the bodily functions which is self-regulating. The mother undisturbed by this function, keeps the child clean and waits for her own child's rhythm to become established. From the first month's three to five bowel movements a day occurring usually soon after nursing, the infant's stools become fewer and firmer. When this change occurs the child may show some measure of excitement before the movement, either squirming, or stiffening his limbs; his breathing becomes more rapid or he holds his breath, at times fixing his eyes on his mother with an expression of considerable attention. His mother senses after the movement that her infant is relieved of a disagreeable tension and that he has a sense of well-being.

Although some mothers at times, with the advice of their pediatricians make some effort to induce movements with finger or suppository and use of potty as early as the second month, they find that such efforts at toilet training are apt to be premature. They are less apt to retain such 'training' later and difficulties in acquiring more stable habits of self care with regard to stools are more likely. Gradual assumption of responsibility for such cleanliness by the child himself is much easier sometime after the end of the first year when he begins to be able to speak and to sit alone on the potty chair. Hence to achieve more lasting results, the mother waits for the period of greater muscular control and readiness of the child for such adaptation to family life, being observant, but entirely permissive. She then gradually gives the child an opportunity to sit on the potty-chair once or twice a day. Under these circumstances when the child experiences from his mother no disgust, impatience or coercive tension, he acquires this skill at his own rate. This acquisition then contributes its measure to the child's growing sense of autonomy, of self-reliance.

Emotional Needs after the Fourth Month

In the first three to four months of his life the infant's needs for mothering care are expressive of his complete helplessness, of his physiological hungers and primarily of the state of development of the near-distance sensory organs of touch, taste, equilibrium, temperature, pain, pressure and so on. From about the fourth month, the healthy, growing infant's needs are progressively those which express the maturation of the distance receptors of vision and hearing and of the muscular system and its coordination. The infant begins to focus his eyes upon the mother's face, to listen to her voice, to raise and turn his head towards her as she approaches. He relaxes and falls asleep after feedings more readily when he sees and hears her beside his crib. Around six months of age a growing awareness of his own body and of himself comes with his increasing ability to move his body about, to roll over, to reach and grasp objects often to put them into his exploring mouth, eventually to sit up. He grows more tolerant of being alone with a few toys for short periods. However, during the increasing periods of wakefulness and such activity he is obviously more content in such play in a play-pen in her presence seeing and hearing her movements or voice. He is soon able to make calling sounds, to pull himself and look in the direction of his mother's usual approach. Although his feelings are still centred primarily in himself and his satisfactions, he is more attentive and more responsive to his mother as well as his father who has shared somewhat in his care earlier. Gradually as his need for contact with his parents is fully satisfied, he shows not only eager anticipatory movements towards them, but also becomes able to respond and relate to others in the family.

In such a family the infant's dependence is not feared but is as fully gratified as possible by both parents as a continuing and essential phase in his eventual greater development of secure independence with the maturation of locomotion, creeping, crawling and then walking. Sharing his pleasurable experiences of such personal contact by both parents and at times with others tends to reduce any tendency on the child's part to fixate too exclusively upon his relationship to his mother, even though she may remain a more central person to him. In such personal and bodily contact with the child neither parent hesitates to express his affectionate warmth in cuddling, hugging or otherwise romping with him. In such play there is no impulse to overstimulate the child's erotisms particularly in the region of the genital and anal area while giving him full opportunity for his own general exercise naked in a warm room before his bath. They evince no anxious horror if they observe an erection in the young son. If they see any auto-erotic play they gently divert him to some other activity. They realize as a matter of fact that such affectionate attention so expressed towards their baby reduces his need for compensatory self-stimulation whether by thumb-sucking or by play with genitals.

His mother continuing breast feeding or breast and supplementary bottle feeding observes his teeth begin to appear between the fifth and seventh month. She encourages him to bite and chew hard bread and other solid foods even perhaps before this. In this way she is less likely to be suddenly startled and to frighten her child by being bitten in the breast. She certainly does not slap him in such an event having no wish to introduce any negative elements into their relation, nor to run any risk of his developing any inhibitions about his biting and chewing. Her only interest is in guiding this new skill into its appropriate relation to eating rather than being associated with frustration and anger. She is similarly permissive about kicking as an exercise in preparation for walking and only gently restrains it when necessary during diapering and dressing.

Although all this growth makes the child somewhat more independent of her, the mother still responds promptly to his ever more insistent calling to attend to his hunger, to any bodily discomfort or to his need for her presence. She senses that such attention reduces the possibility of his anxiety about his inner feelings (which he is still too helpless to assuage himself) developing into acute and severe fears. For the same reason she leaves a dim light in his room at night to prevent his acquiring any paralysing fears of the dark. In short she realizes that her promptly supplying the needs he cannot yet give himself only fosters his growth of trust in people and eventually in himself as his body matures and he ever more confidently explores the world and practises each skill. Under such circumstances the child is less likely to develop a tendency to those disorganizing reactions called tantrums since such rage is clearly a reaction to acute and severe disappointment, frustration or thwarting.

In this period the well-mothered child begins to vocalize, to gurgle and coo. Her delighted repetition of these early sounds in turn obviously delights him as he repeatedly replies. Such early lalling is in itself a pleasurable new activity based on previous mouth, tongue, palatal and respiratory functions having been satisfyingly exercised especially in sucking with additional coordination of the vocal chords. His play with such phonation again with tongue against palate or through lips leads to the primordial syllables of *da*, *na* and *ma* and *ba*. Mother's and father's additional pleasurable and even excitedly eager response increases the child's pleasure still more. He hears himself, he hears her. He has an audience, a sense of communication and an expanding sense of self. His face is expressive of his feeling wreathed in smiles. Word building has begun with these few syllables and proceeds rapidly as his brain matures, records and connects the elements of these experiences and speech becomes progressively an organ of the mind.

This mind, incidentally, is assumed to have begun operating even before this, presumably in the formation of visual images of past experience elicited by some felt inner need and connected with some external stimulus such as the sound of mother's approach. What, of course, can be seen of any such possible subjective mental function is the evidence of excitement, obvious sense of well-being with whatever movements of approach towards the mother which have to that point matured and been developed through practice. It is probable, too, that in such reactions memories of pleasurable sensations of being held, cuddled, warmed and suckled are evoked. These all probably do not last long unless mother's action soon occurs. Nevertheless, it is also evident that in these months anticipation and capacity for attention and evident response to the person of mother and father and towards objects desired appear and progressively increase. Furthermore persistence in seeking more clearly definable and discernible goals and objects through his own efforts or with the help of mother and father is likely to be greater when previous experiences have been satisfactory. Thus his energies are more and more directed and his awareness clearly increases and appropriate action more often follows. He not only manifestly wants what he wants but begins to do something about getting it.

Thus Ribble[4] on the basis of studying a large number of babies and the kind of parental care they received summarizes the development observed. Children of parents who are emotionally mature with a capacity for consistent personal adaptation in their own lives—as those thus far described in this section—developed mentally much more rapidly and in a definitely more integrated manner. Such parents far from using their child as a play object or necessary companion, intuitively and through study recognized and respected his actual personal needs. They showed no evidence of being obsessed by fears that the child's mentality was inadequate, that his erotic expression was precocious or that he might become too much attached to them. If some anomalous behaviour arose temporarily, these parents did not hesitate to seek expert advice.

There was a marked contrast to these more fortunate situations among those children reared by parents, particularly mothers, who were emotionally more detached or absorbed more in social or professional pursuits. Such children were manifestly unhappy, retarded in speech or locomotion and often with a variety of dissociated activities, and with an exaggerated tendency to auto-erotic practices. These babies generally sleep too little, tend to be hyperactive in a disorganized way and frequently have eating problems and disturbances of elimination. The child kept emotionally detached because of fears of exaggerated dependency is more apt to become either much more helplessly, irritably dependent upon his mother or more detached and self-preoccupied with some kinds of repetitive activities. He may be extremely distractable, with a chronically poor appetite along with constipation or diarrhoea or else may become overweight.

Frustrated in his appetites and longings such a child is poorly equipped for further living and has little impulse to love. He may show a tendency towards croup, asthma with irregularities of breathing and disturbed vocalization. Centring this attention on himself that otherwise would be directed towards the parents, the deprived child may have difficulty in focussing general and specific bodily movement. At six months of age he does not reach for the bottle offered him, nor suck steadily, holding the bottle. Instead he interrupts his sucking frequently, looking elsewhere, moving restlessly as if indifferent to the bottle. The hunger sense is diffuse and the pleasure and comfort to direct and integrate his feeding activities is obviously absent. Security in relation to the mother as a basis for smooth physiological functioning and for the smooth beginning of mental development and educability are wanting.

Thus it is clear that the ability to love is a highly complicated potential which is evoked only through the tender care given to the infant at birth regarding his physiological needs and his subsequent more general emotional and psychological needs. It does not appear automatically at some stage of maturation but depends on his total, outside experiences. The pleasure offered by attentive, loving parents in satisfying his hunger for food and other bodily needs is essential in his developing an eager response to external realities. This is particularly so when these needs for food and then for parents is gratified passively and eventually by his own increasing efforts. The abstract intelligence comes later. The drives to love and to learn, their intensity and their mode of expression are deeply rooted in hunger and personal dependency of infancy. The tender skill of the mother has much to do in maturing their fullest development.

4
The Views of Spitz

The views expressed by Spitz in a recent volume[6] deserve special consideration.

In this volume this eminent student of infancy summarized lucidly his numerous studies and close observations of many groups of infants, in their own homes, in a variety of institutions and in different cultures. From the observational data he elaborates his view of the psychological and psychodynamic development of the infant from the 'objectless stage' to that of the establishment of the 'libidinal object'. He examines the maturational processes of primitive prototypes of affective and primitive cognitive responses, and of distance perception 'coenesthetic' to 'diacritic', and the role of experience in their development and in the development of the ego.

He draws an analogy from embryology by using the concept of the 'organizer' in this review of the psychological-personality development of the infant in his stress upon the importance for integration of an orderly progression in this mental development. For this purpose he uses data from examples of maldevelopment in a variety of syndromes. The essential role of the mother and her own psychological state—in the 'dyad' of mother-child—in such mental development of the infant is emphasized throughout this presentation.

He distinguishes three 'organizers' of the infant psyche, three 'concomitant critical modal points', the outcome of each of which is a 'restructuration of the psychic system on a higher level of complexity' (p. 118). They are periods of integration, a process, delicate and vulnerable. If successfully established and consolidated at the appropriate level, each of these turning points, or organizers, are signs that the infant's development can proceed in the direction of next organizer. If 'the consolidation of an organizer miscarries, development is arrested' (p. 119). Although maturational processes, far less susceptible to external influence than developmental processes, continue at a steady rate, a disturbance in the unfolding of the infant's personality follows. In short an imbalance arises in the equilibrium between the forces of development and those of maturation.

The first of the three organizers is said to occur at about three months of age; its indicator is the smiling response only to the need-gratifying sign gestalt of the nodding upper portion of the human face. The rudimentary ego at this age is limited to perceiving, recognizing and responding with the smile but it cannot discriminate between friend and stranger nor protect the child from danger. As long as mother acts as an auxiliary external ego, this rudimentary ego, despite its limitations, operates adequately.

The second organizer appears at from six to eight months of age and its indicator is a variable degree of anxiety at the approach of strangers. The libidinal object, the image of the mother, is becoming established; the capacity for diacritic perceptive differentiation is well developed. 'The child now clearly distinguishes friend from stranger' (p. 150). This anxiety is considered not a response to a memory of an unpleasant experience with a stranger, but a response to the perception that a stranger's face 'is not identical with the memory traces of the mother's face' (p. 155). It is the operation in which a percept in the present is compared with memory traces from previous experience, an operation of apperception. The mother has become his love object since she is distinguished from all others. The child modifies his ways of dealing with, and acquires greater mastery of, his environment. He has acquired the capacity to judge and to decide, which represents an ego function of a higher, intellectual level of mental development and opens up for him new horizons. Thus there are crystallization of affective response, greater integration of the ego and the consolidation of object relations. Also there is progression of development in the somatic sphere (sensory-motor), in the mental apparatus (increasing number of memory traces and growing complexity of mental operations and hence more diversified directed action sequences) and finally in psychic organization (with ego organization enriched, boundaries between psychic instances being established, and boundaries between self and non-self delineated). A beginning capacity for imitation and identification becomes manifest as well as a shift from passivity to activity.

The appearance of the third organizer is indicated by acquisition of the 'no' gesture and word just after the beginning of the second year. According to Spitz this is a momentous achievement, of a capacity for judgment and negation. It is the child's first abstraction, 'the first abstract concept in the sense of adult mentation' (p. 189). He calls it the beginning of human communication, as result of a process of identification with the frustrator or the aggressor (i.e. with the mother who prohibits after locomotion makes it so often necessary). It is a change from the child's expressions of his affects in contact and in action to the beginning of semantic messages and distance communication. The head movement from side to side in avoidance of food, spoon, nipple, occur from about the sixth month when the child is satiated. However, it is not till the fifteenth month that this motor pattern becomes invested with ideational content by the infant, as a message addressed to another person and is integrated into a communication system.

Of considerable importance for the understanding of the needs of the child during the first year are the studies of Spitz and his co-workers of a number of disturbances in infant development. For the convincing wealth of observational data upon the number of infants and their mothers the reader is urged to read for himself the chapters in the book referred to above. Space here permits only very brief mention of these findings.

Spitz states that, since the mother is the dominant active partner in the dyad of mother and child, disorders of her personality will be reflected in the disorders of the child. Such pathogenic relations he divides into two categories: (*i*) a qualitative or 'improper mother-child relations', and (*ii*) a quantitative or 'insufficient mother-child relations'.

For the first category, the qualitatively disturbed mother-child relations, he does not claim exclusive psychogenic etiology. He states that in some of the diseases some congenital elements could be demonstrated. Nevertheless he emphasizes that neither the congenital nor the psychological factors alone but only the conjunction of two would lead to the onset of the disease in question. In these instances, the mother's personality 'acts as the disease-provoking agent as a psychological toxin' (p. 207) and thus he came to call the diseases the psychotoxic diseases of infancy. He lists six different conditions in this group each of which he related to particular maternal behaviour patterns.

Coma in the Newborn

The first of these diseases is coma in the newborn characterized by, in addition to coma, Cheyne-Stokes type dyspnea, extreme pallor and reduced sensitivity. The appearance of shock required treatment with saline enema, intravenous glucose or blood transfusions. After recovery, these infants need to be taught to suck by repeated and patient stimulation of their oral zone. Both Ribble, who first described the condition in 1938, and Spitz related this condition to primary overt rejection by the mother, who may have milk obtainable by manual pressure, but who states that she is unsuccessful in nursing at times saying she has no milk. In some of the few instances studied, Spitz was of the opinion that the rejection of the mother was not directed against the child as an individual, but against the fact of having a child. In less severe instances in which the mother was both passively and actively rejecting the child, the response was infantile vomiting.

Three Months Colic

The second 'psychotoxic disease' listed by Spitz is a condition known as three months colic in which the infant after the third week of life begins to scream in the afternoon. He may be temporarily calmed by feeding but shows symptoms of colicky pains in a short time. Changing his feedings from breast to bottle or the reverse, or changing the formula, and the use of drugs like atropine seem futile. Although some of these infants have some diarrhoea the stools are generally not pathological. The pains last for several hours, stop and begin the next afternoon. This condition continues until toward the end of third month inexplicably disappearing as it appeared.

After reviewing the work of others on this condition, Spitz concludes that there are two factors responsible for this condition: (*i*) a congenital hypertonicity (of both skeletal musculature and of increased peristalsis); and (*ii*) primary anxious overconcern on the part of the mother. The latter emotional condition of the mother leads her to feed her child at his every sign of distress as if to overcompensate for her unconscious hostility towards the child. Her feeding the child repeatedly increases the infant's excessive intestinal activity beginning a vicious circle since he is unable to rid himself of his tension in the course of nursing. The suggested use of a pacifier by Levine and Bell interrupts this vicious circle in that the infant relieves his tension by sucking without introducing the irritant food into the digestive system. Spitz also suggests rocking the infant which has in many families become an outmoded means of soothing him. The self-termination of this disorder in the third month, this author suggests, comes about as the result of the infant's being then able to provide himself with discharge of his tension through active movements of his own body.

Infantile Eczema

The third condition in this category of 'psychotoxic diseases' infantile eczema appearing in the second half of the first year and tending to disappear between the twelfth and fifteenth month. Some dermatological authorities use the term atopic dermatitis for this self-limiting condition 'predominantly on the flexor side, favoring skin folds (inguinal, axillary, popliteal, cubital, crease behind the ear, etc.) with a tendency to weeping and exfoliation in the most severe cases' (p. 225). In the institution in which Spitz and fellow workers studied this condition there was an unusually high incidence of 15 per cent (among 203 infants) as compared to 2 to 3 per cent among infants reared in their own families or in the usual institutional environment. The attending physician made a variety of therapeutic efforts: modifying the food; prescribing vitamins; topical applications of salves, medicated and unmedicated talcum; careful search for possible allergens in the toiletries of the children, in the substances used for the laundry, etc. All of his efforts proved futile.

Following this Spitz studied 28 infants with eczema and their mothers comparing them to 165 infants free of eczema and their mothers in the same institution. He studied all of them with respect to many developmental and behavioural indices and their condition at birth, the vicissitudes of the mother-child relations including the child's behavioural reactions to them. The results of these studies was the presence of two factors: (*i*) a congenital predisposition of the infants who later developed eczema in the form of an increased cutaneous excitability as evidenced by a statistically significant higher skin hyper-reflexia at birth (rooting and cremasteric reflexes): and (*ii*) an attitude of manifest anxiety about their children in the majority of the mothers of the eczematous infants which anxiety on psychiatric exploration was found to conceal unusually large amounts of unconscious repressed hostility.

Since this was a penal institution to which pregnant, delinquent girls from mainly rural regions were committed for a year after coming into conflict with the law for various reasons such as theft and even murder, it was not surprising that this group of mothers of eczematous children were manifestly infantile personalities. This group of mothers did not like to touch their children, and were concerned about the fragility and vulnerability of their children while often exposing them to real danger of injury. The eczematous infants were thus not only deprived of cutaneous contact of which they had greater than the usual need, and exposed to the unconscious hostile behaviour of their mothers, but also showed lessened socio-psychological functioning in that much fewer of them than of the non-eczematous control group of infants manifested eight-months anxiety. To Spitz this indicated a marked delay in psychic development as far as the appearance of the second organizer was concerned. Successive tests of the eczematous infants also showed a deterioration of social and learning sectors which to Spitz indicated that social relations on the one hand and memory and imitation on the other were influenced. He surmised that permanent traces were left on the later psychic development of these children. Again he thought that after the first year as the eczematous child acquired locomotion he becomes more independent of the chaotic affective signals of the mother and becomes more capable of seeking contact and obtaining satisfactions with things and other persons on his own. Thus his special need may be otherwise satisfied and tends to reduce and remove one of the etiological factors of the eczema.

Space permits only brief mention of the last three of the disorders that Spitz placed in the category of psychotoxic diseases. These three are (*i*) rocking in infants; and (*ii*) fecal play and coprophagia; and (*iii*) the hyperthymic child.

Rocking

The result of his study of those infants who rocked violently and as their principal activity was that these children were exposed to marked oscillation between pampering and hostility on the part of their mothers

These mothers were extrovert, infantile personalities with a lack of control over their aggressions as expressed by frequent outbursts of negative emotions and violent manifest hostility. The babies 'were exposed alternately to intense outbursts of fondling, of "love", and to equally intense outbursts of hostility and rage' (p. 233). They were found to be retarded in the sectors of social adaptation and of manipulative ability. Their mother's inconsistent, contradictory behaviour made the 'establishment of adequate objects relations impossible, and arrests the child at the level of primary narcissism, so that he is limited to the discharge of his libidinal drive in the form of rocking' (p. 249).

Fecal Play and Coprophagia

Spitz gives an excellent description of his observation of a child making pellets of feces from her diaper, smearing them on sheets, offering handfuls of feces to the observer's mouth, passing the fecal pellets from one of her hands to the other, putting them in her mouth and chewing them (p. 250). In a study of 16 such infants, he found the syndrome to occur as early as eight months of age with most falling between the tenth and fourteenth month of life and that in the great majority fecal play was accompanied by coprophagia. Studies of these infants and their mothers compared to infants not showing this syndrome and their mothers revealed a significant positive correlation between depression in the mother and fecal play in the infant. The bulk of the psychoses among the mothers in this institution (which were relatively rare) was concentrated in the group of mothers whose children manifested the syndrome. These mothers showed marked intermittent mood changes toward their children, varying from extreme hostility with rejection to extreme, exaggerated, compensatory oversolicitousness. A large number of the coprophagic children suffered injury at the hands of their own mothers such as burns, scaldings or near-drownings during bathing or being dropped on their heads. The only two instances of actual genital seduction by the mother in the study occurred in this group. In some instances mood reversals appeared in the mothers up to four times in course of one year.

Spitz concludes a detailed discussion of the psychodynamics of the coprophagic child and of his depressed mother by a hypothesis that the mother is lost as a 'good' object to the child upon her depressive withdrawal from him. This blocks the infant's usual fusion of the 'good' and 'bad' object into a normal libidinal object. The infant is said to follow 'the mother into the depressive attitude' (without being depressed himself) acquiring 'her global incorporative tendency, attempting to maintain what he had already achieved in the way of object relations' (p. 261). The fact that the child at the end of the first year of life is at the transition from the oral to the anal phase makes it 'more plausible that the coprophagic infant chooses feces for his incorporative behaviour. . . . In this phase, therefore, an "object" becomes available to the child who has just suffered an object loss; it is an affectively charged object, for it was part of the child's body' (p. 262).

The Hyperthymic Child

The last of the psychotoxic diseases of Spitz's list is a syndrome of which he had the least number to study and belongs in its more full-blown form after the first year of life. It is a syndrome characterized by the child's manipulative proficiency and cleverness with inanimate objects, by a conspicuous retardation in the social sector of their developmental profile, and with a tendency in their second year to be hyperactive, not very sociable, and destructive with toys, uninterested in human contact, becoming hostile when approached. Mothers of these children generally among intellectual and professional circles, have a conscious conflict in their feelings towards their child. The infant is not loved, but serves as a satisfaction for 'narcissistic and exhibitionistic impulses'. The mother, however, feels guilty about this attitude and consciously compensates 'by a subacid, syrupy sweetness'. The fathers of these children, aggressive and successful, tend to be hearty, loud, exhibitionistic in relation to the child, may frequently frighten him by rough handling often over the protests of the concerned mother. Spitz mentions having seen a few of these children almost crowded out of their play pens by masses of toys as the effort of the parents to compensate for their guilt.

Emotional Deficiency Diseases

The second category of Spitz's classification of illnesses of infancy related to emotional factors, as mentioned previously, are the consequences of a quantitative deficiency of mothering. He distinguishes two conditions, anaclitic depression and hospitalism, although he stresses that the first may be a transition to the second depending on whether the deficiency of mothering is prolonged beyond three or five months, and on whether the affective deprivation of the event is partial or total.

Anaclitic Depression. In an institution Spitz called a Nursery in which it was frequent that mothers took care of their infants for at least the first six months, he observed normal good relations with their mothers and good developmental progress during this time in some 170 children. Then, if between the sixth and eighth month a child was deprived of his mother for at least three unbroken months—as happened in the case of 34 infants—the child developed progressively a characteristic disorder. The syndrome did not occur in the children whose mothers remained with the child in the institution. The syndrome was characterized in the first month after separation from the mother by the child's weepy, demanding behaviour with a tendency to cling to an observer who succeeded in making contact with him. All this was in marked contrast to their previous happy outgoing behaviour. In the second month, the weeping of the child changed into wailing; he often became insomnic, his weight decreased and his development was arrested. During the third month of the mother's absence, the child tended to refuse contact with the adult, to lie prone in his cot most of the time (a pathognomonic sign), and to lose more weight. His insomnia set in or increased, his tendency to contract colds was augmented; his motor retardation became generalized; and there was a beginning of facial rigidity. After the third month the facial rigidity—reminiscent of adult depression—became more established; weeping ceased and was replaced by whimpering; motor retardation increased further often replaced the lethargy and the developmental quotient (on Buehler's tests) decreased.

If the mothers returned within two months after the third month of the child's illness, or if the child was supplied with an adequate substitute mother, most of the children with anaclitic depression recovered. Spitz expresses doubt that recovery is complete; he suspects that further study would reveal scars the presence of which would be evident in special susceptibilities. Spitz carefully distinguishes 'anaclitic depression' from depression of adult life, from M. Klein's 'depressive position' and from Bowlby's concept of mourning. He emphasizes too that this syndrome is much more frequent and much more severe if the separation followed good mother-child relations.

Hospitalism. When, however, the separation of the child from the mother lasted longer than five months, the symptomatology of anaclitic depression changed radically and seemed to merge with that of the condition Spitz called Hospitalism with a much poorer prognosis. This was also true if the child was deprived of 'all object relations' during his first year for the same period no matter what the pre-existing mother-child relations had been. The symptoms of increasingly serious deterioration, which seemed in part at least irreversible, were at first those described for anaclitic depression following one another in rapid succession in the first three months. Then a 'new clinical picture appeared': motor retardation was marked, the child became completely passive and lay supine in his cot. He did not achieve the capacity to turn to the prone position; his face became vacuous; eye coordination was defective and expression often imbecile. If motility reappeared it was in the form of spasmus nutans; other infants showed bizarre finger movements resembling decerebrate or athetotic movements. There was a progressive decline in the developmental quotient and by the end of the second year the average quotient in these children was 45 per cent of normal or at idiot level. Some of these observed till the age of four, with few exceptions, were unable to sit, stand, walk or talk. Mortality was high: 34 of 91 had died by the end of the second year.

Spitz concluded that 'absence of mothering equals emotional starvation' (p. 281).

In a concluding chapter this author states (p. 300): 'The misery of these infants will be translated into the bleakness of the adolescent's social relations, deprived of the affective nourishment to which they were entitled, their only resource is violence. The only path which remains open to them is the destruction of a social order of which they are victims. Infants without love, they will end as adults full of hate'.

Appendix

THE GENEVA SCHOOL OF GENETIC PSYCHOLOGY AND PSYCHOANALYSIS: PARALLELS AND COUNTERPARTS

By W. GODFREY COBLINER

Spitz's collaborator in this volume, W. Godfrey Cobliner, supplies a fifty-five page appendix lucidly outlining some of the propositions of Piaget's *psychologie genetique* relevant to the subject of the entire volume. This appendix was added because the authors had occasion repeatedly to refer to the work of Piaget and his associates as 'the only developmental psychology that has succeeded in constructing a coherent network' of principles which, besides psychoanalysis, 'accounts for psychological unfolding and explains behaviour'. This account of Piaget's principal findings and ideas on cognitive development and on the constitution of the permanent object, admittedly brief, incomplete, modest and limited to the first eighteen months of the infant's life, was also added because it was thought to be more useful to the reader of the volume than footnotes or references to passages in systematic expositions of Piaget's work by other authors.

There will be here no effort made to summarize or outline the contents of Cobliner's appendix. The present writer will content himself with an indication of its main topics.

A basic point is made at the outset of the parallel and difference between psychoanalysis and the Geneva School. Both assert that the incentive for adaptive performance arises from the psychological unfolding predicated upon a balanced interplay between intrinsic maturational factors and experiential factors. Piaget's system has virtually no dynamics; conflict of forces is not envisaged as in psychoanalytic theory. Cobliner holds that it is precisely because of Piaget's emphasis on psychological *structures* as the constituent elements of mental functions, that the latter's work 'has yielded data which complement findings by psychoanalysts on child development'.

As a mere indication of Cobliner's consideration of the parallels and counterparts of the similarities and differences, between the two schools beyond this basic point, the sub-headings of the remainder of the appendix will be listed. They are as follows: 'Some Basic Assumptions of Piaget and His Concept of the Psyche', 'The Concept of Stages in Ontogenesis'; 'Piaget's method', 'Developmental Mechanisms in Piaget's System'; 'Piaget's Contact with Psychoanalysis'; 'The Three Concepts of Object in Contemporary Psychology'; 'The Discovery of the Non-I'; 'Object Formation and Object Relations', and 'Indicators of Object Formation'.

The last four sections are a particularly detailed summary of Piaget's data and theoretical inferences about the steps in object formation and contain a closer comparison with psychoanalytic contributions particularly from more recent studies of ego psychology. For these reasons they are especially useful to the student of infantile mental development.

Cobliner closes the last section with the statement that Piaget is not concerned with abnormalities in thinking, cognition, etc., and 'links the origin of mental functioning to the displacement of the individual in the objective environment'. The difference between this and Freud's theory is that the latter 'holds that psychic functioning owes its rise to interindividual relations on the one hand and to derivatives of internal processes on the other'. He thinks that the two system builders encompass the scaffolding of all other schools and that the scope of their 'panoramic view of psychic functioning and development remains unsurpassed to this day'. He concludes finally that Freud's system is the more comprehensive. It includes consideration of psychic spheres beyond the conscious and those of psychopathology.

In a concluding section, Cobliner points to the current trend of the narrowing of horizons in scientific exploration. Much time, talent and collective effort are spent on ferreting out 'piddling details with the expectation that they will lead to the disclosure of great truths'. He laments that 'current psychological efforts are drowned in an ocean of data' and that 'instead of acquiring diversity we have drifted into conformity'. He calls for 'balanced return to the study of the system makers' with the avowed purpose 'to synthesize data instead of merely collecting them'. In this way the natural scientific urge would be revived.

5
The Needs of the Toddler and the Young Child

As in the early months of infancy, the needs of the young child from about the end of first year through the next one or two years are to a considerable extent those expressive of the incompleteness of his bodily maturation particularly of his nervous and muscular system. At the same time whatever degree of maturation of his body has occurred and whatever the development of motor-sensory and mental abilities from experience and practice has appeared, his needs are also those of a budding and unique, individual human person. The former implies that his dependency upon his parents to provide for his bodily comforts is still considerable and his increasing autonomy and independence quite unstable. The latter implies in his greater active, self-assertion about all his emerging wishes that he be regarded with affectionate consideration and tact for his developing self-feelings. It implies, too, his need for gentle but firm guidance to help him learn gradually to obtain satisfactions for as many of these wishes as possible, progressively more and more by his own efforts, in ways which take account of the needs and wishes of others. It is a long road for both child and parents but one traversed by most families with considerable success and satisfaction for all of them.

The wise mother however much she enjoyed the helpless dependency of her baby, comes to enjoy equally his emerging skills for manipulation, for locomotion and for increasing speech. She has changed his cradle, if she used one, to a crib when the baby began to be able to move his body about. She has provided a playpen as he began to creep, climb and manipulate his first toys as an aid to his practice of these skills safely and as much as possible in her presence. She has enlarged his freedom from the playpen to the full room of the nursery gradually and in her presence as he began to walk. These changes were to give him still further opportunity to practise and acquire good nervous integration and muscular coordination on which his sense of freedom is based rather than the amount of space allowed him. The mother in short arranges his play space in which he is safe and the objects in it are his and not those which have to be repeatedly taken away from him by tense adults.

Spoon and cup have been available for him to play with, to manipulate at meals. Self-feeding is permitted and encouraged when his ability is clearly present. This may occur between the eighth and twelfth months. She remains undisturbed if for a time in this learning he is not very neat and even if he puts his hands into his food and into his mouth. She knows his mouth is an important organ for exploring and learning. She feeds him alone apart from the family perhaps past his twelfth month to avoid mutual disturbances of child and family until he has fully mastered the skill of feeding himself.

The mother has gradually lengthened the periods of his play with his toys alone after waking in his crib up to half an hour. However, she does not exclude him if he is awake while she has company or is busy. She has observed that his being alone for long periods or with a new nurse are painful to him before he is two years old. Yet from the time he has begun to talk and walk he has been provided with a room of his own. Thus he does not experience, as he might later, this separation as a rejection. It provides him also with an opportunity to acquire a greater sense of his own possessions and to avoid his becoming sometimes disturbed by being aware and overstimulated, or his feeling excluded and jealous, by sound of parental sexual activities or sights of their naked bodies. His need for the sensuous contact especially with mother is lessened from that of the early months of life when they were vital.

The need for contact with mother and father is of course still intense. But this contact progressively is replaced by contact through the increasing communication between them, through the growing medium of speech, through games of 'pat-a-cake', romping play and the like. The parent's presence in or near the room where the toddler plays with his own toys, close enough to respond verbally, or to soothe a hurt or to reduce any momentary sense of loneliness become gradually more sufficient satisfactions for this need.

Tendency to Regression

During these early two to four years there is a strong tendency to reversibility, a sign of the instability of maturational and developmental processes. As Ribble[3] says, 'much of the baby trails along in the toddler, who frequently needs the privilege of "being a baby" '. Under the stresses of being in pain or hungry too long or too frequently, or of being alone, his tendency to revert to previous behaviour, to lose temporarily or for longer periods skills and abilities acquired, may appear in his behaviour. A child unattended to may suck his thumb, or refuse to eat something especially prepared for him, or show he cannot drink from a cup. Ribble[4] gives some examples. On a walk with a father a toddler may protest being carried across the street, only to demand to be carried if father meets a friend to whom he begins to talk and give his attention. Even a four-year-old feeling somewhat excluded after a day of visitors in the home may climb into her mother's lap in the evening asking to be rocked because she 'ain't big'.

Such regressions may at times develop insidiously, becoming more obvious only after a time in forms of disordered behaviour. This is particularly likely to happen when another child is born and if the older child happens not to have been well-prepared, and if he is not included in some ways by mother and father in their attention to the new born, and if he is not given as much attention, affection and compensatory praise for his own abilities. Such an event to a two- or three-year-old may be a shock and may even go unrecognized by the parents until evidence of its results are noticeable in increased destructiveness, if not direct hostility to the baby, and in eating or sleeping difficulties, in general hyperactivity and increased demands for more parental care and attention.

Sexual Interests and Sensuality

More and more parents are gradually coming to be more clearly and unembarrassedly aware that young children as they grow manifest lively interest, and evidence pleasure, in the sensations and functioning of their own bodies and those of others. The earliest of these are in the sensations in and around the mouth, in the free exercise of their muscles, later in the functions of elimination, urination and eventually also in the pleasurable sensations of their own genitals. They show pleasure in exposing their own bodies and curiosity about the sight of the others. How much of these sensual, erotic interests and tendencies come in to full open expression in activities and in their speech to their parents depends a great deal on their actual experience in regard to them and in regard to their own other impulses for activity, learning and for affection.

While naked or during his bath the one-year-old child's fingers may wander over various surfaces of his own body, nipples, navel and into the genital region. If his hand is not slapped, roughly removed by mother, and if she does not with embarrassment or anxious tension say, 'No! No!' but if she gently diverts the child with a loved toy, such sensuous explorations do not become exaggerated trends nor tend to be pursued in secret. The absence of strong disapproval or anxiety permits the child further expressions of bodily feelings, allows his relation to his own body and to his mother to remain undisturbed. Under these circumstances guidance by the parents remains easier. The other danger of the child's increased interest in his sensual activity is also avoided if parents, from an overreaction to previous generations forbidding attitudes, do not permit free sex play without directing the child to other modes of pleasurable activity.

Similarly if full freedom to roll around naked on a blanket before bath has been in any serious degree thwarted during infancy, the child may later show intense interest in naked dolls, a distressed dislike of being dressed or undressed and have little sense that the body is good.

The pleasurable sensations of elimination and his interest in his feces may likewise not become excessively intense interests in the second year if the mother undertakes toilet training gradually, gently and casually. His enjoyment of being wiped, washed, taken to the potty chair can be an aid to his learning cleanliness if all this is introduced pleasantly without maternal stress. Any interest to play with his own stools can be similarly gently diverted to play with pliable materials such as modelling clay, finger paints, soft rubber toys, or permitting him to play with pieces of dough, or to smear some of his semisolid food, such as cereals, at meal times. Such messing for a time at this age is a natural interest. If the child's interest in 'what the body makes' or in how he can urinate is not too quickly suppressed, these interests are not as likely to become overemphasized. In short if training in cleanliness is pursued by the mother without hurried tension, the child acquires the necessary skills more willingly, though more leisurely, with his active participation and with less distortion of interest in the abruptly forbidden.

Erotic play with siblings or playmates is also better not permitted—with an attitude on the part of the parents as calm as the one previously described in regard to auto-erotic play—so that the child's further development is not disturbed by too-absorbing a learned interest in such sensuality.

Between the ages of three and five the child's sensual interests tend to become more clearly centred in the genitals and self-stimulation occurs quite frequently if it has not been too rigidly prohibited earlier. The child is helped a great deal if he is helped calmly and quietly by his parents not to indulge in such activity in public or with children of other families. During this period in such children there is quite evident interest in the parents' bodies, in their activities together, especially there may be questions about why they sleep together, about how babies are made. If parents reply straightforwardly, simply, without tension in a manner which the child can understand, the child acquires no shame or fear about such functions and experiences little if any obsessive interest in their secret or furtive pursuit. In such situations, too, between the ages of three and six the child may display more openly a strong love of the opposite sex with an urge for caressing and bodily contact.

There is then also an intense rivalry with the parent of the same sex with evidence of an effort to an exclusive relation with the other parent. Statements by the little girl that she will marry daddy and that she will take care of him if mother goes away will be heard. The converse declarations of love from the little boy towards his mother are also common. He may evince a wish to demonstrate to her his ability to urinate or to have her fondle his penis or help him in urination. Since children also continue to need the affection of, and admire the parent of the same sex, the conflict in the child's feelings about each of the parents is not unduly intensified if both parents understand the child's problem. Such understanding consists of simple, sympathetic acceptance of the child's declarations of love, of simple explanations of both parents' feelings and quiet firm non-participation in behaviour which could be construed by the child as a response to his wish. Any resentment of the child about the disappointment of his wish for exclusive possessiveness is similarly discharged and dissipated by the tranquil, non-retaliatory acceptance by the parents of the child's feelings and by their quietly firm restraint of any violent actions.

During the varying phases of these oedipal manifestations any surgery, such as circumcision, tonsillectomy or other painful medical treatment, if not absolutely necessary are best postponed. Any fears about mutilation, particularly of the genitals in either sex, especially if they should follow seeing the genitals of the opposite sex are best relieved by giving the child full opportunity, perhaps repeatedly if necessary, to express them. Even fuller relief to such fears may be afforded by giving simple explanations of both the anatomic facts which he can comprehend and of the parents' understanding the child's retaliatory fear of being threatened with genital mutilation (in the case of the boy) or of having been mutilated (in the case of the girl) by the parent of the same sex for their erotic impulses towards the other parent. Similar attitudes of the parents during this period will often help reduce phobias of animals or of other dangers such as the sight of deformed or crippled persons, or nightmares of monsters symptomatic of the displacement of such retaliatory fears from the parent to such other objects.

Such frank, unembarrassed acceptance of the child's pleasure in his own body, of his feelings toward the parents, giving timely simple and direct answers to questions about sex, birth, sexual differences does much to reduce the intensity of the child's conflicts and helps him to live through to the renunciation of his miniature love affair and jealousy. It helps him as his own bodily and mental capacities mature and other interests develop to identify firmly with the parent of the same sex and with a deeper trust in both of them. Such experiences promote a more integrated attitude on the child's part towards general bodily sensuality, sexuality and learning undistorted by crippling inhibitions on the one hand or by a precocious and exaggerated drive to erotic activity on the other. It also minimizes any chances of the child's *fixation* of inhibited erotic interests to members of his own family, particularly perhaps to the parent of the opposite sex. All this is also promoted by the child's having the privacy of his own room, and by the parents' avoidance of undue fondling, caressing of the child and of their exposure of their own bodies to him.

Aggressive Assertiveness

Whether or not one accepts Freud's assumption that there is an innate, aggressive destructive drive in addition to a libidinous one, there is no question that the behaviour of most, or of many, children after the first year after locomotion is established manifests progressively aspects of an aggressive assertiveness, an obvious delight in the exercise of increasing muscular strength and coordination and a greater readiness (in the change from the passivity of infancy to the activity of the toddler) to revengeful destructiveness in reaction to obstacles and to frustration. The toddler runs and rarely walks. He pushes things about, he snatches them. He builds blocks into towers and knocks them down. He sweeps away his dishes energetically. If thwarted in any of these impulses to activity, he bites, screams and kicks without restraint. Together with increasing speech and mental maturation, the exercise of his muscles brings progressive development of his sense of bodily and mental self and of their boundaries and a gradually increasing autonomy of self-direction and of separation from parents and especially from the mother.

Although progressively able to play with toys and objects more and more on his own, he, of course, still needs his mother's presence or proximity when lonely, her comfort when hurt, her giving him food when hungry. All objects which attract him, but particularly his toys (as well as his mother), are his alone and exclusively. He is also if invited gradually and without anxious, rigid insistence able to participate in his own learning where to deposit pleasurably, and eventually proudly, the products of his body. After two years of age he begins to be ready first to play alongside of, and then later, with other children of his own age.

In the case of most children the mother (as well as the father when he is there) provides ample opportunities, things, places and gently firm direction to all this surge of energetic activity to explore and manipulate things and toys safely. A comfortable toilet chair to accustom him to sit on even when not defecating leads gradually to his using it willingly for its purpose. Large light blocks to build with, empty boxes to play in, and rubber balls to throw, sturdy objects to climb on to in his room satisfy his demanding possessiveness. Kitchen utensils to bang with at mother's side while she works relieves moments of loneliness. Instead of mere insistent prohibition of pulling down destructible things his mother offers him alternative toys or activities. When some activity is difficult or beyond his strength or coordination, she offers help or a substitute to reduce his sense of impotent rage or frustration. If his fretful clinging is born of fatigue she gives him some moments of attention or puts him down firmly for a nap. If it is due to loss of interest in the toy or activity which had for some time absorbed him, she suggests and demonstrates another toy or game. In short wherever it is possible instead of an angry or anxious, 'No! No!', the toddler hears, 'Try this', or 'Try it this way', or 'Like this', before enraged frustration either possesses him, or before he has done some irreparable harm or an unwitting nuisance. Similar attentiveness is given him even when friends and visitors are present to preclude his angry whining from loneliness or of being dispossessed from his parents' attention. To the limit of his gradually increasing comprehension, all problems are discussed, 'talked over' with him and slaps or angry prohibitions then may occur less often.

When playmates at home or in a nursery school are introduced he will receive watchful attention to help him learn not to strike, bite, kick or push too violently such a playmate either when he wants the toy, swing or some other plaything or when he is being dispossessed of it. Instead the mother or nursery school teacher helps both to take turns and thus gradually learn some ways of each getting his wish without violence, hurt and subsequent revengefulness. Similarly when a pet scratches or bites after too much and too painful teasing hurtfulness, his mother will explain after his tears dry firmly, clearly but without blame the sequence and of his part in it. Similarly she will quietly and unhesitatingly restrain and discourage any impulse to bite or strike her or to pull her hair whether this is semi-playful or in reaction to some frustrating prohibition by her. Together with as many opportunities to spend his growing strength in satisfying play such assistance from parents and other adults about how to obtain his wish when this is possible rather than receive punishment for damage done permits him to acquire with many repetitions discrimination as to how, when, where, with whom to expend his energy safely and with satisfaction. Frustrations to his wishes, rage about thwarting, revengefulness about disappointments will then be less frequent aspects of his experience, behaviour and of his subjective state.

One source of outbursts of revengeful aggressiveness in the child two, three or four years of age is the coming of another baby into the family. The threat of losing the exclusive possession of his mother's attention which arouses jealousy is probably very frequent if not universal. What the overt reaction of the older child is in this situation depends on several factors. It depends on his experience and the nature of his relations with his parents before such an event. It depends in some measure upon how he has been prepared for it. It depends a good deal upon how he is treated after the event, in particular whether he is actually a loser in the amount and appropriate kind of affectionate attention and regard for his actual needs and abilities from his parents and especially from his mother. It depends, too, upon whether to the extent of his abilities he is included by the mother in the care of the baby. It depends as well upon whether he receives some 'babying' he might indicate he wishes—even indirectly or in some disguised form—from both parents, again especially from the mother. Furthermore it depends also upon whether he is firmly restrained in any potentially harmful gestures, squeezes, pinches, etc., he makes towards the baby without anxious blaming or punishment. In the latter event it may be important that his parents express clearly their understanding of the natural result of his fear, resentment and of his wish to revenge himself upon the intruder so that no suppression of such feelings leads to a false affectionate pretence in his attitude towards the baby. The development of symptomatic regressiveness in the older child's behaviour may thus be avoided or greatly reduced. Similar alertness and directness on the parents' part may have the same effects upon any displaced hostile attacks upon younger playmates who are not his siblings or upon his own somewhat older siblings.

In summary if the energy of the aggressive surge in second, third, and fourth years of life—perhaps particularly in boys—receives opportunity for exercise in constructive activities which enhances the growth, co-ordination and development of his body; if alert watchful guidance of parents reduces frustrations to such exercise and learning; if the urge to such activities becomes more and more self-directed with progressive mastery of skills; if the anger and revengefulness following some probably inevitable disappointments and frustrations is itself neither condemned, nor anxiously and with vacillation permitted in overt action; but if it is redirected, diverted to other activities or submitted to 'rules of the game' with playmates, or if need be firmly restrained; then the development of hostility, of anxious angry revengefulness, towards self, others or objects need not become a major problem. Instead the flow of aggressive initiative in the service of eager curiosity will flow towards mastery of skills and lay a firm foundation for more intellectual learning later and for vigorous bodily health, growth and development. The general trait of exclusive, demanding possessiveness—whether of mother, of her attention when father or visitors are present, or of his toys or any plaything which attracts him—

may also fade as his development proceeds successfully to his becoming progressively self-possessed in skills and in his learning that he need not lose his turn with playmates, nor that mother is lost to him when he actually needs her. His anxiety about mother particularly is gradually reduced when both father and mother demonstrate their readiness to attend to his real needs without creating any divisive tension between the parents and therefore between each of them and himself.

The Beginnings of a Sense of Self

With the development of locomotion and of progressive mastery of his own body and of motor skills of manipulating objects in his environment, and with the acquisition of speech, there begins in about the second half of the second year the appearance more and more clearly of an integrative trend, of a sense of self, of autonomy, of being a person. As Ribble states it, ' "Me do it" now becomes insistent. Self-knowledge leads to clearer awareness of other selves—of parents as more distinct persons. It paves the way for better self-direction and for making choices in the course of action. Later on it will lead to recognition of cause and effect and to discrimination between what is real and what is make-believe'[3].

When past experience begins to manifest itself as *memory* which leads to evidence of reasoning and this in turn leads to anticipatory action towards a currently desired goal, we may speak of one of the aspects of this integrative trend oriented towards adaptation to reality. In addition to the achievement of general bodily coordination, of hand-eye coordination, the experience of actively participating in his own toilet training is an important part of such self-direction. The increasing capacity to self-expression in speech is another and very important milestone in what can now be called mental growth. This is accompanied by a sharper sense of personal relatedness and this brings a marked progress towards self-awareness. A basic part of this mental self is that of his own body image. This develops not only from tactile, sensual and visual self-explorations, from seeing his own image in a mirror, but also from its use in the described activities with toys, objects, from contact with the differences in the feel of the bodies of his two parents and with playmates or siblings. Learning the names of the parts of his own body is incorporated into this body self image.

Acquiring the skill of self-feeding, of toilet habits, or observing differences in bodily structures of other children, of animals, all add discriminating details to this image. Experience with sensual sensations in his genitals if not associated with frightening prohibitions from parents contribute to this self-knowledge. Any fantasied misconceptions, that there is only one sex, or that the child himself can be both sexes, may become openly expressed verbally to parents when trust pervades the relationship. If such fantasies are listened to with sympathetic, serious attention and not laughed at or ridiculed, if they are answered simply, frankly with gentle correction, a more realistic self-appraisal results and still greater sense of trust and assurance is added to his feeling about himself and his parents. This adds to his eagerness to identify more solidly with the parent of the same sex in his playful imitation of that parent's activities. Such recognition and support in his search for information, knowledge from parents in his experimental play aids the child in his growth towards independence, rationality and self-understanding.

Also important in the interest of the fullest possible growth of such a sense of self and autonomy in the child are opportunities to talk, to ask questions, and opportunities to make choices, decisions, to think for himself. The latter is particularly germane when he is in conflict between his wish to please his parents, to win their approval and his wish to assert himself. When such decisions do not involve matters of any danger to himself, it is integrative for him to experience his parents' acceptance of his decision even when it is contrary to their judgment about its wisdom. If, instead of any anxious coercion to an opposite course, he learns from the consequences of an unwise choice, his sense of independence and capacity for wiser judgment is enhanced for the future. Such tact and restraint on the part of parents, together with enthusiastic approval of his wiser decisions in which his own interest is even better served, adds greatly to his ability to think clearly. If such experiences predominate over those in which he submits out of anxiety of disapproval and those in which he feels a need to rebel defiantly and often self-destructively, his self grows stronger and more assured as he experiences more consistently such opportunities for free self-expression and for self-consideration. Then outbursts of greed, jealousy and possessiveness will lessen in frequency and consideration of others will develop much less ambivalently. On this more solid, internal foundation the child acquires progressively more pleasure from social activities, from the approval of parents and others. He will then find it less and less necessary to cling anxiously to more infantile, bodily satisfactions and to erupt in crude, aggressive self-assertiveness or revengefulness in defence of them.

All such learning by the child is the more thorough, of course, when parents are watchful for clues of readiness for it and responsiveness to it from him. Any impatient imposition of their demands particularly if such demands are in effect abrupt interruptions of any absorbing constructive play on his part may destroy or diminish his pleasure in the new activity demanded by the parent. Although parental direction of the child through his day's programme of activities, meals, rest, bedtime and so forth is necessary, gentle, patient reminders beforehand even of a few minutes often, if not usually, prevent reactions of angry defiance, the tears of impotent rage, or the sullen, dawdling compliance. Such attitudes of the parents coupled with helpfulness to put away the toys, to assist the child in learning skills of self-care in bathing, washing, dressing, undressing, brushing of teeth and so on, and to give the child encouraging attention in *his* doing these or other chores for himself as his coordination makes it possible eventually and gradually builds into his feelings pride, pleasure and satisfaction in their mastery and regular, habitual execution. Learning, the solid growth of the self, in these ways becomes spontaneous, eager, gratifying—a positive urge.

Deviations in Development

In these three or four years such self-development is subject to regressions or slowing in reaction to a variety of untoward events. Physical illness of the child, the necessity for hospitalization, a change of nurses if they are present, the mother's longer absence from the home, the birth of a sibling all may be followed by not only a loss of acquired skills and habits of self-direction but may be complicated by even more severe signs of emotional disturbance. The child's appetite may decrease or become finicky. Sleeping habits may be disrupted. Usually pleasurable toys, games or other play may lose their interest for him. Thumbsucking may recur and toilet habits acquired may be lost or training in toileting may become more difficult. The child may become irritable or unresponsively absorbed in phantasy and withdrawn.

Perhaps a more insidious and possibly a more frequent source of disturbances in development of the child is the occurrence of anxious tension in the parents. Such tension in them may have a variety of causes in their own lives. Threats to their economic security, extra stress at work for the father for any reason to which he is susceptible, his or the mother's illness, or illness or death in the families of the parents, the need to assist financially or to house a grandparent in their home, even a prolonged visit of a relative which disrupts the family's routine or poses an emotional stress for the mother are a few examples of the great variety of events any one of which alone or in some combination may in varying degree be or become with time disturbing to the parents. Even when the stress is primarily experienced by the father and he tries to solve it on his own without 'troubling' his wife about it, he may be sufficiently affected in his usual mood or responsiveness to his wife or child at home so that both and especially the wife may react with some measure of anxiety, emotional turmoil, sleeplessness, decrease of sexual responsiveness or some other more or less neurotic reaction. Such tension in her may then decrease her alertness, responsiveness, attentiveness or patience with the child and his needs. Her guilt about such changes in her attitude or behaviour towards the child only further complicates and generally intensifies the resulting difficulties between them.

It occurs with tragically great frequency that the relatively regressive symptoms and behaviour of the child are then met with some measure and form of punitiveness. Such a tendency to punish as a strained effort to be firm becomes in effect an attitude of inconsistency when the mother overwhelmed by a sense of guilt for punishing the child seeks to redress it by seeking to appease the child in swinging to the other extreme of excessive indulgent permissiveness or removing her expectations of his performance. The child's continuing or increasingly disturbed behaviour and functioning in reaction to such inconsistency tends to intensify his mother's turmoil and may add another measure to her tension: a sense of failure as a mother. Finally, unless the family crisis passes, the child's disturbance may itself contribute to any already existing tension between his parents. Such developments may add a quality of self-perpetuation to the turmoil in all three of them which may continue beyond the period of the duration of the extreme difficulty which gave the episode its origin.

It is likely that perhaps most of such episodes of trouble in the family and in the child's behaviour are relatively minor, of short duration and self-limited. The integrative, realistic efforts of father or of both parents to solve the problem or the threat to their security are in such instances effective and the turmoil in each of them subsides. There may be even something learned from the trouble so that they become better prepared to prevent or to avoid similar possible difficulties in the future or be able to react to them with greater equanimity.

On the other hand in some instances the results of such stress are not so fortunate. This may be so particularly if stresses are recurrent, if one follows another before the effects of previous ones are gone, recovered from, or are not integratively solved. This is especially true if there have been brought in to the marriage neurotic or character difficulties by one or by both parents. The picture then may be different. The disturbance in all three may become a chronic one with only relatively minor periods or degrees of recovery. Or, in the case of premarital personality problems on the part of one or both parents, the occurrence of such stress as previously described during these years of the child's life may serve to exacerbate such personality problems of the parent or parents. Such stresses may even be in part precipitated or self-induced by the personality or character difficulty of the father, the mother or of both. In such situations the intercurrent stress may be less possible for them to solve as quickly or as thoroughly. The vicious circles within each member and between them indicated above tend to continue longer perhaps with fewer periods of relief or lessened tension. The effects upon the child's personality development are easily imagined. Various kinds and degrees of neurotic symptomatology or of behavioural character deviation may persist for longer periods, interfere with integrative development in later life or become more or less crippling characteristic traits for a lifetime. Reduction of such difficulties with professional assistance to the child and preferably to all members of the family is neither always easily available nor always very completely successful even with intensive and quite prolonged therapeutic work.

Development of Character Traits

To the extent that one distinguishes the sense of self, or ego, discussed above from what is rather generally called character as a separate aspect of the personality it may be an advantage to consider the development of such traits more discretely. These traits include those attitudes which are often referred to as standards of behaviour particularly in relation to others: namely, love of truth, honesty, consideration for the rights of other persons, personal modesty and other describable tendencies. In the years from two and one-half to four or five the roots of these character traits gradually become fairly well established.

It is quite evident to most students of human development and behaviour that these more durable characteristics have their origin in those phases of bodily and mental maturation that enable the child in a sense to participate in experiences beyond those of immediate personal and physiological needs. Of course the manner in which these personal and physiological needs are obtained and satisfied are a part of these experiences. As Harry Stack Sullivan put it 'culture invades physiology'[8]. How, when, where one eats, or empties his bowels and bladder, how and when one washes and bathes, and so on become regulated as a result of experience with parents, other adults and other children. These matters become invested with the feelings resulting from such experiences which form the core of the system of self-attitudes and of self-regard. In addition, however, the experiences of the satisfaction and pride of parents and others in what the child learns to do and to know, and how he conducts himself with them, and in play with other children reinforces his own satisfactions in such achievements. The rules of fair play which emerge from these experiences become incorporated into the system of self-attitudes and become an internal criterion of self-esteem.

It is possible to generalize these processes by the statement that character grows within the child through the process of identification with the attitudes of other persons, of course primarily with those of his parents whose affection and approval, or the converse profoundly evoke corresponding feelings in the child. In other words how he is treated by them with regard to all aspects of his spontaneous impulses and behaviour determines in large measure how he will come to feel, regard, evaluate and judge his own impulses and behaviour. How parents react to their child's behaviour naturally is an expression of their own self-attitudes toward similar impulses and behaviour in themselves. These self-attitudes of parents expressed in their reactions to the child's impulses and acts will, of course, convey the degree of integration and mastery of non-destructive modes of obtaining satisfaction for such human needs that they have achieved. This means that any measure of conflict about such impulses for example, as sex, truth, honesty, modesty, or hostile revengeful aggression, persistence in pursuing goals and so forth will also be expressed in the totality of their reactions to the child's behaviour. It is a matter of common experience, particularly clinical experience, that, whether or not such evidences of conflict are clearly in awareness of either the parents or the child, the child's self-attitudes and his behaviour are affected by such conflict. How much the child's character is affected by such conflict is determined by various factors; such as, whether both parents or only one of them has similar or different conflicts, whether one or both have conflicts about the same impulses, whether such conflicts of the parents are persistent or change towards integration and so on.[9, 10]

An example of such dynamic relations between the development of character traits in children and the attitudes and behaviour of parents and others which the writer has found particularly striking and dramatically illustrative comes from Erickson's studies of the child-rearing practices among the Sioux Indians[1]. This example concerned the inculcation of generosity in the children. This was a trait of great importance to social survival when the Sioux roamed the great plains in nomadic bands hunting the buffalo. The satisfactions of many of the basic subsistence needs of these tribes were dependent on the successful and timely kill of this animal. Not only much of their food, but their clothing, housing from the hide and other articles as well and even their fuel from the dried dung came from the buffalo. Thus sharing the fruits of the skill and luck of the best hunters with the rest of the band was not only a matter of high necessity for the group but also a trait of great personal virtue. This was also true of other property in the circumstances of their living.

Erickson's investigations led him to trace the beginnings of the trait of generosity to the earliest periods of the child's experience in life. Nursing at the breast was continued up to from three to five years of age and the child was allowed to nurse and play with the breast whenever he whimpered day or night. Even father's sexual privileges were not allowed to interfere with his wife's concentration on this need of the child. There was no systematic weaning; the child in effect weaning the mother by becoming gradually interested in other foods. As he grew older all his toys and possessions were sacredly his. Even the products of his body were his to do with as he pleased as far as his parents were concerned. Only when he could walk was he taken by the hand by an older child to places designated for such functions, thus being allowed himself to reach a gradual compliance with the rules of cleanliness and modesty.

Even in the days of the tribe's limitation to the reservation by the white government many of these practices concerning generosity continued. The parents did not touch the child's possessions until the child had enough of a will of his own to decide what to do with them. Traders near the reservation reported repeatedly incidents of Indian parents coming to town for long needed supplies with long awaited money, only to grant their child every whim with a smile even to the extent of the child's taking a gadget apart. The parents often returned home without the supplies.

Thus as Erickson concluded, generosity in the Sioux child's later life was not sustained by prohibition but by the examples his elders set in their attitude towards property in general (in giving it away to those who admired or needed it) and towards the child's property in particular.

In general terms any culturally and personally important traits of character in any social and ethnic group are best and most solidly inculcated in the child by his experiencing at the hands of his parents, teachers and other adults those very traits in their behaviour towards him. Hence instead of demanding courtesy (Say 'Please' or 'Thank you') a child learns courtesy and consideration from the experience of being treated courteously and considerately. If he is told the truth whether about sex or any other matter in which he shows interest, he learns to be simply truthful. If a parent acknowledges he has been frightened, hurt or angered by some incident, whether or not of the child's doing, the child learns to be honest, rather than ashamed, evasive or denying, similar feelings of his own. If he observes his parents' persistence in accomplishing a difficult task; if he is given patient considerate help in *his* doing something a little beyond his ability or strength, he acquires the characteristic of persistence. If his privacy is respected by his elders, he comes to respect theirs. If all this occurs rather than shaming, derogation or ridicule; if he experiences justice according to his age, ability and needs as between himself and his siblings and playmates, his self-confidence, his self-respect for his actually attained abilities develops.

Learning to Love

Under such circumstances his self-attitudes will be less coloured by self-doubt and anxiety about his worth. His early jealousy, greed or other aspects of egocentricity will gradually fade. A more benign and optimistic attitude will pervade his character from which his interest in the satisfactions of others will eventually become almost as important as in his own[8]. Love can then more probably predominate over hateful revengefulness and disappointments may than be less likely to devastate him.

It should be emphasized that this more fully developed capacity to love does not appear in the child till probably after the end of the first decade of his life—and then probably it is more likely to be directed towards a chum, a friend of the same sex, rather than towards his parents or his siblings[8]. The fact that the child between two and five or six years of age shows signs of what appears like affection towards parents does not need to seem contradictory. Such feelings of the child are apt to be of rather short duration and quite apt to give way to other interests, or even hurt, anger and even revengefulness the next moment if evoked by some intercurrent provoking event. In short the child at this age is quite distractable in his feelings as in his attention. His displays of affection may be spontaneous and parents may find them charming but they are brief.

He is enjoying himself in activities and in the experience of his own feelings. He is still incapable of constancy towards others, but needs theirs to acquire a similar trait slowly.

The parents' reward is not therefore anything similar to more mature love and affection on the part of the child towards them. It is in his growing alertness and healthy maturing. The capacity of affectionate loyalty on the child's part comes later when he has become more certain of himself and capable of thinking with ease and understanding. It is a considerable achievement in the five-year-old when he acquires some restraint of his hostile aggressiveness and of any sexual urges, and when he can begin to show some affection towards both parents and others in the family. And such development depends in no small measure on: whether there has been a good deal of freedom in the exercise of his growing muscular strength and coordination; whether there has been as much self-direction as possible permitted in toilet training; and whether there has been a minimum of anxious-hostile coerciveness or painful punishment in the early years of this period.

Fears and hatreds of doctors, of medical examinations, of painful procedures and injections and of illness are also possible to reduce with repeated truthful explanations, demonstrations and unanxious soothing by parents. Avoidance of situations which arouse anger and jealousy by parents are of similar importance, as well as their permitting their free full expression verbally by the child when such feelings are aroused. All such experiences reduce the possibility that repressed hatred of the dangerous giants against whom the child feels helpless will develop. Such repressed hatreds—of anxiety, anger and revengefulness—undermine and reduce his genuine love of self and hence for love of others.

6

The Needs of the Child from Six to Twelve—Latency

The needs and interests of the child after the sixth year gradually change in most instances rather markedly. Prior to this period much of his play is an effort to duplicate the behaviour of adults. The games the child plays with his toys are in building towers, bridges and skyscrapers and so on with blocks and boxes; he pushes his toy car as if he were driving it, and rides his tricycle as if he were a fireman or motorcycle policeman. In dramatic play representing family life the boy imitates his father's behaviour; the girl, her mother's behaviour including such details as the inflection of her voice, the occurrences of a coffee klatch, a tea service, or the treatment of her dolls as her children. This occurs with both siblings and other playmates whether at home or in a nursery school.

After the age of six with further maturation of the intelligence the child in most literate cultures begins to spend a large proportion of his waking time away from home satisfying a new interest in school. This is the interest in, and growing capacity to grasp, impersonal and abstract concepts, namely letters, words, ideas and numbers. It is not that some rudiments of spelling short words or even his name with block letters or the counting of familiar concrete personal objects as the parts of his own body or toys, possessions or clothing cannot and has not been learned before the school experience. But progressively there appears a fascination in and increasing understanding of the formal, the symbolic, the abstract, and the relational, aspects of numbers, letters, words, maps and diagrams. There is also a growing evidence of absorption in such real but more impersonal matters like the growth processes of living things, the functioning of machines, and the nature of the universe.

With these changes in interests and drives there appears also a shift of personal behaviour from generally imitating, and wishing to please, the adults closest to him to a greater impulse to conform to the behaviour of his peers, schoolmates and friends. How he dresses, which clothes he prefers and how he wears them now are much more subject to the social dictates outside of the home. The way the hair is worn, cut, or whether it is even combed are much more apt to conform to the style of the child's group of age-mates. Similar slipping away from conformity with the parental standards may be the practice of table manners, of cleanliness, of keeping his room tidy and of dropping clothes and possessions about the house. Instead of the pride in use and mastery of words and verbal styles heard in the parents' speech of the earlier years, there is often a studied avoidance of adult modes of speech. Occasional lapses are heard into the expressions usually considered obscene or impolite if the child dares to use them at home. If not, there is persistent, often seemingly uncorrectable preference for the ungrammatical (even if mastered before) or the slang of his gang.

Personal habits tend to change in a similar direction often irritating to parents: picking of the nose, head scratching, kicking the legs of chairs at table, slamming doors or leaving them open, loud belching and the like. Even firm corrections of these matters by parents arouse surprised attitudes of innocence, or of a sense of mistreatment, or protests of the rigidity of mother's and father's standards. Often too the behaviour continues for long periods as if either totally unaffected or reluctantly changed to be repeated again.

Outside of school, games and play become more impersonal, subject to rules and emphasizing skill and competitiveness. Imitation of mother and father fades and disappears. Instead, dramas of the life of the world, of society at large outside of home are more often played out, such as war, crime and police, secret societies, clubs, cliques and the like.

All this partial overt defiance and rebelliousness against the rules and interests of parents is an aspect of loosening of the more intense libidinal ties to parents, especially with the one of the opposite sex, and of freeing the mind of the child for more academic, impersonal learning. It is an aspect of the renunciation of the more exclusive, possessive and dependent relation to the parent which is generally thought to be more marked in the boy than in the girl. Although it often appears to parents and other adults as if this transformation of interests in this phase (which has in psychoanalytic theory been called the latency period) as if it were an almost dangerous and destructive one, this is usually not the case. The boy progressively identifies with particularly his father, and the girl with her mother, but both express it more and more in the world of their own peers. Standards of behaviour, gossip, criticism of their fellows are quite frequent subjects of absorbing discussions among themselves about members of their group. Efforts to maintain their own self-esteem and the esteem of their group by appropriate conduct—apparently self-imposed—are on close examination often quite strenuous and unremitting.

The sexes tend to separate with apparent overt mutual derogation as a sign of striving to control, if not repress the sensual sexuality. That this striving is not wholly complete is often clear. Evidences of yearnings towards a particular age-mate of the opposite sex kept secret or denied to the group are not uncommon. Apparently hostile teasing of girls by boys, the loud whispering and giggling of girls in the presence of boys are also frequent indications of the underlying continued interest. Secret phantasies of great future achievements of skill and daring are not unconnected with the winning of a particularly attractive and even secretly loved person of the opposite sex. This may be associated with an obviously exaggerated indifference to, or pointed avoidance of, direct personal contact till later years.

Psychoanalytic theory postulates that some of the processes of libidinal transformations are the roots of the drives to learn, to create, to find satisfactions in work. As Spock phrases it[7] '. . . The noblest things that man has thought and made are partly the product of his longing for and the renunciation of his beloved parent'. As a part of this process in the fortunate instances of development, the eventual identifications with the parent of the same sex includes a pattern of the 'spiritual, idealistic and chivalrous aspects of human love'[7] of the grown boy towards the grown girl. Otherwise, if such identifications in fortunate, stable family circumstances do not occur, or occur only with partial integration, sexual drives may be less fused with tenderness, loyalty and with an eagerness to learn to work and to create.

Thus, in the effort of the child in the latter part of his first decade of life to increase his mastery of new skills, to learn and accept as his own rules of interpersonal conduct among his peers may for a time be accompanied by some degree of defiance of parental authority and the setting of some distance between himself and them. This is, of course, not wholly complete except in those instances in which the first six years of life were full of conflict and turmoil within the family. Nevertheless the steps towards autonomy and greater independence of parents indicated previously may be for a time accompanied by a greater strictness of conscience than before or afterwards. Criticism of parents' slips in their speed and manner of motoring, or the correctness of their statements or information may be irritating signs of the striving towards an inner authority. Some of the literal mindedness, the black or white quality of the child's judgments of such parental lapses betrays the sternness of this conscience as well as perhaps some glee that the previous all-powerful authority is in the child's view a law-breaker. It may as in common compulsions of this age—such as not stepping over cracks in sidewalks or counting steps, fence posts etc.— also reflect an effort to ward off from open and direct expression or conscious thought some revengeful hostility towards a parental crossness, impatience or actual injustice.

The Latency Child's Need for Continued Firm Parental Guidance

Even though the child between six and twelve years of age is making strenuous efforts to consolidate an internal mode of self-direction chiefly among his peers, to learn new skills, to systematize his knowledge and often collections of things, his manner of seeking some independence of his parents poses a problem for them. This occurs perhaps more often in the case of the boy than in that of the girl as previously indicated. The child has a tendency to express the more integrative aspects of his development in the world of his age-mates of his own sex and even to keep them rather secret from his family. He has a simultaneous tendency to express his striving toward autonomy in relative non-conformity to the parents' expectations and teachings. This makes it difficult for some parents to see the amount of their child's energy engaged in the more positive and integrative aspects of his personality growth. The behaviour of the child at home, his general attitude and even his complaints to them about their rigidities, unfairness or disregard of his impetuous interests provide a constant stimulus to some irritation, strain and even doubt in both parents but perhaps especially in the mother.

Under such provocative circumstances there may be some oscillation particularly in the wearied mother between a tendency to be excessively insistent about each infraction of a rule of behaviour and a tendency to let slip without correction or reminders too many rebellious acts or omissions of self-care, or of considerate behaviour towards others. Depending on their own earlier childhood experience with their own parents, or on their conflicted and perhaps distorted recollections of these experiences, both mother and father may react in a variety of ways to the contrary, or negative, aspects of the behaviour of their own child. Each may find some different aspect of the child's behaviour as particularly difficult to bear or condone, or on the other hand, as understandable, natural for the child's age and permissible. Such different aspects may be representative either of what is remembered by each parent as a particularly pleasant and useful, or a particularly unpleasant and destructive experience in their own childhood. Each parent may then wish to have it repeated or avoided in the experience of their own child. Such preferences of each parent may or may not be realistic as to the actual need of their own child on any given occasion for his guidance towards integrated development.

It is probably a common occurrence in many families that there is some difference between the parents in emphasis or intensity of reaction to the child's attitudes and behaviour during this period. What matters, of course, is how frequently, how deeply felt, how persistently and how these differences are expressed between the parents and towards their child. If these differences contribute to some already existing tension or estrangement between the parents, or to some strained tension of conflict arising from a source other than the child's behaviour, the variety of malintegrative solutions in the family is legion. Communication between the parents which can lead to mutual understanding, to an agreement both about each instance of the difficult behaviour of the child and what they will each do about it may be partial, inadequate and result in little or no resolution of the problem. Varying degrees of strain, estrangement or violent, open or silent disagreement between them occurs, flares up recurrently or smoulders more or less continuously. Each may be alternately hurt, angry and revengeful toward the other, and be partially shaken in his judgment about the problem presented by the child's behaviour, or self-justifyingly hardened in his own attitude towards it. All this may lead to, or aggravate any existing, difficulties in their sexual relation, in their agreements about other common family matters such as finances, plans for family activities and the like.

In such periods of untoward tensions between mother and father, the child may become more anxious, more confused and alternately perhaps less able to concentrate and learn, or more resentful and rebellious and then even less certain of himself. If the conflict between the parents is prolonged or frequently recurrent, one or the other may tend to win him as an ally in the divisive struggle. The child himself may for a variety of reasons contribute to the formation of such divisive alliances predominantly with one of his parents, or oscillate uneasily between them. In either instance his own development and learning may suffer. If the tense estrangement continues even without divorce or other break-up of family living, one of the parents, often the father, especially if he is particularly preoccupied with his vocational interests, may more or less withdraw from participating in parental decisions about the problems the child's behaviour in the home presents. To the extent this happens temporarily, irregularly or more continuously the child in effect loses the advantage of having two parents interested in him and learning from each. In this event he may acquire a confused conflictful sense of his own sexual identity, of similarly difficult tensions about relations between the sexes or about the likelihood of any fortunate development of marital relations.

Naturally any such unfortunate conflictful development within each and between the parents—or some variety and degree not described above —results in some lessened capacity to assess the actual need of their child for firm guidance, for tolerant acceptance of his intense wish to be part of his own world, and for enthusiastic approval and pleasure in his actual learning and achievements. Perhaps it is true that in the majority of families such conflicts between parents are minimal, rare, or if occasionally occurring, capable of fairly prompt resolution because of the strength of their love for each other, their sense of mutuality and the general similarity of their attitudes towards important matters in life. In these families there is then possible mutual, patient support of each other (especially by the father of the mother at the end of the day) at times of strain and trial in reaction to the repetitive provocative behaviour of the child. With relief of such accumulated tensions in discussions pervaded by a sense of mutual trust, there may follow some renewed sense of capacity to deal with the child fairly, with firm and even with humorous, patient expectations.

Some of the child's wishes are indulged: such as to wear his hair or such clothes as are common fashions of the day for his age-mates, or to participate in some group activities which are potentially constructive experiences—if none of them are too extreme or too intrusive on his other interests, work or obligation. To the extent of the family's actual financial potentialities some of his desire for possessions or opportunities similar to those of his friends are afforded him.

Any exaggerated claims for what his playmates have are carefully discriminated by actual determination, discounted and quite firmly denied. Certain at least minimal rules of behaviour at home are clearly, repeatedly delineated and compliance with them consistently expected: being on time and clean for meals; regular bathing; the consistent care of his clothes, of his bed and room; adequate table manners; courtesy to company in the home; regular times for retirement and arising; and sufficient time with school work. Courtesy and consideration for his preferences whenever possible are extended to him and in turn expected of him, although his tendency to some rebelliousness, defiance and distortion of his parent's attitude is recognized as an aspect of drive towards independence from them.

Any actual act of meanness or destructiveness is firmly countered by correction in discussing with him the actual facts. His independent strivings are encouraged as with money for an allowance with clear stipulations as to what are his responsibilities with it for his own needs. Despite his grumblings or repeated neglectful omissions of them, certain regular chores within his abilities about the house are assigned and he is consistently, courteously reminded about their performance. Opportunities to earn extra money for extra work about the home or outside of the home are welcomed if they are not beyond his ability or his other schedule of activities. Occasional work on tasks beyond his own ability *with* the parent of the same sex may be an important integrative experience, if not too long, arduous and done in an atmosphere of friendly cooperation.

All such experiences with parents in which the child's reluctance and rebelliousness in verbal form is accepted calmly but with a quiet expectation of compliance in deed is greatly reassuring to the child in this phase of development. It is not uncommon for a child who senses some hesitation, uncertainty or deeper conflict of the parent to become more uneasy and unconforming and defiant. It seems at times as if he were by such behaviour demanding clearer definition of his own independence. Although it may never be acknowledged by him openly he may come to experience parental vacillation and inconsistency as evidence that their love for him and interest in him are deficient. Also important to the child is to experience an even-handed justice at the hands of both parents as between himself and his siblings[10]. This is important not only as regards possessions, privileges and interest and affection from each parent but also as regards differences, quarrels, or even fights which arise between siblings. The usually wise parent discriminates carefully which differences and disagreements are best permitted to be settled by the contestants themselves, when to intervene, if at all, in actual physical contests and when to examine carefully the contribution of each to the disturbance. It is not rare that in such events neither child has the status of being the wholly innocent victim of totally unprovoked, revengeful, hostile aggression of the other.

Gradually, very gradually, such attitudes of parents begin to bear fruit in the child's development of acceptance of their attitudes towards him as his own towards himself. This development in his more spontaneous behaviour may first become evident outside of the home with his peers, at school, in the homes of his friends, or friends of the family. Finally courteous and considerate behaviour may be more evident at home in the presence of company. Eventually as his own sense of achievement in learning at school, in the development of his own skills in sports and hobbies, in the winning of his own status in his group and a more solid self-regard, he may show gradually somewhat more regularity of orderliness and considerateness in his life at home towards his parents and siblings. But it may simultaneously be true that as he approaches adolescence his confidences, greater intimacies, deep and more open expressions of friendly interest may be reserved for one or a few chums of his own age and sex.

7

Summary

In our present state of knowledge, the needs of children for their emotional health vary in kind and degree from the newborn phase through infancy, early and later childhood. These needs vary at bottom with the characteristics of the given stage of biological maturation. These maturational processes continually require responses from the human environment—primarily the child's parents, but others as well—which promote, enhance and give direction to them. This interaction of the biologically given potentialities with the nature of the human reactions results in what is known as development of personality. Some of these interactions of the child with his family members have been described as operating either in the direction of his progressive integration of personality functioning and others, in the direction of maldevelopment. It is not claimed that factors other than these biologically given potentials and the human response to them are the only ones, or always the most important ones, which determine the degree of mental health of the child. Genetically determined factors as well as acquired, impersonally determined disease have been excluded from consideration. In the absence of these last named factors, which perhaps is at least frequently the case, the maturational and developmental processes discussed are in all probability the significant ones—even if additional future information and knowledge may modify them from those described herein in one or another respect, direction or combination.

One final point made in the discussion throughout—is that the developmental process of the earlier phases affects those of later periods of life. This, too, is no news to the student of biology and no surprise to the student of human development.

REFERENCES

1. ERICKSON, E. H., 1950. *Childhood and society.* New York, W. W. Norton and Co.
*2. FREUD, A., 1965. *Normality and pathology in childhood; assessments of development.* New York, Internat. Univ. Press.
3. RIBBLE, M. A., 1955. *The personality of the young child; an introduction for puzzled parents.* New York, Columbia Univ. Press.
4. RIBBLE, M. A., 1943. *The rights of infants.* New York, Columbia Univ. Press.
5. ROSS, J. B., and McLAUGHLIN, M. M., Eds, 1949. *The portable medieval reader.* (Salimbene, Part 3, 'The Emperor Frederick II'.) New York, Viking Press.
6. SPITZ, R. A. (in collaboration with W. G. Cobliner), 1965. *The first year of life.* New York, Internat. Univ. Press.
7. SPOCK, B., 1964. *Dr. Spock talks with mothers—growth and guidance.* Greenwich, Conn., Fawcett Publications.
8. SULLIVAN, H. S., 1940. Conceptions of modern psychiatry. *Psychiatry*, 3, 1.
9. SZUREK, S. A., 1949. An attitude towards (child) psychiatry. *Q. J. Child Behav.*, 1, 22, 178, 375, 401. To be published in Volume II of Langley Porter Child Psychiatry series entitled *Therapeutics and Training in Child Psychiatry.* Palo Alto, Calif., Science and Behavior Press.
10. SZUREK, S. A., 1948. The child from two to ten. *Nursery J.*, National Society of Children's Nurseries, London.

* This volume came to the attention of the writer too late to be read and digested. Its author's prominence in the field leads the present writer to include it in the above list to call it to the reader's attention.

VII

DEVELOPMENTS IN PSYCHOANALYTIC THEORY AS APPLIED TO CHILDREN*

S. Lebovici

Director of the Centre Alfred Binet, Paris

1
Introduction

Psychoanalytical theory has contributed considerably to our knowledge of normal and pathological development in childhood. Sigmund Freud showed in his early work the advantage that could be derived from the psychoanalysis of adults in reconstructing childhood experiences. After believing, at the beginning of his career, in the stories told by his patients of fantastic traumatic experiences, usually sexual, Freud drastically revised his early theories, for he came to understand that our knowledge of the past as reconstructed by psychoanalysis is based on fantasies elaborated from our childhood experiences[12].

At the same time, at the beginning of this century, Freud described the case of little Hans, a first attempt to apply psychoanalysis to a child aged 5 years suffering from horse phobia[9]. In the following years, in various clinics, psychoanalytical treatment of children was initiated, studying at the same time its indications and methods. After the first world war, differing theories were developed by two schools of child psychoanalysis. Melanie Klein's school extended the indications for psychoanalysis to numerous cases of younger children, whose play activities were studied. The other school, that of Anna Freud, limited psychotherapy to the few cases where it was indispensable and where it could be carried out taking into consideration the particular characteristics of the child's

---

* Translated by Maria-Livia Osborn, Research Assistant, The Institute of Family Psychiatry, Ipswich.

psyche, and its dependence on the family; psychoanalytical treatment, in consequence, had to be modified. One might say that the development of child guidance clinics in the Western world was the result of these attitudes. In a large number of cases psychotherapy derived from psychoanalysis is carried out, while at the same time helping the parents by the 'social casework' method, which is also partly dependent on an understanding of the dynamic relationship which develops between the social worker and her client.

After the second world war, some psychoanalysts became interested in the direct observation of infants in their family and in institutions. Thus they showed the dangers of early maternal deprivation, but at the same time they were able with other psychoanalysts, to attempt to integrate psychoanalytical principles and theory in our biological and psychological knowledge of children. This movement led to the description of an analytical psychology of the child in England and in the U.S.A. (Anna Freud[6], Hartmann, Kris and Loewenstein[14]). In France the attempts to integrate psychoanalysts into our neuro-biological knowledge are known under the name of genetical psychoanalysis (Ajuriaguerra, Diatkine and Badarraco[1]).

Although the direct observation of children by psychoanalysts does not contradict our general knowledge of childhood development, and although psychoanalysis has clearly shown the interactions between maturation phenomena and childhood experiences, one should not forget that psychoanalytical theory insists on the economic aspect of the organization of personality, i.e. the way in which early impulses become elaborated. This constitutes the essential aspect of Freud's metapsychological theory, to which it is essential to refer if one wishes to grasp the importance of the contribution of psychoanalysis to our knowledge of children.

Thus, rather than give numerous examples of the application of psychoanalytical theory to children it seems to us preferable to choose a few limited examples. First, we will devote our attention to a detailed account of the contribution of psychoanalysis to our knowledge of object relations in childhood. We will then show how psychoanalysts can understand and use the child's fantasies in psychotherapy. Finally, we will examine the clinical applications of psychoanalytical theories to our knowledge of child development and child pathology.

2

Object Relations in Children

There is scarcely any recent publication more or less directly inspired by psychoanalysis which does not make some reference to object relations. Psychiatric nosography, whether concerning adults or children, has certainly been renewed and made more precise by these studies, which have introduced a *relational dimension* to the classical description of symptoms. It has given new meaning to the idea of historical continuity and to personality organization. It is the basis of a dynamic typology, and is of the greatest value in structural studies.

Child psychiatrists with a psychoanalytical training were naturally interested in object relations. Through a full understanding of its origin they showed how external reality, which has a structuring role, intervenes in the development of behaviour and explains the maturation process and the integration of the developing functions of the nervous system. It is through a study of object relations that psychoanalytical knowledge can be integrated into a general biological study of child development. Interest in psychoanalytical studies of object relations is probably not as recent as is generally believed, for Freud realized the importance of the problem, and was not content to simply define the psychological object as the goal of our impulses. From his earliest metapsychological studies, Freud realized the great importance of the object. In the chapter devoted to the destiny of the impulses in metapsychology, he shows how the infant begins, gradually and in proportion to his development, to distinguish between internal sources and external sources of stimuli. This is the basis of recognition of objects which may be defined as follows: *the object is 'cathected' even before being perceived*.

A certain number of publications have been devoted to a study of this fundamental hypothesis, and we will now present a systematic appraisal of them (Spitz[18], Ajuriaguerra, Diatkine and Badarraco[1], S. Lebovici[16]).

In order to do this it is necessary to consider the condition of the newborn infant, which Spitz describes as relatively isolated from the outside world, owing to a raised threshold of perception. Its state is characterized by what has been called the *pre-objectal stage* and corresponds to the primary narcissistic stage as defined by psychoanalysts. In order to define it, one may refer to the term of *non-differentiation* used by Spitz. The infant is not differentiated from its surroundings, and can feel maternal care only as part of itself. Ajuriaguerra, Diatkine and Badarraco described in the following way the neurological state of the infant at this stage.[1]

1. The muscle tone consists mainly of hypertonicity of the limbs, which are in flexion, contrasting with the axial hypotonia.

2. A certain number of external or internal stimuli may bring about movement of the limbs in a longitudinal direction. Two hypertonic reactions may be demonstrated:

- (*a*) diffuse tension states, with movements of extension and flexion of the limbs, which correspond in fact to a sort of displeasure reaction;
- (*b*) Moro's reflex characterized by opening of the arms in an embracing attitude, and a temporary axial hypertonia which may be triggered off by a certain number of sudden stimuli, especially by a vertical fall or falling backwards.

3. A certain number of reflexes show that external stimuli may act only under certain conditions, thus the bucco-lingual reflex which is not prominent until a long time after the previous meal. It disappears when the infant is fully satiated, which shows the influence of external events on the most primitive reflexes.

Thus at the beginning of life the infant's responses depend on its needs and requirements, internal and external stimuli are only perceived when they break the barrier of tranquillity. One may therefore speak of a state of dissatisfaction, in order to contrast it with the normal requirements of rest and quiet.

The responses of the newborn seem already to correspond, according to the laws of conditioning, to the stimuli arising from the environment. It is therefore right to say that the first stimuli come from the object, not so much as a libidinal object in the psychoanalytical sense, but as an object acting on deep sensibility: for example, the modifications of equilibrium which have been observed by Spitz: 'If, for example, after the eighth day one lifts a breast fed child from the crib and places it in one's arms in the nursing position (that is in a horizontal position) the infant turns its head in the direction of the chest of the person, male or female, who is lifting him. By contrast, if the same infant is lifted from its crib in a vertical position the turning of the head does not take place.' The cues become more and more specific, but up to the beginning of the second month the infant recognizes food only when hungry.

At the end of this period, the human being commences to take his place in the infant's surroundings. From then onwards he is perceived visually, and what we have called the narcissistic stage gives way to the following stage: thus if an adult approaches a crying baby at mealtime, it will calm down and offer its mouth.

The hypothesis of this initial stage, which we have called the narcissistic stage, is derived directly from psychoanalytical theory and the writings of Freud. In *Metapsychology*[10], this author has contrasted the narcissistic stage with the objectal stage.

'Let us imagine ourselves in the position of an almost entirely helpless living organism, as yet unorientated in the world and with stimuli impinging on its nervous tissue. This organism will soon become capable of making a first discrimination and a first orientation. On the one hand, it will detect certain stimuli which can be avoided by an action of the muscles (flight), these it ascribes to an outside world; on the other hand, it will also be aware of stimuli against which such action is of no avail and whose urgency is in no way diminished by it—these stimuli are the tokens of an inner world, the proof of instinctual needs. The apperceptive substance of the living organism will thus have found in the efficacy of its muscular activity a means for discriminating between "outer" and "inner".

'Originally, at the very beginning of mental life, the ego's instincts are directed to itself and it is to some extent capable of deriving satisfaction for them on itself. This condition is known as narcissism and this potentiality for satisfaction is termed auto-erotic. The outside world is at this time, generally speaking, not cathected with any interest and is indifferent for purposes of satisfaction. At this period, therefore, the ego-subject coincides with what is pleasurable and the outside world with what is indifferent (or even painful as being a source of stimulation).'

The important footnote to this text must also be remembered: 'More, the primal narcissistic condition would not have been able to attain such a development were it not that every individual goes through a period of helplessness and dependence on fostering care. . . .'

The narcissistic stage thus corresponds to an early period of life, when the newborn lives in a state of relative indifference to the outside world, against which it is to some extent protected by a high excitatory threshold. It is thus internal stimuli which reflect its needs and which express themselves during its periods of waking and crying, which take on a rhythmic character linked to the early stages of conditioning. There is no object which can be distinguished; the outside world and in particular the mother are not objects, although she feels herself requested personally by a child whose reactions begin to take on a specific character in her eyes, as she hears and understands its crying.

It is important to underline here, in connection with crying, that if the mother is not an object for the newborn babe, the latter is, however, a significant object for the mother. For her the manifestations of her child take on a communicative value.

Early Precursors of the Object: the Smile

During the whole period from birth to the age of 3 months the activity of the mouth plays an important role. Spitz[20] and Andre Thomas[21] studied by direct observation the behaviour of newborn infants. The whole outer part of the oral region responds to stimuli by movement of the head towards the stimulus, combined with movement of the mouth. The function of this response serves to introduce the nipple into the baby's mouth, thus 'the inner part of the mouth, the oral cavity, fulfils the functions of participating in perception, both from the inside and from the outside'. All perception commences here in the oral cavity, which serves as a bridge from inner perception to external perception. In this unique organ many senses are represented, and grouped together in a single area. Here we have touch, taste, temperature, smell colour as well as deep sensitivity involved in the act of swallowing (Spitz[20]). At the same time, and in some way projected on this primitive function of the oral cavity, three subsidiary functions participate in the act of feeding.

(*i*) The hand by its continuous movements of the fingers which seize, scratch and claw the breast.

(*ii*) The labyrinth. The newborn feels the placing in position for feeding as an interoceptive stimulus, with all the vagueness, the diffuseness and lack of localization characteristic of protopathic sensations.

(*iii*) The external skin surface, the importance of which will be realized by reference to our knowledge of those stimuli which can provoke irritation and disquiet in the newborn.

Thus the primitive and complex intra-oral experience consists of absorbing food whilst enveloped in the arms of the mother and grasping her breast. This series of factors, which become organized from feelings triggered off by a physiological need, bring about a perceptual experience during feeding. Distant perception, which is the origin of cognitive processes, is probably organized in the same way.

We will now see how, as it grows older, the newborn infant is able to understand the significance of waiting for its food. *The mother's face*, which it now recognizes, signifies, as he knows, *the bringing of food to its mouth*. Perception of distance becomes both the mother's face and the food which she brings; the child becomes vaguely conscious of its oral and manual activities.

In the elaboration of this *perceptual function* thus intervene:

(*i*) *Perception of what is outside* through our senses and nervous system.

(*ii*) *Intero and proprio-ception* instinct is associated with these functions.

It is the presence of an affect which gives value to the experience. At this time, i.e. at age 3 months, the newborn probably does not perceive either a playmate or any other person, because individuals are interchangeable. He perceives only a stimulus; it is not the whole human face which forms this stimulus, but a 'gestalt' that Spitz calls a 'gestalt signal', which is made up of the forehead, eyes and nose, the whole in movement. This has been proved by the fact that the child ceases to smile when the face is slowly turned into a sideways on position, and is then no longer recognizable by him. In the same way one may obtain the same significant smiling response in the conditions which have just been described with a paper mask. Spitz has called this gestalt a *pre-object*. Already, at the age of two or three weeks, the child when approached by a human face will follow its movements with concentrated attention. When the child is at the breast, it fixes its eyes invariably on its mother's face, during the period of suckling, but its interest in the human face is crystallized around the third month with a specific and significant smile, which proves that the newborn child attaches a particular importance to the approach of a face.

At this time the relational means of the newborn have evolved: the hypertonia has diminished while some degree of axial tonicity has appeared. Organizational activities become more marked, and are less dependent on need than they were previously. Unpleasant stimuli, which were until now inoperative, begin to provoke more and more specific reactions. Towards the fourth month coordination between vision and hand-movement appears.

Recognition of the Object and Anxiety at Eight Months

After the third month, the child shows its displeasure when the human partner abandons it, but not when it is deprived of a toy. The latter deprivation only incurs displeasure from 6 months onwards.

From this age the affects of pleasure and displeasure come to play a more and more intricate role in the organization of various psychic processes. Between the sixth and eighth month the diacritical discrimination having improved, the child no longer replies with a smile to anybody and everybody; he distinguishes between the people he knows and strangers. If one approaches him in an active way and he does not know the person, he manifests his displeasure by a characteristic form of behaviour, either he cries or screams, or he hides himself completely and hides his eyes, remaining quite inhibited.

Spitz describes this behaviour as the prototype of anxiety. It occurs after the affects of displeasure have provoked successive and various effects:

(*i*) During the first weeks of life, one may note very primitive manifestations of displeasure, which are states of physiological tension in response to internal disturbances. As we have seen in connection with crying, they take on an expressive value for the people around and especially for the mother.

(*ii*) During the second trimester of life, fear reactions appear. It is directed at an object in the child's immediate environment. It represents flight before a true object.

(*iii*) Anxiety proper corresponds to the phenomenon described above, and may be observed from the sixth to the eighth month. When a stranger approaches, the child is disappointed not to see its mother, and the anxiety which he manifests is not due to a previous unpleasant experience with a stranger, but is due to an intra-psychic perception of the non-identity of the stranger with its mother, of whom he is therefore deprived. It is therefore a response to an intra-psychic perception and the reactivation of a desire tension.

It is therefore possible to say that during the second half of its first year, when its mother ceases to be only a value for the child, and becomes the one who is progressively recognized as the person who gives or refuses care, object relation is created, the beginning of which characterizes the foundation of the psychic organization, i.e. the power to imagine an absent object. From this point of view one can say that the invested object founds the ego, its recognition allows the organization of the rudimentary mechanisms of identification.

This decisive advance in the relationship between mother and child, this beginning of a differentiated object relation, occurs at a time when the development of the child is considerable. The muscle tonus becomes modified, the original hypertonicity has practically disappeared and the axial tonic activity enables the sitting position and eventually the standing position to be adopted. The primitive reflexes have entirely disappeared. At this point the activity of the hands becomes quite marked, owing to the fact that the primitive reflexes have disappeared.

The body image organizes at this period the somatic framework for our projections and perceptions, integrating the sensory phenomena into a wider whole, which is constantly renewed, as Schilder[18] has shown. It is precisely at this time that the child begins to recognize itself in a mirror. The joyful reactions to this self-observation suggest that the recognition of the permanence of the object and of one's self occurs at precisely the same time as the appearance of anxiety, associated with the discovery that a stranger's face is not that of the mother. One could continue to show how progress in the recognition of outer reality continues to play a fundamental role in the organization of the child's personality, but at the moment when one may speak of a specific and differentiated object relation, there appear the characteristic signs of the elaboration of what psychoanalytical theory calls the Ego.

The Origins and Beginnings of Semantic Communication

Rene Spitz has particularly studied this problem in his monograph, *No and Yes*[19]: 'during the whole first year of life, although its relationship with its mother is very active, the child does not use semantic symbols and even less words'. Until the sixth month the child perceives messages coming from the mother mainly through the sense of touch, but after the changes which occur under the influence of the second organizer, the perception of the object, certain messages from the mother are understood at a distance. On the child's side appear the first pre-linguistic phases, which may be divided into two periods.

(*i*) That of the cry and moan. This is an articulated expiratory noise, which accompanies the tonic reaction to displeasure.

(*ii*) Lallation appears from the second month onwards. These are articulated sounds which become more and more numerous and are emitted particularly during periods of euphoria, whilst the reactions of displeasure cause a regression to the primitive scream, which as we have already seen, is a significant sign for the people around.

(*iii*) After the sixth month the lallations take on a more harmonic character, which the infant separates into true phases. There is a playful element, which the keen observer will not miss. At the end of this first period one may see the first elements of a significant recognition of other people's language but it consists of simple groups of sounds, which are significant only in a given situation with the mother. True language is not yet present, but the sound symbols take on a value related to satisfaction.

It is then remarkable to note that during the first early months of this reciprocal communication which establishes itself between mother and child, the mother produces symbols, both verbal and extraverbal which become gradually significant for the child. In the case of the latter they organize certain linguistic manifestations which take on significance for the mother. The significance which she gives them will influence the course of the object relation.

In his monograph Spitz shows how the mother, little by little, uses language in her relationship with the child. The 'no', which means prohibition, is first of all accompanied by gestures, until the infant understands the verbal prohibition. Very often he then imitates the negative shaking of the head, which is part of the mother's action. For the child this gesture becomes a symbol and a vestige of the maternal frustration action, whereas the words which the child first of all uses represent what he wants, whether his mother or his bottle, the negative sign and the word 'no' constitute the first concept that the child himself can use, that of negation and refusal in the strict sense of the word. Spitz considers it as the third organizer in the development of the child's personality, and explains it by a dynamic process of identification. Each time the mother says 'no', the libidinal object inflicts frustration on the instinctual drives of the child and provokes its displeasure. The somewhat specific affective charge which accompanies it ensures the permanence of the memory trace of the gesture and of the word 'no'. The infant does not tolerate without resistance being forced to return to the state of passivity, and the affective charge of displeasure separated from the presentation which first accompanied it, provokes an aggressive tendency, which will be caught up between the opposing forces of activity and passivity, of displeasure and of aggression. The infant will use the method of defence by identification, which is essential at this age, particularly the form described by Anna Freud[6], with the term 'identification with the aggressor'. This identification with the mother saying 'no' is a milestone in the development of the individual. It is the beginning of reciprocal changes of intentional communications directed with the help of semantic symbols.

It is also possible to find the first traces of this symbolic movement of negation when one studies the reflexes of rotation and sucking, to which attention has already been drawn. In the young infant, a few weeks old, asymmetrical stimulation of the lips sets off a rotatory movement of the head. If the stimulation becomes symmetrical the mouth closes and sucking commences. Rotation and sucking are mutually exclusive. At six months these rotary movements reappear in a different situation; the 6-month-old infant, once fully satiated, turns its head from one side to the other in order to escape from the nipple, the spoon or from its food, using the same rotatory movement which it used as a newborn infant, but now the movement is transformed into a flight gesture or gesture of refusal.

This behaviour, although expressing refusal, is not directed at any person specifically. It is the expression of a state of satiety in the infant.

At the semantic stage of the 'no', which becomes organized at about the fifteenth month, the congenital motor pattern of this rotatory movement is used for the abstract concept of negation. The motor pattern, the genesis of which has been retraced, becomes therefore integrated in a system of communication.

By studying the first smile, the organization of a specific and differentiated object and the beginning of semantic communication, we have tried to show how recent psychoanalytical studies link the progress in development and the influence of the environment, both specific and non-specific, represented by giving or denying by the mother. The relationship between the mother and her child, at first non-specific and pre-objectal, becomes objectal and is then a direct relationship with the most subtle factors, which can have decisive or even disastrous consequences. The psychoanalytical studies which followed the second world war have emphasized the consequences of maternal deprivation, from the time when there is a differentiated object relation, i.e. especially from the sixth month onwards. Rene Spitz has described the anaclitic depression of hospitalism[19], whilst John Bowlby has made a more systematic study of the consequences of deprivation of maternal care[3]. The popularization of these studies has certainly contributed to important changes in the organization of crèches and day nurseries; at any rate certain criticisms have become manifest concerning the theoretical ideas of Bowlby. Thus in the collective publication of the World Health Organization on the re-evaluation of effects of maternal deprivation[23] Margaret Mead defines the critical point of view of the cultural anthropologist. She shows that a continuous and exclusive relationship between the mother and the newborn child is possible only under the very artificial conditions of urban life, in which the practice of production of food outside the family home is associated with contraception. In primitive societies the mother is forced to help outside the home, which causes an interruption of this relationship[1], she has to look after other children, and participate in the collection of food for the family group.

Under these conditions one can confirm Bowlby's thesis according to which separation from an exclusive maternal figure has a negative effect on character. But Margaret Mead refers to other types of society and shows that group care as practised in the kibbutz in Israel does not have the negative effects which one may suppose. However, certain studies seem to indicate that children brought up under these conditions present both an excessive sensitiveness to the behaviour of their parents, and a disturbing dependency on their companions. On the other hand, a study of large families of the Chinese or Indian type, where numerous women and even young girls and elderly women share in the care of the children, seems to confirm the observations made on so-called primitive societies, that this way of bringing up children offers a feeling of security and encourages fertility.

As is well known from other sources (in particular the researches of Harlow[13] on the results of raising two groups of monkeys in contact with artificial nursing mothers, one group supplying the food, by a system which deprived the newborn of skin contacts by covering the mother monkeys with wire netting, and the others allowing skin contacts, with dummies covered with velvet), it is possible to note the importance of sensory stimuli in the organization of the object relation.

The large number of experiments that have been carried out on animals have led some authors to use ethnological references, e.g. in the case of Bowlby, who in his study[3] of the nature of the links between mother and child insists on the fact that the child is attached to its mother right from the start and the emotional attachment becomes differentiated during development. The development of the successive processes occurs when conditions are satisfactory, according to the ethnological laws of internal release mechanisms. When conditions are not satisfactory the development of these processes may be arrested. Previous stimulations cannot activate development or can do so only with great difficulty. Thus, in his most recent publications, this author has partly given up the theory that progression in differentiation of the object relation is a consequence of the dependence of the newborn on its mother and on its environment. Here, in this second theory, the mother is the essential source of stimulation which enables the instinctual drives to be set off. This theory supposes that there exist from the start some links between mother and child, and Bowlby declares himself in agreement with those holding this psychoanalytical theory, which was particularly well illustrated by Ferenczi in *Thalassa*[5], where he expresses the idea that the whole sex life of man is characterized by an attempt to return to the original fusion with the mother; and again by Balint[2] who described a phase of primary union between mother and child.

The study of child fantasies through their play activities will show, however, that a theory of development of relationship is essential to understand them, and to eventually use them in psychotherapy applied to children of this age.

3

Child Fantasies

Child psychoanalysts often use in therapy various play methods, which may shed light on their functions. Many authors have insisted on what these games may reveal to the observer; whilst playing, the child reveals himself spontaneously, and is unable to hide his feelings.

An activity which has an obvious importance in the eyes of the child must be considered both as an expression of the ways in which his personality has become organized and as a basis on which it will subsequently become organized. Freud studied a case in his essay on psychoanalysis entitled *Beyond the Pleasure-Principle*[11]; a play sequence which he followed in a boy aged 18 months, it was his first game, and Freud, who lived in the same house, studied this child over a period of several weeks. This child was playing with a reel which he held by a thread; he held the reel with considerable skill over the end of his bed, and when the reel disappeared he pronounced the sound 'O-o-o' which sounded rather like the word 'fort' (far). When he pulled on the string and made the object come back again he pronounced the sound 'A-a-a' which recalled 'da' (there). Freud gave the following explanation for this game:

'It was related to the child's great cultural achievement—the instinctual renunciation (that is, the renunciation of instinctual satisfaction) which he made in allowing his mother to go away without protesting. He compensated himself for this, as it were, by himself staging the disappearance and return of the objects within his reach. It is of course a matter of indifference from the point of view of judging the effective nature of the game whether the child invented it himself or took it over on some outside suggestion. Our interest is directed to another point. The child cannot possibly have felt his mother's departure as something agreeable or even indifferent.'

A study of this play sequence, which has already given rise to numerous commentaries, shows clearly the evolution of object relations as explained previously. To the extent that the child only perceived the object when he needed it, whilst he could see it, one may say that the game consisted of making the object disappear whilst secure in the knowledge that he could make it come back again. This is evidence that the child was aware of the permanence of objects. As the game becomes inscribed within the framework of a symbolic activity, it is of course not necessary for an adult to be present for the child to be fully satisfied. With the progress of object differentiation, the game becomes more and more a symbolic procedure in order to master the painful relations with introjected images.

This single example shows that it is essential to place the understanding of games and of their underlying fantasies within the context and progress of the organization of the personality and of the ego of children.

This is not the position adopted by Melanie Klein and her pupils, according to whom the child's play allows him alone to understand the content of its fantasy life[15]. According to Melanie Klein, the play content is in fact identical with masturbatory fantasies which are in this way satisfied. It may be in this way compared with dreams, and like them have the same function of satisfaction of infant desires. Thus, the personalization of play is a sign of non-inhibition of fantasies; the objects of personalized play are, according to Melanie Klein, the projection of objects partially internalized. Melanie Klein in fact believes that in the development of its aggressive and libidinal instincts, the very young child feels the desire to destroy, and the fear of being destroyed by the objects which are partially incorporated in this circular process. Thus, she demonstrates that the game is not only a means of satisfying desires, but also a triumph and mastery of a painful reality, through a process of projection on the outer world. Whence the aphorism 'the game transforms normal child anxiety into pleasure'. The game then, according to Melanie Klein, becomes a direct representation of the struggle of the survival instinct against death, of the struggle between good and bad objects.

The above author has the merit of having shown us how the cruelty of certain games, typical of children, lead us to understand their fantasies, where both aggressive and libidinal drives are mingled. The mother is, in fact, conceived as a closed fortress which it is necessary to tear open and break up, in order to seize the precious contents, whilst at the same time the child fears the same attack on himself. When the games continue during psychoanalysis of a so-called precocious child, i.e. about 3 years old, the patient often gives this reciprocal aggression an excremental content. He imagines that his mother is refusing him a precious food, which becomes transformed within him in excrement, because she is bad.

From these child games and subjacent fantasies Melanie Klein, in the later years of her life, described a position which she called central depressive, within evolution, during the later part of the first year of life, divided into two stages: the first called paranoid stage, where the child is afraid because of its aggressiveness, that its mother will make it suffer its own wishes, i.e. to be torn to pieces, and a second depressive stage, when the child is afraid of having disturbed its mother's integrity and attempts to reconstruct it. This central depressive position, which all children go through, becomes the kernel of all later psychoses, and justifies the frequent use of psychotherapy.

In a study which we carried out with Diatkine a few years ago[17] on the genesis of child fantasies, we showed that the fantasies, described by Melanie Klein, and which concern the partial object, brought us back to various early stages of object relations like we have described. As it is possible to understand the genesis of object relations, one can understand the genesis of these fantasies by comparing their evolution to that of neurobiological development, which necessitates that the maternal object should become differentiated according to certain vicissitudes, which are linked to the conditions of pre-maturation in the newborn.

However, contrary to what Melanie Klein says, this does not of course imply that the infant is conscious at this time of a parental couple responsible for its extremely precocious Oedipus complex. In this same study we have attempted to place what one might call 'oedipification', i.e. the moment at which the child is able to grasp the importance of the father's role in his life. When it is capable of differentiating between father and mother, one may imagine that the child invests its father with its own desires, i.e. those where it seeks to unite itself with its mother as closely as possible on the oral and anal levels. The child, then, no longer feels frustrated by its mother, but by its father, and experiencing within himself, if a boy, a phallic impulse, attributes the frustration which he is suffering to the phallic power of his father. This is the moment when the Oedipus complex becomes organized, and becomes, from now on, the central core of his fantasy organization.

The knowledge on the nature of children's fantasies obtained during psychoanalysis of children through their games does not in any way allow us to discover their origin. We have attempted to show only that our knowledge of the development of the object relation enables us to understand the particular character of these fantasies. The methodological error committed by Melanie Klein is to conclude that the nature of the fantasies indicates their origin. To begin with, we are able to place the probable start of the child's fantasy life, at least such as we understand it in our adult psychology; it is the moment when, becoming conscious of himself because he has become conscious of the permanent nature of the object, the child is able to hallucinate, i.e. to manipulate its image in the same way as he probably does during the period of anxiety at 8 months as we have previously described.

A whole series of publications of the American structuralist school (Hartmann, Kris, Loewenstein[14]) have shown that the organization of fantasies depends on the progress of development of the ego. These functions of the ego become manifest only at a relatively late stage. The earlier stages of object relations correspond to the stage of non-differentiation. At the pre-object stage the child learns to differentiate between what is himself and what is not himself; the self of the outside world. The ego only begins to function at the end of the first year. The systems of defensive organization evolve in chronological order, but become systemized only from the moment when the Oedipus complex appears. It is at the acme of the latter that morals and prohibitions, the super-ego, become organized. The changes in the structural organization of the personality, which finally rests on the tripod, described by Freud in the first part of his work[6], the id or instinct reservoir, the ego or homeostatic state, and finally the super-ego, appendix of the ego, which plays the role of censor, prevent us to manipulate during psychoanalysis, child fantasies, as if they remained, quite apart from any historical or developmental contest, in the earliest stages of personality development.

In practice, the child psychoanalyst must be very careful in his play interpretation. The picture of a closed fortress may not necessarily be recalled by early relationship with the mother, but may represent a desire of the child to protect itself against the curiosity of the psychoanalyst. The drawing of fighting scenes may be understood in various ways; in its deeper aspects it is possible that a combat may be the representation of a fantasy of what the child imagines about the sex relations of his parents, but the combat also represents an activity which causes both fear and pleasure to the child, when in order to fight against the anxiety that determines aggressiveness in his fantasies, he uses the mechanism of identification with the aggressor. These various considerations are not only of technical interest in stressing the care necessary in the interpretation of child games and fantasies; they also show that the depth of the regressions which express themselves in fantasies is not necessarily due to events which occurred at the earliest stage of our lives. This idea has already been discussed at length by Freud when he attempted a reconstruction of infantile neurosis, which he described in 'The Wolf Man'. The fantasies, which express themselves in child games, have been elaborated throughout their history, but are also re-elaborated during the therapeutic relationship which cannot fail to play a role because of the attitude of the adult, who watches the child's game without participating. We must here recall Winnicott's maxim, according to which the depths of the fantasies do not bear any relationship to their early organization[22].

Psychotic children provide an example which makes this clear; it is common in such patients, quite apart from games, to see fantasies expressed very crudely. Some verbalize their anxiety in ways which recall the fantasies of tearing up, as described by Melanie Klein. Often they see themselves torn apart and cut in pieces, and express at the same time their sadistic aggressiveness in the form of a desire to tear up, pull to pieces and rip open. They do not hesitate to say that they have been submitted to such treatment by their own mothers when they were babies. The richness of these fantasies enables us, in the absence of ego organization to understand the nature of the relationship between mother and child, when this relationship does not evolve normally. Nothing, however, enables us to postulate that these fantasies are linked to certain periods of life, and that the child had organized these reciprocally destructive fantasies at the end of its first year. The fantasies of the psychotic child enable us, however, to reconstruct some of the experiences that have occurred between mother and child during the first few months of its life.

In various meta-psychological descriptions Freud had already distinguished between the secondary system of functioning when the thought becomes elaborated in fantasies, and the primary system which characterizes the function of the Unconscious, and becomes established in the undifferentiated relationship between mother and child at the time when the child and the mother nourishing it constitute a single unit. The psychosomatic physicians, who, in France, have recently become recently interested in child psychology, have noted in the children they have examined a remarkable poor fantasy life, which they describe with the term 'operative thinking' (Fain[4]). These children are incapable of imagination or dream production, and can speak of themselves only with reference to practical things, such as the time table of their day, the regularity of their physical life etc. The operative thinking of psychosomatic patients is the proof that they are not able to organize their fantasy life, to the extent that their instinctual drive is not expressed in their fantasies. It is thus to some extent through their bodies that they express their impulses, hence the changes in psychosomatic function. This very recent theory tends, therefore, to focus on the importance of the moment when fantasies become elaborated, i.e. the moment which we have defined in the object relation as the time when the child organizes its ego from its knowledge and manipulation of the maternal object.

Thus, through the most recent theories, if one wishes to understand the psychological development of the child, one is led to attach importance to the earliest phenomena of development and their vicissitudes. It is for these reasons that we have decided to present in the third part of this chapter some recent publications devoted to the study of child development from a clinical viewpoint.

4
Recent Psychoanalytical Studies of Child Development

It is not necessary here to stress the contingent nature of symptoms in child psychiatry. The study of conflicts is no longer necessary in diagnosis unless one refers to the types of organization through which they express themselves. Similarly, when one observes children's play for diagnostic purposes, the display of crude products of fantasies shows that they are not fully integrated, but does not enable one to assume the existence of a pathological state. In all events, it is necessary to know the stages of development, which have been explored in several recent psychoanalytical publications. Anna Freud devoted herself particularly to this problem in her recent book: Normality and Pathology in Childhood: Assessments of Development[8]. In another paper published at about the same time[7] this author studied how psychoanalysts can help in the diagnostic field of child psychiatry. Anna Freud showed the danger of child psychoanalysts concentrating too much on the understanding of the deeper layers of the mind. Numerous children, for example, are able to reveal their dreams, which express very directly their desires (fulfilment dreams). Fantasy (day dreams) also give us information about libidinal development, for example, this is the case when a boy reveals his heroic fantasies as the translation of his male desires. The fantasy of being abandoned and adopted (family romance) indicates a disillusionment with the parents. Certain fantasies of being beaten lead us to understand the sado-masochistic fixations at the anal level of infantile sexuality.

This material could lead psychoanalysts to discover the unconscious content of child games. Although they have to be careful as therapists to obtain the complete cooperation of the patient, i.e. overcome his resistances, before revealing to him the content of his unconscious, the same flair should lead the psychoanalytically orientated psychiatrists to abstain from brutal analysis in order to arrive at a diagnosis and in attempting to determine the deeper significance of play activities.

Since the description of defence mechanisms as defined by Anna Freud, the diagnostician generally becomes interested not only in the deeper content of the material, but also in the derivatives of the unconscious which express it. It is well known, for example, that certain tendencies are repressed and that the absence of difficulty in some sectors (for which the parents should be congratulated) does not exclude the question of repression. When, for example, the parents declare that a child is particularly affectionate with its brothers and sisters, one may ask oneself whether he is not repressing his jealous aggressiveness towards them.

But at the same time the existence of systemized defence mechanisms expressing themselves in the form of a reaction should not be considered, at least in children, as specific of a particular pathological organization. For example, when a child is examined by psychiatrists of the psychoanalytical school and the parents complain of his excessive meticulousness, of his fear of being dirty, of his tendencies to collect things, etc., one is in the presence of an obsessional organization which constitutes a reactional formation against repressed sadistic anal tendencies. It is then necessary to ask oneself if these tendencies do not express certain stages in development; it is also necessary to carry out a complete examination, because such obsessional tendencies may co-exist with impulsive or uncoordinated manifestations, or other symptoms of a psychosomatic character which may constitute other personality tendencies.

In the light of psychoanalytical studies on child development, diagnosis must take into consideration the reaction formations, which become obvious through anamnestic reconstitutions (in particular during the preliminary interviews with the social worker) and by direct observation of behaviour. In her study, Anna Freud gave as an example the timidity which may appear as a reaction formation against exhibitionist tendencies, which could have developed at the phallic stage. Inversely, an exaggerated and aggressive pseudo-virility (manliness) may be a compensation for the fear of castration.

But it is also a good thing to study the history of these various reaction formations. Certain are long lasting, only because they are encouraged by the parents (for example, excessive cleanliness when the mothers suffer from the same reaction formation to cleanliness). Others are only temporary, and seem to depend on the normal history of the organization of the ego (for example, at the age of 3 years, when the anal fixation becomes developed, one may often observe true rites of cleanliness, which are of passing character and without significance).

In games a similar behaviour, or similar interests, do not have the same significance at different ages. To take only one example, the way in which a child plays trains, or plays with a small car, may reveal many things. If he enjoys pretending that an accident has occurred, one may say that he expresses his aggressive concept of sex relationships, as Melanie Klein has pointed out; but one can also say that he is attempting to express symbolically the danger which he feels as a result of his aggressiveness, if he has already reached the stage that psychoanalysts call the latency period. Later, by repairing the cars that he has broken, he may show his attempts at sublimation of aggressive tendencies, which have become more social.

Similarly, a particular interest which expresses itself in the behaviour may not necessarily be the result of a fixation. One may take as an example feeding habits which often have different meanings. Some refuse to eat, and can lead to a study of difficulties at the anal level, when the child refuses certain articles of food because of their colour, or their odour etc. The refusal of everything which is not of vegetable origin may be due to the existence of a struggle against cannibalistic fantasies.

The graph of the development of the child is not always regular or linear; certain regressions are normal, or even desirable. When during an illness for example, he refuses to behave reasonably, becomes capricious, and reveals his need of his mother. If he remains a very good child, if he accepts without complaint unpleasant medicines, painful injections, he may simply reveal how his feelings of guilt are relieved during his illness, which is considered as a punishment.

It is not possible to multiply examples, and remain within the limits of this chapter, but it was useful to mention a few in order to show how the psychoanalyst can use the results of his observations for diagnostic purposes, by avoiding to attach to child behaviour, either observed or reconstituted with the help of his parents, a significance which does not take into consideration the variations in development.

One can even go so far as to say that observation of the child gives the analyst certain information which is best obtained directly. The way in which the child starts to play, and especially the way in which he accepts the end of play, shows how he separates pleasure and fantasy from reality. Psychotic children continue to play during the period of latency, in the same way as much younger children, without taking into consideration either the reality or their surroundings.

Psychoanalysts of the structuralist school have shown how certain autonomous functions of the ego became clear through a history of conflicts and vicissitudes of the instincts. Children who are seriously disturbed express their conflicts directly in a mixture of colours in a drawing, although other children, whose mental function is much more normal only obtain an aesthetic pleasure (autonomy of the ego).

These few examples show how psychoanalysts, without abandoning the study of intrapsychic conflicts, have learnt to take into consideration the different stages of development, and use the findings of diagnostic observation which can be prolonged and repeated in order to derive the maximum value from them.

5
Conclusion

At the beginning of this century psychoanalysts revealed the importance of sexual instincts first, and aggressive instincts later, thanks to a laborious reconstruction during the psychoanalysis of adults. Later psychoanalysis was applied to children and confirmed these studies of the richness of the instinctual life of children.

In this study we have tried to show the efforts of psychoanalysts to integrate their knowledge with that obtained in child development:

1. *On the genetic plane* psychoanalysis shows how the environment acts very early on the development, which cannot be understood simply by reference to a process of maturation.

2. *A study of fantasies in children*, in particular through their games, has enabled us to reconstitute the cruel world of their early experiences, elaborated through secondary processes, but in order to understand them in the clinical field it is necessary to refer to the various stages of development.

3. *Observation of children* is essential in diagnosis, in order to avoid giving a definite value to symptoms and games without taking into consideration particular modalities which are linked to the particular way in which the child has developed.

REFERENCES

1. AJURIAGUERRA, U., DIATKINE, R., and BADARRACO, G., 1956. Psychanalyse et neurobiologie. In *Psychanalyse d'aujourd'hui*. Paris, Presses Univ. de France.
2. BALINT, 1949. (English translation.) Love for the mother and mother love. *Int. J. Psychoanal*, 30, 265-73.
3. BOWLBY, J., 1952. *Maternal care and mental health*. Geneva, W.H.O.
4. FAIN, M., 1966. La médecine psychosomatique chez l'enfant. *Psychiatr. Enfant*.
5. FERENCZI, S., 1938. *Thalassa, a theory of genitality*. Albany, New York.
6. FREUD, A., 1948. *The ego and the mechanism of defence*. London, Hogarth Press.
7. FREUD, A., 1965. Diagnostic skills and their growth in psycho-analysis. *Int. J. Psycho-anal*, 46, 31-38.
8. FREUD, A., 1965. *Normality and pathology in childhood, assessment of development*. London, Intern. Univ. Press.
9. FREUD, S., 1950. *Collected papers*, vol. 3. London, Hogarth Press. Analysis der Phobie einer fünfjährigen Knaben. *Ib. psychoanal psychopath Forsch*, 1, 1-109.
10. FREUD, S., 1925. *Papers on metapsychology. Collected papers*, vol. 4. London, Hogarth Press.
11. FREUD, S., 1955. *Beyond the pleasure principle*, vol. 18. Standard edition of the complete psychological works. London, Hogarth Press.
12. FREUD, S., 1954. *The origin of psychoanalysis*. London, Hogarth Press.

13. HARLOW, H. F., 1962. The heterosexual affectional system in monkeys. *Am. Psychologist*, **17**.
14. HARTMANN, H., and KRIS, E., 1945. The genetic approach in psychoanalysis. In *Psychoanalytic study of the child*, vol. 1. London, Intern. Univ. Press.
15. KLEIN, M., 1932. *The psychoanalysis of children* (translated by A. Strachey). London, Hogarth Press.
16. LEBOVICI, S., 1961. La relation objectale chez l'enfant. *Psychiatr. enfant*, **3**, 1. Paris, Presses Univ. de France.
17. LEBOVICI, S., and DIATKINE, R., 1953. Etude des fantasmes chez l'enfant. *R. franc. Psychan*, **18**, 108-55.
18. SCHILDER, P., 1950. *The image and appearance of the human body*. New York, Intern. Univ. Press.
19. SPITZ, R. A., 1957. *No and yes; on the genesis of human communication*. New York, Intern. Univ. Press.
20. SPITZ, R. A., 1965. *The first year of life*. London, Intern. Univ. Press.
21. THOMAS, A., 1954. Ontogenèse de la vie psycho-affective. *L'encéphale*, **4**.
22. WINNICOTT, D. W., 1954. Transitional objects and transitional phenomena. *Int. J. Psycho-anal.*, **34**, 89-97.
23. World Health Organization, 1962. *Deprivation of maternal care* (A reassessment of its effect). Geneva.

VIII

SOME RECENT DEVELOPMENTS IN CHILD PSYCHOANALYSIS AT THE HAMPSTEAD CLINIC*

JOSEPH SANDLER

M.A., Ph.D., D.Sc.

Research Psychologist and Psychoanalyst, The Hampstead Child-Therapy Clinic; Senior Lecturer, Department of Psychiatry, Institute of Psychiatry, London; Senior Lecturer in Psychopathology, Academic Department of Psychiatry, The Middlesex Hospital Medical School

AND

JACK NOVICK

M.A., Ph.D.

Research Associate, The Hampstead Child-Therapy Clinic

The Hampstead Clinic (or more properly, the Hampstead Child-Therapy Course and Clinic) is a psychoanalytic centre in London devoted primarily to training, therapy and research in the field of child study. Training and research are extensively integrated, and the Clinic provides diagnostic evaluation and intensive psychoanalytic treatment for a substantial group of children.

The Clinic differs from the traditional child guidance clinic in that its orientation is wholly psychoanalytic. It is unique in that the bulk of the treatment provided takes the form of full psychoanalysis. In this each child is seen individually five times a week for sessions of 50 minutes, over an extended period of time. Work with parents occurs in a variety of contexts

* This Chapter is based on material from a number of sources, including the Clinic' unpublished Annual Reports. The function of the authors in respect of Parts 1 and 2 ha been principally to collate and organize this material, but they are responsible for th report on Clinic publications in Part 3.

simultaneous analysis of parent and child is frequently undertaken where necessary and as part of a research project; advisory interviews with parents whose children are not in analysis may be the chosen method of work; or parents may be seen at suitable intervals where the child is in analysis. Very detailed records are kept at diagnostic and therapeutic levels, and these records form the basis for psychoanalytic research, in which both staff members and students participate (A. Freud, 1959[16]).

The contributions to psychoanalytic theory and practice made by the Hampstead Clinic cannot properly be evaluated in terms of publications alone. As a highly active institution its influence on psychoanalytic views and work is spread in many ways—through the ongoing development of its staff members (many of whom also have appointments elsewhere), through its teaching activities with special professional groups (e.g. paediatricians), through those individuals who receive specialized training in child psycho-analysis and in the techniques of psychoanalytic research, through its impact on the many visitors who spend varying periods of time at the Clinic or who bring their own research problems for discussion, and through the circulation of many unpublished reports as well as those which find their way into print. It follows that any description of the Clinic's scientific contributions should, if it is to set the work in its proper perspective, include a historical account of the Clinic's development as well as an indication of its present organization and structure.

1

Historical Development

The Hampstead Clinic as it is today can be seen as a direct descendant of the war-time Hampstead Nurseries, directed by Anna Freud and Dorothy Burlingham. The Nurseries provided war-time homes for children whose family life had been broken up temporarily or permanently owing to war conditions (Burlingham and Freud[7, 8]; Freud and Burlingham[33]). Attached to this war nursery was a theoretical and practical training course for children's nurses and teachers. The Nurseries closed in 1945, and a number of those who had worked there undertook further training as psychologists or as psychiatric social workers in order to qualify for work in the increasing number of child guidance clinics being set up in Great Britain after the war. They were given work in various centres, and because of their earlier experience at the Nurseries felt that the additional training in psychology or in psychiatric social work they had obtained was insufficient preparation for the child therapy they were called upon to do. They felt an acute lack of a more thorough and comprehensive training in child psycho-therapy (including personal analysis), and as a consequence brought pressure to bear on a number of senior psychoanalysts for the formation of a formal child therapy training course.

As a consequence of this, and with the help of Dr Kate Friedlander (then in charge of the West Sussex Child Guidance Service), Miss Anna Freud founded the Hampstead Child-Therapy Course in 1947. Eight students enrolled, most of them former Hampstead Nursery Workers. Personal analyses, lectures, and seminars were provided by a group of psychoanalysts (members of the British Psycho-Analytical Society) who had been associated with Miss Freud in her previous work.

Since the beginning of the course, a new group of some four to eight students has enrolled nearly every year. The Course has changed in a number of respects over the years, but the essential requirements of a personal analysis during training (five sessions a week), supervised child analytic cases, attendances at case conferences, and lectures and seminars (both theoretical and practical) remain as basic requirements. Students have come from many countries besides Great Britain.

With the increase in the number of students and the growth in the scope of the Course, an urgent need was felt for a Clinic in which students could treat children psychoanalytically and which would serve as a centre for the research projects arising out of the consideration of various clinical problems. In 1951 a sum of money was donated and a house bought. This new building opened early in 1952, and at the time of opening, the Clinic staff included Miss Anna Freud as Director, and Dr Liselotte Frankl as psychiatrist-in-charge. Drs A. Bonnard, J. Stross and W. Hoffer acted as honorary Consultants. With the qualification of the first group of child-therapy students, a number joined the Clinic staff (as part-time therapists, educational psychologists, and psychiatric social workers).

The major concern of the new Clinic was the referral and selection of suitable cases. From the outset, cases were accepted for treatment on the basis of students' needs and the research interests of the Clinic. Initially these included studies of the interrelation between the mental disorders of mother and child, the comparison of analytic findings with the observed facts of early development, and the analytic investigation of children deprived of their parents' care from an early age. In the following two years a number of special research projects developed. Among these were the analysis of borderline children and analytic observation of autistic children; the analysis of children with some constitutional organic defect (such as bodily malformation or blindness); and studies of problems of diagnosis, not merely as a preliminary to treatment but also as a means of working towards the establishment of a more precise classification of childhood disorders.

With the expansion of the work of the Clinic, another house was acquired in 1956, and opened on 6th May, on the occasion of the Freud centenary commemoration. A further house was acquired in 1967.

An extensive community service, based in three houses in Maresfield Gardens is now available for research and training. The financial support for these services comes from a number of research foundations*; small sums are donated by parents of children in treatment and other donors. The services are not part of the National Health Service.

2

The Clinic

Clinical Services

The Clinic is under the medical direction of Dr Liselotte Frankl and Dr Clifford Yorke, assisted by other psychoanalytically trained psychiatrists. The staff includes 17 trained child-psychotherapists, two psychiatric social workers, and two psychologists. A number of psychoanalysts work part-time, attached to specific research schemes.

The majority of accepted cases, usually 50 to 70 in treatment at any one time, are seen five times weekly. Less intensive treatment is offered to a few selected cases (child guidance and mother guidance). Treatment is carried out by both staff and students, the latter under the supervision of trained analysts and child therapists.

While all other schemes and projects of the organization work in comparative independence of one another, the Clinic serves, and is used by all departments. The diagnostic service of the Clinic is at the disposal of all other services and all research projects depend on the Clinic for their case material. The diagnostic formulation on each new case is presented at the weekly diagnostic conference.

As far as work on the clinical cases is concerned, the double purpose of giving service (through therapy) and of increasing knowledge and experience (through research) is guaranteed by the fortunate circumstance that in psychoanalysis the method of therapy is identical with a method of investigation. Consequently, every case accepted for treatment, for whatever reason, becomes automatically a case also serving research, and the

---

* The Hampstead Child-Therapy Clinic has been supported by the following foundations: American Philanthropic Foundation, New York City; Annenberg Foundation, Philadelphia, Pa.; Gustave M. Berne Foundation, New York City; Lionel Blitsten Memorial, Inc., Chicago, Ill.; H. Daroff Foundation, New York City; The Division Fund, Chicago, Ill.; Field Foundation, New York City; Ford Foundation, New York City; Foundation for Research in Psychoanalysis, Beverly Hills, Cal.; Foundations' Fund for Research in Psychiatry, New Haven, Conn.; Freud Centenary Fund, London, England; Grant Foundation, New York City; The Estate of Flora Haas, New York City; Lita Hazen Charitable Fund, Philadelphia, Pa.; A. and M. Lasker Foundation, New York City; Leslie Foundation, Chicago, Ill.; Walter E. Meyer Research Institute of Law, New Haven, Conn.; National Institute of Mental Health, Bethesda, Md.; New-Land Foundation, New York City; Old Dominion Foundation, New York City; Overbrook Fund, New York City; Pack Kahn Foundation, New York City; Psychoanalytic Research and Development Fund, New York City; William Rosenwald Family Fund, Inc., New York City; William Rosenwald Foundaton, New York City; William Sachs Foundation, New York City; J. and M. Schneider Foundation, New York City; Philip M. Stern Foundation, Washington, D.C.; W. Clement and Jessie V. Stone Foundation, Chicago, Ill.; Taconic Foundation, New York City.

Q

material derived from it is used as such systematically, without the two purposes interfering with each other.

The fourfold orientation of the Clinic towards training, therapy, prevention and research is reflected in the selection of cases for psychoanalytic treatment, which fall roughly into four categories:

(i) Children with typical infantile neuroses, suitable for treatment by students as part of their clinical training under the supervision of senior analysts or child therapists.
(ii) Children with gross but incipient disturbances treated to prevent the development of severe abnormality.
(iii) Severely ill children sent for skilled therapy by other clinics where psychoanalytic treatment is not available.
(iv) Cases serving research projects such as adolescents, handicapped, blind or orphaned children, and mother-child couples.

In both the diagnostic and therapeutic work with children we are primarily interested in the ways in which the child has departed from the normal course of development, and in the possibilities of restoring the child to a developmental path that will ensure his progression through all the stages necessary for successful development. The therapeutic approach adopted is therefore oriented towards removing, as far as possible, the hindrances to progressive development and adaptation.

Preventive and Educational Services

*Nursery school.** The Nursery School is intended primarily for a small group of normal children from 3 to 5 years of age, but it is sometimes attended by children who are in treatment at the Clinic. Intake is becoming increasingly geared to the assistance of families whose external circumstances are likely to impinge detrimentally on the development of their children; e.g. where housing conditions are inadequate. The development of normal children, the first signs of pathology, and the conflicting demands of education on the one hand, and therapy on the other, are discussed regularly in the Education Unit (a discussion group which nursery school and clinic staff attend jointly).

Nursery Group for Blind Children.† In keeping with the research interest of the Clinic in the development and psychoanalytic understanding of blind children, nursery and pre-nursery groups have been established for these children. We have found that no mother is normally equipped for the task of raising, unaided, a child with a severe physical handicap such as blindness. The service helps mothers to understand the different needs of their young blind babies and to observe them as they go through the various stages of development.

* Teacher in Charge: Mrs M. Friedmann.
† Teacher in Charge: Mrs A. Curson.

Well-Baby Clinic.* A medico-psychological service is offered to mothers and young children with special regard to aspects of preventive work. Guidance is directed to relieving of important early tensions arising between mother and child, in the areas of the child's sleeping and feeding habits, the processes of weaning and toilet training, and the repercussions of these bodily experiences on the infant's mind.

Play Group for Toddlers and their Mothers.† Provision is made for a group of children under 3 to attend regularly once a week with their mothers. This project was started with the aim of studying the problems involved in the young child's transition from home to community life and for parents and staff to cooperate in a closer examination of the psychological meaning of school entry for the individual child.

Research Projects and Study Groups

Miss Anna Freud is Consultant to all research groups and is available to participate in the discussion of problems as they arise. The theoretical and clinical areas being investigated by study groups are the following.

Profile Research Group.‡ This research is concerned with a new approach to the assessment of pathology in childhood with special regard to the variations of normality and the imbalance of lines of development. The intensive study of childhood disturbances at the diagnostic stage and at subsequent points of children who come into treatment is carried out on the basis of 'developmental profiles', a formal method of assessment originated by Anna Freud and described in her book *Normality and Pathology in Children*[28].§

Index.|| One of the duties of psychoanalytic child therapists and analysts who have cases in daily analysis at the Hampstead Clinic is documentation, for the psychoanalytic material collected there is the property of the Clinic as a whole, and is meant to be available for research. A weekly report has to be written for each case, sufficient to give the important features of the week's work; in addition, a further and rather more comprehensive report is composed several times a year.

As more and more cases have been treated, the quantity of recorded reports has grown, and the Clinic was, some years ago, faced with the problem of making use of all of this material for the purposes of research. It became apparent that the accumulation of records, however accurate and illuminating, did not in itself constitute research.

Two real problems had to be faced; problems which could in time become acute. The first of these was that of finding the best way of making this material available to research workers, and the second that of providing

---

* Paediatrician in Charge: Dr J. Stross.
† Staff Member in Charge: Mrs J. Robertson.
‡ Chairman: Dr H. Nagera.
§ See pp. 245-50 for a fuller discussion.
|| Chairman: Dr J. Sandler.

the therapists themselves with the very necessary feeling that their efforts in preparing these reports were not wasted. A solution to these problems was suggested in the form of a proposed Index to the Hampstead case material. The Index project, as it was originally conceived, had two major aims: the first was to make the Clinic's vast mount of analytic material more readily accessible for research, and also for teaching and reference purposes, while the second aim was to open up new lines of research by assembling analytic data in such a way as to facilitate comparison among cases.

The Index was to be constructed on the same basis as an index to a book might be assembled, but in devising a scheme of classification it was felt to be essential that the uniqueness and individuality of each case be preserved, while being at the same time comprehended within a common theoretical framework.

The Index procedures have been evolved during the course of a pilot study in which therapists, together with an Index working party, classified the analytic and other relevant material of 50 cases which were in daily analysis. From this preliminary work it was possible to construct a set of common categories and an indexing procedure which was aimed at retaining the flexibility of therapists' reports, but which at the same time would provide a comprehensive system of classification. The material drawn on from the Index consists of all the therapist knows about the child, and considers to be of importance and interest in the case. Most of this is on record in the Social History and in the Weekly and other reports on the case.

This material can be classified under two main headings. The first, the *General Case Material*, contains information of a factual or psychological nature referring to the external reality of the child (for example, parental attitudes, family history, illnesses, etc.). The second, and by far the greatest division in the Index, contains the *Psychoanalytic Material*. Each division is further subdivided into a number of clinically or psychologically meaningful sections and subsections. Thus the information in the Social History of a case can be classified under a number of subheadings such as *Background* and *Biographical Data*, and the psychoanalytic material is ordered under the various subheadings of the sections: Object relationships, Instinctual material, Fantasies, Ego (Defences), other Ego material, Superego, Symptoms, and Treatment Situation and Technique.

An essential part of the Index project has been the construction of a number of Index Manuals* to help the therapists in their indexing. The manuals explain what kind of material is to be indexed in each section. They also define the use of terms for the purpose of the Index. The manuals are used for teaching purposes in connection with material from the Index and are designed to help the research worker to orientate himself in the Index.

* Only extracts from the Manuals have been published (Sandler *et al.*[72]; Bolland and Sandler[1]).

The Subject Index is not a scheme prepared on purely theoretical considerations, but is continually being revised on the basis of the clinical material gathered in the course of child analyses, material which is then classified in accordance with psychoanalytic theory. The various research projects also have the secondary effect of causing new headings to appear, and the diagnostic research has in particular stimulated a number of changes in the manuals.

During the establishment of the system of classification it has become clear that a number of psychoanalytic concepts require more accurate definition, and as a consequence a substantial degree of conceptual research has emerged as a by-product of the Index work—research into such problems as the concept of the superego, the nature of the mechanisms and processes of phantasy formation, the concept of the ego ideal, sublimation, trauma, etc. The work published in these areas is reported in pp. 245-50.

*Concept Research Group.** This project aims to clarify the historical development and present-day usage of psychoanalytic concepts. As a result of this study, based on an intensive working over of concepts as used by Freud and his collaborators, a manual of basic psychoanalytic concepts is in the process of being prepared for publication with the help of an International Editorial Committee, whose task it will be to check the formulations and contribute suggestions and criticisms.

*Clinical Concept Research Group.** This group has initiated a number of clinical studies on neurosis and related phenomena through the systematic study of the clinical case material of a large number of cases treated at the Clinic.

Development of Blind Children.† Psychoanalytic theory of child development has provided a much needed basis for the study of handicapped children amongst whom blind children have special interest for us. The development of these children, which is often deviant, merits study in its own right so that suitable help may be given.

Research‡ is carried out through observation of totally blind and partially sighted children in a Day Nursery School, through psychoanalytic treatment of some children where necessary, and through home visits to those of pre-nursery school age. Contact with parents is maintained in all cases.

Study of Adolescents in Psycho-Analytic Treatment.§ Using the method of pooling material from cases currently in treatment the Group studies problems arising from the case material presented.

Certain features of adolescent development, as they affect psychoanalytic technique are given special attention. Among these are the

* Chairman: Dr H. Nagera.
† Chairman: Mrs D. Burlingham.
‡ See pp. 236-38.
§ Chairmen: Dr I. Hellman and Dr L. Frankl.

repercussions in the transference of the process of loosening the infantile ties to the parents, the role of secretiveness during certain phases of treatment, the anxiety aroused by the revival of infantile feelings etc.

On the basis of the case material available from adolescents at the point of choosing their career, the motivations influencing their choice and elements of success and failure in it are studied.

A long-term follow-up programme is in progress in an attempt to assess the degree of success of psychoanalytic treatment.

*Study Group on Problems of Delinquency.** This study group was started some years ago, with a research programme for the study of the following three analytic concepts: acting out; the pathology of object relationships; frustration tolerance.

Theoretical and clinical work are involved in elucidating genetic, environmental and dynamic factors relevant to the problems of the patients under consideration. Case material is selected from indexed cases showing delinquent behaviour either at referral or during analytic treatment; from overtly delinquent cases under intensive treatment by members of the group and from weekly interviews with parents.

Modification of technique are discussed as necessitated by the structural characteristics of the delinquent patient specially concerning gratification and abstinence, and transference and counter transference.

Research Group on Borderline and Psychotic States in Children.† A number of borderline children, some of them treated over a period of many years, are studied in this group.

The group has devoted itself to a study of criteria to be used for the differential diagnosis between neurotic borderline and psychotic states in children, and to a reconsideration of how far therapeutic methods appropriate for neurotic children can be applied to the graver conditions. A variety of exploratory methods have been tried out and evaluated. As a result of this work, clinical and theoretical formulations have been made on the special types of anxiety and defensive measures characteristic of these children; the divergent types of primitive object relationship employed simultaneously; the relationship between anxiety and the self-representation and the notable absence of pleasure typical in extreme states.

A further group‡ has been concerned with the study of some severely disturbed children resident in a psychiatric unit for borderline and psychotic children, the High Wick Hospital,§ a number of whom have been brought into intensive treatment. The clinic staff is concerned as well in assisting in the training of the child care staff of this hospital, whose intensive observation of the children forms part of the study.

* Chairman: Miss H. Schwarz.
† Chairman: Mrs S. Rosenfeld.
‡ Under the direction of Miss Ruth Thomas.
§ Medical Director: Dr G. Stroh.

Simultaneous Analysis of Parents and Children.* Children and their parents are analysed independently of each other, by different analysts, and the work is coordinated by a third analyst. A variety of interests (e.g. the interaction of parent and child in creating psychopathology) are served by this research.

Community Education

Discussion Group for Nursery School Teachers and Matrons of Residential Nurseries.† The method employed to bring psychological insight to bear on a variety of special problems arising in both day and residential nurseries has been that of free and relatively unstructured discussion in this group. Problems such as the hospitalization of children, foster-home placement, and the behaviour disorders of individual children are discussed.

Discussion Group with Paediatric Consultants.‡ The integration of paediatrics and child psychology is a relatively recent development in England. However, for a number of years a group of consultant paediatricians has met regularly to discuss problems as they occur in daily paediatric work.

Liaison with the Paediatric Units of General Hospitals. In response to a request some years ago by the consultant paediatrician to the Woolwich Group of Hospitals and the Royal Alexandra Hospital at Brighton, the Clinic provides the services of a staff member§ to the hospital teams on a part-time basis. In addition to introducing and maintaining the psychoanalytic point of view within the special problem-case conference conducted at the hospital, the therapist has joined the consultant's ward round for postgraduate students and takes part in discussion of the social and psychological aspects of the in-patient's condition. Her activities accordingly concern both the in- and out-patient cases seen at these hospitals.

Lectures to Professional Organizations. Following invitations by various Government departments, a substantial number of lectures have been given‖ to such groups as the staff of children's institutions, child welfare workers, nursery school teachers, public health workers, probation officers, house-parents, social service students, and tutors engaged in training the staff of children's homes. Intensive educational work has been carried out at the High Wick Hospital¶ and at the Wellgarth Nursery and Training College.**

---

* A number of analysts and child-therapists function in this project either by conducting treatment or by acting as co-ordinators.
† Conducted by Mrs E. M. Mason.
‡ Miss Anna Freud, assisted by Mrs E. M. Mason.
§ Mrs B. Gordon.
‖ Mainly by Mrs E. M. Mason.
¶ By Dr M. Goldblatt, Miss R. Edgcumbe and Mrs L. Weitzner.
** By Mrs J. Robertson.

3
Review of Clinic Publications

This report is limited mainly to clinic books and papers which have appeared since 1960. In so doing we are not only omitting the important publications prior to 1960 but also those which, at the time of writing this chapter, have not as yet been published. Even with this limitation the volume of material is such that the authors can only touch on certain major points in some of these publications.

General Studies of Normal and Abnormal Development

Anna Freud's book *Normality and Pathology in Childhood*[28] is both a summary and extension of her life's work. A central contribution is a detailed presentation of a relatively unique method of childhood assessment, one which is aimed at freeing psychoanalysis from the static, rigid, descriptive diagnostic categories currently in use. To this end, Anna Freud devised the 'metapsychological profile' referred to earlier. Profiles can be drawn up at various points (such as at the diagnostic stage, during analysis or at the terminal stage), and are aimed at assisting the clinician organize the material so as to produce a comprehensive metapsychological picture of the child, i.e. one which contains dynamic, developmental genetic, economic, structural and adaptive data.*

The major headings of the Profile are as follows:

A. Reasons for Referral.
B. Description of Child.
C. Family Background and Personal History.
D. Possible Significant Environmental Influences.
E. Assessment of Development.
   1. Drive Development.
      (*a*) Libido: (*i*) Phase Development; (*ii*) libido distribution; (*iii*) object libido.
      (*b*) Aggression: (*i*) according to quantity; (*ii*) according to quality; (*iii*) according to direction toward either the object world or the self.
   2. Ego and Superego development: (*i*) intactness or defect of ego apparatus; (*ii*) intactness of ego functions; (*iii*) defence organization.
   3. Lines of development.
F. Genetic Assessments (regression and fixation points) may be

---

* The basic elements of the profile had been outlined by Miss Freud previously[19, 21], and a draft first appeared in 1962[22]. A case illustration of the use of the profile was published by Nagera[48].

determined by: (*i*) certain forms of manifest behaviour, (*ii*) phantasy activity, (*iii*) symptomatology where the relations between surface and depth are firmly established.

G. Dynamic and Structural Assessments (conflicts). Conflicts are classified as: (*i*) external conflicts; (*ii*) internalized conflicts; (*iii*) internal conflicts.

H. Assessment of some general characteristics: (*i*) frustration tolerance; (*ii*) sublimation potential; (*ii*) overall attitude to anxiety; (*iv*) progressive versus regressive tendencies.

I. Diagnosis. There are six categories of diagnosis ranging from behaviour disturbances which fall within the range of variations of normality to the diagnosis of destructive processes at work of organic, toxic or psychic origin.

In the Diagnostic Profile many of the major headings summarized above are accompanied by annotations which enable the diagnostician to make finer discriminations[22]. For example, in the subsection on the status of the defence organization ($E\ 2\ (iii)$) the following factors are considered: 'whether defences are employed specifically against individual drives or, more generally, against drive activity and instinctual pleasure as such; whether defences are age-adequate, too primitive or too precocious; whether defence is balanced, i.e. whether the ego has at its disposal the use of many of the important mechanisms or is restricted to excessive use of single ones; whether defence is effective, especially in dealing with anxiety, whether it results in equilibrium or disequilibrium, lability, mobility, or deadlock within the structure; whether and how far the child's defence against the drives is dependent on the object world or independent of it (superego development). Finally a note is made on any secondary interference of defence activity with ego achievement, i.e. the price paid by the individual for the upkeep of the defence organization.'

The profile was originally developed for use with neurotic child patients but has subsequently been applied beyond the scope of the neuroses. In so doing, a number of sections were amplified in order to assess those aspects relevant to the specific pathology. Nagera and Colonna[52] report on a study using the profile on six blind children. The section on phase development, fixation and regression was amplified as a consequence of this study. Thus it was noted that the signs of oral fixation in normal or neurotic children had to be interpreted differently in the blind, in whom mouthing, for example, can be seen as an auxiliary exploratory ego function. This study suggests that the profile may be used as a way of organizing material on a group of children and comparing the pathology of non-neurotic with neurotic children; and the necessary amplifications for special groups highlights the differences between various types of pathology. Thus Laufer[44] found that, in order to assess the characteristics of the adolescent upheaval, the profile had to be widened to encompass variations of superego development, ideal formation and identity problems. Many points previously made by Laufer in a paper on the ego ideal in adolescence[43] are incorporated in the adolescent profile. Similarly, the application of the profile to borderline children required additional distinctions in the sections referring to cathexis of self and objects (Thomas et al.)[79]. The profile has also been modified for use with adult patients (Freud, A., Nagera, H., and Freud, W. E.)[34]. This was found especially useful in cases when the child and parent were in simultaneous treatment.

The concept of developmental lines was first outlined by Anna Freud in 1960 and published later[23]. As a prototype of a developmental line Miss Freud presents in detail the line of development from dependency to emotional self-reliance and adult object relationships. Eight steps are listed, starting with the move from the biological unity between the mother-infant couple to the need-fulfilling anaclitic relationship, and proceeding further to the stage of object constancy followed by the ambivalent relationship of the pre-Oedipal, anal sadistic stage. This is followed by the completely object centred phallic-Oedipal stage, then the latency period, with its post-Oedipal lessening of drive urgency and the transfer of libido from the parental figures to contemporaries. This goes on to the pre-adolescent prelude to the 'adolescent revolt', i.e. a return to early attitudes and behaviour, especially of the need-fulfilling and ambivalent type. The final stage is the adolescent struggle around denying, reversing, loosening and shedding the tie to the infantile objects, defending against pre-genitality and, finally, establishing genital supremacy.

The other developmental lines described are: (*i*) areas of ego development related to body independence—from suckling to independent eating; from wetting and soiling to bladder and bowel control; from irresponsibility to responsibility in body management; (*ii*) from egocentricity to companionship; (*iii*) from the body to the toy and from play to work.

It should be noted that the developmental lines are more than a subsection of the profile. The concept serves as a background for the assessment of childhood disturbances and as a basis for making clinical decisions and practical suggestions. The lines provide the practitioner with a hypothetical norm of development and by assessing a particular child against this norm, and by taking into account harmony or disharmony between developmental lines, the evenness or unevenness of progression rate, and the permanency or temporariness of regressions, the clinician is provided with a set of criteria for judging the severity of disturbance.

The profile assessment of a child, especially at the diagnostic stage, is dependent to a large degree on data obtained outside the analytic session, from the direct observation of what Miss Freud terms, 'the surface of the mind'[29].

In this article Miss Freud notes that it is increasingly certain that direct scrutiny of the surface of the mind can penetrate into the depths, especially in relation to child development. This is in line with the results of Anna Freud's earlier observations on the relation between readily observable surface manifestations (observed both within and out of analytic sessions) and the hidden structures, functions and contents of the mind. Thus in *The Ego and the Mechanisms of Defence** (1936) she had directed the analyst away from an exclusive focus on the id and emphasized the importance of paying equal attention to the elements of the ego, super-ego, and reality. In stressing the observation of behaviour for the purpose of the assessment of development, she notes that her attitude in this is similar to that of Heinz Hartmann (A. Freud)[30]. The extension of the legitimate areas of analytic observation and interest, first (1936) within the analytic session to the unconscious elements of the ego and superego, and now[28] to observations outside of the analytic session, can be viewed as revolutionary turning points in the history of psychoanalysis. In the first chapter of her recent book[28] Miss Freud describes the historical development of the changing relationship between analysis and surface observation and details those areas in which the relationship between surface observation and the 'hidden depths' have been established and can now be used for diagnostic assessment. However, she warns the analyst against the therapeutic interpretative use of such signs and to respect the limits within which the sign- and signal-function of behaviour operates legitimately.

In a paper on the place of psychoanalytic theory in the training of psychiatrists[31] Miss Freud states that no picture of a human being is complete unless seen within the comprehensive framework of metapsychology; metapsychology being 'the language of psychoanalysis'. She goes on to examine the steps by which the psychiatrist in training may pass from the initial encounter with manifest data to the acquisition of teh language of psychoanalysis. In this context the metapsychological profile can serve as a training device.

The profile is more than just a method of assessment, a research tool, and a training device, but also represents, in concrete form, Miss Freud's general approach to the entire area of childhood development and functioning. A profile is intended to be a comprehensive view of the child, taking all aspects of the personality and their interrelationship into account. It is aimed at countering the tendency to overemphasize isolated areas of the total personality and to omit the rest. Miss Freud applies a similar point of view in her approach to the varied services available to the child. She argues against the current compartmentalized, unintegrated approach in which the child is seen as only a body to be treated by the physician, only as a mind to be taught by teachers, only as a lawbreaker handled by the courts, etc., and sees the current state of affairs as one which splits up the child's life into parts, each of which is catered to by specialists who are ignorant of the interrelationship between their area of interest and other areas in the child's functioning.

At a national conference of the nursery school association ('Why

* Reprinted in 1964[26].

children go wrong')[17], Miss Freud highlighted the variation which can occur in normal child development, emphasizing that these should be understood before considering problems of pathology, and illustrating the developmental approach to such problems as the requirements for entry into nursery school. She describes the various stages leading to the ability to separate from the mother, to tolerate group life and enjoy it, and to tolerate frustration, and emphasizes the normality of temporary regressions.

At a conference of the Society for Psychosomatic Research held in 1959, Miss Freud answered questions put to her by a group of paediatricians. Some of these related to such topics as the effect of rectal manipulation, the effect of injections, the question of cuddling, the crying infant, sleeping and eating disturbances, etc. In her responses Miss Freud[20] expressed her hope that, at a future time, medicine will have a double orientation, one directed simultaneously towards the body and the mind.

For a number of years Miss Freud has participated in seminars on the Family and the Law at the Yale law school in the United States. In *The Family and the Law*[27] Miss Freud contributed three brief discussions which illustrate the contribution which psychoanalytic developmental considerations can make to the court's handling of child cases.

Although the efforts of Miss Freud and others to provide a common ground for all those who work with children have had noticeable effect, the current situation still leaves much to be desired. In 'Interactions between Nursery School and Child Guidance Clinic'[32], Miss Freud presents 'a vision of future training for children's services'. She states '... it is not too difficult to envisage future training schemes by means of which a revolution in the field can be brought about. What is needed above all is a basic training in child development which is common to all professions and concerned with children of all ages, in all conditions, in whatever role. This would have to include the principle facts of neurological, physiological, instinctual, emotional, intellectual and moral growth with their age-adequate and phase-adequate interactions; the child's gradual mastery of his external and internal world and the means by which this is brought about; the child's advance from emotional and moral dependency to independent status; the environment's tasks with regard to the immature individual's need for body care, affection, stimulation and stability. Where specialized professional training will make its departure from a common basic course of this nature, the professions, instead of being closed off hermetically against each other, will retain the possibility of lively interchange.'

There are many highly condensed sections in Miss Freud's 1965 book which stimulate further thought and raise questions which can only be answered by more detailed study of the issues involved. One such area is her classification of conflicts as external, internalized and as 'truly internal', and the relationship of these conflicts to the infantile and adult neurosis.

Nagera[51] in his monograph *Early Childhood Disturbances, The Infantile*

Neurosis, and the Adulthood Disturbances: Problems of a Developmental Psychoanalytical Psychology explores some of these questions in detail.

Following Anna Freud, Nagera approaches the problems of childhood disturbances within the framework of a developmental psychoanalytic psychology, and proposes a developmental scheme running from the early infantile disturbances up to the adult neuroses. In this scheme a distinction is made between:

(*a*) *Developmental interference* which can be defined as any factor which disturbs the typical unfolding of development, but which refers in particular to conflicts between the child's drives and his environment. They are what Anna Freud[22] has described as 'external conflicts', in contrast to 'internalized conflicts'.

(*b*) *Developmental conflicts*. These are experienced by every child to a greater or lesser degree, either when certain specific environmental demands are made at the appropriate developmental phases (e.g. toilet training at the appropriate time and in reasonable form) or when the child reaches certain developmental and maturational levels at which specific conflicts are created (e.g. the conflicts of the phallic Oedipal phase). Frequently a combination of both factors is involved. Typically, developmental conflicts are specific of certain phases or stages in development. Under ideal conditions they should disappear as soon as the next stage is reached.

(*c*) *Neurotic Conflicts*. These are frequently the continuation of a developmental conflict that has not resolved itself properly at the appropriate time. Neurotic conflicts can be considered to be simple units. They result from component instincts pushing for gratification and other aspects of the personality opposing such gratification.

(*d*) *The Infantile Neurosis*. The infantile neurosis is an attempt to organize all the previous and perhaps manifold neurotic conflicts and developmental shortcomings, together with all the conflicts typical of the phallic Oedipal phase, into a single organization. This compromise formation is possible at this point because of the relatively high degree of development reached in several areas, particularly in that of the ego's integrative and synthetic functions. For these reasons the phallic Oedipal phase is in fact an essential turning point in human development.

Nagera stresses the importance of examining manifest symptomatology and expressions of disturbance against a background of a developmental scheme. He had presented this point of view previously in a paper on 'Autoerotism, autoerotic activities and ego development'[50]. In this paper he also makes a distinction between the *phase* of autoerotism and autoerotic forms of sexual activity and expression; the latter may be normally seen in phases other than that of 'autoerotism'.

In a paper 'On arrest in development, fixation and regression'[49] Nagera re-emphasized that, despite frequent assertions to the contrary, it is often possible to distinguish how much of the drive manifestations seen at a particular pregenital stage is present owing to the existence of an arrest at that level and how much to regressive processes. Some analytic workers had previously held that no such distinction is possible at the diagnostic stage. Nagera put forward the view that this distinction is of prognostic importance, for it is unquestionably easier to help the forward movement of libido which has at some point of development reached the higher stages and has then regressed, than that of libido which has always been arrested at the earlier stages. Here Nagera makes use of some of the distinctions made by Anna Freud. In a group of her publications[24, 25, 28] Miss Freud proposed a number of important distinctions in regard to the processes of fixation and regression. She notes that a differentiation should be made between those regressions which are temporary and spontaneously reversible, and those which are more permanent in nature. Regressions of the instinctual drives as well as of the ego and superego are normal processes which have their origin in the immature individual's flexibility. They are useful responses to the strain of a given moment and are always available to the child as an answer to situations which might otherwise prove unbearable. They serve adaptation and defence simultaneously, and both functions help to maintain the state of normality. Occasional returns to more infantile behaviour should be taken as normal, and temporary regressions are in fact more appropriate to healthy psychic growth than steady progressive moves.

Specific Studies of Abnormal Development

Anna Freud has outlined some of the clinical investigations in progress at the Clinic[16]. She comments that the analytic technique as such precludes the setting up of formal experiments, but notes that this embargo on experimentation can be compensated for by the selection of cases for treatment in which either nature or fate has caused the elimination or the exaggeration of one specific innate or environmental factor. These could be termed 'experimental situations provided by nature or fate'. A series of such studies have been undertaken at the Clinic and the area most extensively explored is the study of congenitally blind children.

Studies on Blind Children. Dorothy Burlingham's 'Some notes on the development of the Blind'[3] makes use of material collected on congenitally blind children at the Clinic to contrast their development with that of sighted children. From birth the mother-child relationship is disturbed owing to the effect that the birth of a blind child has on the mother. As a consequence blind babies often receive less maternal stimulation than their sighted counterparts. Excessive restriction of the child may be associated with the development of gross autoerotic and autoaggressive activities, including head-banging, rocking, sucking or masturbation. The lack of external stimulation, due both to maternal attitudes and the absence of the visual modality hinders development by the reduction of normal incentives; consequently retardation, particularly in regard to motor development, frequently occurs. Hearing does not appear to be an adequate substitute for vision in stimulating the child to develop normally in the sphere of motility and in the gaining of motor skills.

In 'Aspect of passivity and ego development in the blind infant' Anne-Marie Sandler[59] explores the factors contributing to the abnormal passivity to be found in congenitally blind children. This is seen to be not only a direct consequence of the absence of vision but also as an indirect effect of failure in development due to blindness. The role of vision in normal development is discussed, with special reference to the part it plays in removing the child's centre of interest away from direct bodily stimulation. This causes the child to remain fixated to the very earliest phase of development in which the passive experiencing of direct bodily gratification is dominant. It seems likely that whatever the degree of maternal care received by the child, a basic pull towards self-centredness and the modes of gratification characteristic of the first half-year of life will always be present.

In 'Hearing and its role in the development of the blind'[4] Mrs Burlingham discusses the role played by the mother in furthering, or in failing to further, the blind infant's innate developmental possibilities. Some of the developmental deviations and the reduction in the ability of blind children to enjoy experiences are attributed to a lack of interaction between child and mother. Mrs Burlingham describes the various ways in which blind children attend to auditory stimuli. Motionless attention is sometimes mistaken for withdrawal. The way in which blind children imitate sounds and voices is discussed, as is the role of auditory 'feedback' to the child's own activities.

On the basis of the observations reported in the paper, Mrs Burlingham concludes that the mother's failure to understand the world of her blind child may lead her to expect too little in the areas where he functions well and to fail to encourage where it would be necessary.

In a further paper on 'Some problems of ego development in blind children, Mrs Burlingham[5] explores the (usually unrecognized) positive achievements of the child who is born blind. Motor restraint is discussed from the point of view of the achievement of control in the interests of safety. Repetitive behaviour and the use of the body for non-active purposes are discussed with reference to the functions they serve. Major sections of the paper deal with problems of orientation, the recognition of objects, and with the problem of verbalization in the blind.

Anne-Marie Sandler and Doris M. Wills in 'Preliminary notes on play and mastery in the blind child'[60] point out that the blind child meets with special difficulties when attempting to respond in an active fashion to passively received stimuli, and for this reason his attempts to master his world follow a different course from that of normal sighted children. With the help of observations made on blind children at the Clinic the authors discuss the baby's early difficulties in moving away from passive instinctual aims to exploration of the world around. The degree to which interest goes via the mother and her body is stressed. The blind child's representational world remains fragmentary, and its further exploration is hindered by a degree of inhibition of motor activity. Hearing and sound are, however, highly invested and are much used in the child's further attempts at mastery.

In 'Some observations on blind nursery children'[80] Doris Wills presents observations on six blind nursery children to test the supposition that blind children understand their world later and in a different way from the sighted child. The author finds that the blind nursery children showed difficulty in distinguishing reality and make believe and reality and fantasy. They had a partial understanding of common objects and differences in the way they reasoned about them. Wills goes on to discuss the role of the mother in helping the child overcome their difficulties in conceptualization.

Humberto Nagera and Alice B. Colonna report the results of applying Anna Freud's diagnostic Profile to six blind children in 'Aspects of the contribution of sight to ego and drive development'[52]. They attempt to single out the aspects of personality and development which appear specific to blind children, organizing the material under the relevant Profile headings.

Borderline and Psychotic Children. Marie B. Singer describes, in 'Fantasies of a borderline patient'[75], the analysis of a boy of ten who appeared to be on the borderline between neurosis and paranoid psychosis. The patient brought an abundance of fantasy material, expressed in many different forms, and the relationship between the content of the boy's fantasies and his disturbance is traced in some detail. Although the analysis differed in many respects from that of a neurotic child, the technical orientation throughout treatment was modelled on the approach usually adopted with neurotic children. After eight years of treatment the boy was able to achieve a precarious foothold in normality.

The special problems to be met with in the diagnosis of borderline conditions and in the therapy of borderline cases led to more systematic research on these cases by the Research Group on Borderline and Psychotic States, and to the publication by Sara Kut Rosenfeld and Marjorie P. Sprince of 'An attempt to formulate the meaning of the concept "borderline"'[57]. Because of wide divergencies in the use of the term 'borderline' the research group examined the common features in a number of cases and collated their findings with formulations found in the literature. The suggestion is made in this paper that 'borderline' children, while having special peculiarities, are not necessarily moving along the path towards psychosis. It is felt that the fact of ego deviation is of significance, but that in addition the crucial area for assessment and prediction is the child's capacity for internalization and the creation of inner representations based on his object relationship. The type of treatment chosen would relate to the capacity for maintaining a particular level of object relationship for a period of time.

Certain specific characteristics of borderline children were found. These are: (*i*) a tendency for the cases not to have attained the developmental level of phallic dominance, with any Oedipal material having an 'as if' quality; (*ii*) the presence of a fault in the ego apparatus, which may be due to inherent or traumatic factors. There is evidence that the fault occurs very early and is related to a disturbance in the capacity to select and inhibit stimuli; (*iii*) anxiety characterized by primitive feelings of disintegration and annihilation. Signal anxiety is itself experienced as an overwhelming threat rather than being restricted to a warning function, as in neurotic and normal cases; and (*iv*) a weakness in object cathexis linked with instability of the object representation.

In her paper 'A contribution to the study of homosexuality in adolescents'[77] Sprince applies the formulation of the concept of 'borderline' to the differentiation between those aspects of adolescent pathological homosexuality which refer to the characteristic qualities of the adolescent upheaval and which are transitory in nature, from those features which reflect true pathology.

In a further paper entitled 'Some thoughts on the technical handling of borderline children'[58], Rosenfeld and Sprince report the conclusions of the Research Group in regard to the techniques used in the initial phases of the treatment of borderline cases. Stress is laid on the fact that the level of ego development and object relationships differs from child to child and a variety of different psychopathologies exist. There is a need to follow the child into his own psychic world in order to make meaningful contact with him, and the therapist may have to adopt a more active role than is customary. The treatment relationship with these children is governed by their proneness to acute anxiety and their low level of object relationship. The methods of dealing with acute anxiety at the beginning of treatment are discussed with special reference to the use of ego-supportive techniques and the timing of interpretations. Some of the special countertransference problems arising in the treatment of borderline patients are delineated and discussed.

The papers quoted illustrate a shift in emphasis over the years as more experience was gained in the handling of borderline children. It is clear that the procedure suitable for the analytic treatment of neurotic children have to be modified (particularly at the beginning of treatment) in accordance with the special needs and difficulties of the child.

Studies of other Handicapped Children. Intensive clinical investigations have been undertaken in other areas in which nature or fate have provided material for experimental isolation of crucial factors.

In 'The analysis of a boy with a congenital deformity'[47] Andre Lussier reports on the analysis of a 13-year-old boy born with malformed shoulders and abnormally short arms terminating in hands having only three fingers and no thumbs. The boy had shown emotional difficulties in the form of the continual creation of a complex fantasy life and an inventive evasion of factual truth. Analysis dealt initially with his denial of his deformity and his use of compensatory mechanisms. He aimed in his fantasy-stories to prove to the world that he was a normal boy, and in fact placed himself in a number of highly dangerous situations. The link between his deformity and his intense castration anxiety was traced. The author describes the special technical problems involved in the analysis of a disabled patient.

In 'The search for a sexual identity in a case of constitutional sexual precocity'[78] Ruth Thomas and her colleagues report on a case of early sexual precocity. Susan's analysis extended from the age of 3 to the beginning of her tenth year. One of the findings was the evidence that constitutional sexual precocity is a major problem for both the child and her family, in which psychological help for a considerable period may be needed. In the case studied, the parents' continued anxiety over her precocity added a special quality to Susan's object relations and complicated the problem of her identifications. The analysis afforded no evidence that Susan's physical precocity was accompanied by the quantitative increase in sexual drive which we associate with puberty. Susan's precocious physical development and her early onset of menstruation (at $6\frac{1}{2}$ years) resulted in no increase of psychic sexual drive. The possession of secondary sexual characteristics gave a particularly intense quality to her phallic Oedipal conflicts. She saw herself as a real rival to the mother with omnipotent powers of retaliation. The possession of these secondary sexual characteristics accentuated castration anxiety and functioned to aggravate the castration complex of the males in her environment.

In 'The analysis of a young concentration camp victim'[46] Edith Ludowyk examines the links between early, traumatic separation and later pathology. The case presented is that of a girl taken to Auschwitz concentration camp without her parents, probably at the age of 2. Medical examination at the time of liberation established Elizabeth's age as approximately 4 years. Ludowyk discusses both the pathology and the technical problems in the treatment of a person whose object relations did not proceed beyond the identifications of early infancy and whose repeated traumatic separations occurred at a time before object constancy had been achieved. She notes that the pathogenic factor in this case was not the objective horror of the concentration camp but the fact that her innate needs remained unsatisfied and that no lasting object relationships could be made. Ludowyk illustrates the way in which analysis enabled Elizabeth to make the step from imitation of external objects to identification proper, and to the formation of internalized object representations.

Twin Studies. The Clinic has accumulated material which allows for the comparison of observational data with data obtained from later analytic treatment. This material can be used to study such problems as the formation of cover memories, the developmental distortion of memories, processes of inner elaboration of external events, etc. Burlingham and Barron's paper 'A study of identical twins'[6] is a report on this type of comparative study. This paper presents a developmental account of a pair of identical twins, Bert and Bill, based on evidence obtained from (*i*) detailed nursery observations from their fourth month to their fourth year (see Burlingham, D.)[2]; (*ii*) enquiry into their external life from their fourth to twelfth year; (*iii*) direct observation in a home for maladjusted children covering the period from age 12 to 13½; (*iv*) material from their analytic treatments (Bert: 13-16 years, Bill: 13-15 years); and (*v*) follow-up data.

In their detailed presentation the authors summarize the comparison of material under the headings: identity of appearance, mirror image, struggle for their own identity, excitability, anti-social development and differences in personality. This article contains substantial data referring to the development of the twins from infancy to adulthood, and to the comparison of early observational with later analytic data.

Follow-up Studies. The follow-up studies being carried out are exemplified by a report by Ilse Hellman[35] who compares the detailed nursery observations on a child with the material concerning her development into adulthood.

The study reports the case of a girl who entered the Hampstead Nursery at 2 years 8 months under unusual and especially traumatic circumstances. The report focuses on the relationship of her present personality (at the age of 23) to a very traumatic separation experience in her third year of life. Jane was a fatherless, homeless, illegitimate child. The circumstances of the separations were that the mother had accompanied a friend to the Nursery and decided on the spur of the moment to leave Jane there also. Jane had not been prepared for the separation but because of the dangerous wartime conditions it was decided to accept Jane. The little girl's reaction to the sudden separation was overwhelming.

In the follow-up study it could be seen that in her instinctual development, in her ego and superego functioning and in her object relationships, Jane functions on an adult level with apparently little interference from inner conflict. The observations of her development and the assessment of her present personality show that the trauma had neither stopped her ongoing development nor had it left a disturbing mark on her adult life. In her paper Dr Hellman discussed the various factors which have enabled Jane to reach adulthood with apparently little damage.

Studies on Mothering and Early Development. The Well-Baby Clinic provides a valuable source of material on the early mother-infant relationship. In a series of articles, Joyce Robertson presents the results of detailed observations on this early relationship. In 'Mothering as an influence on early development'[53] Robertson attempts to show: (*i*) even when the child is in the sole care of a devoted mother, defects in the quality of the mothering can result in emotional needs being unfulfilled, (*ii*) deficient mothering in the first year causes poor general development which can look similar to, but is not to be confused with, retardation due to organic defect, (*iii*) the impairment resulting from the experience of deficient mothering will persist after the first year, but may become partially obscured by neurotic factors. The paper reports a study of 25 mother-infant pairs observed by the author from the baby's first months of life.

Robertson suggests three criteria for assessing the adequacy of mothering in relation to the adaptation of the mothers during the post-natal period from birth to 8 weeks. The outcome of the adaptive period is successful when, on balance, the mother (*i*) feels and expresses pleasure not only in owning her baby but in the activities of mothering, (*ii*) is aware of her baby's affective states and able to respond to them, and (*iii*) uses the heightened anxiety which is normal during this period in the service of her baby.

In a later article Robertson[54] takes up another aspect by seeking to show that what might appear to be minor and transient disturbances occurring at an early stage in the mother-infant relationship can influence the course of an infant's development. Material for this paper is derived from direct observation of two mother-infant pairs. She suggests that the difference between the two children reflects the trends imposed on their development during the first few months, differences which are likely to persist.

In 'Three devoted mothers'[55] Robertson describes a study of three mother-infant couples. In each instance the mother was devoted to her child, attended the Clinic regularly and had a positive relationship to the Clinic Staff. Although it was a situation in which maximum guidance could be given to the mother the article highlights the way in which the mother's personality hinders or furthers the guidance efforts.

Studies of some General Variables. In 'Some observations on the development and disturbance of integration in childhood' Liselotte Frankl[10] discusses processes of psychological integration and their pathology. The aim of integration can be considered from the aspects of the formation of the body ego, the self, the mental representation of the most important objects, the world we live in, and of identity. Frankl states that the sequence of these aims could be regarded as representing a hierarchy from the developmental point of view. She suggests that it is of the greatest importance to diagnose and treat children who suffer from disturbances in these areas promptly, for if treatment is successful future phases of development may proceed normally; whereas if treatment is not instituted at the right time the future development of these children might be seriously impaired. The various points are illustrated with clinical reports. In a later paper on 'Self preservation and the development of accident proneness in children and adolescents'[12] Frankl sees a possible role for psychoanalysis in preventing accidents, a major medico-social problem. Frankl considers accidents as related to failures in the function of self preservation. In considering the development of self preservation she notes that the capacity for it does not exist in earliest infancy. For a considerable period after the child's birth it is the mother who retains this function. The problem of self preservation arises when the toddler gradually separates from his mother. It is during this phase that attempts at self preservation are clearly observable and individual variations can be noted. The self-preservation function is gradually taken over by the child from the mother. Frankl states that the persistence of expression through action rather than through phantasying or thinking, for whatever cause, is a major element which contributes to the development of accident proneness; and in this the defence mechanism most frequently employed is that of turning aggression against the self. The paper is illustrated with examples drawn from observations of normal children in the Nursery Group and from Clinic patients.

Adolescents. Ilse Hellman's paper 'Psychosexual development in adolescents'[37] is a condensed but illuminating discussion of this complex subject. In her paper she comments on the reaction of boys to their first nocturnal emissions. The anxieties reported lead back to childhood fears and to experiences connected with loss of control over urination and defecation in childhood. Aggressive phantasies add to the fear. The first experiences of orgasm may also revive earlier anxieties of emotional loss of control, so often connected with outbreaks of rage. Hellman also describes some of the difficulties encountered in the attempt to establish the relationship needed for the psychoanalytic treatment of adolescents. In a paper entitled 'Observations on adolescents in psychoanalytic treatment'[36] she elaborates on the difficulties encountered in the psychoanalytic treatment of adolescents. She notes, for example, that with many adolescents the analyst is deprived, to a great extent, of those means of access to unconscious processes on which we rely most in the treatment of children and adults. She comments on the fact that adolescent patients can rarely fulfil the basic requirements of psychoanalytic treatment for any length of time. Hellman distinguishes between those cases which come with a disturbance which has been firmly established from childhood onward, and those adolescents whose childhood picture did not seem to show a well defined neurosis and who have dealt with their anxiety in such a way as to enable them to pass through latency without any apparent trouble. She notes that the first group does not present the analyst with specific problems in treatment, at least until they have been freed to enter into the adolescent struggle for independence. It is the latter group which is usually referred to in discussions of the technical problems in the treatment of adolescents. Rosenblatt's case of a severe neurosis in an adolescent boy[56] could be taken as an example of the first type of case, i.e. the adolescent who comes with a disturbance which has been firmly established from childhood. Rosenblatt's paper is a detailed case report of the analysis of a 13-year-old boy who had numerous disturbing symptoms including the poking of faeces out of his anus with his finger, together with great anxiety that the faeces would not come out. Among the many striking features in this case that were emphasized by the author is the manner in which the patient formed a positive relationship with the therapist and used the analytic method as a vehicle for progression rather than regression.

General Technical Problems. In their paper 'The ego's participation in the therapeutic alliance'[14] Frankl and Hellman comment on the fact that although much has been written on problems of *interpretation* in the treatment of adult patients, such problems have not as yet been studied with all their implications where children are concerned. They outline some of the developmental considerations which must be taken into account in the formulation and timing of interpretations, and discuss a case of a 10-year-old girl who was brought to treatment against her will. They trace in details the steps which led to a treatment alliance and ultimately to a favourable result. They note that in the case of those children who tenaciously resist treatment, a great amount of work is needed to arrive at a point where the child is able to face the fact that the disturbance and suffering in his life are located within him and not only in the external world. They comment on the relationship between the early experience of 'good' mothering and the capacity for forming a therapeutic alliance.

Simultaneous Analysis of Parent and Child. Following the paper on 'Simultaneous analysis of mother and child' by Dorothy Burlingham, Alice Goldberger and Andre Lussier[9], several reports have appeared of simultaneous analyses conducted at the Clinic. Kata Levy's paper on 'Simultaneous analysis of a mother and her adolescent daughter'[45] is introduced by Anna Freud, who points out that the 'Simultaneous Analysis' project not only highlights points of interaction, but also traces the indirect as well as the direct effects of the mother's pathology on the child.

In her paper 'The child guidance clinic as a centre of prophylaxis and enlightenment'[18] Anna Freud referred to the fact that young children have primitive pathways of communication with the Unconscious of the mother. This can render the child sensitive and vulnerable to the mother's unconscious libidinal and aggressive impulses and phantasies. She put forward the view that simultaneous treatment is necessary when the pathogenic agents from the mother's side do not remain in the realm of thought and phantasy but are reinforced by actions of the mother which tie the child to her as a result of pleasurable or painful excitations. Kata Levy's paper[45] illustrates these points by reference to the analyses of an adolescent and her mother who showed a great deal of mutual interaction in their personalities and symptoms. The daughter showed all the upheavals characteristic of adolescence, but had no urge to detach herself from her parents and her home. Her peculiarities could be understood better by viewing the mother's difficulties in relation to her anxiety in rearing a child, to her need to make the relationship to her daughter a body-related and sado-masochistic one, to excessive guilt feelings which prevented her from standing up to her daughter and loosening the tie from her side. The main conflicts were understood in both cases by coordinating the vicissitudes of the Oedipal conflicts of both mother and child and their interaction. A fuller and further account of the simultaneous analysis, with particular reference to the child's material, is given in a paper by Marjorie P. Sprince on 'The development of a pre-oedipal partnership between an adolescent girl and her mother'[76]. On the basis of material not available in the earlier report Sprince places special emphasis on excessive oral and anal stimulation of the child, beginning shortly after birth, and traces the influence of these factors on her later Oedipal and genital development.

In 'Simultaneous analysis of mother and child'[38], Hellman, Friedmann and Shepheard report on the simultaneous analysis of an 11-year-old boy and his mother. A striking feature of the interaction between mother and child related to mutual anxieties about the boy's health, and to the way in which the mother's preoccupations and neurotic conflicts affected his development. Particular attention is paid in the report to the meaning of food in the analyses of both mother and child and to their mutual sexual tie. The mother's influence on her son is considered in both its pathogenic and beneficial effects.

The treatment of this case was continued throughout adolescence, and Frankl and Hellman later report on the difficulty in loosening the infantile tie to the mother[13]. Through the psychoanalytic treatment of both mother and son, insight was gained into the dynamics of the mutual ties, and the reaction of each partner to the other partner's attempts at gaining freedom. The anxiety aroused in both mother and son led to the intensification of the libidinal and aggressive demands on each other and to subsequent regression and reunion on a more primitive psychological level. This case, treated from late latency into puberty, shows the inner struggles of the loosening of the tie to his mother in a boy whose development had been partially arrested, particularly in regard to his relationship to her.

This case is referred to again by Frankl as one of three illustrating the varied meanings of bodily symptoms ('The child and his symptom'[11]). She discussed how the boy's bodily symptoms are related to the close mother-infant tie.

Studies from the Hampstead Index

The procedure of indexing described in Part 2 created a need for the clarification of a number of psychoanalytic concepts, and a series of papers has emerged on various aspects of psychoanalytic theory. The first of these was 'On the concept of superego' (Sandler)[61] in which the relevant literature was reviewed and a theoretical model of superego functioning put forward in order to resolve a number of problems which had arisen in the classification of material relating to the superego. The superego was conceived of as having two main aspects. First, it includes a system of authority figures (either real persons or introjects); second, it embraces certain ego responses to these authority figures.

The approach adopted was designed to take into account difficulties in assessing superego functions in the actual therapeutic situation. More specifically, it has been found necessary to consider the reactions of the ego not only to the introjects, but also to real authority figures in the environment, as well as to externalized representatives of introjected authority figures.

Introjection in this context is regarded as consisting essentially as a transfer of authority from the perceived real object to its internal representative. Introjection in this sense is quite different from identification which is regarded as an ego activity which begins early in life and represents the internalization of an aspect of an object representation into the child's self representation. The superego introjects were seen as having a supportive role as well as being a source of anticipated internalized criticism.

The revised Index manual relating to the superego is described in 'The classification of superego material in the Hampstead Index' (Sandler et al.)[72]. The various Index headings are illustrated by clinical examples taken from the Index.

In two papers 'Psychology and Psychoanalysis' (Sandler)[63] and 'The concept of the representational world' (Sandler and Rosenblatt)[74] some of the formulations in the earlier papers on the superego were expanded into a general theoretical model, in which the concept of a developing body image was generalized in terms of the development of a whole world of self, object, thing, word and feeling representations. The influence of the various psychic structures on the representational world was discussed, particularly in relation to problems connected with the psychoanalytic theory of narcissism. The regulation of the feeling of well-being within the representational world was seen as being an important factor in both ego and superego functioning.

Although the concept of the ego ideal is closely related to that of the superego, problems of classifying material relating to ideal formation led to a detailed examination of the ego ideal, and a paper on 'The ego ideal and the ideal self' embodied the conclusions drawn by an Index working party on this topic (Sandler, Holder and Meers)[65]. It could be shown that the term 'ego ideal' had different meanings for Freud at different times, and it was found necessary to make use of the concept of 'ideal self' and 'ideal object' as auxiliary theoretical notions.

Problems arising in the classification of phantasy material in the Index led to the publication of 'Aspects of the metapsychology of phantasy' (Sandler and Nagera)[73]. The following conclusions were reached:

(*i*) As ideational content (representations) may originate from a number of sources (early unorganized sensations, organized thoughts, percepts, memory images, imaginative constructions, etc.), it would appear to be inappropriate to use the term 'phantasying' for the primary-process elaboration of these into the content of instinctual wishes. It is only when the ego takes a hand in the organization of content into wish-fulfilling imaginative products, that we should speak of phantasy formation.

(*ii*) It would appear to be correct to speak of the content of the system *Unconscious* as unconscious phantasy only when that content has been derived from repressed phantasies. In using the term 'unconscious phantasy' it should always be made clear whether the term is used to refer to those contents of the *Unconscious* which have been derived from phantasying, or in its broad descriptive sense.

(*iii*) The process of phantasying can be regarded as an ego function, resulting in organized, wish-fulfilling imaginative content, which may or may not be consciously perceived. The phantasy may then be a derivative, a compromise constructed by the ego between that wish and the demands of the superego introjects. Knowledge of reality may be partially or completely suspended in the formation of the derivative, or it may be utilized and influence the phantasy to a marked degree. The phantasy content may be repressed soon after it has been created, or defended against in other ways.

(*iv*) The phantasy is only one of many derivatives which the ego can construct.

(*v*) The possibility exists that some phantasies represent wish-fulfilments, when the wish in question arises neither from the id nor the superego, but from the ego itself.

Two papers, 'Notes on childhood depression' (Sandler and Joffe[68]) and 'Notes on pain, depression and individuation' (Joffe and Sandler[39]) report a study of the clinical manifestations of depressive reactions in children and a subsequent reconceptualization of the psychoanalytic theory of depression. A central feature of the views presented is that depressive illness of the 'melancholic' type does not occur in young children, but that various forms of depressive affective reaction can be discerned. The depressive reaction was seen as being a response to any sort of painful state in which feelings of helplessness and hopelessness supervened. While loss of self-esteem is painful, this is not the same as a depressive reaction; nor are feelings of guilt always present. It was suggested that normal development involves a process of gradual detachment from past ideal states of the self and that failure to achieve such detachment (individuation) can lead to a predisposition to experiencing depressive reactions.

The concept of mental pain was further explored in relation to depression and to bodily pain of organic or psychogenic origin in a paper 'On the concept of pain, with special reference to depression and psychogenic pain' (Joffe and Sandler[40]).

In 'Notes on obsessional manifestations in children' (Sandler and Joffe[67]) the varieties of obsessional phenomena recorded in the Index were reviewed, and following a discussion of the psychoanalytic literature, certain theoretical propositions were put forward. It was suggested that in obsessional neurosis proper (in both children and adults) a drive regression to anal fixation points takes place, but this is itself an insufficient condition for the development of an obsessional neurosis. Changes on the side of the ego occur as well, and these can be understood in terms of a *functional ego regression* to a mode of ego functioning which is itself normally characteristic of the anal phase. The existence of functional fixation points on the side of the ego can be discerned in the cognitive and perceptual style of the individual. The functional ego regression brings into operation the defence mechanisms which are characteristic of the neurosis and which represent a natural development of the individual's particular style of ego functioning. Varieties of obsessional phenomena other than obsessional neurosis are also discussed.

The problem of categorizing and classifying material relating to disturbances of narcissism was considered in some detail in 'Über einige begriffliche Probleme im Zusammenhang mit dem Studium narzisstischer Störungen'* (Joffe and Sandler)[41], and an approach to the resolution of certain difficulties inherent in the theory of narcissism was suggested. Emphasis was placed on the role of conscious or unconscious feeling-states and on the relatively neglected field of the psychology of values. The supplementary notion of 'affective' or 'feeling' cathexis was introduced and discussed.

The need to reach a clearer understanding of the concept of sublimation resulted in a number of formulations which were embodied in 'On skill and sublimation' (Sandler and Joffe[69]). Difficulties in regard to the concept of 'transformation of energy' were discussed and an alternative formulation considered. It was felt necessary to make a distinction between activities and skills on the one hand, and the employment of these for purposes of sublimation on the other. An essential component of sublimatory activity is that the 'demand for work' imposed by the instinctual drive is reduced in ways which are much more 'distanced' from the original forms of drive discharge and which are accompanied by feelings of pleasure removed from crude instinctual pleasures. In addition, the activity itself receives what could be called a 'value cathexis' of the sort which distinguishes object relations beyond the level of simple need satisfaction, i.e. the person invests the activity with a value similar to that which he attaches to his love objects or to his own self.

Further work on regression and allied problems has led to the formulation of a concept of 'persistence'. This concept is discussed in 'Persistence in psychological function and development, with special reference to fixation and regression' (Sandler and Joffe[70]). The paper presents an approach to problems of id-ego interaction from the point of view of the distinction between structure and function, and both drive and ego regression are discussed in the light of this distinction. The concept of 'persistence' embodies the view that primitive modes of functioning actively persist in the present in the form of 'trials' which are normally inhibited. All forms of regression can then be regarded not as simple 'going back' or revival of the past, but as processes of release and disinhibition of earlier modes of functioning.

In 1964 the Index project was asked to contribute to a symposium on 'Trauma' held in New York, and the conclusions drawn from Index work

* Some conceptual problems involved in the consideration of disorders of narcissism.

on this subject are embodied in 'Trauma, strain and development' (Sandler[64]).

In this study the theoretical definition of the term 'trauma' was compared with the ways in which the term was applied in clinical practice, and as a consequence it was found that a number of difficulties emerge in the application of the concept. In the discussion of these difficulties emphasis was laid on what was called 'ego-strain', and the conclusion was drawn that the child's adaptation to states of ego-strain (which may or may not follow traumatic experiences) is crucial from the point of view of his subsequent development, rather than the experience of the trauma itself.

A similar study on the concept of transference, with special reference to psychoanalytic work with children is reported in 'Einige theoretische und klinische Aspekte der Übertragung'* (Sandler et al.[66]). Here again difficulties in reconciling the theoretical and clinical meanings and usages of the term are considered, and the conclusion was reached that 'transference' is not a metapsychological concept but a clinical one. The various 'dimensions' of transference in the psychoanalytic situation are regarded as paralleling the various dimensions of *relationships* in general.

In 'Kommentare zur psychoanalytischen Anpassungspsychologie mit bezonderem Bezug auf die Rolle der Affekte und der Innenwelt der Repräsentanzen'† (Joffe and Sandler[42]) an outline was given of a general theme which had run through many of the Index publications—but now pulled together for the first time. Crucial to this presentation is the view that the ego bases its adaptive manœuvres on the basis of a continuous process of scanning its (conscious or unconscious) feeling-states, and that it responds to both the instinctual drives and the external world on the basis of the changes which occur in this central feeling-state. The view was also put forward that the ultimate guiding and regulating principle in ego functioning was its need to attain or to maintain a feeling-state of well-being. The relationship of this view to the psychology of ego autonomy was discussed in a further paper 'On the psychoanalytic psychology of autonomy and the autonomy of psychoanalytic theory' (Sandler and Joffe[71]).

The value of indexing as a method of research is described in 'The Hampstead Index as a method of psychoanalytic research' (Sandler[62]) in which the general notion of 'concept testing' is explored and elaborated.

The Hampstead Psychoanalytic Index. A Study of the Case Material of a Two-Year-Old Child (Bolland and Sandler[1]) is the first of the monograph series of The Psychoanalytic Study of the Child. It contains a full account of the analysis of a very young child, together with the subsequent indexing of the case, and is an illustration of the way in which the case and analytic material is dealt with in the process of indexing. The volume contains

* Some theoretical and clinical aspects of transference.
† Comments on the psychoanalytic psychology of adaptation, with special reference to the role of affects and the representational world.

extracts from all the Index manuals and shows the way in which the content of the Index cards is related to the weekly reports and other case material on the one hand and to the definitions in the Index manuals on the other.

REFERENCES

1. BOLLAND, J., and SANDLER, J., 1965. *The Hampstead psychoanalytic index. A study of the psychoanalytic case material of a two-year-old child.* New York, Intern. Univ. Press.
2. BURLINGHAM, D., 1952. *Twins: a study of three pairs of identical twins.* New York, Intern. Univ. Press.
3. BURLINGHAM, D., 1961. Some notes on the development of the blind. *Psychoanal. Study Child*, **16**, 121-45.
4. BURLINGHAM, D., 1964. Hearing and its role in the development of the blind. *Psychoanal. Study Child*, **19**, 95-112.
5. BURLINGHAM, D., 1965. Some problems of ego development in blind children. *Psychoanal. Study Child*, **20**, 194-208.
6. BURLINGHAM, D., and BARRON, A., 1963. A study of identical twins: their analytic material compared with existing observation data of their early childhood. *Psychoanal. Study Child*, **18**, 367-423.
7. BURLINGHAM, D., and FREUD, A., 1942. *Young children in war time: a year's work in a residential nursery.* London, Allen and Unwin.
8. BURLINGHAM, D., and FREUD, A., 1944. *Infants without families: the case for and against residential nurseries.* London, Allen and Unwin.
9. BURLINGHAM, D., GOLDBERGER, A., and LUSSIER, A., 1955. Simultaneous analysis of mother and child. *Psychoanal. Study Child*, **10**, 165-86.
10. FRANKL, L., 1961*a*. Some observations on the development and disturbances of integration in childhood. *Psychoanal. Study Child*, **16**, 146-63.
11. FRANKL, L., 1961*b*. The child and his symptom. In *Psychosomatic aspects of paediatrics*. Eds, MacKeith, R., and Sandler, J. London, Pergamon.
12. FRANKL, L., 1963. Self-preservation and the development of accident proneness in children and adolescents. *Psychoanal. Study Child*, **18**, 464-83.
13. FRANKL, L., and HELLMAN, I., 1963. A specific problem in adolescent boys: difficulties in loosening the infantile tie to the mother. *Bull. Phil. Assn Psychoanal.*, **13**, 120-29.
14. FRANKL, L., and HELLMAN, I., 1964. The ego's participation in the therapeutic alliance. In *Child psychotherapy*. Ed. Haworth, M. W. New York, Basic Books.
15. FREUD, A., 1936. *The ego and the mechanisms of defence.* London, Hogarth.
16. FREUD, A., 1959. Clinical studies in psychoanalysis: Research project of the Hampstead Child-Therapy Clinic. *Psychoanal. Study Child*, **14**, 122-31.
17. FREUD, A., 1960*a*. Why children go wrong. In *The enrichment of childhood*. The Nursery School Assn of Great Britain and Northern Ireland.
18. FREUD, A., 1960*b*. The child guidance clinic as a center of prophylaxis and enlightenment. In *Rec. Dev. Psychoanal. Child Therapy*, **1**, 25-38.
19. FREUD, A., 1961*a*. Four contributions to the psychoanalytic study of the child (reported by Sachs, D. M.). *Bull. Phila. Assn Psychoanal.*, **11**, 80-87.
20. FREUD, A., 1961*b*. Paediatricians' questions and answers. In *Psychosomatic aspects of paediatrics*. Eds, MacKeith, R., and Sandler, J. London, Pergamon.
21. FREUD, A., 1962*a*. Assessments of normality and pathology. In *Clinical problems of young children*. National Association for Mental Health.

22. FREUD, A., 1962b. Assessment of childhood disturbances. *Psychoanal. Study Child*, **17**, 149-58.
23. FREUD, A., 1963a. The concept of developmental lines. *Psychoanal. Study Child*, **18**, 245-65.
24. FREUD, A., 1963b. Regression as a principle in mental development. *Bull. Menninger Clin.*, **27**, 126-39.
25. FREUD, A., 1963c. The role of regression in mental development. In *Modern perspectives in child analysis*, Eds, Solnit, A., and Provence, S. New York, Intern. Univ. Press.
26. FREUD, A., 1964a. The ego's defensive operations considered as an object of analysis. In *Child psychotherapy*, Ed. Haworth, M. W. New York, Basic Books.
27. FREUD, A., 1964b. On the difficulties of communicating with children—the lesser children in chambers; Jean Drew; Cindy. In *The family and the law*. Eds, Goldstein, J., and Katz, J. New York, The Free Press.
28. FREUD, A., 1965a. *Normality and pathology in childhood: assessments of development*. New York, Intern. Univ. Press.
29. FREUD, A., 1965b. Diagnostic skills and their growth in psychoanalysis. *Int. J. Psychoanal.*, **46**, 31-38.
30. FREUD, A., 1966a. Links between Hartmann's ego psychology and the child analyst's thinking. In *Psychoanalysis—a general psychology: essays in honour of Heinz Hartmann*, Eds, Loewenstein, R. M., Newman, L. M., Schur, M., and Solnit, A. J. New York, Intern. Univ. Press.
31. FREUD, A., 1966b. Some thoughts about the place of psychoanalytic theory in the training of psychiatrists. *Bull. Menninger Clin.*, **30**, 225-34.
32. FREUD, A., 1966c. Interactions between nursery school and child guidance clinic. *J. Child Psychother.*, **1**, 40-44.
33. FREUD, A., and BURLINGHAM, D., 1943. *War and children*. New York, E. Willard.
34. FREUD, A., NAGERA, H., and FREUD, W. E., 1965. Metapsychological assessment of the adult personality: the adult profile. *Psychoanal. Study Child*, **20**, 9-41.
35. HELLMAN, I., 1962. Hampstead nursery follow up studies: 1. Sudden separation and its effect followed over twenty years. *Psychoanal. Study Child*, **17**, 159-74.
36. HELLMAN, I., 1964. Observations on adolescents in psychoanalytic treatment. *Brit. J. Psychiat.*, **110**, 466.
37. HELLMAN, I., 1965. The psychosexual development in adolescence. In *Psychosomatic disorders in adolescents and young adults*, Eds, Hambling, J., and Hopkins, P. London, Pergamon.
38. HELLMAN, I., FRIEDMANN, O., and SHEPHEARD, E., 1960. Simultaneous analysis of mother and child. *Psychoanal. Study Child*, **15**, 359-77.
39. JOFFE, W. G., and SANDLER, J., 1965. Notes on pain, depression and individuation. *Psychoanal. Study Child*, **20**, 394-424.
40. JOFFE, W. G., and SANDLER, J., 1967a. On the concept of pain, with special reference to depression and psychogenic pain. *J. psychosomatic Res.*, **11**, 69-75.
41. JOFFE, W. G., and SANDLER, J., 1967b. Über einige Begriffliche Probleme im Zusammenhang mit dem Studium narzisstischer Störungen. *Psyche*, **21**, 152-65.
42. JOFFE, W. G., and SANDLER, J., 1967c. Kommentare zur psychoanalytischen Anpassungspsychologie mit bezonderem Bezug auf die Rolle der Affekte und der Innenwelt der Repräsentanzen. *Psyche*, **21**, 728-44.
43. LAUFER, M., 1964. Ego ideal in adolescence. *Psychoanal. Study Child*, **19**, 196-221.

44. LAUFER, M., 1965. Assessment of adolescent disturbances: the application of Anna Freud's diagnostic profile. *Psychoanal. Study Child*, **20**, 99-123.
45. LEVY, K., 1960. Simultaneous analysis of a mother and her adolescent daughter: the mother's contribution to the loosening of the infantile object tie. With an introduction by Anna Freud. *Psychoanal. Study Child*, **15**, 378-91.
46. LUDOWYK, G. E., 1963. The analysis of a young concentration camp victim. *Psychoanal. Study Child*, **18**, 484-510.
47. LUSSIER, A., 1960. The analysis of a boy with a congenital deformity. *Psychoanal. Study Child*, **15**, 430-53.
48. NAGERA, H., 1963. The developmental profile. Notes on some practical considerations regarding its use. *Psychoanal. Study Child*, **18**, 511-40.
49. NAGERA, H., 1964a. On arrest in development, fixation and regression. *Psychoanal. Study Child*, **19**, 222-39.
50. NAGERA, H., 1964b. Auterotism, autoerotic activities, and ego development. *Psychoanal. Study Child*, **19**, 240-55.
51. NAGERA, H., 1966. *Early childhood disturbances, the infantile neurosis, and the adulthood neurosis*. New York, Intern. Univ. Press.
52. NAGERA, H., and COLONNA, A. B., 1965. Aspects of the contribution of sight to ego and drive development: a comparison of the development of some blind and sighted children. *Psychoanal. Study Child*, **20**, 267-87.
53. ROBERTSON, JOYCE, 1962. Mothering as an influence in early development. A study of well-baby clinic records. *Psychoanal. Study Child*, **17**, 245-64.
54. ROBERTSON, JOYCE, 1965a. Mother-infant interaction from birth to twelve months: two case studies. In *Determinants of infant behaviour III*, Ed. Foss, B. M. London, Methuen. 111-24.
55. ROBERTSON, JOYCE, 1965b. Three devoted mothers. *Samiksa*, **18**, 10-26.
56. ROSENBLATT, B., 1963. A severe neurosis in an adolescent boy. *Psychoanal. Study Child*, **18**, 561-602.
57. ROSENFELD, S. K., and SPRINCE, M. P., 1963. An attempt to formulate the meaning of the concept 'borderline'. *Psychoanal. Study Child*, **18**, 603-635.
58. ROSENFELD, S. K., and SPRINCE, M. P., 1965. Some thoughts on the technical handling of borderline children. *Psychoanal. Study Child*, **20**, 495-517.
59. SANDLER, A.-M., 1963. Aspects of passivity and ego development in the blind infant. *Psychoanal. Study Child*, **18**, 343-60.
60. SANDLER, A.-M., and WILLS, D. M., 1965. Preliminary notes on play and mastery in the blind child. *J. Child Psychother.*, **1**, 7-19.
61. SANDLER, J., 1960. On the concept of superego. *Psychoanal. Study Child*, **15**, 128-62.
62. SANDLER, J., 1962a. The Hampstead Index as an instrument of psychoanalytical research. *Int. J. Psychoanal.*, **43**, 287-91.
63. SANDLER, J., 1962b. Psychology and psychoanalysis. *Brit. J. Med. Psychol.*, **35**, 91.
64. SANDLER, J., 1967. Trauma, strain and development. In *Psychic Trauma*, Ed. Furst, S. New York, Basic Books.
65. SANDLER, J., HOLDER, A., and MEERS, D., 1963. The ego ideal and the ideal self. *Psychoanal. Study Child*, **18**, 139-58.
66. SANDLER, J., HOLDER, A., KAWENOKA, M., KENNEDY, H. E., and NEURATH, L., 1967. Einige theoretische und klinische Aspekte der Übertragung. *Psyche*, **21**, 804-26.
67. SANDLER, J., and JOFFE, W. G., 1965a. Notes on obsessional manifestations in children. *Psychoanal. Study Child*, **20**, 425-38.
68. SANDLER, J., and JOFFE, W. G., 1965b. Notes on childhood depression. *Int. J. Psychoanal.*, **46**, 88-96.

69. SANDLER, J., and JOFFE, W. G., 1966. On skill and sublimation. *J. Amer. Psychoanal. Assn*, **14**, 335-55.
70. SANDLER, J., and JOFFE, W. G., 1967a. Persistence in psychological function and development, with special reference to fixation and regression. *Bull. Meninger Clin.* **31**, 257-71.
71. SANDLER, J., and JOFFE, W. G., 1967b. On the psychoanalytic psychology of autonomy and the autonomy of psychoanalytic theory. *Int. J. Psychiat.*, **3**, 512-15.
72. SANDLER, J., KAWENOKA, M., NEURATH, L., ROSENBLATT, B., SCHNURMANN, A., and SIGAL, J., 1962. The classification of superego material in the Hampstead Index. *Psychoanal. Study Child*, **17**, 107-27.
73. SANDLER, J., and NAGERA, H., 1963. Aspects of the metapsychology of fantasy. *Psychoanal. Study Child*, **18**, 159-94.
74. SANDLER, J., and ROSENBLATT, B., 1962. The concept of the representational world. *Psychoanal. Study Child*, **17**, 128-45.
75. SINGER, M. B., 1960. Fantasies of a borderline patient. *Psychoanal. Study Child*, **15**, 310-56.
76. SPRINCE, M. P., 1962. The development of a pre-oedipal partnership between an adolescent girl and her mother. *Psychoanal. Study Child*, **17**, 418-50.
77. SPRINCE, M. P., 1964. A contribution to the study of homosexuality in adolescence. *J. Child Psychol. Psychiat.*, **5**, 103-17.
78. THOMAS, R., FOLKART, L., and MODEL, E., 1963. The search for a sexual identity in a case of constitutional precocity. *Psychoanal. Study Child*, **18**, 636-62.
79. THOMAS, R., EDGCUMBE, R., KENNEDY, H., KAWENOKA, M., and WEITZNER, L., 1966. Comments on some aspects of self and object representation in a group of borderline children: the application of Anna Freud's diagnostic profile. *Psychoanal. Study Child*, **21**, 527-80.
80. WILLS, D. M., 1965. Some observations on blind nursery school children. *Psychoanal. Study Child*, **20**, 344-64.

IX

SEPARATION AND DEPRIVATION
Parent-Child Separation as a Therapeutic Procedure

John G. Howells
*Director, The Institute of Family Psychiatry,
Ipswich and East Suffolk Hospital, Ipswich, England*

1
Introduction

Much of the confusion about 'separation' and 'deprivation' springs from the fact that the two words are used interchangeably and it would seem to be essential to have a clear definition of each. 'Separation' of child and parent, by common usage, means that the child is physically parted from its parents and has an existence independent of them.

'Deprivation' is a term which indicates that a loss is suffered and when applied to the child it is used in the following two senses:

1. Occasionally it is used to denote that the child suffers the loss of its *parents*, or permanent parent substitute. This usually coincides with physical separation of parent and child. To prevent confusion with the term 'separation', this usage should be avoided.

2. Frequently, it is used to denote that the child is deprived of the necessary care for its emotional growth, and so suffers the loss of *parenting*, i.e. qualities including love, affection and security. This form of deprivation can occur with the parent, or apart from the parent.

'Separation', then, involves the physical loss of the parent, but not necessarily of parenting. 'Deprivation' involves the loss of parenting, but not necessarily of parents; the quality offered to the child, parenting, is differentiated from the object, parent, which supplies it.

Thus, separation and deprivation are not synonymous terms. Also, parents as an entity are distinguished from another entity, the emotional care given by them, i.e. from parenting. Separation of a child from its

INTRODUCTION   255

parents may result in deprivation or non-deprivation of parenting depending on the situation. Equally non-separation of a child from its parents may result in deprivation or non-deprivation of parenting depending on the situation. The commonest occurrence of deprivation of parenting is with non-separation, i.e. due to stressful situations at home between parents and children; separation of children and parents may sometimes be the best way of bringing non-deprivation, i.e. adequate parenting.

This chapter is concerned with some of the issues surrounding separation: clarifying the meaning of separation from that of deprivation; reporting a direct study on separation; reviewing some more direct studies of separation; and emphasizing the value of separation as a therapeutic procedure in certain circumstances. Deprivation, i.e. the lack of the right parenting is accepted to be a matter of major concern in child psychiatry, but is not the subject of this chapter.

Contemporary Child Care

An apt illustration of damaging prevalent opinions on separation is to be found in a statement in an authoritative publication by the British Ministry of Health[30], which was written to encourage the family doctor to take an interest in the Mental Health Services, and gives the following warning:

'On the purely psychological side there is evidence that separation from the parent, or parent substitute before the age of five may have a serious effect on the emotional growth of children and may form the basis of neurotic reactions in later life.'

In this statement two postulates are implied:

1. That child-parent separation is harmful under the age of five and causes the child to lack the ingredients essential for its emotional growth, i.e. separation is synonymous with deprivation of the right emotional care.

2. That separation experiences may lead to mental ill-health later on.

Faced with this and similar statements, there is a reluctance to use separation procedures and indeed great efforts are made to maintain children with their parents, *whatever the cost to the children*. Responsible authorities will often support the adage that 'even a bad natural home is better than any other home'.

The author believes, as the result of clinical experience and research evidence to be given, that the damaging agent is not physical *separation* per se; he holds that *deprivation* of the right care is the damaging agent. Deprivation of the right care, i.e. inadequate parenting may be present without the separation of child from its parents; indeed, the commonest situation surrounding children who come to child psychiatric clinics, suffering from emotional illness consequent on deprivation of the right care, is that they are living with their parents, i.e. are not separated. In Great Britain, only one child in 2,000 lives away from his parents as revealed by the report[39] of the Children's Department of the Home Office.

S

Non-separation in a happy home can be beneficial, but so can separation; many children live in happy foster and adoptive homes and are not deprived though separated. The truth of the matter is that separation is not synonymous with deprivation. Separation, or non-separation are important to child care depending on whether or not they lead to deprivation of the right kind of care. Deprivation is the damaging factor.

The importance of clarifying this issue lies here. As separation has been claimed to be the damaging agent, authorities have adopted the policy of regarding it as a danger. Thus a child in a deprivatory situation in his own home is not separated from it because of the alleged greater dangers of separation. But separation is not damaging in itself—only if it leads to deprivation; it can lead to non-deprivation. Thus, the child is denied the advantage of all those procedures by separation which would give it compensatory beneficial care. It is a curious commentary of contemporary child care, that it can be unmoved at the suffering of a child in its own home, while moved to compassion at the sight of a child deprived when away from its parents. While both are to be deplored, one is greatly more common than the other, and both equally deserving of amelioration. This single fallacious attitude of regarding separation as synonymous with deprivation is the most damaging single liability in contemporary preventive psychiatry.

Once the fallacy is exposed and accepted, it will be a matter of surprise that it was ever held. But it is held, though contrary to everyday behaviour and experience—held by the experts and by a puzzled public. The bias springs from lack of systematic investigation in this field, the considerable difficulties of researching in it, and possibly also from inherent prejudices in the researchers. The field of child care, it can be supposed, may attract those who have suffered deprivatory experiences, and who identify with the deprived. But such deprived individuals may have suffered anomalous upbringing which may lead to misconceptions on family care and, amongst other distortions, to an excessive idealization of parents.

Our knowledge of parental care, in its important emotional aspect, is still rudimentary. Not only is there ignorance, but often an extraordinary distortion of facts which in itself must be the subject for study. One instance is the overemphasis given to maternal care, with the neglect of fathering, and of the neglect of the even more important truth that the child is brought up in a group situation, the family. Views expressed about the hazards of separation have almost exclusively concerned themselves with separation from the mother who, by implication, is regarded as the sole giver of parenting to the infant. But maternal care is but one ingredient in the family group care of children. Maternal care is often beneficial; it may also be destructive. Mothering may be found in the natural mother, but it may be absent and found in another female figure. It may well be that it is more important for a child to have *a* mother, than *the* mother. In a particular instance, maternal care may lack the quality of care offered by a

FIG. 1. Deprivation at home.

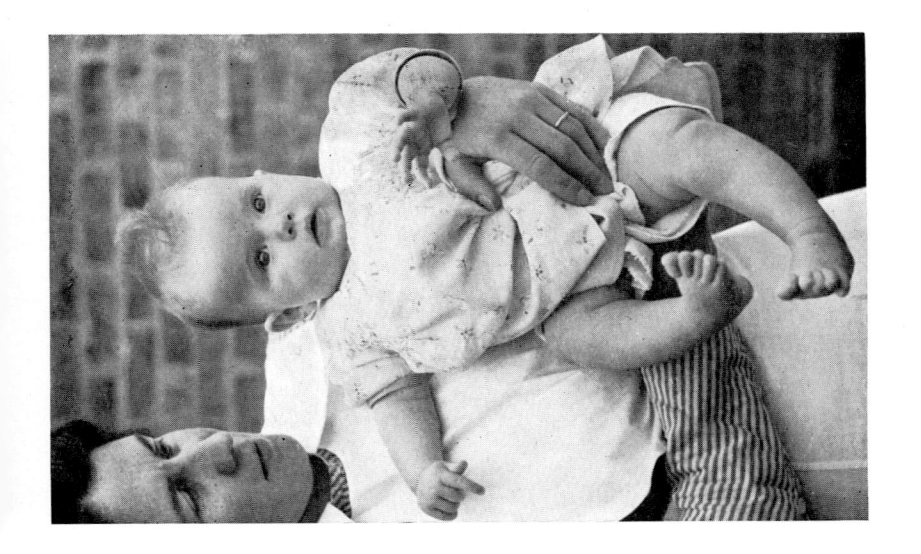

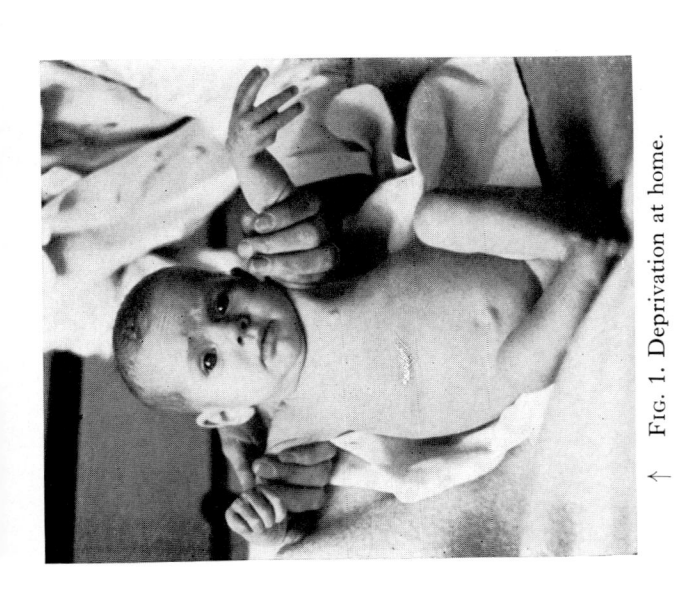

FIG. 2. Improvement after separation.

father, a sibling, a relative, a foster or adoptive parent. Most parents are capable to a reasonable degree of giving satisfactory parenting; some have suffered such deprivation of emotional care as children that they cannot manifest parenting.

Parenting is more important than parents. Nature provides for the upbringing of the young of each species, and to do this it employs a variety of procedures, of which the use of the natural parents, father and mother, is but one. Other procedures are multiple parenting, maternal care alone, paternal care alone, foster care, group care, and care dependent on the physical surroundings alone. For the young of *Homo sapiens* the method of choice is group care, in a family group. Here again nature is flexible, as is revealed by historical and anthropological research. The need to bring up the young is more important than the methods employed. Thus, depending on the demands of the situation, it may employ multiple parenting, foster care, exclusive maternal or parental care, or community care. In regard to group upbringing Mead[29] states:

'At present, the specific biological situation of the continuing relationship of the child to its biological mother and its need for care by human beings are being hopelessly confused in the growing insistence that child and biological mother, or mother surrogate, must never be separated, that all separation even for a few days is inevitably damaging, and that if long enough it does irreversible damage.' 'Actually, anthropological evidence gives no support at present to the value of such an accentuation of the tie between mother and child. On the contrary, cross-cultural studies suggest that adjustment is most facilitated if the child is cared for by many warm, friendly people.'

For a number of reasons, western culture has tended to overlook that the child is brought up in a group situation, the family, and given undue emphasis to one element in the group, maternal care. It is an unusual situation for an infant or child to relate to his mother alone, even in the first few days. In the nuclear family, it relates to father, mother and siblings; but nuclear families are often not as small as this, and in addition often have within them grandparents, parental sibs, friends, servants, and the children's peers. The contribution of each member of a group to the infant is variable; mother may be paramount in giving care; less often father may have the major role—or a grandparent, a relative, or a sib. The care given by any family member, including mother, may be constructive or destructive, depending on their personal qualities and the meaning of the child to them. Paternal care in nature is, of course, as distinct, early and real an entity as maternal care and can manifest the same ingredients of tenderness, kindness and love. To be part of a group gives the child protection; what one member of the group lacks in his care may be supplied by another; for *Homo sapiens*, nature did not 'put all its eggs in one basket'.

The author now proceeds to describe a direct study, employing a control group; this fails to support the view that separation is a considerable mental health hazard. He will then outline some of the few direct studies on separation. Studies on a related but distinct matter, deprivation, will not be reviewed. He will then show how a number of procedures dependent on the utilization of separation can overcome deprivation and make a significant contribution to the promotion of emotional health.

2

A Direct Investigation of Separation

General

The investigation reported here compares separation experiences in a random sample of emotionally sick children attending a child psychiatric clinic with similar experiences in a control group of school-children of average emotional health. The children of both groups were living at home and the separations are brought about by the normal happenings of everyday life. The clinic group was an unselected random group of emotionally ill children and will be referred to as the 'neurotic' group.

Each group contained 37 children, and the two groups were made as similar as possible. The sexes in the two groups were nearly equal, there being 19 boys and 18 girls in the control group, and 20 boys and 17 girls in the neurotic group. The average age in the two groups was approximately equal, i.e. 6·5 years in the control group and 6·9 years in the neurotic group. The questionnaire method was employed. The parents were asked for details of each occasion that the mother, father, or child had been away from home for a night or more until the child's fifth birthday. The information was collected shortly after the child's fifth birthday while the parents' memory was likely to be accurate. The first five years were investigated as the protagonists of the danger of separation view-point regard this as the most vulnerable age-group.

The main investigation explored (*i*) the incidence of separation experiences in the two groups. Should separation be responsible for mental ill-health in children, then it would be expected that there would (*a*) be a high incidence of separation in the sick group and (*b*) that the incidence would be significantly higher in the sick than healthy group. The investigators also explored (*ii*) the effects of separation in both groups; (*iii*) the causes of separation; and (*iv*) the care of the child during separation.

Incidence of Separation

The figures of the separations in the control group and the neurotic group have been tabulated and will be compared and considered from three angles—namely, (*a*) the number of children involved in separations, (*b*) the number of occasions of separations, and (*c*) the total length in time of the separations. The length of each separation is then considered (*d*) and is followed (*e*) by a short study of separations in children under one year of age.

The first six tables have three sections. The first section gives all separations of one day (24 hours) and over, the second gives separations of three days and over, and the third gives separations of one week and over. Thus separations of short duration can be ignored if it is considered that it is unlikely that they have any effect upon the child. Three age periods are investigated, under one year, under two years and under five years.

In addition to the figures given in the tables of separations from fathers, there are in both control and neurotic groups four fathers who are working away regularly for not more than four nights. Night duty for the fathers has not been included.

TABLE I

Number of Children separated from their Mothers

	Under 1 year Control Group	Under 1 year Neurotic Group	Under 2 years Control Group	Under 2 years Neurotic Group	Under 5 years Control Group	Under 5 years Neurotic Group
Over 1 day	2	3	14	17	29	32
Over 3 days	2	2	14	14	28	29
Over 7 days	2	2	14	12	24	26

Table I shows the number of children who have been separated from their mothers. This has entailed either the mother or child leaving home. In both groups separation under the age of one year is uncommon. About a third of the children in both groups under the age of two have been separated from their mothers for more than seven days. This indicates that in only a third of the neurotic group could separation from the mother at this early age have influenced the neurosis; and in fact no more of the neurotic group than of the control group have been thus separated. By the age of five, approximately three-quarters of the children in both groups have been separated from their mothers for at least a day, and about two-thirds of the children have had a separation of one week or more. There is no significant difference between the two groups in this. By the age of five, there were five children in the neurotic group who had experienced no separation from the mother.

Table II shows the number of children who have been separated from their fathers. This has entailed either the father or child leaving home. It can be seen that more fathers than mothers are separated from their children in the first year. It appears that five of the 74 fathers were serving in the Forces for the first few months of the child's life. By the second and fifth year there is close similarity between the incidence of the child's separation from the mother and the father. Under one year there are twice as many of the neurotic group separated as the control group for 24 hours. But it must be remembered that such a short period of separation is hardly likely to be significant. There is still a tendency for neurotic group fathers

TABLE II

Number of Children separated from their Fathers

	Under 1 year		Under 2 years		Under 5 years	
	Control Group	Neurotic Group	Control Group	Neurotic Group	Control Group	Neurotic Group
Over 1 day	5	10	14	19	30	29
Over 3 days	5	8	14	17	28	26
Over 7 days	4	7	13	15	25	24

of children under two to be away, but if separations of under one week are disregarded then there is no significant difference, for 13 control group and 15 neurotic group, i.e. about two-fifths, have been separated from their fathers. Similarly, the number of children under five years involved in the two groups are nearly equal.

TABLE III

Number of separations of Children from their Mothers

	Under 1 year		Under 2 years		Under 5 years	
	Control Group	Neurotic Group	Control Group	Neurotic Group	Control Group	Neurotic Group
Over 1 day	2	4	18	23	71	69
Over 3 days	2	3	18	19	59	53
Over 7 days	2	3	17	15	49	46

The figures in Tables III and IV indicating the numbers of separations from mother or father in each group show little difference from those showing the number of children involved in separations. The number of separations from their mothers of children of all ages was similar in both groups, and few occurred to children under the age of one year. Twice as many separations from their fathers of children under one year occurred in the neurotic group as in the control group, but they apply to a minority. Under two years each group has about the same number, but under five years they have reversed their positions, and the control group has half as many again as the neurotic group. As will be shown later, the reason for

TABLE IV

Number of separations of Children from their Fathers

	Under 1 year		Under 2 years		Under 5 years	
	Control Group	Neurotic Group	Control Group	Neurotic Group	Control Group	Neurotic Group
Over 1 day	5	12	22	26	86	60
Over 3 days	5	10	22	23	73	48
Over 7 days	4	10	20	21	64	42

the greater number of separations in the control group, is that these fathers have more short periods of work at a distance from their homes. There is nothing to indicate why this should be more common in the control group.

TABLE V

Total Amount of Separation from Mother in each Group

	Under 1 year						Under 2 years						Under 5 years					
	Control Group			Neurotic Group			Control Group			Neurotic Group			Control Group			Neurotic Group		
	months	weeks	days	months	weeks	days	months	weeks	days	months	weeks	days	months	weeks	days	months	weeks	days
Over 1 day	1	0	0	2	0	1	11	3	0	15	3	4	29	0	0	54	3	2
Over 3 days	1	0	0	2	0	0	11	3	0	15	2	5	28	1	0	53	3	6
Over 7 days	1	0	0	2	0	0	11	2	5	15	0	3	25	3	4	40	1	1

Tables V and VI give the total length of time of the separations. The periods of separation of all the children are added together for each group. They show that, although there is little difference in the two groups between the number of children involved and the number of separations, there is an appreciably greater total duration of separation from both mother and father in the neurotic group. It will be seen later (Tables VII and VIII) that a small number of cases of long duration account for the difference. In the case of the mothers the difference was accounted for by a small number of long separations due to the illness of the mother. In the case of the fathers a break in the parental relationship and the death of a father

TABLE VI

Total Amount of Separation from Father in each Group

	Under 1 year								Under 2 years								Under 5 years							
	Control Group				Neurotic Group				Control Group				Neurotic Group				Control Group				Neurotic Group			
	years	months	weeks	days	years	months	weeks	days	years	months	weeks	days	years	months	weeks	days	years	months	weeks	days	years	months	weeks	days
Over 1 day	11	2	5	4	3	1	2	3	1	2	2	8	3	2	5	10	10	1	3	17	9	0	2
Over 3 days	11	2	5	4	3	1	0	3	1	2	2	8	3	2	2	10	9	2	2	17	8	1	5
Over 7 days	11	2	0	4	3	0	0	3	1	1	1	8	3	1	2	10	8	3	1	17	7	3	2
Total (disregarding 2 cases where child had never seen father)					2	3	1	2					4	3	2	5					7	9	0	2

TABLE VII

Each Separation from Mother Classified for its Length

| Length of Separation | Under 1 year || Under 2 years || Under 5 years ||
	Control Group	Neurotic Group	Control Group	Neurotic Group	Control Group	Neurotic Group
0–2 days	0	1	0	4	12	16
3–6 days	0	0	1	4	10	7
7–27 days	2	2	13	9	42	32
1–3 months	0	1	3	5	6	8
3–6 months	0	0	1	1	1	5
Over 6 months					0	1

accounts for ten years of separation from the fathers in the neurotic group. Hence the neurotic group figures are also given excluding the two children who have never seen their fathers. Under one year there is more than twice as long a separation from the fathers in the neurotic group. Under two years the control group have caught up to three-quarters of the neurotic group, and under five years they have overtaken the neurotic group by one-third as long again. Average duration of separation from mother under two years in the control group is 9·5 days, and 12·8 days in the neurotic group.

TABLE VIII

Each Separation from Father Classified for its Length

Length of Separation	Under 1 year Control Group	Under 1 year Neurotic Group	Under 2 years Control Group	Under 2 years Neurotic Group	Under 5 years Control Group	Under 5 years Neurotic Group
0–2 days	0	2	0	3	13	12
3–6 days	1	0	2	2	7	6
7–27 days	2	2	11	10	39	22
1–3 months	0	2	5	4	19	6
3–6 months	2	6	4	7	6	7
Over 6 months					2	7

Tables VII and VIII classify the length of each separation from mother and father respectively, and are the most revealing and important tables. Out of the 74 children under one year only five were separated for more than three days from the mother, only one for more than one month, and none for more than three months. Under two years there were four separations of more than one month in the control group and six in the neurotic group. In each group, one child was separated for more than three months. Thus the number and length of the separations from the mother are small in children under two years in both groups and there is no significant difference between them. With children under five years there is again no significant difference between the two groups in the length of separations, except for periods of more than three months; but there was one separation of such length in the control group compared with six in the neurotic group (involving five children). Of these long separations, three lasted over four months, and one over six months. With one exception, the separations of over three months were due to the mother's illness.

There is a similarly greater proportion of long periods of separation from father in the neurotic group. Under one year of age there are two control group and six neurotic group separations of over three months. Separations from the father of less than three months, in children under five, are more common in the control group (78 separations as against 46 in the neurotic group). In the control group, however, there are only two separations (affecting one child) from the father of over six months, compared with seven such long separations (affecting six children) in the neurotic group. The causes of these long separations in the control group were that the father was serving in the Forces and later there was a break in the marriage. The causes in the neurotic group were: in three cases father was serving in the Forces, in two cases the marriage broke down (in one the separation being for five years), in one case a death caused a separation of five years, and in one case the child was transferred to the care of the Children's Officer because of the mother's illness.

In children under one year there were in the two groups six occasions of separation from the mother of at least 24 hours, only one being caused by the infant's illness and admission to hospital. Of the other five, three such separations were caused by the mother's illness, one by a relative's death, and one by moving house. During these five separations the infants were cared for by two grandmothers, two sisters-in-law, and one friend. The mothers reported no ill effects from the separation in children cared for by relatives and friends; there was adverse comment on the one instance of hospital admission.

Discussion. The major finding of this part of the investigation is the striking similarity in the pattern of separation experiences in the two groups, as well as the equally low incidence of separation in both groups. Separations from the mother under the age of one year were rare in both groups; there was only one separation of over a month in the 74 cases and only five of over three days. In both groups two-thirds of the children under two had not experienced separation of more than two days from their mothers. One-third of the children, at the age of five years, had not experienced a separation of over a week from their mothers. The pattern of the findings in the two groups relating to the child's separations from the father largely agreed in the same way. But there were more separations from father than mother. These findings support our clinical impression that in the great majority of children mental ill-health springs from processes arising from being with their parents rather than away from them.

It might be suggested that the neurotic process is set up in susceptible children by a separation which would leave another child unharmed. Later, however, it will be seen that the mothers noted as many favourable reactions to separation in the children of the neurotic group as in the control group and that unfavourable reactions were no commoner in the children of the neurotic group. It is uncommon in clinical practice to be able to relate the onset of a neurotic disturbance to a separation experience.

The differences that do exist in the pattern of the separation experiences in the present study are minor. The most important differences relates to the *length of separation*. Authorities do not agree about the minimum length of a separation period which is likely to cause damage. Spitz and Wolff[41] believe 'that there is a qualitative change after a period of three months after which recovery is rarely, if ever, completed'. Lewis[28] takes three months to two years as a period of 'temporary' separation and a period of two years as a period of 'lasting' separation. Bowlby[4] takes six months as a period of prolonged separation; Burlingham and Freud, quoted by him (1951), state that 'whenever it is more than that (separation of a day's length) they tend to lose their emotional ties, revert to their instincts and regress in their behaviour'. We accepted the very strict standard of one day.

The difference between the two groups in regard to the length of separation is that in the neurotic group there were a greater number of periods of separation from mother lasting over three months—six occasions as compared with one. The six occasions involved only five children and they were all over two years old. These long periods of separation in the neurotic group were caused by the illnesses of the mothers. There was only one continuous period of separation of over six months and this occurred in the neurotic group.

The position is similar with separations from the father: while the two groups differ very little, there is a greater proportion of long separations from father in the neurotic group; again they affect only a small number of children. In the seven periods of separation from the father lasting more than six months, two were due to a break-up of the marriage, one was due to the mother's illness, three were due to absences in the Forces and one was due to death of a father. The first two of the factors involved in these separations may relate to the emotional state of the parents and the third factor may be related to it with less certainty.

It is important to relate these prolonged separations to their causes, and it is significant that the minor differences between the two groups reflect on the quality of the parents. In the case of the mothers the differences are accounted for completely by the greater amount of illness among the mothers in the neurotic group. With less certainty, the longer separations from father in the neurotic group reflect on the quality of the fathers. The mothers of the neurotic group children rarely visited the child if he was admitted to hospital, whereas the mothers of the control group children always did. The neurotic group fathers, when ill, were away for twice as long as the fathers of the control group children. The poorer quality and inadequacy of the parents of the neurotic children is significant. Such parents not only have a greater tendency to become ill for long periods, but also create emotional disturbances in their children when with them. The prolonged separation arising from the mother's illness is a further strain for the already disturbed child unless he is more fortunate in his substitute parent than in his natural parent. Thus a history of long separation, in the few instances when it occurs in a neurotic child, should not be assumed to be the root cause of the disturbance, since the emotional disturbance may have taken place before the separation, and both the separation and disturbance can be consequences of parental inadequacy. In our experience the parental inadequacy springs from a parental neurosis. That this is so is supported by a study in which Rutter[36] compares children referred to the Maudsley Hospital with children referred to a non-psychiatric clinic. The parents of the Maudsley children had twice as much chronic illness and parental psychiatric illness was three times as common.

There is, however, a small group of children in the community who have a permanent break from their parents or a lengthy temporary break which is spent in institutions. As such children are relatively accessible, they have been the subject of many studies. These children, however, do not suffer from separation per se: they suffer from deprivation of affection resulting from inadequate substitute mothering, or deprivation arising from adverse home experiences prior to the separation.

Some children enduring adverse home environments will clearly gain from separation from their parents. Separation is not synonymous with deprivation. Separation has come to mean being 'deprived of normal home life', without reference to the fact that the home life of these children is already far from 'normal' and the home far from a true home. A good natural home may be better than any other home. A good substitute home is better than a bad natural home. The number who gain from separation is not known, and they are less conspicuous than the children who, because of deprivation consequent on bad placements, come to the notice of the various child welfare agencies.

Nevertheless, as has been said, some children do suffer if deprivation is a consequence of separation, and it is of great importance to minimize this danger by retaining a child in a good home whenever possible and placing him in a good substitute when separation is inevitable. It would be erroneous, however, to imagine that by solving the problem of this small group of children who suffer prolonged separation, we would greatly influence the general problem of mental ill health in children, for the great majority of disturbed children suffer from being with their parents.

Various writers have disagreed about the *age* at which the child experiences greatest deprivation consequent upon separation. Bowlby[4] emphasizes the importance of deprivation under the age of three or four years, and the vital importance of the first year: 'deprivation occurring in the second half of the first year of life is agreed by all students of the subject to be of great significance and that many believe this to be true also of deprivation occurring in the first half. . . .'

We find that only two children in the control group and three children in the neurotic group could have experienced deprivation through separation from the mother in the first year. The care of the child while mother was away appeared adequate. Only one experienced a separation of over a month. Of the 37 neurotic children, 34 had experienced no separation in the first year. By the end of the second year two-thirds of the neurotic children had not experienced separation from their mothers for more than two days, and they had not suffered any worse in this respect than the children in the control group. No mothers reported ill effects in a child for a separation of two days or under up to two years of age. By the end of the fifth year a third of the neurotic group had not experienced a separation of more than one week from their mothers, and they had not suffered more in this respect than children in the control group. By the end of the fifth year five neurotic children had experienced no separation whatever.

There is, however, a small number of children in the neurotic group—five—who experienced a separation of over three months between the second and fifth year, as compared with only one child in the control group. This fact need not have causal significance in the mental health of the child. It probably reflects on the inadequacy of a small group of mothers of children between these ages, the separation experience and the mental ill-health of the child springing from the same source.

Our neurotic group of children was not broken up into *clinical categories* and it is not known whether there is a relationship between separation experiences and a particular clinical pattern.

Summary. 1. A group of neurotic children and a control group of average children were compared as to their separation experiences under five years of age. The separation experiences of the two groups were found to be very similar and differences were minor.

2. There was little separation of the child from his parents in the first two years, and there was no significant difference between the two groups.

3. Long separations from mother and father, although few in number, are commoner in the neurotic group. In the neurotic group they are often due to the inadequacy of the parents; illnesses are a common cause of long separations from mothers.

4. Though separation may cause temporary suffering for the child, it does not, in most cases, lead to mental ill-health.

5. It is suggested that most disturbed children suffer emotionally from being with their parents. Deprivation springs most commonly from inadequate parental care.

The Effects of the Separation Experiences

Our investigation also considered the effects on the children of separation from their homes. The separations were brought about by the happenings of everyday life. The mothers were asked to reply to the following question 'Can you comment on the general effect that leaving home had on him on the various occasions?' The replies to this question will be analysed and the responses compared in the two groups.

The replies given by the mothers were divided into four categories—1. No comment. 2. No effect. 3. Harmful effect. 4. Separation enjoyed and the chlld happy. It will be seen in Table IX that in the two groups combined, out of 92 occasions of separation there were nine 'no comments', 20 'no effects', 36 unfavourable comments and 27 favourable comments. In the control group, out of 47 occasions of separation, there was one 'no comments', nine 'no effects', 25 unfavourable comments, and 12 favourable

TABLE IX

Incidence of Comments by Mothers

	Both Groups	Control Group	Neurotic Group
No comments	9	1	8
No effect	20	9	11
Unfavourable comments	36	25	11
Favourable comments	27	12	15
Totals	92	47	45

comments. In the neurotic group, out of 45 occasions of separation there were eight 'no comments', 11 'no effects', 11 unfavourable comments, and 15 favourable comments. It is noted that the neurotic group mothers offered no comment eight times as often as control group mothers—another indication of the fecklessness of the mother of neurotic children.

Separation does not necessarily lead to harmful effects as in 61 per cent of the total occasions the separations were enjoyed or did not give rise to comment. If the 'no comments' are excluded from the total, it can be seen that the separations did not give rise to unfavourable comment on 57 per cent of occasions—i.e. 47 out of 83 occasions of separation. Remarks describing the ill-effects of separation most commonly referred to an emotional response in the child and accounted for about 40 per cent of the remarks, e.g. quiet, anxious, crying, shy, subdued, nervous, miserable, insecure, frightened. About 20 per cent of the remarks applied to physical changes in the child, e.g. change in habit training, enuresis, colds, nail biting, and loss of appetite. About 15 per cent of all remarks applied to the child's tendency to forget the mother and all these remarks applied to children of 18 months or under, except for one child of 24 months. This is understandable as children have a small memory span in this age group. Another small group of remarks applied to the tendency of the child to cling to the parents and to be reluctant to be away from them. A small minority became more difficult in their behaviour.

There would not appear to be any difference in the quality of the ill-effects in the two groups studied. The groups were too small to notice the effects of age on the child's response to a separation, except for the greater and understandable tendency for the child to forget the parents in the first two years. The ill-effects of hospital and non-hospital separations appeared to be the same in character. Four examples from the complete replies will be given.

Example 1. A child of 14 months was in hospital for three weeks for a hernia operation and was visited by the parents. 'Apparently forgot about parents. Did not appear to recognize them when visited.'

Example 2. A child of 20 months went to the grandparents for six weeks because of the birth of a sibling. He was visited by his father. The comment is combined with a later separation at the age of four and a half. 'Enjoyed immensely the attention he received but welcomed me joyously on my return'.

Example 3. A child of two and a half went into hospital for ten days for a hernia operation and circumcision. He was not visited. 'Bewildered and chronically frightened.'

Example 4. A child of four went to a grandmother for various week-ends. The mother explained that it was to give her a break as he was a very trying child. 'He was very excited about it. He always likes to get away from home. It did a lot of good for him and us.'

Discussion. The unfavourable and favourable comment will be discussed in more detail. The influence of the hospital setting, the non-hospital setting, and of age on the separation experiences will then be discussed. It is of interest to compare the replies of the mothers in the control and the neurotic groups. Finally, comment is offered on the practical implications of the findings.

There were *unfavourable comments* on 39 per cent of the occasions of separation in the two groups combined—36 occasions out of 92 occasions, (Table IX). Even some of the healthy control group children had suffered harmful effects from the separation, i.e. 25 out of 47 occasions of separation in this group. The parents were not asked how long the harmful effects lasted. The general inference of the replies is that they were temporary effects and some mothers actually say so, e.g. 'several weeks', 'for a while', 'several days', 'two days'. Five replies suggest that more permanent effects ensued. The separations were for less than two weeks in four of these five replies. Further investigation would be necessary before finally blaming the separations for the permanent effects in these five cases as some of the separation disturbance can be due to previous or coexisting events, e.g. the birth of a sibling. As has been said, the mothers' comments suggest that the upsets, when they occur, are temporary, and do not necessarily lead on to mental ill-health later. Should the upsets have led to mental ill-health, a higher incidence of harmful effects at the time of separation in the children of the neurotic group would have been expected. This was not the finding in the investigation. Indeed, there were more unfavourable comments by mothers of the control group. Furthermore, a higher incidence of separation would be expected in the early histories of neurotic children. The incidence of separation experiences was found to be the same in both groups. In evaluating a clinical history it is as well to bear in mind that parents are liable to blame ill-health, mental or physical, on any outstanding event, such as separation, in the child's past.

There were 27 *favourable comments* out of 92 separations and the two groups gave favourable answers in approximately the same number of cases (Table IX). In every case a favourable comment concerns a visit to relatives or friends. This finding suggests that the child is happier with people he knows and that the parents are aware of this. In the younger age group the separation tended to be unavoidable, e.g. caused by illness in the family, and in this event the child was invariably visited by a parent and probably benefited by this. Over the age of two, separations were often due to the parents taking holidays. The break was planned, the child went to relatives or friends and he was not visited. The children may have enjoyed the separations either because they like the people they were with, or because the environment was more favourable than in their own homes.

That *hospital separations*, even of short duration, are particularly upsetting is suggested from a comparison of the comments on the children's separations due to hospital admission and the comments on the children cared for elsewhere. In neither the control group nor the neurotic group is there a favourable comment on hospital admission (Table X). There is a total of 18 unfavourable comments and six without comment, i.e. 70 per cent of occasions of hospital admission received unfavourable comment. This finding, no doubt, reflects the child's unhappiness with strangers and the traumatic experiences the child undergoes in hospital, such as operations and strange happenings. It is of interest that while their children were in hospital the parents of the neurotic groups only visited once in the course of ten admissions (10 per cent), while parents of the control group visited 13 times out of 16 admissions (81 per cent). Such neglectful parents hurt their children at all times—before separation, during visiting and after separation.

In the *non-hospital separations* harmful effects occur in 18 out of 66 occasions of non-hospital separations, i.e. on 27 per cent of occasions (Table X). From the foregoing it is clear that non-hospital separations of short duration are only harmful on a minority of occasions. It became apparent that the mothers had noted more harmful effects of non-hospital separations when the period of separation lasted more than two weeks. Forty-seven per cent are then said to be definitely harmful.

It took 66 non-hospital separations to lead to the same number of unfavourable comments as 26 hospital admissions. This finding suggests that in determining whether or not the child is deprived of his emotional needs, the environment during the separation is more important than the fact of separation per se. Again, separation is not synonymous with deprivation.

It is of some interest to *compare the replies of the mothers* of the neurotic group and the control group. Analysis of the results (Table IX) suggests that the parents in the neurotic group comment less often and when they do comment they do not observe harmful effects as often as the mothers in the control group. Further analysis showed that the difference was even greater when separations are of short duration and occur in the first two years of the child's life. A striking difference between the two groups in the incidence of hospital visiting has already been noted. The difference is probably not a matter of lack of memory because the neurotic group mothers

TABLE X

Comments on Hospital and Non-hospital Separations

	No effect	No comment	Favourable Comment	Unfavourable Comment	Totals
Hospital Separations	2	6	0	18	26
Non-Hospital Separations	17	3	28	18	66
Totals	19	9	28	36	92

are able to remember the occasions of the child being away, but yet do not comment upon any ill-effects. Furthermore, the mothers are not unco-operative as they were prepared to give information about the child under the other headings of the questionnaire. There appeared to be three possible explanations of the difference that has been noted: (*i*) The mothers of the neurotic group children may be less sensitive to the effects of separation on the child especially when the child is under 2 years of age. When the effects are more evident due to longer separation even they notice them. Less interest in their children is suggested by their reluctance to visit their children in hospital. (*ii*) A number of the children may have already been disturbed before the separation. Accordingly the mother did not notice the ill-effects as easily and would register no comment or 'no effect'. (*iii*) The children of the neurotic group may have gained more from separation as the new environment may have been less adverse than the old. All the explanations, if applicable, imply a lower standard of mothering by the mothers of the neurotic group children.

Practical Considerations. In estimating the effect that separation may have on a child, attention must be paid to the preparation that was given to the child before separation, the presence of an emotional disturbance before the separation, and the age of the child. In addition, attention must be paid to the conditions relating to the separations themselves, e.g. the length of separation, whether the child visited the parents, whether the parents visited the child, the quality of the substitute care and the incidental happenings during the separation, such as the birth of a sibling or operation trauma. The reception by the parents after the separation is a further important factor.

Often no harm results from separation. Should it occur the findings suggest that the maximum amount of harm would appear likely to occur when a child experiences separation of over two weeks under two years of age, and in strange surroundings, such as a hospital. The minimum amount of harm occurs when the child experiences separation for short periods over two years of age and in the care of relatives or friends.

Much has yet to be learned on how effective recuperative measures can be in diminishing or mending the harm done. The comments of some of the mothers suggest that the effects are often short lived once the child is restored to the parent. It appears that the child, returning to its warm, accepting home, repairs the damage done. Our findings suggest that hurtful separation experiences are compatible with subsequent mental health. Even should it be possible to mend the harm done and prevent permanent changes to his personality, there is every reason for taking steps to protect the child from hurtful separation experiences.

Sometimes, the separation trauma may be an additional factor in an emotional disturbance already set in motion by a disturbed relationship with the parent. Clinical experience suggests that the disturbed and insecure child suffers most initially from separation experiences, but he may still be the one who gains most from the separation experience when fortunate in his substitute care.

Hospital admissions have been shown to be particularly harmful. The hospital setting is a controlled situation which should be readily modifiable. Attention needs to be paid to such matters as the preparation of the child for hospital, reception of the child in hospital, maintaining contact between mother and child by frequent visiting or admitting mother and child together, reactions of the child to pain, emotional relationships amongst a group of children, reactions to anaesthesia and producing a more homely atmosphere by suitable arrangement of ward and furniture. Perhaps the greatest need of all is to recruit and train the right type of nurse able to meet the child's emotional needs. Much greater use should be made of part-time nurses who have proved themselves with their own children. Each nurse in a ward should be encouraged to 'mother' a small group of children. There should be competition, not to produce the cleanest and tidiest children but to produce the happiest group of children. The child is not being adequately nursed unless there are prolonged, intimate contacts between nurse and child. A panel of voluntary workers prepared to offer substitute mothering could greatly benefit children in long-stay hospitals when mothers are unable to visit. The World Health Organization[43] has reviewed the literature on the care of the child in hospital.

Summary. 1. Mothers of a group of neurotic children and a control group of healthy children were asked to comment on the effect that leaving home had on their children when they were under five years of age. The ill-effects produced in the children by their separation experiences are described and analysed.

2. Many children did not necessarily suffer harmful effects from separation and some enjoy benefit from the separation.

3. Some children, both healthy and neurotic, experience harmful effects on separation from their homes. There is a greater tendency to report harmful effects on children when the duration of separation is over two weeks and the child under two years of age. Children under two years of age experiencing separation tend to forget the parents, a matter to be expected at this age because of the short memory span. The harmful effects are probably temporary in most cases and they do not necessarily play a major part in subsequent mental ill-health.

4. Hospital admission, even of short duration, appears harmful to children on the majority of occasions. Non-hospital care is harmful on a minority of occasions.

5. The findings suggest that the conditions applying before, during and after the separation are more important than the fact of separation in determining whether or not there will be harmful effects.

6. There is less comment, less unfavourable comment and less hospital visiting by the mothers of the children of the neurotic group. It is suggested that this is explained by the poorer standard of mothering by the mothers of the children of the neurotic group.

7. The conditions which play a part in the ill-effects of separations are outlined; suggestions are made on the care of the child in hospital.

Causes of Separation

It is convenient to consider the causes of the separations in three categories: the mother being away from home; the father being away from home; the child being away from home.

In both control and neurotic groups the greatest length of time that the *mother spent away* was caused by their illnesses (Table XI). The greatest difference between the two groups lies in the extent of the mother's illnesses. Whereas in the control group the mothers of 10 children, on 11 occasions, are away from home owing to illness, for eight months in all, in the neurotic group the mothers of 17 children, on 23 occasions, are away for two years nine months. The average length of each separation is approximately three weeks in the control group, and six weeks in the neurotic group. The greater length of illness of the mothers in the neurotic group accounts entirely for the longer duration of their absence from home and is caused chiefly by five of the mothers. The totals due to the other causes, births of siblings, holidays, illness or death of relatives, and the miscellaneous reasons such as moving house, giving evidence at court, and obtaining a divorce, equal eight in both groups. The control group mothers have been away for nearly twice as long as the neurotic group for the births of siblings but they have also had nearly twice as many births. The greater absence in the neurotic group on account of the illness of a relative is due to one mother who was away for three months for this reason.

TABLE XI

Causes of Separation—Mother Away

	Control Group					Neurotic Group				
	Duration				Occasions	No. of Children	Duration				Occasions	No. of Children
	years	months	weeks	days			years	months	weeks	days		
Illness	8	0	2		11	10	2	9	1	6	23	17
Birth of sibling	6	0	5		13	9	3	1	2		7	7
Holidays	1	3	0		10	9	2	0	0		7	4
Illness or death of relative		1	1		2	2	3	2	0		4	4
Miscellaneous		1	3		4	2				4	3	3

Work is the commonest cause of a *father's absence* from home (Table XII). Work (including service in the Forces), accounts for approximately four years' absence in both groups. Illness is the next most frequent cause of absence and it affects the same number of children in both groups with the same number of separations. But as with the neurotic group mothers, the average length of each absence of the neurotic group fathers is more than twice that of the control group. A breakdown in marriage, leading to separation or divorce, affects three children out of the total of 74. Of the causes for the total of 22 separations of over three months from fathers, work (including service in the Forces or attendance at college) accounts for 12, the illness of father for four, a breakdown of marriage for three, and death for one.

A DIRECT INVESTIGATION ON SEPARATION 275

The commonest cause of the *child's absence* from home is his own illness and the figures are approximately equal in both groups (Table XIII). But the greatest duration of the child's absence from home is caused by the mother's illness. In the neurotic group nine children were separated

TABLE XII

Causes of Separation—Father Away

	Control Group							Neurotic Group						
	Duration				Occasions	No. of Children		Duration				Occasions	No. of Children
	years	months	weeks	days				years	months	weeks	days		
Work	1	3	2	6	13	7			3	3	0	3	3
Forces & Z reserve	2	8	0	1	3	3		3	9	0	0	5	3
Attended college or university	3	6	0	0	2	2						0	0
Illness		4	3	0	5	4			11	1	3	5	4
Separation from mother	1	2	0	0	1	1		5	6	0	0	2	2
Death of father					0	0		5	0	0	0	1	1
Holidays			3	6	6	5				2	5	4	4
Illness of mother or birth of sibling			2	0	1	1			1	3	0	1	1
Illness or death of relative			2	0	2	2						0	0
Miscellaneous				1	1	1					3	2	2

for 13 occasions for a duration of two years four months as compared with six children on six occasions for six months in the control group. It can be seen that on nearly every occasion that the mother goes away owing to her illness, the home is upset and the child also has to go away. For the child there are clear advantages in the mother being nursed at home whenever possible. However, it will be seen later that the trauma is reduced by him generally being cared for by relatives (Table XIV). The illness of the father is not as disrupting a force for the family as is the mother's illness.

TABLE XIII

Causes of Separation—Child Away

	Control Group					Neurotic Group				
	Duration				Occa-sions	No. of Children	Duration				Occa-sions	No. of Children
	years	months	weeks	days			years	months	weeks	days		
Illness or Convalescence	5	3	4		16	12		5	2	0	11	11
Illness of mother	6	2	3		6	6	2	4	0	0	13	9
Birth of sibling	4	0	3		5	5		1	3	0	2	2
Holiday of parents	1	0	5		4	4		1	3	3	8	3
Holiday of child	4	1	0		14	9		2	0	4	5	4
Illness or death of relative		2	0		1	1			1	2	3	3
Miscellaneous			4		1	1		2	1	5	3	4

Summary. 1. The greatest length of time that the mothers spent away from home was caused by their illnesses. Illness is more frequent and lasts longer in the mothers of the neurotic group.

2. Work is the commonest cause of a father's absence from home.

3. The commonest cause of the child's absence from home is his own illness. The greatest duration of the child's absence from home is caused by mother's illness.

Care of the Child during Separations

Separation of mother and child can be caused by the mother leaving home or by the child leaving home. Thus it is convenient to consider: (*i*) the care of the child when mother is away from home; (*ii*) the care of the child when away from home.

In considering the care of the child when the *mother is away*, the two groups can be taken as a whole (Table XIV). It appears that parents make the separation as little traumatic as possible, and residential care is uncommon. The child has gone to relatives and friends on 58 occasions, he

TABLE XIV

Care of Child when Mother Away

	Control Group	Neurotic Group	Total
Grandparents	14	15	29
Other relatives	10	8	18
Friends or neighbours	3	8	11
Father with either siblings, relative or home help	13	9	22
Residential nursery or home	0	4	4

has stayed at home with father on 22 occasions, and experienced institutional care on only four occasions. Three of the four occasions were caused

TABLE XV

Care of the Child when away from Home

	Control Group Occasions	Neurotic Group Occasions	Total
Hospital	16	10	26
Grandparents	13	15	28
Other relatives	15	10	25
Friends and neighbours	3	6	9
Institutional care	0	4	4
Totals	47	45	92

by the mother's illness and the fourth by the birth of a sibling. The importance of relatives, grandparents in particular, can be seen from the table. The child gains from a good clan spirit. Neurotic parents tend to be deficient in this, and their relatives to be neurotic themselves. Thus the children of neurotic parents may not be as well served by relatives. Our figures are too few to throw light on this possibility.

The care of the *child when away* from home can be seen from Table XV. The child had hospital care on 26 out of 92 occasions. The traumatic effect of hospital care has been discussed previously.

Summary. When separation is inevitable, the parents in the great majority of cases reduce the emotional trauma by making use of a relative or friend.

Summary of Whole Investigation

1. A group of neurotic children and a control group of average children are compared as to their separation experiences under five years of age.

2. The incidence of separation in the two groups was found to be very similar and differences are minor.

3. There is little separation of the child from his parents in the first two years, and there was no significant difference between the two groups.

4. It is concluded that though separation may sometimes cause temporary suffering for the child, *it does not, in most cases, lead to mental ill-health.*

5. It is suggested that most disturbed children suffer emotionally from being with their parents. Deprivation springs most commonly from inadequate parental care.

6. Long separations from mother and father, although few in number, are commoner in the neurotic group. In the neurotic group they are often due to the inadequacy of the parents; illnesses are a common cause of long separations from mother.

7. The ill effects produced in the children by their separation experiences are described and analysed.

8. Many children do not necessarily suffer harmful effects from separation and some enjoy and benefit from the separation.

9. Some children, both healthy and neurotic, experience harmful effects on separation from their homes. There is a greater tendency to report harmful effects on children when the duration of separation is over two weeks and the child under two years of age. Children under two years of age experiencing separation understandably tend to forget the parents. The harmful effects are probably temporary in most cases and they do not necessarily play a major part in subsequent mental ill-health.

10. Hospital admission, even of short duration, appears harmful to children on the majority of occasions. Non-hospital care is harmful on a minority of occasions.

11. The findings suggest that the conditions applying before, during and after the separation are more important than the fact of separation in determining whether or not there will be harmful effects.

12. There is less comment, less unfavourable comment and less hospital visiting by the mothers of the neurotic group children. It is

suggested that this is explained by the poorer standard of mothering by the mothers of the neurotic group children. Inadequate parents upset their children both before and after separations and this must be borne in mind in evaluating the effects of separation.

13. The conditions which play a part in the ill-effects of separation are outlined.

14. The greatest length of time that the mothers spend away from home is caused by their illnesses. Illness is more frequent and lasts longer in the mothers of the neurotic group—again a commentary on the inadequacy of these mothers.

15. Work is the commonest cause of a father's absence from home.

16. The commonest cause of the child's absence from home is his own illness. The greatest duration of the child's absence from home is caused by mother's illness.

17. When separation is inevitable, the parents in the great majority of cases reduce the emotional trauma by making use of a relative or friend.

3

Additional Studies on Separation

Failure to distinguish between separation and deprivation has led to the misinterpretation of the findings of many investigations. This will be illustrated by reference to a few well-known studies. Direct studies on separation are few.

Goldfarb's[13] work has sometimes been quoted as showing the ill-effects of separation. However, his main studies, have been comparisons between groups of separated children. He has conclusively shown that separated children flourish according to the quality of care they are given following the separation. In one separation situation they may be deprived of adequate care, as for example, in a bad institution, whilst in another situation, for example, a good foster-home, the care may be adequate. He has shown how children removed from the first situation will improve when placed in the second. His work would appear to demonstrate that the heart of the matter is not the mere fact of the child being separated from its parents, but whether or not the child is deprived of the right care. Similarly, Clarke and Clarke[10, 11, 12] found an improvement in the IQ of the feeble minded, who had been placed in institutions, especially if they came from adverse home backgrounds.

Moore[31], conducted an important investigation on children who had had separations from their mother during the day, but given substitute care. As a by-product, he investigated a group of children who had experienced episodic separations, i.e. not short periods of separation during the day, but continuous breaks from the mother of one week to two or three months. Comparing this group with a group of children who had had exclusive mother care, he found no signs of permanent harm, if anything, they seemed more healthy—despite the fact that several of the children were distressed at the time of the separation.

Some of Moore's findings in regard to periods of separation during the day from mother are of interest. It should be noted that the factor explored was mother-child separation only, i.e. father-child and family-child separations were excluded. The differences in the state of the children who had received mother care or stable substitute care (not more than one change of caretaker) was minimal on the mothers' reports and nil by the psychologist ratings. The difference between children, however, who had had stable substitute care and those who had had unstable substitute care (change of substitute mothers and change of nurseries) was striking. The two above findings put together suggest that the determining adverse factor is the quality of the substitute care, i.e. deprivation rather than separation per se. Moore is also careful to make the point that in the care of children, who had unstable substitute care, the home background of these children was less satisfactory, i.e. conditions in the home that may cause a child to have unstable substitute care arranged for him may also cause disturbance in the child. Moore then compared all the children who had had substitute care with those who had had exclusive mother care; it should be noted that the substitute care group contained a number who had experienced unstable substitute care. Some differences now appeared between the two groups, e.g. at the age of six, at level of significance of $P = <0.05$ there was a difference on four items in 70 for boys on the mothers' reports, but nil differences for girls, e.g. on ratings by psychologists there were five differences between the groups, but not all to the disadvantage of the substitute care group—more excitable, more aggressive, more active but less guilty and less nervous. The investigator believes that some, but not all, the observed differences between the substitute care and maternal care groups may be attributed to differences in maternal attitudes and methods of handling, rather than to daily separation as such.

As a result of this investigation Moore sets up some interesting hypotheses; their implications, if correct, are that the quality of care (or absence of deprivation), maternal or substitute, which is important, rather than separation or non-separation from the mother. He also points to possible benefits in separation. The hypotheses were:

1. Full-time uninterrupted contact with the mother to the age of five fosters superego development (with its advantages and disadvantages).

2. Stable daily substitute care starting after three, especially in a nursery school, tends to toughen the child, strengthening the ego perhaps at the expense of the superego.

3. Instability of regime, commonly one aspect of a generally unsettled life, weakens or retards ego development by inducing frequent regression, causing many problems of adjustment.

Stott[42] compared a group of backward children who had separation histories of at least ten weeks during the first four years with a group of less separated children and found no significant difference in their scores on a social adjustment scale. Schaffer[47] compared two separated groups of children, one deprived and the other not, and found that the deprived group produced lower scores on scales of development—pointing to the importance of deprivation and not separation. Nye[33] compared child adjustment in (*i*) unbroken, but unhappy homes; (*ii*) broken homes; (*iii*) happy broken homes. (*i*) caused most disturbance in children. In their work neither Lewis[28] nor Holman[18] found support for the view that child-parent separation played a significant part in the etiology of maladjustment. Andry[2] did not find separation to be a significant antecedent in delinquency. Naess[32] came to similar conclusions in regard to delinquency. Yarrow[44,45,46] and O'Connor[34] have drawn attention to the need for more precise definition of 'deprivation' and for caution in attributing separation as a cause for maladjustment.

In contrast to the above workers, Bowlby[3] has given much significance to the effects of separation experiences. His first investigation concerned the high incidence of separation experiences in a group of 44 juvenile thieves, and this high incidence, he maintained, has a causal connection with their disturbance. He concluded that prolonged separation caused a variety of personality disturbances, of which the 'affectionless character' might be the most characteristic and the most serious. However, less attention was paid to the possible effects of the deprivation of the right care. From the case histories it appears that both before and after the separation experience these children suffered a loss of the right kind of care. This investigation did not eliminate the variable of deprivation and it would seem difficult therefore to draw valid conclusions about the effect of separation per se. Again separation is assumed to be the damaging agent; in fact it is deprivation. It will also be noticed that those children whose experience of separation was a happy one, would be unlikely to attend Bowlby's clinic, and therefore unlikely to be included in the investigation; a selection factor operated.

In 1953 Bowlby[5] gives his views on separation at that time. He presents a case history of Desmond, who has had five mother-figures. There were four mother-figures under five years, and from five years to 11 years he had the care of his step-mother and father. Following a period of psychotherapy, the prolonged therapy offered (surprisingly in view of the theories held) was a separation experience by admittance to a boarding school. That the child was removed from the continuous care of the step-mother, suggests that in practice significance was given to her adverse care. It would seem that in a condition of non-separation Desmond was deprived; separation had to be employed to overcome deprivation. Deprivation was the damaging agent. In the rest of the paper the author states his theoretical position. He states in regard to mother-child separation: 'we can now be reasonably sure that it is experiences such as these which can set in train the uncontrollable and contradictory impulses which haunt the psychopathic and neurotic character'.

A planned investigation entitled 'The Effects of Mother-Child Separation'[6] compared a group of sanatorium children with a control group of school children. The nature of the study is defined as follows: 'In order to test and refine hypotheses regarding the ill-effects in personality development of separation from mother in early childhood . . .' and when separated and non-separated groups are compared 'common effects are found to follow separations characterized by widely differing associated variables that it is permissible to conclude that the responsible influence is in fact separation'. In five out of 28 items on a teacher's report form, the sanatorium children showed traits which indicated maladjustment. The differences were not as great as had been expected. On the first assessment there was no difference between the two groups. Bowlby summarizes the situation thus: 'It is concluded that some of the workers who first drew attention to the dangers of maternal deprivation resulting from separation have tended on occasions to overstate their case. In particular, statements implying that children who experience institutionalization and similar forms of severe privation and deprivation in early life, *commonly* develop psychopathic or affectionless characters are incorrect. The results of the present study, however, give no grounds for complacency.' Later in correspondence in 1958[7], again in 1966[9], he seemed to return to his former position of regarding separation as a 'serious mental health hazard'. The limited positive findings of the investigation, however, appear to be nullified by the fact that the effects said to be due to the separation from mother alone, cannot be distinguished from those effects due to other factors, for example, the deprivation of the right care in a sanatorium. Again, the limited effects could have been due to father-child separation. The lack of definition of the concepts employed may have resulted in the defective formulation of the investigation. Although the investigation, as the title states, is concerned with separation, the use of this term and of the word 'deprived' are ambiguous, as for example, in a paragraph that contains 'children who for any reason are deprived of the continuous care and attention of a mother', i.e. using the term deprived to mean loss of parent and not loss of parenting, and emphasized by the use in the same paragraph of 'deprived' to mean physical separation.

In another paper[8], it is apparent that the same author still did not find it necessary to differentiate between separation and deprivation. 'For many of the cases in which there has been no episode of actual separation . . . there is often evidence that there has, nevertheless, been separation of another and more or less serious kind. Rejection, loss of love . . . and similar situations all have a common factor—loss by the child of a parent to live and to attach himself to. If the concept of loss of object is extended to cover loss of love, these cases no longer constitute exceptions.' It would seem unwarranted to mix quite different elements of experience, namely loss of object and loss of love, i.e. loss of parent and loss of parenting, in this way. Loss of parents need not lead to deprivation of the right care; loss of parenting does. Recently, Ainsworth[1], a collaborator of Bowlby, in discussing confusion caused by the term 'maternal deprivation' agrees that 'it does not follow that separation necessarily implies deprivation' and that the term 'mother-child separation' is best reserved for discontinuity in a relationship. The term 'deprivation' is defined as 'insufficiency of interaction'. Thus Ainsworth's definitions begin to approximate to those suggested at the start of this chapter.

Separation from parent due to death of the parent can occur in childhood. It was natural that the possibility that such absolute separations might lead to mental ill-health later on should be investigated. The matter has been reviewed by Gregory[14] and findings treated by him with caution. Investigations give conflicting results. Again, they illustrate the difficulty of isolating the effects of separation from the effects consequent on separation, such as deprivation of the right care. For instance, Hill and Price[17] found that depressed patients had lost more fathers, but not mothers, before the age of 15, than had non-depressed patients. But the positive findings cannot be explained necessarily by separation from father as there are many other factors consequent on loss of father, which may be more significant, e.g. loss of father may have led to deprivation of care from a stepfather, or deprivation consequent on break up of the family, or institutional care, etc. as well as many possibilities that may have sprung from the same causes that gave rise to the separation experiences, e.g. inadequate care before they died by fathers, whose disturbance predisposed to death by suicide, illness, etc. Many possible significant factors exist which cannot be controlled in these retrospective investigations.

In recent years, ethological workers have turned their attention to infant care. This with a number of safeguards, may help to throw light on basic mechanisms common to animal and man. Safeguards include care in adjusting findings from animals to a much more complex organism, man; care in interpreting animal behaviour in the artificial conditions of the laboratory; care in projecting into the experiments some of the misconceptions in current human work. That the latter is not completely successful can be seen from an interesting experiment by Spencer-Booth and Hinde[40], where the variables separation and deprivation were not isolated. In the experiment on separation using rhesus monkeys the mother was taken away from the infant. Thus the infants were separated from the mother and also deprived of maternal care; there was deprivation consequent on separation. The changes noted might have been quite different if separation had not led to deprivation by substituting a kindly, loving, solicitous monkey aunt for mother. Spencer-Booth and Hinde's study on monkeys had elements in common with the careful and valuable study by Heinicke and Westheimer[16] on children admitted to residential nurseries for brief periods and compared with non-separated children. The differences noted are not due to separation from mother per se, but deprivation consequent on separation. If, for example, the fathers had moved to the residential nurseries with the children instead of visiting once weekly, the changes noted would have been reduced or eliminated.

Seay and Harlow[38] conducted a similar investigation on monkeys. The emotional disturbance noted indicate that 'sheer physical separation is the crucial aspect of maternal separation for monkeys'. This was a curious comment. Had the infants been separated but not deprived, e.g. by the provision of a monkey aunt, the change would be minimal. It was deprivation consequent on separation that did the damage! Striking evidence of the importance of deprivation rather than separation comes from another study by Harlow and Seay[15] on rhesus monkeys. Four monkeys had suffered a deprivatory upbringing. Later when they became mothers they were totally inadequate as parents and 'none of their infants would have survived had not the experimenters intervened'. The infants were not separated but were deprived of care to the point of death. They were saved by separation and substitute human parenting!

It is understood, of course, that the author agrees wholeheartedly with the view that deprivation of the right care has an adverse effect, sometimes severe, on the developing personality of the child. This deprivation may be consequent on separation or non-separation. Thus the extensive literature on maternal deprivation will not be reviewed here. Bowlby's review[4] of the literature on maternal care and mental health was concerned with deprivation of the right maternal care and should be distinguished from his own investigations on mother-child separations. The general neglect of work on deprivation consequent on defective paternal or family care is noted. The author believes that, in certain circumstances, separation can be used to overcome deprivation consequent on non-separation. Before instituting such separation procedures it was necessary to establish that separation was not in itself responsible for mental ill-health in children. Statements made about effects of separation experiences were so contrary to our clinical work that some years ago an investigation[25, 26, 27], was undertaken to test some of the formulations. This has been reported above. Consequent on this, confidence grew to the point when separation was employed to overcome deprivation. The principles concerned will now be outlined.

4

Parent-child Separation as a Therapeutic Procedure

Deprivation of the right emotional care is the hazard to children. It can arise in conditions of non-separation with the child at home, due to stress from the mother, from the father, or from both parents, or the family collectively. Deprivation can also occur in conditions of separation by inadequate care by substitute parents in the form of relatives, foster parents, adoptive parents, or staff of institutions, etc. Both conditions of deprivation, with separation or non-separation, are to be deplored. Clinical experience suggests that the latter is much commoner.

Separation will now be discussed as one means of overcoming deprivation produced by home care. There are strong emotional prejudices that deny the existence of deprivation by parents and the need for separation. The bond between parent and child, it is said, is different from that between any other person and child, yet parenting can only differ in degree from other relationships. Furthermore, there are degrees of adequate parenting; some parenting is of a quality that few substitutes could emulate, some parenting is of a quality that it is unlikely that substitute care would improve on it, some parenting is damaging, and a small percentage of parenting is actually extremely damaging. Parents, by virtue of being parents, do not magically lose the results of harsh experiences in their life experiences that handicap them in relationships. That handicapped parents exist is a fact of life; that some handicapped parents sorely damage their children is another. It would be a happy situation if the instruments of psychiatry were so powerful that the parental handicap could be overcome; this is seldom the case. Even when possible, the extent of the facilities is such that only a minority of parents can benefit. Meanwhile, the children are deprived. One of the bars to using separation procedures is the reluctance to hurt parents by implying their failure to bring up their own children. Unhappily, the tendency to feel guilt is encouraged by the overemphasis by the community of the importance of parental responsibility and the alleged damage of separation. In fact, parents need not feel guilt at taking steps to help their children and themselves. They can be made to feel the virtue of positive action and pride at the success of measures freely taken.

It is suggested here that a child is normally brought up within a family. There are good reasons for taking the family as a unit in psychiatric practice—hence family psychiatry. Separation may be employed in vector therapy of the family.

Family Psychiatry

The great mass of humanity flowing through time appears at first glance to be made up of a multiple of isolated individuals. But from time to time individuals coalesce into groups which have separate identities and functions—the family, the neighbourhood, the community, the culture. In its emotional aspect, the most meaningful unit in society is the family, as it is responsible for the emotional nurturing of the individual. Because of its size, it also has the advantage of being a manageable unit in clinical practice. Hence family psychiatry[20] adopts it as the unit in systematic clinical practice.

Family psychiatry[20, 23, 24], whereby the family is the functional unit, is a practical and theoretical system for psychiatry. Individual psychiatry, taking the adult as the functional unit (adult psychiatry), the child as the functional unit (child psychiatry), or the adolescent as the functional unit (adolescent psychiatry) is obsolete. Individual psychiatry is replaced by family psychiatry, taking the family as the unit applies throughout the system of practice—it applies to the referral service, to the systematisation of symptomatology, to the procedures of investigation, and to the processes of management or treatment.

Family therapy includes two main procedures. (*i*) Family psychotherapy utilises the direct influence of the therapist on the psyche of the individual or collective psyche of the family by procedures such as individual psychotherapy, dyadic therapy, family group therapy, or multiple family therapy. (*ii*) Vector therapy, as described below. The two procedures are complementary.

Family psychiatry in its theoretical system is a revolt from the present tendency to over-concentrate on individual intrapsychic events alone. It restores balance by giving significance also to events outside the individual; the most cogent are within the family, and others lie in society. Thus account is taken of the individual intrapsychic, family and social events.

Vector Therapy

Within families there are powerful emotional forces that affect all its members for good or evil. A vector denotes a quantity which has direction. Force, including emotional force, is a quantity with direction and therefore can be represented by a vector. Furthermore, as direction is a property of a vector, and direction implies movement, it results in a dynamic situation. *Vector therapy readjusts the pattern of the emotional forces within the life space to bring improvement to the individual or family within the life space.*

The forces in the life space can be thought of in terms of fields of forces. These fields of forces are (*a*) within the individual, (*b*) outside the individual and within the family, (*c*) outside the individual and the family and within the community, (*d*) outside the individual, family and community and within the culture, (*e*) outside the individual, family, community and culture and within society.

Vector therapy can involve:

1. A change in the *magnitude* of the emotional force, e.g. father's aggression may be diminished.

2. A change in the *direction* of the emotional force with no change in its magnitude, e.g. father abuses mother instead of child.

3. A change in the *length of time* during which the emotional force operates, e.g. father works away from home, spends less time at home and his aggression has less duration.

4. A change in the *quality* of the emotional force when one force replaces another, e.g. father treats his son with kindness instead of aggression.

To effect these changes, the sources of the emotional force may have to be moved, e.g. by father going out to work; or the object of the forces may have to be moved, e.g. the child goes to a boarding school to avoid father's aggression.

Faced with an emotionally disintegrated individual or family, reintegration is possible by mobilizing a set of influences in the present that may still nullify the effects of the previous adverse influences. This can be done (a) by the mobilization of intense, precise, beneficial emotional influences from a therapist acting over a short period of time in the interview situation, i.e. by psychotherapy; or (b) by mobilizing less intense emotional influences of a general nature known to be beneficial over a long period of time outside the interview, i.e. by vector therapy. Thus, for example, a child damaged by being deprived of the right kind of care, instead of being subject to psychotherapy, is placed in a foster-home for its ability to provide the right care. In the latter case, benefit comes from a new set of beneficial influences able to act over a long period of time.

In a given instance, psychotherapy and vector therapy are complementary. As an example at a simple level, consider the young infant of a highly anxious, ill-adjusted mother, put to the breast and because of the disharmonious influence from mother being unable to feed. Direct psychotherapy might effect a change in the mother's personality, so that in time she may be able to mother her infant adequately. The situation can also be broken into by a simple rearrangement of the people who provide the emotional influence playing on the child in the feeding situation. The stable young father who stands by little imagines that he has a part to play in the feeding situation; but, by placing the infant on the bottle, and allowing the well-adjusted father to feed him, the infant can have a happy and satisfying feeding experience. By the use of vector therapy, a change of forces has been effected and a disharmonious situation has become harmonious. Psychotherapy is worthwhile for the mother as a long-term project. The infant is best served by the immediate satisfying relationship in the arms of his father. Thus, both psychotherapy and vector therapy have a part to play: they are complementary.

One way of repatterning adverse family situations to the advantage of a child is to employ a variety of separation procedures. The first step in an ideal situation is to build a relationship between worker and family through family group diagnosis. Through the relationship, the family gains insight into its predicament. Through insight, it can see the measures likely to help itself. From the therapist, it gains the support to take action and through him also is introduced to the facilities that can make separation possible.

Therapeutic Uses of Separation

As a result of the investigation and our clinical experience we now have sufficient confidence to concentrate on taking measures against deprivation when it occurs in the presence of the parents[21]. When deprivation was caused by the parents, we formulated ways by which separation could be utilized to reduce trauma, but, of course, we applied the safeguard that separation must not be allowed to cause deprivation, separation must supply what is lacking in the parents' care.

Before turning to some of the therapeutic utilizations of separation, it may be as well to draw attention to its *prophylactic* value. Short periods of separation for children under the care of familiar friends, relatives or neighbours assure the child that living with strangers need not be unpleasant and that the parents can be relied upon to reappear after being away from them for a short time. Such children, of course, accept more readily unexpected periods of separation from the parents, like those due to admission to hospital as pointed out by Osborn[35]. So widespread and exaggerated has been the propaganda about the dangers of separation, that many parents are now fearful of leaving their children under any circumstances, for however short a period. This amounts to a virtual enslavement of the parents and brings an artificiality to the lives of both parents and children.

Either complete or partial separation can be utilized therapeutically. Only some of the facilities can, because of space, be mentioned here.

Partial separation procedures allow the child to live at home, but they arrange his life in such a way that there is a minimum of contact between the disturbed parents and himself. This can be organized within the home by the utilization of a home-help to look after the children, while both parents go out to work, or in wealthier families by employing a nanny for the children. Mothers, however, must be guided not to select a nanny in their own image. Little attention has so far been given to the contribution made by the nanny to the care of children. A partial break between parents and children can also be effected by measures which allow others to give special care to the child, outside the home, during the day. These facilities include day foster care, nursery schools for maladjusted children, day schools for maladjusted children, day hospitals and therapeutic clubs. In the space available, it is intended to say a little more about the use of the day foster care and of therapeutic clubs.

Day foster care[19, 22] is the planned, temporary separation of an emotionally deprived child from his parents during the day, in order to supply him with the right emotional care. This can be effected in at least three ways. First, the attendance of the child at a special day nursery whose staff are carefully selected for their ability to supply the positive parenting which is absent from the home. During the separation, the child is, as it were, in a power house of affection. The second method is to arrange for the child to stay during the day in a selected foster home. A third way is for a small number of mothers to band together to form a nursery club, whereby for one day a week, each mother in turn looks after all the children. Such groups are very helpful, but they should not have more than one or two disturbed children within them.

Therapeutic clubs supply positive emotional care for children during those hours after school when the child would otherwise be in a hostile and negative emotional climate. They supply similar care during weekends and the long holiday periods. Their principal condition of membership is that the child is very difficult and unacceptable to orthodox clubs. The clubs actively create warm relationships between their staff and the children and the staff encourage the children to accept parenting. A high ratio of staff to children is required. Club activities are planned to bring staff and children continuously together by the employment of creative endeavours.

The most *complete* separation is the assumption of parental rights by another family. Less complete, simply because it can be reversed more easily, is the placement of a child in a foster-home. Another less complete separation procedure is the use of hostels for maladjusted children. These hostels provide a great intensity of contact between staff and children, do not undertake schooling facilities themselves and tend to have short holiday periods. They are therefore particularly valuable when a great intensity of parental care is required. Special boarding schools again involve a complete separation from the parents. Here schooling facilities and parental care are supplied under the same roof. They sometimes suffer the disadvantage of being educationally orientated and of having long holidays. In-patient care, in a psychiatric ward for children, involves not only the application of diagnostic and therapeutic procedures within the ward, but also separation from the family. Usually children admitted to in-patient units have a degree of disturbance which is beyond the therapeutic facilities of the agencies previously mentioned.

5

Conclusion

A direct study of separation experiences in young children, reported here, shows that separation per se does not lead to mental ill-health later on. The same study shows that deprivation of the right emotional care, and not physical separation, is the hazard to the emotional nurturing of the child. Unclear definitions of the terms employed may have led to misconception; in particular, the use of separation as synonymous with deprivation.

Emotionally handicapped parents are stressful to children who, in time, also become emotionally handicapped parents. The lack of emotional health in the community cannot be improved unless we can break into this vicious circle. Not all emotionally handicapped parents can be healed. But in most cases it is possible to persuade them to take measures to help their families, including separation procedures. It is urgent for professional workers to accept that separation is not synonymous with deprivation, but that it can be a powerful instrument of health promotion by overcoming deprivation, the enemy of emotional health.

REFERENCES

1. AINSWORTH, M. D., 1962. In *Deprivation of maternal care*. Geneva, W.H.O.
2. ANDRY, R. G., 1960. *Delinquency and parental pathology*. London, Methuen.
3. BOWLBY, J., 1946. *Forty-four juvenile thieves*. London, Baillière, Tindall and Cox.
4. BOWLBY, J., 1951. *Maternal care and mental health*. Monogr. No. 2. Geneva, W.H.O.
5. BOWLBY, J., 1953. Some pathological processes set in train by early mother-child separation. *J. ment. Sci.*, **99**, 265.
6. BOWLBY, J. et al., 1956. The effects of mother-child separation. *Brit. J. med. Psychol.*, **29**, 211.
7. BOWLBY, J., 1958. Correspondence. *Lancet*, i, 480.
8. BOWLBY, J., 1961. Childhood mourning and its implications for psychiatry. *Amer. J. Psychiat.*, **118**, 481.
9. BOWLBY, J., 1966. Correspondence. *Brit. med. J.*, i, 297.
10. CLARKE, A. D. B., and CLARKE, A. M., 1957. Cognitive changes in the feeble minded. *Brit. J. Psychol.*, **45**, 173.
11. CLARKE, A. D. B., and CLARKE, A. M., 1959. Recovery from the effects of deprivation. *Acta psychol.*, **16**, 137.
12. CLARKE, A. D. B., and CLARKE, A. M., 1960. Some recent advances in the study of early deprivation. *J. Child Psychol. Psychiat.*, **1**, 26.
13. GOLDFARB, W., 1955. Emotional and intellectual consequences of psychologic deprivation in infancy: a revaluation. In *Psychopathology of Childhood*. Eds, Hock and Zubin. New York, Grune and Stratton.
14. GREGORY, E., 1958. Studies in parental deprivation in psychiatric patients. *Amer. J. Psychiat.*, **113**, 743.
15. HARLOW, F. L., and SEAY, B., 1966. Mothering in motherless mother monkeys. *Brit. J. soc. Psychiat.*, **1**, 63.
16. HEINICKE, C. M., and WESTHEIMER, I. J., 1965. *Brief Separations*. London, Longmans.
17. HILL, O. W., and PRICE, J. S., 1967. Childhood bereavement and adult depression. *Brit. J. Psychiat.*, **113**, 743.
18. HOLMAN, P., 1953. Some factors in aetiology of maladjustment in children. *J. ment. Sci.*, **99**, 654.
19. HOWELLS, J. G., 1956. Day foster care and the nursery. *Lancet*, ii, 1256.
20. HOWELLS, J. G., 1963a. *Family psychiatry*. Edinburgh, Oliver and Boyd.
21. HOWELLS, J. G., 1963b. Child-parent separation as a therapeutic procedure. *Amer. J. Psychiat.*, **119**, 922.
22. HOWELLS, J. G., 1965. Organization of child psychiatric services. In *Modern perspectives in child psychiatry*. Ed. Howells, J. G. Edinburgh, Oliver and Boyd.
23. HOWELLS, J. G., 1968a. *Theory and practice of family psychiatry*. Edinburgh, Oliver and Boyd.
24. HOWELLS, J. G., 1968b. Family psychiatry. In *Modern perspectives in world psychiatry*, Ed. Howells, J. G. Edinburgh, Oliver and Boyd.
25. HOWELLS, J. G., and LAYNG, J., 1955. Separation experiences and mental health. *Lancet*, ii, 285.
26. HOWELLS, J. G., and LAYNG, J., 1956a. Childhood separation: its causes and care of the child during separation. *Medical Officer*, **96**, 269.
27. HOWELLS, J. G., and LAYNG, J., 1956b. The effect of separation experiences on children given care away from home. *Medical Officer*, **95**, 345.

28. LEWIS, H., 1954. *Deprived children.* Toronto, Oxford Univ. Press.
29. MEAD, M., 1954. Some theoretical considerations on the problem of mother-child separation. *Amer. J. Orthopsychiat.*, **24**, 471.
30. Ministry of Health, 1964. *The part of the family doctor in the Mental Health Service.* London, H.M.S.O.
31. MOORE, T., 1964. Children of full time and part time mothers. *Intern. J. soc. Psychiat.*, **2**, 1.
32. NAESS, S., 1959. Mother-child separation and delinquency. *Brit. J. Delinq.*, **10**, 22.
33. NYE, F. L., 1957. *Marriage and family living*, **19**, 356.
34. O'CONNOR, N., 1956. Conceptual perspectives on the early environment. *J. Amer. Acad. Child Psychiat.*, **4**, 168.
35. OSBORN, M. L., 1964. Time off for mum. *Nursery J.*, **54**, 6.
36. RUTTER, M., 1966. *Children of sick parents.* Maudsley Monograph No. 16. London, Oxford Univ. Press.
37. SCHAFFER, H. R., 1965. Changes in developmental quotient under two conditions of maternal separation. *Brit. J. soc. clin. Psychol.*, **4**, 39.
38. SEAY, B., and HARLOW, F. L., 1965. Maternal separation in the rhesus monkey. *J. nerv. ment. Dis.*, **140**, 434.
39. *Seventh Report on the Work of the Children's Department, Home Office.* 1955. London, H.M.S.O.
40. SPENCER-BOOTH, Y., and HINDE, R. A., 1967. The effects of separating rhesus monkey infants from their mothers for six days. *J. Child Psychol. Psychiat.*, **7**, 179.
41. SPITZ, R. A., and WOLFF, K. M., 1946. *The Psychoanalytical Study of the Child*, **2**, 213. New York.
42. STOTT, D. H., 1956. The effects of separation from mothers in early life. *Lancet*, i, 624.
43. W.H.O. Bull., 1955. *The child in hospital.* Geneva, W.H.O.
44. YARROW, L. J., 1961. Maternal deprivation: toward an empirical and conceptual re-valuation. *Psychol. Bull.*, **58**, 459.
45. YARROW, L. J., 1964. Separation from parents during childhood. *Rev. Child Devel. Res.*, **1**, 89.
46. YARROW, L. J., 1965. Conceptual perspectives on the early environment. *J. Amer. Acad. Child Psych.*, **4**, 168.

X

CULTURE AND CHILD REARING

MARVIN K. OPLER

Ph.D.

Professor of Social Psychiatry, School of Medicine, and Professor of Sociology, the Graduate School, State University of New York at Buffalo

---

1

Introduction

The way in which culture affects child rearing and, consequently the manner in which the enculturation of children in culture influences their adult personality form a chain reaction discussed in this small chapter. Most anthropologists refer to this field of interest as being the study of culture and personality. Social psychiatrists often call the same topic by the words, ethnopsychiatry, transcultural psychiatry, or more simply as the cross-cultural analysis of the epidemiology of mental disorders.

Just as the special subfield of child psychiatry developed much later than the general field of psychiatry proper, so studies in culture and personality according to models of national or tribal personality type—national character, as they were called—preceded more careful studies of child rearing and its effects. Physicians like Leo Kanner[35] and child psychologists like Piaget[61-64] or Arnold Gesell[25] were influential in building up a body of information on child development, the former in the sense of children's pathology, and the latter in terms of their normative growth processes[35]. However, rather than trace this founding of the various subfields in the context of institutes and clinics in various countries, the present author prefers to trace the issues theoretically as they developed in only two disciplines, anthropology and psychoanalysis. Our central terms for this discussion are, therefore, culture on the sociodynamic level, personality on the psychodynamic level, and child rearing which, of course, relates to both levels.

INTRODUCTION

Let us begin with the psychological point of view, the Freudian. In the second decade of this century, Freud was writing essentially in two areas. In his perceptive analysis of cases, such as the paranoid schizophrenic jurist named Schreber, for example, he was tracing out the way in which homosexual trends used defensively against immature infantile desires of an Oedipal sort might in turn lead to paranoid projections and ego disorganization. In the last decade of the 19th century, about 18 years earlier, Freud and J. Breuer explored the ego adaptation involved in hysteria through the analysis of the famous patient of Breuer, Miss Anna O.[6, 7] As a doctor, Freud's thinking and writing on the level of individual case analyses, whether Anna O.[5], the phobia of little Hans[16], Dora's hysteria[15], or the obsessional neurosis of the 'rat man' case[17], had crystallized to a large extent in his theory that early and often infantile psychosexual development is the prime mover determining an individual's later adjustments. Freud's later book, *Totem and taboo*[18], represents his incursion into the field of cultural anthropology, for which he lacked adequate anthropological training. Nor was the field of psychological anthropology sufficiently developed at the time of his exploration into it for him to find ready-made a proper analysis of the relationship of culture to personality. Instead, Freud was forced to fall back on still earlier literature, such as the highly fanciful work on primal origins and primitive law of A. Lang and Atkinson[39]. The latter was an evolutionary fantasy which related how, ostensibly in aboriginal Australian society totemistic rites began when sons in some mythic patrilineal horde rose up in revolt against their fathers, slew them and overcome by remorseful feelings of guilt promptly began to worship ancestral totems while at the same time setting up taboos against eating the forbidden animals. Freud's parallel account of the primal parricidal myth and the symbolic injunctions against 'cannibalism' of the ancestral totem is a more sensitive elaboration of the earlier story, but one for which there is of course no real scientific sanction.

These criticisms of *Totem and taboo*[18] did not pass unnoticed in the reviews of the volume written by the anthropologists A. A. Goldenweiser and A. L. Kroeber. In addition, it was not very long before B. Malinowski wrote his own book called *Sex and repression in savage society*[44] which attempted to modify Freud's doctrine by pointing out that the Trobriand Islanders whom Malinowski studied did not even recognize a father as a biological paternal and socially authoritarian person, but instead vested disciplinary and controlling functions in a child's mother's brother. While it is true that Malinowski[43] recognized repression as possible in this second setting where the father was a mere friendly 'stranger' in the village (even living elswhere) he called the culturally variable phenomena of family organization by the alternative term of *nuclear complex*, refusing to accept the universality of Oedipal and Elektra complexes.

It is true, then, that Malinowski introduced the concept of cultural variability into studies of the roots of repression in different societies. This is, of course, a correction of the idea that all family types and social organizational forms as viewed by the anthropologist are bound to have the same psychological effects in child rearing. Yet, Freudian readers of Malinowski were quick to point out that the substitution of a mother's brother for the father figure is really not much of an extension of basic Freudian theory. Indeed, both sides were right. Malinowski was correct in noting that the Oedipal family of Grecian or Western European Viennese models did not in the slightest exhaust the structural forms of social organization around the world which are known to every anthropologist. However, the Freudians could note, as did even Goldenweiser and Kroeber in their reviews of *Totem and taboo* that this slight revision left intact Freud's more basic doctrine as to the defence mechanisms used by the species in ego or personality adjustments and adaptations. To enter into this old debate, which, as a consequence, was never resolved, the present author can state in criticism of Malinowski that a nuclear complex which merely substitutes one relative for another does not even begin to touch the larger and important issue of how a culture comes to favour or promote one kind of defensive mechanism over another, nor does it even begin to tell us anything about the typical balances or imbalances in human behaviour as this is discovered in the typical forms and functioning types of human social organization.

At the same time, one may criticize both Kroeber and Malinowski for the incompleteness of their position. To say that the defence mechanisms operate in an entire species, like man, and then add that the cultural settings vary is to overlook the entire question of what kind of defences are most used and, indeed, overused in various kinds of cultures. The present author, in an earlier book called *Culture, psychiatry and human values*[50], and in its sequel called *Culture and social psychiatry*[58] has pointed out that a more thoroughgoing theory of cultural relativity is necessary. For one thing, epidemiological studies discussed in both books show clearly that both the form and the amount of mental disorders vary with such cultural differences. This can only mean that the mechanisms of defence, while they may generally be said to have some existence cross-culturally, nevertheless must exist in different amounts of balance or imbalance depending on the culture. Secondly, even within one historical or vertical time sequence in a given culture, the forms and amounts may change with the changes in conditions within the culture. Thirdly, the concepts of health and illness, as an accompaniment of the values orientations in any society may likewise change with cultural conditions[54, 55]. Finally, there are concomitant shifts to be noted when we discard the static doctrines of invariable defences of Malinowski, Kroeber or Goldenweiser, or the invariable idea of a universally Oedipal-structured form of society which plagued Freud's earlier work and still plagues the parrot-like repetitions of many of his followers.

While Freud himself was unable to provide information on the models of cultural variability and intrapsychic differences according to anthropological data in the first half of the century, he nevertheless did respond to the anthropological critics whom he read commenting on *Totem and taboo*[18] by writing a much better book called *The ego and the id*[19] in which he stated quite clearly his feeling that 'the heir of the Oedipus complex' was the superego, further defined as 'the ethical conditions' surrounding mankind. The reader should note, however, that while Freud made this polite bow to cultural anthropology, he had no way of expressing descriptively or analytically how the problems would change. Our feeling is therefore that Freud provided a kind of Newtonian theory of the possibly relevant forces at work, without being able to go on with the theory of cultural relativity and its consequences. For this reason his followers have scarcely bothered to notice the remarkable change in his system occasioned by the substitution of 'superego' for 'Oedipus Rex'. Nor is my suggestion at all like Ruth Benedict's[1,3], namely that 'anything can happen' in an extension of the Freudian system to one of absolute and uncontrolled psychological relativity. The actual case is much simpler in human societies since the evolution of culture itself provides a more limited number of structural models, while at the same time the limited number of balances and imbalances available in human defence systems as these actually become formed and operate are likewise limited by the types and forms of culture produced in cultural evolution on this planet to the present time.

Other sciences, like physics, are concerned with multivariables, which in research must often be controlled to gauge the effectiveness of certain specific ones claiming the attention of the experimentalists. Physical research of this type is, of course, complex and highly quantitative. Because cultural and behavioural sciences deal also with related and sometimes even patterned phenomena, it was inevitable that the first approaches to national character studies tended to be influenced, in the United States, not only by a preference for Freudian theory, but its preference over such bankrupt European approaches as the racist or the geographical determinist explanations. Besides Freud, as a conveniently simple and even oversimplified psychological approach, in the United States Gestalt concepts were beginning to influence the science of psychology because of obvious gaps and lacks in the models provided by behaviourism and reward-punishment schools or movements[76]. The interest in Gestalt concepts fitted in well with the ideas of pattern provided by leading anthropologists like Ruth Benedict, who in turn was influenced by Durkheim's strong formulations of social and cultural conditioning and Dilthey's equally strong depictions of regional and historical epochs. While Benedict, in *Patterns of culture*[1], was driven to epitomize her cultural examples in a style which derived them from what she called 'a principle of psychological selectivity', she claimed such a form or quality in an entire cultural tradition[1,3]. Thus while beginning perhaps as Gestaltist interested in form and feeling that culture determined all else, Benedict paved the way for similar epitomizations by such students as Margaret Mead who were interested in the Freudian claim that 'infantile training disciplines' were the chief item in a psychological theory of causation.

By this time, it should be clear that the theory of culture in relation to personality had changed into one whereby it was thought that some Freudian process in personality formation determined culture. During World War II, a fantastic series of such culture and personality analyses appeared, chiefly influenced by Ruth Benedict and Margaret Mead. While Ruth Benedict's book, *The chrysanthemum and the sword*[3], on the pattern of Japanese culture down through the ages was an attempt to give a modern instance of the picture she had presented for non-literate people in *Patterns of culture*[1], it evoked great criticism because it overlooked changes in economy and in social structure which had occurred in Japan over the centuries. Japanese scholars began to write about their people 'without the chrysanthemum and the sword'. American orientalists, while recognizing much that was true in Benedict's description, likewise felt it was only loosely analytical and often forgetful of changes occasioned in the cultural evolution of Japan.

The national character studies which derived personality from infant disciplines included work of G. Gorer, G. Bateson and also short papers by Benedict on Slavic speaking cultures. Gorer's on Japanese evoked strong counterstatements during the war and after. Benedict's on Russians was similarly greeted. Mead's emphasis on toilet-training and weaning came under the same criticism, too widespread to give in detail here.

It is clear that the first attempts in anthropology to place heavy weight on child rearing in determining personality were psychoanalytic in emphasis. While psychoanalysis was used to explain the behaviour of groups, the early description of primitive cultures and of national character was regarded by most anthropologists as overly simple psychodynamic theories. Malinowski was the first to stress the need for comparative ethnological studies to correct such oversimplifications. He emphasized the structural relations between the parts of a culture and the necessity of studying it from a functional point of view beginning with human needs. But while Malinowski corrected the tendency to describe cultures as results of child rearing, his own tendency to start with any institutional category of behaviour (whether economic as in *Coral gardens*[45] or social organization as in *Sexual life of the savages*) did not help in demonstrating what in culture was basic. His ever widening list of relevant and interconnected factors in a cultural system simply meant that institutions are a kind of merry-go-round with each part connected to the next. Another British anthropologist who called his method functional was A. R. Radcliffe-Brown who emphasized social relationships in social structure and who likewise tended to emphasize the study of culture and society outside of the contexts of psychology and history.

2
Neo-Freudian Influences

We shall omit in this discussion the alternatives to Freudian theory which had developed on the continent with Jungian and Adlerian influences since the major thrust of child rearing studies occurred in the United States among anthropologists and psychiatrists who modified the strictly Freudian viewpoint. The scene was set by dissidents like Erich Fromm, Karen Horney[34], and others. Erich Fromm, both in *Escape from freedom*[22] and *Man for himself*[23], expressed the dilemma by which terms like 'normal' or 'healthy' may mean quite different things. From the point of view of the functioning society, fulfilling the social role or roles one takes, or participation in social productivity and social reproduction constitutes normalcy or health; whereas from the individual standpoint the optimum of individual growth and happiness marks this result. In this view, creativity, spontaneity, freedom, productivity and expression of one's highest potentialities are selected as the aims of mental hygiene. Indeed, in one sense they are. But the error of Fromm, or the dilemma he does not wholly solve, is implicit in the failure to analyse dynamic processes as parts of recognizable social situations or 'fields' of cultural influence.

Both Karen Horney and Erich Fromm, in separate ways, proposed orientations to psychoanalytic theory which reversed Freud's contention that sexual development determined character, and instead contended that character guides all behaviour, including the sexual. Horney, in her discussions of reaction formations in female patients, or in tracing widespread evidences of neuroticism in contemporary American culture, indicates points at which the perpetuation of faulty neurotic solutions to the problems of the feminine role or the competitive role, occur because of invariant conditions in cultural environment.

Fromm therefore created a more cross-cultural concept of 'social character' and also a parallel idea of 'socially patterned defect' without stressing child rearing as such. Horney while recognizing the general importance of culture, confined her criticisms to pitfalls in contemporary American society which she treated of as a general culture, ignoring both its ethnic and subcultural varieties and its differentiations in social class. In the meantime one could find specific analyses of culture only in Horney's overgeneralized picture of America or in Erich Fromm's earlier published work on authority and the family in pre-Nazi Germany. Anthropologists, instead, preferred to work closely in teams with specific psychoanalysts. Perhaps the earliest such collaboration was the theoretical work of Harry Stack Sullivan[82], an American psychiatrist critical of the kinds of social relationships he found common in the United States, and Edward Sapir, an anthropologist, who also sensitively viewed urban America.

A less theoretical collaboration involving a novel approach was represented by the work of Kardiner and Linton in seminars at Columbia University which led to two books, one in 1939 and the second in 1945[36, 37]. In place of the earlier term, 'national character' or tribal ethos, they proposed the terminology of 'basic personality structure' and also 'modal personality type'. Curiously, however, their method was to have a culture described in detail in seminars whereupon the psychoanalyst, Kardiner, proceeded to analyse it. From one culture to the next, there was developed a picture of child rearing practices which, of course, varied in each culture. The modes of nursing and weaning, infant handling and disciplines were found to set and determine a personality configuration shared by the majority, or at least by those in each sex group for each culture. Thus, although Freud was generously criticized in theoretical chapters, one could notice that child rearing determined 'basic personality' which according to the authors moulded the social patterns and institutions. Kardiner further maintained that the types of maternal care were of major importance in determining personality in culture, and consequently, variations in child rearing alone explained why people differed from one society to the next. It is true that much of value was added to this method by perceptively looking at myth, folklore, and religion as if these were the Rorschachs of every culture. Nevertheless, this method does not strongly emphasize values in a culture as being themselves determinative of behaviour; nor does it stress economic organization or even cultural evolution as having a determinate weight. It is obvious that real values in a culture may be controlled by the conditions under which the culture itself exists, and these points are minimized in favour of what turns out to be infantile-discipline determinism.

Another famous collaboration was that of E. H. Erikson and A. L. Kroeber. Erikson, the psychoanalyst, in *Childhood and society*[13] pictured the aboriginal Sioux Indian's hostility and bravado in warfare as a function of the stored-up restrictions of the cradleboard, long nursing interrupted by the eruption of milk teeth, and biting thwarted by duly irritated mothers. This account has graphic persuasiveness extending to the long pent-in motility bursting forth in long expeditions over the Plains within fancy-determined hostility and aggression. The effects of the horse or of such other acculturation phenomena as White encroachments are simply not mentioned.

In Ute studies[48, 49], however, the author reported an almost identical cradleboard stuffed with dried, powdered sage bark to absorb waste. Motion was inhibited. Ute mothers nursed even longer than the Sioux, sometimes with classificatory sisters continuing the suckling after solids were added to the age of 4 or even 6. Like their linguistic cousins, the peaceful Hopi, the Ute aboriginally feared warfare, had 'talking peace chiefs' and held to mountain camps for safety from Plains or Apache marauders. Their culture is distinct from the Sioux at every point. With ceremonies for infants and children intended to promote health, vigour and beauty, they attain protective supernatural power to which young adults later add through dream experience an increased religious rapport or personal supernatural gifts. There is no pattern of medicine bundles in religion, no societies in warfare and no counting of *coup* for prestige. The annual Bear Dance ceremony is again for protection in the mountains and equally to facilitate in-group social contacts and promote courtships. With only defensive warfare, dual standards of Plains peoples are lacking and women not only choose in social dances, but encourage male clandestine visits to camps. Traditionally, marriages were breakable by either spouse. Such patterns as trial marriages up to the birth of a child or decision to hold a marriage ceremony; the custom of *couvade* to indicate a husband's responsibility towards children; adoption by a host of relatives; these techniques all insure child-centred marriages and families. In their system of relationship, any age and experience distinctions link with authority, but such authority is obviously diffused and shared up to the grandparental generation. The protections and privacy attending the family at the time of a birth were so little understood by white health and hospital officials that confinements held in a brick hospital led to all unrelated male patients, in various stages of all illnesses, gathering their blankets about them never to return.

Any account of neo-Freudian influences should include the experimental work of Freudians themselves who attempted to elaborate upon Freud's classic formulations with various kinds of studies going beyond individuals to groups. René Spitz[78, 79], a psychoanalyst, focused his attention upon the results of inadequate mothering among groups of infants. Taking two institutional hospital situations, in one of which the babies were hygienically handled but at the same time neglected in the sense of being handled only occasionally by busy personnel, Spitz contrasted this with institutional treatment elsewhere where mothers visited the institution and spent more time in the actual handling and cherishing of their infants who happened to be illegitimate offspring.

In comparison, the hygienic but isolated treatment proved to be inadequate in safeguarding the babies in the antiseptic and colder environment of the first institution. There the infants suffered such conditions as slower weight gain, slower increase in size or stature, and, as a matter of fact, they succumbed in larger numbers to epidemics of childhood diseases than their more robust comparison group of much-fondled illegitimate babies. However, Spitz's comparison included a psychological theory to account for the severe problems in the more hygienic environment. Noting that the institutionally and antiseptically isolated babies exhibited psychological differences, he characterized these as including greater apathy, a passive listlessness and a relative disinterest in their coldly efficient environment. In fact so marked were such symptoms as time went on that Spitz applied the term, anaclitic depression, to these phenomena[77]. There have been criticisms of the generally descriptive plane of this study and its lack of control over various factors that may have been operating in the two situations. Indeed, Spitz has utilized film technique to describe the two groups, but we hasten to add that the films are strikingly and convincingly full of the kind of detail that answers such stereotyped methodological criticisms.

Anaclitic depression does seem to occur in non-mothered infants, and its existence has been substantiated in further clinical observations of such eminent pediatricians as Dr Julius B. Richmond[66] who has added detail on the signals or signs whereby such infants may be denoted in hospital wards. One may add that the difference between the anaclitic depression baby and the normal infant is not just simply a product of 'psychological causes' since obviously early infantile socialization processes or social identity is fundamentally at stake.

The same style of explanation applies to certain animal experiments with rhesus monkeys carried forward by the psychologist Harry Harlow in Wisconsin. Harlow published in 1959[27] extensive accounts of comparison groups of rhesus monkeys, one of which received adequate mothering in infancy while the other groups were studied under conditions where a wire apparatus and terry-cloth surrogate for a larger monkey provided the milk required by the infants. Those deprived of mothering showed breakdowns of normal behaviour in respect to inter-animal confrontations including a breakdown of normal heterosexual behaviour in both male and female monkeys as these 'matured'. An interesting additional experiment occurred, however, when one previously non-mothered sample received opportunities for reparative peer-group contacts with playful monkeys of the same young age. In the latter, socialization processes were repaired, as it were, and such infants were able later to enact heterosexual behaviour, and a female to achieve adequate mothering behaviour with their own infants—something which isolated and non-socialized females could not achieve[28]. Again, film technique is used to substantiate other types of recorded data and such films, like Spitz's, are exceedingly convincing.

To the above may be added the important work of John Bowlby in England on maternal care which eventuated in 1952 in an important monograph published in the Monograph Series of the World Health Organization[4]. Bowlby particularly gave wide circulation to the impairing effects of hospitalization and isolation on infant development. Somewhat earlier Margaret Ribble in the United States, in a controversial work called *The rights of infants*[65] had made claims of the importance of certain kinds of petting and head-stroking for proper child development. The work of Bowlby like that of Spitz on infants and institutions stood up much better since it utilized extreme poles of care and of neglect in a far more general analytic model than one which was limited to such a factor as petting the head. But the more pinpointed nursing and weaning, or toilet-training models of the early 'national character' position of certain American anthropologists, together with parallel brash claims from certain studies in paediatrics led to a counter-movement of equally extreme scepticism. In psychology, one American author, Harold Orlansky, in 1949 published a psychological bulletin called *Infant care and personality*[60]. Surveying the literature including that of the national character school of child rearing and the now abundant tests of single practices by various psychologists, Orlansky concluded that the literature did not support the thesis of personality determination by infant care. It is interesting that although single trait analyses like nursing and weaning or toilet training fell by the wayside, the studies of more global attitudes and total patterns affecting infants' lives—more in the fashion of Bowlby, Spitz and others—continue to prove their worth. Moreover, while Orlansky in 1949 could conclude that there was no evidence to support a conviction that breast feeding is necessarily superior to bottle feeding, later studies by the psychologist Robert R. Sears in 1950 and 1957[69] demonstrated that such matters as abrupt weaning or the feeding situation in general actually involved more than a quick superficial analysis of between-group differences and required increased understanding of some of the possible meanings of the behaviour being studied. For example, children weaned early might not have a feeding problem, but at the same time protracted sucking does probably strengthen the oral drive or motivation.

Various current studies in paediatrics add weight to the idea that child rearing practices exist in a complex of behavioural attitudes about children. For instance, in contrast to the mere mention of an infantile discipline or training process there are questions about the severity of the training, its timing, the amount of insistence upon it and matters of pressure, irritability, impatience and even punishment.

It is curious that positions stressing the importance of meanings and values in interpersonal behaviour took so long to find experimental proofs. Theoretically, they were foreshadowed in the heyday of Freud's own time of writing and publication, in 1916, by E. B. Holt, whose book *The Freudian wish*[32], dealing with its place in ethics showed how the handling of children's desires and impulses always had meaningful interpersonal connotations. For instance, an adult could block off or protect a small child from some danger by forceful methods of inhibiting him; but the difference between a meaningless and non-insightful act of repression, such as a simple 'thou shalt not' or a senseless act of punishment without explanation (like a slap or blow) and some other inhibiting mode which produced greater insight in the child was essentially the contrast between repression because of punitive sanctions or fears and inhibitory behaviour which might produce mastery. Of course, this analytic model just given is simplified because adult inhibitors or punitive agents always deal with children. In other words the struggle is not only between the infantile *id* or libidinal wishes and some vague sort of ego-control principle, but between actual models of living persons such as an infant and given parental figures or their surrogates. Such interpersonal theory, rather than a more depersonalized account of intrapsychic forces had the consequence of leading more realistically to concrete studies of actual parent-child relationships, of actual forms or styles of family organization according to cultural or subcultural samples and also to studies of generalized patterns of childhood disciplines.

It is this author's opinion that books like Holt's[32, 33] and also various collaborations between anthropologists and psychiatrists (such as Kroeber and Mekeel, Edward Sapir and H. S. Sullivan, and C. Kluckhohn and H. A. Murray) helped considerably in changing abstract Freudian formulations into cross-cultural studies of an exploratory nature. It is also our view that current theory has been negligent in following up E. B. Holt's realistic reassessment of Freud. Freudianism, if truly modernized and brought down to date, would cease to be a theory of mere intrapsychic functioning. In place of such overly simple pronouncements as: 'where the *id* was, there should be the *ego*', or the time-worn emphasis upon the recapitulation of the past, one could substitute more functionally active concepts stemming from actual interpersonal processes. Thus, besides libidinal psychosexual and aggressive drives, there may be qualitatively and quantitatively different forms of mastery which combine libidinal enjoyments, delayed or sustained gratifications, impulse-control and even aesthetic or ethical forms of restraint.

One difficulty with such a Freudian work as *Civilization and its discontents*[21] is that it assumes sublimation can take place, but only with some loss in creativity. Or it assumes that love and aggression are the only drive states. Freud's later inclusion of a death instinct or *thanatos*, to be combined with libidinal love and aggression, is the static view of possible drives. His idea of sublimation comes closest to ideas of mastery; but there is really little attention paid to the many cultural forms and child rearing practices which promote the various kinds and degrees of *mastery*, which in its learned forms are simply ways of talking about 'learning a culture', the enculturation and 'socialization' of children, and the development of special flairs or talents in real people. In brief, there is a tendency for Freud's writing to emphasize the pathological rather than normal development and to assume that one model of development applies to all human beings.

Within neo-Freudian movements, there were certain attempts to move in the direction of the concept of cultural learning or 'mastery' as outlined above. For example, new leadership in psychoanalysis in the United States, notably with such figures as H. Hartmann and E. Kris, emphasized ego-adaptation in development. Another shift in theory could be noted in papers on ego-identity (by Heinz Lichtenstein and in a recent series of publications by Erik Erikson)[14]. Since we have discussed Erikson's early work in *Childhood and society*[13] above, it is only fair to discuss his more recent and current work, for instance his essay, 'Growth and Crises' in *Symposium on the healthy personality*, edited by Milton J. Senn in 1950[70]. At this time Erikson began to develop an evolutionary sequence of stages in the self-identification process. In *Childhood and society*[13] he had begun to trace such a development through the following eight stages: (*i*) oral-sensory, (*ii*) muscular-anal, (*iii*) locomotor-genital, (*iv*) latency, (*v*) puberty and adolescence, (*vi*) young adulthood, (*vii*) adulthood, and (*viii*) maturity. Each of these stages was accompanied by 'phases and crises' in the psycho-social development of personality. For example, the most famous pictures of opposites are the trust *versus* mistrust of the first or oral-sensory period, or the identity *versus* self-diffusion of puberty and adolescence. A final growth stage like 'maturity' was expressed in terms of integrity *versus* disgust or despair. It is obvious that Erikson felt that a firm sense of identity could be contrasted in adolescence with a conflict in roles, making for self-diffusion. When he describes childhood proper coming to an end and healthy adolescence taking over, he begins with intelligence and insight to comment upon the establishment of good relationships to the world of skills and to the teachers and older adults who share such newly acquired skills. Then says Erikson, dramatically: Youth begins.

Much of this evolutionary series in the development of the individual is reminiscent of Harry Stack Sullivan's stages in development from infancy to maturity[82]. As a matter of fact, the initial dichotomy of trust *versus* mistrust can be found again in papers from the Washington or William Alanson White school of psychiatry with which Sullivan was associated as a leading figure. One paper for example which attempts to trace depressive state psychoses to childhood roots does so through depth-analytic studies of depressives in whom it is claimed the fatal lack was of any real relationship in infancy with an adult who could instill a sense of basic trust or security.

It will be recalled parenthetically, that there were other studies from this early period which again implicated the persons rearing children in our society, chiefly mothers in the American scene. For example, famous in its day as was Erikson's writing on adolescence was David M. Levy's earlier work on the theme of childhood overprotection as one important form of actual rejection of the child[40]. The lesson to be learned from Levy was that a maternal attitude of extreme overprotectiveness could mask a virtual rejection of the idea that a child must grow and gain in independence in order to achieve his own life. On the continent, the famous work of M. Sechehaye on symbiotic dependencies of the immature or infantile schizophrenic pointed again to a lack of the achievement of gradual independence and autonomy in stages of growth. Sechehaye's work on her famous female schizophrenic patient reminds one of a whole series of studies by Frieda Fromm-Reichmann and others on fearful schizophrenics who had failed to achieve autonomy, let alone a firm sense of self-identity.

Missing in all of these formulations, and even in the most sensitive case-discussions was any clear development of identification theory beyond the limits of ego or self-identification. While indeed, self-identification adds something to the earlier sexual-identification, the missing theme throughout is lack of a concept of social-identification being developed at the same

x

time. If one refers, above, to Erikson's discussion of the beginnings of a stage like Youth, it is obvious that these references to the teaching and learning of new skills in society must refer not only to self-identity being established, but social-identity being involved all the more.

In summary, the gradual shift we have been describing under the heading of neo-Freudian studies and influences was a shift in the direction of cultural factors, such as types of family or kinship structure and functioning, or one involving the meaningful relationships of children with the adults empowered to exert child rearing disciplines larger in scale than nursing, weaning, or toilet training. Yet, while studies gradually broadened and approached this more social direction, it cannot be said that cultural factors were truly reached in psychiatric and psychological reports. This is, however, to be expected. A more complete degree of attention to such cultural factors could only be developed through anthropological studies in various parts of the world.

3

Cultural Factors

Child rearing practices, of course, vary from one culture to another. If we refer back to the Kardiner-Linton studies[36, 37], discussed above, the Marquesans whom Linton described did not indulge their children in nursing and breast feeding continued for only a short time. Linton's description claims that Marquesan mothers feared breast-disfigurement, and consequently weaned infants within the first year. (The accuracy of this ethnographic description is not wholly satisfying to the author of this chapter since a great many modern cultures could be described as practising weaning within the first year.) At any rate, nonliterate peoples tend to nurse children for a longer period, especially where other elements in food supply may be uncertain. For a few examples, the Chenchu of India nurse children till the age of 5 or 6 and the Lepcha of India did not wean children until 3, but in families with many other children to feed solids they are said to nurse the youngest until puberty. The Ute Indians of Colorado, whom the author studied, occupied a middle ground, nursing many children to 4, 5, or 6 years of age even after solid supplements had been added, and also letting such young children suckle occasionally with 'wet nurses' or nursing mothers who were not always their own mothers[48, 49].

Nevertheless, the Marquesan data of Linton was presented as an example of adult values which might affect child rearing, and in the total description the period of time devoted to nursing, while it is not strikingly different from practices found in our own modern culture, is connected with other attitudes descriptive of how the child will be handled. There were other studies in our own society which went beyond the question of duration of nursing. For instance, Daniel Miller and Guy Swanson, reporting on a study called *The changing American parent*[46], in 1958, stated that the entrepreneurial middle class composed of the self-employed should be distinguished in child rearing practices from the bureaucratic middle class employed mainly on salary in large organizations. The former segment of the middle class was said to possess values of the Protestant ethic more noticeably than those whose economics were constrained by fixed salaried position. In the analysis of the differences in child rearing practices, a greater emphasis was placed on self-control and self-denial among entrepreneurs[47]. A somewhat parallel theoretical interest is reported in a series of papers by B. C. Rosen[68] in the *American sociological review* which finds that in Brazil, boys from the bottom of the social class ladder have much stronger achievement needs than those from the highest class, because the latter occupy a guaranteed ascribed status which includes excessive spoiling and deference by servants, teachers and tutors, etc. About the same time, F. Kluckhohn and F. Strodtbeck, in *Variations in value orientations*[38], pointed out that the American middle-class values emphasized not only accomplishments but the development of achievement needs. They characterized the American middle-class as teaching children to consider the future and to outstrip the occupational level of parents—or in other words as stressing both an activist or 'doing' orientation and also a 'future' orientation in respect to outlooks on temporality.

We have purposely juxtaposed studies of feeding practices and studies of more global values orientations in order to point up the fact that there is, as yet, no real consensus concerning the kinds of factors to be included in research design on the relationships of cultural background and child rearing. Yet anthropologists know that cultures and subcultures ordinarily form a consistent pattern of themes, values and practices in which such an item as the rearing of children could not be developed within the total cultural matrix in some utterly inconsistent or surprisingly unusual way. In our view, such cultural and psychological adaptations have a way of running together so as to produce consistency. Cultures as adaptational modes of gaining greater or lesser adjustment have, of course, built within them ways of handling various kinds of human problems, for instance man's beliefs and practices connected with adaptation to the larger world or cosmos (as in religious, scientific or philosophical methods of gaining rapport). There are also, of course, adaptational techniques in culture for achieving control over the environmental setting (as in economics, political economy and technology). One could even say that all cultures provide aesthetic and recreational release (as in arts, folklore, or even games). But the area of culture that we are here concerned with, in child development and personality functioning is obviously that area of man's relationship to fellow-man (as exemplified in social organization, kinship practices, education, and the like). A key concept in regard to the latter forms of cultural expression is, of course, those techniques by which the human or interpersonal relationships within the culture are learned.

A connected concept of importance is how the individual not only 'learns' his culture and its expectations, but the ways in which he is encouraged to achieve mastery or is prevented, also in the culture, from so doing[51]. Such an approach in anthropology goes beyond the earlier Freudian position concerned with the achievement of controls in respect to such simple biological processes as the intake of food, the excretion of waste, or the handling of sexual tensions. Early in this chapter where we discussed the recent elaborations of the Freudian system by Hartmann, Kris and Loewenstein[30], we might have noted with Hartmann his idea of the existence of 'conflict-free avenues of reality-adapted development' in addition to the usual ego-id conflicts of the earlier Freudian position. Within this 'conflict-free ego sphere' Hartmann placed such ego functions as 'perception, intention, object comprehension, thinking, language, recall phenomena, productivity' and even such well known forms of motor development as grasping, crawling, walking, and so forth. It will be noted that most of ego-adaptation, as defined above, is more than likely tinged with cultural effects[29]. Thus, indeed, whether it is typically acknowledged or not by neo-Freudians, cultural laboratories ought to furnish the greatest variety of conditions for studying ego-adaptations that could be possibly imagined.

The fact that thorough analyses of child rearing practices in cultures are rarely made accounts for the inconsistencies in the findings of certain investigations for the past few decades. The classic study of A. Davis and R. J. Havighurst in the 1940's[12] reported the finding that middle-class parents were stricter and made larger demands on children than lower-class parents. In the next decade E. E. Maccoby and P. Gibbs found just the opposite, namely that middle-class parents were more permissive than were those in lower-class status. The same authors, Davis and Havighurst, also found in a study of white and Negro mothers using intensive interviews with 200 women that permissive feeding and weaning characterized the lower-class more than the middle-class group. They summarized that more lower-class children were breast fed and for longer periods on self-demand schedule and that Negro mothers tended to be lenient in procedures including more gradual weaning. The Maccoby and Gibbs study at Harvard[42] which followed denied this later; they found few differences between social classes in infantile feeding with confirmatory studies following from the Pacific Coast and in the Detroit study of Daniel Miller and Guy Swanson which we have mentioned above.

The American pediatrician, Dr Benjamin Spock[81], and the social psychologist, U. Bronfenbrenner[8], have both suggested that child rearing practices are likely to change in segments of society having the easiest access to the recent permissive literature and the closest connections with the educated sources of information for change such as books, journals, clinics and physicians.

Besides these changes, which are responsive to education and information there have been no indications that this single factor, taken alone, wholly determines later adjustments. To cite just a few factors influencing socialization after infancy, there is the question of how the culture organizes inter-generational relationships, how it limits or extends the size of the effective family unit, and how it structures authority within the family as for example between the sexes or in terms of greater or lesser amounts of patriarchal or matriarchal 'rule'. One excellent study which is a follow-up on the sample of children originally studied by John Dollard and A. Davis in New Orleans is the work by M. Edmondson, an anthropologist, and J. Rohrer, a psychologist. This book, called *The eighth generation grows up*[67], which is a study of a sample of Negro children from the original work called *Children of bondage*[11], is a remarkable account in contrast to the more limited studies of nursing, weaning and the like, because it carefully assesses the quality of parent-child relationships both in childhood and later in the life cycle to determine what total balances and imbalances are achieved. In an adaptational process which is able to consider early influences as well as the community and peer group relationships, the broader area of social identification becomes important.

As Rohrer and Edmondson point out, most aspects of child rearing in the 'Eighth Generation' are reflections of the matriarchy in the Negro society of New Orleans, and the matriarchy itself is reflective of the problems of segregation and prejudice because of which the husbands desert the families. Such happenings in turn cause mothers to develop overprotective attitudes toward male offspring who are selected to compensate for an absent father-figure, or to be, on the other hand, extremely neglectful and inconsistent towards children if the female role and its problems are oppressive. Girls are too often saddled with substitutive housekeeping roles if working mothers find them available for younger siblings. Such hazards may become common if, as with American Negroes or lower-class Puerto Ricans, employment opportunities are less secure for men than for women. In the Puerto Rican case, we have noted both in the island and on the mainland that the male economic role is vulnerable, that women are accommodated with steadier employment and often better pay in occupations like the garment industries, and that these factors in employment history, like the Negro mother's role as domestic, solidify unnatural conditions for the perpetuation of a combination matriarchate and broken home[53].

It is interesting to speculate on how different such family structures and psychological histories might have been if poverty, segregation, and prejudice had not been developed in such particular segments of population. For example, studies conducted both in Los Angeles, California, and in Buffalo, New York, have shown that the economic and social processes of rapid industrial expansion brought about conditions whereby, as the cities became industrialized, segregation of ethnic minorities developed increasingly along with such factors as increasing employment of women[73]. These processes of urbanization, found from city to city, have consequences in child rearing and psychological adaptation in ethnic minorities.

The American sociologist, W. J. Goode[26] has attempted to relate the factors of cultural breakdown, social anomie and rates of illegitimacy in a series of cultures ranging from northwestern Europe, urbanizing sub-Saharan Africa and the Deep South of the United States. In his European examples, he maintains the community retains control and, as happens in Scandinavian countries, the children though technically illegitimate are not regarded as socially illegitimate. In urbanizing Africa, by way of contrast, he claims that Western culture has undermined native social and cultural systems. Too little attention has been paid in such studies to the actual contexts of cultural change. The simple claim that there are parallels between the emergence of a matriarchate among Negroes of the United States, among Puerto Ricans, on the Latin American mainland and in urbanizing Africa may relate to illegitimacy rates, but at the same time may blur the cultural variations in actual family systems and in child rearing practices.

If one selected social factors other than illegitimacy, the analysis might reach quite different conclusions. As concerns segregation, for example, one could note a period in American Negro history in northern cities before the Civil War when there was no segregation and Negroes lived anywhere in the city. A study in Buffalo, New York from 1855 to 1875, conducted by Laurence Glasco, finds that ethnic group segregation and stratification, affecting Negroes, set in during a period of rapid urban industrialization and growth around the time of the Civil War. Similarly, the study of Los Angeles, alluded to above (M. Williams and E. Shevky, *The Social areas of Los Angeles*)[73], points out that as this Californian city likewise grew and modernized such indices emerged as the increasing appearance of women in the labour force, the growth and development of ethnic and minority group segregation, and the tendency of the city to promote stratification and social differences. Such factors ordinarily work in opposition or counter to what has been loosely termed, in the United States, 'the melting pot' and the assumption that ethnic and cultural factors are eliminated in such social processes as urbanization is erroneous.

If one continued these comparisons in Latin America and the Caribbean, it would be clear that historical, economic and cultural differences would emerge[53, 56]. For instance, such a slum as La Perla in San Juan, Puerto Rico, contains sub-areas reflecting different periods and types of economic dislocation on the island; in the upper reaches of the steep hill on which La Perla is located, one can find displaced 'Jibaros', or former villagers from highland regions who have come to San Juan and often have marginal employment at times outside the settlement, and in the less choice areas near the water or built out over it, one finds the displaced urban derelict population types. Contrasted with this are the inner areas of certain blocks in Lima, Peru, where there are segregated, often in different sections, the displaced highland Indians, and also the highly organized criminalistic elements. A third contrast, brought to our attention by Dr Richard W. Patch, an anthropological expert on Bolivia, is represented in lower-class districts in the cities of that country, which, following the agrarian reform and revolution in Bolivia, are often points of total assimilation of Indians who are not ethnically segregated or even separately designated as in Peru by the term for Indians (or the terms for *Mestizos* or *Cholos*). Peru, on the other hand, had no such agrarian revolution and consequently the lowly position of its Indian population has been perpetuated both in the latifundia, or large feudal estates of the highlands as well as in the slums of lowland cities along the coast.

In our analysis, we are therefore in agreement with a number of investigations which have suggested that ethnic and cultural factors are still influential in social processes. M. Gordon, reviewing the literature on *Social class in American sociology* (1950) argued that ethnic groups in America maintained their 'subsistence at all class levels' and thus are continued in the American scene. S. Lipset and R. Bendix in their book on *Social mobility in industrial society*[41] stressed the importance of the ethnicity factor in promoting or in discouraging the vertical mobility of populations. Finally, N. Glazer and Moynihan have stressed the continuity of American subcultural groups in a volume called *Beyond the melting pot* (1963). Obviously, cultural differences may be seen cross-culturally, while at the same time, ethnic groups may be forced to perpetuate a cultural pattern under conditions of segregation and prejudice. In this sense, the cultural continuity, where it exists, must be based upon a stabilization of cultural conditions affecting child rearing practices over time[53, 56].

A second factor, besides ethnic or cultural group, is, of course, social class. Actually, both factors of culture and class may interweave to produce a single kind of subcultural experience[51, 71]. In American sociology, the interest in social class influences on childhood personality has been considerable. In 1961 the literature on class differences in child rearing patterns was ably summarized by an American sociologist, W. H. Sewell[72]. Sewell began with three assumptions, namely the ubiquity of social stratification systems (which we believe is not substantiated everywhere by the anthropological literature), the position that the family's place in stratification determines the child's range of social learning influences and opportunities, and the third assumption that early learning will affect later personality adjustments. Sewell's conclusions from various studies in Chicago and New England, and also including his own in rural Wisconsin, were somewhat disappointing. First, there appeared to be a relatively low correlation between the child's position in stratification and such aspects of personality as measures of adjustment. Nevertheless, some variation by class did occur. Possibly crude techniques for measuring both the class variable and the adjustment accounts for the quality of the correlation found. Secondly, middle-class children did not commonly exhibit more neurotic personality traits than did children of lower-class origins. Indeed, the evidence supported the notion of greater hazards in the lower class. Thirdly, although the Chicago studies argued for class-connected differences in infant training, these studies were earlier, and as we have noted above later studies found increasing permissiveness in feeding and toilet training by middle-class mothers. The same was found for less impulse control, less punitiveness and strictures, and less controls in sexual behaviour and aggression on the part of middle-class mothers. Fourth, the infantile disciplines such as weaning, toilet training, and the induction of schedules had little relationship in general to children's personality traits and adjustments.

On the other hand, low correlations were found between patterns of punishment or permissiveness, degrees of the mother's affectional feelings for the child, and such personality factors as dependency, aggression, or feeding problems. The fifth and last finding relates to the point that such studies show not only weak correlations or relationships but also poor conceptualization concerning both the class and personality variables as such.

Most studies of social class effects on personality are remarkably deepened when the class factor as such is combined with some ethnic or cultural factor that affects the actual lives of people more deeply. In order to test hypotheses concerning the relationship of socio-cultural backgrounds to daydreaming, a questionnaire on fantasy was submitted to a large sample of middle-class students who stemmed from a series of cultural backgrounds, Negro, Irish, Jewish, Anglo-Saxon, Italian and German subcultures[74]. All six groups revealed significant differences in frequency and content of reported daydreams. Of the list, obviously, the more insecure or recently emigrated communities (such as the Negro, Jewish and Italian in the United States) showed considerably more daydreaming behaviour than the more readily assimilated community groups (such as the Anglo-Saxon, German and Irish). The former also showed less identification with fathers and likewise less similarity between their notion of an ideal self and fathers than did the latter groups. This research by J. L. Singer and V. G. McCraven involves, of course, conceptual models that derive from the simultaneous consideration of two processes, one in culture, and one on the psychological level of adjustment.

An earlier conceptual model for these studies was developed in 1956 by the author in a book called *Culture, psychiatry and human values*[50]. Later in that year, after publication of the book, Opler and J. L. Singer published a series of papers on Irish and Italian schizophrenics in which differences predicted on the basis of cultural and family constellations were tested in samples of patients drawn from the Midtown Manhattan Mental Health Research Study[52, 59, 75]. For one variation, the mother's role was more central in the Irish family and the father's in the Italian. The fantasy and daydreaming characteristics in that sample of lower-class and second generation patients was higher in the Irish than in the Italian sample. Emotional lability and acting out was more characteristic of the Italian lower-class patients whose families stemmed from South Italy or Sicily. In the later Singer and McCraven studies the Italian group employed is of college and graduate level or upwardly mobile so that the fantasy and motility factors in these normal middle-class students become reversed.

It is probable that most cultures, or more correctly subcultural groups, have different 'paths' of such role sequences depending on the class membership of persons in the culture. This happens because the cultural patterns of modern groups have a socio-economic structure within them. In the Midtown Manhattan Studies with which the author was associated, a pile-up of pathology could be discerned in the lower-class Manhattan slums where a series of ethnic or subcultural groups had settled. Thus, we found that lower socio-economic status statistically had pathological consequences. But it would be an oversimplification to call these results simply a derivative of poverty, since despite the statistics, there were in all cultural groups very healthy and well-balanced individuals and families. Moreover, and this factor seemed crucial, the specific cultural groups that were most poorly established in Midtown Manhattan, the Puerto Rican and Hungarian communities, yielded the greatest amounts of pathology[56].

It is obvious from the facts just mentioned that culture in-the-abstract does not produce pathology, but that very specific conditions existing within a culture are prime causative agents. It is likewise true that poverty in-the-abstract does not act alone in producing pathology, but that the conditions which are psychological and which accompany poverty can be statistically most potent. We have therefore adopted the position that the combination of poverty and the kind of rapid acculturation which destroys stable human values and disrupts culturally-based forms of family organization constitute the chief causes, taken together, of mental pathology[50, 58]. Such a position extends and amplifies the concept of what is learned in family or in parent-child relationships. We, therefore, do not blithely assume that rapid change is the real agent underlying pathology, but that negative conflicts and deprivations arise only where the change is destructive of real human values in families and in those relationships obtaining between adults and children. One requires a special term for such *negative* forms of acculturation, be they rapid or slow in tempo. Poverty, of course, while it does not operate singly as a cause, is nevertheless *always* a negative factor in the modern scene since it promotes cultural deprivations and dislocations. A key concept relating both to *negative* forms of cultural change, or dislocation, and also to poverty is the concept of culturally induced stress.

It is important to determine how cultural values become obsolete. In negative acculturation the socialization of children may involve conflicted models of the ideal cultural values and the contrasting imperfections of actual cultural conditions. While studying the Puerto Rican community in

New York it became obvious at every point that the male values of *machismo* (or masculine roles of husband and progenitor along with father, or protective provider) were not being served under economic conditions where the women, not the men, had better job placements and job continuity. The older and somewhat Spanish oriented ideals succumbed to family disorganization and to unwelcomed intrusions upon older forms of child rearing practices. Ideal values might be stated about such sex-role and age-role beliefs, but the harsh realities of cultural instability produced a strain between such ideal value concepts and the virtual impossibility of obtaining them in reality[53, 58].

Recently, anthropologists in the United States, like Jules Henry[31] and Ashley Montagu have claimed that the American *ethos* of pecuniary material success in a competitive struggle affects not only child rearing practices, but the underlying cognitive and emotional understandings which standardize and dehumanize the psychological product. Earlier, E. H. Erikson also spoke of this standardization as one which may develop a 'reliable mechanism' prepared to adapt to the competitive exploitation of our machine world. The anthropologist Ralph Linton also noted differences between the influences that might be emphasized in childhood as contrasted with those we experience as adults, and he viewed the resultant as a disorganizing factor in cultural change, common in many acculturation studies. Ruth Benedict, even earlier, wrote on discontinuities in cultural conditioning productive of such conflicts.

There have been attempts to widen the application of such concepts beyond the well-known parameters of major modern societies. Erikson also wrote of the Yurok Indians of California as requiring restraints upon those very elements in modern American society which connote having economic success. In his description, the Yurok with their more limited economy have less opportunity for complete oral gratification, and therefore Yurok mothers feel it is bad for infants to have unlimited optimism. Further, Yurok men have to 'yearn' to catch fish; again it is bad for a man to be easily satisfied with the amount of his catch. In Erikson's view, Yurok culture makes constant use of such oral restraints and remembrances of the need for food intake. Again, there may be much simpler explanations in the cultural conditioning devoted to these ends that must take place throughout all stages of the life cycle in Yurok culture, granted the limitations of their economic base[13]. What distinguishes this type of explanation, either in Erikson's terms or in our own, is that Yurok culture shows a fundamental integration and simplicity about such restraints in ingesting or acquiring food, whereas our own culture contains stresses and conflicts, or as J. M. Yinger calls it, a 'contraculture', especially on the lower-class and poverty levels. Yinger holds that persons in the lower class are subject to propaganda for a value system (for instance, of success and material benefits) which their deprived and alienated connection with society prevents their attaining in reality.

The most ambitious cross-cultural study of positive and negative conditioning in children was reported by J. W. M. Whiting and I. L. Child in their book *Child training and personality*[84]. A cross-cultural study of the effects of childhood experiences does of course have a certain advantage over single cultural studies, but it also presents certain difficulties. On the positive side, there is a larger range of child rearing practices which may be tested in a broad sample of societies. Secondly, some of these practices which may occur only rarely in deviant cases in our own culture occur naturally within other societies, as for example in the protracted breast-feeding patterns we have mentioned above for the Ute Indians of Colorado[48]. But on the other hand, studies in depth of one culture, if properly done through excellent anthropological field methods, possess the firm advantage of being reliable. The Cross-Cultural Index developed at Yale University is an instrument for transcultural studies dependent upon a variety of ethnographic accounts in the literature of unequal reliability. Stated simply, one is not dealing with uniformly excellent studies based on observations or experiments achieved by the same ethnographic techniques. In the parlance of statisticians, such so-called 'samples' may contain a 'mixed bag' of different cultural units, much as a 'sample' of apples and oranges may qualify as being fruits, but fail to qualify on more discriminating taxonomic levels.

A cultural evolutionist, for example, would prefer studies which group cultures of a similar typology rather than one which might include expansive states or settled horticulturalists along with simple hunting and gathering societies which are certainly less densely populated. Nor are these distinctions merely abstract. Clyde Kluckhohn, for example, has written most persuasively about the diffuseness of authority experienced by children in a culture like the Navajo who have contacts as children with an extended range of relatives and hence, says Kluckhohn, have less authority problems and reactions centred in single sets of relatives like parents in our own modern nuclear family structure.

With these methodological cautions, let us return to the Whiting and Child study[84]. The study notes that children are not immediately transformed at birth into adult models of behaviour, and in fact nursing may be rewarding as pleasurable sucking even when it does not relate directly to quieting pangs of hunger. The adult way of eating after being weaned can only contain satisfactions or rewards at some optimum time, distinguished from child development. Consider also their point that a child's attempts to nurse may be punished at a certain time. At any rate, they distinguished gentle methods of weaning as being *positive fixation*, and the punitive methods as constituting *negative fixation*[20].

Freud also wrote about negation resulting from parental influences, but he distinguished further two forms of this process, one being harshly repressive while the other Freud felt lay at the root of cognitive processes. René Spitz also, in 1957, in his book, *No and yes: on the genesis of human communication*[80] deals with the way in which a child may develop drive-inhibitory constraints or restraints as opposed to unhealthy methods of repressive negativism. Such positions are consistent with E. B. Holt's book *The Freudian wish* published much earlier in 1916. Obviously Holt, Sullivan, Erikson and others have placed centrally in their concepts of child development the differentiation of the self from the object world; and what Sullivan calls the development of a general sense of malevolence (lying both within and without a sick human being's self and object conceptualizations) would be possible. But whether it does become possible, we feel, is not just a matter of a single set of conditions producing such stress in one life cycle. While every case of mental disease has roots in an individual's experience within his culture—and every disorder *happens* to one person alone—the student of psychiatry who knows anything at all about epidemiology of psychiatric illnesses in the plural and of their history, knows immediately that there are distinct forms or types of disorder which are not distributed at random in cultures around the world. Conversion hysterias occur more often in some cultures than do the character disorders and paranoid schizophrenias which A. B. Wheelis, in *The quest for identity*[83], typified as our modern American disturbances. Catatonias and often sub-types such as those with wax-limbs inflexibility or passive flexibility, are rarely seen today but were once far more common in European and American culture. In short, the epidemiology of disorders has changed both in form and in amount in different human societies, and as the cultures themselves have changed, so have their child rearing practices.

If we return to our conceptual model of a child's developing ego identifications, it is clear that these are shaped, on the one hand, by parental notions of child rearing and of ethical standards of human value, and secondly, by the already internalized parental ego aspects along with the cultural standards which Freud later termed superego. Obviously, the already existing epidemiology in a culture, as it exists on either neurotic or psychotic levels must again become important in child rearing since parental ego formations, or those of other adults like teachers, nurses, etc., comprise exactly those persons 'at whose tender mercies' the child experiences the object world. Even in animal studies, if H. Harlow's non-mothered rhesus monkeys are a serviceable example, the lack of live models in the wire-and-cloth surrogate figures prevented the baby monkeys from obtaining a furry palpable and moving mirror of their own existences. We are really here arguing against the delimiting and, we think, false conception that child rearing models of the nursing and weaning sort actually begin in a causative sense simply with the infant and his mother. We feel that if one properly weighted culture as pre-existent and affecting the epidemiology of adult disorders, then the importance of the superego as Freud generally conceptualized it in *The ego and the id*[19] would have connotations producing either a smooth interplay of adults and children, of adolescents and the adult society they begin to experience and of ego maturation and social maturation—or else psychological and social breakdown occur together in the system. Children are indeed the products of their cultures, and not individually the creators. Yet because of the very fact that they enter into the developing chain of events later than adults, and in turn will some day meet the challenges of the adult role, they are culture's most precious product and in point of longevity its most lasting.

It is already apparent in our conceptual model that the Freudian terms of love or libido and aggression ordinarily transformed into the terms, sexual identity and self-identification respectively, require some amplification which includes the factor of social identification in addition. We have commented on this necessity elsewhere. In the paradigm of child development we have used, self and object world differentiation appear to be the root of a sense of self-identification. This evolves in stages, but requires at the outset that the substitution of some sense of control and mastery exists or begins to germinate in embryonic form possibly dependent upon early or infantile notions of human contact and mirroring. Erikson and others have referred to basic trust in order to present some idea of an actively developing ego identification. Our tendency, in this essay, has been to include ideas of mastery and autonomy, not as finished products, but in some seedling stage. We do so because our idea of epidemiology includes not only an emphasis on pathological lacks in development, but rather on the more or less durable assets which may be built up in cultures and in people. We are thinking also of Spitz's dependent and passive children with anaclitic depression or of Harlow's macaques who sought maternal contact from non-mothered rhesus monkeys only to be disappointed and deconditioned in their quest. In other words, embryonic notions of mastery include forms of assertion, play and exploration in their turn. But we hasten to add that sexual identification and also social identification must be guaranteed in the developing life cycle. The latter, social identification, has been ably explored by students interested, like Piaget and his followers, in the development of communicative forms in children, in their acquisition of language, of cognitive skills, and even of moral values.

Not all of the controversies concerned with developing or correcting Freudian doctrines occur on the level of early infancy. Whiting, Kluckhohn, and Anthony in 1958[85] attempted by use of cross-cultural data to present evidence that strong, primary identification with mothers, if not transferred later to fathers, will create persistent antagonism or estrangement between fathers and sons. This is reminiscent of the standard Freudian notion that early and strong attachments of males to mothers produce later male sexual insecurities. These three authors subscribe to the universality of that idea as well so that male maternal attachments led in their belief to institutional arrangements intended to cope with such widespread male anxieties. Their work is, of course, of a different variety from Durkheim's view of ritualism, and especially different from the work of Van Gennep[24] who described initiation rites as marking three steps in the individual's formal movement from one social stage to another (*rites de passage*). In one sense Van Gennep's idea of a separation from an earlier status, a movement to the next position, and finally social consolidation in the new status was intended to distinguish between physiological puberty and social initiation rites. Whiting and his colleagues felt that they had found a strong correlation between close relationship of mother and baby, and the harsher or more brutal forms of adolescent initiation rituals. Burton and Whiting[9] extended the hypothesis to mean that such matters as a child sleeping with his mother, but followed by living with his father's people, required painful rites of initiation to complete a firm masculine identification. They argued further that where female identification is culturally instituted through sleeping with a mother as well as through matrilocal residence, the culture would have to furnish some symbolic way of enacting dramatically the existence of the female role. The researchers here selected the custom of the couvade, in which the husband retires to bed and undergoes maternal taboos observed by his wife during her act of childbirth.

To comment on the second set of observances, the couvade, the author will briefly state the nature of this custom among the Ute Indians of Colorado whom he studied. The Ute do not institutionalize matrilocal residence, although the Eastern Apache Indians, whom he also studied, did observe matrilocal residence. Contrary to the Burton-Whiting thesis, the Apache Indians have no couvade at all, but the Ute Indians who favour no set residence role and who may be, therefore, classed as favouring either ambilocal or independent residence happen to have an extremely elaborated couvade rite. In the Ute couvade moreover, the custom includes both the husband's 'lying-in', and also subsequent ritual acts symbolizing his role as a hunter and provider. In all of these customs the Ute greatly resembled a wide range of Great Basin peoples. As for initiation rites, it is the Apache who most strongly emphasize these, but with an elaboration and urgency in such matters only for adolescent girls!

Another anthropologist, Y. A. Cohen[10], has challenged the Whiting position on initiation ceremonies, also using statistical cross-cultural technique. A most important function in such ceremonies, says Cohen, is their tendency to act in the interests of social manipulation of the child in relation to family and kin group. While denying that initiation ceremonies function to resolve conflicts in sexual identity, Cohen feels that they exist to implant social and emotional identities and values. The present author also has noted that films of Australian subincision rites reveal both the boys and the elders to be proud and euphoristic, depite the brief periods of surgical pain. Put together with our own observations on the couvade, it is obvious that economic and social functions appear side by side with psychological ones, in a wide variety of rituals, suggesting that sexual identification is not the only factor, but that along with it, a composite of self and social identification is a cultural value[57, 58].

4
Summary

We have reviewed the theory and data on the relationship of culture and child rearing. Both in anthropology and in psychiatry, or in psychoanalysis, the earliest theories derived cultural and personality models from effects of child rearing. Yet in reviewing studies on either level, psychodynamic and sociodynamic, while we concede with Sapir that personality is always partly individual and partly cultural, the author has added that sociodynamic events have had the greater weight, that is, they affect psychodynamic balances in families, in intergenerational conflicts, in learning experiences, and, on a wider scale, in cultural evolution[58]. Besides the theory of personality conflicts having their roots in childhood and infancy, we require a concomitant theory of cultural learning, mastery and assertion to balance pathologies arising in certain individuals as seen epidemiologically for any society. The Freudian foreshadowing of this in the theory of negation, with both positive and negative outcomes, or the Neo-Freudian shifting to a doctrine of ego-adaptation, is an accommodation to cultural study which began with Freud's *The ego and the id*, but which has continued with studies of culture and mental health in subcultural groups of our own society and cross-culturally around the world. Human behaviour may now be glimpsed in cultural evolutionary adaptations, and child rearing practices are one set of evidence of that adaptation[58]. While not a *primum mobile*, then, child rearing may be viewed as social, as self, and as sexual identification— dependent upon the cultural conditions of existence that weigh so heavily on the adults, and hence children of the world.

REFERENCES

1. BENEDICT, R. F., 1934. *Patterns of culture*. Boston, Houghton Mifflin.
2. BENEDICT, R. F., 1938. Continuities and discontinuities in cultural conditioning. *Psychiatry*, 1, 161.
3. BENEDICT, R. F., 1946. *The chrysanthemum and the sword*. Boston, Houghton Mifflin.
4. BOWLBY, J., 1952. *Maternal care and mental health*. Geneva, World Health Organization, Monograph No. 2.
5. BRAM, F. M., 1965. The gift of Anna O. *Brit. J. Med. Psychol.*, 38, 53.
6. BREUER, J., 1893. Case histories. Case I: Fraulein Anna O. In *Studies in hysteria*. 1950. London, Hogarth Press.
7. BREUER, J., and FREUD, S., 1893. On the psychical mechanisms of hysterical phenomena. Preliminary communication. In *Studies in hysteria*. 1950. London, Hogarth Press.
8. BRONFENBRENNER, URIE, 1958. Socialization and social class through time and space. In *Readings in social psychology*. Eds, Maccoby, E. E., Newcomb, T. M., and Hartley, E. L. New York, Holt, Rinehart and Winston.

9. BURTON, R. V., and WHITING, J. W. M., 1960. *The absent father: effects on the developing child.* Unpublished manuscript. Washington, National Institute of Mental Health.
10. COHEN, Y. A., 1964. The establishment of identity in a social nexus: the special case of initiation ceremonies and their relation to value and legal systems. *Amer. Anthro.*, **66**, 529.
11. DAVIS, A., and DOLLARD, J., 1940. *Children of bondage.* Washington, The American Council on Education.
12. DAVIS, A., and HAVIGHURST, R. J., 1948. Social class and color differences in child rearing. *Amer. Sociol. Rev.*, **11**, 698.
13. ERIKSON, E. H., 1950. *Childhood and society.* New York, W. W. Norton.
14. ERIKSON, E. H., 1956. The problem of ego identity. *J. Amer. Psychoanal. Assn*, **4**, 56.
15. FREUD, S., 1905. Dora, an analysis of a case of hysteria. In *Collected papers*. 1950. London, Hogarth.
16. FREUD, S., 1909. Analysis of a phobia in a five-year-old boy. In *Collected papers*. 1950. London, Hogarth.
17. FREUD, S., 1909. Notes on a case of obsessional neurosis. In *Collected papers*. 1950. London, Hogarth.
18. FREUD, S., 1913. *Totem and taboo.* 1950. London, Routledge and Kegan Paul.
19. FREUD, S., 1923. *The ego and the id.* 1927. London, Hogarth.
20. FREUD, S., 1925. Negation. In *Collected papers*. 1950. London, Hogarth.
21. FREUD, S., 1930. *Civilization and its discontents.* London, Hogarth.
22. FROMM, ERICH, 1941. *Escape from freedom.* New York, Holt, Rinehart and Winston.
23. FROMM, ERICH, 1947. *Man for himself.* New York, Holt, Rinehart and Winston.
24. GENNEP, A. L. VAN, 1909. *Les rites de passage.* Paris, E. Nourry.
25. GESELL, A., and AMATRUDA, C. S., 1941. *Developmental diagnosis: normal and abnormal child development.* New York, Hoeber.
26. GOODE, W. J., 1961. Illegitimacy, anomie, and cultural penetration. *Amer. Sociol. Rev.*, **26**, 910.
27. HARLOW, H. F., 1959. Love in infant monkeys. *Sci. Amer.*, **200**, 63.
28. HARLOW, H. F., and HARLOW, M. K., 1962. Social deprivation in monkeys. *Sci. Amer.*, **207**, 138.
29. HARTMANN, H., 1958. *The ego and the problem of adaptation.* New York, Intern. Univ. Press.
30. HARTMANN, H., KRIS, E., and LOEWENSTEIN, R. M., 1946. Comments on the formation of psychic structure. In *The psychoanalytic study of the child*, vol. 2. New York, Internat. Univ. Press.
31. HENRY, JULES, 1963. *Culture against man.* New York, Random House.
32. HOLT, E. B., 1916. *The Freudian wish (and its place in ethics).* New York, Holt, Rinehart and Winston.
33. HOLT, E. B., 1931. *Animal drive and the rearing process.* New York, Holt, Rinehart and Winston.
34. HORNEY, K., 1937. *The neurotic personality of our time.* New York, W. W. Norton and Co.
35. KANNER, L., 1955. *Child psychiatry.* Springfield, Ill., Charles C. Thomas.
36. KARDINER, ABRAM, 1939. *The individual and his society.* New York, Columbia Univ. Press.
37. KARDINER, A., LINTON, R., DUBOIS, C., and WEST, J., 1945. *The psychological frontiers of society.* New York, Columbia Univ. Press.
38. KLUCKHOHN, F., and STRODTBECK, F., 1961. *Variations in value orientations.* New York, Harper and Row.
39. LANG, A., 1898. *The making of religion.* London, Longmans, Green and Co.

40. LEVY, D. M., 1943. *Maternal overprotection.* New York, Columbia Univ. Press.
41. LIPSET, S. M., and BENDIX, R., 1959. *Social mobility in industrial society.* Berkeley, Calif., Univ. Press.
42. MACCOBY, E. E., and GIBBS, P. K., 1954. Methods of child rearing in two social classes. In *Readings in child development.* Eds, Martin, W. E., and Standler, C. B. New York, Harcourt, Brace and World.
43. MALINOWSKI, B., 1927. *The father in primitive society.* New York, W. W. Norton and Co.
44. MALINOWSKI, B., 1927. *Sex and repression in savage society.* London, Routledge and Kegan Paul.
45. MALINOWSKI, B., 1935. *Coral gardens and their magic.* London, Allen and Unwin.
46. MILLER, D. R., and SWANSON, G. E., 1958. *The changing American parent.* New York, Wiley.
47. MILLER, D. R., and SWANSON, G. E., 1960. *Inner conflict and defense.* New York, Henry Holt.
48. OPLER, MARVIN K., 1940. The southern Ute Indians in Colorado. In *Acculturation in seven American indian tribes.* Ed. Linton, R. New York, Appleton Century-Crofts.
49. OPLER, MARVIN K., 1955. The influence of ethnic and class subcultures on child care. *Soc. Prob.*, **3**, 12.
50. OPLER, MARVIN K., 1956. *Culture, psychiatry and human values.* Springfield, Ill., Charles C. Thomas.
51. OPLER, MARVIN K., 1956. Entities and organization in individual and group behavior. *Group Psychother.*, **9**, 290.
52. OPLER, MARVIN K., 1957. Schizophrenia and culture. *Sci. Amer.*, **197**, 103.
53. OPLER, MARVIN K., 1958. Dilemmas of two Puerto Rican men. In *Clinical Studies in Culture Conflict.* Ed. Seward, G. New York, Ronald Press Co.
54. OPLER, MARVIN K., 1959. *Culture and mental health.* New York, Macmillan.
55. OPLER, MARVIN K., 1959. Cultural perspectives in research on schizophrenias. *Psychiat. Quart.*, **33**, 506.
56. OPLER, MARVIN K., 1964. Socio-cultural roots of emotional illness. *Psychosomatics*, **5**, 55.
57. OPLER, MARVIN K., 1965. Anthropological and cross-cultural aspects of homosexuality. In *Sexual inversion.* Ed. Marmor, Judd. New York, Basic Books, Inc.
58. OPLER, MARVIN K., 1967. *Culture and social psychiatry.* New York, Atherton Press.
59. OPLER, MARVIN K., and SINGER, J. L., 1956. Ethnic differences in behavior and psychopathology. *Int. J. soc. Psychia.*, **2**, 11.
60. ORLANSKY, H., 1949. Infant care and personality. *Psychol. Bull.*, **46**, 1.
61. PIAGET, J., 1932. *The moral judgment of the child.* New York, Harcourt, Brace and World.
62. PIAGET, J., 1951. *Play, dreams, and imitation in childhood,* New York, W. W. Norton.
63. PIAGET, J., 1952. *The origins of intelligence in children.* New York, Intern. Univ. Press.
64. PIAGET, J., 1954. *The construction of reality in the child.* New York, Basic Books Inc.
65. RIBBLE, M., 1943. *The rights of infants.* New York, Columbia Univ. Press.
66. RICHMOND, J. B., and CALDWELL, B. M., 1963. Child rearing practices and their consequences. In *Modern perspectives in child development.* Eds, Solnit, A., and Provence, S. New York, Intern. Univ. Press.

67. ROHRER, J. H., and EDMONDSON, M. S., 1960. *The eighth generation grows up: culture and personalities of New Orleans Negroes.* New York, Harper.
68. ROSEN, B. C., 1962. Socialization and achievement motivation in Brazil. *Amer. Sociol. Rev.,* **27**, 612.
69. SEARS, R. R., MACCOBY, E. E., and LEVIN, H., 1957. *Patterns of child rearing.* New York, Harper and Row.
70. SENN, M. J., 1950. *Symposium on the healthy personality.* Supplement II, *Problems of infancy and childhood.* New York, Josiah Macy, Jr. Foundation.
71. SEWELL, W. H., 1952. Infant training and the personality of the child. *Amer. J. Sociol.,* **58**, 150.
72. SEWELL, W. H., 1961. Social class and childhood personality. *Sociometry,* **24**, 340.
73. SHEVKY, E., and WENDELL, B., 1955. *Social area analysis.* Stanford, Calif., Univ. Press. *Cf.,* SHEVKY, E. and WILLIAMS, M., 1955. *The social areas of Los Angeles, analysis and typology.* Berkeley, Calif., Univ. Press.
74. SINGER, J. L., and MCCRAVEN, V. C., 1962. Daydreaming patterns of American subcultural groups. *Int. J. soc. Psychiat.,* **8**, 272.
75. SINGER, J. L., and OPLER, MARVIN K., 1956. Contrasting patterns of fantasy and motility in Irish and Italian schizophrenics. *J. abnorm. soc. Psychol.,* **53**, 42.
76. SKINNER, B. F., 1948. *Walden II.* New York, Macmillan.
77. SPITZ, R. A., 1946. Anaclitic depression: an inquiry into the genesis of psychiatric conditions in early childhood. In *The psychoanalytic study of the child,* vol. 2. New York, Intern. Univ. Press.
78. SPITZ, R. A., 1946. Hospitalism: a follow-up report. In *The psychoanalytic study of the child,* vol. 2. New York, Intern. Univ. Press.
79. SPITZ, R. A., 1954. Hospitalism. In *The psychoanalytic study of the child,* vol. 1. New York, Intern. Univ. Press.
80. SPITZ, R. A., 1957. *No and yes: on the genesis of human communication.* New York, Intern. Univ. Press.
81. SPOCK, B., 1957. *Baby and child care.* New York, Pocket Books.
82. SULLIVAN, H. S., 1953. *The interpersonal theory of psychiatry.* New York, W. W. Norton and Co.
83. WHEELIS, A. B., 1958. *The quest for identity.* New York, W. W. Norton and Co.
84. WHITING, J. W. M., and CHILD, I. L., 1953. *Child training and personality.* New Haven, Yale Univ.
85. WHITING, J. W. M., KLUCKHOHN, R., and ANTHONY, A., 1958. The function of male initiation ceremonies at puberty. In *Readings in social psychology.* Eds, Maccoby, E., Newcomb, T. M., and Hartley, E. L. New York, Holt, Rinehart and Winston.

XI

CHILD REARING IN THE KIBBUTZ

Louis Miller
M.D.

*Director, Mental Health Services,
Ministry of Health, Jerusalem, Israel*

The Kibbutz Community

In Israel there are about 80,000 people living on about 230 collective agricultural communes which are known as kibbutzim. While their inhabitants comprise only 4 per cent of the Jewish population of Israel, they have played a cardinal role in the resettlement of the country, in its defence and in the establishment of its social values and institutions.

The kibbutz farm is situated on national land leased for all practical purposes in perpetuity to the colonists. The first kibbutz appeared as a unit of Jewish land settlement in the Jordan Valley at the end of the first decade of this century. It was settled by a group of young unmarried Jews from Eastern Europe who had returned to Palestine as Zionists. In so doing they were living out the belief that only by a national revival would a dignified future life be assured for Jews. They believed such dignity could only be attained in a socialist society based on personal labour, on the soil, with complete sharing and equality for all.

These kibbutz farmers suffered many severe privations. They were unused to agriculture. The land provided for them by the National Funds were bought from absentee Arab landlords who had allowed it to degenerate into marshland, or the land consisted of rocky or desert tracts which had never been farmed. Malaria maimed and killed the settlers. They were poorly protected from the elements and exposed to attacks by Arab bands. For many years their diet was exiguous, the proverbial bread and olives; at times they were on the border of starvation. They were carried forward by the joy of their sense of freedom and companionship and profound conviction of their historic destiny and purpose.

The kibbutz is a society in which there is no private ownership. It provides for every need of its members. All means of production and the products of labour, the services, finances and facilities are communally held and administered. The kibbutz member's time and activity are organized by the whole group. Kibbutz government and institutions are elected and set up by community decision through a show of hands at the regular assembly of all the adult members of the community. Work and roles in the community used to be rotated so as to avoid the crystallization of unchanging specialist functionaries and leaders. While specialists in fields of work have begun to appear now, the kibbutz remains a voluntary, classless society with built-in safeguards against the reappearance of privilege.

The Kibbutz Family

Although the parents of kibbutz families are increasingly of the first kibbutz-born generation, most parents were born outside of the kibbutz and the country. The parents who founded the kibbutzim were actuated by Zionist aspirations which were directed as well towards a socialist society, and the rehabilitation of the personality and the image of the Jew. The young unmarried men and women who chose the kibbutz as a way of life were also animated by attitudes to the type of families in Europe from which they came. They expressed resentment of its authoritarian father, of the dependency of the mother and of the neurotic conflicts in its overprotected and overburdened atmosphere.

The plan which was evolved for the kibbutz family called for a relationship of complete equality between husband and wife and for the economic independence of the woman. This was to be ensured through her equality with the man in roles at work and in the kibbutz community. As far as possible she was to be relieved of all social and personal disadvantages such as the elements of drudgery in the maintenance of the family home or in the care of the children.

It was felt that the emancipation of the woman from the authority of the male partner and from economic dependence on him would permit marriage based on love and compatibility rather than on other considerations. The rituals of the traditional marriage ceremonies which were seen as a canonisation of the bondage of women were therefore abandoned. They were replaced by personal agreement by two members that they would live together. However marriage bonds were maintained by a strict code of sexual and social behaviour fully in accord with the ascetic quality of the spirit and life of the kibbutz. Today, marriage ceremonies have reappeared. Where once parents did not own even their personal clothing, now rooms are comfortably furnished, frequently with personally owned effects or those allocated by the kibbutz for private use.

It was felt too that the education of the child from its tenderest years should be outside of the family and in the hands of people expert in that field. Rearing of the child away from the family would avert many of the conflicts which had been evident in the parents' families. Education of the child in the group would engender in him the values of group loyalty rather than the egotisms produced in the family and the society of individualism from which the adults of the kibbutz had come. There was a deep conviction that the future of the kibbutz and its collective philosophy would be decided by the generations born on the kibbutz. The raising of the children should not only be directed to the happiness of the child but to produce in him a personality which would be at one with life on the collective and its humanitarian and socialist ideals.

Children therefore do not live with their parents. All child care, rearing and education take place in the setting of the children's houses where the children live. Education of children has been since the inception of the kibbutz and remains to this day a communal function. Nevertheless, the forms of collective child care which are described here were arrived at through a long process of historical development and one of trial and error. Child care methods vary to some degree among the Kibbutz Federations and even among the kibbutzim of a particular Federation.

Although the principles of communal living on the kibbutz are adhered to strictly, slight modifications have appeared in recent years. These have been less in evidence in the kibbutzim of the two left wing Federations, than in those adhering to the Federation which is less Marxist in its ideology.

Collective Child Care and Education

The care of all the infants and children is organized according to age groups. Each age group lives and sleeps in a 'children's house' accommodated to its requirements. The full responsibility for the care of the children in each age group is placed in the hands of a children's nurse who acts as a house mother. She is designated by the Hebrew name 'metapelet' (plural 'metaplot'). She is responsible for the physical care of the children; feeding, bathing, toilet, dressing, well-being and general health. The nurse is with the infants or toddlers most of the day, watching over them, playing with the individual or the group, serving them, meeting their needs or mediating between the child and others.

From the kindergarten age the metapelet is joined by a nursery school teacher who shares the care of the children but is increasingly concerned with their intellectual and social development and later with their formal education.

When the mother returns with her newborn infant from the hospital the nurse receives the child into her care at the nursery. The mother who is freed from her tasks for a period of about two months, breast feeds her child in the infants' house, bathes and dresses it and puts it to sleep. Weaning is commenced about the third or fourth month and is completed gradually, usually by the ninth month. As the feeds are reduced in number the mother returns for longer periods to her role at work. By the time that the feeds are reduced to those at morning and evening she is fully back at work. In the infants' house one nurse cares for about five or six children. The infants remain in their special house for a period of a year—sometimes for a few months longer.

After the infants' house the group, which is now composed of children at the toddlers stage, is moved to a house suited to its needs. Until about the age of 3 to 4, the children are cared for in groups of four by a metapelet. There are two such groups to a toddlers' house. At about the age of three the metapelet is joined by a nursery-school teacher who a year or so later will go across with the eight children to a building for the children of kindergarten age.

The kindergarten house is again the product of two toddlers' groups and caters for about sixteen children. In this important group the child remains until the end of its school years. In the kindergarten the children have a new metapelet who is attached to the house and the kindergarten teacher who has accompanied them from the toddler stage. This house contains in addition to the facilities for living a specially organized play area with an abundance of toys of educational and social content. This school room is combined with the dining area. The children remain in this house, usually until the end of the first grade. They move together to a house designed for children in the primary school years at the age of 6 or 7. In this house there is a classroom in which most of their lessons are given by their teacher or *M'chanech* who is their counsellor and guide until the completion of primary school.

The Child and the Metapelet

During the first year of the kibbutz infant's life, his mother spends a great deal of time with him in the common nursery. She is the central figure in his life. The metapelet plays the part equivalent to that of a children's nurse in any European middle-class home. However, with the passage of the months, the mother begins to return to work while the metapelet takes over the care of the child at its first mealtime and after the mother has visited the child to bath him and put him to bed. There may be two or three metaplot caring for twelve infants.

The toddler is now transferred to a new house and becomes one of a subgroup of four. He has a new metapelet.

The place of the metapelet as a complement to the mother during the child's first development has been given much attention as she certainly represents for the child a further mother figure. Problems may have arisen from frequent changes of metapelet in a particular age group, in infancy and later.

In the toddler stage visits of the mother and father to the child are less frequent. They come after work to take him to their room and later, in the children's house, bath him and put him to bed.

The position of the metapelet has become central in the child's life.

The second year of life is one of training and socialization with the metapelet as the agent for discipline. She is responsible for toilet training, eating habits and the social behaviour of the group. The metapelet employs each occasion which presents itself to educate the toddlers. They may 'assist' her in household chores or in washing or dressing themselves. Much of the education takes place in the play area around the children's house or in the walks through the kibbutz.

At the age of 3, two toddlers' groups join to form a kindergarten. The children acquire again a new metapelet but they move to the kindergarten with a nursery school teacher who joined them at the toddler stage. The metapelet in the kindergarten group remains an important figure in the child's life. She provides protection, comfort and affection and is the socializer and educator. The kindergarten group is generally composed of children of different ages, from 4 to 7 years.

The last year of kindergarten is equivalent to the usual first grade of school. It is seen as a transitional year from the educational point of view. Formal education therefore begins essentially at 7. The group of 16 children at school is given a different metapelet who will remain with it for all the school years.

At school the children's group receives an educator (mechanech) who will remain with it throughout the school years. This teacher plays an important formative role in the education and social development of the children and acts as their confidant and counsellor. The metapelet is responsible for the housekeeping and for the welfare of the primary school children. She, however, has a crucial role in fostering and mediating group relations, in discipline, in sexual education in the preparation for puberty and in the development of social responsibility.

Spiro[36] summarizes the functions of the metapelet: She is first of all a 'caretaker' responsible for physical care; for the feeding, bathing and clothing of the children. She is the housekeeper as well in the children's house. For the nurse working with infants this will take up most of her time. The metapelet also provides 'nuturance'; love, warmth and comfort. Busy as she is the nurse has many opportunities to react affectionately or comfortingly to the infants and children. At times she may be deeply involved emotionally with them. Spiro did not find any evidence of overt rejection of children by the nurses, but he did note the existence at times of favouritism of attractive babies or of the children of attractive parents. He found the nurses generally permissive and objective in their techniques of socialization but harassed by the weight of their housekeeping duties. With the advent of the nursery school teacher, Spiro notes the nurse could concentrate largely on house-keeping and the teacher was free to serve creative functions with the children such as supervising their behaviour and directing it into productive and creative channels. A further function which the metapelet fulfills is in the field of 'discipline and values'. In the nursery this is in the behaviour system of eating. In the toddlers' house the toilet training is begun. The nurse is also concerned with teaching the child to dress and to attain other motor skills, and with the control of crying and aggression. At the nursery school level kibbutz values such as sharing, living as a member of a group, love of nature and work, and love of the nation are consciously instilled. Elementary intellectual skills are introduced at this time and formal instruction such as in reading and writing are introduced in the transitional class (equivalent to the first grade) at the end of the kindergarten period.

The system of child rearing on the kibbutz has undergone gradual development since its inception and still varies to some degree from farm to farm. So too the role of the metapelet has evolved over the years and her image and function changed in the constellation of child care and education.

Even in the earliest period it seems that women were drawn to this role by their affection for babies and children. Training was provided for them, if informally, especially in physical child care. The care of the youngest children generally tended to be in the hands of qualified nurses and the education of the kindergarten and older groups to be the responsibility of qualified teachers. Selection of suitable or even qualified nurses was hampered at times by the need of the kibbutz for workers in more 'productive' fields. The priorities of child care were at times neglected and the occupation received a lower status than other forms of work.

On the whole, until recently, training of the metapelet was negligible except in the case of the nurses responsible for infant care. Even in their case, training was largely restricted to nursing and physical care. Nurses were shifted in their placement among the age groups and were unable to specialize in the needs, behaviour and problems of a particular development period. Nurses who showed special devotion and aptitude were at times sent to kibbutz seminars for training as nursery teachers. The teacher was accorded higher status than the metapelet.

Nevertheless, with the passage of time, the metapelet often acquired skills and status through her own efforts and interest and by virtue of occasional courses provided for her in child psychology and child rearing. The kibbutz, as it became aware of the possible dangers to the children of frequent changes of metapelet, fostered greater continuity of the relation of the metapelet to a particular group. In the last two years courses in child rearing and education have been planned for metaplot at kibbutz seminars which are staffed by specialists in child guidance and child care in the kibbutz.

The Child and his Peer Group

In the second year of life the kibbutz child finds himself in the almost constant company of a small group of equal age. This immediate group may be of four or five in number in the care of a particular metapelet. Generally two nurses are responsible for eight children.

No definite and organized information is available on the earliest development of group feelings and relations in the toddlers' group. The earliest personality processes in the individual toddler in relation to the group appear to be a continuation of the weaning and separation from the mother and 'individualization' (to use Mahler's term), of infancy. In the establishment of his personal identity the infant experiences his own bodily activity and develops mastery of it. In creating his own identity, he is in effect attributing identity to objects around himself though separating himself from them; identification with them occurs and emotional relations to them develop.

Lewin[19] conceives the earliest group life in developmental terms. Before the phase in which the group life of youngest children is *socially* regulated there may be a phase which is *emotionally* directed. Lewin feels that there may be even an earlier phase before the age of 1 year which he would call one of 'perceptual group relations'. Emotional ties in this stage are as yet limited. This is expressed by the recognition by one child of others in his group. Nagler[24] does not question close relations between children even at the age of 1 year, but he doubts that such a relation could exist between the child and the whole group.

The increasing web of individual relations and their changing quality may provide a key to the establishment of the relation of the individual to the group as a whole. Rot[32] establishes with anecdotes from her experience that in the second year children demonstrate sympathy for and console each other and cooperate. She[32] assesses the earliest relation as identification on the part of one child with another. The child may attempt to influence the other to make progress or fulfil regulations. Nagler[24] thinks that this identification is mutual and that it is based upon the fulfilment of mutual need.

It may be suggested that the processes of the differentiation of self, with which the child is involved in his first year of life, while structurally concerned with perception of himself, are linked to profound emotional contents, tensions and satisfactions. Awareness on the part of the child of other individuals in his environment may be constructed as percepts which too must be linked to emotional content and hence relation and identification supervene. In such a view the perceptions by the child, which have a biological developmental basis, become the frame for the emotional relations they generate. Perception and relations must be virtually contemporaneous and hence reciprocal. It is from the extension of percepts of and identifications with further objects that the manifold of co-existing relations, referred to as 'social' or 'group' supervenes.

The kibbutz peer group makes available abundantly the possibility for rapid extension in number of object relations beyond the first infantile dyadic relations with the mother and those which have developed with the metapelet. Such extension on the one hand may limit the depth of the relations to individuals in the group and on the other may hasten the percepts by the child of the group qua group and deepen the emotional attachments to it.

The development of the individual's identification with the group as an entity may have further elements based on his individual primitive reactions to near total group events. Such reactions are seen in an infant's response to the crying of others or its imitation of their vocal or motor behaviour.

Stimulation of an individual by a group may result in early percepts of the group as such and give rise to imitation and emotional identification with it. Relations of identification in the group and with it may be preceded by imitative activity. Imitation may be seen as an early form of identification during a phase in which the percepts, and hence the emotional projections into them, are not yet clarified.

Perception of the group by the individual and his relations to it will be accompanied by its reflex, the perception by the group of the individual's actions and feelings. The group may then attempt to modify or support such behaviour or feeling.

Biber[4] in summarizing material brought to the seminar on child rearing in the kibbutz, reflects opinions on the central value of the group processes in kibbutz society. The advantages of relieving the individual child of a single, dominating authority figure, by investing the whole group with authority, was weighed against the possible disadvantages of having group controls and sanctions become so strong that the processes of individualization of the personality are thereby weakened. She, however, recalls that the concept of individualization within the group-orientated education was important to the kibbutz educators who encouraged initiative and originality through differences in the children's houses, in the variety of toys and in individualized learning methods.

Peer group pressure, according to Ben Israel[2], controls aggression in the group, which may be displaced from that felt towards adults and is preferably expressed there. The group may be supportive, according to her, because actions and the responsibility for them are shared. Kris[18] feels however that while shared experience among 2-year-olds may be good, they have not yet acquired the ability to supply each other. They cannot supply the love like that which flows from a mature-object relation. The adult is therefore necessary she stresses, to give love to the children and limit their drives. She is convinced that as long as there is a warm metapelet, providing the 'appropriate emotional supply', both in quality and quantity, there is *no deprivation for the child*.

Spiro[36] describes and analyses in extenso the behaviour of peer groups of different ages in the early stages. He perceives in the earliest years (1-2) imitative behaviour for example in following the actions of a particular member of the group. He saw in such imitation the beginnings of conscious or unconscious group solidarity, sharing and identification. (A child about to be given a blanket asks if the others are covered with blankets—a desire to share a common attribute.) Nagler[24] states that 'in the kibbutz the need to conform, or rather the fear of not conforming, is much more prevalent than it is in outside societies'.

Hurwitz[13] notes social differentiation of the sexes in their play at an early age—1½ years. Primal scene play according to Nagler, may represent actual eye-witness experience. He discussed the play of children in his therapeutic practice where aggression and anxiety are expressed as well as the representations of the mother and father relation.

Nagler[24] describes children in his practice who were noncooperative and aggressive or on the other hand extremely apathetic. Mothers refer to these children as 'individualists'. These are passive slow developing children who require the support of an adult. The responsibilities of the metapelet do not allow her time to deal with such cases. Some children may be bullied because they are the 'prey of . . . need for satisfaction on the part of their fellow children'.

Faigin[7] in examining kibbutz children aged 19-36 months, notes that in the youngest groups aggressive responses are more frequent than affectionate responses. Nevertheless, the absence of one particular child is noted by the others. Dependency in the young groups is significantly more in evidence than aggression. The children tend to control each other's behaviour and to conform. Problems of discipline, she feels, were negligible and toilet and eating habits are learned with little conflict. She concludes that group identification, sharing and group control of individual behaviour can be learned by very young children.

Lewin[19], like others, feels that the group life makes for a more gradual solution of the Oedipus complex and a lengthening of the Oedipal phase. He sees certain bodily activities, his reference is to autoerotic activities, as agents of maturation in the formation of body image and self. No deviations in autoerotic activities are found as reported by Spitz, Provence and Lippton in institutionalized children. Rocking is rarely seen and no faecal play is encountered after the first year.

At the kindergarten stage the group may be composed of a greater age range. It may extend from 3 to 6 or 7 years. Sibling rivalry may call for placement of the blood siblings in separate groups. In every case the kindergarten group remains together until the end of the secondary school years. Identification with the group remains a profound feature of the individual's personality and life. Group solidarity and loyalty are such that the individuals tend not to compete in the group, but through their groups with other groups. Group pressure for individual conformity increases with the years, but group support is an important feature, especially in the sense that a feeling or wish is shared by the group.

The peer group is composed of both sexes. In many kibbutzim separation of the sexes for sleeping arrangements are instituted, sometimes at the request of the group, before puberty. In a considerable number of kibbutzim (those adhering to the left wing of the movement) separation is not effected until the age of 18. At the request of the children, however, showering arrangements are separate. Young adults from such groups feel that the other members of the group are like brothers or sisters and the general rule is to select a marital partner from outside of the group. On the whole marriages occur between children of different kibbutzim.

The Child and his Parents

In the first months and before the weaning is fully accomplished the mother sees and cares for her child in the infants' home as intensively and more so perhaps than mothers in the open society. Parents are free to visit their children whenever they wish or when their work allows. In the first few weeks, on many kibbutzim, mothers may sleep overnight in a room adjacent to that of the infants. Anxious mothers may be permitted on some kibbutzim to have their children in the parental home for several weeks after returning from the maternity ward.

Toward the end of the first year of infancy, the mother is already back at work for the whole day. Especially at the toddler stage the child may visit its mother at work in the company of the group and the metapelet. Each afternoon, after work, the father or mother go to the toddlers' home to bring the child to their room. The child remains there for about two hours. It is then returned by one of its parents, who baths the child, dresses it for bed, feeds it and puts it to bed, and to sleep after telling it its bedtime story. The parent does not leave until the child is asleep. Anxious parents may return to reassure themselves that the child is indeed asleep and warmly covered and has not reawakened.

Parents are little involved in the socialization or the education of the child. Their hours together are spent essentially with the parents' full attention on the child, meeting all of his demands for the limited period. A corner of the parental home is devoted to the child's toys, drawing materials and so on. On the sabbath the child spends most of the day with its parents, but it is returned to the children's house for lunch and for the afternoon sleep. If there is more than one child the parents tend each to concentrate on a particular child.

The father on the kibbutz may see his infant and growing child more frequently than his counterpart in the city. The rural ecology of the kibbutz allows a closer contact, generally, between father and child. The father may visit the child frequently, feed him and put him to bed. Educators have stressed the need to introduce male teachers earlier at school.

Spiro[36] confirms that kibbutz parents frequently are not involved in the disciplining, training and socialization of the child. Children of the kibbutz identify their parents as the socializers in only 18 per cent of cases, as compared to 32 per cent for the educators (nurses and teachers) and the peer group itself. Spiro quotes Havighurst and Neugarten who maintain that children of a Midwest community see their parents as the socializing figure in 45 per cent of cases.

Parents on the kibbutz according to Spiro[36] tend to play the role of comrades rather than authoritarian figures. Their educational impact has the quality of the transmission of collective and humanitarian, political and general emotional values in the abstract, rather than in day to day relations in the peer group, which are the field of the metapelet and teacher.

Spiro[36] notes that the collective system of education permits kibbutz parents to be absent from home for longer periods on the whole than the average middle-class family in the city. Mothers and fathers attend outside courses fairly frequently and may be absent from the kibbutz at work, on leave or on service.

It is generally felt that the kibbutz parents are deeply involved and devoted to their children. Spiro[36] explains this universal child-centredness by stressing the sociological nature of the kibbutz itself as a society planned for the future generations, and the feeling of guilt and frustration of the parents as a result of their agreeing to the collective system. Insecure feeling of this sort in the parents could lead to anxiety vis-à-vis the care of their children and possibly a disturbed relation with them.

Insecurity may exhibit itself in the parents in relation to the metapelet and in doubts about the care which the child is getting. These ambivalent feelings are certainly at work in the younger kibbutz mothers, who in many cases are demanding more and more of a share in the care of their children. At times this demand is sharply expressed as a wish to rear their own children at home.

The Child and the Kibbutz Community

From the time the toddler is able to walk out with his nurse and group, he develops an increasing knowledge and personal contact with the kibbutz. He sees more and more of the work in the fields, in the barns and livestock enclosures. He invariably is welcomed by the various workers in the branches of kibbutz labour and sees his parents at their daily tasks. As he grows he begins to participate in the miniature 'farm' which belongs to the children. His imitative activity grows there into productivity, working in the patch or animal house for which the children are responsible. Altogether the children are regarded by the kibbutz as being members of a children's 'kibbutz', a children's society modelled on kibbutz structure and values, having its own government, programme and sanctions.

The children in the later years of primary school are already required to contribute work in some daily measure to the general kibbutz economy. In the high school the adolescent's day is already divided equally between formal education and work in the fields.

At the age of 18 the youths perform their own initiation ceremony which consists of a meeting held in the field with the participation usually of only one older member. The group analyses the personal behaviour and relationships of its members and their fitness for kibbutz membership in the light of the group and kibbutz standards and patterns.

At this age too the young man and woman appear before the general meeting of the kibbutz for election as full members of the community.

It seems that the kibbutz community has for the developing child qualities of the family. His emotional relations to the members of the kibbutz are much deeper than those of a child to other inhabitants of a normal Western village and have something of the qualities of the feeling for kin. The kibbutz also appears to the child with something of the nature of the supervening forces of the general society such as the government, the law and so forth.

Spiro[36] maintains that the kibbutz child grows up to become deeply attached to his particular kibbutz seeing it as home, and bound to its values. The child may see the whole world as a kibbutz and expect kibbutz values and institutions there. The kibbutz-born have a marked tendency to conform and are most sensitive to criticism by members of their group or of the kibbutz. While they are intensely devoted to work, to their children and to the kibbutz institutions, Spiro[36] found that they were inclined to avoid participation in committees and other communal roles. He relates this to the surfeit of group living. His data suggests that the young child wishes to own possessions privately, but by dint of cultural training, he is weaned from this drive.

'Familistic' Trends on the Kibbutz

It would appear that the demand by young kibbutz-born mothers to raise their children in the family home is growing steadily and that it takes several forms. The demand to have children sleep at the parents' home has been raised frequently and with insistence and resisted with equal vigour. Manor[20] speaks of an experiment with children sleeping at home on her kibbutz. She says the parents were happier than those whose children continued to sleep in the children's house. However, she feels that if parents accept the common sleeping arrangements made by the kibbutz, conflicts are not raised in the mind of the child.

In one or two kibbutzim infants are now brought directly from the maternity ward to the mother's room where they are nursed and cared for a limited period. In others there is greater readiness to allow the mother to have her infant at home for some time, if she demands it, or if the infant seems to require particular attention or care.

There are clear trends of opposition to mothers' demands for personal care of the children at home. As early as 1924 Smetterling in his article 'The Family', quoted by Hurwitz[13] says that 'the kibbutzim struggle with the family as with a difficult adversary . . . as compared with love in general, the love of two people for each other is a matter of private choice. That is what separates couples from the rest of the members, and encloses them as an 'isle of the happy' against whose shores beat the waves of collective living'. Hurwitz herself continues, 'With the coming to maturity of the *Kvutza (commune)*, the family became rooted in the life and consciousness of its members. Nevertheless, the conflict between family and collective still continues. . . . The role of parents in cooperative education became accepted only after much deliberation and experience . . . the relationship between parents and educational authorities is being constantly reshaped and revised.'

Talmon-Garber[38] in her anthropological researches in the kibbutz notes the emergence of a 'familistic trend' in the kibbutz. She finds women more family-minded than men. General observation shows that women have progressively left the branches of agricultural activity for those of house-keeping and childcare. Gerson[8] quotes Talmon-Garber as indicating that the source of the familistic trend is their dissatisfaction with communal education and their basic criticism of its 'ideological indoctrination'. He says that the reasons, which he does not find well based in all cases, for the reappearance of the demand for family after 'a long period of equilibrium' are:

1. Charges that the parents' share in communal education is insignificant.
2. Doubts concerning the well-being of the children in communal care and education.
3. Complaints about impoverishment of family life.
4. Lack of trained children's nurses.
5. Widespread dissatisfaction of women with their work.
6. Weakness of identification with kibbutz values due to changes in Israeli society.

He questions whether this tendency is really 'a revolt of human nature against artificially imposed solutions to a human problem'. He does not deny his ideological involvement and says that research has shown that there is a negative correlation between 'the strength of familistic trends and the strength of socialist and national values in kibbutz life. There is a positive correlation . . . between the strength of familistic trends and the growth in a kibbutz of a *private-consumption* approach.' Knowing this he says 'we are not prepared to surrender to these familistic trends. We reject the proposal to restore the rearing of children simply to overcome dissatisfaction; in the light of the tasks of the kibbutz movement we must regard this as a regressive tendency.' On the other hand Messinger[21] says, 'what we see happening today is the giving up of antifamilistic trends. Can the kibbutz stop such a development? It cannot.' Nagler[24] remarks: '. . . some of them (*the changes*) seem to me to endanger the principles of the kibbutz'. Winnik[39] remarks: 'There is a basic ideological difference between two types of kibbutz; one stays as it was from the beginning and the other shows new and different trends . . . the demand to go back does not mean the end of the kibbutz'. Biber[4] compares the situation of the mother on the kibbutz to that of the working woman elsewhere: 'Often a professional woman faces her most difficult moments when her children are young: the deficit of substitute care for her children and the loss of the full depth of mothering experience for the woman'. However she feels that mothers of adolescents who are at work with satisfaction have an advantage in the child-parent relationship. Winsor[41] recalls the fact that elsewhere children are also cared for in two orbits. Sometimes they are cared for in an 'extended family' arrangement by relatives of working-class mothers or in a day-care programme for children from the age of 3 until the school age. Professional women turn to nursery schools, which are expensive. The professional woman if she has her children before her training may not get to work until she is forty.

In the present author's view the movement away from the technical roles by women on the kibbutz and the reduction of her emotional involvement with its idea have played a part in the return of the familistic trend. The change of occupational status probably has a bearing as well on the demand which mothers make that their daughters acquire a profession, rather than give themselves over to the routine tasks on the kibbutz.

Finally, it seems that the mother's position on the kibbutz is fraught with the problems and conflicts of many working women. It appears that the history of the kibbutz, of agricultural pioneering in settling dangerous and desert country and its social and psychological ideology, has forced and justified an alteration of the role of women and mothers in the kibbutz society and family. The tendency to 'normalization' of the kibbutz existence, economically and from other points of view, has set in motion force especially in the woman and mother herself for a return to biological and cultural roles based foremost in the family.

Theory of Kibbutz Education

In his early remarks on collective education on the kibbutz, Segal[33] sets out its values: Many see its chief value in the freeing of the woman, but others would stress the equality of educational opportunity for all children and the right of each child to develop according to his capacities. He himself stresses the pedagogical advantages of collective education over that in the family. Family rearing has for generations, Segal avers, profoundly marked children psychologically. The child is raised in great dependence on authoritative parents. The product of this family is the mass man who values power, has little independence and reacts through rebellion. While the family has lost or abandoned many of its positive features, which provided for the child continuity of care and affection, and thus a sense of the essential and the traditional and of mastery, these family values are to be incorporated into the kibbutz children's home. In addition to the family other formative, value-transmitting spheres in society are the street and the school. The street is important to provide the child with learning experiences through its realities. Learning at school is more abstracted from everyday life and has not been sufficiently a source of social or emotional development. The children's home in the kibbutz combines the positive influences of the family, the outer world and the school in one frame for the child.

In these early remarks Segal notes the possible lack of continuity of the figures with which the younger children of the kibbutz are in contact and the instability of the kibbutz educational environment. He stresses the need for age differences in the groups in order to promote interaction and learning. At least, he insists, contact should be promoted between children's houses (*of different age groups*) lest, 'the whole process of education be saddled with an irremediable defect'. In an earlier essay (1937) Segal[33] notes the evidence of 'conservatism' in the kibbutz children. They oppose every change such as moving to a new children's house or the replacement of worn-out articles. These difficulties are the result of the lack of constant educational figures in their lives. He felt that in the kindergarten stage the group should be composed of 20-25 children in subgroups from $1\frac{1}{2}$ years to 7 years of age. Thus there would be only three children's houses until the age of 14-15 years. Segal defines the educational and rearing aims of the kindergarten as 'control by the child of his body and of his immediate environment, (*and*) training in daily habits and in social ways'.

In a later paper (1947) Segal[33] says that it was not the kibbutz which has removed the function of education from the family, but conversely it is the kibbutz which has found a framework which returned the lost values of the family. The essential value of the kibbutz is the equality of all its members. Kibbutz education is designed to provide equality of educational opportunities and hence transmit the kibbutz value of equality to the generations to come of kibbutz society. Without the liberation of women there would be no real justification for the kibbutz. Women working in the children's homes and education, which is the major function of women on the kibbutz, cannot be compared to mothers caring for their children at home. Women in the children's homes, as in the case of all workers on the kibbutz, are selected for their work rationally, and on the grounds of suitability and ability to succeed with different age groups. The belief that mothers are the best educators of their own children does not bear objective examination. Education in modern life is based on techniques of work and psychological knowledge. The kibbutz should invest greatly in producing the best of conditions for professional workers capable of fulfilling this task.

While the children's house inherits much from the family home, a very definite and important function remains, Segal maintains, to the parents. Since the daily practical concerns of child-rearing no more weighs upon the parents, they may give their time to the fostering of love for their children, a love which is untrammelled by concerns. Hence the relation between children and parents is of infinite importance. All the child's feelings of security depends upon the love of his parents, a love which constitutes the first of all things and the basis for his future life.

The child, he continues, requires only a short period each day with his parents. He needs in that time to reassure himself of their affection. A short, serious conversation and a lively interest on the part of the parents is to be preferred to an extended period with exaggerated expressions of affection or 'aggressive' attempts to educate the child. The love of the parents for the child, Segal feels, is like a still centre to the wheel. All turns about that centre. However, the centre does not interfere with the rim of the wheel. The children's house places the love of the parents in a place where 'it cannot disturb'.

In a discussion in 1964 on the theory and aims of the kibbutz education Segal[34] indicates that it is a planned system. It has, however, roots which go back to the ancient history of Jewish education. Kibbutz education too has a socialist inheritance and its societal content links with education.

It has, too, organic links with modern 'progressive' education. He stresses that the aims of the kibbutz are to produce a kibbutz type of man, fit for kibbutz life. The kibbutz has been conscious of communes that have arisen and disappeared. It is determined to remain in history. The equality for women has been obtained through freeing her from the daily child-rearing tasks. The kibbutz is not a monastic institution. It is in profound contact with the culture, science and society around itself.

He sees the psycho-pedagogical assets of kibbutz education as stemming from three sources: First, the new socializing factor, the children's home, with its rich content and activity—work, social, study, play etc.; secondly, the integration of education and environment; 'filling the gap between organized education and home, and between school and society'; thirdly, it is believed that the 'multiple mothering' involved in shared child rearing between a family and children's home brings about a healthier child life.

Golan[11], too, stresses the significance of child rearing practice on the kibbutz for the problems encountered universally in modern society. In the trend which produces the small family each child grows up essentially as an 'only child'. Moral and educational influence of the family diminishes as a result of the lowering of the age at which organized education begins. The family, burdened with psychological conflicts, is unable to meet the emotional needs of the child. These social developments are irreversible social and objective phenomena. There is a lack of coordination between the educational influences in the child's life that defeats efforts to remedy the situation. Hence delinquency and psychological disturbance reach threatening proportions. The problems in the modern family call for an integration of education on a higher level.

The Adolescent on the Kibbutz

The adolescent is discussed in this paper since he represents the outcome of the earlier child rearing and a continuation of it.

The period of adolescence, in the eyes of the kibbutz parent, is crucial for the development of the kibbutz personality in his children. Alon[1] states that the older generation on the kibbutz looks to its sons and daughters for the continuation of the kibbutz. At the same time kibbutz members and educators feel that the acceptance of kibbutz values and way of life should not simply be the result of conformity but should rest upon real identification. Stern[37] feels that he would not like the children to continue on the kibbutz simply because he himself would like it, and Gerson[8] says he would not be satisfied if the children continued on the kibbutz simply because they 'felt at home there'. The problem of the 'second generation' and its attitude to the kibbutz is an important concern and he accents the fact that the kibbutz cannot accept the view that the second generation must be different from the first, pioneering, generation.

Almost without exception observers feel that the life of adolescents on the kibbutz is too highly structured and leaves too little time for individual activity and relationships. Nagler[24] sees this as a difficulty for girls and also for sensitive boys who feel that their lives are too highly organized, that they are constantly with a crowd, and cannot do things they like to do or 'just do nothing'. He feels that this impairs the search for identity of the youth. There seems to be general agreement that the problem before the kibbutz educator is that of promoting individual activity and independence of thought within the group educational framework. Biber[4] reflecting feeling on the question of individuality states 'they are encouraged to think critically, (*and they*) are exposed to a relatively narrow range of experience to think critically about. For others, there is a grave question of how much critical thinking about the kibbutz society the kibbutz can tolerate.' Bernard[3] has the impression that the kibbutz child is under constant observation. This may be an invasion of the psychological privacy of the adolescent who should not be deprived of the time in which he is apparently doing nothing, but is in reality 'growing'.

The relation of the adolescent to his parents is also thoroughly structured. The time at which the adolescent sees his parents is fixed according to the schedule organized by the kibbutz since his childhood. This may restrict the communication between the child and its parents, as Gilan[10] maintains. While on the one hand there has been an increase in intimacy between parents and children, Alon[1] says, on the other hand, on sex matters youths are much more inclined to speak to their groups and educators than to their parents. He finds that 30 per cent of girls talk to their mothers about sex questions, while only 3 per cent of boys talk to their fathers. Redl[30] analyses the possible effects of the kibbutz organization and values on the relations of the adolescent. The kibbutz adolescent may have a lesser libidinal involvement with his parents and hence less conflict about sex and dating issues when talking to them. Since the parents, however, represent not only authority in the family but the values of the kibbutz as well, there may be more inhibition in speaking to parents about decisions such as vocational choice, or leaving the kibbutz.

The need for rebellion on the part of the youth takes on a special colouration in the kibbutz. Gilan[10] feels that this revolt may be seen in the fact that the youth is not as much concerned with the ideology of the kibbutz, as with the practical matters of everyday life.

The kibbutz is a homogeneous society which sees itself as an ideological island set in a society of vastly different values. Miller[22] remarks that before the establishment of the State of Israel the values of the kibbutz on the whole were admired and imitated by the general community. Recently the situation has changed and a reversal has set in. Pressure from the country on the kibbutz that it should accept the general values has grown. Leadership which before statehood was overwhelmingly drawn from the kibbutz is now drawn increasingly from the city. Irvine[15] sees the problem of adolescent rebellion in terms of the thesis of kibbutz society. Socialist society produces new syntheses out of the confrontation of thesis and antithesis. She asks whence the antithesis to the present thesis of kibbutz society will come, and whether the kibbutz can contain its own antithesis. Or does the antithesis to the kibbutz consist in leaving the kibbutz for the outside world?

Messinger[21] maintains that criticism, as far as it exists on the kibbutz, is directed against the outside society. It is not directed against the kibbutz movement but against the immediate kibbutz. This dissatisfaction with the local kibbutz he feels, arises from social sensitivity and ideals and still permits identification with the kibbutz movement as a whole and opposition to the society which surrounds the kibbutz. Collectivization of kibbutz opinion, he thinks, still permits, on the kibbutz, great individualization of personality.

The expression of aggression in this tightly knit and conforming society takes on particular, everyday forms which are still short of what the society evaluates as delinquent or requiring treatment. Kaffman[17] says 'it is quite certain that we do have aggression, and we probably have the same amount of it as in any other society'. Children of pre-school age fight and snatch toys. In later years aggression is expressed in criticism of leaders, the group and teachers. There are verbal expressions of aggression and also all kinds of acting out—*but according to the social values of the group*. . . . 'They do something like taking a tractor. . . . Sometimes they do steal, but it is not called stealing in the kibbutz society. . . .' In Kaffman's opinion there is no need to encourage aggression on the kibbutz, because it exists. He speaks about the method of control and sanctions by the group. This is performed by group decision. The group meets, the deviant child talks about his problem, the other children give their opinion and then assign the punishment.

It seems to be generally held that if the kibbutz child does lack something in childhood he grows up to be a most successful adolescent and young man. This judgment is made not only by the standards of the kibbutz, but by those generally obtaining. Messinger[21] tells that the kibbutz youth is most successful as an officer, in other specialized roles in the army and in Israel's society. Spiro[36], however, states that kibbutz youth seem to be 'enveloped in a shell, feel inferior and avoid emotional relations'.

Demands for education other than that for kibbutz life have been a source of concern to the kibbutz movement. The kibbutz is unequivocally opposed to concepts of formal intellectual attainment especially in fields unrelated to kibbutz living and ideals. While education is intensive and devoted to the social development of the child, the kibbutz has not subscribed to the concept that the children should automatically take a formal Matriculation examination at the end of their schooling. It is opposed to general university education for its members and attempts to reserve that for individuals who will through it be able to fulfil the better their roles on the kibbutz. This has indubitably led to conflict between individual children, their parents and the kibbutz. The demand for higher education on the basis of individual demand is seen by the kibbutz as 'careerism'. The present author has noted the demand particularly by girls for professional roles which are not accredited by the kibbutz. Recent information seems to indicate that mothers support the girls in their demands and links the role-disappointment of founding mothers with a demand that their daughters assure their personal future through a profession. It would appear that the readiness of boys to accept the roles which the kibbutz provides for them is greater. But their choice of roles is much more extensive and from the point of view of status closer to the values of the kibbutz and the general society. The readiness of the boys to accept the kibbutz roles may also relate to their personality and need to conform. While the impression which Spiro gives above may be biased, there is the impression that the personality of the kibbutz youth is inwardly directed and uncommunicative. This has been expressed to the present author in the opinion of a kibbutz girl; 'in spite of the stimulating education they have had they are not free'. Messinger[21], in seeing the need for relating the kibbutz to the outside world, feels that the time has come to consider new functions in it such as 'education, welfare, the outside world'. His point of view, which is quite novel, stands in contrast to that of Gerson[8] who describes the possibility that kibbutz-born children should go out and found new kibbutzim . . . 'When we reach the stage of decision this will be one of the best and most important ways of giving our young adults the feeling that there is something they can start anew, something through which they can become individuals'.

The Study of the Kibbutz-reared Child

Because of its special social structure and methods of child rearing, the kibbutz may supply information against which theories of personality and group development may be examined. Research into the personality of the kibbutz child has significance as well in establishing criteria for mental health action in the spheres of child care, discipline and education and of social and human relations.

An increasing amount of relevant information is becoming available in the field of human relations and child life in the kibbutz. This information has been subjected to a certain amount of research and organized study, which has supplanted the tendency to express opinion based on impressions or on limited clinical material.

In the field of the earliest development of the ego, Lewin[19] maintains 'that there are two emotional centres (*the mother and the metapelet*), that strengthen the infant ego. Identification with more than one object mitigates frustrations and conflicts and compensates for the sufferings from the separations that are due to the necessities of life'. The infant is encouraged to use all of his abilities while attention is given equally to somatic and psychic development. After gradual weaning the child develops a concept of self. This is followed by the phase of disciplining. The metapelet then takes over increasingly. Since habit training is not being carried out by the mother it leaves the child with a conflict-free relation to the mother.

The fact that the affectionate attachments of the child are divided between the biological mother and the house mother ('intermittent mothering') has stimulated research. Psychological tests, administered by Rabin[28] confirm that the kibbutz child is retarded in his early ego development compared to infants from non-communal villages in Israel. These tests do, however, demonstrate that the kibbutz child at the age of 10 has an unimpaired ego. The retardation of the kibbutz infant is in the area of social and personal responsiveness. In Rabin's view this may be due to the comparatively *high child to adult ratio* in early infancy rather than lack of continuous mothering. Gewirtz[9] reports on his study of the frequency of smiling of infants from four Israeli child rearing environments—town family, kibbutz, residental institution and day nursery. The mean frequency of smiling in the town family and kibbutz reach their peaks at 4 months and in infants in residential nurseries later. All three categories show a decline in frequency of smiles after the initial peak; the reduction of frequency of smiling among kibbutz children after the peak is relatively greater than for the children from the town families.

Rapaport[29] stresses the absence of sufficient data and study comparing the children of the kibbutz with those of other situations in Israel. He did not find evidence of 'separation'. Bowlby[5] refers to the problem of 'multiple mothering', its advantages and problems which may arise from conflicts between children's nurse and mother, change in nurses and their personality difficulties. He sees less 'maternal deprivation' than is supposed but believes the 'regime to be a mistake'. Spiro[36] analyses generally the relations of the child to the many adult figures around himself, feels there is a trauma involved in moving from the nursery to the toddlers' home. This may be accompanied by 'dethronement' of the toddler from the affections of the parents if a new child is born.

In comparing the young child's relation to his parents and to his nurse, Spiro[36] feels that the child responds with more joy, affection and pride to his parents than to his nurse. The intensity of his attachment to the parents is demonstrated by his reaction to their absence and to the birth of a sibling and as shown by the emotional reaction of a child in a group whose nurse is also his own mother. The present author has noted such cases of extreme dependence and demanding behaviour in the natural children of nursery school teachers who are taught in their own classes.

Faigin[7], as stated above, reports on her study of the behaviour of the youngest children from two kibbutzim. She did not employ a control group. In comparing two kibbutzim, she observes that, where there is a greater degree of deliberate educational stimulation, development of speech and environmental awareness are faster but tend to level off. Children in the structured environment appeared to show more dependence on adults, whereas those in the freer environment exhibit more thumbsucking. Spiro[36] observes that the motor development of young children on the kibbutz resembles that as standardized by Gesell for the United States.

Lewin[19] believes that the Oedipus complex lasts longer in kibbutz children. This conflict may be at its climax at 6 to 7 years. He believes this to be the outcome of more tolerant education. The group life, according to the informant, tolerates freer expression of all kinds of genital play, acting out and genital curiosity in the younger age groups. Nagler[24] reports that he has observed play in these children which is expressive of their relations in the family and their anxiety and aggression around them. In spite of the different sleeping arrangements the primal scene appears frankly or in symbol in their play. Ilan[14] sees that they are able to displace their hostility from the family on to the group. This is used as a defence mechanism.

Nagler[24] stresses the powerful pressures for conformity operating in the individual child in the kibbutz group. Unlike the child in groups outside the kibbutz, the kibbutz child has no other group to which he may 'escape'. The threat of being excluded from the kibbutz group may revive strong anxieties which may have lasting effects on the personality. The kibbutz child therefore in Nagler's view is afraid to be different from others. In the present author's experience with some kibbutz youth, Nagler's observation is borne out in the sense of hurt or loss experienced by children who have been removed from the kibbutz either by their parents or for other reasons. It raises the question of the difference in quality of the child's need for his group and his parents, since the latter relation does not, one infers from Nagler, compensate for the loss of the group relation.

Caplan[6] observes that whereas children of the kibbutz below the age of 5 reveal a great amount of thumbsucking and aggressive behaviour, they have a much smoother adolescence, and are stable, cooperative and brave. Golan[12] in a comprehensive description of child-rearing in the kibbutz, compares it to the child-parent relation in the traditional family. Restriction of contact with the parents, and entrusting the care and training of the child to the metapelet has a favourable influence.

Kaffman[16] states that 6 per cent of the total child population, 403 children aged 7-12½ from three kibbutzim, reveal disturbances of behaviour. Twenty-four per cent of those of the children between 2½ and 6 years show enuresis. Thumbsucking is seen in 43 per cent of the children aged 3-6 years. Temper tantrums occur in 12 per cent up to the age of 6 years and 6 per cent in the age group 7-12½ years. Kaffman also states[17] that his experience in the child guidance work of the kibbutzim shows a constant referral of 12-15 per cent of the child population. At the pre-school level the preponderance of boys is 3 : 1, but at the secondary school level the ratio for the sexes is equal. There is a 20 per cent referral of children (of the total referrals) at the high school level but it 'may not reflect the reality'. Kaffman explains the apparently high rate of incidence of emotional disturbance in kibbutz children on the basis of the constant observation of the child, the adequacy of the services and the search for the problems. There is no evidence, he feels, that there is a greater incidence of emotional disturbance in kibbutz children. In referring to his study of the 403 children Kaffman says there was no evidence of unusual incidence of behaviour problems and tantrums and excessive aggression. He observes that the transfer of toilet training to the metapelet has not reduced enuresis, even though theoretically a conflict-free relation should have been beneficial. Faulty training of the metapelet and her emotional problems may cause about 50 per cent of the enuretic problems before the age of 6. In one kibbutz, where advice was given to the metapelet, enuresis in children after the age of 3½ was reduced from 13 per cent to zero. There was a very high incidence of thumbsucking. It was twice or thrice as frequent as in American children, viz. 41 per cent of kibbutz children from the age of 3-9 years. When however thumbsuckers were compared to those without the habit no difference was found in the frequency, or intensity of behaviour problems.

Experience with older kibbutz children reveal the usual percentage of children requiring treatment. Nagler's[23] more recent summary of his clinical work with kibbutz children bears out that impression. He found that emotional problems among them are no different in nature and probably similar in incidence. He felt that the frequency of psychic disturbances, about 10 per cent, was comparable to that in England and the U.S.A. He, like Golan, notes the absence of homosexuality and the 'relatively few cases of delinquency'. Among the frequently encountered disturbances he finds behaviour disorders. Nagler finds that etiological factors of disturbance in the kibbutz child are much more frequently found in the parental relationships than in relationships in the children's house. Parents therefore remain 'effective' parents and the emotional ties to them are strong—this in spite of the fact that the child spends only two hours a day with them.

Nagler notes the most important pathogenic factors in the lives of the children treated:

1. Frequent change of metapelet in early infancy.
2. A practice (now discontinued) requiring non-nursing mothers and mothers who have weaned their babies to leave the feeding to the metapelet.
3. Noisiness in the nursery; lack of concentration by the mother on the child at feeding time.
4. A strict nursing schedule.

These factors have largely disappeared today from the infants' houses. He stresses in addition the pathogenesis of conflicts in parent—educator, (metapelet, teacher), relationships and of poor personalities in the educators.

Nagler does not note (possibly because of the nature of his clinical material) any particular modification of the Oedipal phase of conflict. However its connection, as with sibling rivalry, may be transferred to the metapelet and the group. He noted particularly problems of learning at school, feeling that these may be due to the multiple role of the teacher in child care and her involvement with the child's conflicts.

Tensions in the kibbutz child, in Rapaport's view[29], are inevitable in the process of socialization of the child's instinct, as in any except 'hot house' child rearing. Golan[11] stresses the fact, as does Rapaport, that these phenomena are easily observed in the kibbutz, whereas in the private home they are usually concealed. Rabin[26] does not find evidence in his research tests that the discontinuous mothering has any deleterious effect on the subsequent personality of the kibbutz children. On the contrary they show greater maturity than the controls from family oriented villages. The research does not support the notion that the personalities of the kibbutz children are more uniform.

Rosenfeld[31] writes that research in the kibbutz is impeded by the anxiety aroused in the kibbutz member when values and a way of life to which he has dedicated himself are in question. Investigators of kibbutz society are themselves subject to conflict or guilt, which may result in over-identification with the kibbutz community or a bias against it. Research on the kibbutz therefore should be safeguarded by teamwork and requires time. According to Schwarz[35], the kibbutz may best be studied ethnographically by living in it for a prolonged period. It should not be compared with social forms in other countries, but with other forms of agricultural settlement in Israel. Before the formation of the State and until the present time, the kibbutz member was an idealized figure in the eyes of most of the Jewish population. Research may well have been delayed by this fact and tended to take on an emotional colouring.

Lewin[19], quoting from Golan, stresses that collective education of children of the kibbutz is not a psychological and pedagogical experiment as one that is carried out in ideal laboratory conditions. It is part of real life in a social movement which has had to face great economic hardships and insecurity. Rabin[27] sets out several hypotheses in relation to the child's personality for future research in the kibbutz 'laboratory'. For example the proposition that the kibbutz child is less strongly attached to the parent of the opposite sex than the child reared in the conventional family, should be tested. Problems of social psychology and group dynamics may be readily tested in the kibbutz setting. Winograd[40] suggests research into the Oedipus complex of the child and generally into his libidinal development and conflict solutions.

Neubauer[25] feels that for a person from America, discussion of children in the Israeli collectives raises certain issues which are important for general society. They are:

1. Group living of children. The age of 3 has been considered as the earliest age appropriate for the commencement of group care. Should it be commenced earlier, especially in view of the needs and conditions of certain families? If group care is started earlier than 3 years, what should the size and structure of the group be?

2. Multiple mothering. Social conditions make it imperative at times that others should complement the care which the mother gives, or supplement the deficiencies in the nurturing of the infant or young child. How may one set up a system of collaboration between the child-care nurse and the mother?

3. Mental health planning for the community. The trend towards comprehensive mental health planning for communities and regions may see in the kibbutz a situation where such planning and its implementation may be studied and assessed. Questions of the care of the disturbed members in the community and tolerance of them may be studied there. An important area of demonstration might be the manner in which education, health and social planning may be integrated for mental health and care.

REFERENCES

1. ALON, M., 1965. In *Children in collectives*. Ed. Neubauer, P. B. Springfield, Ill., Charles C. Thomas.
2. BEN ISRAEL, N., 1965. In *Children in collectives*. Ed. Neubauer, P. B. Springfield, Ill., Charles C. Thomas.
3. BERNARD, V., 1965. In *Children in collectives*. Ed. Neubauer, P. B. Springfield, Ill., Charles C. Thomas.
4. BIBER, B., 1965. In *Children in collectives*. Ed. Neubauer, P. B. Springfield, Ill., Charles C. Thomas.
5. BOWLBY, J., 1963. Children in the Kibbutz. *The Guardian*, 3rd July. London.
6. CAPLAN, G., 1953. Problems of infancy and childhood. *Transactions 7th Conference*. New York, Josiah Macy Jr. Foundation.
7. FAIGIN, H., 1958. Social behaviour of young children in the Kibbutz. *J. abnorm. soc. Psychol.*, **56**, 117.

REFERENCES

8. GERSON, M., 1965. In *Children in collectives*. Ed. Neubauer, P. B. Springfield, Ill., Charles C. Thomas.
9. GEWIRTZ, J. L., 1965. In *Determinants of infant behaviour*, vol. 3. Ed. Foss, B. M. London, Methuen.
10. GILAN, J., 1965. In *Children in collectives*. Ed. Neubauer, P. B. Springfield, Ill., Charles C. Thomas.
11. GOLAN, S., 1958. Collective education on the kibbutz. *Am. J. Orthopsychiat.*, 28, 549.
12. GOLAN, S., 1959. Collective Education in the Kibbutz. *Psychiatry*, 22, 167.
13. HURWITZ, E., 1965. In *Children in collectives*. Ed. Neubauer, P. B. Springfield, Ill., Charles C. Thomas.
14. ILAN, E., 1965. In *Children in collectives*. Ed. Neubauer, P. B. Springfield, Ill., Charles C. Thomas.
15. IRVINE, E. E., 1965. In *Children in collectives*. Ed. Neubauer, P. B. Springfield, Ill., Charles C. Thomas.
16. KAFFMAN, M., 1957. Inquiry into the behaviour of 403 Kibbutz Children (in Hebrew). *Ofakim (Tel Aviv)*, 39, 339.
17. KAFFMAN, M., 1965. In *Children in collectives*. Ed. Neubauer, P. B. Springfield, Ill., Charles C. Thomas.
18. KRIS, M., 1965. In *Children in Collectives*. Ed. Neubauer, P. B. Springfield, Ill., Charles C. Thomas.
19. LEWIN, G., 1965. In *Children in collectives*. Ed. Neubauer, P. B. Springfield, Ill., Charles C. Thomas.
20. MANOR, R., 1965. In *Children in collectives*. Ed. Neubauer, P. B. Springfield, Ill., Charles C. Thomas.
21. MESSINGER, J., 1965. In *Children in collectives*. Ed. Neubauer, P. B. Springfield, Ill., Charles C. Thomas.
22. MILLER, L., (1966). Social change, acculturation and mental health in Israel. *Israel Ann. Psychiat.*, 1, 1.
23. NAGLER, S., 1963. Clinical observations on Kibbutz children. *Israel Ann. Psychiat.*, 1, 201.
24. NAGLER, S., 1965. In *Children in collectives*. Ed. Neubauer, P. B. Springfield, Ill., Charles C. Thomas.
25. NEUBAUER, P. B. (Ed.), 1965. *Children in collectives*. Springfield, Ill., Charles C. Thomas.
26. RABIN, A. I., 1957. Personality maturity of kibbutz and non-kibbutz children as reflected in Rorschach findings. *J. Projective Techniques*, 21, 48.
27. RABIN, A. I., 1957. The Israeli kibbutz as a laboratory for testing psychodynamic hypotheses. *Psychol. Rec.*, 7, 111.
28. RABIN, A. I., 1958. Infants and children under conditions of 'intermittent mothering'. *Am. J. Orthopsychiat.*, 28, 577.
29. RAPAPORT, D., 1958. The study of kibbutz education and its bearing on the theory of development. *Am. J. Orthopsychiat.*, 28, 587.
30. REDL, F., 1965. In *Children in collectives*. Ed. Neubauer, P. B. Springfield, Ill., Charles C. Thomas.
31. ROSENFELD, E., 1958. The American social scientist in Israel. *Am. J. Orthopsychiat.*, 28, 563.
32. ROT, M., 1965. In *Children in collectives*. Ed. Neubauer, P. B. Springfield, Ill., Charles C. Thomas.
33. SEGAL, M., 1955. Masot B'Hinuch (in Hebrew)—*Essays in education*. Tel Aviv, Hakibutz Hameuchad.
34. SEGAL, M., 1965. In *Children in collectives*. Ed. Neubauer, P. B. Springfield, Ill., Charles C. Thomas.

35. SCHWARTZ, R. D., 1958. Some problems of research in Israeli settlements. *Am J. Orthopsychiat.*, **28**, 572.
36. SPIRO, M. E., 1965. *Children of the Kibbutz.* New York, Schocken Books.
37. STERN, S., In *Children in collectives*. Ed. Neubauer, P. B. Springfield, Ill., Charles C. Thomas.
38. TALMON-GARBER, Y., 1956. The family in collective settlements. *Transactions of the 3rd World I.S.A. Congress*, **4**.
39. WINNIK, H. Z., 1965. In *Children in collectives*. Ed. Neubauer, P. B. Springfield, Ill., Charles C. Thomas.
40. WINOGRAD, M., 1958. The development of the young child in the collective settlement. *Am. J. Orthopsychiat.*, **28**, 557.
41. WINSOR, C. B., 1965. In *Children in collectives*. Ed. Neubauer, P. B. Springfield, Ill., Charles C. Thomas.

Note: The following publication has been of considerable help to the author.

HORIGAN, F. D., 1962. *The Israeli Kibbutz.* Psychiatric Abstracts No. 9. National Institutes of Health, Bethesda, Md.

XII

PARENTAL ATTITUDE AND FAMILY DYNAMICS ON CHILDREN'S PROBLEMS IN JAPAN

Kiyoshi Makita
M.D., D.Med.Sci.

*Associate Professor, Chief of Children's Psychiatric Service,
Keio University School of Medicine*

AND

Keigo Okonogi
M.D., D.Med.Sci.

*Lecturer of Psychology, Keio University
and Assistant Psychiatrist (teaching analyst), Keio University School of Medicine*

1
Introduction

In the clinical practice of child psychiatry, treatment involves not only the child itself, but, inevitably, also its parents and other family members. The child's behaviour cannot be understood without taking the parents into consideration, nor can the parents be treated without understanding their interrelation and their interaction in the family. The parental attitude is always subjected to the quality of the family, and the quality of the family has to be evaluated in terms of its historical process and of its position in the surrounding socio-cultural environment. Parental attitude, and the child's reaction to it, may be understood in the framework of universally valid principles, but the origin of the attitude is to be ascribed to certain situations specific of some socio-cultural environment. The material of this chapter is based on observation in a particular culture, that of Japan, which usually is considered to be quite different from the average Western culture. Each individual parental attitude, family patterns, family structure and dynamics, significance of roles, and interrelation and interaction of family constellations will be schematically discussed in their relevance to the sociocultural determinants. The postulated significance may be applicable also to the understanding of other cultures, or even helpful in reviewing familiar Western situations.

2

General Consideration on the Parental Attitude and its Response

The importance of the influence of parental attitude on the personality development of children is today universally accepted in the study of child psychiatry. Even though genetically determined elements should not be disregarded, personality development is largely dependent on parent-child relationship, particularly in the child's early years.

It is not necessary to mention the prominent works of Spitz, since it is generally recognized that a wholesome parental attitude is as necessary for the healthy development of a child as proper food, clothing and shelter are. A human being is happy when he feels that he is liked by others, but unhappy when he feels that he is not liked. This is true with human beings from birth, and applies even to mentally retarded children whose intellectual development has been severely arrested. Being the primitive organism he is, the infant tends to behave almost instinctively in a way that will make others like him, and particularly and primarily his parents, since they are the first humans with whom he comes into contact. Parental attitude, therefore, creates a most potent influence in the formation of a child's personality.

As in any organism—plant or animal—there is always an optimum environmental climate for development, and emotional climate is no exception. Plants cannot survive in too cold or too hot climates; similarly the child cannot be expected to develop normally if raised in an inadequate emotional climate. The optimum emotional climate for the wholesome development of a child consists of the three 'A's: affection, acceptance and approval.[53] A child develops a normal personality when he feels he is loved, accepted and approved by his parents, even when he is somewhat intellectually or physically handicapped.

Fortunately, most children are being raised under these conditions. In spite of the increase of emotional casualties in children's clinics and a number of highly publicized cases of delinquency in juvenile courts, it is apparent that most children still remain intact and enjoy wholesome development. But we must focus our attention on the minority of children raised in undesirable emotional climates. In such cases pathological reactions are deeply rooted.

Fujio Shinagawa, a Japanese clinical psychologist, divides parental attitudes into sixteen factors, divided into eight sets of positive and negative attitudes[66]. To simplify, pathological parental attitudes can be divided into two major deviations—positive and negative. The positive deviation is overprotection, the negative is rejection. A deplorable quality, called parental perfectionism comes between the two. Protection, per se, is a sensible measure by parents to save their beloved child from disaster. It is not only important, but indispensable for parents to be protective. But when they are too anxious, or oversolicitous and give their child an 'overdose' of protection, it may produce as noxious an effect as an overdose of drugs, and may even effect a pathological influence on the personality development of the child. The outcome, usually, is a child with a dependent or anxious personality. On the other hand, rejection can be divided into open hostility and neglect (which sometimes appears in the form of overindulgence) and produces aggressive tendencies often imitated or self-taught. This may nurture the growth of delinquent behaviour or the development of a psychopathic personality.

The child can react to parental perfectionism in three ways. If he surrenders unconditionally, he could turn into a perfectionist like his parents and thus become a victim of obsessive, compulsive reactions. The child unable to surrender either withdraws so completely that he presents a pseudo-autistic picture, or he falls into a rebellious behaviour pattern similar to that of an aggressive child.

Although this schematized relationship between parental attitude and the personality development of the child seems to be clear-cut and simple, the real clinical situation with which we are confronted is not so simple, since we are presented with so many conflicting combinations: one parent against another, parents against grandparents, parents against a single grandparent, one parent against grandparents and so forth, with each constellation having a different attitudinal feature. In other words, we may have a combination of a perfectionist mother and a neglecting father, a perfectionist father and an overprotective mother, overprotective parents and rejecting grandparents, etc. The interaction of these differing attitudes, therefore, makes the influence on the child more complicated and conflictual[41].

These reaction patterns of children to different parental attitudes seem, at least to the authors, to have world-wide validity, and hence the reactions of Japanese children can, by no means, be excepted. Nevertheless, since this article is focused primarily on the problems of Japanese children and the thinking of the authors is based mainly on treatment of these children and their parents, the discussion will be confined to the spheres of some specific features of Japanese children's problems compared, whenever possible, to those of Western children, of which one of the authors has had some experience.

3
Determinants of Parental Attitude in Japan

It must be noted that the variety of children's problems brought into children's psychiatric services does not differ essentially from that in western countries, except for reading disability. The factors pertaining to parent-child relationship are essentially the same in Japan as in the West. On the other hand, because of the cultural differences, there are specific differences in day-to-day living conditions. These differences are the characteristic features at the heart of children's problems in Japan. The conflict between child and parents could be a result of the conformity of parents to Japanese society, which they, in turn, force upon the child.

Japan's cultural background, therefore, must be taken into consideration. Formerly, traditional Japanese culture was of an extremely autocratic nature. In its social hierarchy the Emperor stood at the top, followed by court nobles and warriors. Then, mainly as consultants to the rulers, came priests, scholars, engineers and technicians. Merchants, farmers, fishermen and other workers were at the bottom. Through this interrelationship consistently ran the vertical relationship of master and servant. The values of social stations and the roles to be played by individuals were so rigidly prescribed that it was vital for a subordinate to be accepted by his superior.[54]

In such a society to attain social status was a primary goal for any man; his family life was of secondary value since his dependants, including his wife and children, were of less importance than his family status. The same hierarchy was observed in his own domain, the family; the man was at the top as the head of the house. Rather than share the responsibilities of the household with her husband, the wife was expected merely to serve him. She was completely subservient to her husband in their intrafamilial life and did not, of course, take any part in extrafamilial society.

Many marriages were arranged not for love, but to promote the prosperity of one or both households; similarly many love matches were sacrificed to promote the prosperity and benefit of one household. In such cases it was usually the woman who made the sacrifice since she was of less importance. The young child was fondled as if he were a cute doll or a pet animal; he was treated more like a lovable plaything, or even as a personal belonging rather than a human being with emotions. Often an eligible girl was given as a reward or prize to a young man for his services, or to ensure his loyalty in the future. In other words, a girl was considered a chattel to be disposed of by the father for the family's welfare regardless of the girl's feelings towards the match.

The only child given any consideration was the eldest son. On many occasions his status was higher than his mother's since the eldest son was responsible for perpetuating the family name. Often the wife was looked upon as a mere biological machine, designed to produce a male heir rather than to be a wife in the Western concept who would share the husband's responsibilities. Thus traditional Japanese culture could be called a culture of predominance of man over woman.

In feudal days the family unit was large and the various relationships were closely knit. Therefore, to maintain her precarious status, the wife had to make herself acceptable not only to her own family, but also to her in-laws. In other words, the wife always had to be sensitive towards every kind of relationship. She had to observe the proverb, 'Mono ieba kuchibiru samushi'—that is, 'beware of expressing your opinion'. *Ninju*, tolerant submission, was considered to be a virtue in women. It was also a virtue to help her husband advance in society—as long as she stayed in the background. This was called *naijo no kō*. A wife with chapped hands from domestic chores was more valued than one who spent time in society with her husband. She was called *sokō no tsuma*. It was the duty of the wife to raise children while the husband acted as if it were none of his responsibilities.

In those days three generations often shared one roof. Thus, the actual sovereignty of the household often remained in the hands of the grandparents, even when the second generation took over the formal succession and responsibilities of the household. At least the privilege of enjoying their emotional superiority was left to the grandparents and the submission to this grandparental superiority was a matter of social acceptance. Thus the traditional Japanese family structure may be called a culture of vertical relationship augmented by collaterality, as Caudill puts it. In other words, in most instances vertical parent-child relationship was stronger than the horizontal tie of married couples.

This traditional Japanese family culture became less stringent after the Meiji Restoration when, about 1868, the door was opened for cultural exchange between the West and Japan. Though democratic thought was imported, the autocratic pattern still persisted in Japanese family life. After World War II the Japanese were strongly influenced by democracy and exposed to Western culture by the Anglo-American occupation forces and the subsequent close relationship with the United States.

This superficial Westernization took place so rapidly, particularly in urban areas, that some democratic or liberal ideas were misunderstood and a reactionary tendency resulted, which condemned anything traditional as inferior or obsolete. In spite of this Western trend, it cannot be denied that to a large section of the population, traditional Japanese family culture was still ego-syntonic. It could be said that contemporary Japanese culture is in the cross current of two cultures—Western and traditional.

Overprotection

Western observers often praise the Japanese culture for being child-orientated. This may be true since the rearing of children has been left to the mother as a matter of course, and it was the mother's most important role to accomplish this task as best she could, otherwise she would not be accepted by her superiors, including her husband. In other words, a mother is good to her child not only for the sake of the child but also for the sake of her own acceptance and security. To a Japanese mother, to love her child means also to love herself and this motivation of killing two birds with one stone serves as a suitable matrix to foster symbiotic relationship between mother and child. This mother-child relationship is something quite different from the attitude of some Westerners who look upon a baby as an addendum to their marital life, and sometimes even as an intruder who disturbs their privacy. In Japan, parents who take good care of their children are often praised just for acting properly. One common reason for parents, particularly mothers, to be good to their children is a desire for praise. Conversely, this could also be a measure to protect themselves from adverse criticism.

On the child's part obedient submission to parents has been observed; that the child is well behaved and is submissive to his parents is now an accepted attitude in the average Japanese community. This submissive mother-child relationship serves to gratify the child's need of maternal acceptance and, at the same time, to endorse the mother's own acceptance by her superiors and collaterals. To achieve this aim the child must be good. As a result the mother overtly intervenes to control his behaviour, and the father sometimes joins in.

When the mother is unable to assume this role, the father must act as her substitute. In either case, such an attitude could easily foster overt intervention from the parents, since such intervention serves as defence and protection not only for the child but also for the parents themselves. When this protective intervention becomes exaggerated the child may not have the opportunity of becoming independent but is compelled to be dependent. Should this dependent relationship become critical, or tend to be critical, the child could easily become anxious. This could easily result in lack of confidence and a dependent behaviour pattern.

According to a comparative transcultural study made by Caudill, Pavenstedt and Wolf, 3-month-old Japanese babies are getting more attention and care from their mothers than the average American baby of that age[13]. This may be advantageous, since it might reduce the baby's chances of experiencing psychic trauma. However, there are other disadvantages. Too much care could foster the child's pathological dependency, thus interfering with the wholesome development of his independence.

Caudill and Doi point out that 'to be dependent' is more socially accepted in Japan and consequently is more ego-syntonic for the average Japanese[16]. This again may be a result of traditional Japanese culture as previously explained. Doi also stresses that a feeling of *amae* is a very specific feature of the average Japanese by pointing out that he finds in no other foreign language a term that is synonymous[21-31]. Doi explains that *amae* is a noun derived from the verb *amaeru* which means approximately 'to depend and presume upon another's benevolence'. *Amayakasu* is a verb meaning to give *amae* to a person; that is 'to overindulge in accepting dependency of others' or 'overindulge in spoiling', as we put it.

Although *amayakasu* is not an acceptable attitude on the part of the parent, it is likely to be socially less criticized than parental rejection, even if it often has a similar effect on the child. In fact, many dependent behaviour patterns in children which are commonly accepted in Japan are objects of curiosity to occidental observers. For example, most Japanese children not only share their parents' bedroom but are even allowed to sleep in the same bed. Many children are often carried on their mothers' backs. This custom has prompted some foreign psychiatrists to study the significance of this body contact between mother and child. It is common for Japanese mothers to choose and buy underwear for children going to college.

This culture of compliant dependence seems to be transforming into a virtue the tendency of parental overprotection. As a result the child is so lacking in self reliance that at all times he looks for help from his parent, or some other adult, becoming anxious and even disturbed if help is not forthcoming. Overprotection can do more harm than good. Spoiling the child (even when inspired by parental affection) could produce the same result as parental neglect, which is a negative emotional attitude. In Japan undesirable behaviour by children results probably more from lack of discipline, than from lack of care.

It is often said that Japanese culture is child-orientated, and, as mentioned before, it is true that it is common for adults to be lenient with children. The younger the child, the less he is restricted and often adults are permissive to very young and cute children even in the face of misbehaviour. Infantile behaviour is nurtured by the permissive smiles of adults, including the parents. A parent may tell the child to stop his naughtiness without meaning it.

As pointed out by Ruth Benedict, Japanese culture is a culture of shame rather than guilt[3]. In the presence of other adults the mother scolds the child, not for his own good, but to save her face. Other adults may accept this, or pretend to accept it with an ambiguous smile as if the child's age or cuteness was a good enough excuse. But they will not join the mother in reprimanding the child because this would automatically imply that the mother should be ashamed.

Thus children grow up without the basic training to postpone the gratification of their pleasure. As they grow up, they cannot cope when they encounter various situations where they cannot get what they want. Some children may withdraw, while others may act out their aggression. Such lack of discipline is causing many children to become delinquent, or at least, to present undesirable, behaviour patterns. A brief illustration may suffice. A college student steals a car. The mother is summoned and appears before the judge with a huge diamond ring on her finger. She appeals for her son at great length apologizing with tears in her eyes for his misconduct. Telling how sorry she feels about the whole matter, she ends her plea with this comment: 'If only I had bought him a good car, he wouldn't have had to steal one'.

Of course, the rapid increase of delinquent children after the war, unfortunately a universal phenomenon, does not permit any monistic explanation. Undoubtedly the lack of family discipline, particularly in young children, is playing an important role.

The undercurrent of this lack of discipline may be attributed, partially at least, to the rapid change of social values in Japan brought about by defeat in World War II and by exposure to Western cultures during the allied occupation. In pre-war Japan, parental attitude was more consistent even though it was of an autocratic nature. To play the correct parental role in the framework of a democratic family structure was something which Japanese parents had never experienced; they had to face their own anxiety not knowing whether they could take advantage of, or adjust themselves to, this rapid social change.

Democracy was offered to us as a precious gift from the outside; it was not as if it had been won by our own sweat and blood as in the case of Western nations. Many Japanese did not realize that effort was required from every individual in order to maintain a democratic society. Democratic freedom was often misinterpreted as unlimited freedom without control, and the result was chaos.

For those helpless parents, accustomed to a traditional autocratic code, the transition was difficult. They did not know, and still do not know, how to bring up their children within a democratic framework. They lost confidence in handling their children and were greatly concerned about criticism from other people. They were afraid of being considered old-fashioned autocrats or rigid disciplinarians and hesitated to discipline properly their children. A flood of psychological or pseudo-psychological publications overwhelmed their common sense. In the U.S.A. psychoanalytically oriented psychiatrists and psychologists generally urge American parents, who tend to be disciplinarian, to show more outward affection to their children and even to be 'accepting' and 'permissive' at times. This emphasis seems justified since Western culture could be called adult-orientated. However, it is doubtful whether such emphasis should be stressed in Japan where the culture is primarily child-orientated, and where it could result in laxity of necessary discipline. However, this does not necessarily contradict the basic accepting attitude required in handling children's problems. Briefly, it is the authors' opinion that an overprotective parental attitude would be more likely to create behaviour problems in Japanese children.

Rejection

However, this parental anxiety and resultant laxity in proper discipline must not be regarded simply as an expression of overprotection. It is, in fact, only one aspect of the ambivalence existing between overt affection and rejection. When a parent does not discipline properly it must be called a neglectful attitude which seems to correspond to an overall rejecting attitude.

It could be said that, with a few exceptions, brutal parental hostility toward children has already disappeared. In this respect the so-called child-orientated culture of Japan might have checked the emergence of open hostility or aggression toward children. In fact, the authors have discovered that in Japan feelings of rejection from the mother are more rarely expressed than in the West.

Of course, there are a number of narcissistic dictatorial fathers who happily indulge themselves in what they think is a Spartan way of training children, but most of them are motivated by their perfectionism and seldom by primary rejective motivation. Neglect is the more predominant expression of a negative feeling. Parental neglect can be divided into lack of care and lack of guidance or discipline. Substantial lack of care may be seen sporadically in the lower socio-economic population, while lack of guidance or discipline is seen in the lower socio-economic population, as well as in higher socio-economic families. This occurs mostly in the case of fathers. They do not fulfil their roles and indulge themselves in the face-saving justification that their occupational or social extrafamilial roles keep them so busy that they do not have time to assume a father's role at home. They claim—and it is a socially accepted practice—that they must, therefore, leave the training of children to the mothers. Such fathers only punish their children in the role of an 'executioner' when the mothers are unable to control the children. Nevertheless such an expression of recollective resentment as, 'My parents didn't even spank me when I was a child', is rarely heard in Japan.

Perfectionism

At this point, it must be noted that what makes the child feel rejected does not necessarily correspond to parental rejection. A negative parental attitude can cause the child to feel rejected, but, on the other hand, a positive parental attitude can also make the child feel rejected, as in the case of parental perfectionism, which is often a face-saving justification of parental rejection. When the child does not come up to the expectations of the parents he is rejected. However, it should be pointed out that many perfectionist parental attitudes are also derived from primarily positive emotions. It is natural for a parent to want his child to be well and happy and live under better social and economic conditions.

Social reality in Japan is growing much more competitive; to live a better life, one needs a higher education with increasingly higher scholastic standing. Striving to meet these needs create mental health stresses. From kindergarten to university, children must be pushed and prodded by parents to prepare for highly competitive entrance examinations. The strain is even harder on the parents than the children themselves; they spare no effort and will do almost anything to prepare their children for a secure position. It is such a life and death matter that the parents feel any decision relative to their children's education and future should rest solely in their hands. This pressure—conscious or unconscious—creates a negative feeling between parents and children, often regarded by the latter as a negative parental attitude. Thus, parental intervention originating from a positive motivation often results in a negative effect.

Although there may be no difference between East and West in parental perfectionism producing a negative result, it may be pointed out that it is a Japanese characteristic that most cases of parental perfectionism are primarily motivated by positive parental emotions. The underlying dynamics, as explained earlier, is a vigorous vertical parent-child relationship. Although the dependency of the child has been emphasized to explain the pattern of overprotective dynamics, the dependent relationship actually is mutual. While children depend upon their parents, the latter are also consciously or unconsciously motivated to depend on their offspring.

Most Japanese parents expect to be well taken care of in their old age by their children, as a reward for having bestowed affection upon them in their childhood. *Oya-kōkō*, filial duty, has been considered one of the highest moral virtues; it is the rare parent who does not, in his heart expect benevolent treatment from his children and even from their spouses. Parental slogans expressing their all-out good intentions towards their children's happiness and success can be cynically interpreted as secret expectations for a favourable return on investments—with interest. Herein, apparently, lies one important cultural difference between Japan and the West. It seems to be more ego-syntonic for the average Western parents to remain as independent as possible in their old age, rather than to be taken care of by their children.

Although the variety of parental attitudes that help create children's problems and clinical manifestations in Japan may not differ from that of the West, it must be noted that there are, at least a few characteristic differences pertinent to the underlying dynamics, which inevitably are combined with national cultural backgrounds.

4

Determinants of Family Dynamics in Japan

It must be emphasized here that family organization within a sociocultural framework determines parent-child attitudes and relationships; moreover parents themselves are factors in the determination of the atmosphere within the family. As stressed by Howells[38, 39], child psychiatry must develop into family psychiatry. But before discussing family dynamics, we will briefly review some psychoanalytic orientated transcultural studies on the underlying psychodynamics of the Japanese. During World War II Ruth Benedict wrote *The chrysanthemum and the sword* in an attempt to describe the mentality of the Japanese mainly from a socio-anthropological approach[3], and after the war a monograph entitled *Understanding of the Japanese mind* was written by a psychoanalyst, Clark Moloney[58]. Although these publications provided an introductory understanding of the Japanese from a Western point of view, the authors had done little research in Japan itself. In the past five years, however, substantial contributions have been made in this field by Caudill[4-17], Doi[21-31], Wagatsuma[75-77], DeVos[20], Vogel[73-74], Pavenstedt, Wolf and others. A comparison of individual psychoanalytic psychotherapy was made between Japanese and Western patients; socio-anthropological studies on human relationships were undertaken in kindergartens, mental hospitals, etc. Comparative research by psychological test methods was carried out on the subjects of marital relationships as seen in the family courts, and on juvenile delinquency. The workers in these investigations differed from Benedict and Moloney in that their observations are based on experiments conducted in Japan.

Method of the Study

In our psychiatric department at Keio University School of Medicine an extensive research project on family dynamics has been under way since 1961; the object of the research is the Japanese family, which is examined with systematized and integrated methods based upon psychoanalytic concepts. The case material ranges widely from early childhood to adulthood. The project is roughly divided into four stages[56]:

1. Observation of dynamic psychotherapy or play therapy and the combined treatment of the family (in the children's psychiatric service).

2. Observation of intensive individual psychotherapy of adult outpatients with parallel treatment of the family, including some conjoint family therapy (in adult out-patients department).

3. Psychological testing of each individual family constellation by projective techniques such as the Rorschach test, TAT, inventory, CMI and others. (Appraisal of tests was based on our modification of psychoanalytic interpretation by Schafer and Rapaport.)

4. Comparison of findings obtained through the aforementioned procedures with Ackerman's family diagnosis scheme[1].

Through these four procedures, we are attempting to understand the integrative family dynamics and evaluate the interrelationship of family members on each level of personality, role, and identity (including striving, expectation and value orientation) with special emphasis on marital and parental relationships. The project is featured by (*i*) the abundance of case materials, (*ii*) application of Ackerman's scheme, which seems to have world-wide validity, as the basis of evaluation, and (*iii*) the fact that all the participating psychiatrists, clinical psychologists and social workers in this

TABLE 1
Objects of the Family Study

	Kinds of families						
	Hebephrenia	Early Infantile Autism	Neurosis	Child Neurosis	Delinquency	Healthy Children	Total
Numbers of families	30	6	6	10	5	6	61
Psychological test { Families	25	6	3	10	5	6	55
Family members	107	12	11	28	15	22	195
Individual psychotherapy	15	4	6	8	5	—	33
Family interview	28	5	6	8	5	6	58
Home visit	12	—	—	2	—	6	20

project are receiving psychoanalytic training, in the hope that they will be better qualified for further comparative studies. Further elaboration on the tentative results of this research will be published separately[56, 57]. However, it can be said that new views on the psychopathology of Japanese family dynamics arose from our observations, and hence, the rest of this chapter will be based primarily on the observations schematized in Table 1.

Family dynamics inevitably involve the process of chronological transition, and consequently the study carried out by our department in 1965 emphasized the *family history*. To understand the family dynamics of a certain family, we approached the problem from a number of angles. Each family member was interviewed to evaluate his present mental attitude and personality. A psychological test battery was given to each individual. In addition, there were home visits and conjoint interviews to determine the interaction or interrelation of the family members. Furthermore, individual psychotherapy, as well as family therapy, was utilized to understand the history of family dynamics.

On the basis of these findings our study then concentrated on the family dynamics in the present and in the past. Applying Ackerman's scheme to this material, patterns of family dynamics are clarified through an historical family process, divided into two periods. The first is comprised of the circumstances under which the parents were married: the matching of their personalities, their complementarity, non-complementarity, common identity, and role-taking. The second includes the growth and development of the marital and parental relationship and its adjustment or adaptation to the child's birth and its development. The tentative results of our family study suggests a correlation between a few specific psychiatric disorders and types of family dynamics.

The study also helped to understand general trends of contemporary Japanese family life, which can be roughly divided as follows:

1. The age of adult schizophrenic patients in this study ranges between 45 and 60. Consequently, the marriages of the parents took place prior to World War II and their way of thinking was consistent with pre-war autocratic philosophy. Hence, those families had to make socio-cultural and ideological adjustments to the post-war Japanese society in their maturity. This group, therefore, was a good example of a generation with a family makeup which could be traced back to the pre-war era, and fell under the impact of the post-war transition.

2. On the other hand, the age of the majority of parents who brought their children to the clinic for child psychiatric treatment ranges between 30 and 40 years; they became parents in the post-war years, when social modernization was already under way. In other words, as far as child psychiatry is concerned, they may be regarded more representative of contemporary Japanese family life than the parents of the schizophrenics.

The classification of family dynamics patterns observed through our

Table 2
Patterns of Family Dynamics
(especially in terms of parental and marital relations)

	Integrative and Stable Family		Immature	
Family Patterns	Paternally dominant pseudo-integrative family of hebephrenics	Integrative and stable family of children with school phobia	Immature family of hebephrenics	Immature family of children with early infantile autism
Family Processes	fixed and rigid		pseudo-integrative of disintegrative	same as left
Identity of Parents	mother assimilated uncritically with father's identity	joined	original family centred	same as left
Role Relations	fixed role structure	depend upon the identity of parents	mutual withdrawal	maladaptive to marital and parental roles
Perception of Family Relation	distorted	father expects mother to fulfil wife's role rather than mother's role	vague	same as left
Basic Personality — Father	lack of sympathy thought disorders	normal	timid dependent	more withdrawal
Basic Personality — Mother	neurotic	slightly neurotic	timid dependent	same as left
Children	disturbance of self-realization	separation anxiety	identification disturbance	same as left

family research is summarized in Table 2. Evaluation was based on the following criteria:

1. Stability and integrity of parental relationships.
2. Fitness and adjustability (i.e., readiness and maturity) of parents to assume parental role.
3. Personality suitability of parents—their complementarity and common identity, which are necessary for the stability and integrity of their

Family	Disintegrative Family		Healthy Family
Immature family of delinquent	Disintegrative hebephrenics family of	Disintegrative family of a patient of obsessive compulsive neurotics	Integrative family of normal students
always struggling	unstable and conflictual	same as left	stable and integrative
opposing	same as left	same as left	own individual identity of each member and joined family identity
same as left	father, a role allocator, mother, maladaptive to allocated role	same as left	successful role allocation
parents blame each other	father disregards his family members, mother criticizes husband	same as left	realistic
weak-willed	autocratic, dogmatic	same as left	healthier
emotionally labile	emotionally labile and complaining	same as left	
disturbance of super-ego formation	attachment to the pathological father	ambivalent and conflictual	moderate and rational criticism self-realization

parental relationship. How the above requirements are distorted and to what extent the distortion causes emotional conflict within the family.

Partial Results of the Family Study

Within these criteria, we found a distinct difference between the pre-war family (represented here by the families of adult schizophrenic patients) and the post-war family (represented by the families of child patients).

Though specimens of the pre-war family are highly selected, this difference is none the less quite significant.

While the family patterns of the pre-war adult schizophrenic families were of a pseudo-integrative or disintegrative (i.e., opposing-contentive) nature, the patterns of post-war child psychiatric families—such as families of autistic children, of children presenting with school phobias, juvenile delinquency and other emotional problems—indicated a common immaturity. From a socio-cultural point of view, however, there are other important and even more basic factors to be considered as causes producing pathological family dynamics: the existing concepts and values in society regarding the marital and parental role in the family; value orientation as to who in a family should take the leading role.

We will now list changes in these pre-war and post-war socio-cultural concepts of the family, and compare them with the findings of our research.

The Pre-War Autocratic Family Pattern

In the traditional pre-war Japanese family system, the achievement of one's family role—father, mother, husband, wife, eldest son, second son, youngest child, bride, etc.—was of more importance than the expression of one's individuality. In other words, the family as an organic unit playing its adjusted role in society was more important than any one single member. The contact of the family with society was possible only through the head of the family who dominated the personality of each member. Consequently, each family member was rarely allowed to assume a role suitable to his own personality; but had to try blindly to fit himself within the family role structure with its expectations, strivings and values.

Each family member, therefore, was merely part of the organic totaily of the family; and his mental development was only superficially influenced by the logic, ethics, and emotions of the extrafamilial society. This pattern of family structure seems to have resided, more or less as a matter of course, in the deep psychology of each individual. This ideology was subconsciously and unconsciously adhered to even in such social groups as business and the army. As a result, each social group carried a secondary family implication. In other words, each individual, as he entered a social group, tried to reorganize it psychologically in his family pattern.

Tenno (the Emperor) stood at the summit of the autocratic family-type social structure, what Freud calls the *Ur-Vater*. As pointed out by Benedict, *this pre-war autocratic family concept, combined with militarism and the Emperor-myth to arouse the Japanese to complete dedication of themselves to Tennoism by patriotically performing any duty designated by the emperor even at the sacrifice of happiness or life.*

At the same time, however, this dedication created considerable aberration among the Japanese. It produced a distorted perception of the Emperor and other superiors (including the head of the family) and induced a 'false conviction'—almost a delusion—which governed the life of the people. This autocratic family tendency was seen in various forms among pre-war Japanese families. It is noteworthy, however, that it is disappearing rapidly in the post-war family group in our study, and the pre-war autocratic type family has been found among the families treated in our children's psychiatric service. However, even in such families, modernization is only superficial and the cores of family conflict are based on cultural conflict, since one or both parents were raised in a pre-war autocratic family environment. Parental attitude depends upon how the parents themselves were treated in pre-war days. Either they act in the same way as they had been treated by their parents, or act against them. In order to understand the remnants of old Japanese culture, we will comment on the families of adult patients in our study who are under full influence of this culture. It was interesting to discover the autocratic family structure was typical among the pre-war schizophrenic family groups (pseudo-integration families) which we treated.

Lidz and others divided the parental marital relations of schizophrenic patients into marital schism and marital skew, also differentiating them between paternal dominance and maternal dominance[47]. In our study we found that in families with schizophrenic patients, the typical family pattern coincided with the paternally dominant marital skew of Lidz. Frequently, the father of such a family was dogmatic, autocratic and domineering with poor emotional contact, and might be classified as a schizoid personality.

The results of the Rorschach test of such a father indicated a schizophrenic tendency. His wife and child considered it good to respect him, and blindly adapt themselves to any role structure he designated; they considered it bad to be unable to adjust themselves and suppressed their respective individualities. *Consequently, the child denied his father's inhuman coldness and violence with distorted perception and tried to maintain only a good father image.*

Extrafamilial logic or emotion were rejected as 'bad' if they did not agree with the thinking of the father. The family role structure was fixed and resembled what Wynne called pseudo-mutuality[81]. However, in pre-war days such paternally dominated autocratic family dynamics were syntonic in Japanese society from the socio-cultural point of view. In most families the father was important just because he was the father (i.e., because he took the role of the father) and his wife was considered a good wife and mother just because she was the wife and mother. Expectation and reality were often confused and the child viewed the parents as they should have been, not being allowed to examine the picture of parental reality.

It is interesting to note that this type of family gives the impression of formidable integration and stability, whereas in reality it is one of rigid pseudo-integration. In most cases the father is a successful member of society, his schizophrenic child is considered a 'good child' and the family itself is considered wholesome, successful and happy, at least by its members. This type of family sustains its rigidity and pseudo-integration without being influenced by post-war socio-cultural modernization.

Children raised in such a family, and particularly those who become schizophrenics, reach their adolescence without maturing and learning to consider social independence as a measure of self-realization. From early adolescence through their teens, while developing self-consciousness, they become frustrated in their attempt to separate themselves from their parents and adjust to extrafamilial society.

For instance, it is taken as a matter of course that the father in this autocratic family gets extra and better food, selects his child's career and picks his marital partner arbitrarily. The child obeys and he and the mother even think that it is 'good' and virtuous to bow to the father's autocracy.

The pattern might be described as overdoing or overdomineering rather than overprotective. Even when it is taken into account that these findings are based on a series of exceptional cases from schizophrenic families, it can be concluded, in general that in the pre-war autocratic family structure, *a dynamic structure could be similar to the schizophrenic family as far as levels of identity and role-relation are concerned showing a difference on the psychiatric level only in regard to the pathology of parental personalities.*

The paternally dominant autocratic family structure may present another aspect of psychodynamics. Again, some families of schizophrenic patients are assuming a pattern similar to the one described by Lidz as marital schism. In the United States, for instance, there are some schismatic marital relationships which are based on differences of philosophy, race, religion and other traditional identities between husband and wife. This type of disintegration, however, is rarely found in Japanese families and most specimens were of paternal dominance.

According to Lidz maternally dominant skew and schism are common in the United States, but such marital relationships seldom occur in pre-war Japanese families. This fact impresses us as another feature of the traditional Japanese family structure as seen from a transcultural point of view.

In post-war Japan maternally dominated families are not uncommon. However, historical studies of such families usually show an interesting shift of dominance. The mother plays the dominant role and the children submit themselves to her dictates. The personality of the father is usually inadequate, socially incompetent, depressive, or lacking in volition, whereas the mother's personality is socially competent and she is of an unyielding, self-assertive character.

When such marital relationships occurred in pre-war Japan, pseudo-integration was ostensibly preserved in the form of paternal dominance as long as the paternally dominant, autocratic family structure was socially accepted as 'good'. With the decline of paternal autocracy after the war, the role of the mother went through socio-cultural changes and brought about unbalance between the paternal (husband's) and maternal (wife's) personalities—formerly repressed by paternal autocratic ideology—which led to a disintegrative relationship. Familial evolutions like this were usually accelerated by socio-economic changes caused by losing the war, wholesale repatriation from Manchuria, Formosa, Korea, etc. The change of economic balance between husband and wife was caused by repatriation, unemployment of the husband, the increase of the wife's earning power, and the loss of inherited property, which had supported the paternally dominant autocracy.

With the introduction of American democracy came the wife's awareness of women's rights and the children's growing self-consciousness, resulting in overt criticism and resistance to the old autocratic family system. It is noteworthy that some families maintain pseudo-integration, while others show a remarkable shift to maternal dominance with a complete decline in the paternal autocratic pattern. At any rate, the family structure in general departed from the pre-war paternally dominant autocracy. While it did so, it depended, apparently, on (*i*) the social adaptability of the paternal personality, (*ii*) the balance of socio-economic capacities between spouses, and (*iii*) the extent of socio-economic changes experienced.

The Post-War Modernized Family

Research was undertaken on the psychodynamics of families with a code of marital relationship started only in the post-war era after Japanese society had accepted—at least superficially—democracy and modernization. A sample was selected from families whose younger members were treated in our children's psychiatric service. The paternally dominant autocratic family pattern which was so common among pre-war families, can rarely be seen in Tokyo where modernization came more rapidly and decisively than in other parts of Japan. Typical features found in our case studies of what can be termed the 'immature family' included early infantile autism, school phobias, enuresis, juvenile delinquency, and other neurotic manifestations.

The Japanese 'immature family' often gives the appearance of a nuclear family unit, but the husband and wife have not received an individualistic education according to Western standards and their early childhood was spent in the paternally dominant autocratic family structure typical of the pre-war era. Therefore, their own needs for dependency and subordination are much stronger than their Western counterparts. Hence their struggle to identify themselves with the image of the idealistic nuclear family, which has already been accepted in Japan by the younger generation. Unfortunately, these young people have assumed the burdens of parenthood before attaining psychological independence from their own parents. Ironically, their dilemma is quite similar to that of the young couple in the pre-war paternally dominated autocratic society, where it was taken as a matter of course that the husband was 'great' and the wife a good wife and mother.

The perception of family reality is favourably distorted in the expected image in the mind of each family member whereby interpersonal adjustment is more easily attained. These psychodynamics help to sustain the pseudo-integration of the family as a whole. The efforts by the family members are not motivated by inner need but are the result of their unrealistic attempts to identify themselves with the image of the marital relationship (parental role) as it appears to outsiders. This trend is an expression of perfectionism of the parents themselves in their feeling of dependency upon their parents during their own childhood. The efforts of these people to meet parental or social expectation often result in the emergence of obsessions and compulsions. What we termed an 'immature' marital relationship is featured by the discordance of conceptual striving and capacity of the husband and wife.

The characteristics of the immature family can be clarified by comparing the pattern of adjustment of marital pairs in a two-generation family, representing the nuclear family, and the three-generation family, where the face-saving appearance of traditional family autocracy is more or less sustained. In the two-generation family structure the marital pair is better adjusted. Anxiety, due to lack of dependence upon their own parents, may result in compensatory interdependency between husband and wife, Unfortunately, however, neither is mature enough to satisfy his mate's dependency and hence both become easily frustrated.

This marital combination is subject to latent difficulties even when problems are tentatively suppressed or compensated by superficial adjustments and a sense of security is obtained by conforming to society, and sexual satisfaction derived from sexual freedom. With the arrival of a child, however, the couple is confronted with the burdens of parenthood. At this point such compensations vanish and the difficulty of adjustment to the parental role appears with manifold manifestations. These new psychodynamics are projected in their attitude toward child rearing. The cultural background of each of the original families is more directly felt on this level, causing the child to lose his way toward socialization, since he has become involved in the identity conflict of both parents. The frustrated child does not get the chance to learn how to assume his extra-familial social role when the mother indulges herself in reactive overprotection of the child as a compensation of her own dependence on her husband, or when the husband is incompetent and neglects to train the child properly in social responsibility and duty.

For example, a child who refuses to attend school cannot have been encouraged by his parents with proper guidance and with mature flexible attitudes to adjust himself to his extra-familial social role. In short, this type of immaturity on the part of parents serves as a fertile matrix to produce psychodynamics such as parental overprotection, infantile separation anxiety, paternal incompetency maternal hypochondriasis and so forth.

Mutual withdrawal, as Lidz puts it[47], was observed when the parents were not self-sufficient and emotionally immature because of their own subordination to their parents. It is obvious that such a marital pair cannot carry out a parental role even with the biological event of the birth of a child, since they have by no means attained parental maturity. Those parents, however, are convinced—superficially or apparently in their reality —that they have successfully formed a well-adjusted two-generation family centring around the marital pair. Because of the conflict between their subjective image and reality, the child is raised in a harsh environment and receives little emotional warmth. It was extremely interesting to discover that such an immature family pattern was almost always seen in families with early infantile autism (Kanner[41]) as well as families with the simplex type of schizophrenia. The former families, incidentally, were of the two-generation type while the latter were of the three-generation type[56].

In traditional Japanese culture three-generation families were predominant and represented the general family pattern. The large family generates more complicated psychodynamics since its constellations contain numerous interactions and interrelations, which make the adjustment of each member of the family difficult and, indeed, may lead to chaos and panic. The large family, however, has the advantage that latent tension and conflict within each family member can be blocked, or hampered, by the assurance of role structures, or exchangeability of roles. The immaturity of a daughter-in-law, for instance, could be compensated by the mother-in-law's assistance in the rearing of a child. The neurotic mechanism created between the marital pair could be diluted in the emotional climate of the family as a whole, and this, in turn, could generate more emotional interchange between children and other family members. A large family could remain more consistent in value orientation and striving in one way or another, and since the child could be raised with concomitant expectation, the formation of social identity would become more feasible for him.

It must be added that in the era when three-generation families were more common, society in general had a more consistent, unified and consolidated value orientation outside the family. This value orientation was similar in quality to the intrafamilial orientation influenced by a paternally dominant autocratic philosophy. This is one reason at least why the problems of refusal to attend school and juvenile delinquency did not become major social issues in the pre-war era as they have in the Japan of today.

In the two-generation family, research has revealed that in spite of superficial appearances the marital pair is living psychologically in a latent three-generation family setting, lacking only the physical presence of the older generation. Equilibrium could easily be lost, and the family brought to disintegration and tragedy once the older generation—on whom the marital pair has become so dependent—disappears from the scene psychologically or physically.

Thus the advantage of the three-generation family is completely lost in the two-generation family. The latter becomes a loose aggregation—an 'immature family'. In turn, the pseudo-integration of the solid paternally dominant autocracy, as frequently witnessed among the pre-war families of schizophrenic patients, becomes a rarity. This presents a cultural shift of family psychodynamics.

5

Summary

Culture and family determinants on the personality development of the child were discussed on the basis of experience in child psychiatry in Japan, where traditional culture and induced family structure differ sharply from Western countries. To understand the psychopathology of parent-child relationship in Japan, attention should focus on an overprotection-dependency axis, which has been culturally more predominant in Japan, and around which the psychodynamics of the family fluctuate. Patterns of each parental attitude may not differ essentially from those in Western cultures, but nevertheless their motivating factors are deeply rooted in the specific socio-cultural matrix of Japan.

The material used in this chapter is based mainly on a Japanese sample and may not be broad enough for direct trans-cultural observation, but it must be remembered that Japan itself went through a remarkable socio-cultural evolution after World War II, and its post-war culture, particularly in urban areas, is becoming more like the average Western culture. Democratic philosophy was imported and is gradually replacing the traditional autocratic philosophy, thus decreasing the gap between the two cultures. Post-war Japanese culture could be regarded as a projection of Western culture, while pre-war Japanese culture represented traditional Japanese culture as clearly demonstrated in the comparative study of families from both eras. Differences found in pre- and post-war family dynamics may be interpreted as a replica of comparison between the two cultures, and, therefore, the characteristic family dynamics discussed here may encourage Western investigators to undertake comparative studies.

Modernized as it is, contemporary Japanese culture still retains remnants of her traditional culture and it could be said that today Japan is oscillating between the two cultures, causing many childhood emotional problems in those families which are unable to adapt to the new situation.

REFERENCES

1. ACKERMAN, 1958. *The psychodynamics of family life*. New York, Basic Books.
2. BELLAH, R., 1957. *Tokugawa Religion*. Glencoe, Ill., Free Press.
3. BENEDICT, R., 1946. *The chrysanthemum and the sword*. Boston, Houghton Mifflin.
4. CAUDILL, W., 1952. Japanese American personality and acculturation. *Genet. Psychol. Monogr.*, **45**, 3.

REFERENCES

5. CAUDILL, W., and DEVOS, G., 1956. Achievement, culture and personality—the case of the Japanese Americans. *Amer. Anthrop.*, **58**, 1102.
6. CAUDILL, W., 1958. *The psychiatric hospital as a small society.* Cambridge, Mass., published for The Commonwealth Fund by Harvard Univ. Press.
7. CAUDILL, W., 1958. *Some effects of social and cultural systems in reactions to stress.* New York, The Social Science Research Council's Committee on Preventive Medicine and Social Science.
8. CAUDILL, W., 1959. Observation on the cultural context of Japanese psychiatry. *Culture and mental health.* New York, Macmillan.
9. CAUDILL, W., 1961. Around the clock patient care in Japanese psychiatric hospitals: the role of the Tsukisoi. *Amer. sociolog. Rev.*, **26**, 204.
10. CAUDILL, W., 1961. *Some problems in transcultural communication (Japan-United States).* New York, Group for Advancement of Psychiatry.
11. CAUDILL, W., 1962. Patterns of emotion in modern Japan. In *Japanese culture: its development and characteristics.* Eds, Smith, Robert J., and Bearsley, Richard K. Chicago, Aldine Publishing Co.
12. CAUDILL, W., 1963. Sibling rank and style of life among Japanese psychiatric patients. In *Proceedings of the Joint Meeting of the Japanese Society of Psychiatry and Neurology and the American Psychiatric Association.* Eds, Haruo Akimoto *et al.* Supplement of Folia Psychiatrica et Neurological Japonica, Tokyo.
13. CAUDILL, W., (Unpublished manuscript). Maternal care and infant behaviour in Japan.
14. CAUDILL, W., 1964. Thought on the comparison of emotional life in Japan and the United States. *Seishin-Igaku (Clin. psychiat.)*, **64**, 113.
15. CAUDILL, W., and SCARR, H. A., 1962. Japanese value orientations and culture change. *Ethnology*, **1**, 53.
16. CAUDILL, W., and DOI, L. T., 1963. Interrelations of psychiatry, culture and emotion in Japan. In *Man's image in medicine and anthropology.* Ed. Gladstone, Iago. New York, Intern. Univ. Press.
17. CAUDILL, W., and DEVOS, G., 1957. Achievement, culture and personality: The case of the Japanese Americans. *Amer. Anthrop.*, **58**, 1102.
18. CORNELL, J. B., 1961. Outcaste relations in a Japanese village. *Amer. Anthrop.*, **63**, 282.
19. CORNELL, J. B., 1963. Individual mobility and group membership—the case of the burakumin. Paper prepared for Second Conference on the modernization of Japan.
20. DEVOS, G., and WAGATSUMA, H., 1961. Value attitudes toward role behavior of women in two Japanese villages. *Amer. Anthrop.*, **63**, 1204.
21. DOI, T., 1954. Some aspects of Japanese psychiatry. Paper presented at the Neuropsychiatric Conference, FEC, U.S.A. Army Hospital, 8168th Army Unit.
22. DOI, T., 1956. Japanese language as an expression of Japanese psychology. *Western speech*, **20**, 90.
23. DOI, T., 1956. *Seishinbunseki (Psychoanalysis).* Tokyo, Kyoritsu Shuppan Co.
24. DOI, T., 1960. Psychopathology of Jibun and Amae. *Psychiatr. Neurol. Jap.*, **62**, 149.
25. DOI, T., 1960. The theory of narcissism and the psychic representation of self. *Seishinbunseki Kenkyu*, **7**, 7.
26. DOI, T., 1961. Sumanai and Ikenai. *Seishinbunseki Kenkyu*, **8**, 4.
27. DOI, T., 1961. *Psychotherapy and psychoanalysis.* Tokyo, Kaneko Shobo.
28. DOI, T., 1964. Psychoanalytic therapy and 'Western man'. *Seishinbunseki Kenkyu*, **10**, 6.
29. DOI, T., 1964. Discussion. *Seishin-igaku (Clin. Psychiat.)*, **62**, 119.

30. Doi, T., 1965. *Psychoanalysis and psychopathology.* Tokyo, Igaku-shoin.
31. Doi, T., 1962. Amae: a key concept for understanding Japanese personality structure. In *Japanese culture: its development and characteristics.* Eds, Smith, R. J., and Beardsley, R. K. Gren Foundation for Anthropological Research.
32. Donoghue, J. D., 1957. An Eta community in Japan: the social persistence of outcaste groups. *Amer. Anthrop.*, **59**, 1007.
33. Embree, J., 1945. Cultural patterns. In *The Japanese nation—social survey.* Ed. Embree, J. New York, Farrar and Rinehart.
34. Embree, J., 1950. The people. In *Japan.* Ed. Borton, H., Ithaca, N.Y., Cornell Univ. Press.
35. Fleck, S., et al., 1957. The intrafamilial environment of the schizophrenic Patient, II. Interaction between hospital staff and families. *Psychiatry*, **20**, 343.
36. Gibney, F., 1953. *Five gentlemen of Japan.* New York, Farrar, Strauss and Young.
37. Goerer, G., 1943. Themes in Japanese culture. *Trans. N.Y. Acad. Sci.*, **2**, 106.
38. Howells, J. G., 1963. Child psychiatry within a department of family psychiatry. *Proc. the Joint Meeting of the Japanese Society of Psychiatry and Neurology and the American Psychiatric Association*, **103**.
39. Howells, J. G., 1963. *Family psychiatry.* Edinburgh, Oliver and Boyd.
40. Jackson, D. D., 1957. The question of family homeostasis. *Psychiat. Quart. Suppl.*, Part I, **31**, 79.
41. Kanner, L., 1957. *Child psychiatry.* Springfield, Ill., C. C. Thomas.
42. Kato, M., 1964. On the problem of anthrophobia in Japan. *Seishin-igaku (Clin. Psychiat.)*, **62**, 107.
43. Kerlinger, F. N., 1951. Decision making in Japan. *Social Force*, **30**.
44. Kondo, A., 1953. Morita therapy: a Japanese therapy for neurosis. *Amer. J. Psychoanal.*, **13**, 31.
45. Kondo, A., 1964. On mutual care, a pattern of Japanese culture, as reflected in 'shinkei-shitsu' type of neurosis. *Seishin-igaku (Clin. Psychiat.)*, **62**, 97.
46. Lidz, R., and Lidz, T., 1949. The family environment of schizophrenic patients. *Amer. J. Psychiat.*, **106**, 332.
47. Lidz, T., et al., 1957. The intrafamilial environment of schizophrenic patients; marital schism and marital skew. *Amer. J. Psychiat.*, **114**, 241.
48. Lidz, T., et al., 1959. The familial environment of the schizophrenics. On the differentiation of the personality and symptoms in uniovular twins. *Psyche*, **13**, 345.
49. Lidz, T., et al., 1959. The intrafamilial environment of the schizophrenic: the father. *Psyche*, **13**, 268.
50. Lidz, T., et al., 1956. The role of the father in the family environment of the schizophrenic patient. *Amer. J. Psychiat.*, **113**, 126.
51. Lidz, T., et al., 1957. The intrafamilial environment of the schizophrenic patient, I. The father. *Psychiatry*, **20**, 239.
52. Lidz, T., 1963. *The family and human adaptation, three lectures.* New York, Intern. Univ. Press.
53. Makita, K., 1958. A few considerations on child psychiatry. *Jap. J. Psychoanal.*, **5**, 1.
54. Makita, K., 1964. Development and difficulty of social psychiatry in Japan. *Internat. J. Soc. Psychiat.*, special edition No. 3.
55. Makita, K., Nakamura, M., et al., 1965. Statistic survey of children's psychiatric service at Keio University Hospital. *Jap. J. Child Psychiat.* (in press).

56. MIURA, T., MAKITA, K., and OKONOGI, K., 1966. Comparative family study. *Psychiatry*, **8**, 4.
57. MIURA, T., and OKONOGI, K., 1966. Family psychopathology of hebephrenia in terms of comparative family study. *Psychiatry*, **8**, 4.
58. MOLONEY, J. C., 1954. *Understanding the Japanese mind*. New York, Philosophical Library.
59. MURAKAMI, H., 1964. On the Japanese characteristics of neurosis. *Seishinigaku* (*Clin. Psychiat.*), **62**, 87.
60. NAGAYASU, A., et al., 1965. Study group of psychological test. *Jinkaku Test Jirei Shu* (*Case Studies on Personality Test*). Tokyo, Japan, Nippon Bunka Kagaku Sha.
61. OPLER, M. K., 1959. *Culture and mental health*. New York, Macmillan.
62. PASSIN, H., 1955. Untouchability in the Far East. *Monumenta Nipponica*, **2**, 27.
63. PELZEL, J., KLUCKHOHN, F., 1957. A theory of variation in values applied to aspects of Japanese social structure. In *Bulletin of the Research Institute of Comparative Education and Culture*. Faculty of Education, Kyushu University, English Edition, March 1, pp. 62.
64. REISCHAUER, E. O., 1950. *The United States and Japan*. Cambridge.
65. ROSENTHAL, M. J., et al., 1959. A study of mother-child relationship in the emotional disorders of children. *Gen. Psychol. Monogr.*, **60**, 65.
66. SHINAGAWA, F., and SHINAGAWA, T., 1953. *Oyako-kankei Shindan Test No Tebiki* (*Manual for testing parent-child relationship*). Tokyo, Japan, Nippon Banka Kagaku Sha.
67. SMYTHE, H., and NAITO, Y., 1953. The Eta caste in Japan, *Phylon* (Atlanta University Review of Race and Culture), **19**, 157.
68. SUZUKI, T., FROMM, E., and DE MARTINO, R., 1960. *Zen buddhism and psychoanalysis*. New York, Harper.
69. TAKAGI, R., et al., 1965. Nuclear type of school phobia. *Jap. J. Child Psychiat.*, **6**, 146.
70. TAKUMA, T., et al., 1964. Investigation of the practice of mothers' lying with their babies in Japan. *Jap. Women's Univ. J.*, **11**, 1.
71. TAKUMA, T., et al., 1964. A survey on ONBU (carrying babies on mother's back). *Clin. Pediatr.*, **17**, 1072.
72. THAVER, F., et al., 1964. Conceptions of mental health in several Asian and American groups. *J. soc. Psychol.*, **62**, 21.
73. VOGEL, E. F., and VOGEL, S. H., 1961. Family security, personal immaturity and emotional health in a Japanese sample. *Marriage and family living*, **23**, 161.
74. VOGEL, E. F., 1962. Entrance examinations and emotional disturbances. In *Japanese culture: its development and characteristics*. Eds, Smith, R. J., and Beardsley, R. K. New York, Wenner-Gren Foundation for Anthropological Research.
75. WAGATSUMA, H., 1956. Japanese values of achievement—the study of Japanese immigrants and inhabitants of three Japanese villages by means of TAT. Unpublished M.A. Thesis, Department of Far Eastern Studies, University of Michigan.
76. WAGATSUMA, H., 1964. *Jigano Shakai-shinri* (*Social psychology of ego*). Tokyo, Seishin Shobo.
77. WAGATSUMA, H., and DEVOS, G., 1963. The outcaste tradition in modern Japan: a problem in social self-identity. Paper prepared for Second Conference on the modernization of Japan.
78. WAHL, C. W., 1954. Antecedent factors in family histories of 392 schizophrenics. *Am. J. Psychiat.*, **110**, 668.

79. WATTS, A. W., 1953. Asian psychology and modern psychiatry. *Amer. J. Psychoanal.*, **13**, 25.
80. WATTS, A. W., 1957. *The way of zen.* New York, Pantheon Books.
81. WYNNE, L., et al., 1958. Pseudo-mutuality in the family relationships of schizophrenics. *Psychiatry*, **21**, 205.

PART TWO

CLINICAL

XIII

TRENDS IN THE INVESTIGATION OF CLINICAL PROBLEMS IN CHILD PSYCHIATRY*

G. K. Ushakov
Professor of Psychiatry
Department of Psychiatry, 2nd Moscow Medical Institute
Moscow, U.S.S.R.

1
Historical Introduction

The first step in the successful solution of a scientific problem should be the correct definition of the object of the investigation, and in particular of its essential elements.

In child psychiatry, the selection of clinical problems for investigation has been greatly influenced, not always to its advantage, by the historical development of this field.

The scientific stage in the development of clinical psychiatry came into existence in the middle of the nineteenth century. In the early period, psychiatry was mainly based on symptomatology. But by the end of the nineteenth century, many modern notions in the diagnosis and treatment of mental diseases had been formulated; whilst descriptions of mental disorders in children started to appear in the second half of the nineteenth century. At that time, however, they consisted only of superficial descriptions, and indicated only the start of child psychiatry as a specialty. Specific studies on mental disorders in children, which appeared in the first decade of the twentieth century, were events of paramount importance,

* Translated by Mrs Ushakova, Moscow, U.S.S.R., and Maria-Livia Osborn, Research Assistant, The Institute of Family Psychiatry, Ipswich, England.

as they laid the foundation for subsequent developments in child psychiatry. The first propositions formulated in this field allowed the rejection of the idea that the psychic organization of the child is a phenomenon different in essence from the psychic organization of an adult; also the belief that mental disorders in children are identical to similar disorders in adults became tenable. After the well known work by Emminghaus[1], a complete systematization of what was known of neuropsychiatric disorders of children and adolescents was presented in a manual by Homburger[2], which marked the beginning of precise systematization of information in the field of child psychiatry.

Up to the beginning of the twentieth century, psychiatrists had attempted to prove, by their clinical observations, that psychosis might occur in children; in the first decade of our century they started to publish their clinical observations indicative not only of such a possibility, but also of diversity in variants and forms of mental diseases in children; then, in the second and third decade their publications revealed the existence of a variety of forms of disorders, and their clinical characteristics, in children of *different* age groups.

Comparison of corresponding stages in the history of adult psychiatry and of child psychiatry, shows clearly the way in which the latter developed. The history of psychiatry shows that child psychiatry developed later and was influenced by preconceptions originating in the traditional adult psychiatry, and utilized, in this connection, many ideas which had been axioms in adult psychiatry. This determined a number of peculiarities in the development of child psychiatry:

(*i*) Describing the clinical aspects of mental disorders in children and adolescents, many psychiatrists used psychopathological terms and notions from adult psychiatry and frequently transferred them automatically to child psychiatry.

(*ii*) The phenomenological-descriptive method of investigation was transferred into child psychiatry without sufficient grounds (phenomenology is comprehension by way of description according to Jaspers[3] and others). Moreover, it was not taken into account, at that time, that the psychology of adults had been more or less understood, whereas phenomenological studies in child psychiatry had not yet been confirmed by sufficient knowledge of child and adolescent psychology.

(*iii*) The tendency, established in adult psychiatry, to estimate the clinical aspects of a patient by a description of his presenting symptoms, without considering the whole course of the disease, had brought about elements of clinical nihilism. An automatic shift of a similar approach to the psychiatric appraisal of the child proved to be inefficient as well as erroneous.

(*iv*) The idea that psychological abnormalities of childhood and adolescence are caused by the various stages of development has brought about attempts to explain mental disorders in children by the characteristics of immaturity of the psyche. It is known that psychological development, most active in childhood, adolescence and youth, is not completed by the age of 20 to 40 years; it influences the whole life of an individual. Many investigators defined this 'immaturity', which again stressed the psychological difference between child and adult, as an imperfect, inadequate, weak or easily disrupted mental organization. This appraisal was done from the point of view of an adult observer and included biological and teleological elements. However, clinical data prove that this approach is wrong. At every ontogenic stage the harmony of development (biological maturation) strictly corresponds to a stage of development of the individual's psyche. No other stage of 'perfection' or of 'maturity' can be more perfect than that which is right for each particular stage of development.

These, as well as other trends in the development of psychiatry lead to the separation of child psychiatry from the traditional psychiatry of adults, which was based on wider experience and on a richer fund of facts and theories. The division of psychiatry into child psychiatry and adult psychiatry was right from the point of view of organization of health services and for the training of medical specialists, who could render a more qualified and specialized service to each age group. At the same time, such division was not only unhelpful, but even damaging to the field of research in child psychiatry. In psychiatric research such separation resulted in the appearance of 'specific' clinical terms and definitions, and 'specific' opinions on the essence of mental disorders in children and adolescents. Among clinical investigators of neuropsychiatric disorders in children, there were specialists who were often well acquainted with the various aspects of child pathology, but at the same time were little versed in matters of classical, adult clinical psychiatry. Conversely, among research psychiatrists in the adult field, often experienced and inquisitive, many were not skilled enough to recognize the characteristics peculiar to child, adolescent and youth psychopathology.

This situation in psychiatric research reduced the possibilities of research and hampered the longitudinal clinical study of the mechanisms of psychiatric disorders, which should take into consideration all the phases in the life of an individual, and not just his childhood or adulthood.

This fragmentation frequently resulted in unilateral research; the investigator, depending on whether he was a child psychiatrist or an adult psychiatrist, often drawing conclusions about the clinical and pathogenetic aspects of a disease on the basis of findings characteristic only of a part of a morbid condition, a fraction of the developing process. As a rule, the validity of such conclusions was limited, and the conclusions themselves were only partially important, and frequently erroneous in content. Such investigations were inefficient and the results did not justify the amount of staff, the energy and time spent on them.

Research in child psychiatry is made more complex by the fact that separate types of disorders, parts of the total picture of the disease in the same patient, are sometimes investigated by various specialists: neuropathologists—on residual disorders of the central nervous system; psychologists; defectologists; remedial teachers—on conditions of mental retardation; otologists; teachers of the deaf, speech therapists—on ear and speech disorders, etc. Of course, we must not underestimate the value of cooperation with other specialists in the clinical study of mental diseases; their assistance is invaluable in making an investigation complete. Nevertheless, the leading role in the team method of clinical research should be given to the clinical psychiatrist.

The study of important problems in child psychiatry is better and more thoroughly undertaken when the investigator, a child psychiatrist, has clinical experience of classical adult psychiatry, as well as of normal psychological development and of clinical and psychopathological disorders belonging to the field of neuropsychiatry in infants, children and adolescents, and applies, in their study, the method of comparison by age group.

2

Psychiatric Research by Comparison-by-age-group Method

As Applied to Psychosis

Experience shows that in clinical research comparison by age group prevents reaching insufficiently valid and often erroneous conclusions, and offers the right conditions for a complete study of morbid processes embracing the whole duration of the disease with all its characteristics.

By application of the method of comparison by age group in clinical research, it has already become possible not only to revise a number of traditional propositions in psychiatry, but also to define the main trends of investigation.

Application of this method has made it possible to confirm that an overwhelming majority of cases of schizophrenia originates in adolescence, and in childhood, and even in infancy. The dynamic study of the typical development of clinical variants of schizophrenia with different time of true onset induced investigators to change their notion about the clinical essence of this disease; it enabled them to give a different explanation of the manifestations of various degrees of disorders in the disease picture, and to associate them in particular with the time of onset of the psychosis in the different age periods of the individual's development. Within a given form of schizophrenia, the structure of the disorder remains the same irrespective of the age in which the disease is observed. In such cases the differences, typical for childhood, adolescence or adulthood are determined by additional manifestations of the same disorder, these being dependent on the age of the patient, and not by the appearance of separate clinical psychotic disorders.

Side by side with this, the onset of mental disease in childhood and adolescence, and the manifestations which it will present in each age group, leave a mark in the clinical picture of the mental disease during the following periods of its course. As a result, the clinical structure of schizophrenia, for instance, in a 20 to 25-year-old patient, displays, firstly, disorders typical to that particular clinical variant of psychosis; secondly, special characteristics, depending on the time of onset (childhood, early adolescence (10 to 16 years) or late adolescence (16 to 20 years)), and, lastly, it displays characteristics due to changes since the time of the onset of the schizophrenia (childhood, early adolescence and late adolescence). There is great need for further investigation in those disorders which present with different manifestations depending on the age of onset.

Investigations in schizophrenia using the comparison by age group method have demonstrated that, among its clinical variants, are predominant forms with a slow, creeping course; forms with a periodical (remittent) course are rare; and schizophrenia with a malignant course, the so-called nuclear variants, are even rarer and constitute not more than 10 per cent of all schizophrenia cases. This systematization of variants in the course of schizophrenia allows us to revise another belief which has become traditional. In fact, the prognosis for schizophrenia does not conform with established ideas. In schizophrenia with a slow course, the organism often retains a great capacity for compensation. In the periodical variants, spontaneous or therapeutical intermissions (deep remissions) are not accompanied by great pathological changes in the patient's personality. The approach to the study of schizophrenia here, the method of comparison by age group, enabled us to abandon the belief that the severity of the disease is related to the time of its onset, i.e. that the earlier the onset the severer is the course of the disease. Clinical observations give every reason to assert that even in cases of psychosis of early childhood appearing in the first age period the prognosis is not necessarily always unfavourable. Among the variants of early childhood schizophrenia, forms with a slow creeping course amount to no less than one third of all cases. These forms leave a deep mark on the forming personality of the child and, later, of the adolescent, but do not show early on deep disturbance of the personality.

As Applied to Neurosis

Comparison by age group in the field of neurosis has given rise to new ideas. Neurotic reactions observed in children, which seem little differentiated, and yield to systematisation with difficulty, are often the initial symptoms of neurosis-like conditions in adolescents. In their turn, the characteristics of these conditions determine to a great extent the structure of true neuroses in later age groups. Thus the neurotic reactions, neurosis-like conditions and true neurosis are not different diseases in the same patient, but different manifestations of the same disorder, i.e. stages of development of a neurosis taking shape at various ages in the same individual. In this connection, detailed clinical investigations of manifestations of neurotic disorders in different age groups allow us to understand better both the development and the etiology of the neuroses.

Child psychiatrists are familiar with the difficulties of classification of neurotic conditions in children and adolescents; these disorders are often called conditions of disharmonious, pathological personality development in the child or in the adolescent, instead of being given proper differentiation into the respective clinical disorders. At the same time, investigations of the case histories based on a comparison of clinical phenomena by age group, allows one to assert that it is more correct to evaluate multiform behaviour disorders in children and adolescents as true psychopathological conditions. Various forms of neurosis take shape in late adolescence or adulthood, developing from such conditions. Thus, psychopathological conditions, originating in children and adolescents and outside the structure of other nosological forms, should be classified as pre-neurotic conditions. We succeeded in differentiating some characteristics of these conditions, and taking into consideration their properties, were able to predict the possibility of remissions, or the nature of neuroses likely to develop in the future.

The problem of clinical differentiation of various forms of schizophrenia, of neurosis and of behaviour disorders, and the investigation of their development by the comparison by age-group method, is one of the most important fields for detailed clinical research.

3

Comparison by Age-group Method of Symptoms and Syndromes

Investigations by the comparison by age-group method in the pattern of development of psychoses, neuroses and behaviour disorders are possible and have scientific value only when the investigator is clinically experienced and aware of the changing features of mental disorders at different stages of their development and in different age groups.

The changing qualities of delusional disorders in ontogenesis may serve as an illustration. In very young children delusional phenomena are mainly of a motor nature and often do not include other delusional components. At the age of 2 to 3 years, delusional phenomena in the motor sphere are manifest as continuous twitching of the shoulders, opening of the mouth, licking of the lips, intermittent slight coughing, choking, pulling the hair out, finger sucking, nail biting, etc. Another form of delusional phenomena, peculiar to this age, is delusional fears. The content of these fears is common: they are often evoked by fairy tales which the child has heard, and by events he has experienced. These delusional fears are manifested by a monotonous repetition of 'I'm afraid, I'm afraid', by crying, shouting and appealing to the mother, accompanied by gestures and vegetative components.

When the child is 4 to 5 years old the clinical picture of his delusions becomes more complicated. The emotion of fear involves more elements of individual rationalization and imagination, leading to fear of solitude, fear of darkness, etc. The subject of fear becomes richer and more varied: the child may avoid touching things; he is afraid to be infected; sits at the table with his hands up; he eats without touching the plate; he is afraid of books with a frightening plot. His movements and actions often acquire a ritual character: before a play he 'must' touch the floor, or touch the table with his palms, or the table with his chin. He must lick his mother. He cannot eat unless he licks her, etc. Motor compulsions also become complex: compulsive hand-clapping, clenching of teeth, gritting the teeth, twisting of hands, repetitive winking, twitching of shoulders, lifting the shoulders as if 'the bra is slipping down', wrinkling the nose, making faces, shaking the head, etc. Parallel with these compulsions, elementary rationalized delusions occur for the first time, such as: it is necessary to speak with 'bad thoughts' to make them disappear; shoes should be put down in a certain way only, 'otherwise something might happen'. And so on.

At the age of 6 to 7 years, delusions by association become more frequent and elaborated: the child washes his hands often, blows on them in order to 'clean them from dirt'; he is afraid of his own 'bad thoughts', there is compulsive 'guessing of days', counting of days and enumerating; anxiety that a piece of something might fall off and he might swallow it; fear of death, and of quick aging. He understands that his fears are groundless, but cannot rid himself of them.

At the age of 8 to 9 years the explanation of accompanying feelings becomes still more typical. The child may jump up and rub one foot against the other; before he begins to write he puts the pencil on the floor or puts it to his throat; he doesn't know why he does it, he 'can't help doing it'. He pulls out his eyelashes, winds his hair round his finger and pulls out whole locks; he dislikes going bald but 'can't do anything with himself'. He blinks 'as if a fly got into his eye'—there is no fly but he can't help blinking. He doesn't allow anybody to touch his bed, if anybody touches it he 'must' rap on it before going to bed; if he doesn't do this he 'feels bad'. There is compulsive abdomen twitching. 'Of course I can restrain it but after that the twitching increases.' The fears become more complex, developing into 'fear-thoughts'; fear of death, fear of illness, fear of darkness, and of solitude. The child constantly washes his hands and washes all objects before using them; he has to wipe the taps and the wash basin before washing. If anyone prevents him from doing these things, he becomes irritated and is rude to his parents and other people.

In adolescence delusions are still more complex. In fact, they acquire properties typical of the generally accepted form of 'delusions'. Tracing the development of delusional phenomena in children, it is not difficult to observe that, as they approach adolescence, their structure becomes more complete, and motor compulsions are more often replaced by sensory rationalized delusions. At the age of 15 to 16 years, and particularly in late adolescence (17 to 20), we find already those variants of delusional disorders very similar to those characteristic of adult patients. Thus, if we consider only the first stages of motor delusions, without tracing their subsequent development, we can deduce that these disorders are not delusions, as postulated by Christian Viek[9], but a peculiar stereotypy. Comparison by age group of subsequent development of these disorders shows that the above deduction is erroneous. A similar method could be applied with advantage to other forms of clinical disorders. Space does not permit me to enlarge on this particular point, but we will briefly discuss some related matters.

Clinical observation has shown that many well known psychiatric disorders may be detected in childhood. However, at that period they present with different manifestations, generally defined as rudimental forms, aberrations, or latent forms of the corresponding disorders in the adult. But the premonitory signs of these disorders can be originally detected only at a definite age. For instance, rudimentary phenomena of depression, oneiroid conditions, hidden forms of depersonalization, and Candinsky-Klerambo's mental automatism syndrome may be detected in the total picture of a psychosis only in very early adolescence (10 to 12 years old). There is no doubt that their origin in this age reveals a definite stage of development of the mental mechanisms involved in the pathological structure of these disorders. However, it is evident that in the previous period of development (i.e. in early childhood) similar disorders go undetected, not because they are absent, but because they have different pathological qualities and a different expression. The clinical study of the special characteristics of these and other disorders in childhood is an interesting field for research. The knowledge derived from such studies will allow us to follow the whole pattern of development of the disease; moreover they will be an invaluable aid to an early diagnosis, prognosis and the early treatment of mental diseases.

4

Problems in the Analysis of Clinical Syndromes

The evaluation of psychiatric disorders by their presenting symptoms has resulted in the first awareness of mental disease, particularly of schizophrenia, to be regarded as the true onset of the disease, when in fact it is only the stage at which the manifestations of the psychosis are clearly obvious. The comparison by age-group method in the investigation of mental disorders shows that it is erroneous to date the onset of the disease from the period of unfolding of manifestations. The true onset of a mental disease is to be dated much earlier, sometimes many years earlier, than the period of its obvious manifestation. The initial disorders especially in the paranoid and hebephrenic forms of schizophrenia, precede by three to five years, and even longer, the manifestation of the psychosis.

These new concepts on the pattern of development of many psychoses, especially endogenous, make it necessary to revise established notions, such as 'prepsychosis' and 'prepsychopathic conditions', and consider them as initial stages of psychosis, neurosis or psychopathic conditions. The problem of precise differentiation between the notions of 'premorbid' and 'initial disorders' of a disease needs investigating, as there is every reason to believe that the term 'premorbid' can be applied only to those conditions, irrespective of their characteristics, which precede the observation of the first obvious symptoms of the disease. However, the initial phenomena of the disease, from the moment of first appearance of the symptoms to the time when its manifestations are well-developed obvious mental disorders, should be regarded as the initial period of development of the disease.

Changed concepts of the whole pattern of development of psychotic disorders and diseases of the time of their *true* onset present an international challenge for research by psychiatrists, and offer great possibilities for the scientific study of early diagnosis, early prognosis, and early therapy, as well as prophylaxis, of primary and secondary mental disorders.

Moreover, the classic traditional method of estimating the onset of a disease from the time of its actual manifestation, rather than from the time of true onset of the psychosis, compels us to revise the main propositions regarding the etiology of mental diseases. It is obvious that investigations into the primary and secondary clinical manifestations in a psychosis, are not related to research into its etiology; such investigations allow us only to define some causes of transition of a disease from one state to another, and nothing more. Thus, many investigations into the problems of etiology of mental diseases have been invalidated because the investigators did not keep to a strict methodological principle in their work.

Therefore, laboratory investigations in the pathogenesis of mental diseases, are of much greater value and have greater depth if a precise definition of the investigation precedes their execution. In other words, investigation into the mechanisms of a disease means, first of all, a clear understanding of its clinical essence for the whole length of its course with all its qualities.

The correct interpretation of results of laboratory analysis is also essential. Our observations allow us to affirm that often biochemical deviations and other humoral shifts from the norm are assumed, because of an essential defect of interpretation of findings. The detection of a formally 'normal' content of one or another biochemical component does not by itself give ground to assume that this is the 'norm'. The normal functioning of a metabolic chain under investigation assumes not only the content of concrete substances within the range of their normal oscillations but also a normal shift of the contents of these substances influenced by special factors, similar to the shift which takes place in a healthy subject due to the action of the same special factors. For instance, we have found 'normal' contents of gamma-globulinum in the blood of schizophrenic adolescent patients. But, when these patients fall ill with infectious diseases, which in healthy subjects invariably cause an increase of gamma-globulinum content, their blood, on the contrary, shows a decrease of its content. Hence one may affirm that the 'norm' of the component content found was not a 'norm', but a peculiar variant of insufficiency which might remain outside the sphere of the investigator's observation and lead him to an erroneous estimation of the results of laboratory investigations. We have found that such situations are typical for many laboratory investigations and therefore we would like to bring attention to them.

From what has been said, which is not an exhaustive survey of the field, can be deduced the importance and value of the method of comparison by age group in psychiatric research. Many propositions in clinical psychiatry are based on the results obtained by the application of this method. We have only touched on the range of application of this method, which gives rise to many other investigative approaches for the clinical study of the nature of neuro-psychiatric disorders in children and adolescents.

Neuro-psychiatric disorders (oligophrenic phenomena, neurosis-like conditions, epilepsy, cerebral palsy, etc.) are believed to have a 'non-specific', 'undifferentiated', character in childhood; this is not because these disorders present similar manifestations to objective observation but because the clinical characteristics of the course, development and pattern of the disorder, as well as the change of pattern in its various stages, have been inadequately estimated. The interpretations of clinicians, defectologists, teachers and psychologists are complexly intermingled in the estimation of oligophrenic conditions, and this, in our opinion, is one of the causes of insufficient differentiation in the psychopathology of oligophrenia. At the present time, particularly with the discovery of various mechanisms which determine oligophrenic conditions (chromosomal aberrations, genetic impairments, enzymatic disorders, etc.) it is realistic to expect developments towards a more precise clinical differentiation of these conditions. The same applies, as has already been said, to the differential diagnosis of psychopathic-like conditions.

It follows that it is questionable whether it is justifiable to consider that one type of mental disease reappears as another in the same patient (for instance, neurosis developing into schizophrenia, etc.), as well as the validity of the proposition about the 'fluid transitions' of clinical conditions occurring in the picture of residual brain damage in children. With the comparison by age group analysis of development and course of morbid conditions these notions acquire a new meaning, and a new understanding is reached about the significance of disorders lying at the root of each disease entity.

The unity and integrity of the organism, which has been especially well demonstrated scientifically by Pavlov and his followers, also contradicts the possibility of the co-existence of different mental diseases in one individual.

The term used to denote the various mental diseases are only a nosological convenience denoting morbid conditions of the whole organism; these terms have been formulated by physicians to refer, for instance, to neurasthenia, hysteria and schizophrenia, but these conditions are not so well defined in nature. When diseases develop they affect the whole organism, but they may involve in particular one or another of its systems. A combination of disorders of mental activity, following a definite pattern, is given a specific name by doctors. Consequently, the disease is a single entity, and the constant pattern of its development has something characteristic to it, which makes this disease differ from another and attaches to it specific qualities. Therefore, it is at least erroneous to refer to separate stages of a single developing disease by terms denoting other diseases. The nosography, the term by which we refer to a disease, is not all important; the essential is the condition itself, the stage by stage changes occurring in its development, especially in the period of manifestation of the disease. The latter is determined by the whole course of development of the disease. What has been said applies, most of all, to mental diseases, which are diseases affecting the whole organism. The principle of qualifying a disease by the part it affects requires, in this connection, a different logical reasoning.

However, it is necessary to investigate patterns of nosokinesis, the development and course of diseases, particularly complicated in disorders presenting in childhood and adolescence. These patterns cannot be described accurately without a thorough study of preceding and accompanying patterns of syndromogenesis—a definition of qualitative characteristics of mental disorders as estimated by comparison by age groups.

5

Investigation of the Processes of Compensation and Correction of Disorders

The absence of really comprehensive clinical investigations in child psychiatry has resulted in lack of accurate knowledge about the many different factors influencing the development and functioning of the nervous system. We often confine ourselves to references to the high plasticity and compensating nature of the child's brain functions, and we make excursions into the field of reasoning about the connectedness of functions and structures, and their refined mechanism of interpenetration. But, when the structure of a mental disease is thoroughly investigated, nature reveals to the investigator many multiform examples of compensation of clinical disorders. The most common illustration is perhaps the appearance within the limits of every nosological form, of a mental disease both as a variant with a malignant, destructive course and, more often, as a variant with a slow progress and periodical remissions, which has a relatively more favourable prognosis. The study of the laws governing various types of progress of mental diseases, i.e. the explanation as to why in one case the disease develops in a way different from another case, provides the investigator with valuable means of controlling the disease.

Some other characteristics of the course of development of mental diseases are even better illustrations of what has been said. First of all, let us consider the characteristics of the initial development of psychotic and neurotic disorders. We have shown[7] that during the initial period of schizophrenia in children and adolescents the productive symptoms, as well as the pathological alterations of personality, are not of the same type as those found later when the disorder is continuous, but are of an interrupted, unclear nature. We have now observed the same phenomena in clinical models of development of neuroses and psychoses. This meagre symptomatology shows that morbid phenomena, having emerged for a short period, go through a period of spontaneous remission. In the course of mental diseases, these disorders with a prolonged discrete symptomatology are replaced, in due course, by uninterrupted pathology.

The unclear nature of initial disorders may be considered as a natural model, where one can observe not only the conditions of emerging and remitting clinical disorders of a definite quality, but also those mechanisms which provide such unclarity. This is another means by which the investigator may control the morbid process and at the same time gain a deeper knowledge of those mechanisms of compensation of morbid phenomena used by the organism itself. The clinical structure of development and remission of the main syndromes of mental diseases is a model of no less significance, which allows the study of compensation mechanisms. When studying the patterns of syndromogenesis, two main features are immediately apparent. Firstly, the gradual development of a syndrome is not always uniform. Often one, or more, phases of a syndrome may be missing, or may be present in a lighter form, thus changing its whole structure. Or, at a definite stage of development, the syndromes may regress without the disease completing its evolution. Thus, we are right in considering the many variants of gradual development of the same syndrome as a characteristic trait of the first phenomenon. This diversity is determined by complicated co-existence of the features of decompensation and compensation of the respective functional system (or constellation of systems) of the psyche within the dynamics of syndrome development.

The second phenomenon is the simultaneous co-existence, within the structure of a complex syndrome, of several disorders (for instance, depression and delirium, delirium and hallucinosis, etc.), presenting the clinical picture of polymorphisms. Simultaneous impairment of several functional mental systems, or constellation of systems, may be regarded as a distinctive property of this phenomenon.

Thus we can see that by analysing the structure of the syndromes the investigator can gain a still deeper understanding of the essence of compensation mechanisms, which will provide him with a third means of controlling diseases.

These propositions, in their turn, reveal the main aspect of the approach to the therapy of mental disorders. The main mode of therapy in child and adolescent psychiatry should not be by drug therapy, but meaningful developmental therapy, healthy upbringing (*die Heilerziehung*) and remedial teaching (*die Heilpedagogik*).

About 100 years ago, Trousseau, a French physician, carried out a famous experiment; for one year no drugs were given to 50 per cent of all his patients suffering from the same disease, the other 50 per cent were treated with pharmaceutical remedies common at that time. The percentage of patients who recovered was the same in both groups. Despite great achievements in pharmacology, our present clinical practice confirms Trousseau's conclusions.

The main method of therapy for mental disease in the early stages of development should be that of compensation of the impaired functional system from a healthy functional system. To achieve this a great deal of clinical research is necessary, as well as deeper knowledge in the ways in which the organism itself compensates for impaired functions, during the course of a disease. For this purpose our methods of healthy upbringing (*die Heilerziehung*) and remedial teaching must become more selective and single minded. The method of comparison by age groups in this field is one of the main tools for research by child psychiatrists.

6

Main Methods of Clinical Investigation

The thoroughness and depth of an investigation in the patterns of syndromogenesis depends, in particular, on the correct choice and usage of the main techniques and methods of investigation.

The method of perspective study of a disease in a child or in an adolescent is without doubt the best for the collection of sound clinical data. This method provides direct prolonged observation of the characteristics of child development in the period preceding the disease, followed by study of the stage by stage evolution of the disease process, with accurate observation of complex alterations of the structure of psychiatric disorders. The advantages of the perspective method of clinical investigation cannot be overestimated. However, the complexity of its comprehensive application should be taken into consideration; as yet science has not evolved to the point when an investigator can foresee the appearance of a disease in a child. For this reason, this method is frequently used in combinations with other methods, and mainly for the dynamic observation of hospital patients.

Taking into account the advantages of the perspective method of investigation, we should not, however, underestimate the significance and possibilities of the *retrospective method* of disease study. All past achievements, now at the disposal of modern clinical psychiatry, are in fact the result of the retrospective method of study of disease development. When applying this method, it should be borne in mind the importance of consecutive and orderly collection of verified data, which alone will be useful for the application of scientific treatment. The subjective assessment of information from the patient himself, his parents and his relatives may be avoided if every clinical item is checked by gathering data from different witnesses. A rational combination of perspective and retrospective methods of investigation of mental disorders in children and adolescents significantly increases the accuracy of information obtained by an investigator.

The catamnestic method of investigation is another method which could have a wider use in psychiatry. It is well known, that it was the method of catamnestic observation that allowed Kraepelin, for instance, to revise clinical diagnostics in psychiatry and develop his nosological theories after isolating manic-depressive psychosis and early dementia (schizophrenia). The neglect of the catamnestic method of investigation leads to the same erroneous conclusions about the clinical essence of mental diseases; this, as stated above, result from assessing morbid conditions from the presenting symptoms alone. Close contact and collaboration of child psychiatrists with the staff of psychiatric clinics for adults is especially important when applying the catamnestic method of investigation. Experience of investigations in our clinic on a long-term catamnesis (up to 20-30 years from the manifestation of the first signs of the disease) shows that such investigations produce invaluable information about the development of lingering mental diseases, about the characteristics of the stage by stage formation of pathological manifestations in a subject and, moreover, makes it possible to reach essential theoretical conclusions.

In the course of study of mental disorders in children and adolescents the combination of perspective, retrospective and catamnestic methods of investigation remains the most effective and productive. The combined application of these methods, together with constant use of the method of comparison by age groups needs, of course, great cooperative efforts by the specialists concerned, and proves the advantages of a team method in exploring problems in a common field of work.

Epidemiological studies are very important in the investigation of neuro-psychiatric disorders in children and adolescents. Good epidemiological investigations are of special importance in child psychiatry. We need not stress that the complicated process of development of a child's psyche is the result of the many and varied influences of the environment on his life. The epidemiological study of the possible influence of each life situation on the development of the various functional systems in the child's psyche enables us not only to trace the mechanism of events causing pathological manifestations, but reveals the true etiology of mental disorders.

In the past, many child psychiatrists have paid great attention to the infectious diseases of childhood when dealing with the etiology of a number of mental disorders, including endogenous ones. Epidemiological investigations have shown that neither the presence of several childhood infections at the same time, nor the appearance of a 'chain' of infectious diseases bear relation to the origin of endogenous psychosis in children. At the same time, frequently repeated infectious diseases in a child or a 'chain' of infectious diseases undoubtedly modify the structure of his personality considerably, and can influence the development of neurotic disorders and pathological characteristics of personality.

In child psychiatry, great importance is attached to the emotional isolation of the child, to a 'broken home'. Our clinical observations enable us to recognize the importance of 'broken homes'. Statistically, they are certainly more frequent in the anamnesis of children with reactive psychosis, schizophrenia, children with neurotic conditions and pathological development of personality. However, a thorough epidemiological study of the influence of a 'broken home' on a child does not give ground to regard it as the main and single cause of reactive psychosis and schizophrenia.

Thus, epidemiological investigations in this field, carefully and thoughtfully carried out, also allow the assessment of the importance of isolation and the influence of a 'broken home' on the origin and development of mental disorders. It seems to us that such investigations should not be undertaken with a ready preconception. Only a strict scientific analysis of clinical facts offers the opportunity to reach well-founded conclusions on the clinical essence and causal mechanisms of mental disorders. This brings us to another important issue.

It is well known that in psychiatry, especially in child psychiatry, specialists of different countries apply notions and clinical terms the meaning of which is often far from being similar. Psychiatrists, with a legitimate desire to learn more about the clinical essence of mental disorders, plead for a unified criterion in appraisal of numerous clinical facts. Lack of such unified clinical concepts and terms hampers the possibility of using the results of investigations obtained by scientists of different countries, and thus hinders the development of scientific child psychiatry. We believe that one of the international organizations interested in further promotion of child and adolescent mental health, should create a single dictionary which would include not only the periodical list of definitions of mental disorders and their properties, but also a universally recognized meaning of these terms and concepts. Such a complex and important work is needed for coordinating the efforts of psychiatrists of all countries in advancing research in child psychiatry; coordinate research will significantly increase the effectiveness, intensity, economy and control of scientific investigations.

REFERENCES

1. EMMINGHAUS, H., 1887. *Die psychischen Störungen des Kindesalters.* Tübingen.
2. HOMBURGER, A., 1926. *Vorlesungen über Psychopathologie des Kindesalters.* Berlin, Springer.
3. JASPERS, K., 1923. *Allgemeine Psychopathologie* (3rd ed.). Berlin, Springer.
4. KRAEPELIN, E., 1899. *Textbook of psychiatry.* 6th ed. Leipzig.
5. PAVLOV, I. P., 1951. *Complete works*, vol. III., book 2. Acad. Sci. U.S.S.R., Moscow-Leningrad.
6. USHAKOV, G. K., 1959. Material zur Untersuchungen der Atiogenese der Psychosen. *Psychiat. Neurol. med. Psychol.*, 9, 257-67.
7. USHAKOV, G. K., 1965. Symptomatologie der Initialperiode der im Kindes— oder Jugendalter beginnenden—Schizophrenie. *Psychiat. Neurol. med. Psychol.*, 2, 41-47.
8. USHAKOV, G. K., 1965. Clinique de la schizophrenie. *La Psychiatrie de l'enfant*, 8, 1.
9. VIEK, C., 1965. *Schizophrenie im Kindesalter*. Leipzig, Hirzel.

XIV

THE DEVELOPMENT OF ELECTROCEREBRAL ACTIVITY IN CHILDREN

W. GREY WALTER
Burden Neurological Institute, Bristol

1
Introduction

Since the first description of the human EEG by Berger in 1929 the variations in the intrinsic brain rhythms during human maturation have attracted the interest of an increasing number of scientists and clinicians. Unfortunately the problems of technique and interpretation are more frustrating in the study of children than in any other field and few of these have been resolved even with the aid of modern equipment.

Problems Encountered in Obtaining EEGs in Young Children

In order to obtain a satisfactory EEG record the subject must either be completely passive or cooperate to some extent. In young babies and normal older children one or other of these states can usually be achieved, but in young or disturbed children who are too old to submit without question or too young or too inaccessible to understand explanations it is difficult to record for more than a few moments. Furthermore, records obtained during physical restraint or in intervals between active resistance cannot be considered 'normal'. For these reasons many centres rely on sleep records in young children even when these require administration of soporifics or sedatives. When the purpose of the examination is to identify or exclude organic lesions this practice is often an excellent substitute for the usual procedures, but it is of little value in estimating functional variations within the normal range. It is likely that several features regarded as 'normal' in the EEG of young children are really the product of the situation, which must be more mysterious and menacing to a child of 1-3 than to a baby or to one who is old enough to accept and understand explanations and demonstrations. A hospital atmosphere is worrying for most children and the more obvious features—antiseptic odours and white coats are best avoided.

The difficulty of obtaining 'clean' records from restless children is often avoided by limiting the frequency response and sensitivity of the recording equipment, but records taken with short time-constants (less than 1·0 sec.), high frequency 'muscle' filters and reduced gain (less than 50 μv per cm) give a very distorted representation which is difficult to compare with the patterns found in cooperative mature subjects.

When youth is combined with mental disturbance these difficulties and distortions are augmented, often in quite subtle ways. By definition, a child who has difficulty in communicating with other people is harder to put at ease than a normal one of the same age, yet may not be able to convey its apprehension or discomfort. For this reason it is always an advantage to record autonomic and somatic variables as well as the EEG in children—a consistently high or rising pulse rate for example indicates an unusually disturbing degree of anxiety while a high rate which declines to normal suggests progressive adaptation.

Interpretation of Intrinsic Rhythms

Even when an adequate record has been obtained serious problems of interpretation remain and these are still matters of dispute. Everyone agrees that, apart from artefacts, the intrinsic rhythms of the EEG in wakeful children contain a larger proportion of low frequency activity than is commonly seen in healthy adults. Whether these components are in any useful sense slow versions of the normal adult alpha rhythms or signs of separate and distinctive processes is another matter. In many normal young children spatial and frequency analysis reveals components within the normal alpha range (8-13 c/s) together with other features in the delta (1-3 c/s) and theta (4-7 c/s) band. The most useful description of EEG maturation is that during the first decade there is both a rise in frequency of alpha rhythms, from seven to nine or 10 c/s and a prevalence of delta activity from birth to 3 or 4 and theta from 2 to about 7 years.

Such a description is too static to be of much value since all the intrinsic rhythms and transients in the EEG are responsive in some degree to external and internal stimuli. As in the familiar classical alpha blocking reaction, opening and closing the eyes generally affects both the juvenile alpha rhythms and, to a lesser extent, the other features of the resting EEG. Here again, however, strict comparison of age groups is difficult since very young children rarely close their eyes to order for more than a few seconds and babies cannot follow such instructions at all. On the other hand, some events which have no effect on the EEG in adults may produce marked changes in children. The most important of these are fluctuations in theta activity due to frustration, disappointment, annoyance or embarrassment. The common prevalence of theta rhythms in children undergoing EEG examinations is probably due to the generalized annoyance that most children feel in any constraint, and augmentation of this feature can usually be traced to exacerbation of this feeling. For example, if a child has been persuaded to cooperate by being given a toy or sweet, closing the eyes and enforced immobility, or swallowing the sweet, terminates a pleasant experience and this is usually associated with an increase in theta activity which may persist for some time. The same effect can be demonstrated in some adults, but it requires more powerful stimuli to tease the appetite for gratification.

This effect can sometimes be exploited in the study of affective function. The appetitive or aversive value of a particular object or experience can be estimated by observing the amplitude and duration of theta activity when various test objects are presented and withdrawn under controlled conditions. Here again simultaneous registration of autonomic variables can add greatly to the interest of the experiment.

Application of Telemetry

As already emphasized, the simple fact of being restrained in an EEG laboratory may be enough to perturb quite normal children and when there is any degree of psychiatric disturbance this effect may be of paramount importance, overlaying or masking more subtle influences. During the last few years the introduction of miniature transistorized units for multi-channel EEG radio-telemetry has opened a new field and it is now possible to obtain satisfactory records from free-ranging subjects engaged in normal everyday activities, with no mechanical linkage with the recording apparatus. This technique has not yet been applied systematically to the study of children, but since it can be used while they are talking or playing quite freely indoors or out, careful analysis of telemetered records should provide valuable information about the 'natural' EEG (Fig. 1). This procedure will obviously be of special value in the study of disorders of behaviour and where epilepsy is suspected; the incidence of temper outbursts or minor seizures can be monitored without disturbing spontaneous behaviour and related to naturally occurring precipitating factors. Another device of great value in the study of children, particularly when combined with telemetry, is closed-circuit television which permits unobtrusive remote surveillance with greater flexibility than a one-way vision window.

Abnormalities in the EEG

The variations in the patterns of intrinsic rhythms in childhood, and their relation to clinical problems, have been described in detail elsewhere (Lairy, G. C., and Netchine, S.[12], Lairy, G. C.[10, 11], Pampiglione, G.[16], Hess, R.[8], Gastaut, H., and Pinsard, N.[7], Walter, W. Grey[18, 19]). The identification of organic disorders and epilepsy, which is one of the main applications of EEG in adults, is made more difficult by the relative

S.I.M.
7yrs.   FLASH   CLICK

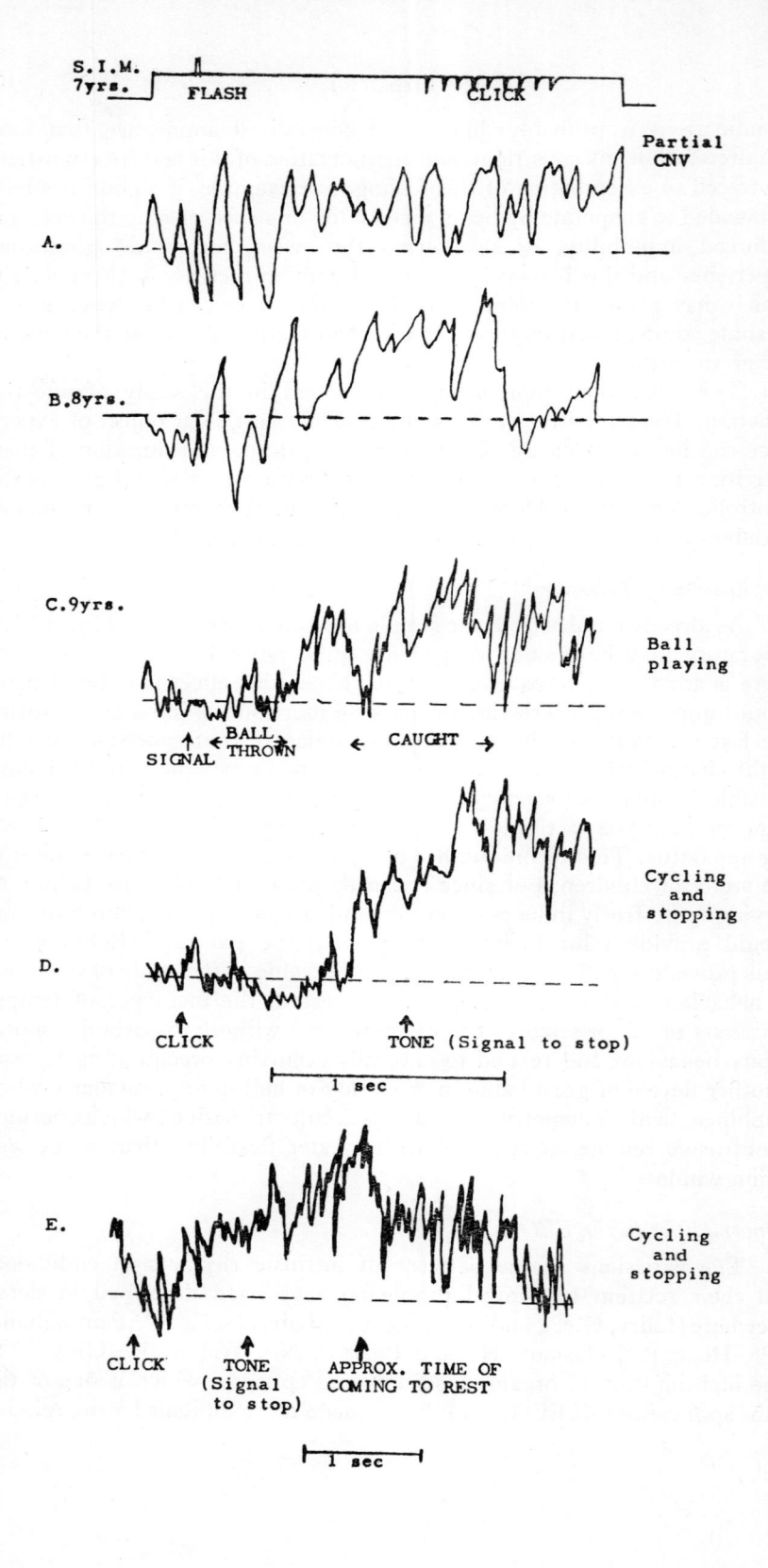

A.   Partial
                                                      CNV

B. 8yrs.

C. 9yrs.   Ball
                                                      playing

         ↑   ←BALL→   ←   CAUGHT   →
       SIGNAL THROWN

                                                      Cycling
                                                      and
                                                      stopping
D.

       ↑   ↑
     CLICK   TONE (Signal to stop)

              |—— 1 sec ——|

                                                      Cycling
                                                      and
                                                      stopping
E.

      ↑   ↑   ↑
    CLICK   TONE   APPROX. TIME OF
            (Signal   COMING TO REST
            to stop)

              |—— 1 sec ——|

abundance in children of slower rhythms which would be classed as abnormal or at least unusual in older people. Persistent asymmetry and paroxysmal features are generally regarded as of ominous significance, but the interpretation of such signs is often debatable. Frequent, rapid transitions between sleep and waking may mimic the abrupt features of epilepsy and the absence of normal slow activity may make an affected hemisphere look more normal by adult criteria. Repeated examination is of the greatest value and indeed the interpretation of any single record should be treated with considerable reserve. Inexhaustible patience and careful electrode placement are the answer to most problems, but these are easier to specify than to achieve.

The most spectacular abnormalities of the EEG in children are associated with the lesions of encephalitis. There is no succinct explanation for the peculiar features of these records, which are recognizable at a glance and appear early in the development of the disease.

Origin and Functions of Intrinsic Rhythms

As in adult studies, the application of the EEG to psychiatric problems is less advanced than in neurological ones. The fact is that the patterns of intrinsic brain rhythms, which constitute 'the EEG' as ordinarily considered, seem to be little related to the mental state except in relatively trivial matters. Since there is still no agreed explanation for these rhythms this is not surprising, but the fact limits the scope of interpretation to conditions in which the clinician is already well-informed. A very simple analogy may help to explain the difficulty. If we consider the intrinsic background rhythms of the EEG as signs of an intricate traffic control mechanism, the traffic lights at brain intersections, so to say, we are not so surprised that the individual vehicles, the neural messages, are imperceptible to us, and that we cannot tell whether they are 'normal' or disordered. An organic lesion may grossly interrupt the free flow of traffic, which we see as an irregularity of the normal rhythms or exaggeration of the slower ones, but anomalies in the vehicles or messages may be present with a perfectly normal and orderly control system. Such an image is quite

---

FIG. 1. (opposite). A. Direct record of average of 12 responses to visual and auditory stimuli with operant response in a normal child age 7. Showing marginal Contingent Negative Variation (CNV) and considerable juvenile intrinsic activity. B. The same, one year later; the CNV is now clearly developed but there are still traces of juvenile rhythms. C. The same subject one year later. Record of average of 12 responses obtained by radio-telemetry while the child was playing outdoors. At the signal (given by another radio channel) an experimenter tossed a ball to be caught by the subject. A series of Negative Variations accompany the decision to catch the ball and persist for over one second. D. The same subject while cycling. A click signal was given as a warning to prepare to stop and a tone to stop. Average of the first 12 trials shows a Negative Variation starting just before the final command and persisting for several seconds. E. The same subject a few minutes later. The average of 12 trials over a longer period shows that with increasing skill the CNV starts at the first warning and begins to decline only when the cycle has actually come to rest.

fanciful, certainly inadequate and probably entirely wrong but any hypothesis is better than none and this one has the virtue of being testable since it engenders detailed predictions.

For example, if we suppose that, as in many road traffic control systems, the stop-go mechanisms have an intrinsic time cycle but can also be operated by the vehicles themselves, then we should expect that when traffic is light there would be a regular rhythm of stop-go at the intrinsic period. When the traffic is heavy the pattern would be disrupted by the local ebb and flow across intersections which would set the mechanism according to the density on any particular path. This would have predicted the familiar observation that the normal alpha rhythms are most regular when the visual traffic is lightest and are disrupted when it is more dense. It would also suggest the tendency for visual signals to 'set' some alpha rhythms and in turn to be regulated by the alpha phase. As a corollary, combinations of signals within certain frequency ranges would be expected to penetrate the system with unusual density; this is the effect known as 'photic activation', in which intermittent visual stimulation evokes large brain responses over wide areas and may lead to epileptic seizures. This phenomenon was predicted many years ago and is now a part of routine EEG procedure. It can happen accidentally as well and has been responsible for many accidents on the road. Some children with petit-mal even give themselves attacks by moving their fingers across their eyes as they gaze at the sky, and 'television epilepsy' is one of the minor hazards of the age.

Techniques for Detecting Evoked Responses

These effects have been the subject of numerous special studies; their discovery attracted attention also to the more general problem—the way in which sensory signals are handled by the brain and integrated to form the basis for perception, learning and action.

Until a few years ago enquiry into the brain mechanisms underlying these higher nervous functions was hampered by great technical difficulties. From animal experiments it was known that the classical notion of the brain as consisting of specific receptor and effector fields was far too rigid; the discovery of the diffusely projecting reticular formations established a new phase of theoretical and experimental analysis. However, the application of these observations and ideas to human brain physiology was only tentative until two technical advances opened the way to new realms of research. These were, first, the development of surgical procedures for the therapeutic implantation of electrodes within the brain and second, the application of electronic computers to the analysis of the very small brain responses to sensory stimuli.

The investigation of patients in whose frontal lobes multiple electrodes had been implanted for selective coagulation disclosed at once that the human frontal cortex is an integral part of the sensory system. All stimuli in any modality evoke electric responses over wide areas, but these responses are highly selective—their distribution and amplitude depend not on the intensity of the stimuli but on their novelty or significance. Furthermore, when paired stimuli are presented the responses to the first of the pair are augmented while those to the second are attenuated. These discoveries suggested that more careful analysis of records from the scalp might also reveal similar effects, but the difficulty was that the amplitude of the evoked responses relative to the background activity is very much smaller with scalp electrodes, which pick up potentials from a large brain area—as well as artefacts due to scalp and eye movements and muscle activity. This difficulty can be overcome by exploiting the redundancy of the brain responses with electronic computation of the average of several trials. As demonstrated by Dawson[4] with this system the background activity, whether cerebral or artificial tends to be effaced, while the responses, being synchronized with the operation of the computer, are steadily enhanced. The signal-noise gain or penetration is a function of the square-root of the number of samples taken; thus with say 12 stimuli the amplitude of the 'wanted' responses relative to that of the unwanted background will be increased by a factor of about 3·5.

With this arrangement, responses to sensory stimuli can be detected with scalp electrodes and these resemble very closely those observed in patients with intracerebral electrodes. Extensive study of these effects in both normal subjects and neuropsychiatric patients has confirmed that the frontal lobes play an important role in normal perception and sensori-motor integration (Walter *et al*[22]). Furthermore, the patterns of the responses to sensory stimulation correspond more closely to variations in mental state than do the various intrinsic rhythms.

Features of Evoked Responses

The principal features of evoked responses in adult subjects may be summarized as follows in order to provide a basis for comparison with observations in children:

1. There are three main categories of response: primary specific, secondary specific and non-specific. The specific responses arise in the region of direct sensory projection (for example in the occipital cortex in the case of visual responses). The primary responses involve only a small area of cortex and are correspondingly difficult to detect on the scalp, but persist unchanged over long periods. The secondary responses, from the specific association areas, are more widespread but tend to habituate with repetition. The responses in non-specific cortex arise over much wider areas, particularly in the frontal lobes, and fluctuate with the conditional significance of the signals.

2. The non-specific responses exhibit 'dispersive convergence', that is, responses to stimuli in all sensory modalities appear in the same widely separated frontal areas.

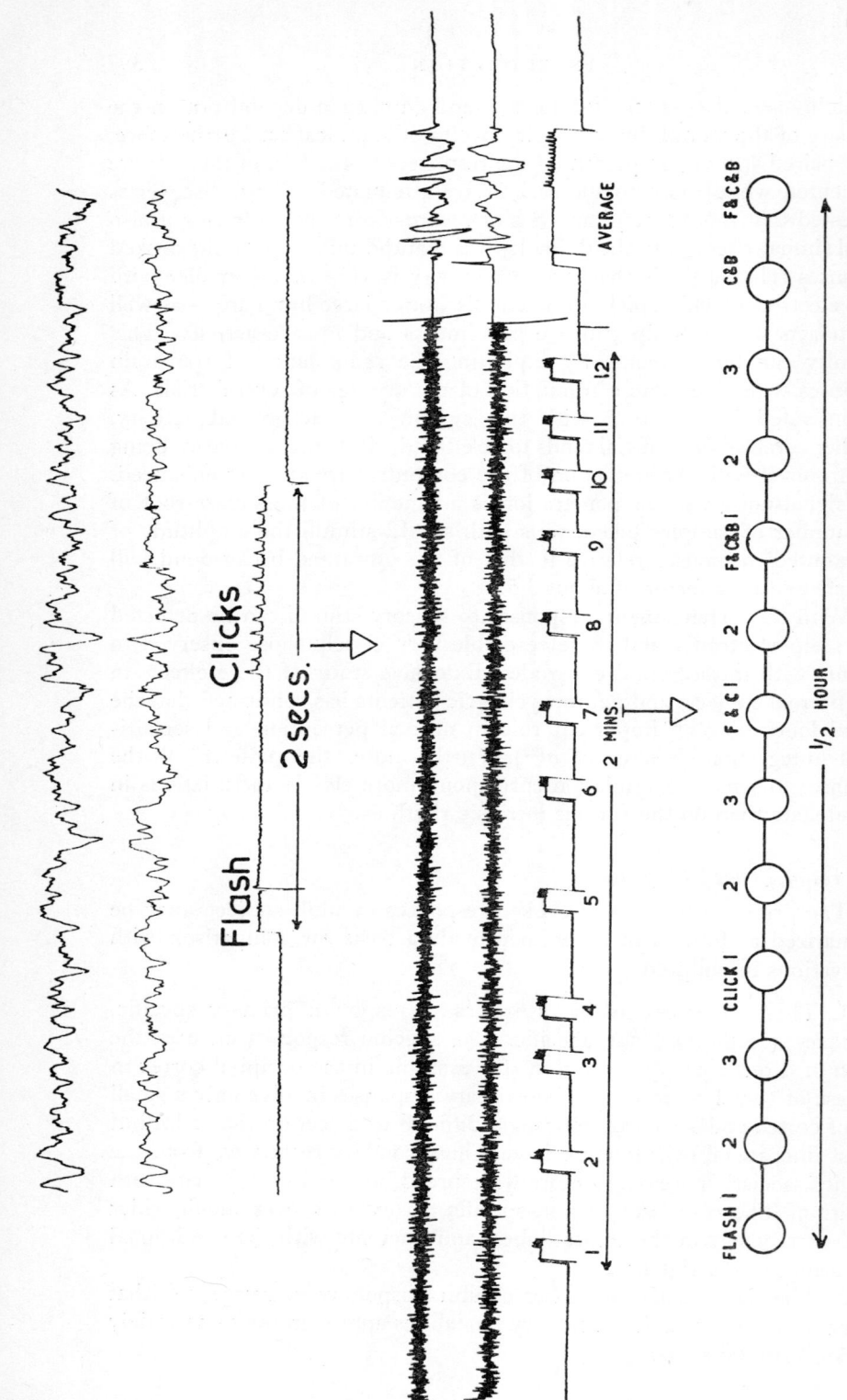

FIG. 2. Schematic illustration of the stimulus program for a standard experiment. Each presentation is during a 2-second epoch over which the signals in 2 EEG Channels are stored in the average computer. Twelve such epochs, at irregular intervals, make up a set of presentations lasting about 2 minutes; the average of the 12 epochs is written out

3. The transmission of signals to the non-specific regions is by 'idiodromic projection', that is each modality has a private line to the frontal cortex. Thus there is no inter-modality occlusion.

4. Non-specific responses have a 'modality signature'; visual, auditory and tactile stimuli from the same brain region have a characteristic waveform.

5. Non-specific responses 'habituate' with monotonous repetition of stimuli, but any change in the character of the stimuli may restore the response.

6. When stimuli are paired in association the responses to the first of the pair tend to increase while those to the second tend to diminish; this is described as 'contingent amplification' and 'contingent attenuation'.

7. When the subject is instructed to respond in some way to the second stimulus of a pair a new effect appears, a slow increase in electronegativity of the frontal cortex, starting just after the first (conditional) stimulus and lasting until the response to the second (imperative) stimulus. This effect has been designated the Contingent Negative Variation (CNV) and is known also as the Expectancy Wave (E-wave).

Contingent Negative Variation

The importance of this last effect, the CNV, is that it is the only clear electric sign of the unique function of the brain, its capacity to form relevant associations between signals. In normal adults the CNV is the most constant and consistent feature of the EEG in a situation requiring attention to conditional associations; it seems to represent the essential link in the brain mechanisms that join one event to another as a basis for decision or action. In order to study this phenomenon special equipment and procedures are necessary. The scheme or paradigm of the experimental arrangement for these investigations is indicated in Fig. 2. This is, in effect, an adaptation of the Pavlovian procedure, providing for the sequential analysis of habituation (or 'extinction of the Orienting Response'), conditional association, operant performance, extinction of the conditional response, equivocation, distraction and so forth.

With this procedure the evoked responses and CNV have been analysed in 90 normal adult subjects, in 70 adult neuropsychiatric patients, and also in 130 normal children and 80 juvenile patients. As already mentioned, the electric patterns of association in normal adults are extremely consistent and take the form shown in Fig. 3. The deviations from this pattern in neuropsychiatric patients are often quite striking even when the intrinsic EEG rhythms are well within the normal range (Walter[21]). In psychopaths the CNV is almost entirely absent although the evoked responses may be quite normal. In patients with chronic anxiety the CNV can be established in a reassuring atmosphere but when the standard tests of equivocation and distraction are introduced, the resulting uncertainty (from which normal subjects recover quickly when association is restored) has a

A.

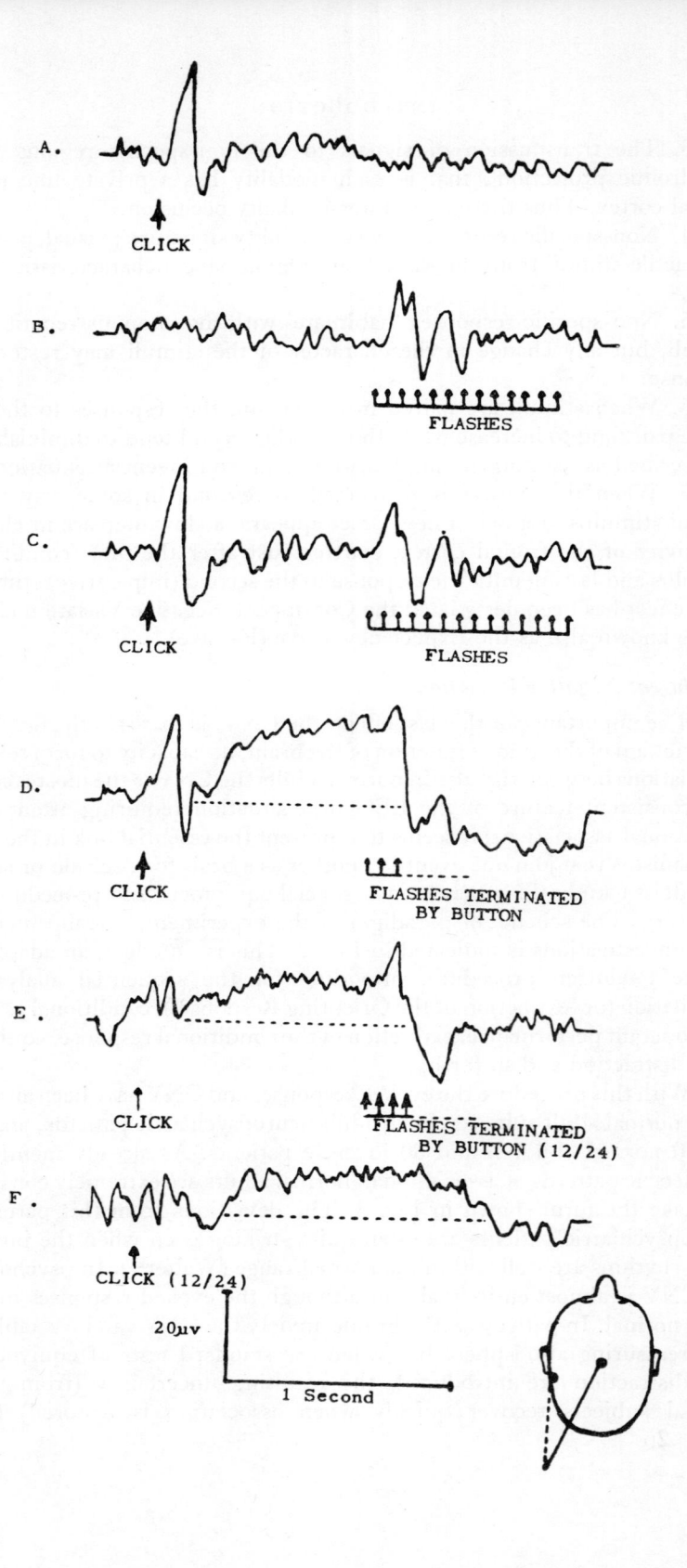

↑
CLICK

B.

↑↑↑↑↑↑↑↑↑↑↑↑
FLASHES

C.

↑
CLICK

↑↑↑↑↑↑↑↑↑↑↑
FLASHES

D.

↑
CLICK

↑↑↑
FLASHES TERMINATED
BY BUTTON

E.

↑
CLICK

↑↑↑↑
FLASHES TERMINATED
BY BUTTON (12/24)

F.

↑
CLICK (12/24)

20μv

1 Second

prolonged effect and the CNV may not reappear for many hours. Compulsive, obsessional states on the other hand are associated with protracted negative variations that long outlast the completion of the operant response, even when this is competently performed.

Origin and Function of the CNV

These observations have shown that whatever may be the brain mechanisms underlying the CNV, they are closely related to variations in mood and mentality. The origin of the effect is still uncertain but measurements with chronic cortical electrodes indicate that the potential difference arises in patches of the superficial layers of the frontal cortex and the obvious inference is that it represents graded depolarization of the feltwork of apical dendrites over this region.

The functional role of the CNV could perhaps be imagined to be as a cortical 'fuse and primer' system, whereby the structures responsible for the initiation of conditional actions or decisions are prepared for discharge at the correct times, in proper sequence and with the greatest economy. It is fashionable at this time to implicate the other main constituent of cerebral cortex, the neuroglial cells, which do seem to contribute in some way to the complex electrochemical transactions in these regions. Of all the electric phenomena in the brain, the CNV seems the most promising candidate for glial intervention because of its slow time-course and wide spatial distribution and also because in appropriate experimental conditions it can vary independently of the evoked responses. This last property suggests that these slow widespread electric waves may in fact be an outward and visible sign of short-term memory; preserving the information contained in conditional or warning signals even when the responses to these are themselves invisible.

The maturation of the higher nervous functions as reflected in these electric responses has not so far been studied longitudinally (partly because they were discovered so recently) but having outlined the general features in adults, the observations on various child populations may now be described in some detail.

FIG. 3. (opposite). Typical patterns of evoked response interaction in a normal adult subject. Each trace is the average of twelve trials. A. Response to isolated clicks. B. Response to isolated flashes. C. Responses to paired clicks and flashes without action by the subject. All these responses diminish by "habituation" if the stimuli are repeated monotonously. D. Responses to paired clicks and flashes after the subject has been instructed to respond to the flashes by pressing a button which arrests the flashes. A Contingent Negative Variation (CNV) or Expectancy Wave appears following the conditional stimulus and submerging the response to the imperative stimulus. E. Responses to paired stimuli with operant response by subject when only 12 out of 24 conditional clicks were reinforced by imperative flashes. The 'Equivocation' is accompanied by attenuation of the CNV and emergence of the imperative response. F. Average of the responses to the twelve unreinforced conditional clicks during equivocation. These signals, being indistinguishable from those that were to be reinforced, also evoke a CNV but this persists until the expectation of reinforcement is dissipated.

2
Evoked Responses and CNV in Children

(The original survey from which this information was obtained was supported by the Mental Health Research Fund, and later by the Medical Research Council and the W. Clement and Jessie V. Stone Foundation of Chicago.)

Subject Material

The first population consisted of 88 children. Of these, 40 were from normal families, 18 were clinically normal but from the Family Homes administered by the Children's Department of the Corporation of Bristol and 30 were disturbed, so-called 'autistic' psychiatric cases. The age-range of the children in these groups was as nearly similar as possible, from 2 to 16. The inclusion of the normal institutional group provided a check on the effects of Institutionalization as such, the majority of the disturbed group being in-patients under Dr Gerald O'Gorman at Smith Hospital, Reading.

Clinical and EEG Features

The patterns of intrinsic EEG activity in the three groups were closely related to the provenance of the subjects, as shown in Table I. Of the 40 Normal children only one had an abnormal record, of the 18 Institutionals 11 were doubtful and three abnormal and of the 30 Disturbed five were doubtful and 22 abnormal. The children with the abnormalities in the Institutional group included two epileptics and one temporal lobe

TABLE I

Distribution of intrinsic EEG patterns, applying criteria used in clinical referrals.

EEG	Normal Family	Normal Institution	Disturbed	
Normal	39	4	3	46
Doubtful	0	11	5	16
Abnormal	1	3	22	26
	40	18	30	88

focus. None of the Disturbed children with persistent abnormalities was epileptic, nor did any show signs of focal brain damage, but eight had very low voltage records of the type seen in so-called 'Athetoid Spastic' children. These findings were in accord with the clinical features in the Disturbed group which included seven children with family histories of mental disorder in one or both parents, one mongoloid, one 'super-female' with three sex chromosomes, one microcephalic, one with both parents deaf and dumb and three whose mothers had been rubella contacts in early pregnancy. Thus only 12 of the Disturbed children were without some clinical indication of genetic or organic anomaly. The heterogeneity of this group is typical of such studies—only rarely can a psychiatric entity be isolated in a population of adequate size, even when it seems to be quite clear cut in discussion or in the literature.

Autonomic Variables

As well as the EEG, the pulse rate, respiration and palmar skin conductance (Psycho-galvanic Response, PGR) were also recorded in these experiments in order to assess the degree of autonomic involvement and its influence on brain responses. In the Normal and Institutional groups the mean pulse rate was 85, with the usual fluctuations during the presentation of stimuli. In the Disturbed group, however, the mean rate was just over 100 and was almost unaffected by stimulation except in one case whose pulse rose from 105 to 170 during the stimulation period. The respiratory rates and PGR patterns showed similar differences between the groups, the Normals and Institutionals approximating to the adult patterns, the Disturbed showing extreme diversity and variability in incidence, amplitude and latency with little relation to the modality or context of the stimuli.

These observations illustrate the importance, already referred to, of recording some autonomic variables in any study of juvenile brain activity. There is a highly significant statistical relation between the autonomic features in these children and the characteristics of cerebral responsiveness to be described below; autonomic excitement is incompatible with orderly cerebral integration. Which is cause and which effect is still a matter for conjecture and experiment, but the significance of anomalies in the electric signs of higher nervous activity cannot be estimated without reference to autonomic function. Taken by themselves the autonomic indicators give the impression that the Normal and Institutional children, although 'nervous' at the outset of the experiments, were easily reassured and encouraged, while in the Disturbed children a randomizing factor had been introduced, affecting all connections with external stimuli and social influences. This could, of course, be a description of the 'autistic' state amplified by the features of the cerebral responses which are the next to be described.

3

Cerebral Responsiveness in Normal Children

Of the 40 Normal children, nine gave responses to visual, auditory and tactile stimuli which conformed with the criteria of mature normality. Eight of these were among the 11 children aged 11-15 but one was only 7. This last was an interesting exception because he was a precocious child, walking at 8 months, talking fluently at 18 months, always top of his class and with a wide variety of mature interests. His autonomic functions were similarly balanced and mature, with a pulse rate of 60 and no signs of endogenous excitement. As well as features approximating to the adult norm all these children retained some juvenile characters. These were: (*i*) A tendency for all responses to all stimuli to be followed by a slow secondary negative component (SNC) irrespective of their context. (*ii*) A

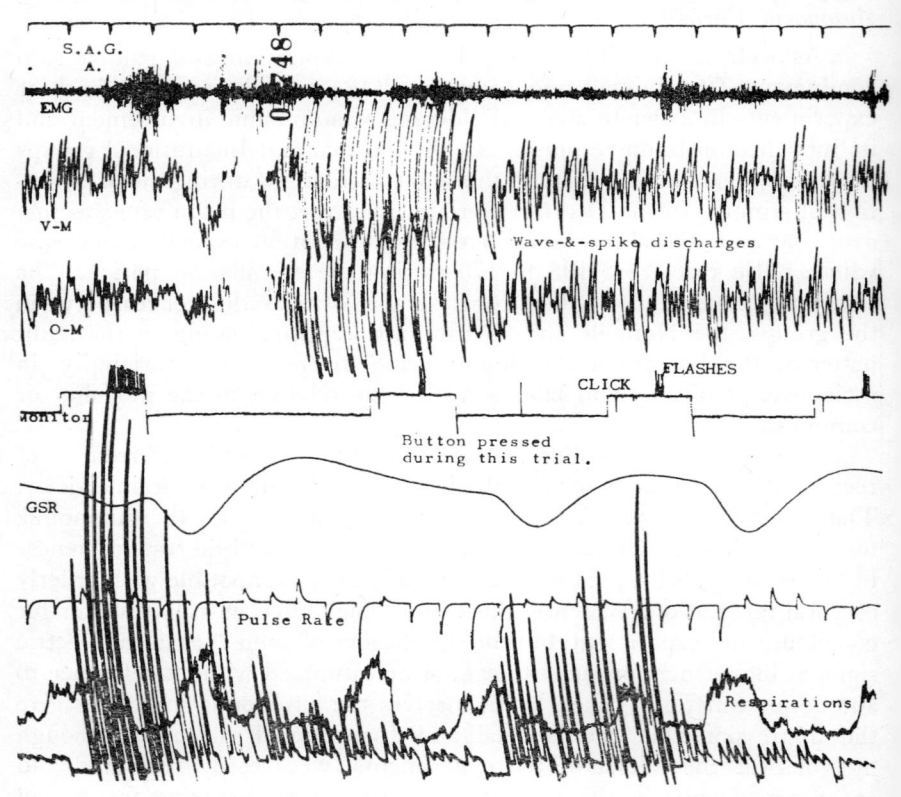

FIG. 4. (A) Persistence of operant response to conditional stimuli during a wave-and-spike discharge lasting 4 sec. The discharge started 2 sec. before the imperative click and lasted throughout the 2-sec. epoch but the button was pressed promptly as indicated by the arrest of the flashes and the EMG of the operant muscles. There was also a PGR to this, to the other trials, suggesting that neither voluntary nor autonomic responses were impaired during the brief seizure, although the PGR latency is significantly prolonged.

wide spatial distribution of the SNC particularly in the parietal region following visual stimuli.

In these children the association of stimuli and instructions to perform an operant response evoked regular Contingent Negative Variations (CNV) only in the older ones, but taking the occasional appearance of a CNV as a criterion of 'latent maturity' the proportion at various ages was 0-4y : 0/8, 5-7y : 6/11, 8-10y : 8/10, 11-15y : 11/11. These figures suggest that from the age of about 6 a conditional association between events begins to evoke an orderly expectancy in the brain even while juvenile mechanisms are still dominant. At this age, of course, the attention of the subjects tended to wander more than with older subjects, and the variability of the CNV reflects the familiar distractability of young children. It also indicates the importance of social influences since the CNV could usually be maintained or restored by repeated exhortation or admonition.

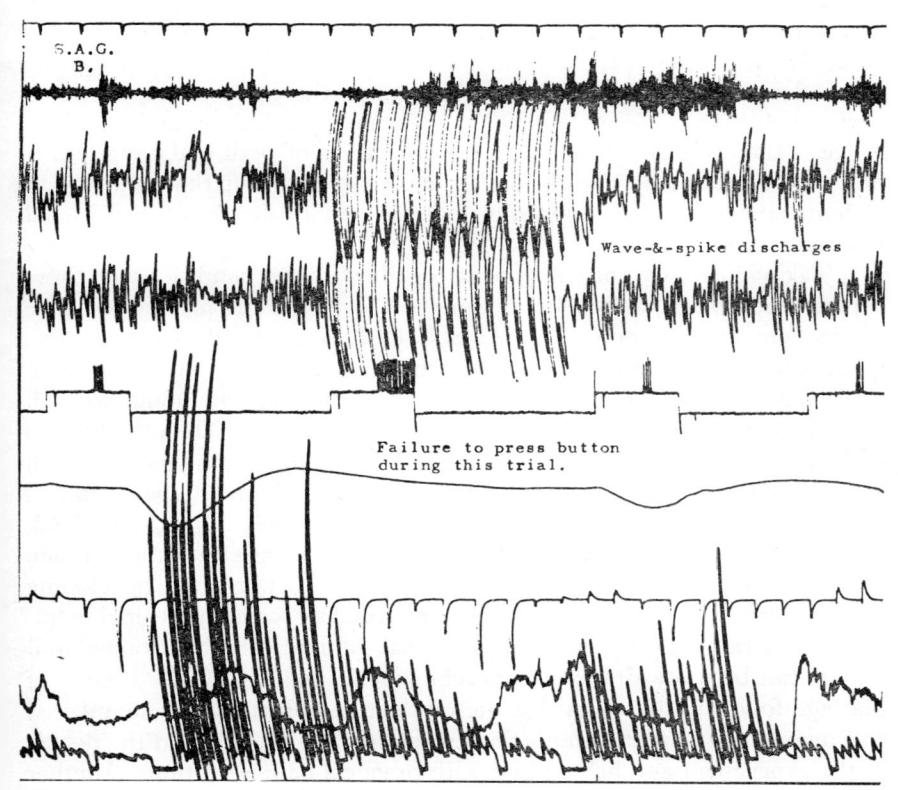

FIG. 4 (B). The same patient, a few minutes later. A wave-and-spike episode lasting 6 sec. prevented both the operant response and the GSR without alteration in pulse or breathing, although the episode began only a fraction of a second before the conditional click. There was a long burst of operant EMG activity during and after the attack following the relaxation when the button should have been pressed, but the operant response to the following stimuli was normal.

In the Institutional group six out of the 18 showed relatively mature interactions, all in the 11-15 age range of which there were 13 from this source. This difference from the Normal group is not significant, nor would it be with the same partition in a population three times larger. However, only one of the five Institutional children below the age of 11 showed any sign of a CNV compared with the 14 out of 24 in the Normal group. Comparison of the 8-15 age groups shows that while 19 out of 21 Normal children showed signs of mature association only 10 out of 17 Institutional ones did so. These figures are statistically insignificant but consideration of the whole picture in individual subjects suggested that the apparent maturity of cerebral integration reflected the extent to which a particular child had been exposed to intimate, varied and sympathetic social influences during his early years.

The two epileptic subjects in the Institutional group provided interesting records; one gave quite well-organized responses while the other gave almost none and had frequent wave-and-spike episodes during the experiment. During some of these episodes the operant responses as well as the cerebral ones were absent, but during others the operant response was performed with reasonable speed and accuracy (Fig. 4A and B). This suggests that the paroxysmal cerebral discharges of petit mal impair cerebral organization only slightly if they are brief and that the tendency to epileptic activity need not interfere with the establishment of conditional interaction in the brain.

Taking the two normal groups together in the conditions of these experiments 14 out of the 24 children aged 11-15 showed mature response interactions and only one of the 34 below 11 did so. It would seem that this procedure reveals in the brain those processes of integration that become dominant and effective rather abruptly at about the age of 11 and are well formed in about 50 per cent of children at the age of 15. When the criteria of 'latent maturity' (that is the capacity to develop occasional although evanescent mature integration patterns) is applied to both groups combined the partition ratios in the various age groups is 0-4y : 0/8, 5-7y : 7/12, 8-10y : 8/14, 11-15y : 21/24. These figures again suggest a rather sudden appearance of transient mature features at the age of about 7, developing rapidly during the next few years unless retarded by social impoverishment. In this age range 7-11y the effects of social influences both sustained and topical can be quite dramatic; one child of 7 showed a CNV typical of that age following the usual laconic instructions but this was augmented and maintained in adult proportions when his father explained the details of the experiment and helped him with practical demonstrations. Another factor that emerged was the importance to children of 'visceral distraction'. In several cases the abrupt subsidence of the CNV was traced to embarrassment by a full bladder, associated with a sudden rise in pulse rate, muscle tension and PGR incidence.

The deliberate lack of detailed instructions and the possibility of visceral distraction may help to explain why the brains of so many children who were obviously quite competent in everyday life seemed incapable of orderly adaptive integration. It is possible that what we may call the '11 plus contingency transition' is related to development of the capacity to learn from independent direct experience. Until this phase is reached the cerebral mechanisms involved are latent, but can be evoked by suitable education and exhortation. This stage of latent integration seems to start at about 7 years: in younger children even explicit and repeated instruction rarely promotes clear-cut and sustained contingent responses.

4
Cerebral Responsiveness in Disturbed Children

The interpretation of responses from disturbed 'autistic' children must evidently be based on these considerations since the definition of their condition practically excludes the possibility of social preparation and reinforcement.

Applying the same criteria of maturity as for the other groups five of the 30 Disturbed children developed a CNV comparable with those in the Normal groups. Two were age 9, two twins were 11 and one was 15. This compares with the 15 children with mature CNVs in the combined normal groups numbering 58. This difference is quite insignificant. However, if the partition ratios of 'latent maturity' according to age groups is considered the contrast is more striking. In the Disturbed group the figures are: 0-4y : 0/6, 5-7y : 1/7, 8-10y : 3/7, 11-15y : 5/10. Excluding the lowest age group, in the combined Normal groups a total of 36/40 had cerebral signs of latent maturity while in the Disturbed group only 9/24 did so. This difference is highly significant statistically.

As well as this striking departure from the normal trend of CNV development the Disturbed children displayed a wide variety of peculiar anomalies. Several had been regarded as deaf and their withdrawal attributed to peripheral impairment. When there is true loss of sensation both primary and non-specific responses are, of course, absent apart from the more subtle interaction effects. In totally blind children, for example (Cohen and Walter[3]) visual stimuli evoke no responses, while stimuli in other modalities often evoke particularly large responses. In the Disturbed children, however, there was a possibility that, as O'Gorman has put it, the perceptual cart has been put before the mental horse. Several of these children did in fact show gross anomalies in their simple sensory responses; four gave no response to visual stimuli and nine none to auditory ones. Not all of these could be tested with tactile stimuli but the proportion of the population exhibiting responsiveness in this modality was about the same as in a normal population. The absence of responses in non-specific cortex to sensory stimuli is all the more peculiar in that all but two children showed clear *autonomic* responses to these same stimuli. Only two patients, one age 3 and one 6, showed no physiological responses whatever. This lack of evoked responses cannot be attributed to youth, since responses can be detected in all modalities in young babies and even in premature infants. One child age 4 showed no responses in any modality but there were large regular PGRs to visual and auditory stimuli with a marked tachycardia as well to the auditory stimuli. There can be no doubt that the sensory signals were reaching the CNS and presumably the hypothalamus but this circuit seemed quite dissociated from the neocortical projections. This patient's speech had been arrested at the 'mum-da' stage since the age of 18 months and she was withdrawn, with psychotic mannerisms. There was no indication of organic disease; the only suggestive feature in her family history was that her father had been treated repeatedly for anxiety and alcoholism. An example of the converse of this dissociation was a Disturbed child age 16, the oldest in the group. She showed clear responses in all modalities with typical contingent amplification and attenuation during conditioning but no trace of a CNV, and in fact a tendency for a surface *positive* component in its place, suggesting absence of participation by the superficial cortical elements. In spite of this clear though limited responsiveness and interaction at cortical level there was no sign whatever of any autonomic response; the pulse rate was completely steady at 70 and there were no PGRs, even to intense stimuli.

Similar features have been seen in a few adults, all delinquents given to repeated acts of violence or depravity 'for the kicks'. It seems possible that when signs of autonomic excitement are absent at ordinary levels of stimulation an action may be exaggerated or extended until some emotion (in the James-Lange sense) is finally aroused. In one such case the equivocation trials produced an *augmentation* of all cerebral and autonomic responses and the patient confessed that she enjoyed the uncertainty of partial reinforcement.

5

Recent Developments

This survey has been followed up by further studies with improved computation and procedures better adapted to children's interests and capacities. The formal operant responses to simple stimuli have been supplemented by more rewarding situations in which the subject can obtain an interesting picture on a television screen by learning to press a button at the right time in relation to the conditional and imperative signals which can also be purely semantic, that is verbal or pictorial (Walter[20]). The results in these conditions are essentially similar to those described above, but interest can be sustained more easily and for longer periods than when crude stimuli are used. The sequence and intensity of the signals are unimportant provided that they convey information of interest to the subject. The effects of fatigue and boredom are naturally pronounced in young children and the CNV can be maintained only by varying the presentations (Fig. 5); for example by arranging for the subject's operant response to project a series of pictures forming a story suitable for the child's age. In older subjects the display can include projection tests, items in an Intelligence test or parts of a formal problem. It is also possible

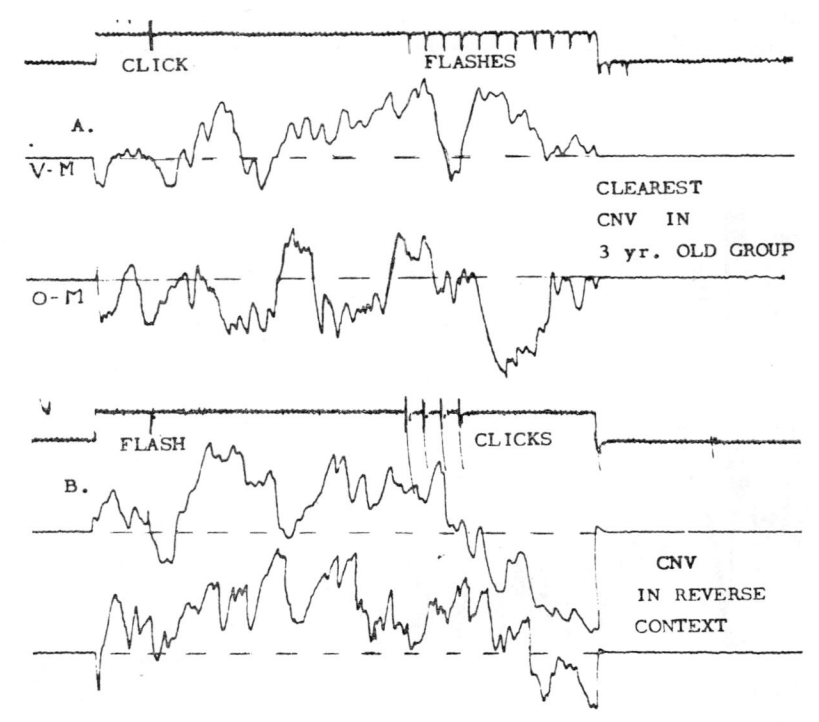

Fig. 5. Interaction of responses in precocious child age 3. A. Presentation of conditional clicks followed by imperative flashes evokes a small CNV for the first set of trials. B. Reversal of signal context also evokes a CNV with a secondary negative component also in the posterior regions following the visual warning stimulus.

for the subject to initiate the process of projection and response computation by his own voluntary spontaneous action. With this arrangement a negative wave *preceding* the voluntary action can be detected, as described by Kornhuber[9]. This 'Intention' or 'Readiness' wave is closely related to the CNV and in fact may be identical with it, the 'Contingency' in this case being association of the events leading to a mental decision with the resultant action.

In adult psychiatric patients these procedures have already opened a new field of investigation and their application to child psychiatry offers hope of re-defining some of the basic questions relating to perception, sensori-motor integration and mentality.

6

Cerebral Responsiveness in Organic Disorders

The familiar application of the EEG to the identification, diagnosis and prognosis in cases of organic brain disease may also be extended by these means. A group of 50 children were referred by Dr Beryl Corner for investigation. They were all between 2 and 3 years of age, and all had

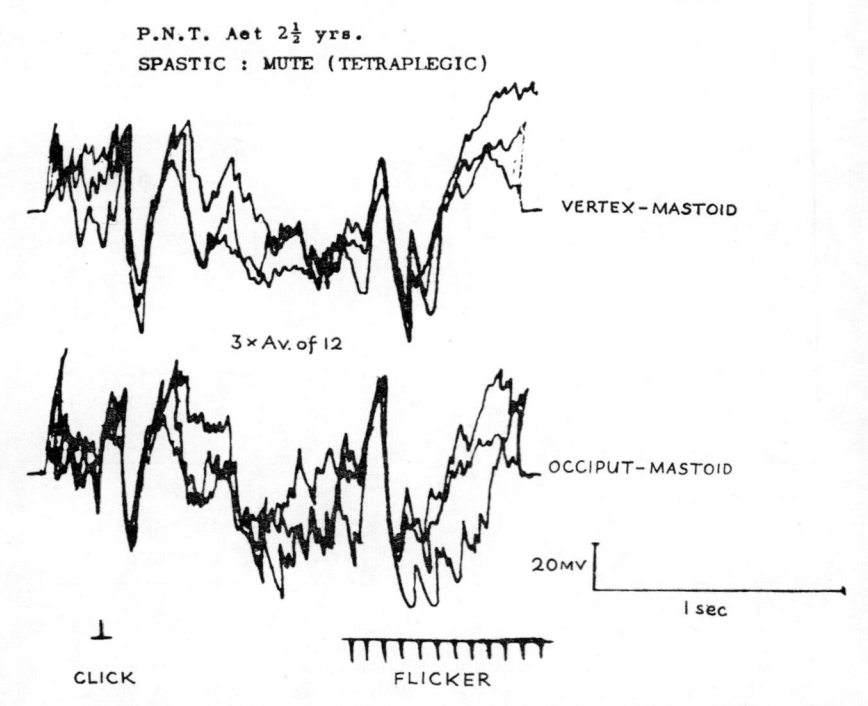

FIG. 6. Superimposition of three averages, each of 12 trials, of responses to clicks and flashes in vertex and occiput of severely brain-damaged child age 2½. The responses were very large and invariant over an indefinite period and showed no spatial differentiation or contingent interaction.

some degree of anoxia at birth. With the exception of two children all were considered to be clinically normal at the time of the examination. One of the two clinically abnormal children, a boy aged 2½, was considerably anoxic when born with some degree of cerebral irritation. At the time of investigation he was tetra-plegic, and died 18 months later. His routine EEG was scarcely outside the normal limits but when subjected to the conditioning procedure he exhibited extremely large, regular evoked responses in all modalities (Fig. 6). These had the typical waveform and latency but they were absolutely constant over hundreds of presentations. There was no trace of habituation, nor did the responses in one modality interact in any way with those in another. The responses to isolated visual stimuli could be superimposed on those following auditory stimuli and vice versa. In this case the frontal cortex, however abnormal, was capable of receiving information in any modality but was unable to process it either for rejection or integration. This case illustrates an important point; the presence of an evoked response to a stimulus is no indication that the stimulus is perceived in any useful sense. It is the modulation of responses by association and action that is related to their functional significance.

Recovery from Encephalitis

Just as the interaction of evoked responses can be used to estimate cerebral maturity during development, so the reappearance of these effects can indicate recovery of function following cerebral disease. This is illustrated by the following case. A boy aged 12 was admitted to hospital in September 1962 after five weeks of headache, photophobia, vomiting and pyrexia, followed by status epilepticus. A diagnosis of encephalitis was supported by EEG and air-encephalograms. He lapsed into unconsciousness with frequent violent movements and grand mal seizures. A cortical biopsy showed evidence of diffuse encephalitis resembling the nodular pan-encephalitis of Pette-Döring. He remained unconscious for six months with several periods of apnoea. Eight months after the original illness he spoke again but without sense and one year after the onset he was almost mute, doubly incontinent, unable to feed himself and flaccid in all limbs. At this time he was brought for special EEG studies according to the procedure described above. These showed normal responses to visual and very large persistent ones to auditory stimuli. The patient could not, of course, cooperate fully and no operant responses were obtained but there were some signs of sensory interaction, the responses to the second stimuli showing contingent attenuation. There was no trace of a CNV (Fig. 7A); in fact there was usually a small surface positive swing between the conditional and imperative responses. These observations suggested that the frontal cortex had retained some capacity for intermodality sensory integration but none for sensori-motor association. This suggested that systematic retraining in very simple sensori-motor activities might help to re-establish some degree of functional recovery.

Similar records were obtained at regular intervals for the next $2\frac{1}{2}$ years, while the patient was undergoing progressive re-education. The liability to seizures was controlled by anti-convulsant medication. Psychological tests were also administered to estimate the level of intelligence and performance. The electrical records, the formal tests and informal observation of the patient's behaviour all showed a steady improvement. The first sign of a CNV appeared in May 1964, 20 months after the onset of the illness (Fig. 7B). At this stage he had relearned to read with good comprehension and it is interesting that two months before, when he could read

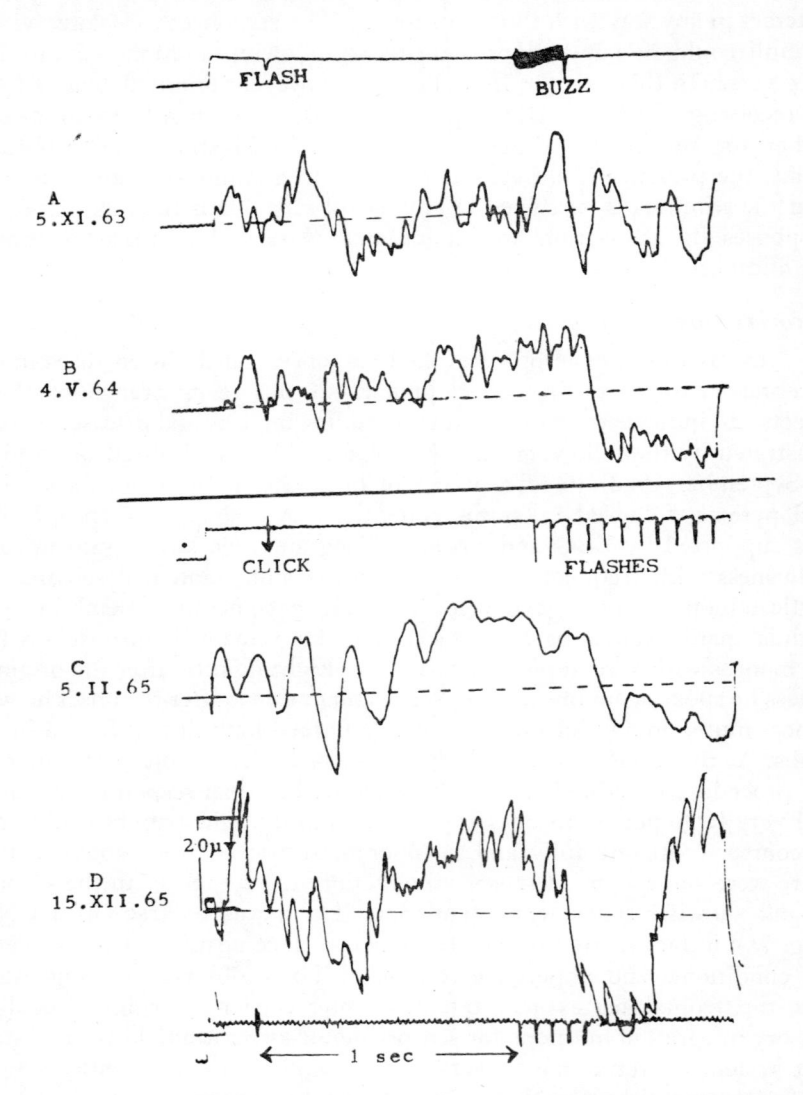

FIG. 7. Growth of CNV during recovery from encephalitis in boy age 13-15. A. Average Responses to associated visual and auditory stimuli one year after acute illness. These were persistent and not interactive and there was no CNV. The patient was mute and incontinent with paresis of all limbs; no operant response could be performed. B. Six months later. The visual responses are smaller and a CNV has appeared, submerging the auditory response. He could now perform the operant response occasionally and was able to read with comprehension. C. Nine months later on the day of discharge. Responses now evoked by clicks followed by flashes. In spite of considerable excitement the CNV is larger and almost within the normal range. He was preparing to return to his old school, with an I.Q. approaching 90. D. Ten months later after three terms at school. He was leading a normal life without assistance. The CNV is within the normal range for his age. This development over two years appeared to recapitulate the normal maturation from infancy to puberty.

accurately but without comprehension, there was still no CNV. From this date improvement was particularly rapid and by December 1965 he had returned to school and his CNV was within the normal range of variation in simple situations (Fig. 7c and D). The only persistent sign of disability was perseveration of the operant response during extinction trials and context reversal. The response patterns were also more dependent on social influences than in a normal child of 15. His physical development was measured by Dr Tanner at the Institute of Child Health in March 1965 when he was 13/8 years. His bone age was estimated at 12/7 and there were few signs of pubertal changes. One year later his growth was considered normal and pubertal development was well advanced.

The striking feature of this case—apart from the simple fact of recovery—is the very close correspondence between the electrocerebral, mental and physical development following the illness. When first seen, the intrinsic EEG patterns, the frequent seizures and the general condition of the patient offered little hope of total recovery, but the presence of cerebral responses to stimuli, and particularly their interaction, suggested that cortical function might be re-established by elementary training, however tedious this might be. The simultaneous appearance of a CNV and comprehensive reading would be expected in normal development at the age of 6-7 years, but this event at the age of 13, 20 months after an illness which must have destroyed much of the cortical fabric, suggests the possibility of some kind of neural regeneration. As already mentioned, there is considerable interest just now in the possibility that some neuroglial element may play an active part in cortical integration. The lesions in the type of encephalitis in this case are mainly glial nodules in grey matter and there is no doubt that neuroglia retains an all too active capacity for growth throughout life. It is conceivable that the dramatic recovery in this case was due to regression of the glial anomalies and normalization of the glial functions during the period of intensive re-training.

7

Relation between Electrocerebral and Psychosocial Development

Attempts to relate objective measures of cerebral maturity to behavioural development have been made ever since the first applications of EEG to clinical problems. Extensive discussion of this problem is one of the prominent features of the four volumes of the proceedings of the Study Group in Child Development sponsored by the World Health Organization[19]. The most promising approach seems to be to use the concepts developed by Piaget and Inhelder, as described in the work above quoted, particularly those relating to transitions between defined mental stages, as landmarks in child development. In this way it is possible to search for features in electrocerebral activity which might also display more or less abrupt alterations and to ascertain whether these two classes of transition are statistically or logically related to one another.

Such an investigation is likely to be conclusive only if numerous longitudinal studies are feasible, since cross-section statistical analyses of populations inevitably blur any sharp transitions with respect to time. Moreover, the apparent objectivity of the EEG is illusory unless some method of impersonal quantification is used. Unfortunately these two requirements are almost incompatible at the present time since refined methods of EEG quantification have not been available long enough to permit longitudinal surveys of adequate extent.

Using various methods of 'eyeball' quantification of the conventional EEG several observers have found that the distribution of the principal EEG features depends not only on the age but on the provenance of the population studied. This was the case in the child population described above, in relation to the presumed intimacy and permanence of family life, but others have found clear differences according to socio-economic level (Brockway et al.[2]), vocation (Liberson[13], Rémond and Lesèvre[17], Béhague et al.[1], Dell and Robert[5], Gastaut[6]), and ethnic origin (Pampiglione[15]). The assessment of the last named factor, ethnic origin, is usually perturbed by other factors; for example children of negroid origin living in London are likely to be of lower socio-economic status than a random selection of the native pinko-grey. However, the observations reported by Pampiglione suggest a significantly earlier maturation of brain rhythm responsiveness in young London children of African origin than in those of European or Indian parentage.

Such differences obviously make interpretation extremely difficult since all the features, both electrocerebral and psychosocial, are multi-factorial and may well be inter-active as well in unpredictable ways. In a careful study of 128 children aged 5-9 y. Netchine and Lairy[14] examined the relation between the frequency and distribution of intrinsic rhythms on the one hand, age and Intelligence (IQ) on the other. The average occipital alpha frequency rose from 8·25 to 9·15 over the five years, with a range from 5·6 to 13·7. The range of variation was much wider in the sub-group of lowest intelligence. Frequencies below 7 c/s were found in 13 out of the 48 with IQ less than 85, in 2 out of 50 in the middle IQ group and in none of the 30 with IQ greater than 105. At the same time particularly *high* frequencies were found only in the youngest group with the lowest IQ This explains why the *average* alpha frequency in a young population does not correlate well with average IQ or with age in a low IQ population. The spatial organization of the EEG rhythms was also studied using an index of ratios between occipital, parietal and central amplitudes. A high occipital frequency combined with restriction of alpha rhythms to the occipital region was associated with higher intelligence, while a low frequency and wider dispersion were associated with lower intelligence.

These findings illustrate the importance of considering the topography as well as the amplitude, frequency and waveform of EEG patterns, in relation to psychosocial factors. The development of alpha frequency and particularly spatial organization in this population showed clear signs of rather abrupt transitions with age; the degree of alpha restriction to the posterior regions falls from the age of 5 to 7 and rises quickly from 7 to 9 years. There seems a possibility that this effect may be related to the transitions in visual perception and thinking as described by the school of Piaget.

In the studies of evoked responses and contingent interactions described above there were also indications of something like critical phases of development. The first phase would seem to be the occasional emergence of the rudimentary CNV with social reinforcement at the age of about 3, the second the establishment of this effect from direct experience at about 7 and the appearance of almost adult patterns at about 15. Even in a normal population of intelligent children the scatter is very wide and, as already explained, it has not yet been possible to follow these developments longitudinally, but the correspondence with the Piaget stages is a tempting inference. The most striking factor affecting the brain responses in these stages is the whole range of social influences; there is a gradual emergence of personal judgement based on direct sensory experience and motor competence. Together with this appears something that may correspond to the 'conservation' and 'reversibility' concepts of Piaget; the child of 10 or 11 begins to regard the stimuli as signs or symbols for action, irrespective of their modality, intensity or sequence, the brain responses involve less and less the specific association circuits and more and more the information-processing mechanisms in the frontal lobes.

These are conjectures, scarcely worthy of the name hypothesis, but with increasing technical refinement and collaboration between medical and scientific disciplines, we may hope for the emergence of a rigorous neuro-physiological theory of human brain development. This will include social factors as well as the material changes in structure and chemistry that more obviously influence the integrative functions of the human brain.

Acknowledgment

The surveys of normal children and young patients described here were made possible by the help and advice of the Parent-Teachers' Association of Henleaze Junior School, Bristol, The Children's Department of the Corporation of Bristol, the Staff and Consultants of the Bristol School for the Blind, the Medical and Nursing Staff of Smith Hospital, Reading, and the Paediatric Department of Southmead Hospital, Bristol. The observations by telemetry were made in collaboration with Dr W. Storm van Leeuwen and Dr T. Kamp of the Institute for Medical Physics, Utrecht, Holland. All the experimental work was done with the skilful assistance of Mrs V. J. Aldridge.

REFERENCES

1. BÉHAGUE, P., RÉMOND, A., ROCHE, M., and LESÈVRE, N., 1959. Étude d'Une population de 440 conducteurs de poids lourds. Rapport entre l'EEG et les resultats obtenus à divers test psychotechniques. *Rev. Neurol.*, **101**, 397.
2. BROCKWAY, A. L., GLESER, G., WINOKUR, G., and ULETT, G. A., 1954. The use of a control population in neuro-psychiatric research (psychiatric, psychologic and E.E.G. evaluation of a heterogenous sample). *Amer. J. Psychiat.*, **111**, 248.
3. COHEN, J., and WALTER, W. GREY, 1966. The interaction of responses in the brain to semantic stimuli. *Psychophysiol.*, **2**, 187.
4. DAWSON, G. D., 1953. A summation technique for the detection of small evoked potentials. *Electroenceph. Clin. Neurophysiol.*, **6**, 65.
5. DELL, M. B., and ROBERT, A., 1959. Routine EEG in aviation medicine. *Aeromed. Assn, 30th Ann. Meeting.* Los Angeles.
6. GASTAUT, H., 1957. Confrontation entre les données de l'EEG et des examens psychologiques chez 522 sujets repartis entre 3 groupes differents. In 'Conditionnement et Reactivité en EEG''. *EEG. Clin. Neurophysiol.*, Suppl. No. 6, 283.
7. GASTAUT, H., and PINSARD, N., 1965. Children suffering from cerebral seizures. *2nd Advanced Course in Electro-encephalography.* Salzburg, Vienna, Academy of Medicine. p. 81.
8. HESS, R., 1965. Children with cerebral lesions. *2nd Advanced Course in Electro-encephalography.* Salzburg, Vienna, Academy of Medicine. p. 52.
9. KORNHUBER, H. H., and DEECKE, L., 1965. Hirnpotentialänderungen bei Willkurbewegungen und passiven Bewegungen des Menschen: Bereitschaftspotential und reafferente Potentiale. *Pflügers Archiv*, **284**, 1.
10. LAIRY, G. C., 1961. Le concept de normalité en électro-encéphalographie. *J. Psychol.*, No. 4, 445.
11. LAIRY, G. C., 1965. Children with behavioural disorders. *2nd Advanced Course in Electro-encephalography.* Salzburg, Vienna, Academy of Medicine, 137.
12. LAIRY, G. C., and NETCHINE, S., 1960. Signification psychologique et clinique de l'Organisation Spatiale de l'EEG chez l'enfant. *Rev. Neurol.*, **102**, 380.
13. LIBERSON, W. T., 1941. Researches biométriques sur les encéphalogrammes individuels. *Contributions de l'Institut Biol. de l'Université de Montréal*, **43**, 1.
14. NETCHINE, S., and LAIRY, G. C., 1960. Comparison of EEG data and intelligence level in children. *Proc. London Conference Scientific Study of Mental Deficiency.* July 24th-29th. May and Baker Ltd., Dagenham, England, 1962, **2**, 378.
15. PAMPIGLIONE, G., 1965. Brain development and the EEG of normal children of various ethnical groups. *Brit. med. J.*, ii, 573.
16. PAMPIGLIONE, G., 1965. Head injuries in children. *2nd Advanced Course in Electro-encephalography*, Salzburg, Vienna Academy of Medicine, 109.
17. RÉMOND, A., and LESÈVRE, N., 1957. Remarques sur l'activité cérébrale des sujets normaux. In 'Conditionnement et Réactivité en EEG'. *EEG Clin. Neurophysiol.*, Suppl. No. 6, 235.
18. WALTER, W. GREY, 1950. In *Electro-encephalography*. Eds, Hill, J. D. N., and Parr, G. London, Macdonald and Co.
19. WALTER, W. GREY, 1956. Electro-encephalographic development of children. *Discussions on child development.* Tavistock Pubs. **1**, 132.

20. WALTER, W. GREY, 1965. Brain responses to semantic stimuli. *Psychosom. Research*, **9**, 51.
21. WALTER, W. GREY, 1966. Electrophysiologic contributions to psychiatric therapy. *Current Psychiat. Therapies*, **6**. (In Press.)
22. WALTER, W. GREY, COOPER, R., ALDRIDGE, V., MCCALLUM, W. C., and WINTER, A. L., 1964. Contingent negative variation. An electric sign of sensorimotor association and expectancy in the human brain. *Nature, Lond.*, **203**, 380.

XV

SLEEP DISTURBANCES IN CHILDREN

MELITTA SPERLING

M.D.

Clinical Professor of Psychiatry, State University of New York, Downstate Medical Centre, Division of Psychoanalytic Education

---

1

Introduction

In any discussion of disturbances of sleep—whether of children or adults—it would be advantageous to define first the function of sleep. In *The interpretation of dreams*[6] in 1899 Freud made a revolutionary explanation of the phenomena of sleep and dreams which for many centuries, although the subject of persistent research, had remained enigmatic. Freud introduced into the phenomenon of sleep an active principle—namely, the *wish* to sleep, that is, voluntary withdrawal from reality into sleep. If for neurotic reasons the wish to sleep is either absent or turned into its opposite, we meet with a neurotic sleep disturbance. Freud has shown that the most common cause of interference with the wish to sleep is anxiety[8]. This anxiety stems from repressed impulses and wishes and is a fear of a breakthrough of such impulses and wishes during the state of sleep. Freud attributed to dreaming an essential sleep-protecting function. By disguised expression of repressed wishes and impulses in a compromise between wish and defence against it, the dream serves the purpose of drive discharge during sleep and protects sleep against disruption by anxiety-evoking unconscious impulses.

It is of particular interest that most recent psychophysiological research into the phenomena of sleep and dreaming seem to fully confirm Freud's early assumption[2, 4]. The findings of dream-deprivation experiments are particularly interesting in this connection. Serious personality changes and even psychotic outbreaks have been shown to occur in subjects who had been deprived of dreaming either by forced awakening, total sleep deprivation or suppression of dreaming by certain drugs[2, 4]. This would indicate that dreaming is not only an essential nocturnal psychological activity as Freud has assumed[6] but perhaps even a physiological necessity.

In 'A bioanalytical contribution to the problem of sleep and wakefulness' Jekels[13] pointed out that sleep on its deepest level represents a danger to the existence of the conscious ego. Awakening, according to Jekels, is not merely a passive occurrence but is achieved actively and with the help of the dream. He ascribes to the dream the function of serving as the waker of the sleeping ego. Dreams, therefore—and this was also proposed by Freud in *Beyond the pleasure principle*[7]—have above and beyond their function of providing hallucinatory wish fulfilment and of guarding sleep, a more basic function, namely: to awaken the sleeper from sleep and to provide a transition from the sleeping to the waking state. Under ordinary circumstances dreams facilitate a gradual transition from sleeping to waking. Under extraordinary circumstances—when there is an acute danger to the sleeping ego, either for physiological or psychological reasons—the dream has the function of *abruptly* awakening the sleeper. This is usually accomplished by a nightmare or an anxiety dream. This aspect of dreaming will be dealt with more fully later in the discussion of pavor nocturnus.

Here again present-day experimental research into the phenomena of sleep and dreaming are most interesting. This research has established that dreaming with its hallucinatory and especially visual imageries takes place during REM sleep (*R*apid *E*ye *M*ovements) and 'that during these phases a quasi-waking level of physiological activity is attained, which does not occur in any of the other sleep stages'[4].

I should like to quote from the paper by Jekels[13] the following passage because it seems to me that this might help us to utilize more adequately the meaning of dreams for our study of sleep disturbances in children:

'It also seems to me that the delicate and cautious process of restitution is evidence of the tendency to protect sleep as much as possible, a tendency to which the wish fulfilling tendencies of the dream may contribute their share. I do not think that the main objective of this function of the dream is to be the guardian or keeper of sleep. It appears rather that the main task of this function consists in its opening up the deepest wells of the life instinct—the wells of infantile sexuality—thus contributing all the libidinal cathexis necessary for the restitution process.' (pp. 184-85.)

2

General Remarks

The subject of neurotic disturbances of sleep was reviewed by Fenichel and others in a symposium in 1942[3]. In his discussion Fenichel re-emphasized that for complete fulfilment of the function of sleep, tensions must be excluded from the organism. These tensions may be determined by external physical discomforts or by psychological conflicts. Impairments of the function of sleep was, he believed, encountered in every neurosis. That sleep disturbances are sometimes relatively slight, Fenichel explained by his observation that some neurotics had learned to render innocuous by secondary measures sleep-disturbing stimuli emerging from repression. He found '. . . that the sleep-disturbing effect is greater for those involved in acute repressive conflicts than for those who have learned to avoid struggles by means of rigid ego attitudes'. Both incipient failure of repression and intensely experienced affects—especially sexual excitement without gratification—apply particularly to insomnia in certain phases of childhood.

As no systematic studies of neurotic sleep disturbances of children have been made as yet, this study represents such an attempt. I have arranged, therefore, the clinical material to be presented in accordance with the phases of the psychosexual development of the child. The basic and characteristic conflicts of each developmental phase are reflected in sleep disturbances which may be considered as typical of each phase. Each successive phase adds its own characteristics to the sleep disturbances of the preceding phases, if the sleep disturbance has not been treated or has not subsided on its own accord.

The occurrence of mild and transient sleep disturbances during the oedipal phase (between 3 and 5 years of age) can be considered a typical feature of childhood in our culture. The severer disturbances of this phase, however, especially the acute exacerbations leading to persisting sleeplessness, are pathological phenomena indicative of serious emotional disorder. A persistent sleep disturbance during this phase can be considered to be the manifestation of the infantile neurosis of this child. There is a definite analogy between these sleep disturbances and the traumatic neuroses of adults with regard to genesis, dynamics, and treatment. This and other aspects of this type of sleep disturbance will be discussed in more detail later in the paper.

I consider a better knowledge of sleep disturbances in children important not only for the purpose of appropriate immediate therapy, but even more so for prognostication of later neurotic illness and for prevention of such illness. I wish particularly to emphasize that disturbances of sleep in children are the first reliable signs of emotional conflicts, and that this symptom precedes any other overt indication of such conflicts in the behaviour of the child.

3

Sleep Disturbances in Infancy

The Oral Phases of Development of the Child During the First Year of Life

A peacefully sleeping infant is the essence of relaxation and tranquillity. It seems inconceivable that infants should suffer from neurotic insomnia, rather than from sleeplessness incident to illness, pain, hunger, and other physical discomforts. Because infants normally require a great amount of sleep, a prolonged and severe interference with it in a very young child should be considered to be of serious import, even in the absence of other signs of distress. The organism of the infant is dependent upon its environment for protection from too intense stimulation which creates in the infant states of excessive tension. According to Freud[8], 'The flooding with excitation of an organism without adequate defences is the model for all later anxiety'. Anxiety is the most frequent cause of sleeplessness in children, as it is among adults. Unless the physical and emotional needs of the infant are reasonably gratified, or until its physical and psychological tensions are relieved, it cannot achieve sleep sufficient for its requirements. As it is not possible to explore the sources of the infant's anxiety directly, it is necessary to examine carefully not only the infant but even more so its environment, particularly its mother and her feelings regarding her child, in the search for the sources which provoke and maintain the state of tension in the infant. Rarely is a psychiatrist or psychoanalyst consulted for such a sleep disturbance in an infant. This is the domain of the paediatrician, and having been a paediatrician myself before training in psychoanalysis I have had rich clinical experience with this problem paediatrically. It is only by chance that I had occasion to see a few cases of severe sleep disturbance in infants in my analytic practice. I should like to present two cases in order to illustrate and to discuss the dynamics and management of such a situation.

In one case, the maternal grandmother was my patient and in her analysis she frequently spoke of her grandchild, an infant of 4 months. She and the entire family were very much disturbed by the fact that the baby cried incessantly, particularly at night, and could not be calmed, even with sedatives. The many paediatricians who had examined the child—even with X-rays—could neither find a cause for this behaviour nor suggest an effective therapy. The grandmother, applying some of the insight and understanding which she had gained from her analysis, arrived at the conclusion that the baby cried and could not sleep because it was very unhappy. 'She sighs like an old person,' my patient would tell me, 'and food has to be forced into her and then she vomits it up. I don't think she wants to live.' Her daughter, the mother of the infant, lived at my patient's house and depended entirely upon her parents who had not allowed her to marry the father of the child whom they considered a fortune hunter. The infant's mother came to see me upon my patient's suggestion; she was very frank about her feelings regarding the baby. In the beginning, she had hoped that because of her pregnancy her parents would allow her to divorce her husband and marry the father of the child. When she realized, however, that they would not agree to this and when she also recognized that this man was a highly irresponsible individual, she would have liked to have an abortion. But she was afraid to do so because of her parents and because of the advanced stage of pregnancy. In the hospital she would have liked to place the baby for adoption but had not dared because of her parents' opposition. Now she felt that the infant was to blame for her unhappiness. She could not look at the child, she could not pick her up and could hold her only with great repugnance. She was aware that the baby nurse was rather forceful with the infant but this did not trouble her; it would be better if the baby were dead anyway. She could not discuss these feelings with her mother, although she felt that her mother also did not accept the child. Her father was so angry that he had not even seen the child yet. Being a genuinely warm person who felt frustrated and bitter about the outcome of her love affair, she was able to accept the interpretation that she was projecting her responsibility for her unhappiness on to the child, and was able to overcome her rejection of the baby. The effect of the change in the mother's feelings upon the child was most impressive. Within a short time, her restlessness disappeared; she was able to sleep and her eating also improved considerably. Contributing factors, it would seem, were also the changed attitudes of the grandparents who began to show affection for the child. Since no other treatment had been instituted and in fact all medication had been withdrawn, the sudden and marked change in the infant's behaviour may justifiably be attributed to the change in the attitude of the environment towards the infant, particularly that of the mother[21].

In the second case, the mother of a 6-month-old girl reported that the child was waking up many times during the night, crying incessantly; even when held by her mother it was difficult to quieten her. During the day her sleep was very restless, and she would frequently awaken screaming and anxious. The child's mother was an over-anxious person who was beginning to show signs of emotional strain which was believed to be caused by the child's insomnia. Investigation proved, however, that the mother's emotional condition was the cause and not the result of the child's sleeplessness and that the mother actually prevented the child from sleeping. Her over-conscientiousness about the child was a disguise for her unconscious hostility. She had a fear that something would happen to the child during sleep and she was constantly watching her. She would listen over the crib to determine whether the infant was breathing and became very apprehensive when it was quiet. She would then fuss with the bedclothes until the child awoke which provided her with a reason for taking the child out of the crib. To advise that the child be permitted to sleep was useless because of the severity of the mother's neurosis which was affecting the child in this way. Treatment of the mother provided an opportunity to follow up the development of this child for two and a half years. The marked improvement of sleep corresponded with changes in the mother's feelings toward her child[26].

4

The Role of the Mother-child Relationship in the Genesis of Infantile Sleep Disturbance and the Role of Infantile Sleep Disturbance in the Etiology of Severe Emotional Disturbance in Childhood

The importance of the mother-child relationship for the emotional development of the child is now generally accepted as a fundamental factor of child psychology. The deleterious effects of a disturbed mother-child relationship have been described from direct observation by investigators such as Fries[11], Ribble[17], Spitz[33], to name only a few. The method of simultaneous psychoanalytic treatment of disturbed children and their mothers introduced by me 20 years ago has opened up new insights for the understanding and treatment of emotional disorders in children[22, 23, 24, 25, 29]. This method permitted me to study (and to modify) the modes of this interaction between mother and child and the subtle ways in which the mother's unconscious feelings are transmitted as well as the child's specific pathological responses. The two cases of infantile sleep disturbance just reported and the material to follow are illustrative examples of the role of such a disturbed mother-child relationship in the etiology of early sleep disturbance of the child. There are no references in the psychoanalytic or psychiatric literature to the role of infantile sleep disturbance in the etiology of severe emotional disturbance in later childhood except for my own contributions to this subject[21, 25, 27]. I have pointed out there, and I am stating again here, that I consider a severe neurotic sleep disturbance in infancy a rather ominous symptom which may be the first and only clinical indication of a psychotic development in later childhood. Adequate assessment of such a sleep disturbance in its incipience and proper management of such a case may forestall a malignant later development. I had occasion to treat a considerable number of children with severely disturbed behaviour in whom sleep disturbance in infancy had been the only manifest neurotic feature of the early life. The atypical behaviour and other manifestations appeared only much later. I should like to present some case material pertinent to this issue:

Case 1. Fred was 9 years old when he was referred to me because of his strange behaviour. After a short period of observation, it became evident that Fred's mother, herself a latent schizophrenic, was in need of treatment and unable to cooperate sufficiently to make it possible to treat the boy in his home environment. He was hospitalized, and while he was receiving psychotherapy in the hospital I worked with his mother. I learned that Fred had had very severe sleeping difficulties, practically from birth. During the first year of his life his mother had had to carry him in her arms almost all night every night without being able to quiet him. Later he suffered from frequent nightmares. According to his mother, Fred had been difficult to manage from infancy but it was at about the age of 6 when he started to school that his peculiarities became most apparent. His sexually uninhibited attitude towards his mother also became apparent then. He shared the parental bedroom and often was in bed with his mother who, on the one hand, was seducing him and, on the other, was very unpredictable and often openly sadistic towards him. While we can only speculate upon his early (first year of life) sleep disturbance, considering it as a result of the intense—psychotic—anxiety stemming from his oral sadistic impulses (this boy later showed definite paranoid trends with severe anxiety), we are on certain ground when we interpret his later sleep disturbance as a defence against overwhelmingly strong sexual-aggressive impulses toward his mother and murderous impulses towards his father. One day, prior to his admission to the hospital, Fred remarked while walking with his mother: 'Don't we look like husband and wife? If you want me to, I could kill father.' To sleep in such a situation meant to expose himself to the danger of being overcome by his impulses and of carrying them out in a state of impaired consciousness. That this was psychodynamically so was corroborated by the change in the nature of his sleep disturbance as a result of his treatment and separation from his home environment. Fred's sleep, on his admission to the hospital, had at first been severely disturbed, but after a stay for several months there he was able to sleep through the night comparatively well. During his week-end visits home, however, he had a very difficult time in falling asleep and developed a ritual. After he went to bed, he would start a discussion with his mother saying, for instance, 'I will fall asleep now. Is it all right?' If she said that it was all right, he would not be satisfied and would reply that she should have answered something else. No matter how she responded to his question, he was not satisfied and it soon became obvious that this was a means by which he wanted to keep her and himself awake. At a later point, he was able to explain to his mother what had forced him to act in this way: 'At first, I was afraid that I might die in my sleep and so I had to stay awake. But then I was afraid that you might die in your sleep and so I had to talk to you to make sure that you were still alive.' Fred because of his belief in his magical powers expected the immediate fulfilment of his destructive wishes, and he tried to cope with them in a way similar to that of the compulsive neurotic. This case illustrates the importance of voluntary withdrawal from the outside world as the active dynamic element in the onset of sleep. In a state of depression and in states of acute influx of aggressive destructive impulses with a decrease in object cathexis, sleep is intentionally avoided because it would mean destruction of the object world and of oneself. According to Simmel[20], in certain neurotic, pre-psychotic and psychotic states, such a danger to life seems to exist from within and sleep has to be avoided for that reason.

Case 2. Mike, a boy of 6½, was referred by the school because of his infantile behaviour which was so disturbing that he had to be expelled from school. From earliest infancy Mike, because of a severe sleep disturbance, had been given sedatives with little effect. According to his mother, he had not slept at all during any night of his first year of life. Between 1 and 2 years of age he became very destructive and unmanageable, but then his sleep improved. At the age of 3, he again suffered from insomnia from which time on he slept with his mother. In this case also, aside from the very pronounced infantilization, the results of maternal seduction were obvious. His mother sometimes allowed Mike expression of his impulses with little restraint and at other times imposed upon him severe deprivations. This inconsistency led to a pathological ego and superego development. The clash with the outside world and society occurred when he entered school. In the treatment, Mike was aggressive towards me, in an openly sexual manner jumping at me, trying to poke at and to touch my genitals. Dolls he would grab, pull their legs apart and poke between the legs. He would pull their arms out, poke at their eyes, tear their hair off, and then throw them to the floor, seeking to smash them completely with his feet.

I learned from the mother that, during this period of his treatment, his sleep had improved remarkably. This could be explained by the fact that Mike was releasing his sadistic impulses during his play sessions. During part of the anal phase, that is, from age 1 to 2, Mike had had a period of comparatively undisturbed sleep. This, as we will hear later when discussing the role of the anal phases in the etiology of sleep disturbances of children, is not what one would have expected in this case. The explanation for this was found in the fact that Mike's mother had allowed him discharge of anal sadistic impulses freely. But she had severely restricted any open expression of phallic (sexual) behaviour and of masturbation. At the same time she was over-stimulating Mike by over-exposure and close physical contact (taking him into bed with her) and thus increasing his sexual tensions.

It is known that the outbreak of a severe neurosis, and particularly of a psychosis, is often preceded by an acute disturbance of sleep. Simmel[20] raised the question: 'Is it not conceivable that the start of a schizophrenic process might be at least associated with a disturbance of the temporary ability to regress by means of sleep?' In this connection again the findings from recent sleep-deprivation experiments are of particular interest[4]. This would mean that under the pressure of intense repressed sexual and destructive impulses sleep has lost its economic function to serve as a refresher for the ego and has to be avoided because of the danger of an imminent psychotic break. It is known that an individual may wake from sleep or rather from a dream with a full-fledged psychosis. The struggle between the psychotic ego, which wants only sleep and which has a strong tendency to regress to its prenatal condition, and the non-psychotic ego can be observed in latent psychotics and particularly in depressed patients. Such patients have a difficult time awakening and getting out of bed in the morning. There is a continuous struggle between the ego which wants to awaken and to turn towards reality and the object world and the other part of the ego which wants to sleep and to turn away from reality.

It is characteristic that such a sleep disturbance initiating a psychosis may show itself resistant to sedatives, even when given in large doses. Illustrative is the case of a 12-year-old boy in whom the outbreak of an acute schizophrenic episode of a paranoid type was preceded by severe insomnia which had lasted many months and resisted all sedation. This boy not only did not sleep but avoided going to bed. He would walk through the apartment all night long spending most of his time in the kitchen where he could keep the light on without disturbing his sleeping parents and sister. This acute and intense insomnia had occurred at the time when his only sister, 19 years old, had become engaged and was soon to be married. Ralph, my patient, had shared his sister's bedroom since he was a little boy. Not only had he shared the room with her, but he had often slept in the same bed with her. When he was ten and had been away with his mother and sister in the country he had shared their room, and he had also had a short period of insomnia then. He had behaved very strangely at this time and was heard mumbling obscene words to himself. He had always been a somewhat peculiar boy, impressing people as mentally retarded (which he was not). He kept to himself, had no friends, and showed an infantile attachment to his mother. His mother rejected him openly; she had not wanted a second child and not a boy. Ralph had been a great disappointment to her. In his case, also, the outstanding feature in his early infancy was a sleep disturbance. Ralph had to be hospitalized and sleep had to be induced by the intravenous use of hypnotics. The topic of sleep disturbance and psychosis will be taken up again in the discussion of pavor nocturnus and sleep phobias.

5

Sleep Disturbances during the Anal Phase of Development between Ages One to Three

Freud ascribed the genesis of neurosis in man to the repression of primitive drives, a factor indispensable for the process of civilization[9]. During the short span of its second and third years, the child in our culture has to accomplish the amazing feat of being transformed from a primitive being into the little citizen of our homes and nurseries. During this period toilet training is at its height or completed, and repression of anal-erotic and anal-aggressive impulses takes place even if toilet training has not been instituted prematurely or harshly. During this period mild sleep disturbances of a transitory nature are therefore a rather common occurrence. Whenever such repressions are excessive and abrupt and additional traumatic experiences aggravate the situation, the effect will be reflected immediately in more severe disturbances of sleep. Additional traumata may be the birth of a sibling (which often prompts the mother to accelerate the training of the older child), surgical operations, and other severe illnesses. Emotional overstimulation and seduction are particularly traumatic because they prematurely stimulate phallic impulses and thus re-enforce anal conflicts and intensify the child's repressive struggles.

B. Bornstein in 1931 demonstrated that the fear of lying down to sleep of a $2\frac{1}{2}$-year-old child was the result of an acute fear of soiling the bed during sleep which had been re-enforced by premature phallic impulses[1]. A similar instance in a child of 18 months was reported in 1927 by Wulff[35]. In this case it was of particular interest that the child's sleep disturbance was relieved through counselling the parents in regard to their handling of the boy's toilet training, that is, by advising the parents to relax their demands for abrupt suppression of anal impulses. More recently S. Fraiberg[5] reported similar observations of sleep disturbance of children during the anal phases of development. These psychoanalytic observations are confirmed as it were by the studies of behavioural psychologists. A. Gesell[12] in his behaviour profiles based on large-scale studies of small children, considered sleep disturbance at this age (from 15 to 30 months) as one of the developmental features of this period.

Management

In the early stages before the sleep disturbance has fully developed treatment may be very rewarding. Very good results can often be obtained indirectly by guidance of the mother. It is necessary to provide substitute gratifications and outlets for anal-erotic and anal-sadistic strivings through physical activity and appropriate play such as smearing (plasticine), tearing, cutting, colouring, etc. It is also necessary to advise mothers to relax their demands for too early and too rigid cleanliness and conformity. In this area one has to be careful to avoid the pitfalls of mothers going into the opposite extreme by not setting any standards for performance. I should like to illustrate this aspect of faulty habit training as it specifically relates to faulty sleeping habits by citing two somewhat extreme cases of this kind, one of a nearly 2-year-old and one of a 10-year-old child.

Case 1. The mother of a 22-month-old boy consulted me because of his severe insomnia from birth which had become progressively worse. From the history and my observation of the boy's behaviour, it was clear that the mother had over-indulged him. She had been afraid to allow him to cry at night because her husband became angry when his sleep was disturbed. She had resorted to hiring someone to sit with the child throughout the night. She was desperate because all these measures including sedatives were not effective. The boy screamed so loudly during the night that the neighbours complained. She then decided to take care of the child herself but soon felt exhausted and unable to cope with this problem. While the mother was giving the history, holding the boy in her lap, he was trying to prevent her from talking, obviously annoyed with me because I was diverting his mother's attention from him. The mother was clearly afraid of him and was capitulating to him, although she seemed at the same time to be annoyed with him. When I told him in a firm tone to keep quiet and to allow his mother to talk, the effect startled his mother. He suddenly became quiet, looking at me open-mouthed, but he did not cry. His mother had told me that he was rather a friendly child, very active and demanding, seldom crying during the day. When I suggested that she let him cry through several nights without attending to him, she raised the objection that even if her husband permitted it, the neighbours would have her evicted. I assured her that I would give her a certificate to the effect that she had taken this course of action upon medical advice, and that if her husband objected she should board him with friends for several nights. This soon proved successful and during the past three years the boy has been sleeping peacefully. This case is a disturbance of sleep from faulty training. That it was rather easily corrected was a consequence of the early age of the child and the fact that the mother was not seriously neurotic.

Case 2. A 10-year-old girl suffered from chronic and severe insomnia to such a degree that she scarcely slept throughout the night. She would fall asleep toward dawn and then could not be awakened. Her father held her while her mother dressed her; when she finally got to school—usually an hour late—she would fall asleep. The school recommended psychiatric consultation. The parents and the paediatrician believed that the child's condition was organic and were sceptical about psychotherapy. The mother told me that the girl had been a very small baby with so 'tiny' a stomach that she believed that she had to feed her hourly during the night. By the age of 2 she would consume a quart of milk in the course of the night. The father had formed the habit of playing with the child while she was awake during the night. When the mother felt that the child was strong enough to do without these feedings, she found that the girl would insist upon having her bottle, clinging to it all night even when it was empty. Sedation, corporal punishment, deprivations had no effect and only contributed to making her a serious problem. She had also, it transpired, shared the parental bedroom from infancy up to her tenth year. She was still usurping her mother's place in the parental bed with the father. The mother slept on a cot.

Returning to the problem of managing such sleep disturbances in children during the anal phases of development, I want to point out that at this stage the counselling of the parents is often the most effective therapeutic factor which also has a preventive value, not only for the specific symptom of sleep disturbance but also for faulty character development. Even when the anxiety resulting from the repressed anal impulses has already led to reaction formation and compulsive traits of character in the child, treatment at this early age is comparatively simple and effective.

Case 3. The case of a 3-year-old boy may illustrate this. At about 1½ years of age he began to have frequent nightmares and occasional night terrors. He appeared to be too much concerned with cleanliness and showed the beginnings of food and sleep rituals. His mother was preoccupied with anal functions, and frequently used suppositories or gave the boy enemas. On his third birthday she gave him a doll and carriage which he had not requested. She was aware that she would have preferred him to be a girl, and could see nothing wrong with the encouragement of feminine traits in him. He had shown a tendency to have temper tantrums at age 2 which she had quickly suppressed. The boy indulged in a form of anal masturbation by sticking his finger frequently into his anus. During a short period of treatment he was helped to release some of his repressed anal aggression. The mother was induced to relax her rigid regime with her son. Her anal practices and preoccupation with the anal functions of her child were explained to her as forms of subtle seduction to be discouraged. It was possible to convince her that she must not take the boy into her bed because she had assumed that this was the only way to get him to sleep after he had awakened from a nightmare.

The practice of taking a child into the parental bed, as a means of restoring sleep disturbed by nightmares, serves only to provide an additional source of overstimulation for the child whose disturbance of sleep itself indicates its inability to cope with its aggressive and sexual impulses. It has the effect of adding fuel to the fire. The remedy is usually to eliminate the source of the over-stimulation which very often emanates from a mixture of parental prohibition and seduction.

6

Sleep Disturbances during the Oedipal Phase between Three and Five Years

The oedipal phase is the classical period of sleep disturbance in children. During this age, from about 3 to 5, almost every child experiences a transient period of disturbed sleep. While most children can surmount this temporary disturbance, we find that some develop a permanent disturbance of sleep, often of a rather severe character. In most of these cases, a very similar setting is found. These are children who, on the one hand, are exposed to sexual over-stimulation, often bordering even on seduction, by their parents. On the other hand, these same parents and with boys especially the father do not allow overt expression of sexual impulses and by their behaviour increase castration anxiety and the conflicts of the oedipal phase.

The repression of the oedipal wishes and the conflicts about infantile masturbation with the resulting fears of castration is reflected in the specific sleep disturbances of this age. In most cases it is mild and temporary, with occasional nightmares and difficulty in falling asleep.

The circumstance under which such disturbances become chronic and pathological I have found always to be a defeat of the child's task of renouncing its oedipal strivings through faulty parental attitudes. Particularly harmful is the suppression of any overt manifestation of sexual feelings, sexual curiosity, and jealousy in the child, with concomitant over-stimulation and seductive behaviour toward the child. This is seldom done in a way which is manifest to the parents, but is sensed as seduction by the child who reacts to it as such. Maids, governesses, relatives are often agents of gross excesses in such pathological over-stimulation of children, dating back to the oral and anal phases of development.

The onset or exacerbation of difficulty with sleeping is often attributed to such various external sources as television, movies, unusual excitement, or frightening experiences. Although many children are exposed to these experiences, only few react to them in this particular way. The fact that only some individuals exposed to the same stimulus develop a traumatic neurosis is an indication that the trauma has activated repressed experiences from the past in those who have a latent predisposition. Precipitating traumata are birth of a sibling, surgery, or illnesses which are interpreted as castration by the child. The following cases will illustrate this.

Case 1. A 6-year-old boy was preoccupied with fears of death for a year and a half. He had had no experience of death in his family. He would cry before going to bed because he was afraid he might die. When finally he fell asleep he would soon wake up in fear. This had become progressively worse. At 5 years of age, when driving past a cemetery, it was explained to him that this was a place where dead people were buried; that their bodies slept there forever while their souls went up to heaven. His mother described him as a model child who was greatly attached to her and very considerate of his baby brother, 1½ years old.

Very soon, during sessions of play therapy, an intense repressed hostility and death wishes toward his brother became evident. This brother had become the immediate rival for the affection of his mother at the time when the boy found himself in the difficult situation of having to renounce the mother as the oedipal love object. His unconscious death wishes against the rival-brother had gained reality with the discovery that there was a special place from which dead people did not return. Fearing he might be punished in like manner for his evil intent, going to sleep became an acute danger which was associated with death in his mind. The mother had in many ways fostered his unhealthy attachment to her, at the same time putting a premium on the repression of aggressive and sexual behaviour. Release and working through of these impulses in play therapy and modification of the attitude of the mother resulted in a striking improvement in the boy's sleep within a short time.

Case 2. Frank, another boy of 6½ years suffered from severe nightmares and difficulty in falling asleep from the age of 4½. The reason for seeking treatment at this point was an acute exacerbation of the sleep disturbance due to an experience in school. The teacher had discussed fire prevention in class, and had given the children a questionnaire to be filled out by the parents. The boy, becoming preoccupied with the fear that there would be a fire in the house, refused to go to bed, walked through the house to see that the gas was turned off and that everything was under control. The mother was also concerned because he was rather timid, did not play with other boys, and was not attentive in school.

Early in his analysis Frank would run out of the office several times during each session to see whether his mother was still in the waiting room and present her with love letters which he either dictated to me or managed to write himself. When later he was convinced that he could reveal his true feelings, he vented an intense resentment against both parents which proved to be connected with having witnessed the primal scene during his nocturnal wanderings, and with the birth of his sister when he was 2. Clinging to his mother was a reaction-formation to unconscious hostility, and his possessiveness of her was his way of taking her away from the father and the sister. The intensification of the sleep disturbance was the result of repressed dangerous aggressive impulses to set the house on fire when everybody was asleep and he himself not fully awake.

7

Sleepwalking (Somnambulism) and Allied Phenomena and their Relation to Neurotic Insomnia

The two cases of acute sleep disturbance just cited are a good illustration for the neurotic type of oedipal sleep disturbance. Both children had a relatively well-functioning ego and superego and were able to handle the intensification of their oedipal conflicts, their aggression, and their sibling rivalry by repression. They were able to maintain repression of these impulses during the day without manifest disturbance of their behaviour. They were able to tolerate the intrusion of derivatives of their repressed impulses in disguised form—in one case the fear of death and of dying and in the other case the fear of fire and of burning consciously, that is, they were able to tolerate a certain amount of anxiety without symptom formation and impairment of their functioning. Sleep, however, to both these children, because they were in a state of acute and abrupt repression, represented a danger, namely, the danger of a breakthrough of these repressed impulses during the state of sleep. They defended themselves against this danger by neurotic insomnia, that is, by trying to stay awake and by awakening *fully* with the help of anxiety dreams when these repressed impulses threatened to overcome the sleeping ego.

I would like to compare the behaviour of these children with that of children who sleep-walk. The essential difference would seem to be that the sleepwalking child is only partially, that is, motorically awake, during the sleepwalking, while the child with neurotic insomnia is fully awake during its nocturnal activities, whatever these may be—getting out of bed, walking through the house, going to the bathroom, parents' bedroom, etc. In contrast to the sleepwalking child, who has amnesia for his nocturnal activities, the child with neurotic insomnia never leaves the house during his nocturnal wanderings, he is at all times fully aware of his actions and has complete recall for the events of the night.

Sleepwalking is an insufficiently understood and inadequately studied phenomenon in children. It is by no means a rare occurrence; to the contrary it is found rather frequently and often in combination with night terrors (pavor nocturnus). I should like to present some clinical material to be used as a basis for the investigation of the dynamics of sleepwalking and for study of the differences and similarities in the dynamics of this syndrome and neurotic insomnia as well as of the prognostic significance and treatment of this type of sleep disturbance.

Sleepwalking children are rarely brought for treatment because of the sleepwalking unless it is very excessive or associated with night terrors. Treatment is usually sought because of other symptoms such as behaviour difficulties, school problems, etc. I have found that sleepwalking children as a rule suffer also from coexisting psychosomatic symptoms, especially from so-called allergic conditions such as hay fever, bronchial asthma, migraine headaches, petit mal, epilepsy, and such. Neither these psychosomatic symptoms nor the behaviour problems, however, are regarded as related to the sleepwalking by untrained observers.

Case 1. Walter was $12\frac{1}{2}$ when he was referred for treatment because of behaviour and learning difficulties. Although he was a boy of superior intelligence, he had consistently failed in most of his subjects but was not left back because the public school rules did not allow this. His parents felt that the best way to handle him was to deprive and punish him. His mother seemed particularly annoyed with him and the father claimed that she behaved in a rather uncontrolled fashion with the boy. I learned from Walter that he was in the habit of waking up several times at night and that he also was an occasional sleep-walker. His habit of waking up nightly and going to the bathroom was considered as quite normal by his parents and since the sleepwalking happened infrequently, they attributed no significance to it. Walter's analysis revealed that he was sexually highly overstimulated and that this, to a very large extent, was the basis for his difficulties. In working with the mother it was found that she had unconsciously identified Walter with her younger brother who had died of acute appendicitis at the age of 8. Walter's mother, who had been an adolescent when this happened, blamed herself for her brother's death because she thought that she had prevented her mother from calling a doctor in time by saying, 'You don't call a doctor for a little belly-ache.' She seemed to have some concern about her son's sleep disturbance, as indicated, for example, by the following remark: 'My brother had nightmares and used to sleepwalk and people say that children who do that die young. I was worried about Walter for that reason and calmed down only when he passed the age of 8.' It was at that time, also, that she gave birth to a little girl and turned her attentions to the baby. Until the early part of his analysis Walter's home environment continued to be a sexually overstimulating one. His mother took showers with him, there was a great deal of sexual play with his little sister, and an unusual physical closeness with the father.

The analysis of his nightmares revealed many homosexual fantasies; e.g., he was run over, crushed by a truck, attacked from the rear, etc. He had had some actual homosexual experiences with boys at camp. At home he would walk around in the nude and sleep in the nude, but he was very much concerned about exposing his body to boys. He claimed that they teased him because he did not have pubic hair and because he looked 'girlish'. Walter had complete amnesia for his sleepwalking. On many occasions he had endangered himself seriously while sleepwalking and leaving the house. Once he was found in the middle of the night sitting in a parked car by a passing motorist, who brought him home. His many perverse and aggressive incestuous impulses could be brought to the fore and worked with therapeutically only after he had stopped sleepwalking.

Case 2. Harry was 9 years old when brought for treatment for a severe school phobia. In the course of treatment it was found that he also suffered from a sleep disturbance which had preceded his school phobia and that he had been sleepwalking during the past year. He also suffered from psychosomatic symptoms beginning with belly aches and diarrhoea and now was sneezing and coughing suggestive of an incipient bronchial asthma. During the past year he had had on a few occasions nocturnal convulsions suggestive of epileptic seizures. The parents, and particularly the father, did not seem to be concerned with any of these symptoms but interested only in getting Harry back to school as quickly as possible. The father had tried every means himself, including severe corporal punishment and deprivation, unsuccessfully before reluctantly accepting psychiatric treatment which he considered a treatment for weaklings. The father had an unusually close relationship with Harry from infancy and had been instrumental in Harry's developing severe reaction formation against anal impulses at an early age. Both parents had been over-concerned when he was little. They had lost one child before Harry was born and another infant when he was 2 years old. It was apparent that the father was trying to shape Harry into some kind of idealized image of himself. Harry was the only child until age 5 when a sister was born.

Harry developed a severe sleep disturbance followed by the school phobia and other symptoms after his father returned home from an absence of two years. Harry was then 6 years old. The psychological records, including a Rorschach taken when Harry was 8½ years old, showed that he was struggling with tremendous repressed aggression and lived in terror of being overwhelmed by his impulses. A tendency to withdraw had been noted, but there were no concrete evidences of disturbed thinking or deterioration of reality at that time. Clinical exploration indicated that a rapid deterioration of personality had taken place in the intervening half year. Harry appeared close to a psychotic break. His nightmares were of such intensity and vividness that he would awaken confused, unable to differentiate between dream and reality. More recently the feeling of reality of his dream images carried over to the daytime. He had amnesia for his sleepwalking. He also had brief lapses of memory during the day which seemed to be the beginning of petit mal. His father had found him on many occasions in the paternal bedroom (the parents slept in separate bedrooms) in the middle of the night. Harry seemed unresponsive, staring at his father, seemingly unaware of his surroundings and actions. His nightmares dealt with violence and death, something terrible happened in them, somebody was getting killed. He had difficulty recalling them and appeared very frightened when talking about them. He had a recurrent nightmare which appeared to be a link to the sleepwalking. This dream dealt with the disappearance of his father, there was a devil in it, and an explosion.

It was found that there was very close physical contact between Harry and his parents, the father being alternately seductive and sadistic. The mother was still bathing him and cleaning him after bowel movements. There was an enormous intensification of both positive and negative oedipal strivings which had to be abruptly repressed because of the intense aggression and murderous impulses against the father. Because of his intense unconscious aggression his castration anxiety was of psychotic proportions. He was turning in masochistic (homosexual) submission towards the father in reality. At the same time he was trying desperately to cope with his repressed homo and suicidal impulses. This was expressed in the sleep disturbance at night and in the school phobia by day. The various somatic symptoms served as emergency outlets for his destructive drives. His main mechanism in dealing with his instinctual drives was to externalize the internal and therefore inescapable danger, which he was trying to accomplish by sleepwalking at night and in the school phobia during the day.

I have dealt with the interrelated dynamics of sleep disturbance of this kind with phobia and paranoia in *Animal phobias in a two-year-old child*[24] and have taken up this problem again in a paper, 'School phobias: classification, dynamics and treatment' (*The Psychoanalytic Study of the Child*, 1967, **22**, 375-401).

When his panic lessened and he was apparently accepting me as his therapist, the father, I believe threatened by this, withdrew him from treatment and placed him in a military school. The father, who appeared to me to be a borderline case with marked depressive and paranoid trends, was inaccessible to any psychotherapeutic intervention. I felt that under the circumstances separation from the sick father was therapeutic in itself.

Case 3. Bill was also 9 years old when he was referred to me because of night terrors and sleepwalking. I will limit myself here to the discussion of his sleepwalking and come back to this case in the chapter on pavor nocturnus. He was the youngest child in the family and the mother's pet boy. He was very much overprotected by her and kept away from boyish activities. Because of frequent nightmares, which he had had from an early age, he had been allowed to come into the parents' bedroom and into bed with his parents. He could never fall asleep when his mother was not at home and, on such nights, he would either go to bed in the parents' bed or wake up shortly after he had gone to sleep and walk into their bedroom while in a sleeping state. The father did not dare to oppose his wife, but did not quite agree with her upbringing of the boy, thought him sissyish and would have liked him to be more aggressive and 'a fighter'. The family standards regarding manners were very high and perfect behaviour was required. On the other hand, the mother exposed herself freely to the boy when dressing or bathing and treated him as the 'innocent little boy'. Bill's acute increase in night terrors and sleepwalking between ages 8 and 9 could be understood as a direct reaction to his parents' being out evenings more frequently than they had in the past. The mother had rationalized her over-concern for Bill in this way: before Bill was born, she had suddenly lost a son at the age of 8 from an acute respiratory infection. Bill, too, suffered from frequent colds and he had hay-fever; and for these reasons the mother had been staying at home most of the time, afraid to leave him, although there was a grandmother, a maid, a 16-year-old daughter and another some ten years older than Bill in the house. When Bill had passed the critical age of 8, the mother became more daring and often left the house. It was then that his night terrors and sleepwalking increased to such an extent that his parents could no longer overlook it. The referring paediatrician who had seen him in several attacks gave me the following description: Bill would either be sitting in his bed, gesticulating and talking, or jumping around on his bed, as though fighting with somebody. Frequently he would jump out of bed, walk around, turn on the water, and perform imaginary fights. When his parents found him near the staircase one night, just attempting to walk down, they became sufficiently alarmed and accepted the paediatrician's suggestion for psychiatric treatment.

In the treatment, Bill at first could not remember anything about his nocturnal activities. After some time he was able to recall some nightmares in which he found himself lost or in danger or—as in one of his nightmares—walking straight into a lake. As treatment progressed he began to remember some of the events which took place during his night terrors and the sleepwalking. The main theme was fights with his father. He also talked in his sleep and would say, for example, 'get into reverse', 'this tackle isn't good'. There was a special sensation attached to his sleepwalking which was always present. It was a feeling that the person towards whom he was walking was coming closer and closer to him and was becoming enormously big. This was very frightening to him. There would seem to be some connection between this sensation and the sensation which epileptic patients experience in their aura. However, Bill did not suffer from petit mal, epilepsy or headaches.

Discussions. From approximately 30 children in whom sleepwalking was a symptom, I have selected those three cases because they highlight certain features which I consider typical of this condition. In my case material the number of boys was far greater than that of girls. It seems to me that this is not an accidental finding but that this type of sleep disturbance may actually be more frequent among boys because of its relation to castration fear. Striking in these cases is the similarity in parental attitudes characterized by a two-faced morality. Under the guise of parental concern these parents permitted themselves release and gratification of pregenital (perverse) impulses of an exhibitionistic, voyeuristic, coprophilic, sadistic nature, at the same time prohibiting any overt expression of such impulses in their children. This leads to a pathological ego and superego development of the child, a subject which I will discuss further in the chapter on pavor nocturnus. I consider this as a specific etiologic factor in the development of sleep disturbance associated with sleepwalking. The oral phases of development are usually satisfactory in these cases but beginning with the anal stage there is a progressive pathological development with intensification during puberty and adolescence. These children in contrast to those who suffer from neurotic insomnia do not have a latency period. The difference lies in the different character structure and the different mechanisms of defence against instinctual drives used by these children. The child with neurotic insomnia by awakening fully from the dream does not permit himself any acting out of forbidden or dangerous impulses in reality. The child with pavor nocturnus and sleepwalking by not awakening fully and by continuing the dream, as it were, permits himself to act out in disguise some of these impulses in reality. I would put the differential emphasis between these two groups on *action*. The sleepwalking child needs to act out in reality without being fully aware of his impulses and actions and with amnesia for them. There is a similarity between this behaviour and that of acting-out patients and perverts. The child with neurotic insomnia, very much like the neurotic patient, can accept fantasy gratification instead of acting-out of impulses in reality.

The dynamic situation, and this is important for therapy, in cases of sleepwalking is similar to the situation encountered in patients with character disorders and acting-out behaviour. As in sleepwalking, so in this type of acting out, repressed memories are not admitted to consciousness and the patient acts them out in some disguised way in real life, without being aware of the meaning of their behaviour. In these cases the patient, only after some amount of analysis and with strengthening of the ego, is able to admit these memories to consciousness and to tolerate them, that is, actually remember them instead of acting them out. In sleepwalking the urge for discharge of these impulses is even stronger while the pressure of the superego does not permit this because they are of a homosexual and sadistic nature and often of a criminal perverse nature. It is of interest that in all these children death, and especially their own death, played a great part in their emotional lives. In most of these cases they were actually a replacement for a dead child which in the fantasy of the patient meant that were it not for the death of the sibling, then his parents would not have wanted him and he would not have been born. This may contribute to an intensification of the self-destructive drives in these children. The sleepwalking child is awake bodily but he refuses to awaken fully and to assume awareness of and responsibility for his actions. The urge to act out destructive impulse seems to be particularly strong and the ability to tolerate anxiety, that is, some awareness of these impulses, very low. It is not coincidence, in my opinion, that all children with sleepwalking whom I have treated had psychosomatic manifestations also, such as asthma, hay fever, allergy, and in one case convulsions—this is rather a further indication of their inability to tolerate tension and their need for immediate—that is, somatic—discharge of their threatening impulses.

Sadger[19] has emphasized the fact that for the sleepwalker the motoric awakening of the lower extremities is characteristic. The legs are used for running away from a danger. Actually, sleepwalkers have a tendency to leave the house. A 10-year-old sleepwalking boy had once walked to a neighbour's house in the middle of the night. He thought that his parents were not at home he said later. Actually, his parents and little sister were all in their beds sleeping. It is erroneous to assume that the sleepwalker is completely unaware of his environment. In this case the boy had very strong destructive impulses directed towards the entire family and in his state it was safer not to acknowledge that they were all fast asleep but to leave the house for their protection, as it were. At another time his parents had found him, again in a sleepwalking state, busying himself at the gas range where he had already turned on the jets. He also suffered from persistent headaches and violent attacks of sneezing which had been diagnosed and treated as hay fever. In the analysis, these symptoms revealed themselves as the distorted and somatically converted expression of severe chronic anger against his stepfather who would often punish him severely by beating and deprivation. Similarly to Harry, this patient too appeared overtly submissive towards his stepfather while his aggressive and homosexual impulses were expressed in his symptoms.

In conclusion, it would seem that the danger from which the sleepwalker wants to run away is an internal one, namely the succumbing to deeply repressed, intense sadistic and perverse impulses which is turned into an external danger similarly to the mechanism used in the dream and in phobias. The close dynamic relation between these conditions and other (hysterical) states of amnesia and epileptic fugues would seem to me to be explicable also on this basis[19, 27].

Typical Fears Associated with the Sleep Disturbances of the Oedipal Phase and Some Remarks on Management

There are typical fears associated with the sleep disturbances of this phase, such as fear of attack, injury, death. These are expressions of the child's fear of punishment for masturbation and his castration anxiety. Typical also are fears of monsters, ghosts, burglars, robbers, kidnappers. These fears on closer investigation reveal themselves as projections of the child's own aggressive impulses directed towards the parents or sibling rivals. The case of 6½-year-old Dick may illustrate this. Up to the age of 5, Dick had been the only child and according to his parents a model child. He was rather timid and passive, openly afraid of his father. He also showed signs of a beginning compulsion neurosis. He had had frequent nightmares from about the age of 3. During the last year, his sleep had been very disturbed and he would come into his parents' bedroom at all hours of the night with signs of great fear. For this reason, prior to the time he started treatment, the boy had been sleeping with his mother while the father slept in the boy's bed. He had fears of the dark, could not stand any noise during the night, and constantly talked of burglars, robbers, and kidnappers. When he was 5, a sister had been born and his parents were delighted with his wonderful attitude towards the baby. The acute exacerbation of his sleep disturbance and his many fears, however, revealed themselves in the analysis as the result of strong sadistic impulses directed towards his sister and mother—at whom he was angry for having had the baby. His fears of burglars, robbers, and kidnappers were a projection of his own aggressive impulses and wishes regarding his sister whom he would have liked to be kidnapped and his father whom he wanted to rob of mother.

Dick's case lends itself also for a brief discussion of some basic principles in the treatment of such sleep disturbances. His anxiety dreams and his night and daytime fears, his timid and effeminate behaviour and his learning inhibitions were related to the excessive repression of aggressive and sexual impulses. In the treatment of the neurotically inhibited child there is inevitably in the course of the treatment a transitory phase of freeing of these repressed impulses from the symptoms in which they are expressed, namely, sleep disturbance and fears. This therapeutic re-education of the child should be carried out preferably in conjunction with the parents so that they do not enforce immediate repression of these freed impulses which the child in the course of his therapy will learn to sublimate, that is, to use constructively. In order to get the child ready for this a part of his neurosis and character deformation has to be removed.

The analyst has to be able to establish a relationship with the child which enables the child to make a positive identification with his analyst in the important therapeutic aspects and to be willing to accept discipline from him. Only then, will the analyst be able to convey the feeling to the child that the child can tolerate his destructive impulses in consciousness without having to act them out instantly. There seems to be a naïve belief that psychoanalytic therapy with a child is permission given by the analyst to the child to act out all of his impulses. If this were so, such a therapy would certainly not only not help the child, but would increase his internal and external difficulties. Being at the mercy of his impulses, he would only get into more serious conflicts with his environment in his attempts to act them out. The child must feel that the analyst, while understanding his urges and his need to release them, will stand by and not let him be overwhelmed by them. If the child does not feel safeguarded in this way by his analyst, he will be anxious and distrustful, looking upon the analyst as a person who seduced him into being 'bad' and thus getting him into conflict with himself and his environment. Also the child always, and rightly so, interprets complete permissiveness of the adult, as weakness, and as a result may become increasingly destructive in order to test how far he can go without being stopped. Every analyst has had the experience in the treatment of children that the analyst's permissiveness is felt as a threat by the child. The child, like the adult patient, wants the analyst to be as afraid as the child himself is of his impulses so that the analyst will not insist upon bringing these dangerous impulses to the fore. The analyst must not fail in this test because it is this specific experience which so many children have never had in actual life with their parents who are afraid of their child's impulses.

Dick's parents were compulsive personalities with very high standards. His training had been strict and discipline in his case meant to deny the *existence* of any 'badness'. After he realized that he did not need to impress me with his gentlemanlike manners and that I neither approved nor disapproved of his actions, his behaviour changed very much in the playroom. He began not only to throw things around but insisted that he could hurt me and that I had to pick everything up for him. While it was necessary to allow him to bring to the fore and to release his repressed aggressive impulses, at the same time his behaviour had to be interpreted and it had to be made clear to him that I wasn't his mother, whom he wanted to abuse and punish for sleeping with father and having the baby. It was necessary to insist that he does not deliberately destroy things, and that he help me clean up the mess. It was also necessary to guide the parents so that they should not restrict him too severely as they had before but yet do not allow unrestrained behaviour. It is the acceptance of the *existence* of such feelings in the child without condemning them which is essential and not the *permission* to *act out* such impulses. To the child such permission means that he is not able to control his impulses, if he is aware of them. Therefore these children operate with excessive repression and denial of such impulses and become overly 'good', passive and generally inhibited. The child has to learn to tolerate them in consciousness and to acquire control over them, instead of either acting them out or repressing them. This is only possible with parents who are tolerant of such feelings but not of such behaviour. Dick, for instance, had never been allowed to smear or to play with finger-paint. He had had a very strict period of bowel training with abrupt repression of anal erotic and anal sadistic impulses. It was then that his sleep disturbance began and became intensified during the oedipal phase with repression of sexual impulses and masturbation. The birth of the sister was an additional trauma which acutely aggravated his sleep disturbance.

Dick's parents, because they felt guilty for having restricted him severely in the past, now tended to go overboard in the opposite direction by not setting any limits and by encouraging release of destructive impulses instead of offering more suitable indirect outlets. This phase of treatment could be managed successfully with the parents. Dick, who remained in treatment long enough after his sleep disturbance had cleared, was able to work through and to consolidate his 'new' personality.

There is a general tendency for misinterpretation of psychoanalytic principles and for mistaking an intermediary phase of treatment for the goal of treatment. In treating sleep disturbances in children one should be aware of the fact that the sleep disturbance is a symptom of the child's neurosis and one form in which the child expresses his neurotic conflicts. It is inadvisable to limit treatment to the removal of the presenting symptom only (in our case the sleep disturbance) because the neurotic conflict, if left unaltered, will seek expression in other symptoms and behaviour. It is also sometimes not desirable to remove the sleep disturbance too quickly because some parents bring the child for treatment only for the inconvenience which the child's sleep disturbance causes them and when other measures have failed to stop it. Such parents will withdraw the child from treatment as soon as the sleep disturbance clears, that is, during the intermediary stage without giving the child a chance to finish treatment. $5\frac{1}{2}$-year-old Roy is such an example. He came for treatment because of a severe sleep disturbance which had become increasingly worse, so that hospitalization was being considered for him. He suffered from nightmares and night terrors and kept his parents up most of the night. His nightmares revealed rather openly his death wishes for his parents;

usually both his parents would be killed in them or disappear in a sewer, etc. Roy would awaken in great fear and, to make certain that they were still alive, he would keep them up with him for the rest of the night. He was afraid to fall asleep because of these nightmares and for that reason refused to go to bed altogether. Roy shared his parents' bedroom from birth. He was resentful of both parents—of his mother who was overstimulating him sexually in many ways, and of his father for being very strict with him and for having intercourse with the mother. As soon as Roy was able to bring to the fore his repressed (sexual and sadistic) impulses, his sleep disturbances cleared up and his parents, mainly concerned with his disturbed sleep and the night-terrors, withdrew him from treatment. I should like to mention one rather amusing feature from Roy's treatment, indicating that he was in the transitory phase. One day he came to my office with a baseball bat which he put down beside himself while we played a game of cards. When I asked him why he needed the baseball bat, he said, 'To hit you over the head in case you win'. He had become outwardly aggressive during this phase of the treatment. That his parents had not given us a chance to work through this liberated aggression was one of the reasons for my regretting his too quick 'recovery'.

I have no follow up on Roy, but I would be inclined to think that he continued in the direction of externalizing his aggression of which his parents at that point apparently were more accepting than of the sleep disturbance. I consider the type of sleep disturbance associated with night terrors, from which Roy suffered, as an indication of a serious personality disturbance, which may become fully manifest in puberty and adolescence.

Four-and-a-half-year-old Ruth was a similar case of sleep disturbance, which had started after a tonsillectomy when she was 18 months old. It was found later that the tonsillectomy had only intensified a sleep disturbance which had been in existence from early infancy on. Since that time, she was up every night most of the night, keeping her mother up too. In the play analysis, it became obvious that there was an additional later trauma responsible not only for the maintenance but for the intensification of her sleep disturbance. When Ruth was $2\frac{1}{2}$, a baby brother had been born. Ruth's envy of this brother was brought out clearly in the treatment. The mother, who felt guilty for her rejection of Ruth and the attentions she gave to the little boy, had arranged that her husband should spend more time with Ruth. The attentions which the father paid to little Ruth only intensified her oedipal conflict. By this time, she had become openly possessive of her father and provocative and defiant towards her mother. Incessantly and with great delight, she played the following game with me: I had to be sick and lying in bed; she was the doctor; she would tell me that I was so sick that I would soon have to die, because I was so tired and did not get enough sleep. In an elaboration of this game Ruth expressed her desire to take her mother's place with the father and to take the baby from her mother. The traumatic effect of the tonsillectomy which

was interpreted by Ruth as a punishment for her oral-sadistic impulses and as an oral castration was brought out in the analysis of her nightmares, especially in one which recurred frequently. In this nightmare she saw a spider crawling on her bed, wanting to take her to the hospital. After telling me this nightmare, she showed me how the doctor had cut off her 'pussy', 'because I'm very bad', she said; and laughing hysterically, she added, 'I and my Mommy have a big one; my brother and my daddy have a little one'. And then she said, 'I could cut my brother's pussy off', and climbing up on me, 'I'm the doctor and I'll cut your nose-pussy off'. A very remarkable change in Ruth's total behaviour took place after this material was worked through with her. Her sleep disturbance cleared up and her parents wanted to withdraw her from treatment. I prevailed upon them to leave her in treatment for three more months during which time I was trying to help Ruth to work through her sibling rivalry and to establish a more satisfactory relationship with her mother. The family then moved. I saw Ruth again when she was $7\frac{1}{2}$ years old. She presented the picture of a fullblown childhood schizophrenia clinically and confirmed by psychological testings, which gave her a poor prognosis regarding accessibility to treatment. I was able to establish contact with Ruth on the basis of the previous treatment experience and to treat her for two-and-a-half years and for two more years during adolescence. She has been able to remain in school, to finish her education, to work and to marry. She has retained contact with me to the present (over 20 year follow up).*
She is an unusual case because of the therapeutic outcome, but she is typical for those cases in whom early and severe sleep disturbance may be the only clinical indication for a later psychotic development. I shall now proceed with a discussion of pavor nocturnus.

8

Pavor Nocturnus†

Pavor nocturnus is so frequently encountered in children that paediatricians and parents have come to regard it as a phenomenon of childhood to be placed in a category similar to certain daytime fears considered typical in children.

If we consider the fact that the wish fulfilment tendency of the dream is to be observed in young children in an almost undisguised way, the occurrence of a pavor nocturnus is a somewhat surprising finding. We assume that in children the ego and the superego are not so strongly

---

* 'The Psychoanalytic Approach in the Treatment of Childhood Schizophrenia,' presented at the Symposium on Childhood Schizophrenia, Annual meeting of the American Psychiatric Assoc., Atlantic City, May 1957.

† Some of this material is taken from 'Pavor Nocturnus', *J. Amer. Psychoanal. Assn*, **6**, 1958.

opposed to the demands of the id as in the adult, and will permit fulfilment of frustrated or warded-off wishes to come through in the state of sleep, with little or no objection.

What then causes children to suffer from the sleep disturbance known as pavor nocturnus?

I should like to briefly review some of the known theories on this subject first, before discussing my findings of my psychoanalytic investigations of pavor nocturnus in children. In *The interpretation of dreams*, Freud[6] makes brief reference to this subject, stating that pavor nocturnus is a nocturnal anxiety attack with hallucinations occurring frequently in children; the anxiety being a result of the warded-off and distorted sexual impulses. In accordance with Freud's view, Jones in his fundamental work *On the nightmare*[14] considers pavor nocturnus in adults as a form 'of anxiety attack essentially due to intense mental conflict, centring around some repressed component of the psychosexual instinct'.

Since pavor nocturnus is essentially a phenomenon of childhood, it is a matter of some surprise that the psychodynamic factors have been almost exclusively reconstructed from adult analysis, and that its investigation thus far has not been approached more directly through study in children. A case in 1935 reported by J. Waelder[34] of a 7-year-old boy who had pavor nocturnus, corroborated Freud's concepts of the sexual nature of warded-off instinctual wishes in the genesis of pavor nocturnus. M. Klein[15] stressed the role of aggressive impulses in pavor nocturnus. J. Waelder and others who have observed pavor nocturnus in children are impressed with the phenomenological differences between this manifestation in children and the nightmare syndrome of the adult. J. Waelder[34] considers pavor nocturnus essentially a childhood phenomenon.

The pavor nocturnus of childhood as I have studied it in children of all ages, from 2 years to adolescence, has manifestations that do not occur in the nightmare of adults. Jones[14] considers three features as being essential characteristics for the adult nightmares: (*i*) agonizing fear; (*ii*) a feeling of oppression with a sense of suffocation; (*iii*) the feeling of utter helplessness and paralysis. These features, although present at times in children, are in many cases missing from the pavor nocturnus picture of childhood. In fact, in most cases, the pavor nocturnus in children is characterized by hypermotility rather than by the paralysis characteristic of the adult. In her detailed account of the psychoanalysis of the 7-year-old boy, J. Waelder[34] describes the pavor nocturnus attacks in which the boy would suddenly awaken, sit up in bed, cry out, scream, thrash about with his body and arms as if he were fighting. He was obviously acting out a dream, and although he was talking and moving about, he was neither completely awake nor actually asleep. In the case of J. Waelder, psychoanalytic study of the pavor nocturnus brought out another major difference between the pavor nocturnus in children and the nightmare of the adult, namely the vivid recall of the content of the nightmare by the adult, and the retrograde amnesia for the pavor nocturnus attack in the child. In some cases, adults' nightmares may have a recurrent theme and, in a way, remain with the patient during his waking state as a conscious memory. Although this type of behaviour does occur frequently in children, the pavor nocturnus in which there is hypermotility and retrograde amnesia is decidedly characteristic for children.

On the basis of clinical observations and dynamic considerations I am suggesting to differentiate between three types of pavor nocturnus in children. I would like to discuss their clinical criteria, their etiology and their dynamics as well as the prognostic significance of this symptom for the future development of the child.

Type I: Pavor nocturnus with hypermotility, psychotic-like behaviour during the attack and retrograde amnesia for it.

Type II: Is characterized by a sudden onset of pavor nocturnus dramatically following a specific trauma. This type is, from the etiologic, phenomenologic and dynamic points of view, closely related to the traumatic neurosis of the adult. In fact, this type of pavor nocturnus may be regarded as representing the initial phase of the traumatic neurosis of the child, and might well be referred to as the traumatic type of pavor nocturnus.

Type III: Is characterized by the occurrence of nightmares with varying contents during sleep, from which the child awakens fully, in anxiety, and with a vivid and often lasting memory of the contents of the dream. Often the parents may not even be aware that their child suffers from this type of pavor nocturnus, because these children frequently lie awake in anxiety for many hours during the night, but do not disturb their parents' sleep. These children suffer comparatively 'silently', as it were, while the children of the first group are rather noisy during the attack and always manage to awaken and to disturb the parents. This form of pavor nocturnus may be called the neurotic type. It is most closely related to nightmare syndromes of the adult. In this group also belong the milder and transitional forms of Type I and Type II.

In Type I, the psychotic type of pavor nocturnus, there is an early and insidious onset of the pavor nocturnus, with marked intensification during the anal and particularly the oedipal phases. Both the positive and negative oedipal strivings are highly intensified with repressed murderous impulses toward both parents, and there is a progressive course during latency, extending into puberty. These children grow up in an atmosphere of varying degrees of continuous sexual over-stimulation by one or both parents, older siblings, or other adults in the child's environment; e.g. they are permitted to witness or even to participate in all kinds of sexual intimacies between their parents. They usually share or have shared the parental bed or bedroom for long periods of time. These parents use the child for gratification of their own perverse sexual needs (coprophilic, exhibitionistic, voyeuristic, sadistic, homosexual) with various rationalizations, while the child's overt sexual expressions and activities are repudiated, often in peremptory and cruel fashion. This two-faced moralistic attitude of the parents leads to a pathological development of the superego with specific structuring of it, namely a 'split of the superego'. The mechanism of the splitting of the superego was first described by M. Klein[16] who considered it to be a mechanism 'analogous to and closely connected with projection'. Otto E. Sperling[32], using the same term, developed his concept of the 'split of the superego' from the psychoanalytic study of perversions in adults. He found that part of the superego of these patients not only condoned but, in fact, demanded the patient's perverse behaviour. The corrupted superego of the child, prevented from unification and consolidation by the inconsistencies of his parents, is not opposed to the breakthrough and acting out of the forbidden impulses in a state in which the child is not asleep and yet not fully awake. The dynamics of this type of pavor nocturnus would bear out the validity of Simmel's ideas[20] concerning the relation of sleep and psychosis. Simmel stressed the disturbance in psychotic states of the ability to awaken during the day. There is a great similarity between this dream state with motoric awakening in pavor nocturnus and certain psychotic states.

Pavor nocturnus, Type I, can be considered as a psychotic episode occurring under the special condition of sleep; it is limited to the night time and is without recall for the events of the night. The interrelation between the pavor nocturnus of this type with somnambulistic states, petit mal, fugue, states of amnesia and psychosis has been pointed out in the section on Somnambulism. It is beyond the scope of this paper to do more than point to the possible transitions between these states. One factor of paramount importance should be emphasized here, namely the prognostic significance of this type of persistent pavor nocturnus as a possible indication for a later psychotic development. Conversely, any study of psychotic behaviour in children bears inquiry into the incidence of an earlier pavor nocturnus pattern as we have seen in the foregoing sections on sleep disturbance in infancy.

Two clinical examples may illustrate these points.

Case 1. 9-year-old Bill, whose sleepwalking has been discussed in the section on Somnambulism, is of particular interest because his development was followed up to adulthood. He was treated by me from age 9 to 11 and then again from age 15 to $17\frac{1}{2}$, and seen for shorter periods until age 20, at which time he started full analysis which terminated after three years. His was a typical case of pavor nocturnus, Type I, with early onset, severe exacerbation during latency and into puberty. All the factors which I consider of etiological significance in such cases were found in almost pure culture in the case of Bill, aggravated by a particularly neurotic mother, a seductive father and a 10-year-older brother. In his pavor nocturnus attacks Bill would be sitting in bed, talking and gesticulating, or jumping around and engaging in imaginary fights. Invariably he would end up in his parents' bedroom and remain there for the rest of the night. In treatment, he succeeded in lifting the amnesia for some of his pavor nocturnus attacks, especially those in which he was duelling with his father.

Since the pavor nocturnus attacks had ceased and the boy appeared to be functioning very well, the parents considered him cured and discontinued treatment when he was 11 years old. Bill was seen by me again at the age of 15. According to his parents, he had done very well until he became excessively preoccupied with his violin and wanted to quit school. His loss of interest in his studies was the primary concern of his parents who were unable to appreciate the boy's serious condition. However, they consented to further treatment.

Bill was withdrawn and distrustful; he appeared very close to a psychotic break. The analysis of his nightmares, of his sadomasochistic fantasies, of his preoccupation with sexual crimes and criminal perverts, and of his fears of homosexuality brought great relief of his panic. The summary of the Rorschach taken when Bill was 16 years old states: 'On the whole, the impression is of a very bright, gifted boy, who is suffering from a paranoid schizophrenia. There is no danger of immediate overt psychotic breakdown, but the schizophrenic process would seem progressive and pervasive.' While I did not share the pessimistic prognosis based on the Rorschach and the opinions of consulting psychiatrists, this Rorschach is here cited in support of my belief of the close interrelation of the pavor nocturnus, Type I, with psychosis.

At 17½, Bill was well enough to go to an out-of-town college and function in a college community. At 20, analysis was suggested so that he could work out many unresolved problems, especially his latent homosexuality and his relationship with women. The outbreak of a frank psychosis in early adolescence in this case had been prevented, I am convinced, through the earlier treatment; it is my belief that the final outcome of untreated severe cases of pavor nocturnus of Type I is psychotic development. I have a twelve-year follow up on Bill. He has been able to chose and to pursue successfully a difficult professional career. He is married, the father of two children, and leads a very satisfactory life.

Case 2. I should like to cite briefly a case of pavor nocturnus, Type I, in another 9-year-old boy whom I did not treat but whose mother was in analysis with me for several years. Her analysis, undertaken for reasons unrelated to her son's disturbance, disclosed a particularly intimate relationship between the boy and herself. She would think of him as her 'little husband' since he looked like her husband, and was lovingly attached to her, while she felt that her husband, who suffered from a chronic depression, was often detached and distant. Arnold was apparently accorded some privileges of a husband by his mother; he could lie down with her and fondle her breasts, tell her what to wear and how pretty she looked. She expressed annoyance about Arnold's excessive masturbation in her presence.

Arnold would awaken during the night, cry and fail to recognize his environment. When he was 3½ years old and a brother was born, there was an increase and intensification of the pavor nocturnus attacks. When he was 5 years old, the parents consulted a child specialist who reassured them and did not advise treatment. At the time the analysis of his mother began, his pavor nocturnus attacks were frequent and frightened his mother. He appeared to be very agitated, would jump out of bed, run around, often saying, 'He'll kill us if he finds us in the nest. I'll kill him'. He was not awake and did not recognize his environment and would fall asleep when his mother would lie down with him. For these attacks, he had complete amnesia. In the analysis of the mother it was found that the reference to the 'nest' was a fantasy which the mother apparently shared with her son, a phenomenon which Sachs[18] has described in *The community of daydreams*. She would repeatedly dream of herself and the members of her family as birds in a nest or in a cage. She had a fantasy in which she imagined herself as a little bird in a nest fed by the mother bird. In actuality, Arnold and his mother owned a pair of parakeets and together cared for them.

The mother was particularly impressed with the marked changes which took place in her son's total behaviour concomitant with her analysis. During the first year of her analysis, his pavor nocturnus attacks had stopped completely. The mother had remained in analysis until Arnold was 11½ years old. He is now 13 and his development seems to have proceeded very satisfactorily. That a 9-year-old boy with pavor nocturnus, Type I, was so decisively influenced by the analysis of his parents (his father was also undergoing analysis at that time) is a suggestive observation which raises *one* very important question and sheds light on *another*. Is it possible to bring about a decisive change in the structure of the superego of a 9-year-old child indirectly by changes in the behaviour of his parents? In this case, it was particularly the behaviour of the mother who, for neurotic needs of her own, had from his earliest infancy seduced the boy into a highly pathological relationship with her which had been changed through analysis.

The phenomenon which this case helps to explain is the following: it is a common experience that the pavor nocturnus attacks of young children may be brought to an end without treatment by the mere fact that the parents carry out consistently the advice not to take the child into bed with them. Friedjung[10] reported such experiences first in 1929. This phenomenon cannot be explained only by the elimination of overstimulation. My impression is that these children are keenly aware of their parents' true feelings and that they cannot be fooled by lip service. They interpret and react to the change in the parental attitude not only as the parents' decision to set limits for the child but to set limits for the parents as well. They need the example of a firm, honest and consistent superego. In the case of Bill, the analyst had no or little contact with the parents, who were patently unwilling to modify their behaviour in any way. In the case of Arnold, the analytic work was with the parents only.

I consider pavor nocturnus, Type I, characterized by hypermotility, hallucinations and retrograde amnesia, to be a specific childhood phenomenon which does not occur in this form in adults. There is an insidious onset and progressive development into puberty, at which time serious character disorders, perversions or even psychotic states may become manifest. The most important etiological factor is chronic sexual traumatization. From a dynamic point of view I consider the structure of the superego as the most significant factor in these cases. I have referred to this as a 'split in the superego'. The pathologically intensified pregenital sexual and the phallic impulses are permitted by the superego to break through and to be acted out in the disguise of the pavor nocturnus attack. Sleepwalking, which as we have seen is often associated with pavor nocturnus, Type I, is the form of sleep disturbance which in some cases may be continued into adulthood. I am referring in this connection to the interrelation of this symptom with fugue states, states of amnesia and certain psychotic states.

The second type of pavor nocturnus, the traumatic type, is characterized by a sudden onset following an acute trauma such as surgery, sickness, accident, death in the family, birth of a sibling, etc. There seems to be a definite analogy between the pavor nocturnus of these children and the traumatic neurosis of adults. This type of pavor nocturnus occurs in children of all ages and is characterized by fitful sleep, crying out during sleep, frequent awakening in anxiety from a dream which represents a repetition of the original traumatic situation, and a need, especially in younger children, to cling to the protecting parent. Very often, this phobic clinging is carried over to the daytime.

I intend to deal with this type of pavor nocturnus more fully here because the findings from the treatment of these children would seem to me to provide a better understanding of the traumatic neurosis in adults. I would like to recapitulate briefly some concepts of traumatic neurosis developed by Freud in *Beyond the pleasure principle*[7].

According to Freud, the traumatic neurosis is the result of a breakthrough of the stimulus barrier. The fact that of those exposed to the same stimulus only some individuals develop traumatic neurosis while others do not, is an indication that the trauma has activated repressed experiences from the past in those who have a latent predisposition. An outstanding characteristic of traumatic neurosis, at least in its early phases, is the tendency of the patient to relive the traumatic situation in nightmares. Freud considered these dreams to be an exception to the theory of dreams which is based on the principle of wish fulfilment. In fact, this phenomenon of recurrent nightmares in traumatic neurosis is used by him in support of the concept of repetition compulsion. Freud explained that the function of such dreams is to help to bring about, by repetition in the dream of the traumatic situation, a belated mastery of the stimulus, the lack of which has caused the traumatic reaction in the first place.

In my opinion, it is difficult to conceive that, for the purpose of mastery, there would be a recall of a danger situation that could not be mastered in the waking state, during sleep when the ego and superego are least prepared to cope with it. To the child in the post-traumatic state when both the narcissistic equilibrium and his object relationships are profoundly disturbed, sleep, due to its withdrawal from reality and from the real objects, may come to represent a danger situation, namely the danger of permanent loss of reality. While the memory of the trauma can be warded off during the day when the mother is present and when motility and other outlets are available, its intrusion cannot be avoided during sleep. In fact, in some cases, the state of sleep itself, because of the immobilization and the separation from the mother, becomes associated with the traumatic situation and may be feared and avoided because of this. It would seem to me that the revival of the traumatic experience in the nightmare has the function of precipitously awakening the sleeper and bringing him back to the reality which, painful though it may be, is preferable to the intolerable psychic state which results from the imminent danger of being overwhelmed by the original trauma. Jekels' concept[13] of the function of the dream as a waker and of awakening as an active process seems especially applicable here. When the continuation of sleep and dreaming becomes a threat to the maintenance of the psychic and possibly of the physiological equilibrium the nightmare serves as the abrupt waker. To be overwhelmed by one's own impulses equals loss of control of one's self which in turn equals loss of one's mind and loss of reality. By awakening, the sleeper now actively extricates himself from the traumatic situation (relieved in the dream) over which he had no control and which he suffered passively when it occurred in reality. Awakening thus represents mastery of the trauma by actively interrupting the traumatic situation of the dream and an attempt to re-establish the shattered narcissistic equilibrium by securing the protective presence of the love object (mother).

The traumatic effect of an experience comes from two sources, mainly: (*i*) the feeling of complete helplessness provoked by the traumatic situation; (*ii*) the specific meaning which the experience holds for the child. In this connection, the psychoanalytic work with adult cases of war and civilian traumatic neurosis of Otto E. Sperling is of particular interest[31]. He found that the traumatic effect of the experience derived from the fact that these patients had interpreted the trauma as a command of their superego—parent(s)—to submit to the ego-alien wishes such as enemy propaganda, illness or even death. This concept of 'The Interpretation of the Trauma as a Command' proved to be particularly applicable to the behaviour of the children with traumatic pavor nocturnus treated by me.

The traumatic type of pavor nocturnus is characteristic of the early phases following a traumatic experience before definite symptom formation has set in. Eventually these children will develop similar sequelae to those studied in treatment of the traumatic neuroses of adults. There will be neurotic, psychosomatic or psychotic disorders, depending upon age, level of fixation, degree of disturbance in object relationship and other factors.

The case of a 4-year-old child, in whom this type of pavor nocturnus could be observed in *statu nascendi* and resolved in the acute phase, might serve as an illustration. Olga developed an acute pavor nocturnus and a very serious anorexia following a tonsillectomy. This child had been very carefully prepared for the operation. Her mother was with her until she was taken into the operating room. Olga remained in the hospital for only one day, during which the mother was with her most of the time. I saw Olga two weeks after the tonsillectomy when she was in very poor physical condition, had lost weight, refused food, even liquids, and hospitalization because of dehydration was considered. She had nightmares in which she screamed. 'Don't, I won't, I can't, no, no, I don't want to leave this room', and screamed for her mother. She would wake up five or six times a night, go into her parents' bed, saying that she was frightened. She appeared depressed, withdrawn and negative, and clung to her mother. At the age of 8 months Olga had exhibited fears of dogs, fire engines, noises and moving objects. At that time, she had been abruptly weaned from the breast and bottle, transferred to her own room, and toilet training had been instituted. Still she developed well until the time her brother was born, when she was not quite 3 years old. At $3\frac{1}{2}$, she was sent to nursery school. She seemed to accept the separation from her mother, but became a 'finicky' and dawdling eater. She seemed to be quite attached to her brother and was heard on several occasions expressing the wish to have a genital like his. Olga's case is very similar to that of 2-year-old Linda, described in 'Animal phobias in a two-year-old child'[24]. Linda developed an acute pavor nocturnus following the birth of a brother. A few months prior to this, Linda had been placed in treatment with me because of a peculiar kind of sleep disturbance: recurrent attacks of nocturnal paroxysmal tachycardia. The relation of nocturnal psychosomatic 'attacks' and sleep disturbance will be taken up briefly later in the paper. The birth of the brother and the onset of the pavor nocturnus occurred while I was on vacation. Play analysis revealed intense repressed oral-sadistic impulses directed against her mother and baby brother. It further revealed that she had interpreted in retrospect a tonsillectomy she had undergone at 18 months as an oral castration and punishment by her mother for her oral-sadistic impulses.

Olga, through her play and by verbalization, revealed that she too had interpreted the tonsillectomy as a punishment for oral-sadistic wishes (directed toward her mother's breast and her brother's penis) and had experienced it as an oral castration inflicted upon her by her mother.

This was brought out very instructively in a game with a clay doll. She was the mother, the analyst was the sister, Olga, and the doll was the baby brother. On one occasion, she got angry with him, grabbed him, hit him, saying that he was dirty and naughty. She then bit off his head, and was furiously cutting his neck with a knife, saying that her tonsils had been cut out by a lady doctor. The analyst restored his head and also put back his little clay penis which Olga had removed several times before, without any interference. When she again took it off, I asked her casually, 'What's that?' She said, 'A little nothing'. I said, 'But this is something. It is his little penis.' She got very angry and said that he had to have his appendix taken out. She prepared him for the operation which she performed by cutting his belly and pulling out clay representing the appendix and the contents of his belly.

That the anaesthesia had been a particularly traumatic experience was brought out in her play and in her nightmares. The 'No, no' and 'Don't' in her nightmares expressed her struggle against being overcome by the anaesthetic against her will, an event she had been unable to prevent in reality, but from which she could escape by waking up when she relived it in the nightmare. The experience of being overwhelmed by the anaesthetic and made unconscious against one's will would seem to be the prototype for the fear of being overwhelmed by one's own impulses and to lose control and contact with reality. In this connection, the case of an 11-year-old girl, who had had a tonsillectomy at age 10, is of particular interest. She remembered her dream while under anaesthesia. She saw coloured circles running around. She tried to push them around the corner, but she couldn't. A mocking voice said, 'Rhoda, you are going crazy'. This was her interpretation of anaesthesia as command, 'You must be crazy, must die'. She was terrified. She didn't want to cry, but she had to when she came to. Since then she has a funny feeling in her dreams. It is like being in another world and a feeling that she couldn't come back as she had thought that she would not come back from the anaesthesia. She came for treatment because of her strange and withdrawn behaviour. She had once tried to choke herself by grabbing her neck with both hands. In Olga's case the preparation for the operation, the covering of the eyes, and the anaesthesia, were a very important part of the surgical game and repeated with precision again and again. She did not know what tonsils actually looked like and was relieved when it was shown to her by shaping them from clay. She said, 'Oh, just two little balls'.

There was a complete resolution of the pavor nocturnus and the anorexia following the release and interpretation of this material in the child's play sessions where she had been doing actively to the clay doll (her brother) what she had suffered passively in reality. For Olga, the tonsillectomy had been the ultimate trauma in a series of traumata, experienced by her as oral deprivations, inflicted by the mother (abrupt weaning, early toilet training, birth of the brother, who was being nursed and who had a penis). Thus, Olga's chronic disappointment in her mother suffered an acute exacerbation at the time of tonsillectomy, to which her mother took her and which was performed by a lady doctor. Her acutely intensified oral aggressive impulses had to be repressed abruptly by her severe superego, and this led to the pavor nocturnus, the anorexia, and the total behaviour which resembled a depression. Olga had interpreted the tonsillectomy as a command by her mother (superego) not to eat the breast-penis and to accept the punishment (castration). She responded to it with the exaggerated unconscious obedience characteristic of the traumatic neurotic.

In conclusion, I should like to emphasize again that Type II of pavor nocturnus can be considered the traumatic neurosis of childhood, from which the later sequelae—neurotic, particularly phobic, psychosomatic or psychotic manifestations—develop. The onset is sudden, often dramatic, following a final trauma in a series of narcissistic injuries. Under the impact of the trauma the aggressive impulses are intensified. Because the trauma is interpreted by the child as a command of the superego to submit —that is to be sick—to die—these impulses are turned against the self.

The third group, the neurotic type of pavor nocturnus, does not need to be dealt with extensively here. It is a frequent phenomenon of an episodic or recurrent nature in children and has its origin in the conflicts of the oedipal phase. To this group also belong the sleep disturbances of the oedipal phase discussed in preceding sections. The concepts developed on the nightmare of the adult by Jones[14] apply to this type of pavor nocturnus in children.

The superego permits the dangerous and forbidden impulses that are warded off during the day to come out during sleep in the disguise of the dream, but insists upon immediate waking up when there is a danger that the ego might be overcome by these impulses and carry them out in reality. The child awakens fully in anxiety, and with a vivid recall of the contents of the nightmare, which may become a lasting memory. It can be revived later in life, either in its original or in somewhat changed form.

Nocturnal Psychosomatic Symptoms, Enuresis and Soiling

The occurrence of a psychosomatic disturbance during the night which awakens the sleeper is a form of sleep disturbance which occurs in children and adults. I am not concerning myself here with psychosomatic diseases in which nocturnal attacks are a frequent occurrence—e.g. bronchial asthma or ulcerative colitis—but what I have in mind are the cases in which the child wakes up in the middle of the night, feeling sick nauseated, or having severe stomach cramps which often necessitate calling a doctor. This occurs repeatedly and examination does not reveal any organic causes for these symptoms. I should like to illustrate this with one case:

Eight and a half year old Erna was referred for treatment because she suffered from many fears and although she did not wet herself during the day, she always had damp panties. Since the age of 4, she had recurrent attacks at night in which she would wake up with a severe stomach-ache, often so severe that a doctor had to be called. During treatment, we learned that Erna still shared her parents' bedroom. Her parents thought that, aside from her attacks, she was a sound sleeper but actually she very often had been up at night and had witnessed parental intercourse many times. She had many fears of a sexual nature. She was afraid to walk up the stairs alone, even in broad daylight, fearing that a man was following and would attack her. She had very sadistic rape fantasies and her damp panties were a result of her constant sexual overstimulation. Her parents were rather annoyed with my suggestion to remove Erna from their bedroom. When they finally did, her mother asked me whether she could sleep in the same room and bed with Erna, rationalizing that she had to have this type of a bed because of her back-ache. On this occasion, I learned that the mother was frigid, always objected to intercourse and had used Erna, in a way, as a protection against her husband's approaches. Erna's idea of intercourse was that of assault and rape; for this was really what it amounted to between her parents. Analytic investigation revealed that, in that symptom, Erna was putting herself in her mother's place, being penetrated by the father, but instead of pleasure, she was experiencing excruciating pain and fear as a punishment for such wishes which are taboo in the unconscious.

In a similar situation, another patient, a boy of 5, also had stomach-aches but his was not a conversion symptom, but intentional; he was simply faking. 'If I say that I have a stomach-ache,' he told me, 'My parents get up. Mother makes tea for me. They fuss around and I wind up in bed between them.' This boy was achieving consciously and deliberately what other children achieve only through a symptom at the cost of anxiety and suffering, namely, to separate the parents and prevent their intercourse at night.

It would seem to me that the cases of enuresis and soiling or diarrhoea at night also belong to this group. While we cannot really consider enuresis as a sleep disturbance since the enuresis serves as a vehicle for the discharge of tensions and thereby rather makes sleep possible, it may be of interest to learn something about the sleep behaviour of children when they are treated because of their enuresis. In my experience most of these cases during their treatment have a transient period of disturbed sleep with nightmares preceding the giving up of the enuresis. Many mothers have told me of their observation of how restless the child's sleep becomes at a certain period of treatment, while this same child during the enuretic phase had been a very sound sleeper. Some children actually stay up for part of the night to make certain that they will not wet. This struggle takes place only as long as the child unconsciously still wants to wet. Once this is worked out in the treatment, these children can sleep very soundly and not wet—e.g. Jean was 8 when, after a year of analysis, she decided that she could give up enuresis. Frequently her mother would overhear her say in her sleep, 'I won't do it. No I won't'[30].

Sleep Phobias, Sleep Rituals, Habitual Waking Up

A frequent form of sleep disturbance is a sleep phobia. A certain amount of sleep phobia is a factor in most sleep disturbances. In the more pronounced cases, the children not only want their mothers to be at home but the mother has to lie down with the child until he falls asleep. The child will often wake up in the middle of the night to make sure that mother is still there and go looking for her through the house and stay awake if she is not at home. Usually these children also show phobic traits and a phobic attachment to their mothers during the daytime. This is indicative of their repressed hostility and death wishes against their mother. This hostility and resentment against the mother stems as we have already seen from the same two main sources—the oedipal situation and sibling rivalry. I would like to give two examples.

1. Six-year-old Miriam would refuse to go to sleep without her mother and would physically resist any attempt of her mother to leave her bed by holding tightly to her mother's breast. This she had done since the birth of her little brother when she was $3\frac{1}{2}$. She had severe nightmares with the typical content of being pursued by wild animals who wanted to devour her, thus revealing her own very strong oral-sadistic

impulses. By holding on to her mother, she was not only taking her away from the brother who slept in the parents' bedroom but also from the father. To separate her parents was one of the aims which she achieved with the sleep disturbance. When I interpreted to Miriam her sadistic behaviour towards her mother and her possessiveness of her, Miriam became very angry and said, 'I won't let you take my mother away from me. I am going to have her in bed with me when I want to, or I'll have so many headaches in the morning that you won't know what to do!' She often complained about headaches in the morning and used this as an excuse for staying home from school. She was able, however, after having understood this behaviour to relinquish her hold upon her mother to a considerable extent.

2. In the case of 12-year-old Charles who suddenly developed a sleep phobia, we were able to study the dynamics very clearly before he had a chance to combat it by compulsive mechanisms. Usually such an acute sleeping phobia is the result of an acute defensive conflict due to a sudden increase or mobilization of aggressive impulses. In his case, a traumatic experience preceded the onset of his phobia. He had witnessed by chance the suicidal jump of a woman from a window. He reacted to it immediately with disturbance. That night he was afraid to go to sleep and, since his condition did not improve but became increasingly worse, he was referred for treatment. In his treatment, it was found that this experience had mobilized his own suicidal impulses; that is, he was afraid to go to sleep lest he be overcome by the impulse to jump out of the window during the night. But he also had—and this was at the basis of his conflict—the unconscious impulse to throw his younger brother out of the window, as he had seen the body of the woman being flung through the window. Not to go to sleep was a defence against being overcome by such an impulse.

Compulsive neurotic rituals of children aimed at counteracting their repressed impulses are common and well known; for instance the need to have bedclothes arranged in a certain way, to have something placed under the pillow, or as one of my patients, a 12-year-old girl did, to have all her shoes lined up in a row near her bedside. These children often spend part of the night rearranging the objects and go into a panic when anyone moves any of them.

Thirteen-year-old Ernest, who suffered from intense castration fears reactivated and intensified by several traumatic experiences, developed a rather unusual sleep ceremonial. Sleepless for many months, he had finally devised an ingenious contraption which made it possible for him to fall asleep for several hours at least during the night. He had attached one end of a string to the knob of his door and the other end to his wrist. To the middle of this string which went over a chair, he had attached a pen knife. He had figured it out very accurately that when anyone who was six feet tall (his father) opened the door, the pull of the string would release the knife which would then directly hit the penis of the person who walked in.

Six and a half year old Barry suddenly developed the following sleep ritual: every night, he was found sleeping on the floor on the doorstep of his mother's bedroom. In his case, this was a very sensible action, as we found out. His father had left the family several months ago, and Barry had often heard his mother say that she was so fed up with everything that it would be best for her to leave also. By placing himself in front of her door, Barry, in a very effective way, planned to prevent his mother from carrying out her threat. Consciously, Barry had not been aware of why he had to sleep in this fashion.

The habit which some children have and which often continues into adulthood—of awaking at a certain time or several times during the night to go to the bathroom—is in most cases a result of the particular methods of toilet training. It is a form of sleep disturbance which yields easily to explanation of its cause[30]. Children often like to delay going to sleep and will use all kinds of delaying tactics. Very often the reason for stalling is a rather harmless one. The child is still full of energy and wants to participate in the family activities. These children as well as those with milder transitory sleep disturbances during the anal and oedipal phases present no real management problems.

This paper focuses on the psychopathology and the differential diagnostic criteria of the more severe neurotic sleep disturbances in children in the hope that early detection and proper assessment will enhance not only our therapeutic but even more so our preventive efforts with children.

REFERENCES

1. BORNSTEIN, B., 1935. Phobia in a two-and-a-half-year-old child, *Psychoanal. Q.*, **4**, 93-119.
2. DEMENT, W., 1964. Experimental dream studies. *Sci. Psychoanal.*, **7**.
3. FENICHEL, OTTO, 1942. Symposium on neurotic disturbances of sleep, *Int. J. PSA.*, **23**.
4. FISHER, C., and DEMENT, W. C., 1963. Studies on the psychopathology of sleep and dreams. *Am. J. Psychiat.*, **119**, 1160.
5. FRAIBERG, S., 1959. On the sleep disturbances of early childhood. *Psychoanal. Study Child*, **5**, 285-309.
6. FREUD, S., 1953. *The interpretation of dreams* (1899). Standard Ed., vols 3 and 4. London, Hogarth Press.
7. FREUD, S., 1955. *Beyond the pleasure principle* (1920). Standard Ed., vol. 18. London, Hogarth Press.
8. FREUD, S., 1936. *The problem of anxiety*. New York, The Psychoanalytic Quarterly Press and W. W. Norton.
9. FREUD, S., 1930. *Civilization and its discontents*. London, Hogarth Press.
10. FRIEDJUNG, J. K., 1924. Beitrag zum Verständnis der Einschlafstörungen der Kinder. *Wien. Med. Wochenschr.*, **74**, 1002-03.
11. FRIES, MARGARET, 1945. The child's ego development and the training of adults in his environment. *Psychoanal. Q.*, **14**.
12. GESELL, A., 1943. *Infant and child in the culture today*. New York, Harper.

13. JEKELS, L., 1945. A bioanalytical contribution to the problem of sleep and wakefulness. *Psychoanal. Q.*, **14**, 169-89.
14. JONES, E., 1931. *On the nightmare.* New York, W. W. Norton.
15. KLEIN, M., 1932. *The psychoanalysis of children.* New York, W. W. Norton.
16. KLEIN, M., 1948. Personification in the play of children. In *Contributions to psychoanalysis.* London, Hogarth Press. pp. 215-26.
17. RIBBLE, M., 1943. *The rights of infants.* New York, Columbia Univ. Press.
18. SACHS, H., 1942. The community of daydreams. In *The creative unconscious.* Cambridge, Mass., Sci-Art Press. pp. 11-54.
19. SADGER, I., 1919. Sleep walking and moon walking. *Nerv. Ment. Dis. Monogr.*
20. SIMMEL, E., 1942. Symposium on neurotic disturbances of sleep. *Int. J. Psychoanal.*, **23**, 65-68.
21. SPERLING, M., 1949. Neurotic sleep disturbances in children. *The nervous child*, **8**, 28-46.
22. SPERLING, M., 1950. Children's interpretation and reaction to the unconscious of their mothers. *Int. J. Psychoanal.*, **21**, 1-6.
23. SPERLING, M., 1951. The neurotic child and his mother. *Amer. J. Orthopsychiat.*, **21**, 351-364.
24. SPERLING, M., 1952. Animal phobias in a two-year-old child. *Psychoanal. Study Child*, **7**, 115-125.
25. SPERLING, M., 1954. Reactive schizophrenia in children. *Amer. J. Orthopsychiat.*, **24**, 506-512.
26. SPERLING, M., 1955. Etiology and treatment of sleep disturbances in children. *Psychoanalyt. Q.*, **24**, 358-448.
27. SPERLING, M., 1958. Pavor nocturnus. *J. Amer. Psychoanalyt. Assn*, **6**, 79-94.
28. SPERLING, M., 1959. Equivalents of depression in children. *J. Hillside Hospital*, April, 138-148.
29. SPERLING, M., 1959. A study of deviate sexual behavior in children by the method of simultaneous analysis of mother and child. In *Dynamic psychopathology in childhood.* Eds, Jessner, L., and Pavenstedt, E. New York, Grune and Stratton.
30. SPERLING, M., 1965. Dynamic considerations and treatment of enuresis. *J. Amer. Acad. Child Psychiat.*, **4**.
31. SPERLING, OTTO E., 1950. The interpretation of the trauma as a command. *Psychoanalyt. Q*, **19**, 352-370.
32. SPERLING, OTTO E., 1956. Psychodynamics of group perversions. *Psychoanalyt. Q*, **25**, 56-65.
33. SPITZ, R., Anaclitic depression. *Psychoanalyt. Study Child*, **5**.
34. WAELDER, J., 1935. Analyse eines Falles von Pavor Nocturnues. *Ztschr. Psychoanal. PAD.*, **9**, 1-70.
35. WULFF, M., 1927. Phobie bei einem Anderthalbjährigen Kinde. *Int. Ztschr. PSA.*, **13**.

XVI

PICA

REGINALD S. LOURIE

M.D., Med.Sc.D.

*Director, Department of Psychiatry, Children's Hospital of D.C.
and Hillcrest Children's Center,
Professor of Pediatric Psychiatry, George Washington University
School of Medicine*

AND

FRANCIS K. MILLICAN

M.D.

Research Associate, Department of Psychiatry, Children's Hospital of D.C.

1

Introduction

Pica is described as an abnormal appetite or craving for inedible substances. Pica has been known since ancient times and found to occur on every continent[1, 6, 11]. It is common in India, Indonesia, Australia, Africa, the West Indies, and some parts of South America; in the United States it is common in the southeastern states, the slum areas of large cities, and in some Indian tribes. Since 1959 there have been medical reports on pica cases from Israel[2], South Africa[5, 10], Sweden[4], and England[3], as well as the United States. Medically, pica is important because it has long been recognized as the cause in most cases of lead poisoning in young children[16]; also children who are hospitalized for accidental poisoning are found to have a high incidence of pica (55.7 per cent)[18].

The etiology of pica has been attributed to various causes, including nutritional, mental retardation or brain damage, cultural and economic, and emotional deprivation.

2
Psychiatric Study

During the 1950s and early 1960s, significant psychiatric studies of pica were reported. A. Van der Sar and H. M. Waszink[21] made a detailed psychiatric study of a 5-year-old boy with pica. They described the boy's frustrations and the neglect he experienced, and the oral aggressive aspects of his pica. Leo Kanner reviewed material on 31 cases of pica[9]. He noted the frequency of organic brain damage and mental retardation and commented on the possible relationship of affectional deprivation and family instability to pica.

R. G. Mellins and C. D. Jenkins[15, 16] studied the epidemiologic and psychological aspects of 46 cases of children with lead poisoning in Chicago. Thirty-two of the children were given psychological examinations. The authors found that when 'motor, language, and emotional control were considered together, it appeared that the group showed an average development in early childhood, a severe setback caused by lead poisoning, and a gradual, but incomplete, trend toward recovery by one-fourth to one-half of the group'. They suggested that the study of the mother-child relationship might well prove to be the key to understanding the psychodynamics of pica, and commented on the possible relationship of pica to aggression.

H. Wortis et al.[22] reported on pica by reviewing their data from a longitudinal study of children who had been born prematurely. They found that the children with pica had suffered more neonatal insults, were slower in motor and mental development, showed more neurological defects, had more deviant behaviour, and had poorer living conditions than did a control group from the same premature population who did not have pica.

Preliminary findings on the first cases of pica studied by the Children's Hospital research team[12, 13, 19] indicated that the major factors in the etiology of pica were: (*i*) emotional; (*ii*) cultural; (*iii*) economic; (*iv*) organic brain damage.

3
Children's Hospital Research Study of Children with Pica

This paper describes the research study of pica carried on at Children's Hospital of the District of Columbia (Washington), United States, together with the implications of the results of the research; outlines clinical treatment procedures, with emphasis on psychotherapy; and suggests preventive measures.

Subjects and Methods

As part of their normal development, children begin explorations via mouthing at about 5 months of age. According to Gesell[8] such hand-to-mouth activity becomes less frequent at about 1 year of age. For the purposes of our research into the psychological aspects of pica, it was necessary to distinguish between such normal oral activity and that which by its duration and intensity indicated that psychopathology in the form of an oral symptom was present. We arbitrarily defined a child to have pica if he was 18 months of age or older and had persistently ingested non-food substances for at least three months prior to the time of the study. All of the children studied showed a remarkable persistence in their pica, seeking out the pica substances in preference to food or candy in many cases. The substances ingested included plaster, putty, paint, paper, dirt, crayons, wood, cigarette ashes and butts, matches, string, cloth and laundry starch.

The research team consisted of a psychiatrist, a psychologist, a paediatrician, a social worker, and a nurse. Two separate studies were carried out by the team: (*i*) psychiatric, and (*ii*) nutritional.

For the psychiatric study the research population comprised 154 children (125 Negro and 29 white), of whom 95 were children with pica and 59 were control cases, 24 normal and 32 psychiatric. In the nutritional study the research population was 54 children with pica, all Negro, and 28 normal control children. The basic data on each case in the psychiatric study consisted of history from the parents, psychological testing of the child, psychiatric playroom interview with the child, and Rorschach evaluation of 115 mothers. Seventeen of the pica cases were also seen in psychotherapy. The nutritional study, in addition to serving its primary aim, which was to evaluate the nutritional status of pica children, gave additional data on other facts of the problem from home visits, social and economic information, psychological testing of the children, and observations of the mother-child relationship through a one-way viewing screen.

The Pica Lead Poisoning Clinic begun at Children's Hospital in 1957, has furnished further data on pica through the more than 500 children who have been seen there. Most of the pica children from the two research studies were followed in the clinic for several years after the initial evaluation.

4

Illustrative Cases

The following cases of pica illustrate the types of problems encountered in the children and their families.

Family A

Case 1. Doris, a $3\frac{1}{2}$-year-old Negro, was hospitalized for lead poisoning caused by eating paint and plaster. The onset of her pica was at 10 months of age, when wall plaster eating began. From 18 months to 2 years, no plaster was available, but shortly thereafter her mother noticed she was passing pieces of coal in bowel movements. The substances being ingested just prior to her hospitalization were plaster, pencil leads, fingers from the doll which she took to bed with her, newspapers, rocks, and sticks.

Doris was the third child of her mother, with two older half-siblings, Hanna, 5 years, who also had pica, and Jack, 8 years, who did not have pica. Doris's father never lived with the family. The household at the time of study included the mother's brother and a male roomer.

Doris was noticeably depressed at the age of 6 months following the death of her maternal aunt, who had been caring for her. The mother worked until Doris was 18 months of age, at which time she accepted public assistance in order to be at home. Both weaning and toilet training were accomplished with difficulty, when Doris was about 3 years, after much vacillation on the part of the mother, the use of threats, and many battles. When first seen Doris had recently been sucking her thumb and biting her fingernails. Her hands were slapped for pica. She had allergies, manifest as eczema and bronchial asthma.

Psychological testing and the playroom interview showed an energetic, active child with a lively imagination, trusting, and able to form relationships with adults easily. Intelligence was slightly below normal, and her speech development lagged. She was quite controlling of the adults, showed a preoccupation with dependency. She was seen in psychotherapy with a male therapist for a period of eight months. She was a trusting, vivacious, bossy participant. Her play emphasized oedipal wishes via doll house play with the therapist. She also continually played a game in which a woman was sadistically killed. As in her relationship with her mother, there was a controlling relationship and oppositional behaviour. Pica stopped, but she continued to chew on her fingernails and her belt.

It was learned from the Rorschach and continuing case work with her family, that the mother was interested in the children, but playfully childish with them. She was unable to set meaningful limits on their behaviour, talking rather gruffly, but the children learned how they could get what they wanted, and control the situation. She was unable to cope with their uncertainties and questions factually; for example, she told them that babies were bought in a store. In certain ways the children were expected to control mother's impulses for her and meet her unmet dependency needs stemming from her own childhood. With the oldest child, Jack, she was very strict. While, as noted above, he had no pica, he did have quite mixed sexual identification for which he too was seen in psychotherapy.

The mother had dull normal intelligence, with a meagre cultural and educational background. Her orientation was egocentric, dependent and passive, but she was also periodically capable of warm, spontaneous expression of affection. She was very compliant with authority, but found it difficult to exert authority herself.

The mother had a habit since 8 years of age of keeping snuff in her mouth, of which the children were aware. She said that without the snuff she would feel dizzy, that she was dependent upon it—it was a companion to her.

Case 2. Hanna was the 5-year-old sister of Doris. The mother did not identify herself as much with Hanna as she did with Doris. She frequently was in battles with Hanna, whipping her for not eating and for pica.

Hanna's parents separated in her infancy. She had pica from 11 months until $2\frac{1}{2}$ years, eating dirt, plaster, toilet tissue, and starch. Following the paternal grandfather's hospitalization when she was 5, she began eating much dirt again. The grandfather was very close to the children, visiting regularly every evening.

Hanna was nursed until 6 months, and was weaned from the bottle at $3\frac{1}{2}$ years, when the bottle was given to Doris. Like Doris she was not toilet trained until age 3, when the diapers were given to Doris.

Psychological studies showed that Hanna had average intelligence, was very immature, showing concerns about aggression and much negativism. She seemed to regard herself and others as bad, with no suggestion of more positive relationships. Sexual concerns were apparent. Immaturity was expressed in a need for infantile dependency and in poor impulse control.

Hanna was seen in psychotherapy with a female therapist for 23 sessions. Treatment focused on establishing a trusting relationship with the therapist within which limits could be set with her when impulses were out of control. She was also helped to repress her sexual concerns, which stemmed from distortions in her family relationships, and she was able to fit into the family more comfortably.

Family B

(Cases 3, 4, 5 and 6, described below were children in this family.)

In this Negro family, four of the eight children had pica at the time of the study, and a fifth child had previously had pica. The father was employed as a truck driver. When the studies of the children began, the mother was found by the research team to be an ambulatory schizophrenic with paranoid ideas, who was suffering an acute psychotic episode for which she required hospitalization for several months. She was preoccupied with considerable rage toward her husband, particularly about his infidelity and his lack of support in caring for the children.

Psychiatric interviews with the mother and Rorschach testing showed her to be a quite immature, excessively dependent woman with an egocentric orientation. She was quite closely tied to her family. Her affect was flat. There was evidence that much of her conflict centred around childbearing, and her psychotic break followed by a few months the birth of her last child, which was accompanied by tubal ligation. Prior to the psychotic break she was reported to have been a very patient mother with her children. Her principal means of coping with anxiety were by the defences of withdrawal and projection.

Both the paternal grandmother and maternal grandparents were actively participating in the care of the children. The father was interviewed to evaluate the possibility of family casework with him while the mother was hospitalized. He was not perceptive of the children's needs or feelings, and was emotionally inaccessible, expressing very little of his feeling or thinking in verbal terms.

Studies of the children were carried out while the mother was hospitalized. The mother was followed actively after her discharge by the study social worker. Although the mother had initial difficulty in utilizing the help offered her, she seemed to rely on the support of talking with the social worker when she felt the need. Her self-esteem improved. She became less vague about the children, and more able to do something about her own dissatisfactions with her husband, mother-in-law and living situation, particularly housing. This family is typical of the treatment approach to most pica families in that the social casework with the mother was of prime importance in helping the mother better meet the needs of the children. When she was able to better meet their needs they could give up the pica.

Case 3. Donna, $8\frac{1}{2}$ years, was the oldest of the children in the family studied. Her pica consisted of eating paper. She was mentally retarded, I.Q. 62, and was in a special class in school. Her contact with reality seemed poor; although she was interested in relationships she seemed to feel threatened by them. She had fears associated with aggression. She used autistic logic, showed confusion, perseverative activities, and had sexual concerns. Her affect was inappropriate and bland. She had a schizoid personality and it was felt she might easily become schizophrenic. Psychiatric treatment for her was pending when the family sent her away to live with relatives.

Case 4. Bobby, $4\frac{1}{2}$ years old, had borderline intelligence. He was sad to the point of depression when interviewed, quite immature, inhibited, unrelated, and anxious. He spoke very little, and his play was quite repetitive. He still sucked his fingers and soiled and wet his clothing.

Case 5. Lee was the youngest, 2 years 2 months, and was the brightest, with an I.Q. of 115. He was still taking four bottles a day. His pica appetites were chiefly for cloth, and he also had a habit of stuffing cotton into his nose and ears. He was passive, compliant, and depressed. As with Bobby, his mother's absence was a contributing factor in his depression.

Case 6. Kim was a $7\frac{1}{2}$-year-old mentally retarded boy with an I.Q. of 64 and suggestive organic brain damage. His pica craving was for string. He had poor control of impulses, marked dependency needs and immaturity and fears of separation. His pica was on a primitive incorporative basis. He was interested in other people, but saw them as bad, threatening and punitive. There was considerable distortion in his perception of reality.

He was seen in psychotherapy for about ten months. The aims achieved in therapy were to provide him with a healthier emotional relationship in which he could learn to express his feelings, handle them in socially acceptable ways, increase his ability to control his impulses, and increase his reality testing. Improvement toward these goals resulted.

Family C

Case 7. Pamela was a 3-year-10-month-old white girl when she was treated for lead poisoning caused by her ingesting paint from the window sills and doors. The age of onset of pica was reported variously as 11 months to 18 months. A younger sister with pica was found also to have lead poisoning, and was treated three months after Pamela.

Pamela's father drank excessively. The parents were repeatedly separated, beginning while the mother was pregnant with the patient. When Pamela was 18 months, the parents were finally divorced, and the mother began working, which continued sporadically. At the time of study, she was on public assistance. For two years the household had consisted of the mother, grandmother, and two girls.

At the time of hospitalization, Pamela's diet consisted chiefly of milk from the bottle, with very little solid food, and she had a severe anaemia. On occasion she would eat a special dish which her grandmother cooked for her. The first attempt to wean her from the bottle was at the age of 20 months. After a week during which the child would not eat anything, the mother 'had to give the bottle back'. This was the first of three such unsuccessful attempts. The bottle was also used as a pacifier, being offered her whenever she fretted about anything. She also sucked her fingers and bit her nails. She had been completely toilet trained at 9 months.

Psychological testing showed Pamela to function at a superior level of intelligence (Stanford-Binet I.Q. of 128). There was no evidence that any organic brain damage had resulted from the lead poisoning. She performed better on non-verbal than verbal tests, and there was an element of passive-aggression in her withholding speech.

The mother and grandmother were both very overprotective of Pamela, and fearful about physical harm to her. The mother readily blamed others for all problems. She was still dependent upon her own mother, who was the dominant member of the family. The mother, usually hostile, was able to bring the children for follow-up in the pica clinic, and they were seen there by the research team over a period of several years.

The mother's attitude toward casework help available in the pica clinic gradually changed with continuous reaching out to her for a year before she could take the initiative in calling the social worker when problems arose.

Pamela's pica ceased immediately after hospitalization for de-leading. In therapy she was able to be tolerant of her mother's limitations, saying that her mother 'never grew up'. Pamela gradually identified more with the grandmother, in being dominant and controlling with her own mother. Pica for her represented an aggressive activity toward her mother, at the same time that it served as a substitute for a satisfactory dependent relationship with her mother.

5
Results of the Research and Implications

The results arrived at in the research studies led to the conclusion that pica has a multiple etiology, with various factors contributing to pica in different degrees in each child. Some of these factors are innate in the child's constitutional make-up and in his normal course of development; some have their source in the child s environment and his interaction with it.

Constitutional Factors

Organic brain damage and mental retardation, it was found, predispose some children to pica. This finding has also been reported by Kanner[9]. In a study of children who had been born prematurely, Wortis[22] found that children with pica had more neurological damage and more mental and motor retardation than the children without pica. The study indicates that these constitutional hazards make extra demands on the parent figures to meet needs which are not always recognized.

The exploration of the environment by mouthing is part of normal development, beginning at the age of about 5 months. Its continuation past its normal phase limits can lead to pica. Children have different constitutionally determined degrees of intensity of oral drives and they differ in their willingness to relinquish these drives. Therefore the type and amount of available parental control particularly with children who have a high level of mouth activity is crucial in the development of pica as a symptom.

Environmental Factors

Cultural and economic factors, it was found, contribute to the occurrence of pica. This finding was supported by a preliminary study[18] undertaken to gain some idea of the prevalence of pica in children from 1 to 6. The prevalence of pica in the United States is not known, although there are indications that it is more widespread in lower socio-economic groups. Lead poisoning in children, despite its neurological effects and mortality, is not a reportable disease in the United States except in a few cities. If it were, it would furnish some clue as to the prevalence of pica in children, because of the relationship between the two conditions.

In the prevalence study three segments of the population known to Children's Hospital of D.C. were surveyed[18]: (*i*) Children from low-income families (clinic patients); (*ii*) Children from middle- and upper-income families (private patients); and (*iii*) All children hospitalized for the ingestion of poisons over a specified eleven-month period. Of the 486 children in Group (*i*), 32 per cent ingested non-edible substances, whereas only 10 per cent of the 294 children in Group (*ii*) did so. Of the 79 children in Group (*iii*), 55 per cent had pica (Fig. 1).

These figures, in addition to their indications about prevalence per se are revealing in that they show a statistically significant difference between the percentage of pica children in the low-income group and in the middle- and high-income group. This difference suggests that cultural and socio-economic factors are involved, particularly in the amount of available mothering.

Cultural factors were found to be particularly important in the etiology of pica in the Negro children who were part of the research population[12]. It should be noted that the Negro families to which this segment of the

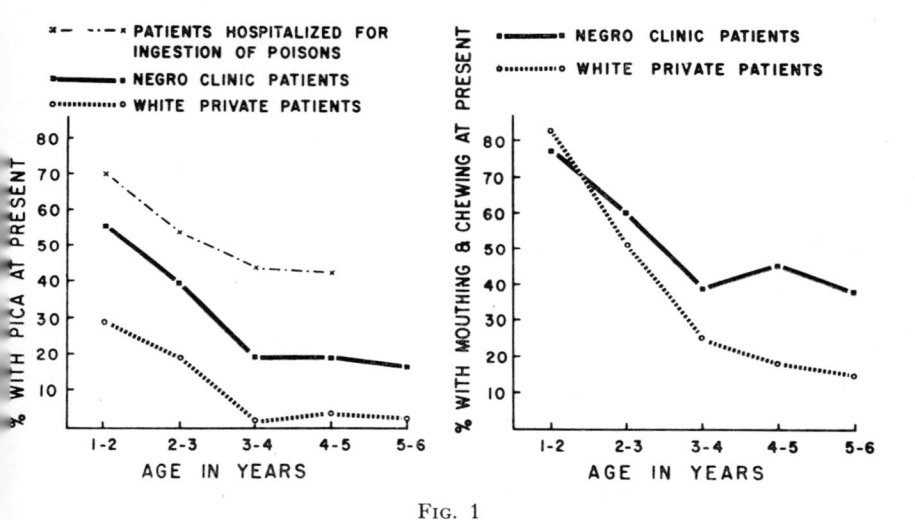

FIG. 1

research population belonged came largely from the southeastern United States, where the eating of clay, dirt, and laundry starch is a not infrequent and accepted custom. Interviews with mothers of children with and without pica led to the following conclusions:

1. Mothers of Negro children with pica more frequently came from communities where clay and starch eating are a part of the culture than did mothers of Negro children with other psychiatric problems.

2. Mothers of children with pica have significantly more pica themselves as adults than have mothers of children without pica. Sixty-five per cent of pica children had mothers with pica.

3. Some mothers teach pica to their children, and some children acquire the habit by imitation of the culturally based pattern found in the mother.

4. On a cultural basis, some mothers encourage the child's use of oral satisfaction as a means of coping with anxiety. This can be important in the choice of pica as a symptom.

2H

Nutritional Factors

Pica has probably been used throughout the centuries to assuage hunger pains when food is not available. The relation of pica to other types of inadequate nutrition[6], particularly anaemia, has been repeatedly suggested, on the understandable assumption that pica is an attempt to supply some essential missing nutrient. Therefore, to clarify the role of nutritional factors in the etiology of pica a nutritional study was carried out at Children's Hospital of D.C.[8a]. In this study children with pica were found to be normal on clinical examination and by anthropometric evaluation. They tended, however, to have less adequate diets, lower levels of ascorbic acid in the plasma, somewhat lower haemoglobin concentrations, more reported respiratory illness, and more recorded days of hospitalization than children without pica. In spite of these findings, two double-blind experiments failed to show that iron given intramuscularly, or a multiple vitamin and mineral preparation given daily for six to seven weeks was any more effective than placebos in curing or lessening the habit of pica.[7, 17]

No evidence was found in these studies that nutritional deficiency is etiologically related to pica. It would seem, rather, that poor economic conditions and inadequacies in mothering and child care contribute both to the symptom of pica and to less than adequate nutrition of the child. It has been shown that the reverse can be true, that pica which involves prolonged eating of large amounts of some substances such as dirt may produce severe anaemia, and even death.

Psychodynamic Factors

The patients studied were largely drawn from the marginal income Negro population of Washington, D.C., in which there is a high incidence of family instability. However, even within this group, major separations from parents were more frequent in the pica group than in normal and psychiatric control groups. In numerous cases the onset of pica was related to such major separations or to the mother's beginning employment. In the normal control group there were more fathers present in the home, and the fathers were more involved in the child's upbringing. In some cases it seemed that the role of the father in the family was decisive in preventing pica, where the presence of all other factors suggested the child might well have been symptomatic.

The incidence of pica (63 per cent) in the mothers of the pica children, was significantly higher than that in normal or psychiatric control groups. The mothers who had pica themselves also showed evidence of other forms of oral fixation: obesity, alcoholism, and drug addictions.

Only one adult male with pica, father of four sons with pica, was known to the study. The wife and daughter of this man did not have pica. Pica is not usually an acceptable masculine activity. In contrast, alcoholism and drug addiction were frequently found in the fathers of the pica children.

In addition to separations from the parents which interfered with consistent nurturing of the child in his earliest years, the personalities of many of the mothers rendered them unable to relate to the child in a satisfactory way. The personalities of the mothers frequently revealed passivity, dependency, narcissism, poor impulse control, manifest anxiety, and neurotic and depressive personality patterns. A few of the mothers in the study were overtly psychotic.

Most important in the choice of pica as a symptom when parental, particularly maternal, deprivation was present, was the mother's fostering of the use of mouth satisfactions as a substitute for themselves in dealing with the child's anxiety. In addition to the pattern for identification supplied by the mother's own pica, such encouragement also occurred in the form of late weaning, i.e., after two years, or vacillating weaning, the use of pacifiers well beyond infancy, and the mother's encouraging the child to put something in his mouth (bottle, pacifier, or substances such as starch or clay) when faced with any anxiety. Rather than find the source of upsetness in the child or awareness of his feelings, the mothers instead shunted the child to oral activities. Thus, if the mother fosters oral activity as a means of handling anxiety, pica is likely to occur if the child is in addition deprived of a secure relation to his parents. It should be emphasized that the mother's attitude toward oral activity does not in itself produce pica, when there is otherwise adequate mothering, as was demonstrated in the normal control children.

Psychopathology Accompanying Pica

The major psychiatric diagnostic classification of the children which pica is given in Table 1. Only the primary diagnosis of each child is presented for the total group of 95 children. The survey of children over 5 years of age with pica shows that these older children had the most severe psychopathology, as would be expected; and in this portion of the Table both primary and secondary diagnoses are recorded. Although pica occurs in children with various psychiatric disorders, certain behavioural characteristics were significantly present in the cases studied when they were compared with normal children. Children with pica had a high degree of other oral problems, including mouthing of inedible objects (in addition to ingestion), thumbsucking and feeding problems. They were as a whole somewhat retarded in their use of speech, and some even withheld speech. They showed conflicts about their dependency needs, also conflicts around handling of aggressive feelings, and considerable negativism. Some showed excessive physical clinging to their mothers, and did not relate as readily as normal children do to other adults.

The children with pica seemed to fall into three main groups:

1. Children whose pica is largely the result of parental deprivation, such as absence of the father, or—even more important—separation or severe personality problems in the mother.

TABLE 1

Diagnosis of Children with Pica

	Major Diagnosis	All Diagnoses		
	Total Group ($N = 95$)	6 years and over ($N = 9$)	5 years ($N = 8$)	4 years ($N = 13$)
None	2			
Brain Damage	14			
Severe		2	4	5
Suggestive		3	3	1
Mental Deficiency	1			
Severe		2	3	2
Mild		4	1	1
Psychosis	9	3	2	3
Psychophysiologic	0			
Neurosis	8	2		2
Personality Disorder	28		6	6
Schizoid		3		
Other		1		
Transient Personality Disorder	33			

2. Children whose pica had as a major etiological factor identification with the mother's pica. As such, the basic psychopathology is not as severe as in the other groups. However, we feel that persistent pica even before the age of 18 months is suggestive of some degree of psychopathology.

3. Children over 3 years of age with pica showed the most severe psychopathology. In these cases, pica occurred most frequently in children with weak or defective egos, often due to organic brain damage or schizophrenic disorders. Among other diagnoses in this group were neuroses and personality disorders especially related to impulse control difficulties.

Of the nine children over 6 years of age studied, two had suffered major separations from the mother by death or desertion, four had schizophrenic mothers, the mother of one child was alcoholic, another child's mother had a paranoid personality, and another was an employed mother with neurotic and somatic complaints.

Among other problems and habits seen as other symptoms in the pica children were rocking, thumbsucking, head-banging, nail-biting, hair-pulling (and sometimes eating). Symptoms in the older children with pica included fears, nightmares, enuresis, encopresis, temper tantrums, uncontrolled aggression, fire-setting, stuttering, and oral-genital sex play. Asthma and dermatitis occurred in two cases. Children followed after the disappearance of pica without therapy had subsequent school problems, behaviour disorders, phobias, compulsive masturbation and neurodermatitis.

Relationship of Pica to Addiction

Pica is one of the earliest forms of oral craving and preoccupation with ingestion as a means of attempting to deal with unmet needs. Although it is not an addiction in the true sense, it has etiological factors similar to many of those described in the later addictions such as alcoholism. Preliminary follow-up studies of children with pica and retrospective studies of adults with addictions have led us to suspect that childhood pica indicates an 'addiction-prone' individual.

6
Outpatient Treatment of Pica

A Pica Clinic established at Children's Hospital of D.C., was initially to provide follow-up of children who had been treated in the hospital for lead poisoning. Added to this in turn were children with pica who needed to be screened for lead poisoning, and children who had been hospitalized for the ingestion of poisons other than lead, who were found to have a high incidence of pica. Later children were included with pica but no lead poisoning. The combined medical and socio-psychiatric approach to the children and their families in the clinic was more acceptable to the parents than earlier attempts to study and treat the children in the Department of Psychiatry.

The staff consists of a paediatrician, a nurse, a psychiatrist and/or psychologist, and a medical social worker. The multiple activities of the clinic are best performed by a multidisciplinary staff.

Medical Evaluation

Medical history included special attention to symptoms and signs of lead-poisoning, including gastrointestinal or central nervous system symptoms, evaluation of behaviour, appetite and pica symptoms. X-rays of the long bones and blood samples were obtained. It has been found that where pica is present, even when there is a negative history from parents for ingestion of lead-containing substances, the blood lead level should be checked. This has been found to be an important method of early case finding of lead poisoning, and prevention of its neurologic damages. The clinic also provides a continuing follow-up of children who have had lead poisoning until there is no longer danger of repetition.

There is a high incidence of pica in the siblings of children with pica. Hence, from the point of view of case-finding, inquiry about pica in siblings of children being treated in the pica clinic should be automatic procedure.

An educational approach was the first step utilized in dealing with the mothers. The harmful effects of lead-containing substances were explained, and the likelihood of pica children in particular ingesting other poisons, such as household cleaners and medicines was discussed. The mothers were encouraged to wean older children who were still taking the bottle, and were advised to try to substitute some activity with the mother when the child was noted eating non-edible things as well as stopping the activity. The fact that the physician, in his role as an authority figure did not accept pica as being harmless acted as a counterforce to the cultural acceptance of pica by many of the mothers, and as a result many of them were able to change their handling of the symptom.

Parents were also given guidance in handling their children's developmental problems. Any feeding problems were explored and the implications of struggles over food explained. Specific dietary advice was given. If anaemia was present, it was treated. Behavioural and other problems which the child had were also discussed with the parent to clarify the nature of the problem and possible ways of handling it.

Where this initial superficial approach to the mother was not sufficient to enable her to stop the symptom of pica in the child a more comprehensive study was undertaken. Where there was organic brain damage in the child, personality problems in the child or the mother, or socio-economic problems at the root of the difficulty an individual approach to meet the needs of child and mother was outlined. Where parents were encountered who are passive, apathetic, or irresponsible at times to the extent of physical neglect of the child, it was found necessary to help the physician and other team members understand their own often hostile feelings about the unavailable or neglectful parent before they could be useful in guidance of the family[20].

When maternal deprivation as a determinant of the pica was caused by economic or marital problems, the social worker on the team was the key person. Utilizing casework approaches, the social worker was able to help families with multiple problems utilize the usual community resources—social agencies for immediate financial assistance or for moving into better housing, visiting nurses associations for help toward better child care, and mental health clinics. Reduction of family problems may reduce some of the family stresses that contribute to the development of the symptom of pica in the child. In many instances, mothers could meet the dependency needs of their children more adequately only when some of their own needs were met. Only then they could use the opportunity of learning new ways of dealing with family problems. Many of the younger children with pica were able to give up the symptom and continue with their normal development when home conditions were changed. The children with more fixed and severe psychopathology, generally the white children and the older Negro children, consistently needed psychotherapy before they could give up the pica. In these children, even when the symptom of pica had stopped, the child often still needed help with other emotional problems.

7
Preventive Measures

Since pica is one of the symptoms produced by emotional deprivation, it is obvious that primary prevention of pica—efforts to remove or alter factors involved in its etiology—must be directed toward improving the mental health of children in infancy and early childhood. Particularly in families with severe economic problems, social welfare programmes are needed to prevent the disruption of family life and in improving economic conditions so that mothering can be consistently available and adequate.

Parents should be educated about the hazards of lead poisoning; such education is particularly necessary for parents whose cultural background makes them accept pica as harmless and even beneficial. In the United States the city of Cleveland has carried on a successful preventive programme along these lines, which might be used as a model in other cities. The programme, initiated in 1958, used pamphlets, radio programmes, visits to homes in slum areas by public health nurses, and exhibits by parent-teachers associations in the schools.

Preventive measures should be instituted when conditions are found in the environment which expose a child with pica to the development of lead poisoning, such as lead-containing paint in housing, on cribs and toys.

In sum, the mental health worker and physicians in general should be alerted to the possibility of pica when the following conditions and situations are present:

1. Inadequate mothering as a result of separation or psychological unavailability of the mother because of her personality characteristics of passivity, dependency, depression, psychosis, or poor impulse control.
2. Economic deprivation.
3. Cultural acceptance or encouragement of pica by the mother.
4. Absent father.

It should be noted that measures designed to remove or to lessen factors known to predispose to pica may also have other long-term benefits. Among these are the elimination of some of the conditions which contribute to emotional problems in later life, such as alcoholism and drug addiction.

REFERENCES

1. ANELL, B., and LAGERCRANTZ, S., 1958. *Geophagical customs*. Upsalla, Sweden, Amquist and Wiksells Boktrycheri Ab.
2. BER, R., and VALERO, A., 1961. Pica and hypochromic anemia. *Harefuah (J. med. Assn Israel)*, **61**, 35.
3. BERG, J. M., and ZAPPELLA, M., 1964. Lead poisoning in childhood with reference to pica and mental sequelae. *J. Ment. Def. Res.*, **8**, 44.
4. CARLANDER, O., 1959. Aetiology of pica. *Lancet*, ii, 569.
5. CATZEL, P., 1963. Pica and milk intake. *Pediatrics*, **31**, 1056.

6. COOPER, M., 1957. *Pica*. Springfield, Ill., Charles C. Thomas.
7. GARDNER, J. E., and TEVETOGLU, F., 1957. The roentgenographic diagnosis of geophagia (dirt-eating) in children. *J. Pediat.*, **51**, 667.
8. GESELL, A., and AMATRUDA, C. S., 1941. *Developmental diagnosis: Normal and abnormal child development*. New York, Paul B. Hoeber.
8a. GUTELIUS, M. F., MILLICAN, F. K., LAYMAN, E. M., COHEN, G. J., and DUBLIN, C. C., 1962. Nutritional studies of children with pica. *Pediatrics*, **29**, 1012-23.
9. KANNER, L., 1957. *Child psychiatry*. 3rd Ed. Springfield, Ill., Charles C. Thomas.
10. LANZKOWSKY, P., 1959. Investigation into the aetiology and treatment of pica. *Arch. Dis. Child.*, **34**, 140.
11. LAUFER, B., 1930. Geophagy. *Field Museum of Natural History. Anthropological Series*. **18**, No. 2. Chicago, Illinois.
12. LAYMAN, E. M., MILLICAN, F. K., LOURIE, R. S., and TAKAHASHI, L. Y., 1963. Cultural influences and symptom choice: clay-eating customs in relation to the etiology of pica. *Psychol. Rec.*, **13**, 249.
13. LOURIE, R. S., LAYMAN, E. M., MILLICAN, F. K., SOKOLOFF, B., and TAKAHASHI, L. Y., 1958. A study of the etiology of pica in young children, an early pattern of addiction. In *Problems of addiction and habituation*. Eds Hoch and Zubin. New York, Grune and Stratton.
14. LOURIE, R. S., LAYMAN, E. M., and MILLICAN, F. K., 1963. Why children eat things that are not food. *Children*, **10**, 143.
15. MELLINS, R. G., and JENKINS, C. D., 1957. Lead poisoning in children. *Arch. Neurol. Psychiat.*, **77**, 70.
16. MELLINS, R. G., and JENKINS, C. D., 1955. Epidemiological and psychological study of lead poisoning in children. *J. Amer. med. Assn*, **158**, 15.
17. MENGEL, C. E., *et al.*, 1964. Geophagia with iron deficiency and hypokalemia—cachexia africana. *Amer. med. Assn, Arch. Int. Med.*, **114**, 470.
18. MILLICAN, F. K., LAYMAN, E. M., LOURIE, R. S., TAKAHASHI, L. Y., and DUBLIN, C. C., 1962. The prevalence of ingestion and mouthing of non-edible substances by children. *Clin. Proc. Children's Hospital of D.C.*, **18**, 207.
19. MILLICAN, F. K., LOURIE, R. S., and LAYMAN, E. M., 1956. Emotional factors in the etiology and treatment of lead poisoning. *Amer. med. Assn J. Dis. Child.*, **91**, 144.
20. SCHOLTZ, B. W., 1962. Medicine in the slums. *Clin. Proc. Children's Hospital of D.C.*, **18**, 345.
21. VAN DER SAR, A., and WASZINK, H. M., 1952. Pica (report on a case). *Docum. Med. Geog. Trop.*, **4**, 29.
22. WORTIS, H., RUE, R., HEIMER, C., BRAINE, M., REDLO, M., and FREEDMAN, A., 1962. Children who eat noxious substances. *J. Amer. Acad. Child Psychiat.*, **1**, 536.

XVII

PEPTIC ULCERS IN CHILDREN

THOMAS P. MILLAR
M.D., C.M.

*Director, Child Psychiatry, Housatonic Psychiatric Centre,
Lakeville, Conn. U.S.A.*

1
Introduction

There is considerable reason to believe that anxiety and emotional problems may play some part in the pathophysiology of peptic ulceration. If this is so, we are not able, at this time, to prove it. Nor can we trace, with certainty, the connection between the life experiences of the individual and the pathological changes in his gastro-intestinal tract. We are not presently able to say why a particular individual reacts to his life stress by developing an ulcer and another individual experiencing similar stress does not. Nor are we able to say why a particular patient develops a peptic ulcer and not asthma or hypertension or some other 'psychosomatic' disorder.

Despite these limitations in our present knowledge the patients present themselves for care and we must try to treat them. If treatment is to be more than the mindless dispensation of pills and reassurance it ought to be organized in terms of some rational formulation, however tentative, of the problem to be dealt with. So it is that we are compelled to make assumptions based upon uncertain knowledge.

The intent, in this presentation, is to explore briefly the present knowledge concerning peptic ulcer in children, to contribute some clinical observations, and from this base, outline an approach to treatment.

2
Incidence

For many years peptic ulcer has been considered to be rare in children, but in recent years sizeable series of cases are being reported in the literature.

Duodenal ulcer has become a disorder to be considered in the differential diagnosis of abdominal pain in the pediatric patient[2, 3, 13, 18].

It is not possible to say, however, whether peptic ulcer is on the increase in childhood or whether increased clinical awareness, coupled with improved radiological technique, is leading to the more accurate diagnosis of the condition.

Duodenal ulcers are more common than gastric and both are more common in boys than in girls. Ulcers in infants make up a considerable proportion of cases; 30 per cent in Tudor's series were less than one year of age[18]. A family history of ulcer is quite commonly reported, but there is disagreement concerning the incidence of such history[22, 7].

3

Diagnosis

The symptoms of peptic ulcer in children tend to be atypical, particularly in younger children[13]. The pain, when reported, may be poorly localized and less clearly related to food intake than in the adult. Less often too, is it relieved by eating. Nausea and vomiting, sometimes following meals, are common symptoms associated with ulcer in children, and are possibly related to the smaller calibre of the duodenum. Anorexia, early morning discomfort and headaches are frequently reported. A considerable number of ulcers in children are first diagnosed when a complication, usually haemorrhage, has occurred[2, 13].

Most clinicians rely upon radiological demonstration of a crater to establish the diagnosis. When the X-ray reveals pylorospasm or irritability of the bulb, the diagnosis of duodenitis is sometimes made. Berg reports that the re-examination of such cases, after a period of treatment has reduced the irritability, may reveal the ulcer crater[2].

It is possible that a number of ulcers in children are going undiagnosed. This author, commenting upon an observed association between peptic ulcer and school-phobia, noted that the gastrointestinal complaints of the school-phobic children had not, in many cases, been investigated[10].

4

Psychopathology: Clinical Reports

In general non-psychiatric observers reporting peptic ulcers in children draw attention to emotional problems accompanying the ulcers, some considering these to be of such character and degree as to have etiological significance. Lipton *et al.* in their recent discussion of psycho-physiological disorders in children provide an excellent survey of these reports[7].

Psychiatric studies of children with peptic ulcer have been few, and, as is inevitable with post hoc reports, they have serious drawbacks.

Perhaps their greatest value lies in making evident some of the dimensions that would be essential to a definitive study of the disorder.

Taboroff and Brown reported on six boys with peptic ulcer. They found significant emotional distress to be present in all cases. They reported that the boy's relationship to their mothers was disturbed in that they were overly dependent upon and markedly ambivalent toward this parent. Mixed rejection and overprotection characterized the maternal attitudes, and the children themselves were tense and shy. The authors felt that dependent desires and a 'felt danger over losing mother' were significant aspects of the observed psychopathology. They concluded that their data 'tended to substantiate Alexander's view . . . of the crucial factor being frustration of the dependent, help seeking and love demanding desires'[17].

Chapman et al. reported in detail upon five children, three boys and two girls, with peptic ulcer. They too found marked emotional problems which they felt to be significantly related to the ulcer. They described the children as tense, subnormally assertive, and having a desperate need to secure affectionate approval from the persons around them. They too implicated unmet needs in the area of affection and emotional security[6].

This author, in a previous publication, reported on five children with peptic ulcer in all of whom some degree of reluctance or refusal to attend school was also present. These children also had conflicts over dependent concerns. However, it was the author's view that the psychopathological configuration seen, i.e. an ambivalent, overprotective mother with a dependently conflicted, ego-immature child was not specific for peptic ulcer. Indeed this pattern is a most common one among latency age children presenting in psychiatric settings and is seen in association with a variety of symptoms, not all of which are psychosomatic.

Lipton[7], reviewing studies of asthmatic children reports very similar characteristics. 'Psychiatrists find almost total agreement on one point, that these patients have an inordinate attachment to their mothers. There is considerable agreement that the mothers are ambivalent toward, if not rejecting of these children, however their overt behaviour is more generally described as overprotective'. Later Lipton et al. conclude that 'the often cited nuclear conflict (in asthmatic children) appears to be the non-specific dependency problem characteristic of many patients with so called psychosomatic or chronic diseases beginning in childhood'.

So, while clinical studies provide evidence of significant emotional conflict in children with peptic ulcer, they do not establish with any clarity, the relationship between that emotional conflict and the ulceration itself. Clinicians, impelled perhaps by the need for a rational approach to treatment, have tended to formulate that relationship in terms of one or another of the theoretical models that have been postulated. There is point perhaps, in reviewing these models briefly, at this time.

5
Theoretical Models

The earliest such model postulated that psychosomatic disorders were conversion reactions and that the symptoms themselves represented symbolic expression of repressed feelings. While this view is generally discredited today, echoes of it are heard occasionally in clinical conferences or journal articles.

Dunbar attempted to correlate particular personality profiles with specific disorders but this view too has not found support from most observers. Attempts to define an ulcer personality were reviewed by Roth[14] who concluded, somewhat euphemistically, that 'the nature, or even the existence of an ulcer personality cannot be considered as established'.

Alexander hypothesized the specificity of conflict, i.e. that each conflict situation is accompanied by a specific pattern of physiologic alteration, and that the organ involved was related to the nature of the conflict situation. While clinicians frequently report strong dependency conflicts in patients with peptic ulcer, similar dependency conflicts are seen in patients with other psychosomatic symptoms. Streitfield[16] compared adults with peptic ulcer to patients with other pychosomatic disorders and found he could not differentiate the patients on the basis of oral-dependent needs.

The concept that psychosomatic disorders result from a regression to physiological mechanisms of an earlier developmental period has been examined by Mendelson *et al.*[8] who concluded that the concept provided but the illusion of knowledge.

Wolff[21] postulates that individuals have a biological reaction pattern which is genetically determined and consistent for that individual. When a particular individual is exposed to stress he will react in terms of his particular biological predisposition, which could result in the disordering of function of a particular organ system. The studies of Rutter, Birch, Thomas and Chess[15] concerning primary reaction patterns in children suggest that the behavioural reactions of children, might be in part due to similar innate predispositions.

The possibility of a physiological predisposition to peptic ulcer is suggested by the findings of Mirsky, as cited by Lipton[7], regarding the tendency to the hypersecretion of pepsinogen. Wretmark's[22] view that a specific familial disposition to ulcer exists might also support the view that a genetically determined biological reaction pattern may play a significant part in determining which individuals will react to life stress by developing an ulcer.

At this time, it would appear that the theoretical position remains unclear, yet it can be said with some certainty, that we now know more of what isn't so, than we did scant years ago.

6
Gastric Function and Peptic Ulcer

Before turning to clinical observations of children with peptic ulcer a brief review of elementary gastric physiology as this is related to emotions and peptic ulcer might prove helpful.

The gastric mucosa secretes pepsin and hydrochloric acid and, under normal circumstances, the mucosa resists the proteolytic activity of these substances. It seems probable that peptic ulceration occurs either when proteolytic activity increases, or when the resistance of the mucosa is diminished, for one reason or another.

The rate of secretion of hydrochloric acid appears to be under vagal and hormonal control, whereas the secretion of pepsin appears to be primarily under vagal control. It is possible that ACTH may render the gastric mucosa more sensitive to these physiological stimuli.

The gastric mucosa, ordinarily resistant to acid pepsin digestion and also capable of rapid regeneration, protects itself by the secretion of mucin. This secretion is stimulated by mechanical means or by vagal impulses. It is possible that ACTH reduces this protective reaction.

It is possible that persons who develop peptic ulcer are natural hypersecretors, and as a consequence their duodenum is their psychosomatic Achilles heel. If under conditions of emotional distress, the gastric mucosa is stimulated to increased secretion of pepsin and hydrochloric acid, it is possible that, for such persons, proteolytic activity within the duodenum may reach pathogenic levels.

There is some evidence that persons with peptic ulcer are hypersecretors of hydrochloric acid, although the post hoc nature of such studies makes it uncertain that they were hypersecretors prior to the development of their ulcer. Weiner *et al.*[19] were able to predict, with some success, which army recruits might react to the stress of basic training with peptic ulcer. They based their predictions upon measures of the blood pepsinogen levels.

There is a considerable body of evidence indicating that gastric functions are sensitive to emotional stress, that increased secretion of acid and pepsin may occur in certain people subject to certain kinds of emotional stress. Lipton *et al.*[7] review the findings concerning the effect of emotions on gastric function and conclude that the evidence, while strongly suggestive, is by no means unequivocable.

While there is evidently a good deal of work still to be done to clarify these matters, we have the elements necessary to establish a linkage between emotional stress and peptic ulceration. At the present time, and for clinical purposes, it seems safe to assume that neural or hormonal linkages between affect states and gastric physiological events exist, and that measures directed toward reducing the emotional distress of the peptic ulcer patient will be of value in his treatment.

7
Clinical Observations

The child psychiatrist probably sees but a small fragment of childhood peptic ulcer cases for, despite the general dissemination of psychiatric information that characterizes our times, not all parents, or physicians for that matter, see psychiatric intervention as a necessary part of the treatment of peptic ulcer. It is the author's impression that the children who are referred may be those with the most obvious emotional problems accompanying their ulcer. Under such circumstances generalizations from clinical data must be regarded as tentative.

The nine children with this disorder that the author has been privileged to study demonstrated a number of similarities in their personalities and life pattern. It is proposed, at this time, to describe a typical case as a basis for discussion of these similarities. Before doing so, it should be pointed out that the constellation of personality attributes and life pattern described is not, as the author has pointed out in a previous publication[10], specific for peptic ulcer. Indeed, these children and their families resemble a number of others, referred for quite different reasons, as much as they do each other.

Presenting Problems

The patient, whom we shall call Peter, is a 9-year-old boy, presently a third grade student. Peter has had intermittent pain and anorexia in the mornings for the past two years. These symptoms have seemed worse in the fall of the year, when school began, and after Christmas vacation. His mother had felt they were related to his recurring reluctance to attend school. They had, she confided ruefully, seemed to go away quickly enough when she gave in and let him stay home.

This summer the boy's father had been involved in an automobile accident, which, while not life threatening, had led to a period of hospitalization. Both Peter and his mother had found this very upsetting and Peter's stomach complaints were heard again. When school resumed the pattern of reluctance to attend, coupled with abdominal pain, anorexia and a suspicion of a black stool took mother to her family doctor.

X-ray investigation revealed an ulcer crater and occult blood in the stools. The child was placed on a bland diet, antispasmodics and antacids. Psychiatric referral was suggested and the mother agreed since she had 'other concerns about Peter besides his ulcer'.

Adjustment Problems

In addition to his ulcer and reluctance to attend school, Peter has problems in all areas of his life. He is a nervous, moody boy, inclined to be apprehensive in many situations. Despite his arrogant belligerence with his mother and siblings, he is quite timid outside of his home.

Peter's relationship with his mother is troubled for she finds him stubborn and wilful. He does not brush his teeth if he is not reminded several times. He is slow to dress in the morning and requires much supervision if he is not to be late for school. He forgets his chores. When he wants something, he wants it immediately and cannot wait. If he does not get it, he follows his mother about the house, whining or demanding, and he persists in this behaviour until his mother capitulates. If attempts are made to discipline him he acts 'as though his rights were being infringed upon'. He seems quite unaware of the rights of others in the household, however.

Peter's mother finds him very aggravating 'at times', but in general she is inclined to extenuate his shortcomings for she feels he is not a very happy boy.

A major concern of mother's is Peter's school difficulties. Even so he has shown some improvement in that setting. In the first and second grades Peter used to disrupt the class by his lack of cooperation and his tendency to talk out inappropriately. He was at that time openly resentful of the teacher's attempts to exercise her authority. At the present time, Peter is quiet in the classroom, but he has become quite withdrawn. He looks out the window, daydreams and seldom finishes the assigned set work. Sometimes he does not even start the work. Despite his above normal intelligence he is in danger of repeating the third grade if he persists in failing to do his work.

Peter's peer relationships are poor. As a pre-schooler and in first grade Peter was egocentric and bossy with other children. Because of these traits he experienced a considerable amount of rejection. Now he isolates himself or plays with children younger than himself. He has but one continuing friendship, with an uncertain, compliant boy who has adjustment problems of his own. In that relationship Peter is an autocratic leader.

At the present time, in settings other than his home, Peter gives the impression of being an inhibited, apprehensive child, lacking in self confidence. His teachers have been reluctant to pressure him to complete his work.

Family History

Peter is the oldest of three children, two boys and a girl. Life in his family is not untroubled for his parents occasionally express their dissatisfaction with each other quite openly. The focus of some of these discussions is Peter's behaviour and its management. However, the parents have never separated, and neither sees their relationship as that bankrupt.

The father is a salesman, at which he is moderately successful. He is absent from his home a good deal. More significant, however, is his psychological absence, for he involves himself minimally in the parenting of his children. The history suggests that, as family problems accumulated he expressed his essential passivity by withdrawing from a situation in which he felt powerless. He feels his wife spoils the boy, but that there is nothing he can do to stop her.

The mother, therefore, is the key parenting figure. She is an uncertain woman, uncertain of her rights as an individual, not only with respect to her husband, but also with her children. Her lack of clarity concerning the difference between adult and child perogatives leads her into ineffectual discharge of her limit-setting responsibilities. She has a continuing relationship to her own mother, one that has strong dependent overtones.

Her ambivalence to Peter is marked. It is possible to elicit, if one is the least supportive and non-critical, an increasingly direct account of her considerable aggravation with the child. Similarly, if one focuses upon Peter's nervousness or unhappiness, she will begin to express increasing concern and solicitude for the child. Her overprotectiveness amounts, at times, to infantilization. It seems to arise out of her solicitude, a feeling which is periodically reinforced by the remorse she feels following an occasion when her accumulated aggravation has led her into an angry explosion. At such times, her desire to 'make it up to the child' leads her into quite inappropriate responses to his behaviour.

Developmental History

Peter was 1 month premature, but he weighed six pounds. Partly perhaps because of this, and partly perhaps because it was her first child and Peter's mother had never been a very self-confident person, her approach to child care was a concerned one. During Peter's infancy his mother was inclined to hover, to anticipate the child's needs and to want to spare her baby the frustration of waiting for gratification, be it for his bottle, or her attention. As a result, weaning, toilet-training, the expectation that the child dress himself, all were somewhat delayed, and when begun, mother tended to continue to involve herself in their supervision excessively. Even after Peter had begun school, mother continued to tie his shoelaces and dress him in the morning quite frequently.

The impression one gets is that Peter experienced a surfeit of dependent gratification. As an infant mother found him to be an easy, pleasing baby, and she addressed herself to his needs with self-effacing dedication. And it was not until he was nearing 3 years of age that he became so wilful and demanding.

It seems probable that a change in mother's attitude coincided with this alteration. She began to feel that it was time he gave up some of his infantile ways. Perhaps this was some emerging awareness on her part of Peter's immaturity. Perhaps the arrival of a second child made it no longer possible to indulge Peter as she had done. It was about this time that Peter began to express some separation concerns. However, this anxiety was not mastered, for mother avoided separation. As she puts it, 'I never went out, so it wasn't much of a problem'.

In reviewing the character of Peter's mothering, two things seem apparent; One, there was an excessive closeness and a surfeit of dependent gratification. Two, mother seemed unable to assist Peter to mature by offering him measured expectancies. The excessive solicitude that led her to indulge him, seemed also to motivate her to protect him from expectancies with which he might not be able to cope.

The Child

Peter is a spare, almost thin child, who is constantly shifting, twisting, tapping or contorting some part of his body. He walks and speaks quickly, sometimes stumbling over his words. He enters the interview situation with his guard up. As his alert eyes take the measure of the playroom and the doctor, his responses are controlled. However, he is not so anxious that he cannot communicate nor respond to a relaxing pleasantry. He is clearly a perceptive child, and he knows there is a good deal more going on than merely chatting with a 'nice' man. As the interview progresses, Peter relaxes his guard, and in the latter portion he is beginning to test the limits of acceptable behaviour in the playroom, and trade roles with the examiner.

In the course of the interview Peter gradually reveals his style of dealing with himself and the world. It becomes gradually apparent, for example, that his braggadoccio, his vigorous declarations of competence and worth, conceal a deeply damaged self-esteem. His declarations to the contrary, it becomes very much apparent that he cares very much that his peers call him 'baby' and other names, and don't want to play with him. While he declares the fault lies in his rejectors, it is clear he suspects, albeit transiently, that there is fault in him.

While he derogates learning, he knows that his peers can tolerate the tedious aspects of classwork better than he, and senses that this too, is an aspect of his incompetence. While he justifies his outbursts of temper on the basis of intolerable provocation, it seems that these too may reflect a personal weakness.

Peter's fragile self-esteem requires constant defence. He sees criticism in the most gentle query, and he may react with arrogant belligerence, that requires careful handling if the relationship is not to be disrupted or rendered sterile.

Another prominent aspect of Peter's personality is his poorly developed tolerance for delay or unpleasure, of which of course, his intolerance for anxiety is most evident. This is evident in the history. In the interview, Peter can become quite scattered. He moves impulsively from topic to topic, or activity to activity as each touches upon some unpleasure within him, or each offers some promise of more immediate pleasure. Yet there are concerns Peter needs to deal with, and if one leads him gently, he will explore those issues.

In the course of Peter's projection of his inner concerns two themes dominate. The first of these is his continuing separation anxiety, and the second is his pervasive concern over his autonomy.

Peter is gradually able to reveal that he worries about accident or injury occurring to his mother and that sometimes, when he is daydreaming in the classroom, he is thinking about his mother at home and wondering whether she is all right. Then he wishes he were home so he could assure himself that she was all right. It is a thought he cannot rid himself of, and sometimes he elaborates upon frightening possibilities. She has, for example, only recently learned to drive, and he wonders maybe if she might not have gotten into an accident. Sometimes, his concern takes the form of wondering whether she might not have just gone away and left the family to fend for itself. When his father got sick, it worried his mother, and that made him worry too. If he didn't have his mother, he says, who would take care of him?

Peter's other major concern is to define his autonomy, that is, to make clear which aspects of his life are his to control and which are subject to the will of others. Peter's approach to this definition is to assert his omnipotence, and to regard all expectations of adults as attempts to deprive him of all self direction. And so he reacts to expectations pridefully. As his mother puts it; 'If you tell Peter to do anything, he gets his back up immediately, but if you ask him nicely, sometimes he will do it'.

When Peter's teacher attempts to exercise her authority with respect to classwork, Peter balks. He says; 'she is bossy, always coming on strong. She can't make me do that work'.

In Peter's play, themes of power and subservience, the boss and the bossed, occupy a good deal of his interest. One of the first questions he asks the doctor, when he has become sufficiently relaxed, is: 'Who is your boss? Can he fire you?' In the interview relationship Peter is constantly setting up situations where struggles for control could eventuate, so it is that he tests limits, or seeks to switch roles and prerogatives with the psychiatrist.

Another aspect of Peter's personality that is evident in the interview situation, as well as the history, is his continued egocentricity, that is his failure to move from a pre-Copernican view of the world, with himself at the centre and events taking their meaning from that perspective, to a beginning of the ethnocentricity upon which social interaction is based. He cannot, in his home or peer relationships conceive of himself as a member of a group, and has, as a consequence, a most limited view of the rights of others.

His concern over accident or injury occurring to his mother is really concern for what might happen to him, if she were not there to care for him. Similarly, in the interview situation, his awareness of the examiner and his concerns is conditional upon how those concerns touch him. He sees, for example, no obligation to answer a question that doesn't interest him, and cannot conceive of a social obligation to respond. It seems evident that it is his egocentricity in his relationships at school and home that leads to his rejection, and equally evident that he cannot understand how he offends. His egocentricity is such that it simply does not occur to him that another child might not want to play the game that he at that moment finds attractive.

Recapitulation

In this typical case history are contained the similarities the author has observed in his experience of children with peptic ulcer and their families. Very briefly recapitulated, they are these:

The peptic ulcer is rarely seen unaccompanied by serious other psychological symptoms of which reluctance or refusal to attend school is common. Some recent aggravant of the child's anxiety in the period preceding the discovery of the ulcer is not uncommon in the history. A particular constellation of behavioural and adjustment problems at home and school is quite frequently seen in these cases.

The fathers tend to be minimally involved in the parenting of their children, and *the mothers excessively involved in an ambivalent and overprotective manner*. The origins of the mothers' ambivalent overprotection appear to be several and to vary from case to case, as will be discussed in more detail later. The effect of these maternal attitudes upon the child rearing practices is such that *the child receives a surfeit of dependent gratification, but is denied gradually paced expectation for increasingly independent function*.

The children tend to be anxious and inhibited outside of the protective milieu of their homes. They reveal considerable *conflict over dependent needs* and experience continuing separation anxiety. They demonstrate *intolerance for delay* or unpleasure, marked continuing *egocentricity*, a major concern over and preoccupation with their personal *autonomy*, and seriously *impaired self esteem*.

8

Dynamic Formulation

In attempting to formulate a comprehension of these children we are confronted with an apparent paradox. While the children are clearly conflicted over dependent concerns, their mothers have offered them, during their infancy, an excess of dependent gratification. They have certainly not experienced the deprivation of dependent gratification that previous theoretical formulations had led us to look for.

Yet this may not be a paradox. It is only one if we continue to conceive of children as needing a certain amount of dependent gratification, which need, once met, frees the child to move on to independent function. Perhaps children, or adults for that matter, have dependent needs as long as they are realistically dependent, that is, until such time as they have developed sufficient adaptive ego strength to essay function independent of the protection of mother.

In this connection Caldwell[4] comments relevantly in her review of the effects of infant care. She concludes that 'studies concerned with oral gratification and oral activities provide little support for the hypothesis that sustained gratification leads to drive satisfaction'. Indeed it is her view that 'continuing gratification seems to heighten the infants emotional response to the transition' (to other techniques of obtaining nourishment). While, in this Caldwell is dealing with oral activities per se, the theoretical implications seem relevant.

It would seem that, for these children, the dependency conflicts arise as a consequence of mother's failure to offer her child the measured expectancies that exercise and nourish his capacity for independence. *The child remains dependent because he is psychologically incompetent to move on to appropriately autonomous function*[10].

In order to understand in more detail, precisely how Peter's personality defects are related to his mother's child rearing practices it is proposed to examine these characteristics in the light of these events.

Intolerance for Delay

In seeking to spare Peter the pain of frustration his mother may also have denied him the experience of unpleasure mastered, of delay coped with successfully. As an infant Peter undoubtedly woke hungry and cried for his bottle. His mother's concern for him was such that she may, as infantilizing mothers not infrequently do, have begun to anticipate his waking, perhaps even sitting by his crib, bottle warmed, waiting for him to awake. By so doing she may indeed have spared Peter frustration, but she may also have denied him the experience of delay mastered to a successful conclusion.

The hungry infant's cry is an expression of his internal unpleasure. In waiting a brief while he learns:

1. Unpleasure is tolerable.
2. It comes to an end.

So it is that the foundation for tolerance of delay is laid. This capacity is an indispensable building block for many later emerging adaptive functions.

Early childhood is replete with situations which require the delay of gratification or the tolerance of unpleasure. Each reasonable such requirement coped with, increases the child's capacity for later coping. The experience of successful coping reassures the child and nourishes his emerging esteem.

The infantilizing mother may see her child's frustrations as overwhelming or excessively painful and be led to spare him, sometimes quite unrealistically. In another publication the author described such a mother whose toddler became extremely upset when the sofa did not move when he pushed against it! To spare him his evident frustration, the mother took to hiding behind the sofa and pulling it when the child pushed, so preserving her child's omnipotent view of the world and easing his psychic pain.

While these may be gross examples, it is apparent that the child whose needs are constantly anticipated, who is protected from minor frustration and unpleasure by an overly concerned mother, has little opportunity to develop a capacity for unpleasure. When such a child is faced with some of the normal anxieties of maturation, such as separation, it is not surprising if he seems overwhelmed by them.

Egocentricity

The 4-year-old believes the sun rises when he does, follows him around all day, and goes to bed when he does. This egocentric conception of the world is, in the normal course of events, eventually disillusioned by the intrusion of discrepant realities.

The interpersonal egocentricity of the child comes up against the rights of his parents, who, if they are self-respecting individuals unwilling to subjugate themselves or organize all aspects of their life around the needs of their child, begin the disillusioning process. It seems probable that, as the child becomes more mobile and communicative, his capacity to dominate the lives of his parents increases, and it becomes increasingly necessary for the parents to communicate to the child some limits with respect to his place in the life of the family. In order to do this, the parent must know, with some clarity, the difference between their prerogatives and that of their child. As this phase is gradually navigated the child is equipped with a beginning awareness of the rights of others which serves him in his essays at relating to his peers.

The parent who, for one reason or another, is excessively concerned for her child, or self effacing with respect to him, may fail to offer her child the input that will lead him away from egocentricity. His infantile egocentricity persists and he remains minimally aware of the rights and concerns of others. Difficulties with peers and his teacher often arise. The child's egocentricity is such that he truly cannot comprehend how he offends.

Omnipotence and Autonomy

An important phase of the ego development of the child is that during which his normally acquired omnipotent view of the world is disillusioned[1, 10, 11]. The perceptual immaturity of the infant leads him to misinterpret the responses of the world as non-elective acts obedient to his will. It is easy to conceive how such an omnipotent comprehension would have profound anxiety-avoiding value for the helpless infant. The disillusioning of this omnipotence is a gradual process arising in part as a result of the growing perceptual maturity of the infant, but largely dependent upon the parents' increasing unwillingness to acquiesce to the will of the infant. The accepted child, who comes to this point having experienced his parents' responsible care, will be able to give up the omnipotent illusion for a belief and trust in the omnipotence of his parents.

The overprotective parent may seek to protect her child from the disillusioning reality, as was the case with the mother who pulled the sofa. She allows her child to persist in his omnipotent illusion concerning the world. Nor does she equip her child with any real competence, the knowledge of which might make it easier for the child to accept his realistic self. Yet his perceptual maturation is providing input that may suggest to him that his faith in his omnipotence is ill placed. So it is perhaps that he seeks to confirm his omnipotence by demonstrating it, by ordering his parent about, by testing whether or not she must not acquiesce to his powerful will. So it is perhaps that the child has an abnormal investment in the omnipotent illusion.

This may be related to his symptoms, e.g. these children are frequently preoccupied with power themes, which appear in their play and also characterize their relationships in and out of treatment. It is the author's experience with school phobias that omnipotent concerns are not infrequently the precipitants of the school refusal pattern. A confrontation between the teacher and the child so threatens the child's omnipotent view of himself that he avoids school rather than accept the devaluation he fears.

It is possible also that the seriously damaged esteem of the child plays a part in his tendency to see limits as affronts or derogations that diminish him. It is as though to define him as a child, without adult prerogatives, is to label him as inadequate or even worthless. Even so, it is the author's experience that once a clarification of adult and child roles has been weathered through, such children experience considerable relief.

Impaired Self-esteem

It seems probable that self esteem arises less out of parental approval than it does out of experienced success. When a child faces an expectancy such as learning to tie his shoe laces, and his efforts to have his mother solve the problem for him are resisted, he will eventually fumble his way through to a successful completion of the job. A few minutes of daily instruction and patient expectation and eventually the child will complete the job himself. The first time he does this on his own his pride and pleasure in the accomplishment will be apparent. It is through multiple experiences of expectancies faced, coped with and mastered, that the child develops a conception of himself as an adequate person[20]. It seems improbable that parental approval, without experiences of coping, can lead to any significant self esteem.

The infantilized child is allowed to give up, things are done for him, and he does not cope nor experience mastery. Just as his capacity for independent function fails to develop, so his self esteem is not constructed. Later, when he leaves the unconditional approval of his home, it will not escape him that his peers cope successfully with situations he cannot handle. His fragile esteem is threatened by this knowledge. So it is that the Peters sometimes hide behind arrogant braggadoccio and declarations of superior worth.

Peptic Ulcers in Children: a Tentative Formulation

In the foregoing the adjustment difficulties and personality characteristics of the child with peptic ulcer have been examined in relation to his parental experiences. This examination suggests that the observed psychopathology might best be understood in the following terms.

The marked adaptive immaturity of these children arises out of maternal overprotection which denies the child appropriate limits and measured expectancies. As a consequence the child is poorly equipped for appropriately autonomous function. Given his adaptive capacity he has little real competence for function outside of the dependent dyad.

At the same time, the child is under considerable pressure, both internal and external, to give up his dependent mode. To varying degree, the child may have learned to be ashamed of his immaturity. While he clings to it, he may resent the need to. A principal source of the considerable hostility these children feel toward their mothers, seems to arise as a reaction to mother's failure to be a wise parent and lead her child to psychic strength. To a considerable extent the child may be internally motivated to give up his dependency.

The external pressures on the child stem from school, his peer group and his mother. His mother, despite her dynamically determined need to perpetuate her child's dependence, may also find this personally onerous and have become aware of its abnormality. In ways which are often ineffectual she may, for brief periods, pressure her child to become more independent.

As a consequence, the child is constantly fighting the same battle, that of separation to achieve some degree of independent function. Yet he never wins. His essay at independent function may founder when his adaptive maturity proves unequal to the task. Or his mother, fearful for his well-being, may invite him back to the haven of her protection. It is an invitation he cannot resist, and so begins another cycle of failed separation.

It seems probable that the child with peptic ulcer is subject to repeated bouts of anxiety over separation. The pathology lies in the unproductive and repeated nature of these episodes. The normal child experiences separation anxiety, but, the separation achieved, masters this anxiety and is less its victim the next time around.

It is possible that the predisposed child may react to particularly intense or prolonged episodes of such anxiety, with altered gastric function which may lead to a peptic ulcer. Yet this does not mean that a specific dynamic relationship between dependency conflict and peptic ulcer is involved.

In the author's experience, this psychopathological configuration is not specific for peptic ulcer. It is seen in relation to such symptoms as school phobia[9], learning and behavioural disorders, as well as other psychosomatic disorders[7]. This is in accord with the findings of others, as reported earlier in this presentation.

Further, it is entirely possible that a group of adolescents with peptic ulcer may be conflicted over some adolescent concern such as the struggle to clarify their identity. All that can reasonably be inferred from these clinical findings is that a considerable degree of emotional conflict, functioning perhaps as a non-specific stress, appears to play a part in the genesis of peptic ulcer.

Assuming then, that this emotional conflict leads to altered gastric function, we need still to postulate some other determining factor, such as a biological predisposition to abnormal gastric function. It is, apparently, only certain individuals who develop such a degree of imbalance between proteolytic activity in the duodenum and the protective capacity of the mucosa, to permit ulceration to occur.

In summary then, children with peptic ulcer are characterized by marked dependency conflict, which seems to be a consequence of infantilization that prevents their developing ordinary adaptive competence. It seems probable that this conflict leads to alterations in gastric function. Some biological predisposition in the child is the final determinant of his reacting by developing a peptic ulcer rather than some other symptom associated with this psychopathological configuration.

The purpose of dynamic formulation is to give direction to treatment, and hopefully to illuminate where therapeutic leverage is possible. We turn now to a consideration of these issues.

9

Treatment Considerations

The preceding formulation suggests both short-term and long-term considerations are relevant to planning the psychiatric treatment of the child with peptic ulcer. The short-term considerations involve the reduction or alleviation of anxiety which may be contributing to the duodenal pathology during the acute phase of the illness. The long-term considerations have to do with promoting the adaptive maturation of the child with a view to equipping him for independent function without excessive conflict.

The Acute Phase

Presuming the child is seen in the acute phase of his ulcer and the psychiatrist is asked to contribute to the total management of the illness, his first concern will be to reduce the level of anxiety in the child. The assumption is that this anxiety may be contributing to gastric hypersecretion and so to the ulcer pathology.

Anxiety may be reduced by tranquillizers, alleviated by exploration and ventilation in interview or projective play, and/or avoided by removal or alteration of its situational precipitants. It is mastered by coping.

It seems rational, on theoretical grounds, to regard acute peptic ulcer as a valid indication for the use of tranquillizing drugs. It would be interesting to know, however, precisely how these drugs effect gastric secretion in peptic ulcer patients.

Frequent interviews at the bedside, or in the playroom, will facilitate the early establishment of a relationship in which the child's anxieties may be given indirect expression. One may discover that some recent increase of the child's separation anxiety has occurred, or possibly that something has aggravated a phase of his chronic ambivalence to his mother. Some real occurrence may have illuminated his particular concerns. For example, the death of a known relative may have endowed his fantasies of accident or injury occurring to his mother, with sudden reality.

The exploration and ventilation of these concerns lessens their affective intensity. Projective play that displaces and drains off either hostile or anxious feelings reduces the conflict within the child. It is doubtful if interpretation to the child of the meaning of his play is of value in this phase of his care.

Information obtained in such interviews together with what one learns of the home situation provide the psychiatrist with a comprehension of the particular dynamic configuration of this child. It is from this base that he may be able to advise changes in the situation of the child that will reduce his conflict.

The decision to hospitalize the child may, for example, involve weighing such considerations along with the medical indications. In this connection the extremities of view-point are represented on the one hand by those who feel that the way to deal with separation anxiety is by 'parentectomy', and on the other by those who regard 'separation' as the villain and its total avoidance as the solution.

The judgment to be made involves a consideration of the child's present capacities in terms of the short-term and long-term goals of treatment. The child can be overwhelmed by an expectance too far beyond his current capacity, but neither are his interests served by an excessive lowering of the sights to accommodate his, or his mother's, estimate of that capacity. It must be remembered that while separation anxiety may be alleviated by avoiding separation, separation conflict is mastered by achieving appropriate degrees of separation.

Promoting the Adaptive Maturity of the Child

It seems evident that finding ways to promote the adaptive maturity of the child is the principal concern of the treating psychiatrist, for not only may the child's future freedom from peptic ulcer depend on this, but also his life style, his effectiveness as a person, depends upon his developing capacity to deal with the vicissitudes of the human condition in a modern society.

It seems, to the author, that this is not necessarily an impossible undertaking. This optimism stems from the following considerations. The child is yet a child. He is still flexible, capable of learning and unlearning if he can be provided with the appropriate experiences. His parent, misguided perhaps, is concerned for the well-being of her child and his problems stem more from distortion than deprivation. His present state may be regarded as an impasse, a blind alley into which his life experience has led him (and his mother). Adaptive psychological growth has stopped or been markedly slowed. If he and his parent can be led from this blind alley and faced in the right direction, the child's innate capacity for psychological maturation will begin to express itself again.

The psychiatrist has three entries to this task. He may work with the parents, helping them to deal with the child in ways that will promote his maturation. He may establish a relationship with the child, and through that relationship assist the child to a more effective use of himself. Finally he may guide the teacher so that she may contribute effectively to building the adaptive maturity of the child.

Work with the parents. Insofar as the parents are still the primary socializing influence for latency age children, work with them has the greatest potentiality for therapeutic gain. And, since it is the mothers of these children who are primarily involved in the difficulties, much of the effort must be directed to helping the mother deal more effectively with her child.

If one reviews with the mother, her patterns of child care, her infantilizing overprotection is often readily apparent. She may, for example, still dress the child in the morning, or tie his shoes for him. She may stay home at night because her child objects to her going out. Her pattern of deferring to her child may be more or less obvious. The point is, that a review of her daily relationship to the child, will immediately suggest changes in parenting behaviour. While there is undoubtedly something to gain by direct guidance to the parent around this behaviour, it is also true that unless we can comprehend the dynamic origin of mother's overprotective attitude and involve that dynamic in our dealings with her, our guidance may well prove ineffective.

Maternal overprotection has many roots, some of which make this attitude more accessible to change than others. Normal parents may overprotect a handicapped or chronically-ill child as a reaction to their special concern for him. Dependent mothers, women who have been unable to solve their own problems with separation and independence, may see the world as a fearsome place, and separation for their child as unthinkable. Frustrated unhappy women sometimes project their unhappiness into their children and seek to succour themselves in their child. Some mothers sacrifice their self respect on the altar of their guilt and so make slaves of themselves to their children.

Some overprotective patterns arise as secondary complications. Not all children, for example, are as easy to rear as others. Some intensely reacting, energetic children may struggle vigorously to dominate their mothers and retain their omnipotent posture, while other more placid children may respond to mildly enunciated expectations with smiling compliance. The mother of the former child may well develop hostile feelings which she may feel constrained to disown. She may then convert these feelings into a compensatory protectiveness, which in turn perpetuates the immaturity of her child and aggravates the cycle.

The classical approach, of course, is to explore with the mother, the roots of her need to overprotect her child, hoping that with insight she will be able to give up this behaviour. It is the author's experience that this is not always the most expeditious approach to guiding the mother to more effective management of her child. If for example one drains off a significant amount of the mother's irritation with the demands of her child, the reduction in her hostility may make it possible for her to approach her child with more assertion and assurance. Similarly, if the guilty mother can ventilate her concern and become less guilty she can, without insight, approach her child with less need to sacrifice herself to his needs. It seems that a change in mother's feelings toward her child, even if she remains without insight into her protectiveness, opens the door to a more realistic child rearing approach. The mother is then in a position to learn from experiences of successful parenting.

At this point, it is often the case that direct guidance to the mother around the management of a specific fragment of her child rearing, may initiate important learning for her and her child. She may, for example, set a limit successfully, because the doctor told her to; i.e. making her child dress himself or lose his T.V. privileges is undertaken, not out of hostility to the child, but because the doctor told her to. When her child eventually responds to this expectation by accepting it, shows pleasure in his capacity to measure up, and proves not to hate her for her firmness, she is led to question some of her previous concerns. At this point she may come back to the psychiatrist with some insight of her own into her prior protectiveness. Not infrequently she will have abstracted from her successful management some fresh principles concerning parent-child relationships.

Many factors enter into determining how effective guidance to the parents will be in altering the overprotective pattern, with some parents much more able to respond than others. However it is the author's experience that significant gains can be made with most intact, middle-class families.

It is the author's view that some mothers who would otherwise slip into overprotective relationships to their children do not do so, because their husband will not permit this state of affairs to continue. The interested and concerned father who sees his wife deferring excessively to or over-protecting the child, interferes on behalf of his wife, or child, or both. Reassured by him, the wife may find the strength to deal more effectively with the child, or the father may himself assume limit-setting responsibilities in areas where his wife seems incapable.

The fathers of these children appear to have abandoned their wives and children to their pathological overinvolvement with one another. Some effort to bring the father back into the situation is warranted and sometimes proves a most effective remedy. The author finds it helpful initially to define the father's area of involvement quite specifically, and to caution his wife not to interfere with her husband's limit setting. A favourite device of such fathers when mother does interfere is to say, 'all right, do it your way', whereupon, absolved of further responsibility, the father withdraws once more from participation. If the father can be nourished until he experiences some success as a parent, his continued involvement can be promoted.

In assisting the parents to set more effective limits and to offer their child appropriate expectancies, it is hoped to promote the child's capacity to tolerate delay, and lead him away from infantile egocentricity. By weathering a confrontation concerning his omnipotence the child may be led toward comfort in his autonomy. With each expectancy met, the esteem of the child is served. The process is a continuing one, and the parents have a crucial part to play in it.

Work with the child. In treating the child directly the psychiatrist establishes a relationship with the child which he utilizes to clarify the child's confusion about himself and the world about him. By allowing the child to ventilate and examine his anxieties, he helps the child to manage them.

It is inevitable, as the relationship develops that the child introduces into it the distortions that are the source of so much of his difficulty at home and school. So it is that the child introduces his conflicts concerning autonomy. He sets up struggles for control, struggles in which the therapist can lose therapeutic ground in two ways. He can, for example, serve the omnipotent fantasies of the child by deferring to him. But in this he must fail, for the child's omnipotent demands will increase until they must be denied, at which point the therapist may have compromised himself out of business. The other way in which the therapist can lose is to counter omnipotence with omnipotence, which only confirms the child's view that there are only two categories of being, that of king and that of slave. But the therapeutic goal was to assist the child to autonomy, the concept of a degree of self direction appropriate to his maturity. If the therapist can succeed in treading the narrow ground between these two errors, with but occasional minor lapses, the child can gradually be led to give up his omnipotent fantasy. If at the same time events at home are providing new input for the child, this process may occur with reasonable dispatch.

Another characteristic of the child which makes itself felt in the therapy is his egocentricity. By presenting himself to the child as a real person with rights the therapist intrudes upon the egocentric perception. The child may resist this intrusion, but if the therapist persists in requiring the child to take him into account, the child will begin to accommodate. Such accommodation is the beginning of ethnocentricity. With it may come some insight on the child's part of his role in his failures with his peers.

The therapist may also serve the child by assisting him to develop a capacity for delay. The scattered child may be assisted to retain his focus by limiting his freedom to move from activity to activity without control. By expecting the child to wait for certain gratifications his capacity to wait may be increased.

By leading the child to persistence and small success in playroom activities, the child is helped to discover the route to esteem.

In all of these activities the therapist's acceptance of the child is the source of much of his leverage. If the therapist can see, behind the omnipotent tyranny, the child struggling to find a way to like himself, he may convince the child that, despite the painful confrontations, he is serving the child's interests.

Work with the teacher. The school has always had an important role to play in promoting the maturation of the child, yet sometimes it seems that the teacher's concern for the child's emotional state, leads her away from the successful discharge of that role. Because children like Peter seem anxious, teachers are sometimes reluctant to reinforce the normal expectations. This, of course, does nothing to promote Peter's tolerance for unpleasure nor does it disillusion his omnipotence or assist him in his peer relationships.

In fairness to the teacher it should be said that the routes to this approach to children like Peter are many. Sometimes the teacher is under considerable pressure from the parents not to expect too much of the child. In order to get Peter to do his work, a good deal more supervision than the teacher is able to offer may be required. Then too there is the teacher's emotional reactions.

When the child challenges the teacher's prerogatives he sometimes leads her into a determination to clarify exactly who is in charge of the class. She feels she must win this battle, or lose control of her class. She may be led into inappropriate measures, or angry actions about which she later feels guilty. After one or two such encounters she may be willing to settle for peace in the classroom and allow herself to forget that the child's interests are not served by accepting his minimal academic performance.

Within the limits of her situation, the teacher can be helped to deal more effectively with the child and so promote his maturity. A consultative relationship with the teacher can do much to serve this aspect of the total therapy of the child. The dynamics of this consultation have been discussed in detail in another publication and need not be more than alluded to here[12].

10

Conclusion

In this presentation the author has explored briefly the present knowledge concerning peptic ulcer in children, contributed some clinical observations and essayed an approach to treatment based on a proposed formulation of the dynamics involved.

It is evident that controlled clinical studies of this and other psychophysiological disorders in children are badly needed, and that no one of us sees a sufficiently representative sample to permit more than tentative generalizations. Yet we must treat these children, and it is in the light of this urgency that the author presumes upon his limited experience.

REFERENCES

1. AUSUBEL, D. B., 1952. *Ego development and the personality disorders.* New York, Grune and Stratton.
2. BERG, R. M., 1961. Peptic ulcers in children. *Southern med. J.*, **54**, 325.
3. BERG, R. M., BERG, H. M., ERIKSON, J. A., and LEVI, W. E., 1960. Peptic ulcers in children. *Lancet*, ii, 43.
4. CALDWELL, B. M., 1964. The effects of infant care. In *Review of child development research*, vol. 1. Eds, Hoffman, L. W., and Hoffman, M. New York, Russell Sage Foundation.
5. CASTENUOVO-TEDESCO, P., 1962. Emotional antecedents of perforation of ulcers of the stomach and duodenum. *Psychosom. Med.*, **24**, 398.
6. CHAPMAN, A. H., LOEB, D. G., and YOUNG, J. P., 1956. A psychosomatic study of five children with peptic ulcer. *J. Pediatrics*, **48**, 248.
7. LIPTON, E. L., STEINSCHNEIDER, A., and RICHMOND, J. P., 1966. Psychophysiological disorders in children. In *Review of child development research*, vol. 2. Eds, Hoffman, L. W., and Hoffman, M. New York, Russell Sage Foundation.
8. MENDELSON, M., HIRSCH, S., and WEBBER, C. S., 1956. A critical examination of some recent theoretical models in psychosomatic medicine. *Psychosom. Med.*, **18**, 363.
9. MILLAR, T. P., 1961. The child who refuses to attend school. *Am. J. Psychiat.*, **118**, 398.
10. MILLAR, T. P., 1965. Peptic ulcers in children. *Canad. Psychiat. Assn J.*, **10**, 43.
11. MILLAR, T. P., 1968. Limit setting and psychological maturation. *Arch. gen. Psychiat.*, **8**, 214.
12. MILLAR, T. P., 1966. Psychiatric consultation with classroom teachers. *J. Am. Acad. Child Psychiat.*, **5**, 134.

13. MUGGIA, A., and SPIRO, H. M., 1959. Childhood peptic ulcer. *Gastroenterology*, **37**, 715.
14. ROTH, H. P., 1955. The peptic ulcer personality. *Am. med Assn Arch. Int. Med.*, **96**, 32.
15. RUTTER, M., BIRCH, H., THOMAS, A., CHESS, S., 1964. Temperamental characteristics in infancy and the later development of behavioural disorders. *Brit. J. Psychiat.*, **110**, 651.
16. STREITFIELD, H. S., 1954. Specificity of peptic ulcer to intense oral conflicts. *Psychosom. Med.*, **16**, 315.
17. TABOROFF, L., and BROWN, W., 1954. A study of the personality patterns of children and adolescents with the peptic ulcer syndrome. *Amer. J. Orthopsychiat.*, **24**, 602.
18. TUDOR, R. B., 1954. The peptic ulcer problem in infancy and childhood. *Lancet*, ii, 189.
19. WEINER, H., THALER, M., REISER, M. F., and MIRSKY, J. A., 1957. Etiology of duodenal ulcer: I. Relation of specific psychological characteristics to rate of gastric secretion. *Psychosom. Med.*, **19**, 1.
20. WHITE. R. W., 1963. Ego and reality in psychoanalytic theory. *Psychological Issues*, **3**. New York, Internat. Univ. Press.
21. WOLFF, H. G., 1950. Life stress and bodily disease, a formulation. *Proc. Assn Res. nerv. ment. Dis.*, **24**, 1059.
22. WRETMARK, G., 1960. Mental and psychosomatic morbidity in peptic ulcer families. *J. Psychosom. Res.*, **5**, 21.

XVIII

THE MANAGEMENT OF ULCERATIVE COLITIS IN CHILDHOOD*

DANE G. PRUGH
M.D.

AND

KENT JORDAN
M.D.

Departments of Psychiatry and Pediatrics, University of Colorado School of Medicine and Dentistry, Denver, Colorado, U.S.A.

"For some patients, though conscious that their condition is perilous, recover their health simply through their contentment with the goodness of the physician."

(*Hippocrates: Precepts*)

1
Introduction

No clinical condition has puzzled and challenged physicians more than that of chronic non-specific ulcerative colitis. This syndrome was first described by White[115] in England in 1888, as an entity distinct from other causes of the 'bloody flux' of antiquity. Although Logan[72] in 1919 reported a single child case, its occurrence in childhood was not generally recognized until the incisive description put forth by Helmholtz[53] in 1923. Since then many cases have been described in childhood in the literature of most Western countries[18, 43, 54, 55, 57, 62, 66, 75, 83, 88, 106].

In this presentation, based on a study of 76 child and adolescent

---

* This work was supported in part by grants from the National Institute of Mental Health, National Institutes of Health, United States Public Health Service, Washington, D.C.

patients, attention will be directed toward the details of management and therapy of this condition. First, however, a brief review and summary will be offered, dealing with the highlights of the somatic and psychosocial aspects of the clinical picture, as well as certain psychophysiologic and etiological considerations. These aspects will be dealt with more fully in a future publication.

2

Epidemiologic Aspects

Ulcerative colitis has been reported in all age groups, from infants to the elderly[1, 81]. The incidence rises in childhood until puberty, with some decrease in frequency during adolescence. There appears to be little difference in incidence between males and females[1, 37, 98]. Reported differences among racial and socio-economic groups are difficult to interpret[1, 81].

Although multiple cases do occur in families, at a higher rate than would be expected by chance[81], sex linked or direct Mendelian inheritance does not seem to be involved. The number of siblings and ordinal position in the family do not seem to be significant variables[37, 98]. A relatively high incidence of other bowel disorders with psychophysiological components has been described in families of patients with this disorder[19, 94].

Actual incidence-prevalence figures are obscure in childhood[81, 98]. Most reports are based upon more seriously ill patients in hospital populations; patients with milder cases are often not hospitalized, and may be more frequent among children than adults.

3

Pathology of the Bowel

Any portion of the colon may be involved, as well as the terminal ileum. In the majority of the chronic cases, the entire colon is eventually affected; the lesions may be restricted to the rectum, however[109]. Acute and chronic phases of inflammation are characteristic. Even in the latter phase, the inflammatory response and the ulcerations are usually limited to the mucous membrane[44, 109]. Recent electron microscopic studies have not indicated any specificity of the histopathological lesions in ulcerative colitis, and have not clarified the question of etiology[44].

4

Somatic Clinical Picture

The majority of children with this disorder have a premorbid history of mild to moderate disturbances in bowel function, including prolonged colic in infancy, constipation and diarrhoea.

2K

Three major types of onset of ulcerative colitis are encountered: an acute mild, an acute fulminating, and an insidious type of onset. The acute mild type typically involves rectal bleeding without systemic symptoms. The acute fulminating involves rectal bleeding, with or without diarrhoea, and is associated with systemic manifestations, such as fever, anorexia, vomiting, and marked prostration. The insidious type of onset occurs over a period of weeks or several months, with the presenting symptoms being mild and variable[18, 54, 65, 83].

Approximately one-fourth of the cases exhibit an initial episode followed by complete and apparently permanent remission[83, 98]. The others go on to a chronic course, of either intermittent (with remissions and relapses) or continuous nature[18, 65, 83]. A small number of the apparently permanent remissions from acute onsets turn out to be very mild cases of chronic intermittent nature, with relapses occurring up to five to ten years after the initial episode[98]. In general, the chronic intermittent course is the one more frequently encountered in children, and is milder than the chronic continuous type[18, 65, 83]. The latter is associated with a relatively high incidence of secondary systemic complications, such as electrolyte depletion, growth failure, and delay in puberty, as well as local bowel complications, including carcinoma[18, 54, 65, 83, 98].

There is by now fairly convincing evidence that chronic ulcerative colitis is basically a systemic disorder, and that the bowel lesions are only the most serious and dramatic characteristics of a more generalized disease process[18, 24, 65, 83]. Extracolonic manifestations are frequently apparent in other organs; various types of arthritis and dermatological disorders are most common, bearing an intimate relationship clinically and pathogenically to the bowel disorder[64, 83].

Ulcerative colitis in childhood is a serious and often life-threatening disease, with an over-all mortality until recently of from 15 to over 25 per cent[57, 66, 82]. Approximately a third of these deaths are due to carcinoma of the bowel, which has an increased incidence in ulcerative colitis[62, 65, 82]. Cases with onset in early childhood and those with chronic continuous courses over ten to fifteen years seem to face the greatest danger of carcinoma[62, 65, 82].

5

Psychosocial Observations

Most of the studies of psychosocial factors in childhood[2, 4, 5, 9, 25, 37, 41, 42, 59, 60, 67, 94, 103] have been carried out on older children who have been hospitalized, and most have been retrospective in nature. Within these limitations, a fairly consistent constellation of psychosocial factors has been described, with considerable similarity to adult studies, as summarized by Engel[29, 30]. Most children with ulcerative colitis have been characterized as exhibiting passive, inhibited, overly submissive, and dependent personality traits, often with pseudo-maturity, obsessive-compulsive, and depressive features and sometimes with strongly manipulative tendencies. They tend to have marked conflicts over the achievement of autonomy[35] and the handling of aggressive impulses, related to the anal psychosexual level[39], as well as underlying conflicts over the establishment of basic trust[35] and unsatisfied oral-dependency needs[39]. Despite the relative consistency in personality descriptions, these do not appear to be type-specific for ulcerative colitis; similar pictures may be found in children with predominantly psychological disturbances or in those with other psychophysiologic disorders[37, 97].

In the authors' series, many of these personality characteristics were seen, and the lack of type specificity was confirmed through comparison with children with other disorders. A wider spectrum of personality pictures than has usually been described was encountered. Approximately one-third of the children fell into a more severely emotionally disturbed group, with limited adaptive capacities and strong tendencies to regress, with the onset of colitis, to a helpless, passive-dependent, depressive position, sometimes combined with manipulation of adults. Another group of slightly over half the children could be placed in a moderately disturbed category, with better adaptive capacities and less regressive tendencies, exhibiting many obsessive-compulsive manifestations with a pseudo-mature façade. Another group, consisting of about one-sixth, were only mildly emotionally disturbed, including children with hysterical psychoneuroses and situational reactions. From various types of evidence, it would appear that such personality disturbances antedated the onset of the ulcerative colitis, although the presence of a severe and often chronic physical disturbance appeared to contribute significantly to the emotional problems[25, 76, 98].

Psychosocial factors involved in the precipitation of the onset of the colitis and in later exacerbations appeared to be of two major types: the actual, fantasied, or threatened loss of a relationship with a parent or other key figure upon whom the child was very dependent, or a situation in which the child felt helpless to cope independently or achieve satisfactorily, especially without parental support or approval. These are similar to those described in the literature for children and adults[6, 8, 9, 14, 16, 17, 29, 31, 32, 38, 59, 67, 96, 103].

Considerable consistency has been seen in the mother-child relationship, again without type-specificity. In the author's series, as in the literature[37, 67, 86, 94, 112], the mothers tended to be the dominating person in the family, and showed unconscious needs to be overprotective, over-controlling, and over-restrictive toward the child patient. They were frequently perfectionistic, often with obsessive-compulsive features, and with many feelings of guilt and inadequacy as mothers. While trying to prove themselves through pressure on the child for achievement, they simultaneously bound the child to them. Many of the mothers in the authors' series exhibited strongly bowel-oriented attitudes, with a high incidence of coercive approaches to bowel training, associated with frequent usage of suppositories or enemas. However, some of the mothers were inconsistent in their control and domination of the child, showing transient overpermissiveness and at times submitting to manipulation by the child. A small number were consistently overindulgent, with a few showing detached or rejecting attitudes. Although a small percentage exhibited severe personality disturbances, of psychotic or borderline degree, nearly one-fourth were felt to be only mildly disturbed, including a few with less dominating relationships with the child patients.

In the authors' series and in others'[37, 67, 86, 94, 112], the fathers were predominantly passive and often withdrawn from the family; some exceptions were noted, however, and a few fathers were warmer and more effective with their children. The siblings have usually been described as less disturbed than the patient[37, 67]; in the authors' series and one other study[58], however, there was some evidence that the siblings were more disturbed than has been generally recognized, occasionally in the direction of aggressive and antisocial behaviour.

Descriptions of the family functioning as a whole[37, 58, 98] tentatively indicate rather severe difficulties in dealing with separations and in communication of affect, with marked social restriction, and a pattern of communication of 'restrictiveness' of spontaneous action from generation to generation has been seen[58]. This, together with the frequently bowel-oriented attitudes in these families, may represent a type of 'psychic inheritance' passed on to the child patient in particular, who appears unconsciously to be singled out, often in relation to conflictful events occurring during the pregnancy[86] and early parent-child interaction. Family characteristics of this nature also do not appear to be specific for this disorder, but much more research in this and other psychosocial areas is necessary.

6

Psychophysiologic Interrelationships

Correlative studies of direct or indirect nature clearly indicate changes in colour, engorgement, secretion, and motility of the colon in response to naturally occurring and experimentally induced emotions in patients and normal subjects[1, 10, 30, 47, 48, 95]. These physiologic concomitants of emotions (largely unpleasant ones) appear to be mediated by the cerebral cortical-hypothalamic-autonomic nervous system interconnections, involving principally the action of the parasympathetic portion of the autonomic nervous system[116]. Such factors, though partially involved in onset and exacerbations, do not appear to be type-specific for ulcerative colitis. They are also present as immediate responses to emotions in patients with mucous colitis or chronic non-specific diarrhoea[19, 114], and thus cannot explain the abnormal tissue response of the colonic mucosa, involving bleeding and the appearance of chronic ulcerations[29, 30, 97]. Less immediate and more lasting effects upon colonic function may be mediated in part by the cortical-pituitary-adrenal axis, though those too are not specific.

7
Multiple Etiologic Considerations

Theories put forth regarding etiologic agents have been legion. These include the possible action of infectious agents, proteolytic enzymes in the bowel, food allergies, autoimmune mechanisms[61], and psychological factors. From a critical review of the evidence[107] it seems clear that no single factor can be responsible for the total picture. The etiology of ulcerative colitis thus appears to be multifactorial in nature, with interrelated determinants functioning as necessary or contributory predisposing, precipitating and perpetuating influences.

Various theoretical models have been proposed to explain the operation of multiple factors in psychophysiologic disorders such as ulcerative colitis. Of these, the most helpful at present is that of Mirsky[85], postulating the existence of predisposing biological factors, developmental psychosocial determinants, and current precipitating factors of social or interpersonal nature. Engel[30] has developed a parallel model for ulcerative colitis.

All such formulations are predicated upon the unitary theory of health and disease[27, 100], in which health represents the phase of positive adaptation and development, and disease a phase of failure or breakdown in adaptation. From this point of view, stressful stimuli (of relative significance for the individual) impinging upon physiological, psychological, or social levels of functioning of the human organism may overwhelm the individual's adaptative capacity, resulting in adaptive breakdown and the appearance of a disease state. These three levels may be said to communicate with each other via complex feedback mechanisms mediated through the 'central regulating system' (brain and mental apparatus) and the neuroendocrine system.

Stressful stimuli at the psychological or interpersonal level may result in unresolved emotional conflict, with persistent physiologic concomitants of unpleasant emotions. These physiologic concomitants may exert a strain upon the physiologic capacities of the organism, and may precipitate or enhance pre-existing or latent pathological processes at the biochemical or organ system level, producing what are currently designated as psychophysiological disorders. These disorders may in turn affect the individual child as a result of the impact of the disease process, producing regression or other psychological responses. They may also arouse social adaptive devices, with their answering reactions on the part of parents and family members to the presence of illness or chronic disability on the part of the child. Thus the nature and degree of response of the child to significantly stressful stimuli are determined by hereditary, constitutional, developmental, and experiential factors.

In regard to ulcerative colitis, the types of predisposing biological influences remain unclear. They might include such factors as an abnormal type of inflammatory response[79, 93], a genetic predisposition to the development of antoimmune mechanisms[1], or the inheritance of an autonomic pattern of reaction to stress involving particularly the gastrointestinal tract[94]. Developmental psychosocial determinants, also of predisposing nature, may include those involved in the parent-child interaction with resulting emotional conflicts for the child. An additional experiential determinant may be related to possible conditioning of the gastrocolic and defaecation reflexes, involving the association of early emotional states and feeding or toilet training experiences[98, 115].

In this view, both biological and psychosocial predisposing factors may be regarded as 'necessary but not sufficient' conditions[30] for the development of ulcerative colitis, unless they occur in combination with precipitating interpersonal events, at times aided by contributory precipitating factors involving various physical stimuli of local or systemic nature. Perpetuating influences may be provided by shifts in biochemical or immunologic mechanisms as a result of the appearance of the basic disease process[1, 30], by the enforced dependence of the child as a result of chronic illness, by the response of family members, or by a combination of such physiological, psychological or interpersonal reverberations.

Any such attempt at formulation of the mode of interaction of complex and still poorly understood etiological variables of multiple character leaves much unexplained, and is speculative. It is possible that a continuum of response is involved, with some children exhibiting heavier 'biological loading' and requiring less intense influence of psychosocial factors, and with others, carrying more limited biological predisposition, developing the picture only in the face of greater weighting of psychosocial factors.

8

Management and Therapy

In this section, medical, surgical, and formal psychotherapeutic methods of treatment will first be considered separately, followed by a discussion of a comprehensive integrated approach which is deemed ideal. Although the psychological and social aspects of these therapeutic approaches will be emphasized, these cannot be discussed without reference to the somatic aspects. Otherwise the attention of the mental health clinician may be diverted by the sometimes dramatic psychosocial phenomena away from the serious and sometimes dangerous physical implications.

In the phase of diagnostic evaluation, the clinician must avoid an 'either-or' approach; he should weigh positively the degree of operation of somatic, psychological, and social factors in the individual case, arriving at an approach to management and a plan of therapy which is balanced appropriately[36, 77].

Medical Aspects

The goals of immediate management of children with acute onsets of ulcerative colitis have as their target the restoration of the physical and psychological equilibrium exhibited by the patient prior to the attack. *Hospitalization* is often helpful in establishing these goals[4, 18, 36, 73, 83]. If the child is markedly ill, hospitalization may be vital in this potentially life-threatening phase. In less severely ill children, in addition to the immediate medical benefits, hospitalization can provide an emotional 'moratorium' for child and parents, both in relation to the frightening impact of the illness and to the emotional and interactional problems so often related to the background and precipitation of the clinical picture. In addition to careful diagnostic evaluation, with the aid of various consultants, opportunities are available for observation of the personality patterns and behaviour of the child and the parent-child interaction, with the help of nurse, teacher, occupational or recreational therapist, and other ward staff. A relationship can be established by the physician with child and parents, and initial therapeutic measures may be undertaken, with gradual preparation for return home.

Although many children with ulcerative colitis respond well to hospitalization and immediate treatment, this is not true for all. A few children with insidious onsets or mild courses have responded, in the authors' experience, to hospitalization with an exacerbation of their symptoms, as if the threat of separation were too great. Others with chronic intermittent courses have not improved or may have worsened in the hospital, even over long periods, but often have responded dramatically on return home; this has also been the experience of others[12, 36]. For the child with milder symptoms, it may be best to handle him on an ambulatory basis[18, 65, 83]. Certainly the decision to hospitalize a child should be made on an individual basis. Guidance for such a decision would include, in addition to the severity of the physical disorder, the degree and type of the psychosocial problem involved.

For the child who is hospitalized in a paediatric setting, the length of stay may at times vary more with the psychological balance in child and family than with the severity of the disease process. Some children respond to the plan for return home with an exacerbation. Occasionally long-term psychiatric hospitalization, with medical consultation and treatment, is necessary for such a child. Such may also be required for the child with markedly manipulative tendencies, who sets the paediatric ward staff and parents against each other, and who simply cannot be managed without specialized psychiatric techniques[36].

In paediatric hospitalization for an acute onset or exacerbation, the *initial approach to management* of the child's illness involves the restoration or maintenance of basic nutrition, the relief of symptoms, the restoration of intestinal functions, and the control of emotional difficulties[18, 83]. Careful attention is necessary to the indications for the use of electrolytes to replace losses of sodium, chloride, and particularly potassium from diarrhoea if long present, since even minimal exacerbations may suddenly deplete marginal supplies of electrolytes[18]. If significant anaemia is found, iron, selected for tolerance[18, 85], or transfusions may be indicated, as may plasma, serum, or protein hydrolysates in the presence of hypoproteinia. Antispasmodics of parasympathetic blocking nature may be helpful in dealing with tenesmus and painful urgency, although codeine may be necessary for adolescents who may be especially upset by such symptoms[99]. Buffered salicylates or occasional gold therapy may be useful for arthritis[18], or various therapies may be employed for other extra-colonic manifestations.

In acute fulminating cases in particular, the use of steroid hormones has recently found much usefulness. In children, cortisone may be more effective than ACTH[18, 24, 83], and adrenal steroid enemas are employed routinely by some[83]. These agents appear to have been effective in many instances in reducing the severity of the individual attack and the length of hospitalization[54]. They do not modify the basic disease process, however, and later relapses occur in about the same frequency as in children not treated with steroids[24, 54]. Cautious usage is important, with small doses employed and with cessation of steroid therapy as soon as possible[18, 24]. The danger of perforation is real[98]; patients on high doses may go into adrenal collapse in relation to surgery[13, 26]; wound healing may be delayed[13], and ulcerative colitis has even been precipitated during steroid therapy[11]. Although their action is not wholly understood and the positive results largely empirical, the anti-inflammatory effect of the steroids is probably the outstanding one. Thus the danger of masking or intensifying infection, if present, is a significant one[18, 24].

Variations in the effect of steroids are not uncommon. In adults, the effectiveness of such agents has been noted to be reduced if the patient feels helpless and depressed[28]. Exacerbations may occur after initial response to steroids in adults[28] and children[96], in relation to plans to return home or in response to the physician's leaving on a vacation. Psychotic responses to steroid administration have been reported in adults[89, 90, 101]. These are infrequent in children, but may occur occasionally in adolescents. Whether the psychosis is the result of the direct effects of the steroid on the central nervous system or to the effects of the illness, with associated realignments in the balance of adaptive forces, or both, is not always clear[97, 101].

The use of tranquillizing agents has been recommended to deal with anxiety or other emotional manifestations[83]. In the authors' experience, these are rarely effective unless a good deal of free-floating anxiety or apprehension is present. In seriously disturbed adolescents, the side effects of the phenothiazines, such as slight drowsiness or dizziness, may occasionally increase confusion and anxiety through the experience of feelings of unreality or depersonalization, which may intensify identity confusion or body image problems.

Although some adult patients are said to respond favourably to a milk-free diet, in spite of the absence of proof of allergic tendencies, the employment of bland or restricted diets, beyond known food idiosyncrasies, is felt to be unnecessary in childhood by many[18, 25, 67]. Indeed, it seems unwise to alter the patterns of living of the patient and family more than is absolutely necessary[18]. A more positive approach, with permission and encouragement for the patient to choose more tempting foods, appears to help maintain appetite and avoid anorexia[18, 67], as well as to aid the patient in experiencing the interest and support of the physician[33]. In adults, free diets have been noted, on controlled study, to cause no more difficulties than bland or restricted ones[63].

Traditionally, bed rest has been recommended for patients with acute onsets or exacerbations of ulcerative colitis. The limitations in this concept, except in seriously debilitating states, have been pointed out for adults, in regard to disruptions in calcium metabolism and other adverse effects, if long continued[22]. In addition, other problems arise for children, in relation to prevention of discharge of energy through play and the promotion of psychological invalidism. Whenever possible, it seems wisest to encourage activity to within normal limits[18, 65, 67].

In addition to antibiotics in the presence of known intestinal or systemic infection, intestinal antiseptics, such as salicylazosulfaperadine (azulfadine), have enjoyed considerable popularity. A double blind controlled study has shown some value to these in adults[21], in spite of the absence of definitive primary or secondary infection. Side effects, such as nausea and vomiting or anaemia, may limit their usefulness. The question of at least a partial placebo effect, related to confidence and trust in the physician, cannot be ruled out when such agents are used clinically. Indeed, such an effect represents a significant component of the pharmacodynamic effect of any drug[97].

Other treatment, such as medico-ileostomy, with the use of a Miller-Abbott tube, may be helpful in fulminant cases. Recently, antimetabolites have been employed cautiously, on the assumption that autoimmune phenomena are involved. Azathioprine has been administered, on the basis of its apparent immunosuppressant effect, to a small series of patients, with some positive effects on the illness and with a striking decrease in lymphoid infiltration of the rectal mucosa[78].

Implicit in the medical aspects of management and treatment is the importance of *the relationship between the patient and his physician*. The necessity for continuity in this relationship with a single interested, calm, confident, unhurried, predictable, and reliable physician cannot be overemphasized[28, 49]. The course of the illness may be more smooth and benign if such a relationship is maintained[33, 54]. Breaks in continuity which are unexpected can lead to exacerbations in the illness or to feelings of rejection or mistrust in psychologically vulnerable individuals[33].

The psychotherapeutic aspects of the role of the paediatrician or family physician begin with the establishment of a positive relationship with the child and parents during diagnostic and early treatment phases. His approach and manner should lead the parents to feel confidence in his competence and thoroughness, as well as to perceive his consideration of the child patient and his respect for them. Careful explanation and preparation of the child patient (and parents), couched in terms appropriate to the child's age level, should be carried out for every new diagnostic and therapeutic procedure. Daily visits for emotional support and discussion of fears or misconceptions by the child are most important. Frequent contacts with the parents, in order to deal with their anxieties and confusions, should be a part of such an approach, as should discussion of coming absences or vacations, with the introduction of a substitute physician to child and parents, and similar measures.

Even such an apparently simple matter as a change in bed arrangements or a move of the patient to another ward should be dealt with in this manner, in order to avoid anxiety and possible exacerbations. In a sense, the physician offers himself during this phase as a surrogate[33] or auxiliary ego, helping to test reality for the child and assuming at first a more omnipotent attitude in the approach to the satisfaction of his dependent needs, later weaning the patient toward greater independence.

In such a supportive psychotherapeutic approach, the physician uses his empathy with the patient and parents as a therapeutic tool. In the phase of diagnosis and early treatment, he will gain valuable knowledge of the child and parents from a psychosocial point of view. Nevertheless, he will be wise not to explore all such details initially; too much early probing may be upsetting to the patient or parents, and may interfere with the establishment of a positive relationship. Data of this nature will become available during the course of his ongoing contacts with the family. Such an approach is of necessity not a deeply 'uncovering' or insight-promoting one. The physician does not ordinarily point out connections between emotions or behaviour and symptomatology, unless these are overtly expressed by patient and parents. (Even in formal, intensive psychotherapy, such insight-promoting techniques are rarely appropriate in the initial phase, for reasons to be discussed.)

The child with ulcerative colitis often becomes readily dependent upon the physician, with remission of symptoms frequently occurring as a result of this dependence as well as other treatment measures[35, 98]. Such dependence, transferred from parental figures, must be accepted and tolerated in the early phases, even if the patient is clinging, demanding, or manipulative. Firm and kindly limits should be set upon unrealistic demands and manipulations, however, and may actually decrease the child's anxiety and guilt. Brief visits, at the beginning and end of the day, may express support and interest toward the patient more effectively than longer, less frequent contacts. Careful attention to detail is important. If the physician must be late, he should let the patient know that this will be necessary, in order to avoid anxiety and interference with the developing dependent relationship in its early stages[33]. Discharge from the hospital should be planned well in advance with the child and parents, with attention to psychosocial as well as physical readiness for return home.

When such patients are intensely manipulative or demanding, it is hard for the physician or other staff members to avoid countertransference reactions, involving feelings of anger or at times helplessness, particularly during regressed phases. These may be dealt with by realising that the patient's transference attitudes do not carry personal implications, but are part of a set of reaction patterns directed toward all parent substitute figures, which may be intensified by the impact of the illness and the related emotional regression. Psychiatric consultation may be of value in this and other connections. Not every patient need be seen psychiatrically, however, if a positive response to such a treatment approach is obtained.

Problems may arise in working with the parents of such children. The employment of some controlled compassion, with avoidance of critical or judgmental attitudes, is frequently necessary on the part of the physician, combined with awareness of the unconscious forces which dictate some of the parents' controlling or ambivalent behaviour towards the child patient. Parents may be overanxious, suspicious, or depressed, or may unconsciously push the child toward unnecessary surgery, even predicting the child's death[36, 67]. A few may deny the seriousness of the child's illness, while a number, particularly the mothers, are over-interested in the details of the patient's colitis and its treatment[2, 67]. Even though the correlations between family interactions and the child's symptomatology may be painfully evident to the physician, he should avoid interpreting these to the child or parents in the early phases of treatment. He must accept at first the fact that the parents and patient see the illness as an exclusively physical one, indeed with serious implications.

When psychiatric consultation is invoked, the parents or the older child may often be helped to understand that the symptoms may be 'aggravated' by emotional tension, with no initial implication that the parent(s) may be involved in such a process. Later in the course of treatment, after a relationship has been established with the physician, a more active counselling approach, still with avoidance of probing techniques, may be adopted. In this phase, the parents may be helped to handle the patient differently, permitting more independence (which the child at first may not be ready to utilize).

In spite of difficulties, visiting should not be interrupted between child and parents, because of the vulnerability of these children to separation. If the child seems upset during visits, parents may be positively helped to cut down the length of time involved. An experienced social worker may be extremely helpful in working with their feelings of guilt and other conflicts. Even if the child seems to be having serious difficulty in adjusting in the home, premature thoughts of placement in foster-homes or other setting should not be entertained. Psychiatric hospitalization or long-term residential treatment may be more usefully invoked.

When the child is not too seriously disturbed, such an approach by the physician, combined with other medical measures and assisted if necessary by psychiatric consultation, will frequently bring the symptoms under control and, in long-term follow-up, will act to promote more healthy adaptation by the child, often with continued remission[18, 36, 66, 83]. Re-evaluation of the colonic status periodically remains important, however, in view of the possible 'silent' progression of the disease process. Medical check-up at least every six months seems appropriate, even in remissions lasting for many years, during which the supportive psychotherapeutic benefits of the child-parent-doctor relationship may be significantly realized.

While not overlooking somatic factors, due caution should be employed by the physician in regard to barium enemas and repeat protoscopy during follow-up. Exacerbations can follow such procedures in children with tenuous adaptive balances[8, 98]. With careful preparation of the child and parents, a barium enema once a year and sigmoidoscopy every two years should be sufficient to guard against 'silent' phenomena. General anaesthetics of short acting, inhalant nature may be necessary for sigmoidoscopy in the preschool child or the more disturbed older child or adolescent, in order to diminish anxiety.

Surgical Aspects

Although radical surgery in children with ulcerative colitis has in the past carried with it a serious mortality rate, modern methods have reduced this remarkably. The classical indications in the chronic patient have been related to the complications of the bowel disorder, including stricture or obstruction, actual or impending perforation, uncontrollable haemorrhage, and carcinoma. To these have more recently been added others, including severe persistent fistulas, marked interference with growth or delay of puberty, and general physical debilitation or emotional invalidism unresponsive to medical and psychological treatment measures[18, 25, 73, 82]. The impression has grown that earlier surgery in chronic and intractable cases carries with it a lower mortality[25, 51, 54, 80], and that such patients are more often symptom-free, with a lower rate of re-hospitalization, than similar medically treated patients[73].

Because of the special developmental problems of children and the greater possibility of carcinoma, the indications for surgery in childhood are currently interpreted more liberally than in adults[25, 51, 73, 80, 83]. Results obtained are often quite dramatic; rapid weight gain is frequent, with greater physical and social mobility, marked growth spurts followed by normal growth, and often, though not always, subsidence of arthritis, major skin manifestations, and other extra-colonic manifestations[18, 54, 73, 83]. If serious growth lag is prolonged beyond 15 or 16 years, the growth spurt may not be obtained, and permanent dwarfism may result[18, 83].

In acute fulminating cases who show overwhelming toxaemia and who do not respond to medical treatment, surgery has been employed in the past as an emergency and sometimes life-saving method. With the advent of steroids, more effective fluid and electrolyte therapy, and other treatment modalities, including psychotherapy, most such children respond adequately and promptly to medical measures, however[18, 65, 89]. In addition, in view of the relatively high surgical mortality under such circumstances, many surgeons are reluctant to operate[40, 69].

For chronically ill patients in childhood, ileostomy alone was formerly the initial procedure of choice, as colectomy was regarded as too extensive and stressful a procedure. With advances in surgical treatment, more extensive surgery has been possible where indicated. Ehrenpreis[25, 26] believes that surgical choice should be a compromise between radical excision and preservation of bowel continuity. He has in a number of cases achieved excellent results with total colectomy and ileo-rectal anastamosis if rectal involvement is slight or moderate, with follow-up to determine if secondary ileostomy and excision of the rectum is necessary. In some cases, total colectomy and ileostomy in one stage have been carried out, with excision of the rectum where involvement was severe. The possibility of future closure of a temporary ileostomy and restoration of bowel continuity by ileo-rectal anastamosis is kept in mind, but the likelihood of such a step is not great[25, 40, 73]. In other series, sub-total colectomy and ileostomy or sub-total colectomy and ileo-rectal anastamosis have given equally good results for the majority of patients[83].

Although total colectomy and permanent ileostomy is the procedure most likely to produce permanent results[18, 25], it has been pointed out that such an operation carries with it the risk for boys of the danger of injury to the parasympathetic control of ejaculation and urination[7], and it cannot be employed for some seriously or acutely ill patients because of the length of the procedure. Vagotomy[20, 104] has been employed in adults; results appear to be good if vagotomy is complete but poor if not. The procedure has rarely been used in children.

In view of the facts cited earlier regarding prognosis, the authors feel that earlier referral for surgery by medical physicians is often indicated than has traditionally been the case. Bleeding can often be brought under control by modern medical measures, and may be a less frequent indication for surgery than in the past[18]. If, however, in spite of adequate medical treatment, including formal psychotherapeutic measures where indicated, a state of total disability continues for more than one year, surgery seems indicated[24, 25, 65], as well as when a state of partial disability persists for five[25] to seven[22] years. Special thought should be given to this possibility if the illness has its onset in the preschool period[18, 73], if the course is a chronic continuous one, or if a chronic intermittent course fails to show a decrease in the frequency and severity of the exacerbations or exhibits an actual increase[18, 73, 83].

Because of the very real danger of carcinoma, some surgeons have recommended prophylactic surgery, particularly if polyposis is extensive or long-standing[40], or if adenomas develop in polyps[73]. In the face of the smaller but still significant operative mortality, ranging from a little over two to nearly ten per cent in various series[25, 54, 73, 83], the necessarily sweeping adjustments by child and parents to the post-operative condition, and the fact that current impressions have arisen from more chronically ill populations seen in hospitals, prophylactic surgery in the absence of other life-threatening or chronic debilitating conditions does not seem warranted, in the opinions of Richmond[99], Ehrenpreis[25], and the authors. Even if carcinoma develops, early diagnosis and surgery may give good results, in spite of the tendency for such lesions to be more highly undifferentiated and malignant in children[84]. If the above criteria for surgical intervention are followed, approximately 20[25] to 25[83] per cent of children may require such steps.

Although dramatic responses to surgical intervention are frequent, results are occasionally fair to poor[18, 83], with the mortality as noted above, particularly if patients are referred late. Post-operative complications are also common. Bowel obstruction, excessive electrolyte loss, major skin excoriations, wound separation, cicatricial hernia, prolapse, ulcerative bleeding of stoma, ileostomy fistula, and retraction and stenosis of the ileostomy have been reported[25, 40, 73, 83]. In a number of chronically ill patients, the extra-colonic manifestations may not be affected even by total colectomy[18]. As many as one out of three patients may have major difficulties following ileostomy[25, 73]. In one series, one-third of the children required repeat operations for revision of ileostomy or adhesions or obstruction; in the children with ileostomies, occasional children required multiple (1-5) re-operations[83]. Frequent bowel movements after ileo-rectal anastamosis are often encountered[25, 83]; these may be well tolerated but at times appear to upset the child in an especially bowel-oriented family. Ulcerative ileitis[29] and ileo-jejunitis[67] are not infrequently reported following surgery.

The psychological aspects of surgical treatment of ulcerative colitis have received limited attention but are of central importance. Indeed, some have felt this to be perhaps the most important feature in the determination of the smoothness and effectiveness of surgical management[33, 73].

Psychological preparation of the child, geared to his level of development, should be always undertaken prior to surgery[25, 105]. The surgeon should do this himself or make sure that it is done, as it is all too easy to assume that someone else has undertaken this step. Preparation of the parents is of equal significance.

Adult patients who have not developed a positive relationship with the surgeon have been known to do poorly[34], and the authors have a similar impression regarding children and adolescents, particularly with those who are seriously depressed. In such instances, psychotherapy undertaken pre- and post-operatively may even be life-saving[34, 98]. Although a high incidence of psychotic decompensation has been reported in adults in relation to surgical procedures[91], this has not been the authors' experience with children; in this series it occurred in one patient. The taking of responsibility by the surgeon may help diminish the ambivalence and guilt in the relationship between child and parents on both sides[36].

Following surgery in children, the severe regression as well as the withdrawn and isolated behaviour often disappears rapidly with returning health[36]. The basic personality problems in the child and the family interactional difficulties often persist, however, though sometimes outwardly in subtle form. In one 15-year-old girl, for whom psychotherapy and medical measures were unsuccessful, colectomy produced marked physical improvement, but the mother continued to sleep with the patient in the context of her marital problems with her husband. Parental overconcern may not cease completely with returning health, with fears of exacerbations or other dangers continuing, and chronically ill children may find the shift to health a difficult one to accomplish after long periods of invalidism, as may the parents[97].

Although some adult studies have suggested that most patients experience little difficulty in emotional adjustment to ileostomy or colostomy[113], other workers have discussed individual problems in adjustment[8, 23, 108]. One survey[68] indicates that a significant number of adult patients seek psychiatric help following surgery, even though this is a smaller number than those who have taken such a step prior to surgery. Ileostomy clubs may offer supportive experiences for adults and older adolescent patients, in addition to professional help[13, 75]. In children, the impressions of some[25, 69] suggest the difficulties are few; the experience of the authors would suggest otherwise, however, in a number of cases. It is true that modern plastic bags and improved methods of ileostomy care have diminished mechanical problems in this area. Nonetheless, previously disturbed children and parents in bowel-oriented families may show hypersensitivity about possible odours. Children with school phobic tendencies often rationalize their continued absence from school with fears of possible rejection by peers. Struggles for control within the family may continue to be centred around the care of the child's ileostomy or colostomy. Occasional children or adolescents may erotize the stoma, to the point of stroking it in an almost masturbatory fashion, a phenomenon reported in adults[34].

The misconceptions of disturbed children regarding the nature of the operation are highlighted by the conviction of a 14-year-old boy that the surgeon's knife had slipped, and that he could never become a man. His school phobia continued unabated, and the family eventually broke up around troubles over his post-operative care.

Although surgery may be life-saving, it should be emphasized that the surgical approach should not be divorced from other aspects of the management of patient and family. Where formal psychotherapy has been in process prior to an operation, it should not be discontinued, as is all too frequent. Indeed, its importance during preparation for operation and the post-operative period may be as great or greater than before, and the effectiveness of psychotherapy may be markedly enhanced by a positive response to surgery[36]. As Engel has emphasized[33], the need for surgical intervention does not necessarily represent a failure of psychotherapy. Psychiatric consultation is often vital prior to operation, particularly in patients who are overly anxious, mistrustful, or depressed, or with parents who are mistrustful or confused.

Formal Psychotherapeutic Aspects

In the section on medical aspects of management and treatment, mention was made of the psychotherapeutic role of the physician. A supportive psychotherapeutic approach was described which, when combined with other medical aspects, can be beneficial to a number of patients[3, 34, 36]. It is proposed in this section to discuss considerations involved in a more formal psychotherapeutic approach by psychiatrists or by psychologists, social workers or other trained psychotherapists with psychiatric consultation.

Other forms of psychiatric treatment than psychotherapy have been tried. Mention has been made of the use of tranquillizing agents, which appears to have limited value in children. Antidepressants, chiefly MAO inhibitors[3], have been utilized in adults, with some positive results, as has prolonged narcosis with amobarbital (Dauerschlaft) during acute exacerbations[52]. Antidepressants are often less effective in children, and have not been useful in this condition in the authors' experience. To the best of our knowledge, prolonged narcosis has not been tried in childhood, nor has prefrontal leukotomy[70], which has been tried in intractable adult cases; the former would seem unwise and the latter contraindicated in children. No reports regarding the use of hypnosis are known to us.

Types of Psychotherapy. Formal psychotherapeutic approaches with adults and children can be located along a continuum. With adults, at one end are those therapists who believe that only a supportive relationship is indicated, with a directive, reality-oriented approach, involving encouragement and environmental manipulation, and with no attempt to utilize expressive, 'uncovering' or insight-promoting techniques[46, 50, 71]. At the other end are those who believe that more expressive, analytic, insight-producing methods are appropriate, including those offered by psychoanalysis[15, 110]. In between are those who feel that supportive methods are indicated early in treatment, at a time when more intensive techniques may actually be contraindicated, since they are likely to stir up too much anxiety, resulting in exacerbations. They feel, however, that a more analytic approach, including psychoanalysis, may be possible with certain patients with adequate ego strength in the later phase[16, 33, 74, 87, 92].

With children, a similar continuum of psychotherapeutic approaches exists. Some feel that supportive measures only, without a significant expressive component, are beneficial or necessary[18, 25] or that intensive analytic approaches are contraindicated[83]. At the other end, some have employed mainly intensive, actively interpretative and insight-promoting types of psychotherapy, principally psychoanalysis[60, 102]. Sperling[102] feels that such an approach is the only means of 'curing' the patient. Even though she regards the majority of patients with ulcerative colitis as exhibiting fragile and impaired ego functions, with 'latent' psychoses, she feels that intensive psychotherapy including psychoanalysis is in no way contraindicated, nor will it precipitate a psychosis. She feels that non-interpretative psychotherapy not only does not cure the patient, but itself militates against the cure by reinforcing the patient's feelings that he cannot understand or control his disease.

Sperling's results in a small series of cases are impressive, and are in accord with Weinstock's[110] in adults. It is clear that, in certain cases, such an approach, if used skilfully, may not be harmful, and can be most beneficial, with results lasting over many years. Nevertheless, other workers[31, 56, 67], feel that such methods are rarely effective or indicated in the early phases of treatment, particularly with acute fulminating cases, with occasional exceptions to be discussed. Finch and Hess[37] feel that the psychotherapy of children with ulcerative colitis can rarely follow strict psychoanalytic principles. They believe that supportive measures are indicated in the early stages, but that a number of patients in the later phase of treatment can be helped through more expressive techniques to become more independent and to express and handle more openly and healthily their markedly repressed hostile feelings. This is a view with which the authors agree, with careful regard for the individual child's ego strength and personality picture, as well as the nature of family interactions, in the selection of patients for this particular treatment approach.

Results. The results of psychotherapy have been given some study, both in children and adults. One attempt to treat adult patients with ulcerative colitis by psychotherapeutic (supportive, ventilative) measures alone, without the use of drugs[45], suggests that such an approach compares favourably on follow-up with reports from a matched group (age at onset, sex, severity and duration of illness, and X-ray changes) treated with diets and a standard medical regimen, as well as with reported results from other studies based on prevailing medical methods of therapy.

In another adult study, with a control group matched for severity of disease, sex, age at onset, and previous use of steroids, it was found that psychotherapy in a group of chronically ill patients showed a demonstrably favourable effect upon the somatic course of the disease[89, 90] over long-term follow-up, as indicated by proctoscopic examination and ratings of symptom severity. Although there was no direct relationship between the degree of psychological and physical improvement in this series, psychological improvement significantly reduced the social and personal disability caused by symptoms of the disease. In this work, intensity and duration of psychotherapy did not appear to be related to the extent of somatic improvement, the incidence of surgery, or the mortality rate, but did seem to be correlated with the level of psychological improvement. Although patients treated with relatively short term therapy of supportive nature showed some positive psychological responses, patients treated with psychoanalysis displayed a considerably greater ability to function effectively in their life situations. Another longitudinal follow-up study[110, 111] supports the above impression that intensive psychotherapy or psychoanalysis is most effective in producing long-term, symptom-free remission if begun when symptoms are mild and the patient is ambulatory.

Statistical studies of the results of psychotherapy in childhood are more limited and have been less systematic, partly because of the greater difficulty in studying and following children. In Langford's[67] long-term study of a group treated medically and psychotherapeutically, along with appropriate therapeutic work with parents, he concluded, on the basis of comparison with a group of children treated only medically, that psychotherapy did not seem to alter the somatic course of the disease. The mortality rate in the group treated by medical measures alone was considerably higher, but the number of patients who improved was greater. In a larger group of 109 children, 63 of whom received psychotherapy, the symptoms of the illness appeared to be less incapacitating, however. There were greater feelings of self-improvement and less severe diarrhoea, even with continuing evidence of disease by proctoscopic examinations, in those who were treated psychologically than those who were not. Some patients were treated by supportive measures, others by more intensive approaches, but no differences in the type of response were reported.

Sperling[102] reported on a group of children previously unresponsive to medical measures, who were treated with psychoanalysis and followed over 10 years or more without exacerbations of the illness. In a series of 6 children who had also not responded to accepted medical regimens, Barron and Spurlock[4] reported that hospitalization for periods ranging from six months to several years, together with intensive psychotherapy or child analysis plus medical measures, resulted in marked improvement at the time of discharge and follow-up with medical and psychotherapeutic treatment.

In the authors' series, exact follow-up has been difficult, because of moves of the families of children and moves of the therapist. Psychotherapy together with symptomatic medical treatment has been undertaken with 34 patients and their parents. Of these 21 children and adolescents between the ages of 3 and 18 years have been treated for varying lengths of time by one of the authors; 13 patients were treated by other therapists for whom one of the authors was the supervisor. In the group of 29 patients for which follow-up data is available, over half of the patients (16) exhibited marked psychological and physical improvement, with return to normal in bowel findings; some showed marked reversal of what seemed in some instances to be advanced structural change. Seven or nearly one-fourth of the patients exhibited considerable psychological improvement and some physical symptomatic improvement; this group, however, showed no alteration of the underlying disease process in the bowel, either showing continuing signs of mild activity or in several instances, signs of 'silent' progression by proctoscopy. The remaining patients (six) showed no positive response to psychotherapy; three of these were referred by one of the authors for surgery, while three families broke off treatment, with the children undergoing surgery later.

No exact correlation could be seen between age, sex, psychiatric diagnosis, degree of regression, ego strength, family pathology, type of onset or course prior to psychotherapy, and the outcome. In general, the less disturbed children with better adaptive capacities and less disturbed families responded to treatment with greater psychological and physical improvement, but some severely disturbed children in chaotic families also responded. With a few older school children and adolescents, the family showed little change, but the child improved markedly.

From the present series, it appears that a little over three-quarters of the patients (23) followed received some significant psychological benefits from the addition of formal psychotherapy to a medical regimen, with over half of these showing complete remission from physical symptomatology, some for a number of years. However, in about one-fourth of the total group of patients treated and followed (7), the basic continuation or, in a few instances, progression, of the disease process in the bowel was not altered. If one adds the group where psychotherapy exerted no effect because of the difficulties of the child or family in establishing a relationship (three cases) or the family in undertaking therapy (three cases), it is clear that in nearly half the patients no immediate effect on the bowel disease was possible from psychotherapy.

In addition, about one-third (five) of the 16 patients showing psychological improvement and complete clinical remission experienced one or more exacerbations after completion of treatment, during follow-up over a period of five to ten years. Since a number of the longer follow-ups were necessarily by telephone or letter (one of the authors moved twice during this period), the nature of the precipitating influences and the degree of bowel disease could not be ascertained with any exactness. In general, these exacerbations appeared to be related to such events as the death or illness of a parent or sibling, a family move, going to college, marriage, and pregnancy. Such exacerbations were generally mild and brief, but one was of an acute fulminating type, responding to strenuous medical treatment. None of the patients in the total group followed up have developed carcinoma up to the present time.

In a relatively small series, these results are not statistically significant. They are sobering, however. They fit with the impression of Engel[33] in adults that many of these patients, however much improved psychologically, still retain vulnerability at the tissue level to significant emotional stimuli in relation to events which they cannot control.

Although it is harder to maintain contact with adolescents and post-adolescents following termination of formal therapy (fairly regular contacts by letters and telephone over a number of years have been kept up by the patients in about one-third of the treated cases), it is possible that if the therapist had remained in the patients' home town, a more continuous and frequent personal contact might have been maintained, with greater benefits therapeutically, as has been Engel's[33] experience with adults. Also the question of spontaneous remissions in a chronic, variable disease process must be considered. The authors have the impression that such remissions are often not truly spontaneous however. Some of them at least appear to be a response to the re-establishment of a key relationship, the development of a new one, or a more positive realignment of the balance of family or other interpersonal forces, permitting the patient to employ a higher level of adaptive behaviour. It must be added that, although the authors' total series contains some less sick patients referred early from practising paediatricians, the patient population receiving treatment was more heavily weighted on the side of the more chronically ill groups ordinarily seen in hospital settings.

From all these considerations, in the literature and the authors' experiences, it can be said in summary that formal psychotherapy for child and family appears to add an important dimension to the total treatment approach, which should be available to a number of children with ulcerative colitis. Although psychotherapy for child and parents can add significantly to the patient's developmental capacities and often may free him from invalidism or aid in his rehabilitation, it seems to have only a limited influence on the basic tissue abnormality at the bowel level. Such therapy may 'immunize' the child and his bowel against some but certainly not all of the potential stressful circumstances which may occur in later life. If both psychological improvement and return to normal of the bowel picture occur, the outlook should be good with occasional exceptions. If psychological improvement and some local symptomatic response result, with, however, signs of continued though quiet activity of the colonic process or of progression, surgery should be considered; if no improvement arises and progression continues, within a reasonable period, as discussed earlier, surgery should be recommended.

In the experience of the authors with this often chronic and at times life-threatening disease, psychotherapy should *always* be combined with medical treatment in the early phases, and should be used cautiously, in severely disturbed or acutely ill patients, in view of the danger of exacerbations. Later, the emphasis may be placed more heavily on the psychotherapeutic approach, but medical follow-up, with surgical consultation when necessary, should always be collaboratively involved. Psychotherapy, like the adrenal steroids, can be a two-edged weapon, and should be used with judgment, as with any other therapeutic tool.

Specific Therapeutic Considerations

In the authors' series, as in that of Finch and Hess[37], the type of therapy used has been in general a supportive one during the early phases, particularly with acute fulminating cases. Later, as the patient improves, it has often been possible to move gradually into a more insight-promoting, expressive approach. This has as its goals the diminution of anxiety, the promotion of greater independence, the achievement of more healthy handling of aggressive impulses, and the strengthening of the child's ego in the direction of dealing with conflicts rather than employing repression or other, more primitive defences[36].

Exceptions to this approach have involved patients whose adaptive capacities or the adaptive equilibrium of their families have been so limited that a continuing supportive approach, with little or no probing, has been necessary. Other exceptions in a different direction have included several adolescents with chronic disease, whose dramatically manipulative behaviour necessitated a confrontational approach, with some interpretation, at the outset of therapy, in order even to establish a relationship within which further therapy would continue. Also, in two cases, a verbal or play interpretative approach was employed during the fulminating phase, when the patients were not responding to medical treatment, and were considered too ill for surgery. These and other special therapeutic issues will be considered in more detail in relation to children and families.

Children. The therapy of a child of course cannot be considered ordinarily as separate from that of the parents, except with older adolescents where the parents can permit but not participate in therapy. Nonetheless, certain considerations regarding the approach to the child in the initial phases of therapy, especially with acute fulminating and often seriously regressed patients, need to be discussed, along with other matters. In particular, the management of regression and the establishment of a dependency relationship are key issues in this early stage. With adults, the emphasis has been laid frequently on the therapist's assuming a directive, omniscient and omnipotent role at first, emphasizing a reality-orientation and encouraging dependency, aiding mastery over helplessness and the restoration of self-esteem by frequent visits, coordinating most aspects of the patient's actual care, manipulating the environment, and providing some comforts personally[33, 49, 87]. A type of 'replacement therapy' as in dealing with acute grief, has been recommended[71]; in this approach, the therapist attempts to provide restitution of a lost or threatened dependency relationship with a key figure through assuming that person's role for the patient and, through shared experiences, encouraging identification and attachment. Margolin[74] has undertaken 'anaclitic therapy' with such patients, often encouraging the patient to regress to the level of a helpless infant, with the therapist attending personally to the patient's physical needs, even to the point of providing sucking gratifications.

With children, many of the above principles are applicable, with some modifications, however. During regression, any kindly, interested, supportive adult tends to be regarded as omnipotent or omniscient by a child, who has some such attitudes towards all adults during health. This approach should not be overdone in the hospital, however, as a child whose demanding and manipulative tendencies are already strong may, in spite of regression, feel guilt over being able to control adults too much around his illness, with the associated 'secondary gain'. A combination of a warm, 'giving' approach with some limits set on the child's demands, in a manner which the parents are frequently unable to accomplish, seems best in most instances with children.

In addition, the assumption by a therapist of the role of a mother calls for much data about the family which may not be available at first, while the frequently intense ambivalence between child and parent makes such a role assumption difficult, especially with the parents close at hand. In this connection, the role of the nurse, as an 'ideal' mother-substitute, assumes great importance in the care of children. The fact that parents may be threatened by and feel rivalrous or guilty toward hospital staff members who are close to their child (and who 'succeed' where they have failed) must also be taken importantly into account. This parallel or tandem work with the parents by the social worker or psychiatrist is often vital.

In regard to regression, the child's developmental level and his current existence in the network of interpersonal relationships within the family must especially be kept in mind. Most school age children and adolescents tend to feel guilty or ashamed if too much regression is encouraged or permitted, and parents may be upset by this also. Sperling[102] in particular feels that the regression should be strongly combated, for reasons mentioned earlier. Langford[67] has recommended encouragement toward early and gradually increasing ambulation as an aid in opposing regressive trends and in weaning the child back to his original level of functioning. In the authors' experience, permitting (but not encouraging) some regression in the early phases, within broad limits, has seemed to be helpful, with gradual weaning after a dependency relationship has been established; the latter often results in prompt diminution of bowel symptoms and a lessening of the regression with returning physical well-being.

As an example, one very dependent, markedly regressed 9-year-old boy asked to be carried around in the arms of the male therapist, saying that this helped his abdominal pain, 'when my mother does it'. The onset of his fulminating picture had occurred during the first night of his father's return from a long absence in military service; the father's sleeping with the mother ousted the boy from her bed for the first time in two years. In this instance, with such clinical data at hand, the therapist offered this regressive satisfaction for brief periods for several days, with marked symptomatic improvement. This function was then transferred to a warmly maternal nurse who gradually encouraged the boy to walk himself, first with support, and then alone, over a period of several weeks.

Although, as mentioned earlier, a supportive psychotherapeutic approach, with brief visits at the beginning and end of the day, and with avoidance of probing, confrontation, or interpretation, is generally best suited to the care of the acutely ill patient, some expression of displaced feelings toward staff persons may occur safely[34]. Ordinarily negative feelings will not be directed toward the parents or the therapist in the early phases, and this should not be encouraged, as conflict or guilt may be intense and may even intensify bowel symptomatology. The elicitation of misconceptions or fantasies regarding bowel or bodily functioning[76] may be a useful approach to dealing with more superficial anxieties, leading later to more expressive methods. An attitude of constructive caution is thus best adopted during this phase; exceptions to this rule have been encountered, however, as in the following examples.

With one $3\frac{1}{2}$-year-old girl who had an acutely fulminating picture, steroid therapy was not helpful, and she was considered too ill for surgery. One of the authors tried to undertake supportive therapy with her. She remained withdrawn and aloof in her bed, however, clinging to her mother during visits, and producing several bloody stools when the mother attempted to leave (see Fig. 1). The therapist knew that her illness had begun the day after the return of the mother from the hospital with a new baby sibling. The mother had given the little girl two goldfish on her return, one of which died when the patient 'accidentally' dropped them on the floor in her room. With this knowledge, in a rather desperate attempt to reach the patient, the therapist set up a doll family scene on the bedside table, with the little girl doll expressing her dislike of the mother's new baby. When the baby doll accidentally fell off the table, the little girl smiled; she then responded with laughter and a beginning relationship when the therapist made the little girl doll repeatedly kick the baby doll off the table. Over several days, with repeated doll play by the therapist, the patient began to talk and engage in the play, showing first rapid subsidence and then complete remission of her symptoms within two weeks time.

In another situation, an acutely ill adolescent boy responded dramatically to the early interpretation that his regressive increase in manipulative and provocative behaviour represented a desperate search for an adult to control his angry feelings before he hurt someone. Such an interpretative

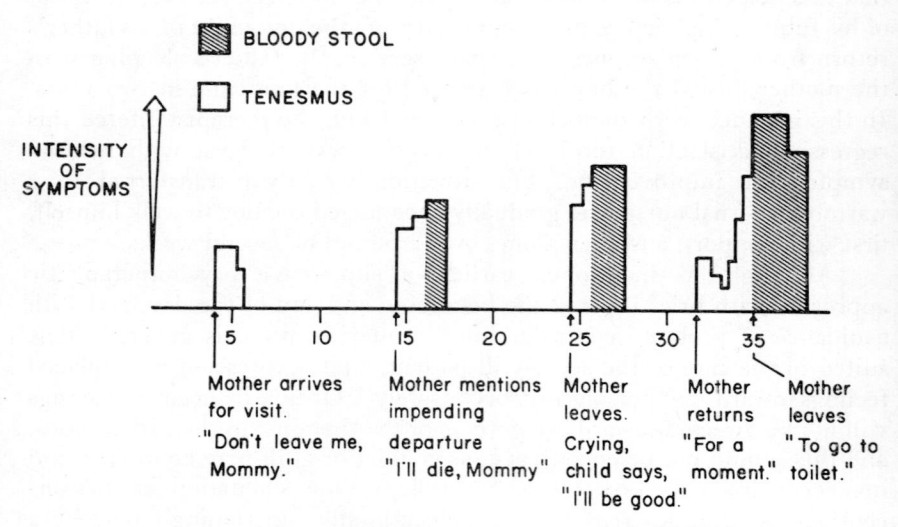

```
         BLOODY STOOL
         TENESMUS
```

INTENSITY OF SYMPTOMS

| 5 | 10 | 15 | 20 | 25 | 30 | 35 |

Mother arrives for visit. "Don't leave me, Mommy."

Mother mentions impending departure "I'll die, Mommy"

Mother leaves. Crying, child says, "I'll be good."

Mother returns "For a moment."

Mother leaves "To go to toilet."

TIME IN MINUTES DURING SINGLE OBSERVATION

FIG. 1.

play or verbal therapeutic approach may occasionally be quickly effective and even possibly life-saving. (Rarely is the patient too sick or too 'toxic' to respond to some extent.) Interpreting a 5-year-old's fear that his parents no longer wanted him when they sent him to the hospital, combined with support, reassurance and the encouragement to get well and go home, resulted in a prompt and virtually total remission of symptoms in a boy who was regarded as fatally ill. In spite of similar reports by Sperling[103], the authors feel that these represent exceptions to the usual approach, however, and should not be used without a good deal of knowledge of the child and family—and then only under serious conditions.

The later phases of ambulatory psychotherapy, after the child has been discharged from the hospital, may involve special difficulties with preschool or younger school-age children in particular. They may show marked clinging or intense separation anxiety, often combined with inability of the mother to separate from the child or with manipulation of the parents by the child. In such situations, the use of a tandem approach, with a therapist for the child and one for the mother in the same room, can be most effective. Gradually the child can be helped to relate to his therapist, with the mother being engaged by hers and, with help, gradually giving the child 'permission' to move off toward a more independent status.

With the $3\frac{1}{2}$-year-old girl mentioned earlier, this approach was necessary after discharge. The child's therapist engaged in solitary play with clay, which the child at first watched with intermittent interest from the mother's lap, where she clung while the mother talked to the social worker. The making of clay 'money' drew the child's interest. Her first step toward separation from the mother took place when, after three weeks, she accepted a gift from the therapist of a 'pile' of round clay money. After two months of weekly interviews, she separated comfortably from the mother, showing less difficulty in this process than the mother herself. The child remained anxious over 'messy' play herself with clay or fingerpaints for some months, however.

As Engel[33] has emphasized with adults, termination often represents a special challenge with the more dependent ulcerative colitis patients, who may show an exacerbation if termination occurs in the usual sense. With children, of course, it is important for the therapist to 'let go' eventually, as the parents must do also, particularly if the adolescent is chronologically ready for a step toward college or work. Tapering down toward longer intervals between interviews may be continued for years beyond the end of formal therapy. The encouragement of telephone calls, letters, or vacation contacts may help the therapist maintain a 'life-line' for an adolescent over a number of years, while encouraging gradual moves toward independence. As indicated, therapy may occasionally be briefer, even crisis-oriented, for some less disturbed children and adolescents, with no necessity for a continuing approach[6, 90]. Caution in termination should be observed, however.

Work with Parents. Certain implications for work in this area have been mentioned earlier. The need for inclusion of the parents in a 'therapeutic alliance' with the hospital staff cannot be overemphasized. Such parents may be difficult to deal with; often the mother in particular may arouse intense counter-transference feelings of irritation, anger, or frustration on the part of the members of the hospital staff or the out-patient therapist(s). The parents may, if sufficiently guilty or rivalrous, project their own anger on to the staff, and may even sign the child out of the hospital against advice or break off out-patient treatment. In the face of such manifest behaviour, their desperate anxiety and guilt may be all too easy to overlook. Anxiety or uncertainty on the part of the staff may affect them markedly, and a kindly, firm, authoritative (but not authoritarian) approach may be most helpful during hospitalization of the child.

In the approach to psychotherapy with such parents, their personality structures and the nature of family interactions are important guides.

With some, whose adaptive capacities are limited or with the few who are borderline psychotic, very limited psychotherapeutic goals may be necessary. The provision of a dependent relationship with a therapist may allow a mother, for example, to make up to some extent for her own perceived lack of mothering. Thus she may gradually come to permit the child to move toward maturity without such a strongly ambivalent need on her part to obtain vicarious satisfactions through their interaction. With parents of greater ego strength, a neurotic involvement of the child in a struggle between marital partners may yield to insight-promoting therapy with both parents, in tandem with the treatment of the child.

With parents, as with children, the therapeutic approach should be tailored to the clinical situation[36]. Surprisingly good psychological results may be obtained at times. Flexibility and appropriate modifications of the usual psychotherapeutic techniques may be necessary, however, in order to avoid stirring up too much anxiety or conflict on the part of the parents, with the possibility of an exacerbation of colitis in the child.

Other Psychotherapeutic Approaches

The authors are aware of no published reports on formal group therapy with children or adolescents with ulcerative colitis. As mentioned earlier, some older adolescents have apparently obtained some emotional support from participation in adult 'ileostomy clubs', involving group discussion of common problems in adjustment[75]. In general, an individual approach seems to be important at least in the early phases of the psychological treatment of children with this disorder. Sharing the relationship to the therapist with others may be especially difficult in this phase for the more disturbed children, with their greater narcissism, dependence, and conflicts over aggression. Activity group therapy for children or interview group therapy for adolescents might have positive benefits at a later point.

Only one published report of family group therapy in this condition is available[58]. Specific results were not reported in this conjoint approach with children and parents, but it is apparent that such techniques can be used safely by experienced people. Although the authors have had no formal experience with this therapeutic approach to the families of children with ulcerative colitis, occasional family interviews with the parents and the child or adolescent patient have been found helpful, during the course of tandem therapy, in clarifying and dealing with particular interpersonal transactions of importance in the current phase of treatment. The authors believe, with Finch[36], that caution in family approaches would be vital, as it is in such therapy in other conditions. If interactional problems are dealt with too early or too interpretatively, the problems in communication[37,58] and difficulties in dealing with aggression[37,58] in many of these families could easily lead to the stirring up of an exacerbation of bowel symptoms in the child or to the premature disruption of unhealthily interlocking family relationships.

The need to employ some environmental manipulation during treatment has been emphasized by some, particularly in adults[50]. This may also be helpful in children, especially around the handling of school phobic patterns in some children and adolescents. The collaboration of practising physicians, teachers, school nurses, social workers, and public health nurses may be most valuable. In the authors' experience, the use of foster-home placement, with rare exceptions, has not appeared to be appropriate or helpful in most instances. Even when family problems are intense, the greater dependence of many of these children and their frequent involvement in close interactional ties with the parents seem to militate against the success of such a step.

A Comprehensive Approach to Treatment

The use of relatively short-term paediatric hospitalization, with combined medical and psychotherapeutic measures, has been mentioned, as has the long-term employment of psychiatric hospitalization in selected cases, with medical and/or surgical consultation. The latter approach can provide appropriate emotional support combined with controls and insights for the child, with opportunities for more effective work with the parents. In addition, gradual steps may be undertaken toward overcoming the secondary gains of chronic illness, which are difficult to deal with on a medically oriented ward.

In the initial phases of study and treatment in paediatric hospital settings, the usual approach has involved a succession of different treatment attempts, by paediatric, surgical, or psychiatric personnel[36]. On an outpatient basis, several different approaches may have been employed concurrently, often without much communication among the staff persons involved; different aspects of treatment may thus be carried on in a 'compartmentalized' or even rivalrous manner. In recent years, the importance of the 'team' or multidisciplinary approach to the treatment of children with ulcerative colitis has been emphasized by Finch and his colleagues[36, 77] and others[56]. In this approach, as used by Finch, a team consisting of a paediatrician, a surgeon, and a child psychiatrist, evaluate[5] each case of ulcerative colitis referred to the hospital, with initial agreement as to the major treatment emphasis. Monthly meetings are held in which each case is jointly discussed, thus promoting communication and collaboration no matter what phase or type of treatment may be involved.

This type of multidisciplinary coordination of diagnosis and treatment is certainly ideal, and indeed is applicable to the handling of many other types of illness. In some settings, however, where fewer cases are seen, such a specialized team may not be possible only for children with ulcerative colitis. In addition, it is important that there be a clearly designated 'captain' or coordinator of the team, who has knowledge of and respect for the contributions of other professional members, in order to promote cooperation and to prevent over-possessiveness toward the patient on the part of any one discipline[77]. This may be harder to achieve in some settings than others.

In the authors' opinion, the initial coordinator should ordinarily be the paediatrician, who supervises the medical aspects of the initial therapy. He can draw upon the consultative help of the child psychiatrist and surgeon, as well as others, including the dermatologist or the orthopaedic surgeon. Decisions can then be made as to whether medical, psychiatric, or surgical steps should be taken, with coordination of follow-up planning. In this way, if indicated, psychiatric hospitalization can be undertaken after initial stabilization of bowel or systemic symptoms is achieved. The emotional readiness of the child and family for surgery can be considered in addition to the bowel symptoms. Continuation of psychotherapy after surgery can be arranged, and the paediatrician can maintain his relationship with the family and patient, regardless of what specialized approaches are involved.

In the experience of the authors, such a hospital team approach can most effectively be implemented through the use of a weekly or semi-weekly *ward management conference*, held in the paediatric ward setting. If a senior paediatrician is available as clinical director of the ward, this is ideal; at least a paediatrician with experience in the team approach to comprehensive management should chair the conference, with the child psychiatrist attending regularly as a consultant and the paediatric surgeon present at least periodically. Other members of the conference are the head nurse and/or nursing supervisor, other members of the nursing staff as indicated, school teacher, clinical psychologist, social worker, recreational therapist, occupational and physical therapists, and other regular members of the ward staff, including semi-professional persons such as, in our setting, 'foster grandmothers'.

With many less severely disturbed children and families, a supportive psychotherapeutic approach by the paediatrician, along with appropriate medical measures, may be the plan of choice. In such instances, the psychiatrist's role is largely a consultative one at the outset, regarding immediate management and treatment planning rather than a formal psychotherapeutic one. Through the medium of the ward management conference, implementation of the following principles, of importance in the handling of other types of cases as well, may be achieved: *communication* among ward staff members, so vital to effective treatment planning; *collaboration* among the various disciplines, with decisions as to who should be involved in various aspects of the management approach; *consultation* from members of the conference with specialized training and from other outside specialists invited for particular occasions; *continuity* of relationships between physician and nurse and child and family, with designation of one physician and one nurse to be involved wherever possible, and with the assignment of a foster grandmother or other semi-professional person to offer continued emotional support if indicated; *consistency* in techniques of ward management, particularly in the setting of appropriate limits on the patient's behaviour, in dealing with the tendency of patient and parents to manipulate and play one staff person against another, and in setting up an atmosphere in which the anxiety, hostility, and other feelings of child and parent may be brought under effective control; *coordination* by the chairman of the ward management conference, which assures that the various other principles are implemented and that a unified and balanced programme of management is achieved.

In addition to his consultative role, which includes help in the promotion of the principles of ward management, the psychiatrist may function as the psychotherapist in a formal sense, if such measures are indicated. He may in some instances supervise a member of another mental health discipline in such an approach. He may continue to function in a psychotherapeutic or supervisory role in an out-patient child psychiatry clinic[56] following the child's discharge, with regular consultative contacts with the paediatrician, surgeon, and other professional persons. Where psychiatric hospitalization is indicated, he may function as both the co-ordinator and therapist, or another therapist may be involved. In other situations, he may act as a consultant or therapist in situations where early surgical intervention is called for[36, 77].

Communication, collaboration, consultation, continuity, consistency, and coordination of the type described are more difficult to achieve on the part of the practising paediatrician, who is handling a child with ulcerative colitis on an ambulatory basis. Nevertheless he can, by using consultation with a child psychiatrist and surgeon who are known to him, achieve a somewhat similar result, including the approach to management during periods of hospitalization if necessary. This requires a considerable amount of time on the part of the paediatrician, but the results are usually worth the effort. Some pediatricians, particularly those in small groups, have invited a social worker to join them on at least a part-time basis. With her help in seeing parents, and with monthly meetings with a consulting child psychiatrist and a child clinical psychologist, together with consultations with a paediatric surgeon or others as indicated, they have been able to handle mild to moderately disturbed children with ulcerative colitis (and with other problems in which psychophysiologic factors are involved) with much success. The more seriously disturbed children whose physical symptoms are under control may be referred to private psychotherapists or to mental health facilities for formal psychotherapy. Continuing communication and consultation as well as coordination may be offered by the psychiatrist in such instances, with medical follow-up provided by the paediatrician and with surgical consultation as needed[56].

9

Prevention

Since certain of the multiple etiologic factors involved in this condition are as yet unclear, no comprehensive programme of prevention is as yet feasible. It is possible that, when certain biological factors involved in the abnormal tissue response of the colonic mucosa or the systemic manifestations are more firmly identified, a biological 'tag' will be available to identify children in early infancy who may develop the condition. It might then be possible to offer specific psychological preventive help or to follow them anterospectively, as has been done with children with high blood pepsinogen levels who constitute the group from whom patients will later develop peptic ulcer[85]. Such a step might lead to specific preventive steps at the physiologic level, such as the alteration of biochemical systems or the prevention of the formation of destructive enzymes released in the antigen-antibody reaction. It could also clarify the interaction of physiologic, psychologic, and social factors, in regard to the possible predisposing effect of experience on tissue vulnerability, as well as the balance of forces involved at the time of onset of symptoms and during the later clinical course.

In the absence of any available means of early identification of potential patients, some indirect preventive effect may be achieved through anticipatory guidance and supportive psychological measures undertaken by paediatricians and family physicians in their work with infants and young children and their families, particularly those of the general nature described. Undertaking such measures during the period of the establishment of trust and autonomy in the infant, in which feeding, weaning, and toilet-training seem to present particular difficulties, might minimize at least some of the predisposing psychological forces. Such help might also prove effective during the preschool and early childhood period in regard to the cushioning of the impact of separation experiences, to which these children later seem so vulnerable. A controlled study[12] indicates that such measures can enhance the adjustment of children during the preschool period. The early employment of other helping persons and agencies in the community, in regard to marital problems, psychotherapy for disturbed parents, family therapy where indicated, and other steps may also be of preventive significance in a broad sense.

10

Summary

1. There appear to be significant influences of psychologic and interpersonal forces upon the onset and course of ulcerative colitis in childhood,

with both immediate and long-range effects upon bowel function and the general state of the patient.

2. These influences, however significant, do not appear fully to explain the nature of the disease, which often assumes a systemic character, nor the abnormal tissues response appearing in the mucosa of the colon, the principle target organ. Multiple etiologic determinants of social, psychologic, and as yet partially understood biological nature appear to be involved, with predisposing, precipitating, and perpetuating influences upon the total picture.

3. The psychotherapeutic approach, geared to the needs of child and family, can be an important, indeed vital component in the treatment of ulcerative colitis in childhood and adolescence. Interdisciplinary collaboration and coordination among paediatricians, surgeons, and child psychiatrists, together with other professional persons, would appear to be the touchstone of comprehensive management of this distressing and often serious illness.

REFERENCES

1. ALMY, T. P., and LEWIS, C. M., 1963. Ulcerative colitis, a report of progress based upon the recent literature. *Gastroenterol.*, **45**, 515.
2. ARAJARVI, T., PENTTI, R., and AUKEE, M., 1961, 1962. Ulcerative colitis in children. A clinical, psychological and social follow-up study. *Ann. Paediat. Fenn.*, **7**, 259, **8**, 1.
3. ASKEVOLD, F., 1964. Studies in ulcerative colitis. *J. Psychosom. Res.*, **8**, 89.
4. BARRON, S. H., and SPURLOCK, J., 1958. Ulcerative colitis: psychosomatic factors. *Med. Sci.*, **3**, 412.
5. BLOM, G. E., 1955. Ulcerative colitis in a five-year-old boy. In *Emotional problems of early childhood*. Ed. Caplan, G. New York, Basic Books.
6. BRESSLER, B., 1956. Colitis as anniversary symptom: emergency psychotherapy with relief of symptom. *Psychoanalyt. Rev.*, **43**, 381.
7. BROBERGER, O., 1964. Immunologic studies in ulcerative colitis. *Gastroenterol.*, **47**, 229-40.
8. BROWN, C. H., 1963. Acute emotional crises and ulcerative colitis. *Amer. J. dig. Dis.*, **8**, 525.
9. CASTELNUOVO-TEDESCO, P., 1962. Ulcerative colitis in an adolescent boy subjected to a homosexual assault. Report of a case. *Psychosom. Med.*, **24**, 148.
10. CHAUDHARY, N. A., and TRUELOVE, S. C., 1961. Colonic motility: a critical review of methods and results. *Am. J. Med.*, **31**, 86.
11. COHEN, N., HOFFMAN, W. A., and SPIRO, H. M., 1960. Ulcerative colitis arising during corticosteroid therapy. *Gastroenterol.*, **38**, 93.
12. COOPER, M. M., 1947. Evaluation of the mothers' advisory service. *Mon. Soc. for Research in Child Develop.*, No. 12.
13. CROHN, B. B., ENGEL, G. L., FLOOD, C. A., and GARLOCK, J. H., Management of ulcerative colitis and transcription of a panel meeting on therapeutics. *Bull. N.Y. Acad. Med.*, **34**, 366.
14. CROHN, B. B., YARNIS, H., WALTER, R. J., and GABRILOVE, L. J., 1956. Ulcerative colitis as affected by pregnancy. *N.Y. State J. Med.*, **56**, 2651.

15. CUSHING, M. G., 1953. The psychoanalytic treatment of a man suffering with ulcerative colitis. *J. Am. Psychoan. Assn*, **1**, 510.
16. DANIELS, G. E., 1948. Psychiatric factors in ulcerative colitis. *Gastroenterol.*, **10**, 59.
17. DANIELS, G. E., O'CONNOR, J. F., KARUSH, A., MOSES, L., FLOOD, C. A., and LEPORE, M., 1962. Three decades in the observation and treatment of ulcerative colitis. *Psychosom. Med.*, **24**, 85.
18. DAVIDSON, M., BLOOM, ALAN, A., and KUGLER, MARGARET M., 1965. Chronic ulcerative colitis of childhood; an evaluative review. *J. Pediat.*, **67**, 471.
19. DAVIDSON, M., and WASSERMAN, R., 1966. The irritable colon of childhood (chronic non-specific diarrhoea syndrome). *J. Pediat.*, **69**, 1027.
20. DENNIS, C., and EDDY, F. D., 1947. Evaluation of vagotomy in chronic non-specific ulcerative colitis. *Proc. Soc. Exp. Biol. Med.*, **65**, 306.
21. DICK, A. P., GRAYSON, M. J., CARPENTER, R. G., and PETRIE, A., 1964. Controlled trial of sulphasalazine in the treatment of ulcerative colitis. *Gut*, **5**, 437-42.
22. DOCK, W., 1944. Evil sequelae of complete bed rest. *J. Amer. med. Assn*, **125**, 1083.
23. DONALDSON, G. A., 1963. Current concepts in therapy; management of ileostomy and colostomy. *N.E.J. Med.*, **268**, 827.
24. DOWER, J. Personal communication.
25. EHRENPREIS, T., ERICSSON, N. O., BILLING, L., LAGERCRANTZ, R., and RUDHE, U., 1960. Surgical treatment of ulcerative colitis in children. *Acta Pediat.*, **49**, 810.
26. EHRENPREIS, T., and ERICSSON, N. O., 1964. Surgical treatment of ulcerative colitis in children. *Surg. Clin. N. Amer.*, **44**, 1521.
27. ENGEL, G. L., 1960. A unified concept of health and disease. *Persp. Biol. Med.*, **3**, 459.
28. ENGEL, G. L., 1961. Biologic and psychologic features of the ulcerative colitis patient. *Gastroenterol.*, **40**, 313.
29. ENGEL, G. L., 1954. Studies of ulcerative colitis: I. Clinical data bearing on the nature of the somatic process. *Psychosom. Med.*, **16**, 496.
30. ENGEL, G. L., 1954. Studies of ulcerative colitis. II. The nature of the somatic processes and the adequacy of psychosomatic hypotheses. *Am. J. Med.*, **16**, 416.
31. ENGEL, G. L., 1955. Studies of ulcerative colitis: III. The nature of the psychologic processes. *Am. J. Med.*, **19**, 231.
32. ENGEL, G. L., 1956. Studies of ulcerative colitis: IV. The significance of headaches. *Psychosom. Med.*, **18**, 334.
33. ENGEL, G. L., 1958. Studies of ulcerative colitis: V. Psychologic aspects and the implications for treatment. *Am. J. dig. Dis.*, **3**, 315.
34. ENGEL, G. L., 1952. Psychologic aspects of the management of patients with ulcerative colitis. *N.Y.J. Med.*, **52**, 2255.
35. ERIKSON, E. H., 1956. *Childhood and society*. New York, W. W. Norton.
36. FINCH, S. M., 1964. The treatment of children with ulcerative colitis. *Am. J. Orthopsychiat.*, **34**, (1).
37. FINCH, S. M., and HESS, J. H., 1962. Ulcerative colitis in children. *Am. J. Psychiat.*, **118**, 819.
38. FRIEDMAN, M. H. F., and SNAPE, W. J., 1946. Color changes in the mucosa of the colon in children, as affected by food and psychic stimuli. *Fed. Proc.*, **5**, 30.
39. FREUD, S., 1940. *An outline of psychoanalysis*. New York, W. W. Norton.
40. GARLOCK, J. H., and LYONS, A. S., 1954. The role of surgery in the therapy of ulcerative colitis. *Gastroenterol.*, **26**, 709.

REFERENCES

41. GARNER, A. M., and WENAR, C., 1959. *The mother-child interaction in psychosomatic disorders.* Urbana, Illinois, Univ. Press.
42. GERARD, M., 1953. The genesis of psychosomatic symptoms in infancy. In *The psychosomatic concept in psychoanalysis.* Ed. Deutsch, F. New York, Internat. Univ. Press.
43. GLANZMANN, E., and ASCH, H., 1937. Colitis ulcerosa in kindesalter. *Jahrbuch v. Kinderheilk,* **158**, 233.
44. GONZALES-LICEA, A., and YARDLEY, J., 1966. Nature of the tissue reaction in ulcerative colitis: light and electron microscopic findings. *Gastroenterol.,* **51**, 825.
45. GRACE, W. J., PINSLEY, R. H., and WOLFF, H. G., 1954. The treatment of ulcerative colitis. *Gastroenterol.,* **26**, 462.
46. GRACE, W. J., and WOLFF, H. G., 1951. Treatment of ulcerative colitis. *J. Amer. med. Assn,* **146**, 981.
47. GRACE, W. J., WOLFF, S., and WOLFF, H. G., 1950. Life situations, emotions, and chronic ulcerative colitis. *J. Amer. med. Assn,* **142**, 1044.
48. GRACE, W. J., WOLFF, S., and WOLFF, H. G., 1951. *The human colon.* New York, Paul B. Hoeber.
49. GREEN, M., 1960. Discussion of Masland, R. P. Ulcerative colitis. In *Symposium on adolescence.* Eds, Meiks, L. T., and Green, M. *Ped. Cl. N.A.* 7, No. 1. Philadelphia, W. B. Saunders.
50. GROEN, J., and VAN DER VALK, J. M., 1956. Psychosomatic aspects of ulcerative colitis. *Gastroenterol.,* **86**, 591.
51. GROSS, R. E., 1953. *Abdominal surgery of infants and children.* Philadelphia, W. B. Saunders.
52. HARPER, E. O., 1952. Prolonged narcosis in the treatment of severe ulcerative colitis. *Gastroenterol.,* **42**, 758.
53. HELMHOLZ, H. F., 1923. Chronic ulcerative colitis in childhood. *Am. J. Dis. Childhood.,* **26**, 418.
54. HIJMANS, J., 1962. Ulcerative colitis in childhood. *Pediatrics,* **29**, 389.
55. HOLOWACH, J., and THURSTON, D. L., 1956. Chronic ulcerative colitis in childhood. *J. Pediat.,* **48**, 279.
56. HUNT, A. D., Jr., *et al.,* 1952. Collaboration between a children's hospital and a psychiatric clinic for children in the treatment of ulcerative colitis. *Am. J. Dis. Childhood,* **84**, 490.
57. JACKMAN, R. J., BARGEN, J. A., and HELMHOLZ, H. F., 1944. Life histories of 95 children with chronic ulcerative colitis: statistical study based on comparison with a whole group of 871 patients. *Am. J. Dis. Childhood,* **59**, 459.
58. JACKSON, D. D., and YALOM, I., 1966. Family research on the problem of ulcerative colitis. *Archs gen. Psychiat.,* **15**, 410.
59. JACKSON, M., and PLAUT, A., 1955. Psychological aspects of ulcerative colitis in childhood. *Archs Middlesex Hosp.,* **5**, 21.
60. JOSSELYN, J. M., LITTNER, N., and SPURLOCK, J., 1966. Psychological aspects of ulcerative colitis in children. *Amer. Med. Wom. Assn,* **21**, 303.
61. KIRSNER, J. B., and GOLDGRABER, M. D., 1960. Hypersensitivity, autoimmunity, and the digestive tract. *Gastroenterol.,* **38**, 536.
62. KIRSNER, J. B., RASKIN, H. F., and PALMER, W. L., 1955. Ulcerative colitis in children. *Am. J. Dis. Childhood,* **90**, 141.
63. KOCH, J. P., and DONALDSON, R. M., Jr., 1964. A survey of food intolerances in hospitalized patients. *N.E.J. Med.,* **271**, 657.
64. LAGERCRANTZ, R., 1958. Extracolonic manifestations of chronic ulcerative colitis. *Acta Paediat.,* **27**, 675.

65. LAGERCRANTZ, R., 1955. Follow-up investigation of children with ulcerative colitis, with special reference to indications for surgical therapy. *Acta Paediat.*, **44**, 302.
66. LAGERCRANTZ, R., 1949. Ulcerative colitis in children. *Acta Paediat.*, supplement, **75**, 89.
67. LANGFORD, W. S., 1964. The psychological aspects of ulcerative colitis. *Clin. Proc. Children's Hosp. (Wash)*, **20**, 89.
68. LENNENBERG, E., 1963. Quoted In Brown, C. H. Acute emotional crises and ulcerative colitis. *Amer. J. dig. Dis.*, **8**, 525.
69. LEVIN, P., FONKALSRUD, E. W., and BARKER, W. F., 1966. Surgical treatment for pediatric ulcerative colitis. *Surgery*, **60**, 201, 211.
70. LEVY, R., WILKENS, H., HERMANN, J., LISLE, A., Jr., and RIX, A., 1956. Experiences with prefrontal leukotomy for intractable ulcerative colitis. *J. Amer. med. Assn*, **160**, 1277.
71. LINDEWANN, E., 1945. Psychiatric problems in conservative treatment of ulcerative colitis. *Archs Neurol. Psychiat.*, **53**, 322.
72. LOGAN, H. H., 1919. Chronic ulcerative colitis: a review of 117 cases. *Northwest Med.*, **18**, 1.
73. LYONS, A. S., 1956. Ulcerative colitis in children. *Pediat. Clin. N. Amer.*, **19**, 153.
74. MARGOLIN, S., 1957. Psychotherapeutic principles in psychosomatic practice. In *Recent developments in psychosomatic medicine*. Eds, Wittkower, E. D., and Cleghorn, R. A. Philadelphia, Lippincott.
75. MASLAND, R. P., 1960. Ulcerative colitis. In *Symposium on adolescence*. Eds, Meiks, L. T., and Green, M. *Pediat. Clin. N. Amer.*, **7**, No. 1. Philadelphia, W. B. Saunders.
76. MCDERMOTT, J. F., 1966. Children with ulcerative colitis: their own perception of the disease. *Psychosomatics*, **7**, 163.
77. MCDERMOTT, J., and FINCH, S., 1964. Ulcerative colitis: physician teamwork in the treatment. *Clinical Pediatrics*, **3**, 75.
78. MCKAY, J. R., WALL, A. J., and GOLDSTEIN, G., 1966. Response to agothioprine in ulcerative colitis. Report of 7 cases. *Amer. J. dig. Dis.*, **11**, 536.
79. MCGOVERN, V. J., and ARCHER, G. T., 1957. The pathogenesis of ulcerative colitis. *Austral. Ann. Med.*, **6**, 68.
80. MEEKER, J. A., Jr., and GOFF, P., 1956. Surgical significance of ulcerative colitis in infants and children. *West J. Surg.* **64**, 545.
81. MENDELOFF, A. I., MOULE, P. D., SIEGEL, C. D., and LILIENFELD, M. D., 1966. Some epidemiologic features of ulcerative colitis and regional enteritis. *Gastroenterol.*, **51**, 748.
82. MICHENER, W. M., GAGE, R. P., SAVER, W. G., and STICKLER, G. B., 1961. The prognosis of chronic ulcerative colitis in children. *N.E.J. Med.*, **265**, 1075.
83. MICHENER, W. M., BROWN, C. H., and TURNBULL, R. B., 1964. Ulcerative colitis in children. *Amer. J. Dis. Child.*, **108**, 230-36.
84. MIDDLEKAMP, J. N., and HAFFNER, H., 1963. Carcinoma of the colon in children *Pediatrics*, **32**, 558.
85. MIRSKY, I. A., 1958. Physiologic, psychologic, and social determinants in the etiology of duodenal ulcer. *Amer. J. Dig. Dis.*, **3**, 285.
86. MOHR, G. J., JOSSELYN, I. M., SPURLOCK, J., and BARRON, S. H., 1958. Studies in ulcerative colitis. *Amer. J. Psychiat.*, **114**, 1067.
87. MUSHATT, C., 1954. Psychological aspects of non-specific ulcerative colitis. In *Recent developments in psychosomatic medicine*. Eds, Wittkower, E., and Cleghorn, R. Philadelphia, W. B. Lippincott.

REFERENCES

88. NELSON, W. E., 1963. Chronic ulcerative colitis. In *Textbook of pediatrics*. Ed. Nelson, W. E. Philadelphia, W. B. Lippincott.
89. O'CONNOR, J. F., 1966. Ulcerative colitis: emotional problems and their management. *Medical Times*, **94**, 106.
90. O'CONNOR, J. F., DANIELS, G., FLOOD, C., KARUSH, A., MOSES, L., and STERN, L. O., 1964. An evaluation of the effectiveness of psychotherapy in the treatment of ulcerative colitis. *Ann. Int. Med.*, **60**, 587.
91. O'CONNOR, J. F., DANIELS, G., KARUSH, A., FLOOD, C., and STERN, L. O., 1966. Prognostic implications of psychiatric diagnosis in ulcerative colitis. *Psychosom. Med.*, **18**, 375.
92. PAULLEY, J. W., 1956. Psychotherapy in ulcerative colitis. *Lancet*, ii, 215.
93. PRIEST, R. J., REBUCK, J. W., and HOVEY, G. T., 1960. A new qualitative defect of leukocyte function in ulcerative colitis. *Gastroenterol.*, **38**, 715.
94. PRUGH, D. G., 1951. The role of emotional factors in ulcerative colitis in childhood. *Gastroenterol.*, **18**, 339.
95. PRUGH, D. G., 1949. Variations in attitude, behavior, and feeling states as exhibited in the play of children during modifications in the course of ulcerative colitis. In *Life and bodily stress. Proc. Assn Res. nerv. ment. Dis.* Baltimore, Williams and Wilkins.
96. PRUGH, D. G., 1960. Emotional factors in the clinical course of ulcerative colitis in children. *Feelings*, 2, No. 5.
97. PRUGH, D. G., 1963. Toward an understanding of psychosomatic concepts in relation to illness in childhood. In *Modern perspectives in child development*. Eds, Solnit, A., and Provence, S. New York, Intern. Univ. Press.
98. PRUGH, D. G., Unpublished material.
99. RICHMOND, J., 1960. Discussion of Masland, R. P. Ulcerative colitis. In *Symposium on adolescence*. Eds, Meiks, L. T., and Green, M. Philadelphia, W. B. Saunders.
100. ROMANO, J., 1950. Basic orientation and education of the medical student. *J. Amer. med. Assn*, **143**, 409.
101. SPENCER, J. A., KIRSNER, J. B., REED, P. A., MYLNARYK, P., and PALMER, W. L., 1962. Immediate and prolonged effects of corticotropin and adrenal steroids in ulcerative colitis: observations in 340 cases for periods up to 10 years. *Gastroenterol.*, **42**, 113.
102. SPERLING, M., 1957. The psychoanalytic treatment of ulcerative colitis. *Internat. J. Psychoanal.*, **38**, 341.
103. SPERLING, M., 1946. Psychoanalytic study of ulcerative colitis in children. *Psychoanal. Quart.*, **15**, 302.
104. THOREK, P., 1951. Vagotomy for idiopathic ulcerative colitis: results in 21 cases. *J. Amer. med. Assn*, **145**, 140.
105. TITCHENER, J. L., and LEVINE, M., 1960. *Surgery as a human experience*. New York, Oxford Univ. Press.
106. WALLGREN, A., 1955. Ulcerative colitis in children. *Deutsch. Med. J.*, **6**, 45.
107. WARREN, I. A., and BERKS, J. E., 1957. The etiology of ulcerative colitis. A critical review. *Gastroenterol.*, **33**, 395.
108. WARREN, R., and MCKITTRICK, L. S., 1951. Ileostomy for ulcerative colitis, technique, complications, and management. *Surg., Gyn., Obstet.*, **93**, 555.
109. WARREN, S., and SOMMERS, S. C., 1954. Pathology of regional ileitis and ulcerative colitis. *J. Amer. med. Assn*, **145**, 189.
110. WEINSTOCK, H. I., 1962. Successful treatment of ulcerative colitis by psychoanalysis: a survey of 28 cases with follow-up. *J. Psychosom. Res.*, **6**, 243.
111. WEINSTOCK, H. L., 1966. Psychotherapy for ulcerative colitis. *J. Psychosom. Res.*, **6**, 249.

112. WENAR, C., HANDLON, M. W., and GARNER, A. M., 1962. *Origins of psychosomatic and emotional disturbances: a study of mother-child relationships.* New York, Paul B. Hoeber.
113. WHITE, B. V., 1951. The effect of ileostomy and colostomy on the personality adjustment of patients with ulcerative colitis. *N.E.J. Med.*, **244**, 538.
114. WHITE, B. V., COBB, S., and JONES, C. M., 1939. Mucous colitis: a psychological medical study of 60 cases. *Psychosomatic Med. Mon.*, No. 1., Washington, D.C., National Research Council.
115. WHITE, W. H., 1888. On simple ulcerative colitis and other rare internal ulcers. *Guy's Hosp. Rep.*, **45**, 131.
116. WOLFF, S., 1966. The central nervous system regulation of the colon. *Gastroenterol.*, **51**, 810.

XIX

PSYCHOGENIC RETARDATION

ANDREW CROWCROFT

B.Sc., M.B., B.S., M.R.S.C., L.R.C.P., D.P.M.

Consultant Psychiatrist, Queen Elizabeth Hospital for Children, London and The John Scott Health Centre

1
Introduction

In our early childhood we have to *learn* to perceive the real world[36]. We have to become aware of events in the environment as separate from events within ourselves[6]. As adults, we are so familiar with things in the external world being arranged as meaningful objects, outside us, in space and time, we can hardly imagine it was not always so for us. As adults, we unconsciously link our immediate sensory perceptions to ideas and memories already in our minds, and in doing so give meaning to our experiences. The infant and young child, lacking an extensive past, is much less able to see the world as we do. There are two aspects to the growth of a child's perceptual ability which must be acknowledged: perceptual capacity, which depends to an extent on the organic maturation of the central nervous system and of the sense organs such as sight or touch and so on; and perceptual learning, in which knowledge is built up about things in the world—including oneself—through the almost endless experiments of childhood. The perceptual learning aspect will obviously be linked to intelligence. The ability to perceive particular things therefore depends on the mental age (cleverness) of the child, as well as on his chronological age. When it came to thinking about intelligence a generation ago, the emphasis, in the United Kingdom at any rate, was on heredity[25a, b]. There is a much livelier appreciation now of the effects of the environment upon the growth of ability in the child[4]. Perception is both part of intelligence and is also the link between the inner and outer world—the inner world of thoughts, feelings, impulses and ideas and the outer world of things and people, to whom the individual relates. It follows then, that while of course it matters what is perceived and how much stimulation, or neglect an infant receives, this is not merely passively recorded by his perceptual systems, but undoubtedly contributes to the growth both of his personality and of his intelligence. It also affects how he feels—secure, or insecure. It is interesting to note, if we regard the brain and its perceptual system as a computor, a very striking superiority of the nervous system over the conventional computor resides in the organic system's ability to be modified profoundly by use. Communication and information theory may help us by an analogy to understand some perceptual and neurophysiological problems[22]. In psychology and psychiatry however, we can never ignore the affective correlatives of cognitive processes. Thus modification by learning, and the existence of powerful feelings should always be taken into account in any outline of human mental development, alongside consideration of the maturation of the central nervous system as an organic qua organic system by itself.

Psychoanalysis has for a very long time acknowledged the distortions that can be imposed on the intellect by emotional factors, but this discipline has tended to under rate, or ignore, the effects of the actual continuing environment until fairly recently. We can reasonably assume, however, that if the environment affects the emotions, and the emotions affect the intellect, then the general as well as the particular here-and-now-situation surrounding children influences their intellectual growth. Lack of intellectual stimulation itself of course can be destructive, leading to low levels of aspiration in the child. Too cerebral an approach by parents, with all feeling split off, can augment schizoid traits in the child, leading gradually to a child who is a stranger to his own real feeling state[23]. Such a child might remain bright, but he may well show ego-constriction, and have severe limits set to the areas in which he can exhibit his intellect, or which he dare explore[12].

2

Severe Subnormality

A much quoted reference to a research project which describes the apparent production of severe subnormality by severe environmental stress is a paper by Bourne[2]. He called his study 'Protophrenia, a study of perverted rearing and mental dwarfism'. It was designed to evaluate the effects of social and psychological adversity in infancy and the effects of these were called *psychogenic amentia*. A further aim was to discover the prevalence and the clinical features of the condition. Bourne noted the long known fact that most *severe* cases of subnormality are due to organic brain disease. There was a smaller number of cases, however, where no organic pathology could be determined and there was no familial pathology. His description of 'psychogenic amentia' was of a physically healthy child, with an uneven backwardness showing from about the second year of life, who exhibited severe behaviour disorders, and whose early milestones had not been delayed. Such a child was not clumsy or impoverished in facial expression. In all these features the group contrasted with other forms of amentia. Such a child would appear remote, even deaf, and would often have monotonous mannerisms such as head banging or tearing out of hair. They might be persistently screaming or destructive. These children, he thought, had suffered an aborted organization of their personalities because of 'perverted mothering'. Bourne did not believe that he was describing psychotic children, but later workers[32] have thought that some of his group were in fact showing what has come to be called, in this country, symptoms of the 'schizophrenic syndrome in childhood'[34]. Even if this were so, I believe the cause of this condition is sometimes 'psychogenic'[6]. The syndrome according to the 'Nine Points Scheme'[34] includes 'A background of serious retardation' and fairly falls therefore under our examination of psychogenic retardation, as do Bourne's other nonpsychotic but severely subnormal cases.

It is interesting to compare the older texts on mental subnormality[25a,b] with the more contemporary ones[20a,b]. These latter are more socially orientated. Emotional and environmental factors loom larger and larger as we approach the present day, in the general assessment of causation, even where organic factors are present. Here one may link the contemporary views as to the cause of subnormality in childhood with well-established observations with regard to Senile Dementia. In Senile Dementia it has long been known that the degree of organic pathology does not parallel the degree of intellectual and emotional dilapidation[29]. A sympathetic supportive environment can keep a person functioning who in fact has quite a severe degree of brain damage. This seems true of children too. A poor environment, on the other hand, maximizes the effects of any organic impairment both in children and in the elderly. It is interesting that whereas in Senile Dementia, acute and chronic confusional states are seen, in brain-damaged children, the clinician sees from time to time a psychotic-like picture as a response on the part of the child to emotional stress. Unlike other child psychotics, this type of child quite quickly responds to improved environmental conditions. He needs a simple, unstressful learning situation in which to develop. He tends to have delirium more easily, when physically ill, than other children. It is difficult to assess his intelligence formally, and the result of such testing shows areas of both high and low functioning[20a].

3

Wastage of Ability

Wastage of any ability at the lower levels of IQ leads almost inevitably to the queue for an institution. There is now massive evidence however that a very considerable wastage also goes on with potentially more gifted children, due to the various kinds of physical and emotional environments they grow up in, and to the different types of class attitudes towards education to which they too are exposed. It has been shown quite unequivocally by Douglas[9] that ordinary children from good homes and schools improve in their test performance between 8 and 11 years, whereas children from poor homes and schools deteriorate. It was felt that the problem goes quite beyond the influence of the primary school itself, and that it is likely that in the preschool years the mental development of many children is stunted by the poverty of their surroundings. Douglas and his colleagues felt that the only way of tackling such a problem would be via nursery schools, which should aim to give small children the stimulus so often lacking in their homes. Douglas was highly aware of the need to know much more about the impact of the family on the early processes of learning and on the acquisition of learning incentives before children reach school. It is now clear that the predictability of the IQ at any given age has been called severely into question[5] and we no longer fixedly think of intelligence as 'general innate cognitive ability'[3]. The IQ does not appear to be constant and some of our compulsory education is probably disastrous for some children, committing them to schools as destructive and stultifying from the intellectual angle, as their own bookless homes. It would be nice to avoid value judgments such as some of the above statements appear to be. However, our educationalists are often committed to expensive programmes of education based on value judgments, which entirely lack the kind of evidence Douglas has amassed to support his own conclusions. Certainly culturally depressed areas can be defined, and apart from setting up of nursery schools, the schools in those areas should either be specially designated, and have much smaller classes, in order to attract and keep good teachers, or in addition, or alternatively, teachers in these areas should be more highly paid. There is evidence that the turnover of teachers in infant and primary schools is of the order of 25 per cent per annum even in London. In the poorer areas of London—in the King's Cross area for example, some schools have teacher turnover figures of more than 60 per cent per annum. This in itself is very upsetting to the young child, disturbing in many cases what is essentially a transference situation, and leading many children into giving up trying to learn from the 'untrustworthy' teacher-figure.

4

Cultural Deprivation

Apart from misguided, if sincere, or accidental mishandling of children, there are then those limitations imposed by a supposedly 'normal' social and family background on the child's intellectual growth. The condition of subnormal intelligence occurs much more frequently in those social strata found at the bottom of any social scale of class than it does at the top of the scale. The use of intelligence tests over the last 50 years has made this fact abundantly clear. As we have acknowledged, earlier accounts attributed the class differences to differing heredity. It was assumed that class differences reflected the genetic composition of each class. Twin studies seemed to support the concept.

In this view, high grade subnormality was merely the tail end of a normal distribution curve, a curve, to be sure, skewed somewhat, since few things seemed to make children brighter, but illness and accident could make them duller. Gradually social and cultural factors came into prominence. As an example, it was shown that negroes living in a northern state of the U.S.A. are brighter than poor whites living in the south, leave alone also being brighter than southern negroes with whom they share the same genetic background[19]. In the U.K., A. D. B. and Anne Clarke showed how the subnormal who have experienced much family deprivation could respond to special training and gain in intelligence, even through their twenties. They suggested that family deprivation retarded intellectual growth and their evidence showed that the worst deprivations could cause the most retardation. It was equally important that they showed the reversibility of deprivation effects by special training[5].

There are two classes of the mentally subnormal. In one, there are clearly important physical defects, metabolic, or neurological. As we have said, most of the severely subnormal belong to the first organic group. About 75 per cent of all cases of subnormality, however, belong to the second non-organic group. This majority have a high grade of subnormality, and again, as we have already seen, belong to the lower socio-economic classes. A study of this second group has been carried out to see if the families in it could be classified by their culture—their systems of values and attitudes, their way of life[35]. It has been found possible to define two broad cultural categories among these families, one of whom showed no signs of evaluation with the middle class, in particular with its values of achievements through education and aspiration. The second category comprised the families who did show signs of evaluation with middle-class values or at least showed aspiration towards them. A homogenous clinical type of subnormality, without detectable organic handicap, was drawn entirely from the families who showed no sign of middle-class evaluation. It seems that high-grade subnormality without brain damage is specific to this group, and the evidence is very suggestive that cultural factors contribute importantly to the handicap. As with the Clarke's experiments, it was found that adults from this group did not have irremediable damage, since their adult intelligence test scores tended to increase beyond their childhood ones. The culture producing such individuals handicapped them in the areas of verbal skills and thinking and in the academic abilities tested by intelligence tests and required for academic success.

Incidentally, it was noted, as it has been before, that boys are ascertained as subnormal more often than girls are. Children of higher social class are more often kept within the educational system, and have special schooling. Lower-class children were more often excluded from school. Children from broken homes were more often ascertained than children from intact homes. This latter feature was particularly striking in the adolescent group who, if they showed any behaviour disorder in adolescence, tended to end up in hospitals for the subnormal. (Of course, there is an enormous shortage of beds for adolescents of any psychiatric category, and this might have been one of the reasons for this.)

The study we have been quoting speaks encouragingly of the results of special training and schooling in the subnormal field. It emphasizes the need for prolonged schooling, because of the continued rise in ability that can attend this. It also pleads for helping vulnerable families, pointing out how poorly adapted the modern, nuclear family is to bear the extra strain of a handicapped individual.

Maternal Deprivation

We can speak then of *cultural deprivation* and by this refer to the group of factors some of which we have just considered. These factors seem to go against a child realizing his full intellectual potential. While it is valid for social anthropologists to avoid saying one culture is better or worse than another, we are examining sub-ethnic groups who have been demonstrated to function worse than the general or other parts of the total population. There is, I believe, an obligation on us to seek causal factors, especially ones we are capable of changing. We are only slowly learning about the issues connected with social change. Social and educational failure can be felt as an extreme humiliation by the individual facing them, as well as by the family producing such an individual. We need not apologize, then, for making both attempts at 'social diagnosis', and suggesting remedies where we can. It has been fashionable latterly to romanticize about the working class in some sociological circles. It is salutory to note studies which describe particular working-class cultures possessing an almost implacable hostility towards education[30]. It has been suggested that many high grade subnormal children can be seen as casualties of such a culture[35].

The first possible deprivation is, of course, maternal. The literature on maternal deprivation is formidable now[15a-e]. The earlier emphasis on the production of delinquents and affectionless psychopaths has rather altered. We must acknowledge for the purposes of this chapter however, the intellectual results of such deprivation. Due to the lack of verbal and other stimulation, maternally deprived children undoubtedly suffer intellectually as well as emotionally[15,e-d]. Whereas a Stanford Binet test will merely show a depressed score for such a child, a W.I.S.C. will often show a marked disparity between Verbal and Performance Scores. All the various measures to keep preschool children with their mothers through social and other crises, have a contribution to make to the intellect of the population also.

5
Language, Learning and Culture

It is surprising how long we have had to wait for studies of language related to cultural phenomena, considering how long 'English' has been a subject in schools and universities. It is also interesting to see how much convergence there is in several disciplines through these studies—sociology, education, psychology, psychiatry, child development generally, and in particular, subnormality. While many worthwhile papers have been published on communication and information theory, and on non-verbal communication, there has been an obsessive interest in the unconscious and non-verbal problems of human interaction—a necessary obsession, since the importance of these factors had only been noted as a semantic problem over the past 70 years. And yet, just as existential psychiatry can still find new things to describe which are directly available to us for examination in our consciousness[22, 23], so there have been new things to say about language per se[27, 7]. *'Speech is the major means through which the social structure becomes part of individual experience'*[1]. It is a link, that is to say, between the cultural factors we have considered briefly, and the end result in the person, bringing cultural enrichment or impoverishment. Luria has shown the importance of the impelling, or starting and planning function of speech for behaviour. *'Language marks out what is relevant, affectively, cognitively and socially, and experience is transformed by that which is made relevant'*. Studies of the language development of institutionalized children show them to be severely retarded in vocabulary, complexity of sentence construction and type and power of abstraction. Bernstein, whom we have just quoted[1], has examined middle-class and working-class language. He has demonstrated how the latter is extremely weak in syntax, in formal construction and in its ability to express—and therefore for the individual to know—generalizations or abstract concepts. Language has an influence on the development of a child as a person, his perception, his relations with other people, his ethical development and on his intellectual growth. A child deprived of verbal communication can be left impoverished not only verbally, but even in the use of non-linguistic symbols—even, say, in his ability to recall past *visual* experiences[26]. This in turn can leave him with a poor imagination, and little ability to phantasize. Thus the language environment of children is of immense importance for the growth of their intelligence and personality. As Freud put it: The Ego wears an auditory lobe.

Bernstein has compared and contrasted two linguistic forms of English. One he calls an elaborated code, the other, a restricted code. With the former, a person can be verbally explicit. He can communicate his individual, unique experiences. A restricted code inhibits these functions and restricts the verbal signalling of individual differences. Bernstein believes that 30 per cent of our labour force is limited to a restricted code and have no other. Middle-class children, on the other hand, in becoming socialized, learn both codes. The restricted code arises, he says, because the original relation between mother and child exerted little pressure on the child to make his experiences relatively explicit in a verbally differentiated way. The Newsons are confirming many of these points in their valuable long term studies of children[33].

'Speech, language and total mental development go together'[28]. Cultural deprivation undoubtedly produces many of its main effects through the kind of language environment with which it envelopes the child. A poor language environment seems clearly responsible for a very large part of a great loss of potentially usable intellect across the whole board of IQs. Operating against the lower levels of potential, language alone can thus drag down to subnormal levels, individuals who might otherwise have gone through normal schools and jobs. Our remarks in an earlier section about nursery schools and so on, appear relevant again, now in the context of teaching a worthwhile language, which would produce social, emotional and intellectual change.

6

Family Studies

There are several convincing research projects now to hand which show the importance of interactions within the family in relation to psychogenic retardation. I have been talking in a broad way of social factors, because I feel these have often been, until recent times, very neglected in psychiatry. Let us turn to more direct psychological influences.

Learning inhibitions in individual children have been found as symptoms which seem to be embedded in the *total family situation*. Authors have commented on the resistance to therapy of the *individual* latency child, for example, and noted how the dynamic interaction of the whole family has to be understood, before this individual resistance can be put in proper perspective. Children can be found clinically, who show learning inhibitions as their major complaint. They can be, as far as any contemporary tests of physical status can judge, healthy and 'normal' organically. The results of intelligence testing can indicate normal intelligence. Yet these children can be several years retarded in academic achievement. These are children who do not seem to have suffered from either cultural or maternal deprivation. Their backwardness is however, also, psychogenic rather than constitutional. Many of the papers are psychoanalytically orientated, and a common theme is connected with the primitive nature of the oedipal problems underlying the inhibitions. These children have sadistic phantasies attaching to the identifications they have with their parents. And, as we so paradoxically say in psychiatry, they are unconsciously aware of unconscious parental prohibitions with regard to learning. It is the presence of unsublimated sadism in these children which is the chief deterrent to successful learning.

An example of a family-orientated research is one called, 'Fathers of sons with primary neurotic learning inhibitions'[16]. Here the authors have studied a number of boys who had severe learning difficulties. They were of at least normal intelligence and came from homes without gross social pathology. Their major complaint was being at least two years behind their chronological age in one major sphere. They had no physical impairment. The fathers tended to regard themselves as failures. Ones who were in fact successful, thought their success due to luck rather than to their own gifts. There were two patterns commonly found in the families. In one the father was passive and dependent on the mother, who held the position of leadership and authority. In the other the father defended himself against feelings of inadequacy by adopting an ineffectual aggressive pattern and it was the mother who was submissive and helpless. She saw her husband (and maleness) as powerful and potentially destructive. Both types of family seemed to confuse hostility with constructive aggression. They seemed to assume, also, that if one marital partner was dominant, the other had to be submissive.

Where the fathers were passive and dependent, the mothers tended to be very competitive with men and to fear males. They had married men who saw themselves as ineffectual, so that they themselves could be in a position of superiority, and be able to deny their own dependency needs. They tended to infantilize both their husbands and their sons. The fathers saw their sons as dangerous rivals for the mother's love and both mothers and fathers saw masculine achievement as dangerous. The parents unconsciously undercut their sons' attempts to learn.

In the other families, in which the mothers seemed helpless and afraid of the fathers, there were strong elements of sado-masochism. The wives had carried out counter-phobic manœuvres, marrying men who were embodiments of the qualities that frightened them. Learning difficulties here were related to the infantilizing behaviour of the mothers, and the view that male assertion was dangerous, and to the need of the fathers that the sons should not succeed. The children felt hopeless and incompetent in the face of their parents, who demanded high performances. The boys could not identify with the competent aspects of their fathers.

An equally interesting study was one in which the term *anti-achievement* was used in reference to poor academic work by children or adolescents, whose intelligence would again indicate a potential for better performance[17]. Again there was a learning inhibition, work inhibition, but not 'moral masochism'. In this group of boys an impairment of the super ego was posited to account for their poor achievement. The study emphasized a dysfunction of the processes of taking in, and digesting, and synthesizing information. The learning inhibition, from the psychodynamic angle, was thought to arise from the disruptive entrance of instinctual needs and conflicts into what should be the conflict-free areas of cognitive function. The problem was a defect in the ability to put forth effort, to accomplish, to develop confidence, to produce, or master events internally and in the environment. The basic objective of the 'masochistic defence' used by these children was the maintenance of an inflexible bond, with a withholding, omnipotent, but potentially protective figure. Anti-achievers contrived to keep this kind of tortured relation with their parents in reality and also with the incorporated images of the oral period. There seemed to be a suspension of specific tasks of the normal super ego, so that without experiencing much guilt, the anti-achiever could evade his social and educational obligations, upset his parents, and sometimes become caught up in aggressive behaviour. There was also an impairment in the ego function of reality testing. The anti-achiever greatly underestimated the self-defeating features of his behaviour. The impairments in super ego and ego functions enabled the under-achiever to overcome two great barriers to his acting out his unconscious impulses through anti-achievement. On the one hand he had first to hurt and defeat his parents, teacher—and therapists, without being overcome by guilt; on the other, he had to hurt himself without being stopped by the pain of this.

7

Individual Studies

Perhaps all psychiatry, in a sense, can be seen as a technique to understand and to deal with psychogenic retardation. Quite well known early writings of Freud dealt with the success or failure of individuals in life[13], and yet it remains a surprise for many patients to discover that they can fear success even more than failure, and therefore have been spending their lives avoiding success. Melanie Klein[21] has dealt at length with the intellectual losses that can attend the process of repression, and how emotional factors can restrict ability, leave the enquiring mind forever superficial, or finally lead it not to enquire at all. All these mechanisms relate to academic achievement—or otherwise. Every psychotherapist is familiar with how much brighter a really successful case can be after treatment and that this increased brightness can be measured by intelligence testing. The subtle descriptions of particular intra-psychic dynamics do not lend themselves easily to summarizing, but I would like to acknowledge them. They are both valid in themselves and also underwrite conceptually much current research in the inter-personal, inter-actional field. Current clinical working hypotheses have moved, on the whole, away from dealing with a single child in a social vacuum. Individuals exist in and are influenced by their family, their peer group, and their culture. In earlier stages of development, the maternal relationship is the critical one for the growth and development of the child. I prefer to see even this as essentially a *social* situation, be it a small one. The infant's ability—and need—to relate to another is every bit as 'real' as his egocentricity[6]. A disinterested mother affects his relating ability, and by her self-preoccupation fails to reward the child's endeavours. This lack of reinforcement can lead to intellectual apathy, or a neurotic over-compensation. The relatively rejecting, ambivalent or constantly hostile mother can make the world seem too dangerous to explore. The depressed mother speaks little to her child and creates about him a joyless world, hardly worth knowing. Immigrant West-Indian children with such mothers have latterly presented the social services with severe problems, seeming almost autistic in the acuteness of their withdrawal, and severely subnormal in their intellectual handicap. As Leo Kanner has said of Child Psychiatry generally, so in the field of child subnormality, much classifying of children can be done by the assessment of parental attitudes alone.

8

Ego Theories—The Vulnerability Factor

We have touched on environmental factors which seem to have effects on the growth of intelligence and we have mentioned studies of family interaction. The latter usually assume a certain (psychoanalytic) view of the structure of mind. Whereas it is possible to produce some hard data concerning environmental factors, this is less easily done through clinical studies. Nevertheless, a systematic clinical examination of small populations is vastly better than a mere guess, given that we know the bias and theoretical assumptions of the observers.

It is, of course, legitimate to hypothesize about mental structures in the individual. It is legitimate, in other words, to try to imagine what kind of mind the child has that gives him his strengths and vulnerabilities[6]. Psychiatry has never been short of hypotheses. On the contrary, they surround the clinician as often in a bewildering, as in a helpful way. Psychoanalysis, for example is not a unitary theory of mind. To say 'analytically oriented' is not an explicit statement. Psychiatry still awaits generally agreed definitions, and a definitive description of mind, satisfactory to its own discipline, and also to the physiologist, the psychologist, the neurologist, and so on.

From good theories, good practices arise, and opportunities for further experiments and conceptualizing. If psychogenic retardation is a common condition, as the evidence suggests it is, it is not enough to assert this fact. I believe we require a theory of the ego, or a combination of theories, which might be more helpful to us than older ones in seeing how it is that the environment acts as it does on the intellect. Such a combination of theories could also suggest to us what parental and educational practices are to be preferred. I am indebted to John and Elaine Cummings for much of this construct[8]. Even though it was devised for a quite different setting, it had a learning situation in mind.

The ego—'The Life Space' as Lewin called it[24]—is the point at which a person meets the situation. It grows through a series of successfully resolved crises, each of which disturbs a temporary equilibrium, but leads to re-organization at a higher level[10]. The 'total' self is always an 'object' to the ego[14]. On the one side we have the impressive literature of psychoanalysis which concerns itself with the *ego-of-conflict*. This describes that mainly conscious part of the self which is at a focus, and is also a compromise between the unconscious, the super ego and the environment. This ego-of-conflict thus has a synthesizing function. This is the 'classical' psychoanalytic view of the ego, very concerned with unconscious phantasies, and the classifying of these phantasies under the rather misleading title of 'mental mechanisms'. But there is also, a *conflict-free part of the ego*[18], a part developed from the natural endowment of the individual, composed of native competences, such as the ability to walk, to talk, to solve problems. We do not teach children to walk, for example. The ability simply emerges. From the conflict-free ego arise capacities of thought, perception, intention, comprehension of objects, motor development, and all those things that have been called the 'executive function' of the ego, and which, in other language, is described by Gesell, Piaget, etc., in their developmental studies.

Certain environmental minimae are required in order for some potential capacities to emerge. Here we may link to the ideas of the *ethologists* with their descriptions of *sensitive, critical periods of learning*. The ego-born-of-conflict, and the conflict-free ego, of course, interact one with another, but I believe it is worth having them as separate descriptive terms. An example of the interaction of the two 'aspects' of the ego, is found in the regressions of traumatically hospitalized preschool children, who may stop speaking, walking, lose bladder control and so on, as the ego-of-conflict becomes too disorganized and affects the normally conflict-free part of the ego. If this should happen at the time when the child was about to master, or had only just mastered a skill, in disrupting the skill, the event will tend to lead to a vulnerability in that instinctual area. Much will depend on the quality of the child's care before, during and after the event, with regard to his recovery from it[15d]. It is worth remarking that some children seem constitutionally fragile. Tiny early mishaps mark them severely. Other children seem incredibly robust. We do not yet know how to identify each group and so commonsense urges the highest standards of care for all. Individuals also vary in other native endowments and in their innate energies. These variations will also contribute to any differences between individuals responding to stress.

We have no satisfactory general theory to account for human instincts, or drives, yet, but we still need one and we can see children acting to reduce tension, to avoid pain, to pursue pleasure, and so on.

We also see them demanding a kind of complexity from life, of disliking boredom and repetition. They want to initiate actions and sometimes even fear passivity and dependency. Some of these aspects of personality appear linked to *ego-identity*, when the 'individual successfully aligns his basic drives and his endowments with the opportunities of his situations'[10]. This feeling of ego-identity appears when there is a harmony achieved by the individual, a confidence that he has an ability to maintain an inner sameness and continuity, matched to a sameness and continuity of his meaning for others. The child who learns to know and master himself and the world has a sense of himself as one who is capable of handling a predictable environment. As a child increases his skills and drives, the culture demands more and more of him. He needs to adapt his ego at various crisis points, such as weaning, toilet training and so on. Each time he solves a problem, he is better able to solve the next one and his ego will be stronger. This is what we mean by ego growth through crisis resolution. If he fails to resolve a crisis, the reverse will be true. His ego will remain weak and less able to resolve the next problem. It is essentially in a social situation that this development goes on, at first as an interaction between the child and his mother, and then via complicated identifications by the child with both parents. It is here, in the first five or six years of life, that environmental upsets and distortions operate most destructively[15a-e]. And we are, of course, not discussing—for once—the standard neuroses, the obsessions, hysteria, or anxiety states. We are discussing learning neuroses.

It is in the classical writings of the analysts that one notes the terms inhibition, repression and so on. It has been repeatedly pointed out how the mechanism of repression drags down into the unconscious a great number of other ideas and tendencies associated with particular complexes and dissociates them from the free interchange of thoughts, or at least prevent them from being handled with scientific reality. 'If natural curiosity and the impulse to enquire into unknown as well as previously surmised facts and phenomena is opposed, then the more profound enquiries (in which the child is unconsciously afraid that he might meet with forbidden, sinful things) are also repressed along with it. Simultaneously, however, all impulses to investigate deeper questions in general become also inhibited.' Thus Melanie Klein, who goes on to discuss how development may be influenced by an 'injury to the instinct for knowledge, and hence also the development of the reality sense. . . '[21].

We must complicate our views of the ego still further if we are to get a closer feel of the vulnerability of the child as a growing intelligence. The ego can be seen as an encounter between the self and the cultural and interpersonal situation. The child—like the adult—is guided in this encounter by what Paul Federn calls 'ego feeling'. By this is meant a feeling or sense of the self which accompanies the state of ego identity. In the small child this may be mere narcissism. As the child becomes socialized and learns to value being identified as himself, he is, paradoxically, more able in a sense to become a different self in relation to another. He partly adapts to his human environment and partly changes that environment, in what we can call the creative act of relating to another. *This the very small child can only do with maternal help*, through, or within his relationship with his mother. Only later is it possible with others. Too great a dysjunction between himself and 'society' produces *ego-diffusion*, subjectively felt in ordinary terms as unhappiness. Freud, Klein and Winnicott describe failures here, when the child feels insecure, in terms of his projected aggression. The child then experiences persecutory anxiety, feeling threatened by the feelings he has referred out of himself and into others. R. D. Laing on the other hand, would describe the experience of insecurity *as a felt struggle to maintain a sense of identity*. These are not, however, incompatible descriptions.

Ego feeling, the experience of the self felt as self, brings with it a sense of the boundaries of the self, physically and mentally. It is feeling at the ego boundary[4]. Objects often experienced at this boundary become part of the ego. This is one way of looking at learning.

Children vary in the extent of their ego feeling. In crisis some only too easily feel alienated, emptied or depersonalized. Repeated, or severe crises make the boundaries of the ego—the inner and outer worlds—seem too dangerous to explore, to learn about, or even to see clearly. Thus is ego restriction and denial augmented.

Through role-taking the boy becomes boy-like, the girl, girl-like, and again, each assignment has its complexities, as parents relive or phantasy through their children. Gradually the child manages the idea of a 'generalized other', someone who is not father, or mother[31]. The child can take on increasingly more roles, being one authentic person in relation to mother, another to father, another to sib[22]. After each growth-crisis successfully managed, his ego is enhanced and his roles diversify. He eventually achieves a 'hierarchy of roles' with different 'ego sets', so that he can swiftly switch from being a brother, a son, an infant in class, a grandchild, and so on[8].

All these are social skills carrying perceptual, cognitive attributes with them. Disruption of learning these skills underly other learning failures.

Even if very brief, a multiple construct seemed necessary here in order to show how psychogenic retardation may come about. This in no way claims to be a comprehensive review. Personal constructs and learning theory also come in, if only to be acknowledged here, as conscious—or unconscious, individual contributions to ego-theory, and the individual vulnerability factor in psychogenic retardation.

9

Conclusion

As with so much in contemporary psychiatry the literature grows apace and we can only attempt to pick out growing points. In a world obsessed with quantity, it seems to the writer of enormous importance that the contributions of psychiatry, psychology and sociology should more and more be concerning themselves with the quality of life. An understanding of how emotional factors can affect this quality is already at some depth, and promises to revolutionize our ideas both in education itself and in psychiatry.

REFERENCES

1. BERNSTEIN, B., 1961. Aspects of language and learning in the genesis of the social process. *J. Child Psychol. Psychiat.*, **1**, 313-24.
2. BOURNE, H., 1955. Protophrenia. A study of perverted rearing and mental dwarfism. *Lancet*, ii, 1156.
3. BURT, SIR CYRIL, 1937. *The backward child*. 2nd ed. London, Univ. Press.
4. CAMERON, T., FREEMAN, J., and MCGIE, H., 1958. *Chronic schizophrenia*. London, Tavistock.
5. CLARKE, A. D. B., and CLARKE, A. M., 1953. How constant is the IQ? *Lancet*, ii, 877-80.
6. CROWCROFT, A., 1967. *The psychotic*, chapter 4. Pelican Original. London, Penguin Books.
7. CROWCROFT, A., 1966. The importance of speech in development. *Maternal and child care*, **2**, 291.
8. CUMMING, J., and CUMMING, E., 1962. *Ego and milieu*. New York, Atherton Press.
9. DOUGLAS, J. W. B., 1964. *The home and the school*. London, MacGibbon and Kee.
10. ERIKSON, E., 1958. *Childhood and society*. 2nd ed. New York, W. W. Norton.
11. FEDERN, P., 1952. *Ego psychology and the psychoses*. New York, Basic Books.
12. FREUD, A., 1954. *The ego and the mechanisms of defence*. London, Hogarth Press.
13. FREUD, S., 1965. *Some character-types met in psychoanalytic work*. Standard edition of complete psychological works. Vol. XIV, pp. 309-32. London, Hogarth Press.
14. FREUD, S., 1946. *The ego and the Id*. London, Hogarth Press.
15. *a.* GOLDFARB, W., 1945. Effects of psychological deprivation in infancy and subsequent stimulation. *Am. J. Psychiat.*, **102**, 18.
    b. SPITZ, R., 1945. Hospitalism: an inquiry into the genesis of psychiatric conditions in early childhood. *Psychoanal. Study Child*, **1**, 53. 1946. Hospitalism: a follow-up report on investigation described in vol. 1. *Ibid*, **2**, 113.
    c. BOWLBY, J., 1951. *Maternal care and child health*. Geneva, W.H.O. Monograph No. 2.
    d. AINSWORTH, M. D., 1962. *Deprivation of maternal care*. Geneva, W.H.O. Public Health Papers, No. 14.
    e. PRINGLE, KELLMER, M. L., 1965. *Deprivation and education*, London, Longmans.
16. GRUNEBAUM, M. G., HURWITZ, I., PRENTICE, N. M., and SPERRY, B. M., 1962. Fathers of sons with primary neurotic learning inhibitions. *Am. J. Orthopsychiat.*, **32**, 462-72.
17. HALPERN, H., and HALPERN, H., 1966. Four perspectives on anti-achievement. *Psychoanal. Rev.*, **53**, 83-93.
18. HARTMAN, H., 1958. *Ego psychology and the problem of adaptation*. London, Hogarth Press.

19. HAVIGHURST, R. J., DAVIES, A., EELS, K., HERRICK, V. E., and TYLER, R., 1951. *Intelligence and cultural difference*. Chicago, Univ. Press.
20. *a.* HILLIARD, L. T., and KIRMAN, B. H., 1965. *Mental deficiency*. 2nd ed. London, Churchill.
    b. PENROSE, L. S., 1963. *The biology of mental defect*. 3rd ed. London, Sidgwick and Jackson.
21. KLEIN, M., 1950. *Contributions to psychoanalysis*, 1921-1945. pp. 31-38. London, Hogarth Press.
    See also KLEIN, M., 1961. *Narrative of a child analysis*. London, Hogarth Press.
22. LAING, R. D., 1961. *The self and others*. London, Tavistock Publications.
23. LAING, R. D., 1960. *The divided self*. London, Tavistock Publications.
24. LEWIN, K., 1951. *Field theory in social sciences*. New York, Harper.
25. *a.* LEWIS, E. D., 1929. *Report of the mental deficiency committee*, Part IV. London, H.M.S.O.
    b. TREDGOLD, R., Editions prior to 7th (1949). *Mental deficiency*. London, Baillière, Tindall and Cox.
26. LEWIS, M. M., 1965. Impairment of language in relation to general development. In *Children with communication problems*. Ed. Franklin, A. W. London, Pitman Medical.
27. LURIA, A. R., 1961. *The role of speech in the regulation of normal and abnormal behaviour*. Oxford, Pergamon Press.
28. LURIA, A. R., and YUDOVITCH, F., 1959. *Speech and the development of mental processes in the child*. London, Staples Press.
29. MAYER-GROSS, M., SLATER, E., and ROTH, M., 1960. *Clinical psychiatry*. 2nd ed. p. 515. London, Cassell.
30. MAYS, J. B., 1954. *Growing up in a city*. Liverpool, Univ. Press.
31. MEAD, G. H., 1934. *Mind, self and society*. Chicago, Univ. Press.
32. Mental Deficiency Section, R.M.P.A. Working party on childhood psychosis, *First report*, 1962.
33. NEWSON, J., and NEWSON, E.:
    (1) Four years old in an urban community. (1968) Allen and Unwin.
    (2) *Some social differences in the process of child rearing*. Penguin survey of the social sciences. 2, (1967), ed. Julius Gould.
34. Schizophrenic syndrome in childhood., 1961. *Brit. med. J.*, ii, 887-90.
35. STEIN, Z. A., and SUSSER, M. W., 1963. The social distribution of mental retardation. *Am. J. ment. Defic.*, **67**, 811-21.
36. VERNON, M. D., 1965. The development of perception. In *Modern perspectives in child psychiatry*. Ed. Howells, J. G. Edinburgh, Oliver and Boyd.

XX

DEVELOPMENT AND BREAKDOWN OF SPEECH

Moyra Williams
D.Ph.

Principal Psychologist, Department of Clinical Psychology, Addenbrooke's Hospital, Cambridge

---

1

Introduction

Considering the importance of speech in all human activity, our understanding of how we carry out this function is still very limited. The mystery does not concern merely our acquisition of a vocabulary; of far greater interest is our manipulation of it—the way we manage to choose each word at each particular moment. Oldfield[43] has calculated that 'the average, reasonably young university educated person' knows between 55,000 and 90,000 different words; yet at any single moment in time he can and does utter only one. How does he know which word to choose and what is he doing with the ones he does not want? In other words, how is the word-stock stored and organized, and by what means do we gain access to the individual items in it?

Until the past few years, man's use of speech has been taken for granted. Controversy has raged over a number of related subjects, such as the association between speech and intelligence, the phonetic properties of speech, and the divergence of different languages. The study of how we use words, based on experimental and quantifiable methods did not really start till about 1950 (Brown)[6] in the branch of science now generally known as Psycholinguistics.

A great deal of the impetus to this study came from communication problems experienced during the last war when the greatest possible amount of information had to be conveyed in the shortest possible time, but in such a way that while it could not possibly be misunderstood by those who were meant to receive it, it remained incomprehensible to the enemy. Communication engineers discovered a series of mathematical rules applying to such tasks which they then found applied to communication in general. It was found, for instance, that a large proportion of the words used in normal speech are unnecessary or redundant. It was found that while long words are less easily confused than short ones, short words are more easily recognized than long ones. Short words are also more frequently used than long ones (Zipf)[69]; common words are more quickly found than rare ones (Oldfield and Wingfield)[44], but the speed with which a word is either recognized or emitted depends on the context in which it lies (Goldman-Eisler[18]; Treisman[61]). In normal language words are not emitted or received in isolation but in sequences or strings bound together by syntax and controlled by grammatical rules. Thus, if we know the language and know the beginning of a string, we can often 'guess' how it will end. Each word restricts the type of word which can follow it. We cannot, for instance, place an adjective after its noun. A sequence of two words restricts those that can follow it even more closely. By the time we have a sequence of seven or eight words, the choice of the next is so closely restricted that we can 'guess' what it must be without even having to hear it. We seem to have a built-in computer working out the transitional probabilities of word strings telling us which word to produce or expect at any moment.

The computer working out these calculations bases its expectations not just on the individual words, but on the structure of whole sentences, their grammar. It knows that if the subject of the sentence is in the singular, the verb must be in the singular too; if one verb is in the past tense, others must be as well. It can expand a sentence by adding relative clauses, and contract three or more separate sentences into one by the use of conjunctions or pronouns. When we start to make an utterance, the whole thing must be ready formed in our minds before we say a single word.

The basic mental mechanisms which carry out this function are still not fully understood, but a model which could account for our use of grammar was put forward by Chomsky in 1957[11] and has given rise to a number of recent experiments and speculations (Rosenberg)[53].

The words and sentences, however, are meaningless unless we know to what they refer. It would do no good hearing the perfectly grammatical message, 'Attack on D-Day' and being able to repeat it accurately unless we knew to what D-Day referred. Words are only symbols for meanings, and knowing the language means knowing the meaning to which each sequence of sounds refers—i.e. cracking the code.

Each language is a different code, and the code is usually acquired in childhood. The question is, how does the child do this? How does he develop his store of words and know how to build them into sentences? And what happens to this whole process if the brain or mind is deranged?

2
Development of Speech in Normal Children

Pre-linguistic utterances

The study of speech development in children is not new, but some of the more recent observations and experiments have thrown a rather different light on concepts of the mechanisms involved from those existing in the past. For instance, it used to be taken for granted that the sounds used in intelligent adult speech were the same as those used by the babbling infant; that speech, in fact was a mere rearrangement or reorganization of innate infantile activity. That this is not the whole story has now been shown by the careful recording and analysis of baby sounds.

Some controversy has centred around the identification of infantile utterances and the methods by which they should be recorded. Phonetic transcriptions do not always agree with spectrographic analyses of infantile utterances; and the interpretation given to a vowel sound depends to some extent on its surrounding consonants (McCarthy)[33]. Despite these difficulties, there is considerable agreement between different observers regarding the general pattern of development and maturation.

All agree with Irwin[24] that with increasing maturation there is an increase of the consonant/vowel ratio. When vowel sounds are considered from the point of view of where and how they are made, considerable changes seem to occur at about the time the child assumes the erect posture. Before this time the predominant consonant sounds are made with the back of the articulatory apparatus, while the vowels are made with the front. As the child sits up and begins to gain greater control of his lips and tongue (which are further exercized as he begins to eat solid food), there is an increase in the front consonants (dentals and labials), and the vowel sounds are pushed back. At these times, French guttural r's and German umlauts occur in the English babbling child as well as in those born on the continent, but the continental phonemes gradually disappear in children raised in English-speaking countries. At about the age of 26-27 months, there also emerges a marked sexual difference, girls forging ahead faster than boys.

With these observations the nineteenth-century notion of speech development as depending on the integration of single elementary units came to be modified. Jesperson, and later Goldstein (see McCarthy)[33] put forward the organismic concept of progressive differentiation in opposition to the previous theory which attempted to explain speech as a gradual accumulation of units. They drew parallels between the development of articulation and that of other motor activities; but this does not explain how different languages come to evolve, nor many other aspects of adult language.

Early Linguistic Utterances

In the child's development of speech proper, two factors have usually been considered as of prime importance: (*i*) imitation, (*ii*) association. Recent studies, while not claiming to discredit these beliefs, are, however, indicating that both may involve a large number of other variables whose nature is still a bit obscure.

Imitation. The part played in the child's development of speech by imitation is still far from clear. The fact that we learn to speak the language of the culture in which we are raised is sufficient proof of the importance of imitation. Moreover, children raised in culturally deprived environments tend to be permanently impaired in their use of language.

Goldfarb[17] in an interesting series of studies evaluated the language of children who spent their first 3 years in an institution. He compared them with children raised in foster-homes from early infancy. Comparisons were made of speech sounds, intelligibility of speech, and level of language organization. Retests were made after 7 months at 6 and 8 years of age, and again in adolescence. The children reared in an institutional environment showed marked language deficiency in all areas assessed. The author summarized their behaviour as being passive and apathetic and their personalities as impervious to environmental stimulation. However, Kellmer-Pringle[26] points out that emotionally unstable children from all types of background show language retardation, so that the defects seen in institutionalized children may well be due to emotional factors.

A large proportion of the speech uttered by children is, however, spoken for their own amusement or entertainment rather than for purposes of communication. In 1924 Piaget[46] first drew attention to the egocentricity of many childhood utterances and remarked on the fact that they seemed to take the form of behaviour accompaniments rather than information exchanges. Piaget also remarked on the fact that these soliloquies nevertheless seemed to have some social function since they tended to occur only in the presence of others; an observation which has been followed up by a number of later workers attempting to define more precisely the 'conversation value' of different situations.

McConnon[34] conducted a study of 28 nursery school children in which two samples of conversation were recorded in each of six different situations; lunch, morning outdoor play period, indoor free play period, table-play, afternoon outdoor play, and an outdoor play situation at home. Twenty-five responses were recorded in each situation for the same group of children. Surprisingly low coefficients of agreement between the two observations in each situation were found.

In a study by Van Alstyne[62] it was found that in only half their time did preschool children tend to talk to other children while working with play materials. Certain materials appeared to have considerably more 'conversation value' than others. Doll play, blocks, crayons, and clay ranked high for percentage of time that their use was accompanied by conversation, whereas painting, scissors, and books were low in conversation value. It is worth noting, in view of the sex differences mentioned between boys and girls that the doll-corner activities and dishes, which are typical girl activities, were among the highest in conversation value. It might be concluded that certain differences in language are due to the effect of the situation, but it must also be remembered that certain situations may attract children of different levels of language development.

Not only does it appear that children practise much of their language alone, but recent studies have shown that when young children are attempting to imitate adults they in fact seldom copy exactly what they hear. Adults, for instance, seldom speak in single words, but usually emit words in strings. The only words uttered singly by them are words such as Yes, No, Good, etc. Yet the first language utterances of children are usually single names for objects which take the form of whole sentences. By degrees more words are added to each utterance, and all modern observers agree that the best single index of language development in children lies in length of utterance. The single-word sentence is replaced by the two-word sentence consisting of a noun and a modifier (Brown and Bellugi)[7]. To this core further words are added as age increases.

Moreover, in what they do actually mimic from their elders, children are extremely selective. They do not start repeating a sentence from the beginning and fade out at the end of their immediate memory span; if a sentence is too long for them to reproduce as a whole they condense it by omitting some words and concentrating on others. Ervin[14] has shown that children tend to select the most recent or the most emphasized words for imitation, but Brown and Bellugi[7] have drawn attention to the similarity between the selection shown by children and those made by adults when each word is at a financial premium, as in a telegram. It is the important words that are chosen, the redundant ones that are omitted. It is noteworthy that when adults suffer from cerebral pathology that makes word production difficult (Nominal Dysphasia) the 'telegraphic speech' to which they are often reduced follows the same principles.

It appears, then, that it is not mere exposure to sounds that provides the basis of language. Children select from all the sounds to which they are exposed those which represent most closely the things which have importance. How do they know what is important?

Association. The most obvious answer would be that the words they hear associated with important events become fixed before others, i.e. that learning of language follows a conditioning procedure. The idea that this was so was put forward by Skinner[56]. Verbal conditioning has never, however, been proved satisfactorily (Spielberger)[57], and certainly in the case of children cannot account for many of their utterances. Once a child learns a certain word, he will cheerfully apply it to a number of objects with which he can never have heard it associated and to which association is not rewarded. The word Dog is used to refer to any furry animal; 'Daddy' to any man; Table to any piece of furniture. It is only as the child learns to differentiate between different objects that it learns different names to associate to each one. Nevertheless, frequency of experience does seem to play some part in acquisition, for the more often words are used in the language of the culture, the earlier they are learned by the child (Rochford and Williams)[51].

No sooner has the child learned to differentiate between objects and their names than it has to learn that the same name can also be applied to numerous different objects. The word 'teeth' can apply not only to a part of the body, but also to parts of the comb; 'hands' to the upper extremities and to the pointers on a clock. It is not surprising that the use of these homonyms are learned much later in their rare context than in their commoner ones (Rochford and Williams)[51].

Learning different uses for the same word does not seem to be so difficult for the child as learning new words. Braine[4] carried out an experiment in which children were asked to associate names to 'nonsense shapes' and showed that the associations were formed to familiar names sooner than to unfamiliar ones. It appears that a new association is learned more easily than a new word. This may be one reason why one of the most frequent causes of change in language as a whole is due to familiar words being applied to new concepts. The confusion resulting from such practice appears to be offset by the economy of effort involved in it.

At the same time as they learn to associate words to objects, children are learning to associate words to one another. There are two ways in which this occurs: (*i*) semantically; (*ii*) syntactically.

Semantic Associations. In adult speech, words tend to be associated because they refer to some common sphere of thought (hot and cold; hands and feet). Hence, if the average adult is asked to respond to one word by saying the first thing that comes into his head, he will usually utter another word of the same grammatical class and from the same semantic field. A noun is responded to by a noun; an adjective by an adjective (cat-dog; deep-shallow). In the same way an adult dysphasic patient who is having some difficulty in finding words can often be helped in his word search if a common association to the missing word is provided. But in children up to the age of 9 years, the associations to a word tend to be either rhyming ones (cat-pat) showing phonetic generalization; or those which might follow it in a common sentence (deep-hole) (see Jenkins)[25].

Semantic association hence appears to be a phenomenon which occurs with maturity, and although once formed it resists disruption in cerebral pathology, it cannot be regarded as the basis for language learning.

Syntactic Association. By habit and convention we string words together, as has already been mentioned, in stereotyped ways so that if the first words of any sequence are established, the choice that can follow is limited.

Yet when children start stringing words together into sentences, they often infringe the syntactic rules, making up such phrases as 'A this truck', 'A your car' (Brown and Bellugi)[7] which they cannot have imitated from an adult.

On the basis of such observations, it is argued (Ervin)[14] that children must develop early in life a set of grammatical rules or logic which, while different from that of adults, enables them to manipulate words in order to express ideas. Two of the first rules they learn are: (1) those for creating plurals of nouns, and (2) those for creating the past tense of verbs. They not only apply these rules to nonsense words (Berko)[2], but also to familiar ones. Long before they know that the plural of mouse is mice or the past tense of do is did, children will form all plurals by adding an 's' or 'z' to the singular (mouses) and the past tense of verbs by adding a 'd' to the present tense (do-ed). Yet, even while they are doing this and making these mistakes, they appear to be absorbing some aspects of adult grammatical form. Bruce and Pugh[8] asked children to repeat sentences approximating to grammatical English, and found that the closer statistically the approximation, the better they were repeated.

Cross-modal associations. Particular attention has been paid recently to the connection between language and other aspects of behaviour, especially perception and motor performance. Bartlett showed as long ago as 1932 (Bartlett)[1] that the way we store and recall a visual stimulus depends largely on the name we give to it at the time of perception. More recently experiments on the association between verbal commands and conditioned reflexes in children have been described by a number of Russian workers and summarized by Luria and Vinogradova[32] and by O'Connor and Hermelin[40]. It is claimed that once a motor behaviour pattern (such as the salivary reflex) has been established to a conditioned stimulus (e.g. bell), it can be elicited by the name of the stimulus as easily as by the stimulus itself, indicating that the links that associate words to objects occur at a deep physiological level. Moreover, as Luria and Vinogradova have further shown, the response is not confined to the name of the stimulus object, but is generalized to all those semantically related to it. Thus, if a response is conditioned to the word 'cat' it can also be evoked to some extent by the words 'dog' or 'kitten', but only in young children or subnormals by phonetic associations (e.g. 'pat').

More will be said about this important field of investigation in the section on Development in Subnormal Children.

Comprehension. All observers agree that comprehension precedes emission of words and that the comprehended vocabulary is very much larger than the used vocabulary in both children and adults. How we learn to comprehend speech and the processes involved in speech comprehension are, however, very little known.

It would seem logical to presume that this must depend primarily on hearing, so that children born with hearing defects would be handicapped to a degree relative to the intensity of their hearing loss. This is not so.

Whetnall and Fry[65] point out that there is little relation between degree of hearing loss and speech retardation in children, the most important single factor in speech comprehension being the age at which training in sound discrimination is begun. If the child is older than two years before an attempt is made to introduce it to speech sounds, it never becomes able to discriminate them adequately. This suggests that (*i*) speech discrimination is a learned act; (*ii*) it depends on exposure at an optimal period. In these respects it parallels visual perception.

Speech discrimination seems to depend on many factors. The phonetic properties of speech sounds can now be recorded and analysed by means of the spectrograph. Then, by cutting out various portions and synthesizing speech minus one portion or another, it is possible to discover those aspects which are essential for speech comprehension. It has been found, for instance, that most of the information comes from consonants but the carrying power or loudness is conveyed by the vowels (Whetnall and Fry)[65]. It is further becoming evident that we do not hear any distinction between sounds which do not have different significance in our own language. To the Russians, who do not distinguish between 'v' and 'w', both these letters as pronounced by an Englishman sound the same. To the Englishman who has no specific meaning to attach to 'u' as opposed to 'ü' the two sounds are easily confused.

Another very important factor in comprehension is our ability to distinguish the order in which different sounds arrive—their time relationship. Although it seems clear that direction is important and that we must take in words in the exact order in which they are uttered, there is a growing suspicion that this may not be entirely so. We may, in fact, store up a chunk of sounds, decode this as a whole, and then start storing up another chunk; it is during this period of storing that the input-order may become confused with disastrous results. To the young child, the sequence of sounds 'winter' and 'witner' are the same. As his speech matures, the child learns to keep the order of input more correct and to divide up bands of incoming sounds into meaningful chunks based on word or sentence boundaries (Bruce and Pugh[8]; Bevers and Fodor[3]). Thus, it seems, as concluded by Brown and Bellugi, that the development of language is more like the biological development of an embryo than the acquisition of a conditioned reflex (Brown and Bellugi)[7]. It proceeds by a process of simultaneous integration and differentiation; not by the mere arithmetical addition of individual items.

3

Development of Speech in the Deaf and Hard of Hearing

It is traditional that a great deal can be learned about the mechanisms of normal mental behaviour from a study of the abnormal. Since speech in normal people is so intimately bound up with hearing, it might further be assumed that much could be learned about normal speech development by comparing the progress of deaf children with that of those who have normal hearing.

In fact, however, the processes of development in both groups show more similarities than differences. Although development in deaf children consistently lags behind that of normal children of the same age, the pattern of acquisition is largely the same (Myklebust)[39]. In both groups, girls mature more quickly than boys; in both groups maturity is related to vocabulary size and length of utterance. In both groups maturation in one of the language functions (e.g. reading) is related to maturation in all others (speaking and writing). In both groups there is a tendency to generate original sentences, even if these do not follow the rules of adult grammar, rather than to parrot those given to them by adults. Indeed, if simple parroting (echolalia) is seen, the child is suspected of mental subnormality rather than of simple deafness (Whetnall and Fry)[65].

The degree to which deaf children learn to interpret the speech they hear depends largely on their recognition of the common syntactical sequences of speech so that they know what to expect and can profit from the knowledge of transitional probabilities. It is to this rather than any other factor that Whetnall and Fry[65] attribute the importance of early learning in deaf children.

Despite their gross similarities, there are, of course, a number of differences between the language of deaf and normal-hearing children. These have been described by Myklebust. Thus deaf children tend to reach a plateau at a level equivalent to that of the normal 11-13 year old and continue thereafter to use shorter sentences with a greater proportion of nouns. Moreover, although the errors they make in sentence structure are by and large similar to those of normal children, consisting of omission (a boy playing), substitutions (a boy will playing), additions (a boy is be playing), and alterations of word order (a boy playing is), deaf children tend in general to be less flexible in their sentence structures than normals and to repeat 'carrier phrases' (I see dog—I see boy) seldom seen in those with full hearing.

What they lose in their speech, deaf children tend to gain in their writing. They tend to make fewer spelling mistakes and are superior to normals in their use of punctuation.

Thus deaf children unlike subnormal, psychotic and aphasic children appear to have the same basic language mechanism for speech comprehension and generation as normals, despite the different experiences to which they must be subjected during this period of acquisition.

4

Development of Speech in Subnormal Children

Before considering speech development in this group, the concept of subnormality itself requires some discussion. The idea that intelligence is a unitary function susceptible to measurement has had to be modified in the light of recent observations. It is now recognized by the majority of psychologists that different aspects of mental behaviour can break down or develop independently of one another; and that whereas there is a close correlation between them all in the majority of people, many exceptions to the rule exist.

In those who are classed as mentally subnormal, there may be poverty of all intellectual functions or of only some. Classification depends primarily on social and educational factors; hence those who fall into this general group vary much in their specific abilities and deficiencies, and not surprisingly, show differences in their use of speech.

By and large, however, three major abnormalities of speech have been recognized in these subjects, who will be referred to hereafter in this paper for convenience as if they were a homogeneous group: (*i*) poor articulation, (*ii*) small vocabulary, (*iii*) lack of cross-modal associations.

1. *Poor articulation*. The articulatory defects concern primarily the enunciation of consonants (Renfrew)[49]. Subnormals tend throughout their lives to use a higher proportion of vowel sounds than do normals, but even when they do use consonants, these tend to be slurred. It appears that the intricate control of the individual muscles necessary to form normal speech never develops to such an extent in some subnormals as in normals; and indeed in this it parallels the poor motor control leading to clumsiness in other aspects of behaviour.

The failure of development in these subjects is seldom restricted to the motor field. In the sphere of comprehension, consonant-identification may also be faulty (Renfrew)[49] especially at word endings. Thus a subject may be able to identify the words 'tray', 'sea', and 'you', but be unable to distinguish 'cart' from 'calf', or 'sheet' from 'sheep'.

2. *Small vocabulary*. It has frequently been noted that subnormal children have a smaller vocabulary than normals and tend to use those words they do know more often. Parallel with this deficiency is the inability to conceptualize objects spontaneously and hence to call different classes by different names. It has already been mentioned that when young children are first learning to speak they apply one noun to many dissimilar objects. 'Bag' applies to anything a lady carries; 'dog' to any animal. Normal children learn to correct these errors at an early age and with little outside assistance. Speech-retarded subnormals continue to make these mistakes long after normals, and may even require expert assistance to overcome them (Renfrew)[48]. They have particular difficulty in grasping the concepts represented by prepositions (down, under, after), and use a higher proportion of nouns in their adult speech than normals.

It is also interesting to note that the speech of subnormals tends to be more imitative than that of normals. Echolalia (the exact and immediate repetition of short sentences) is quite common. Subnormal children will often also pick up and reproduce a phrase they have overheard despite their obvious ignorance of its meaning. Generalization tends to remain at the phonetic level rather than proceeding to the semantic (O'Connor and Hermelin)[40], which may be due to the smallness of the semantic field from which associations can be drawn rather than from inability to draw on those that exist.

3. *Lack of Cross-Modal Associations.* The association between words and other aspects of behaviour has always fascinated students of humanity. Piaget's[46] classical observations of the association between thought and language have given rise to a number of interesting experiments. Recent attention, however, has been focused, particularly by the Russian scientists, on the association between speech and motor learning. Luria[31] found that normal children learned tasks quicker if they accompanied their actions by words than if they did not, arguing that the verbalization reinforced the response. Subnormal children, he argues, learn more slowly because they fail to verbalize in association with their actions to the same extent as normals. O'Connor and Hermelin[40] have reported an extensive series of experiments, many of which confirm this observation. They found that if verbalization could not be used by normals in a learning task (as in the tactile discrimination of meaningless shapes) they learned no more quickly than subnormals. An important additional observation of theirs was that verbalization seems to lead to stabilization of a learned response, after which its reversal becomes more difficult. In demonstrating this, O'Connor and Hermelin trained two groups of children, subnormal and normal, to respond by pressing a key when they saw a blue light, but not pressing it when they saw a red light. Once the response had been learned and practised to a certain criterion, the task was reversed, so that the key had to be pressed to the red light, but not pressed to the blue one. While the subnormal children learned the original task rather more slowly than the normals, it was found, contrary to expectations, they learned the reversal more quickly. The authors then took another group of subnormal children and asked them to verbalize their acts as they carried them out: 'Blue—Press; Red—Don't press'. Under these conditions the subnormals learned as quickly as the normal group and reversed as slowly. The authors summarize their findings by saying, 'While conditioning with the influence of the verbal system takes place quicker than without it, the connections thus developed are less mobile than those established on the basis of direct signals only' (O'Connor and Hermelin)[40]. The authors conclude by suggesting that one of the prime disabilities in the subnormal is the absence of bonds between the verbal system and other systems such as motor performances.

5

Development of Speech in Psychotic Children

Psychotic or autistic children are recognized as a separate group on account of a number of features. These were defined by a working party set up in

1961 (Creak)[12], whose list of the criteria essential to diagnosis has now been generally accepted.

Besides disorders of speech these children demonstrate a lack of the desire to communicate or to form any sort of emotional relationships with other people. They also appear to be unaware of their own personal identities, and show pathological preoccupation with particular objects or parts of them without regard to their accepted functions. Their perceptual experiences appear to be abnormal in that they show either lack of or excessive responsiveness to sensory stimuli. Thus they avert their eyes from other people or dart only flickering looks at them. Objects are examined by touch, smell and taste rather than by vision (Furneaux)[15]. Sounds will often evoke no response at all, as in the deaf; and indeed, although the sleeping EEG and PGR responses of these children are normal, there is evidence that they cannot localize and register sounds in the usual way (Taylor)[58]. Occasionally children exhibiting many of the classical signs of autism are still able to communicate verbally and may then describe a desire to cut themselves off from external stimuli. 'I'm not going to look at you—I don't want to listen.' Repetitive, stereotyped motor behaviour such as rocking is another marked feature of the syndrome, but will not be considered further here.

O'Connor and Hermelin[41, 42] have compared psychotic children with subnormals and with mute but non-psychotic (aphasic) children on tests of word repetition and picture recall (Hermelin and O'Connor)[22]. They found that in contrast to all other groups of children, psychotic children were no better at recalling connected items than unconnected ones, suggesting a fundamental inability to structure experiences or form associations. These authors also compared the same groups on tasks of learning and discrimination involving cross-modal transfer. All groups, when studied before testing responded to verbal commands to the same degree (Hermelin and O'Connor)[21]. On tasks involving transfer from vision to touch psychotic children did as well as the other two groups; but on tasks involving transfer in the opposite direction (touch to vision) they were significantly worse. Moreover, the mute psychotics were worse on these transfer tasks than the children who could verbalize. The authors explain this by suggesting that 'visual encoding' of data is assisted by 'verbal encoding', so that if the latter is absent the former is retarded.

There is some evidence that psychotic children acquire some form of verbal system even while mute and hence in the absence of any feed-back from their own practice efforts. The first words or phrases uttered by mute children when they do start speaking are often fairly mature in form (Furneaux)[15]. One speech therapist described a child of 3 years, who, after some months of therapy started speaking straight away with well-formed adult words instead of going through the normal phases of babbling. Nevertheless, it is rare for these children ever to acquire normal adult speech. The most common residual defects are: (i) referring to the self in the 3rd person (John wants to eat—He's hungry); (*ii*) reversal of pronouns; (*iii*) echolalia; (*iv*) a pedantic over-elaborate form of speech often referred to as 'officialese' (Furneaux[15]; Rutter[54]). The similarity between the picture presented by these children and by adult patients suffering from schizophrenia will be discussed later.

6

Development of Speech in Aphasic Children

The term 'childhood aphasia' is usually used when referring to children whose speech is abnormally delayed or impoverished in the absence of any other defects (e.g. psychotic manifestation, severe subnormality or hearing defect). The term has been objected to by a number of authors on the grounds that aphasia rightly applies to the loss of an established skill rather than the inability to acquire it; but the term 'childhood aphasia' is now so firmly established in the clinical literature that it has undoubtedly come to stay.

Children in this group usually show a number of abnormalities in their response to sounds. Lea[29] noted that they appeared to have difficulty in focusing on single sounds and picking these out from others, which suggests some failure of the 'filter mechanism' which enables the normal person to follow a conversation in a noisy room by cutting out the extraneous stimuli. (See, for example, Treisman[61].) In contrast to their good visual retention, their auditory retention is poor. Eisenson[13] also noted defects of auditory discrimination in aphasic children. Using operant conditioning techniques he found that aphasic children could often be trained to discriminate between single vowel sounds, but not between those same sounds, if they were bounded by consonants; i.e. they could distinguish between 'a' and 'e', but not between 'bat' and 'bet'. Even in those children who have undergone prolonged speech therapy, sequence reproduction remains difficult, e.g. a series 572 might be reproduced as 752—and understanding of speech is restricted to short sentences only (Lea)[29] and is very dependent on context.

The language defects in these children are not, however, confined to speech comprehension. While written material may be understood better than spoken, aphasic children like subnormal and psychotic children usually show defects of articulation and of generalization alongside their severe disorder of comprehension. Moreover, from an early age they exhibit great difficulty in associating sounds with actions. Thus, whereas the normal 3-year-old child can be taught to place a peg in a board at a given signal without much difficulty, the aphasic child has great difficulty in learning to do so, even if his pure-tone audiogram shows no defect (Taylor)[59].

Children who are rendered aphasic by cerebral lesions show a very different picture from the above. Those with temporal lobe lesions usually show much better comprehension than production of speech, but tend to remain quite mute, whereas adults with similar lesions nearly always make some attempt to verbalize even if it is inappropriate.

The most important point to be learned by the linguist from the study of childhood aphasia seems to be the one already mentioned in the section on deafness; namely, that the acquisition of speech interpretation (and hence of its production) does not depend only on the ability to hear single sounds, but on the ability to recognize sound patterns. In order to do this, it seems that one must: (i) be able to select certain 'required' sounds from all others, (ii) store up groups of sound for short periods of time before processing them. Both these functions depend on our expectations derived from past experience.

Comparison between the Acquisition of Speech by Children and Adults

The similarities and differences between the learning of the mother-tongue by a child and the learning of a foreign language by an adult do not seem to have been considered to any great extent, but a brief summary of some obvious points may be relevant here. Both aspects seem to be similar in that:

1. Learning of words and of their grammatical relationships proceed together.

2. Frequency of occurrence plays an important part in deciding which words are learned first. The words most commonly heard and most often practised are learned before others.

3. Length of utterances produced and understood (encoded and decoded) increases with general efficiency.

4. The speed with which sentences are encoded and decoded also increases with general efficiency.

5. Comprehension precedes production in both groups, and the comprehended vocabulary exceeds the used vocabulary in most instances.

Childhood and adult learning are, however, very different in that whereas the child has to learn to conceptualize his environment as well as to talk about it; the adult has (in the majority of instances) only to attach a new label to established concepts.

7

The Breakdown of Languages Associated with Cerebral Lesions

It has long been recognized that lesions in the dominant cerebral hemisphere may be followed by disorders of language functions, but that the loss is seldom total. The sufferer's ability to communicate is severely disrupted due to his difficulty in finding appropriate words at the right moment or in stringing these together in the accepted syntactical sequences.

These disorders of expression may or may not be accompanied by loss of comprehension.

Many attempts have been made to classify and measure these disorders and to find the relationship between them and other mental functions (e.g. Head[20]; Weisenberg and McBride[64]). Many attempts have also been made to discover if specific verbal defects are associated with specific anatomical lesions. Much of this work has led to contradictory conclusions, and it seems that these will only be resolved when more is known about the language functions themselves. Only recently has attention been paid to a study of the basic language function of these patients, and to comparing it with that in unbrain-damaged people (Grewel[19]; Pincas[47]).

Howes and Geschwind[23] studied the statistical properties of the speech emitted by two groups of dysphasic patients: (*i*) those with severe reduction of output but little disturbance of comprehension (expressive dysphasics); (*ii*) those with a tendency to talk jargon, in whom disorders of comprehension were also evident (jargon dysphasics). The first group was by far the larger, and it is this type of patient who will be referred to in the following pages as 'dysphasic'. Howes and Geschwind noted that the speech these patients did emit followed the normal statistical laws, but that there was a severe restriction of vocabulary and a tendency to make greater than normal use of common words.

Schuell[55] compared the speech of a mixed group of dysphasic patients with that of children and noted many similarities between the two. Common, high-frequency words were used by both groups more often than rare, low-frequency words; and both groups tended, if they were unable to find a required word, to use one semantically associated with it. In the dysphasic patients, however, Schuell maintained that the defect is seldom restricted to one function alone (e.g. expression), and that although comprehension is commonly better retained than expression, it is almost always impaired to some extent if expression is grossly abnormal.

A similar conclusion was reached by Rochford and Williams[51], who found a close parallel not only between the word-finding difficulty of children and dysphasic patients, but also between both these groups and normal adults subjected to time-stress, and between psychiatric patients during the stage of recovery after ECT. It seems that certain words have a certain intrinsic difficulty of access which while not usually evident in the normal person is highlighted in abnormal mental states.

Rochford and Williams carried out numerous investigations to discover the factors involved in word accessibility. Using the Thorndike-Lorge Word Count[60] as a measure of word frequency and asking their subjects to give the names for objects presented to them pictorially, they noted that on the whole common words are more easily accessible to dysphasic patients than rare ones, thus again showing a parallel with normal function (Oldfield and Wingfield)[44]; but that the accessibility of the word depended also on the context in which it was required. Using homonyms with common and rare uses (the teeth in the mouth and the teeth of the comb; the bridge of the nose and the bridge over a river), they found their dysphasic patients could find the word in its common context more easily than in its rare one (Rochford and Williams)[51]. Moreover, a word that could not be found spontaneously in response to the request to name an object could often be found if the patient was given a 'cue' consisting of a verbal or semantic association 'We bite with our ....'), or if the word itself was produced in a different context. Thus after naming the teeth in the mouth, a patient would turn to the comb and say, 'Of course, these are called teeth too'.

Rochford and Williams also found that the ability to find composite words (e.g. wheelbarrow, sundial) depended on the accessibility of the first syllable only. Using composite words with rare first and common second, and common first and rare second syllables, they found that the ease with which dysphasic patients named the objects was related to the frequency of the first syllable only, the frequency of the second being irrelevant (Rochford and Williams)[51]. They concluded that the accessibility of words (at least in the name-finding situation) depended on the subject's being given some lead-in to the specific verbal field; that this lead-in can be given in a number of ways, but that by and large commonly used words are more accessible than rarely used ones.

There is one considerable difference between the adult dysphasic patient and the normal child; this is the effect of repetition or practice. The more a child rehearses a rare word, the more accessible it becomes, but in the brain-injured dysphasic, rehearsal or practice seems to have little effect (Butfield[9]; Weigl and Kreindler[63]). It is true that immediately after a word has just been uttered its accessibility is improved (as in the case of the search for the 'teeth' of the comb mentioned above), but once the context has been changed it becomes as hard to find as ever (Rochford and Williams)[51]. The way dysphasic patients can best be helped to find words is by cueing them in to the appropriate field.

The effectiveness of various cues was also studied by Rochford and Williams who found that as with normal adults (in contrast to young children) semantic associations were more effective than phonetic ones. The dysphasic adult has not, it seems, lost his basic word store or its organization, but only his access to different parts of it.

More about this word-store can be learned from a study of the mistakes made by patients when they fail to find a correct word, i.e. an analysis of errors. It has already been mentioned that when dysphasic adults and normal children do not know the name for an object, they seldom remain mute. The tendency is either to describe the subject by its use (e.g. for hands of the watch, 'pointers') or to give a word associated with it ('fingers'). But the words actually given at these times tend to be rare ones; i.e. words not as commonly used by normal adults as the names actually sought. Rochford and Williams tried to account for this apparent anomaly by suggesting that these error-names are never actually dropped from the repertoire when the child learns to correct them, but are rehearsed and rejected each time the correct name is given. This subliminal rehearsal increases their accessiblity so that when the adult's ability is impaired by his cerebral defects, they are the most accessible to him in a given situation. This would also account for the observation that when *children* suffer cerebral injury they, in contrast to adults, remain mute. They have no well-rehearsed and rejected names to fall back on.

After temporal lesions of the dominant hemisphere, it has already been mentioned that comprehension tends in the majority of cases to be less severely disturbed than expression. The patients in whom this is not so, tend to show so many other concomitant disorders—especially jargon speech—that the breakdown of comprehension alone is not easily studied in these cases. However, there are two other groups of patients who show abnormalities of language and in whom disorders of comprehension appear to be as badly disrupted as expression. These are patients suffering from senile dementia and schizophrenic illnesses (Rochford and Williams)[52].

8

The Breakdown of Language in Senile Dementia

It has long been recognized that senile dementia may be accompanied by a breakdown of some language functions, but that the language disorders seen in these patients show many differences from those seen in the dysphasia due to focal lesions. In the early stages speech usually remains fluent and grammatical, even if not always appropriate. There is some difficulty in naming objects and a lack of precision. In the next stage, speech is reduced to simple phrases in which sounds and propositional forms remain intact, but which contain little meaning. Speech tends to go on endlessly and to be repetitive. Patients can comprehend the general trend of a conversation, but miss the details. In the final stage of dissolution speech is limited to one or two sensible utterances among a mass of inarticulate jargon (Mayer *et al.*)[36]. It is in the first two of these stages of deterioration that the defects can best be studied.

Rochford and Williams[52] found that, in contrast to the dysphasic patients, senile patients were often better at naming pictures than at selecting a named picture from alternatives. Equally, they were better at reading lists of words aloud than at matching written words to pictures. Their ability to read aloud indicated that their failure on the matching tasks could not be due to visual defects alone, and indeed their whole behaviour on the matching tasks suggested that they had failed to grasp what they were supposed to do rather than that they were unable to do it. Completely erroneous responses were often accompanied by a loose verbal confabulation. For example, if asked to 'point to the key' among a set of eight pictures of equal familiarity, a patient might point to the book, making a comment such as, 'This is a key on a fine reading day'.

At the same time, the errors made by senile patients when failing to name objects correctly showed some evidence of perceptual defects as opposed to purely linguistic ones. Thus a dice might be called 'A box with seeds in it'. A garden rake might be called 'a brush' and a windmill, 'a coffee pot' (Rochford)[50]. If they were asked to name things which could be identified without difficulty (such as parts of the body) naming errors were fewer than when asked to name random objects or pictures; and difficulty in senile dementia did not in any case correspond to word frequency.

In these cases of senile dementia, it will be noted that breakdown does not show any parallels to normal language function or to the development of language in normal children. It is not accessiblity to words which appears to be at fault, but inability to select the correct word both in expression and comprehension. It appears as if the wrong semantic field is alerted, probably through faulty perception.

9

The Breakdown of Speech in Schizophrenics

The abnormalities of speech demonstrated by some schizophrenic patients have been recognized for years and have usually been taken to reflect the presence of thought disorder. However, as argued by E. B. Williams[66], 'It does not follow logically that if speech is disordered then thought is disordered too'. In some patients who exhibit jargon speech following cerebral lesions, thinking as measured by the ability to solve perceptual problems may be well preserved (Kinsbourne and Warrington)[27], but it is undeniable that in those schizophrenic patients who show abnormalities of speech, there is usually some accompanying inefficiency on perceptual and constructional tasks suggesting disorders other than purely linguistic ones. To talk about schizophrenic illnesses or schizophrenic patients as if they were a single group is, of course, unjustified; but since the patients in this broad diagnostic category who demonstrate abnormality of speech usually show a number of other features in common, and since these are fairly well defined and recognized clinically, the patients under consideration will be referred to in the rest of this paper merely as schizophrenics.

The speech disorders shown by these patients are of quite a different type to those shown by either dysphasic or demented patients. Vocabulary remains large—even over-large for there is a tendency to use long words rather than short ones and to coin new words (neologism) at random. Speech is fluent—even over-fluent, for the patients tend to talk (and write) more profusely than before. An object cannot be given a simple name without elaboration (over-inclusiveness, see Payne[45]). For all this output, the content remains meagre and the normal listener gains little information from it. Sentences tend to change direction in mid-stream (the Knights move) or to peter out without conclusion (thought blocking). If the listener tries to press the patient, he is firmly interrupted and pushed aside.

Many attempts have been made to analyse and define the 'basic defect' in schizophrenic speech. Moran, Mefford and Kimble[38] using factor analysis found little difference between schizophrenics and normals in basic language structure, and other workers (see Yates)[68] have shown that schizophrenics *can* form the same kinds of concepts as normal people if pressed. Nevertheless, although the capacity for normal verbal responses by schizophrenics is not impaired, the fact remains that in the majority of situations they do demonstrate the abnormalities mentioned above.

A more profitable approach to an understanding of the illness seems to be the analysis of the conditions under which schizophrenic patients exhibit speech disorders. It is notable, for example, that they show little abnormality when answering simple factual questions about impersonal events ('What date is it today?'). If the task they are set is well structured and allows for only one answer, they respond as would a normal person. It is only on the more open-ended type of problem (e.g. proverb interpretation) that they begin to break down.

This being so, it might be expected that they would follow the normal syntactical constraints of language fairly well, and indeed Lewinson and Elwood[30] found this to be so. Schizophrenic patients who were asked to repeat from memory sentences varying in grammatical and syntactical accuracy, were found to be somewhat inferior to normal subjects but to follow the same laws. This finding has not been confirmed by two later studies (Lawson *et al.*[28]; Gerver[16]), but Williams has suggested that the trouble may be due not so much to the grammatical complexity of the material which they are unable to deal with as the amount. When normal people are asked to continue a verbal sequence by adding one word to those given ('as he went into . . . .'), it is found that the more words in the given sequence, the more closely is the response constrained. Shannon's technique (see Miller)[37] for producing passages of statistical approximation to English consists of giving one subject the first 'n' words and asking him to add one more; then folding over the first word of the sequence and handing the passage on to another subject with the same instructions, as in the game of consequences.

The greater the number of words (n) in the passage, the closer will a sequence of 100 words so produced approximate to normal English (see Miller[37]). This same technique was tried on schizophrenic patients by M. Williams[67], but in these patients it was found that increase in the length of the passage to be completed decreased rather than increased the passage's ultimate approximation to normal. Williams has described various other experiments in which schizophrenic patients were asked to respond to verbal passages of varying length and has found in each case that they did better the smaller the amount they were given.

This finding raises the possibility that the schizophrenic difficulty is not so much in expression as in comprehension—not so much the encoding as the decoding. There is a considerable body of evidence supporting this conclusion. When schizophrenic patients were compared by Rochford and Williams with dysphasic patients on tests of comprehension and naming, the schizophrenics were found to resemble those suffering from senile psychoses in being comparatively worse at comprehension than at naming. It has also long been recognized that schizophrenic patients show abnormalities on tests of visual perception (see Yates[68]). The difficulty psychotic children appear to have in auditory perception has already been mentioned; and recently Chapman and McGhie[10] have drawn attention to the extreme difficulty adult schizophrenics both exhibit and describe in assimilating multiple stimuli, expecially verbal. The reason they cannot repeat sentences of high redundancy (i.e. including small, unimportant connective words) was thought by these authors to be due to the fact that the redundant words act as distractors instead of supplementers (Chapman and McGhie)[10]. How can all this be explained?

It has already been mentioned that normal hearing depends to a large extent on cutting out (filtering off) irrelevant stimuli as well as on receiving relevant ones. Were we not able to do this, we would never be able to follow a conversation in a noisy room. However, the rejected stimuli are not filtered off entirely (Treisman)[61]. If something in the rejected message is highly important, or if it fits in better with what we are thinking about than the message being followed, we can switch over to the rejected message and let it in. This suggests that we must be able to receive and store two messages simultaneously; one which is being attended to and one which is being rejected.

But we cannot attend to too much at once. As suggested by Broadbent[5] we appear to keep a word in mind for only a short time—until we have understood it—then push it to one side so that we can concentrate on the next. Yet we do not push it away altogether. If necessary we can do a 'double take' and recapture it for a second look. Hence there must be at least a second level at which incoming stimuli are held and dealt with, besides the level dealing with immediate attention and rejection—the short-term memory store.

The normal person, however, does not deal with each word he hears in isolation. He will wait till he has received several words and then process these together in a chunk. One of the main features in development, as we have already seen, lies in the size of the chunk (length of utterance) an individual can deal with. One of the chief characteristics of the speech-retarded child lies in his ability to deal with small chunks only. Is this the trouble with the adult schizophrenic patient? There is some evidence that it may be; that instead of being able to store up and deal with sequences of words in chunks, each word has to be dealt with individually. This may be why redundant words act as distractors, and why schizophrenics have greater difficulty in completing long verbal passages than short ones. Yates suggests that it is not the primary channel capacity which is reduced and causes this disability, but the speed with which information is processed by it. If the channel capacity is restricted as Broadbent suggests, and if the existing information in it is processed too slowly, then as Yates points out, the channel will quickly become overloaded and produce the picture seen in schizophrenics. This conclusion is further supported by Williams' finding that when asked to associate to multi-word stimuli in a word association type of experiment, normal subjects who were put under time pressure produced the same type of response as schizophrenic patients (M. Williams)[67].

A further, and as yet unpublished investigation, however, suggests a slightly different explanation for the phenomenon (Marchbanks and Williams)[35]. Schizophrenic patients were shown a number of pictures and were offered for each picture a number of alternative words. They were asked merely to say for each word whether it was the correct name for the picture or not. The words offered were: (*i*) the correct name; (*ii*) two words associated with it in common use; (*iii*) four words with the same beginnings or endings; and (*iv*) two quite irrelevant ones. For example, one of the pictures shown depicted a small hatchet. The names offered were: finger, tree, prophet, hatching, latchet, hatchet, hatchway, arrow, hacking. While the thought-disordered and acutely-ill patients showed much greater difficulty than the other groups of schizophrenics, all groups tended to accept the associated words to a far greater extent than expected. For example, one patient accepted the names Tree ('because it is used for cutting a tree'), Hatching ('it's used for hatching trees'), Latchet (misread as Hatchet), Hatchet, Hatchway ('just thought it sounded right'), Hacking ('because it hacks'). The irrelevant words were seldom accepted; and indeed, when the subjects were given the same task but told that they could choose only one of the possible words, they chose the correct name in the majority of instances.

This experiment seems to suggest that each word not only arouses the concepts most commonly associated with it, but many others as well; and that the main difficulty for the schizophrenic lies in sorting through this vast pool of aroused associations. When discussing the abnormalities seen in dysphasia, it was suggested that arousal of 'rejected' association occurs in all of us. The speech abnormalities seen in schizophrenic patients corroborates this hypothesis. But in dysphasia the main difficulty lies in the retrieval of words from the basic store and in selecting the appropriate one at the right moment. In the case of senile dementia, it was suggested that perceptual stimuli tended to alert the wrong areas of the word store. It can now be suggested that in schizophrenics too much of the word store is made available at every single moment—the store is over-aroused.

It must be emphasized, however, that these suggestions are purely speculative and highly imaginative. In postulating stores, channels, filters, etc. as a means of systematizing our data about language, we must not forget that these are still only words—or diagrams in text books. We cannot look at a perceptual input channel under the microscope, and we still have little idea what actually operates the filter to cut off unwanted sounds. Moreover, as yet no location for the store has been discovered. Neither Brocas area nor any other part of the temporal lobe in the dominant hemisphere seems to act as a permanent filing system, for although their intact presence is necessary for speech, the removal of a given part does not remove any single words from a person's repertoire; it only makes all words harder to find. We still have a long way to go before we will be able to answer the questions raised in the Introduction to this chapter, but so much work is being done in this field at the moment that the answers to some questions may be provided in the not too distant future.

REFERENCES

1. BARTLETT, F. C., 1932. *Remembering*. Cambridge, Univ. Press.
2. BERKO, J., 1958. The child's learning of English morphology. *Word*, **14**, 150.
3. BEVERS, T. G., and FODOR, J. A., 1966. Gestalt principles and psycholinguistics. *Proc. XVIII Int. Congress of Psychology*, 2.
4. BRAINE, M. D. S., 1963. On learning the grammatical order of words. *Psychol. Rev.*, **70**, 323.
5. BROADBENT, D. E., 1958. *Perception and communication*. Oxford, Pergamon Press.
6. BROWN, R., 1958. *Words and things*. Illinois, Free Press.
7. BROWN, R., and BELLUGI, U., 1966. The child's acquisition of syntax. In *New directions in the study of language*. Ed. Lenneberg, E. H. Ann Arbor, Mass., M.I.T. Press.
8. BRUCE, D., and PUGH, H., 1966. Immediate verbal memory and linguistics in children. *Language and speech*, **9**, 2.
9. BUTFIELD, E., 1958. Speech therapy in aphasia. *Speech Path. Ther.*, **1**, 9.
10. CHAPMAN, J., and MCGHIE, A., 1962. A comparative study of disordered attention in schizophrenia. *J. ment. Sci.*, **108**, 487.
11. CHOMSKY, N., 1957. *Syntactic structures*. The Hague, Mouton.
12. CREAK, M., 1961. Autistic children. *Lancet*, ii, 818.
13. EISENSON, J., 1966. Perceptual disorders in children. *Brit. J. Dis. Commun.*, **1**, 21.
14. ERVIN, S. M., 1966. Children's language. In *New directions in the study of language*. Ed. Lenneberg, E. H. Ann Arbor, Mass., M.I.T. Press.
15. FURNEAUX, B., 1966. The autistic child. *Brit. J. Dis. Commun.*, **1**, 85.
16. GERVER, D., 1965. Linguistic rules in the speech of schizophrenic patients. Talk to Experimental Psychol. Soc., London.
17. GOLDFARB, W., 1934a. Infant rearing and problem behaviour. *Am. J. Orthopsychiat.*, **13**, 249. 1943b. The effects of institutional care on adolescents. *J. Exp. Educ.*, **12**, 106.
18. GOLDMAN-EISLER, F., 1958. The predictability of words in context. *Q. J. exp. Psychol.*, **10**, 76.
19. GREWEL, F., 1963. Linguistic approach to aphasia. *Speech Path. Ther.*, **6**, 24.
20. HEAD, H., 1926. *Aphasia in kindred disorders of speech*. Cambridge, Univ. Press.

21. HERMELIN, B., and O'CONNOR, N., 1964. Crossmodal transfer in normal, subnormal and autistic children. *Neuropsychologia*, **2**, 229.
22. HERMELIN, B., and O'CONNOR, N., 1967. Immediate memory for words and pictures. Talk to Experimental Psychol. Soc., London.
23. HOWES, D. H., and GESCHWIND, N., 1961. Statistical properties of aphasic language. Excerpta Medica Int. Congress, Ser. No. 38, *VIIth Int. Congress of Neurol.*, Rome.
24. IRWIN, O. C., 1947. Development of speech during infancy. *J. exp. Psychol.*, **37**, 187.
25. JENKINS, J. J., 1966. Mediation theory and grammatical behaviour. In *Directions in psycholinguistics*. Ed. Rosenberg, S. New York, Macmillan.
26. KELLMER-PRINGLE, M. L., 1965. Language difficulties among deprived children. In *Children with communication problems*. Ed. White Franklin, A. London, Pitman.
27. KINSBOURNE, M., and WARRINGTON, E., 1963. Jargon aphasia. *Neuropsychologia*, **1**, 27.
28. LAWSON, J. S., McGHIE, A., and CHAPMAN, J., 1964. Perception of speech in schizophrenia. *Brit. J. Psychiat.*, **110**, 375.
29. LEA, J., 1965. Children suffering from receptive aphasia. *Speech Path. Ther.*, **8**, 58.
30. LEWINSON, P. M., and ELWOOD, D. L., 1961. Contextual constraints in language samples in schizophrenia, *J. nerv. ment. Dis.*, **133**, 79.
31. LURIA, A. R., 1961. *The role of speech in the regulation of normal and abnormal behaviour*. Oxford, Pergamon Press.
32. LURIA, A. R., and VINOGRADOVA, O. S., 1959. The dynamics of semantic systems. *Brit. J. Psychol.*, **50**, 89.
33. MCCARTHY, D., 1954. Language development in children. In *Manual of child psychology*. Ed. Carmichael, L. London, John Wiley.
34. MCCONNON, K., 1935. The situation factor in the language of nursery school children. Ph.D. dissertation. University of Minnesota.
35. MARCHBANKS, G., and WILLIAMS, M., 1967. Unpublished experiments.
36. MAYER, GROSS W., SLATER, E., and ROTH, M., 1960. *Clinical psychiatry*. London, Cassell.
37. MILLER, G. A., 1951. *Language and communication*. New York, McGraw Hill Book Co.
38. MORAN, E., MEFFORD, R. B., and KIMBLE, J. P., 1964. Idiodynamic sets in word association. *Psychol. Monog.*, **18**, 340.
39. MYKLEBUST, H. R., 1960. *The psychology of deafness*. New York, Grune and Stratton.
40. O'CONNOR, N., and HERMELIN, B., 1963. *Speech and thought in severe subnormality*. Oxford, Pergamon Press.
41. O'CONNOR, N., and HERMELIN, B., 1964. Measures of distance and motility in psychotic and subnormal children. *Brit. J. soc. clin. Psychol.*, **3**, 29.
42. O'CONNOR, N., and HERMELIN, B., 1965. Visual analogies of verbal operations. *Language and speech*, **8**, 197.
43. OLDFIELD, R. C., 1966. Things, words, and the brain, *Q. J. expl Psychol.*, **18**, 340.
44. OLDFIELD, R. C., and WINGFIELD, A., 1965. Response latencies in naming objects. *Q. J. expl Psychol.*, **17**, 273.
45. PAYNE, R. W., 1961. Cognitive abnormalities. In *Handbook of abnormal psychology*. Ed. Eysenck, H. J. New York, Basic Books.
46. PIAGET, J., 1924. *Le langage et la pensee chez l'enfant*. Reissued in translation (1955). *The language and thought of the child*. New York, Meridian Books.

47. PINCAS, A., 1955. Linguistics and aphasia. *J. Austr. Coll. Speech Therapists*, **15**, 20.
48. RENFREW, C. E., 1959. Speech problems in backward children. *Speech Path. Ther.*, **2**, 34.
49. RENFREW, C. E., 1965. Development of speech in mentally retarded children. In *Children with communication problems*. Ed. White Franklin, A. London, Pitman.
50. ROCHFORD, G., 1966. Organic speech disorders. Thesis offered for D. Phil., Oxon.
51. ROCHFORD, G., and WILLIAMS, M., 1962-66. The development and breakdown of the use of names. *J. Neurol. Neurosurg. Psychiat.*, **25**, 222; **26**, 377; **28**, 407.
52. ROCHFORD, G., and WILLIAMS, M., 1964. The measurement of language disorders. *Speech Path. Ther.*, **7**, 1.
53. ROSENBERG, S., 1965. *Directions in psycholinguistics*. New York, Macmillan.
54. RUTTER, M., 1965. Speech disorders in autistic children. In *Children with communication problems*. Ed. White Franklin, A. London, Pitman Medical.
55. SCHUELL, H., 1966. Aphasia in adults in relation to language disturbances in children. *Brit. J. Dis. Comm.*, **1**, 33.
56. SKINNER, B. F., 1957. *Verbal behaviour*. New York, Appleton-Century-Crofts.
57. SPIELBERGER, C. D., 1966. The modification of verbal behaviour. In *Directions in psycholinguistics*. Ed. Rosenberg, S. New York, Macmillan.
58. TAYLOR, I. G., 1965. The deaf and the non-communicating child. In *Children with communication problems*. Ed. White Franklin, A. London, Pitman Medical.
59. TAYLOR, I. G., 1966. Hearing in relation to language disorders in children. *Brit. J. Dis. Comm.*, **1**, 11.
60. THORNDIKE, E. L., and LORGE, I., 1944. *The teacher's word book of 30,000 words*. New York, Columbia Univ.
61. TREISMAN, A., 1965. Verbal responses and contextual constraints. *J. Verb. Learning and Verb. Beh.*, **4**, 118.
62. VAN ALSTYNE, D., 1932. *Play behaviour and choice of play materials in preschool children*. Chicago, Univ. Press.
63. WEIGL, E., and KREINDLER, A., 1960. *Arch. Psychiat. Nervenkr.*, **200**, 306.
64. WEISENBERG, T., and MCBRIDE, K. E., 1935. *Aphasia*. Oxford, Univ. Press.
65. WHETNALL, E., and FRY, D. B., 1964. *The deaf child*. London, Heinemann.
66. WILLIAMS, E. B., 1964. Deductive reasoning in schizophrenia. *J. abnorm. soc. Psychol.*, **69**, 47.
67. WILLIAMS, M., 1966. The effect of context on schizophrenic speech. *Brit. J. soc. clin. Psychol.*, **5**, 161.
68. YATES, A. J., 1966. Thought disorder in schizophrenia. *Austr. J. Psychol.*, **18**, 103.
69. ZIPF, G. K., 1949. *Human behaviour and the principle of least effort*. Cambridge, Mass., Addison Wesley.

XXI

DYSFUNCTIONS OF PARENTING: THE BATTERED CHILD, THE NEGLECTED CHILD, THE EXPLOITED CHILD

RICHARD GALDSTON
M.D.

*Instructor in Psychiatry, Harvard Medical School, Boston, Massachusetts
Chief, In-Patient Psychiatric Consultation Service, The Children's Hospital Medical Center, Boston, Massachusetts*

1
Introduction

The normal purpose of parenting is the conception, birth and culture of children through a confluence of drives which subserves the perpetuation of the species by the creation of a new individual. A parent must stay alive and sane to attain this goal in any part. Self-preservation commands an obligatory priority in the parent's distribution and utilization of his psychic energies and culture of the child is subordinated to the parent's requirements.

The battered child and the neglected child and the exploited child each represent a by-product of the parent's particular pattern of mental manœuvring to maintain homeostasis in face of an emergent threat to his own psychological integrity.

Culture of children confronts the parent with all of his aspirations for the future and taps into all his emotions from the past. The mere presence of the child serves to activate in the parent any latent conflict between what he is and what he wanted to be, between those emotions he has felt and those emotions he has been unable to accept. Being a parent to a child mobilizes the child in the parent and forces claim that each recognize and acknowledge the other. When this meeting occasions such conflict that open strife ensues, the resultant tension may be discharged on to the child.

The closeness of the child to the parent allows for its use as a means of relief from distress. The fact that the child is derived from the physical substance of the parent makes it eminently suitable for utilization as an extension of the parent's psychological substance. The way in which the child is utilized to afford relief to the parent depends upon a complex of factors. The age, sex, and birth order of the child are important in dictating the corresponding times and issues in the parent's past. The parent's character structure determines the type of behaviour he will bring to bear upon the child in response to his perception of the child and the emotions it evokes. Depending upon the interplay of these forces in their particular cultural context, the battered child, the neglected child or the exploited child will appear as the result of a dysfunction of parenting in which the perpetuation of the species has been sacrificed in some measure to preserve the integrity of the individual.

2

The Battered Child

Definition

The battered child has been physically abused by an adult without provocation in the child's behaviour. The child is usually too young to be considered capable of conscious deliberate acts or of the use of language as an organized mode of communication which distinguishes the syndrome from punishment.

Description

A little boy or girl is brought to attention in a state of morbidity varying from terminal coma to relative health. The combination of fresh and old bruises, recent and healed fractures of the ribs, head of the humerus or the skull with welts or burns are pathognomonic of repeated trauma. The parents may or may not acknowledge their responsibility. Usually their initial story is vague and subject to later revisions. The child may or may not show evidence of neglect. Many of these children are well nourished and dressed.

The acute picture is of two sorts. One is of listlessness, apathy and unresponsiveness to all but painful stimuli. The child displays a blunting of all evidence of vitality akin to that seen in adult cases of shell shock. It appears that the child has attempted to fend off further assault by suspending any signs of physical and psychological animation and feigning death. The other pattern is characterized by flight in fear upon any approach. The child cowers, whimpers and attempts to hide from attempts at contact.

With time and treatment the picture changes as the child follows one of four recognizable courses.

(*i*) Death either with or without demonstrable physiologic cause.

(*ii*) Clinging without discrimination to any and all persons who avail themselves to the child.

(*iii*) Recovery from the sequelae of physical abuse with persistent signs of anxiety and withdrawal at the approach of others.

(*iv*) Recovery from the stigmata of physical abuse and rapid growth of ego skills far beyond the pre-morbid level.

Signs of pleasure in eating are the harbinger of the return of an investment in living. The gradual introduction of persons who respond to the child in accordance with its level of being fosters the accrual of bits and fragments of pleasure which in turn promotes a shift from inertness towards an attitude of activity. Preserving a climate of care which accommodates to the developing initiative of the child allows for the further flourishing of pleasure which is often accompanied by a temporary renunciation of a specific skill. A beaten, debilitated 3-year-old who fed herself with knife and fork and fastidious joylessness upon admission to the hospital responded to treatment by forsaking implements in favour of exuberant finger feeding. Only by turning back the clock of ego development through temporary regression in its skills can the lost pleasures be recaptured and wedged back into the nooks and crannies of experience. It is a regression in the service of the growth of the ego.

Under proper treatment some of these children can make remarkable recovery to levels which appear to exceed their previous maturity. However there are points of no return. It appears that the age of $3\frac{1}{2}$ to 4 mark the point of closure beyond which the ego has great difficulty in utilizing pleasure to correct previous damage to its development.

It is noteworthy that observations of over 100 battered children have failed to detect a single instance of autistic development or childhood schizophrenia although many of the children display periods of auto-erotic activity during their recovery phase.

Parents

There are seven factors which collectively dispose parents to resort to beating a child in order to spare themselves the conscious experience of their own intrapsychic distress. No single element is unique to this syndrome nor will any one alone account for the phenomenon. The presence of each of these items increases the likelihood that a parent will batter a child.

(*i*) Major reliance upon projection as a leading defence against intrapsychic stress:

Clinically this feature is illustrated in the choice of terms used to describe the child. The parent speaks of the child in words appropriate to an adult. Whereas the normal parents on occasion will speak of the child 'as if' he were an adult reflecting the human tendency to project ourselves into our offspring and the present into the future, these parents omit the 'as if' and confuse the child with the adult. There is a defect in their capacity to test the reality of the child. The child functions as a delusion in what is essentially a transference psychosis.

(*ii*) A tendency to translate affect states into physical activity without the intervention of conscious thought:

This impulsivity enables the parent to 'take it out on the child'. The act of 'taking' conveys the literal transfer of affects from the parent on to the child.

(*iii*) The presence of intolerable self-hatred:

This is the 'it' which the parent 'takes out' on the child. The qualities and attributes with which the parent endows the child and for which he abuses it are the very features which he cannot countenance in himself. They are expressions of that affective residue of his life experience which he cannot tolerate acknowledging as his own. He tries to dispose of them by projecting them on to the child and exorcizing them through physical abuse. The child is the scapegoat for the parent's unconscious sense of self-loathing.

(*iv*) Correspondence of the child by sex, age and position in the family to events in the parent's own life which occasioned his great self-hatred:

The capacity to see ourselves in our children is influenced by the extent to which the child's physical presence in time and place correspond to our own affects. A parent who despises his own dependent longings is more likely to beat a young infant. The parent who cannot tolerate his sexual feelings is more likely to abuse an older child. It is the presence of the child of a particular sex, age and position which serves as the seed crystal about which the parent's forgotten unwanted emotions threaten to precipitate out of unconsciousness into painful awareness.

(*v*) Relative lack of available alternative modes of defence against conflict because of environmental factors:

Poverty, illness, domestic demands, social isolation, housing problems all can contribute an increment to the likelihood of physical abuse by reducing the availability of alternative modes for discharging intrapsychic tension.

(*vi*) Compliance with the act of beating by the marriage partner due to dependence and a reciprocal willingness to support projective defences:

The scapegoating phenomenon has considerable power to recruit unconscious collusion among those for whom dependent needs with their attendant guilt have a high priority. Passive compliance spares the partner from the anxiety which would accrue from active intervention.

(*vii*) Relative absence of available authority figures:

The deterrent power of grandparents, religious or social authorities as an antidote to idiosyncratic perceptions and eccentric behaviour is seldom available to the abusing parent. In many cases the parents previously have sought out the influence of such figures without obtaining their response.

In addition to these seven genetic factors there are three noteworthy corollaries.

The reversal of marital roles among the abusing parents is usually gross and long antedates the child. The outbreak of beating often coincides with a breakdown in the role reversal because of external factors. This illustrates the defensive function of role reversal in sparing the parent from the intrapsychic conflict mobilized by the presence of the child.

Jealousy of the child, a common parental affliction, is not a force for beating. Its presence bespeaks the parent's recognition of the child as a separate, albeit more favoured, person. Jealousy of a child is a force for spouse abuse not child abuse.

Neglect and beating the child may or may not coexist. If they do, the course is one in which the parent has attempted to neglect the child without success. Because of the ambivalent quality of the parent's attachment to the child he cannot give it up through neglect and is forced to recognize it in abuse. The parent who beats a child is not the parent who abandons it and few are willing to give the child up for adoption. These are highly wanted children whose existence fulfils a complex of parental needs. Such is the nature of human attachment to children that intense, contradictory and very personal emotions can follow rapidly one after the other. When the child is out of the home these needs are not fulfilled and the missing child is often sorely wanted. When the child is gone the guilt is gone leaving only a longing.

3

The Neglected Child

Definition

The neglected child has not received sufficient attention from his parents to promote growth. His requirements for stimulation have not been met and his development has suffered with resultant retardation in physical and psychological maturation.

The neglected child lives with and is neglected by his parents. His plight differs from that of the deprived child who has been deprived of his parents and is therefore free to forage for the attention of others. The neglected child lives in the solitude of a family prison.

Description

When the condition is marked the neglected child presents as one who has failed to thrive. Below the range of normal percentiles for height and weight he appears emaciated, uninterested in his surroundings and devoid of any but the simplest self-centred activity.

Usually the history is one of fussy eating habits with poor food intake and frequent regurgitation. Often the stigmata of chronic malnutrition are present despite the parent's assurances that adequate amounts of food have been presented to the child. He is not lying. His perceptual grasp of his child is so feeble that both the flesh of his body and the stuff that goes to nourish it lie beyond his ken.

When asked, the parents describe the stools as very foul-smelling, but upon being questioned further they portray most of the child's physical attributes as offensive. A history of chronic diarrhoea is common. A prior diagnosis of coeliac disease or intestinal allergy may have been entertained.

The characteristic feature of the neglected child is his lack of spontaneous activity. The child sits and does nothing. He gives no sign of curiosity, fear, pleasure, or pain. The blank facies, fixed posture, and stilled voice lend him the semblance of a miniature mummy. Usually these children fall between the ages of 3 to 24 months, but they are so much smaller than their chronological age would warrant that the observer may fail to appreciate the peculiarities of behaviour because he views the child as being younger than he actually is.

When left to his own devices the child sits inertly failing to manipulate proffered toys, ignoring the initial approaches of others while rocking, picking at small spots on his skin or the bedding, or humming to himself. Yet the child recognizes other humans, follows them with his eyes and appears quite aware of the persons and events about him. Passive, alert and joyless the neglected child is a psychobiological robot. Neither happy nor sad, without fear or fun, he is and no more. Existence is a matter of physiologic function for the neglected child and no part or process of his body has been surcharged with emotion. Sucking, mouthing, touching, defecating, smearing, seeing and all other vital activities are performed without pleasure or pain. Venepuncture can often be accomplished without protest.

On initial observation the neglected child appears incapable of the motor skills appropriate to his chronological age. With repeated encouragement the child reveals his ability to perform the act in a mechanical fashion. Herein is the nub of his pathology: a primary failure to fuse feelings with his body. Neither eating nor patty-cake, nor piling blocks nor peek-a-boo provide the child with pleasure. There is no joy in doing anything. There is no gratification in any part of his body. Most children respond with uncontrollable giggling when the observer pokes his forefinger to tickle the belly-button while sticking out his tongue to make a flatulent sound. The neglected child stares in disbelief. The constitutent parts of his body with their associated processes and derived functions fail to provide him with pleasure. Their exercise is a matter of automatic necessity commensurate with staying alive. The child fails to thrive because there is nothing in it for him, neither pleasure nor pain.

The treatment of the neglected child requires the provision of stimulation diluted to a consistency which the child can tolerate. Starting with a gruel of mere bodily presence and gradually adding in playing with a shared object, the concentration of stimulation is titrated to the level of the child's current capacity to absorb attention.

The initial absence of appetite for food or contact can be a discouragement for those charged with caring for the neglected child. It requires that the person who proffers herself to the child be comfortable in the face of rejection. She must be able to accept the child's ignoring her even as the child has been ignored. Gradually there follows an activation of appetite for food and for stimulation. Once mobilized, the craving passes from the tentative to the voracious. It is as if a back-log of longing once released, pours forth. The child consumes an enormous amount of food and comes to cling tenaciously and indiscriminately to anyone available. His newly developed activity is awkward and often offensive, poking in the ears and up the nostrils, pulling the hair and besmearing the person who cares. This shift from passivity towards activity may pose a strain on those who are comfortable with an inert passive child but not with an intrusive messy one.

The provision of adequate appropriate stimulation adjusted to the child's changing capacity to receive attention is as specific a therapy for the neglected child as antibiotics are for the child with pneumonia.

The act of feeding is the basis of everything. The pleasure of the one who feeds becomes the child's pleasure. The affect goes with the foodstuff. No bottle-propping, naso-gastric tube feeding or intravenous drip can provide this crucial ingredient which cannot be synthetic. Around feeding, comes holding and touching and seeing. His arms, hands, and eyes become something of value to the child and their exercise becomes a source of pleasure to him in response to the one who takes pleasure in his presence.

If treatment is begun by the age of 24-30 months the neglected child can make great strides in development. Many aspects of the failure to thrive can be overcome with the restoration of normal levels of physical and motor maturity. The child can learn to acquire pleasure from the exercise of many ego skills. However, there is one area of operation which is particularly vulnerable to irreversible destruction. The establishment of a hierarchy of relationships with the dominance of a one-to-one attachment which is characteristic of the healthy child and his mother proves to be beyond the capacity of most of these children. They retain a promiscuous attitude towards all persons utilizing them without regard for their individuality. It is as though the absence and presence of pleasure have been such consuming issues in their early experience that they are left incapable of perceiving beyond the sensory state to recognize the person behind it. It is not pain which causes this failure but rather the absence of pleasure. Observations of children in acute or prolonged pain from accidents or illness indicate that pain, like pleasure, is a sensory state which occasions affects which the child can share with others to sustain a sense of self.

Parents

Parents who neglect a child can be considered in two groups. Those who rely upon projection as a leading defence against intrapsychic distress perceive the child as belonging to them but see it as the embodiment of undesirable attributes. The second group rely heavily upon denial as a defence against intrapsychic distress and they suffer from a primary failure to perceive the child as belonging to them.

The first group of parents share many of the psychological features of the parent of the battered child. However, they do not have the same tendency to translate affect states into physical activity. They are not impulsive. They are compulsive. They are disposed to utilize mental mechanisms to abuse the child and defend against this disposition by putting as much distance between themselves and the child as possible. Such a parent sees his child as bearing the loathsome qualities for which he despises himself. To avoid beating it he relegates its care to others. Herein socio-economic factors play a significant role and account for the apparently greater incidence of the battered child among the poor. The poor cannot hire others to care for their children. If there is an effective extended family they can get someone else to care for it. Otherwise the poor parent is forced into intimate contact with the child he sees as hateful. The well-to-do parent can seek relief by putting physical distance between himself and the child through the use of a nursemaid.

Similarly the presence of authority figures serves as a powerful deterrent against physical beating and tends to reinforce the reliance upon neglect of the child as an alternative mode of relief. In general, society is more tolerant of sins of omission than of sins of commission. Among those instances where the child has first been neglected and then beaten, the loss of a babysitter or the money to hire one, or the loss of a previously available authority figure often precipitates the outbreak of physical beating.

The second group of parents deny the existence of the child. They fail to perceive the child as theirs. They account for those children afflicted with early, severe failure to thrive requiring hospitalization within the first six months of life. Such a mother gives eloquent testimony of her need to deny that the child belongs to her. She says that she had great difficulty in finding a name for the child until it was several weeks of age and then gave it a name chosen by someone else. She may tell of a fantasy that the child is a changeling foisted upon her in the hospital. Complaints that she was never able to 'feel for the child' are common, as are statements that the baby ignores her and isn't interested in the food she has to offer. Often the mother asserts that she noted nothing wrong with the infant and was surprised at the shock expressed by a relative or physician at her child's cachectic state. Only when the child is taken out of her charge and institutionalized as the proper responsibility of others is she able to perceive it in its being.

Such a mother is self-centred by definition. Her sphere of perception is so restricted that it cannot accommodate her child of whom she disposes through denial. Yet in other areas of her life she may well be able to extend her awareness to include others.

It is her knowledge of the very existence of the child which is denied rather than some specific attribute which she perceives in the child. It is not what he is, but rather *that he is* which the mother cannot stand knowing. This mother is highly vulnerable to post-partum depression of psychotic proportions. Knowledge of the existence of her child would fill her with an unbearable sense of unworthiness. She spares herself this burden by denying the existence of the child who in turn fails to thrive. For such a mother the existence of the particular child is a fulfilment of wishes which she has rejected as inadmissible. The reasons for her having reached such a conclusion are deeply rooted in her past and dwell beyond her range of conscious access. As long as the mother harbours her prohibition of this conception she remains vulnerable to severe depression or the child will fail to thrive as a result of obligatory neglect. These mothers, when forced by external circumstances to lay claim to the child as actually belonging to them, are prone to suicide and infanticide

The child should not be returned to the mother until she has been helped to alleviate her own prohibition of this pregnancy sufficiently to allow her to experience the child as belonging to her. This point can best be determined by observing the way in which the mother feeds the child. The act of feeding epitomizes the symbiosis so essential to the early development of the child. As long as the mother needs to see the feeding of her child as belonging to another, he is not safe. Once she can take this act as her due, the acute danger is past.

4

The Exploited Child

Definition

The exploited child lives in a state of partial symbiosis with a parent for whom he provides a specific intrapsychic function which they share. His performance of a particular psychological service for the parent is the basis of his primary value for both parent and child. All other aspects of the child's being are subordinated in their claim upon energies for development. The exploited child functions as a pseudopod extending the parent's psychic structure to fulfil a task specialized in accordance with a preexisting failure in the parent's personal development.

Maturation demands the sequential mastery of developmental tasks each of which involves the resolution of appetites with their corresponding expectations for behaviour. A state of inner conflict will persist if the parent has been unable to bring about a harmonious fusion of his desires and his performance. Under certain circumstances the parent may seek relief by exploiting a particular child as the repository for one of the constituents of his own conflict. The child is made the agent of an appetite or the standard bearer of a prohibition. In either instance he functions as a prosthetic device for the adult. The exploited child has been sent upon a man's mission.

Description

The hallmark of the exploited child is stamped in some aspect of his appearance as a caricature of adulthood. In word, gesture, facies, posture or deed the exploited child conveys his efforts to perform a psychological function suited to an adult. Overall the child does not act his age. His demeanour and countenance may appear to be older or younger than his years but some feature of his being will have the mark of adulthood. This behaviour, this function and this part of his body are strained with the burden of the precocious fulfilment of a requirement for adulthood.

Other aspects of the child's being have suffered a reciprocal inhibition in their development. Attitudes, interests and behaviour appropriate to the child's actual years are missing having been abandoned by the wayside in favour of the adult function in which the child has specialized.

When the charge of his own minimal needs plus the surtax imposed by the parental assignment exceed his capacity the child is liable to break down in certain recognizable fashion. The presenting symptoms and signs to which the exploited child is particularly vulnerable are influenced by the function and the organ which have been stressed with the burden of adult assignment. These can be classified in terms of the desires served and/or the prohibitions enforced.

Certain cases of childhood obesity are due to the exploitation of the child's feeding to satiate the parent's appetite. The adult's eyes are bigger than the child's stomach. These children are enormous. They eat all the time without knowing why. They deny any pleasure in eating. They have no likes or dislikes or any food fads. They eat automatically without gusto or discrimination. They have been fed incessantly like a stuffed Strasbourg goose. Yet when removed from their homes they welcome dieting and weight loss which is usually reversed upon return.

Some children do not master control of their bowel function and persist in defecating when and where they do. Often the history is of sparse and short-lived efforts by the parent to train the child with eccentric practices such as spreading newspapers about the house or rubbing the child's face in his feces. The parental attentions to the child's fecal functions are less in the service of the mastery of continence and more to obtain vicarious freedom from the fetters of self-control through the perpetuation of the child's messiness.

Certain children display a precocious air of interest in sexual intercourse. In word or posture, act or suggestion they invite adult attention towards their genitalia. Many of these children have been directly stimulated by a parent or knowingly have been exposed to the sexual attentions of another adult.

Certain children display disordered behaviour characterized by their repeated involvement in accidents from which they suffer fractures, burns and lacerations. The activities in which they are hurt are appropriate to a much older person. Study of the circumstances of the accident often reveals that the parent had directly invited the child to participate in an act which served to gratify the parent's own desires for violence. The child describes the event in the vernacular of an adult as if he viewed the act as quite consistent with his station. The desires served are as much or more the parent's than the child's. It is not merely that the parent fails to declare a prohibition but rather he issues an invitation to the child to partake of a particular bodily activity.

Conversely there are children who are exploited to subserve a parental need to erect prohibitions against their own instinctual cravings. Many children obtain precocious impeccable control of their bodies. They regulate their mouths, their eyes, their limbs and their sphincters as if their very lives depended upon it. They believe that they do. This performance is not merely to please the parent. It is based upon their appreciation that the parent's psychic integrity and with it their own protection depend upon their sparing the parent from the threat of loosely regulated appetites.

There are children who inhibit their intake of food to the point of weight loss. They have concluded that the food is bad or that the act of eating is bad or that they themselves are bad. The attendant self-deprivation roots out a major source of human pleasure. Often study reveals that the parent had directly asked the child to support efforts at restriction of food because of his own difficulty in mastering the intensity of his appetites.

There are certain children who have imposed such complete prohibition upon the relaxation of their anal sphincters that they develop severe constipation. They pass days without moving their bowels save for overflow incontinence. Usually these children were subjected to early and desperate toilet training that bespoke their parent's anxiety about the act of defecation and whatever pleasures they associated with it.

Certain children, particularly girls, are subject to disorders of urination characterized by burning and frequency without evidence of infection. They occasionally wet themselves during the day but not at night. They go to the toilet many times a day and always need to know its location. These children charge the control of urination with great concern. Their urethral sensations serve to remind them of the threat posed to them by the loss of control.

Some children pass through childhood and adolescence without showing any awareness of their genitalia. They do not touch, fondle or display. They do not masturbate. They behave as if the world were asexual and they had neither genitalia nor erotic sensations. With the advent of pubescence these children are vulnerable to the development of headaches which become preoccupying and a cause for severe restriction in their social intercourse. Often these children come from homes in which sexuality in all its dimensions was denied. The child responds to the parent's stand that the existence of the genitals and their sensations is too dangerous to recognize and he protects that position.

There are certain children whose early attempts to discharge energy through the exercise of their musculature upon their parents failed to elicit a response. It takes two to play patty-cake. These children often grow awkward, inhibited, and passive in their attitude towards the energies of aggression.

Regardless of the appetites served or the standard carried the exploited child has the cast of asymmetry to his development. He is a psychological specialist trained to perform one particular function at the expense of others. He is old in one respect and young in others.

The differential diagnosis of the exploited child lies with the child who has identified with an adult or the child who spontaneously has grown in an asymmetric fashion. The diagnosis is based upon the failure of the exploited child to derive pleasure from the exercise of his skill. Whatever the instinct expressed or the prohibition maintained the child works for the adult. His behaviour aims at the parent's relief and it takes its power from the urgency of that need. The exploited child may derive pride in the exercise of his function but not pleasure. His behaviour is not harnessed to his appetites or his expectations. He is in life's business for another. The nature of his actions is determined by the dictates of his parent's needs rather than taking source from the initiative of his own identifications. His performance is prescribed as obligatory in the priority of prerequisites for parentage.

Parents

Exploitation of a child by his parent is a process of which neither is conscious. The main purpose of exploitation is to spare the parent from conscious knowledge of one element of his intra-psychic conflict, either an appetite or its prohibition. The attainment of this goal requires that neither parent nor child know what they are doing. The resultant motivational vacuum is filled with rationalizations which constitute a contract in which the child and parent agree to exchange psychic service for upbringing. The pact comprises statements describing a relationship. Behind the manifest text is a secret treaty honoured in a private world. The covert clauses are written in the special syntax of a parent speaking to the child as if he were also the parent. Enforcement of the contract is implemented through the threat of abandonment by the parent and betrayal by the child.

The translation of such terms into their unconscious meaning requires the observer to note the words, the way they are spoken, the physical placement of the parent and child, intonation, gesture and what goes unsaid. It is as much how it is done as it is what is done. The mother says to the physician of her incontinent 6-year-old son, 'We are having trouble with *our* bowel movements, doctor!' She means 'His bowels are my bowels!'

The father says of his exhibitionistic 10-year-old daughter, 'I'm afraid she doesn't like psychiatrists, doctor. She doesn't like to make trouble!' He means, 'I don't want a psychiatrist to confront me with my incestuous longings for her'.

The parent says of the child, 'I can read her mind and she thinks just as I do!' He means, 'I will do all the talking for her and don't you talk to the child nor the child to you!'

The parent says to the child, 'All of us Smiths think so and act this way and do that!' He means, 'If you want to remain a member of the Smith family you had better do and be as I tell you!'

The father says to the daughter, 'Now dear, you don't *really* mean that, do you?' He means, 'The reality of your desires is not admissible to me.'

The mother says to her daughter, 'Why must you always try to get your own way?' She means, 'Your own desires are not an acceptable basis for the conduct of your life.'

The father says to his daughter, 'You are a great help to me, dear. I don't know what I'd do without you!' He means, 'If you don't do it for me I will leave you!'

The mother says to her son in desperation, 'If you don't behave and do what I tell you, I just don't know what I'll do!' She means, 'Go ahead and do it—I won't try to stop you!'

The mother says to her daughter recalcitrant at feeding, 'I am going upstairs and when I return I want to see your plate all cleaned up!' She means, 'If you do not eat, I will leave you!'

Such words might be ordinary talk in the mouths of others. But to these parents, spoken in a certain fashion at a particular time with other words unsaid, the sentences convey the charged details of a secret treaty.

Children love secrets. As viewed through the magnifying glass of childhood, secrets are one of the brightest trappings of the grown-up world. The prestige of being despatched upon a secret mission is a source of great exhilaration for the child. It is a bonus he receives in reward for sacrificing the knowledge of his own wants and his own goals in order to serve his parent. Furthermore, the pact is drawn up in the special language of an adult addressing a child as if he were endowed with the psychic equipment of an adult. The vocabulary of adult appetites and morality is used to bully, exhort and ride herd on the instincts of childhood.

If one hunts a fly with an elephant gun, after a while the fly begins to think of itself as an elephant. So too the exploited child comes to view himself as an adult. With his special rewards there are special burdens. But because the true terms of the pact are hidden beyond the reach of consciousness, they are not available for re-negotiation through the direct use of words or actions to express affects.

A re-negotiation of the terms basic to the maintenance of the parentage contract often ensues upon the development of an alteration in the child's body either in locus, function or both. The child may run away from the parent. The parent may send the child away from him. Accidents, fractures, burns, poisonings, feeding disorders, a variety of hysterical afflictions of the motor or sensory functions of the nervous system, the onset of anorexia nervosa, ulcerative colitis, systemic lupus erythematosus and rheumatoid arthritis have been observed to occur in children who had been exploited by their parents. The onset of these conditions was followed by a dramatic though transient change in the nature of the relationship of the parent and the child and the terms upon which they lived together.

5

Summary

The battered child, the neglected child and the exploited child each represent a dysfunction of parenting in which culture of the child has been sacrificed for the maintenance of the parent's psychological homeostasis.

The battered child responds acutely with a pattern of fright or flight into immobility. Recovery is usually prompt with appropriate treatment. The most apparent sequel is the persistence of a sadomasochistic mode of relating to the world. The battered child retains the ability to relate to others. The warmth of wrath appears to sustain his sense of self.

The neglected child responds with a failure to thrive physically and/or psychologically. The isolation imposed by a parent who is present but inaccessible deprives the child of a human with whom to live. His capacities arrive in accordance with his biologic stage but he fails to exercise or develop them for want of another's interest in his presence. The condition is reversible with vigorous and appropriate treatment aimed at providing the child with human contact to evoke pleasure at the exercise of his skills. Defects in the establishment of a hierarchy of relationships persist and the neglected child likely retains a promiscuous attitude towards others. The chill of indifference appears to blight his sense of self.

The exploited child responds by distorting his development to accommodate to his parent's intrapsychic requirements. He fails to harness his behaviour to his appetites in favour of serving his parent's needs. The exploited child appears particularly vulnerable to the development of disturbance in his physical functions. Treatment is aimed at separating the parent's need from the child's function so that each may better serve himself. A frequent sequel is the recurrent liability to exploitation by others as a source of a sense of self.

The parent who batters his child hates some part of himself which he projects on to the child. He beats the child to exorcize that attribute while still retaining that part of the child he loves.

The parent who neglects his child hates some part of himself which he denies. To avoid his self-hatred he must avoid the child in whom he fears to see himself.

The parent who exploits his child attempts to retain ownership of the elements of a personal conflict. He takes the child in partnership assigning to him a function which spares the parent from conscious suffering while preserving his integrity.

REFERENCES

1. ADELSON, LESTER. 1961. Slaughter of the innocents—a study of forty-six homicides in which the victims were children. *New Eng. J. Med.*, **264**, 1345-49.
2. ADELSON, LESTER, 1963. Homicide by starvation—the nutritional varient of the 'Battered child'. *J. Am. med. Assn*, **186**, 104-06.
3. ALLEN, ANNE, and MORTON, ARTHUR, 1961. *This is your child: the story of the National Society for the Prevention of Cruelty to Children.* London, Routledge and Kegan Paul, Ltd.
4. ANDREWS, J. P., 1962. The battered baby syndrome. *Illinois med. J.*, **122**, 494.
5. BAIN, KATHERINE, 1963. The physically abused child. *Pediatrics*, **31**, 895-97.
6. BAKWIN, HARRY, 1956. Multiple skeletal lesions in young children due to trauma. *Pediat.*, **49**, 7-16.
7. BAKWIN, HARRY, 1962. Report of the meeting of American Humane Society. *Newsletter (Am. Acad. Pediat.)*, **13**, 5.
8. BARMEYER, G. H., ANDERSON, L. R., and COX, W. B., 1951. Traumatic periostitis in young children. *J. Pediat.*, **38**, 184-190.
9. BARTA, R. A., Jr., and SMITH, NATHAN, J., 1963. Willful trauma to young children. *Clin. Pediat., Pa.*, **2**, 545-54.
10. BOARDMAN, HELEN E., 1962. A project to rescue children from inflicted injuries. *Social Work*, **7**, 43-51.
11. BRAUN, J. G., BRAUN, E. J., and SIMONDS, C. 1963. The mistreated child. *California Med.*, **99**, 98-103.
12. BRYANT, HAROLD D., *et al.*, 1963. Physical abuse of children: an agency study. *Child Welfare*, **42**, 125-30.
13. CAFFEY, J., 1946. Multiple fractures in the long bones of infants suffering from chronic subdural hematoma. *Am. J. Roentgenol.*, **56**, 163-73.
14. CAFFEY, J., 1946. Infantile cortical hyperostosis. *J. Pediat.*, **29**, 541-59.
15. CAFFEY, J., 1950. *J. Pediat. X-ray Diagn.*, **2**, 684-87.
16. CAFFEY, J., 1957. Traumatic lesions in growing bones other than fractures and dislocations—clinical and radiological features; the MacKenzie Davidson Memorial Lecture. *Brit. J. Radiol.*, **30**, 225-38.
17. CHESSER, EUSTACE, 1952. *Cruelty to children.* New York, Philosophical Library, Inc.
18. Children's Bureau, Welfare Administration, U.S. Department of Health, Education, and Welfare, 1963. *The abused child—principles and suggested language for legislation on reporting of the physically abused child.* Washington, D.C., U.S. Government Printing Office.
19. Children's Division, American Humane Association, 1963. *Guidelines for Legislation to protect the battered child.* Denver, Col., American Humane Association.
20. CLASS, NORRIS E., 1960. Neglect, social deviance, and community action. *Natl Probat. and Parole Assn J.*, **6**, 17-23.
21. COLES, ROBERT, 1964. Terror-struck children. *The New Republic*, May 30.
22. CONNELL, JOHN R., Jr., 1963. The devil's battered children: the increasing incidence of willful injuries to children. *J. Kansas med. Soc.*, **64**, 385-91.
23. CURTIS, G. C., 1963. Violence breeds violence—perhaps. *Am. J. Psychiat.*, **120**, 386-87.
24. DAVID, LESTER, 1964. The shocking price of parental anger. *Good housekeeping*, 181-86, March.
25. DEFRANCIS, VINCENT, 1963. *Child abuse—preview of a nationwide survey.* Denver, Col., Children's Division, American Humane Association.

26. DEFRANCIS, VINCENT, 1963. Parents who abuse children. *PTA Magazine*, **58**, 16-18.
27. DEFRANCIS, VINCENT, 1964. *Review of legislation to protect the battered child: a study of laws enacted in 1963.* Denver, Col., Children's Division, American Humane Association.
28. DELSORDO, JAMES D., 1963. Protective casework for abused children. *Children*, **10**, 213-18.
29. DUNCAN, G. M., FRAZIER, S. H., LITIN, E. M., JOHNSON, A. M., and BARRON, A. J., 1958. Etiological factors in first-degree murder. *J. Am. med. Assn*, **168**, 1755-58.
30. ELMER, ELIZABETH, 1960. Abused young children seen in hospitals. *Social Work*, **5**, 98-102.
31. ELMER, ELIZABETH, 1963. Identification of abused children. *Children*, **10**, 180-84.
32. ERWIN, DONALD T., 1964. The battered child syndrome. *Medico-Legal Bull.*, **130**, 1-10.
33. FAIRBURN, A. C., and HUNT, A. C., 1964. Caffey's 'third syndrome'—a critical evaluation ('The battered baby'). *Med. Sci. Law*, **4**, 123-26.
34. FEINSTEIN, H. N., et al., 1964. Group therapy for mothers with infanticidal impulses. *Am. J. Psychiat.*, **120**, 882-86.
35. FERGUSON, WILLIAM M., 1964. Battered child syndrome. Attorney general's opinion regarding the reporting of such occurrences. *J. Kansas med. Soc.*, **65**, 67-69.
36. FISHER, S. H., 1958. Skeletal manifestations of parent-induced trauma in infants and children. *S. med. J.*, **51**, 956-60.
37. FLATO, CHARLES, 1962. Parents who beat children. *Saturday evening post*, **235**, 30-35.
38. FONTANA, VINCENT J., DONOVAN, DENIS, and WONG, RAYMOND J., 1963. The maltreatment syndrome in children. *New Eng. J. Med.*, **269**, 1389-94.
39. FRIEDMAN, MORRIS, 1958. Traumatic periostitis in infants and children. *J. Am. med. Assn*, **166**, 1840-45.
40. GALDSTON, RICHARD, 1965. Observation on children who have been physically abused and their parents. *Am. J. Psychiat.*, **122**, 440.
41. GILL, THOMAS D., 1960. The legal nature of neglect. *Natl Probat. Parole Assn J.*, **6**, 1-16.
42. GREENGARD, J., 1964. The battered child syndrome. *Med. Sci.*, **15**, 82-91.
43. GREENGARD, J., 1964. The battered child syndrome. *Am. J. Nursing*, **64**, 98-100.
44. GRIFFITHS, D. L., and MOYNIHAN, F. J., 1963. Multiple epiphysial injuries in babies ('battered baby' syndrome). *Brit. med. J.*, ii, 1558-61.
45. GWINN, JOHN L., LEWIN, KENNETH W., and PETERSON, HERBERT G., Jr., 1961. Roentgenographic manifestations of unsuspected trauma in infancy. *J. Am. med. Assn*, **176**, 926-29.
46. HANCOCK, CLAIRE, 1963. *Children and neglect . . . hazardous home conditions.* Bureau of Family Services, Welfare Administration, U.S. Department of Health, Education and Welfare. U.S. Government Printing Office.
47. HARPER, FOWLER V., 1963. The physician, the battered child, and the law. *Pediatrics*, **31**, 899-902.
48. HOUSDEN, LESLIE GEORGE, 1956. *The prevention of cruelty to children.* New York, Philosophical Library, Inc.
49. JACOBZINER, HAROLD, 1964. Rescuing the battered child. *Am. J. Nursing*, **64**, 92-97.
50. JONES, HENRY H., and DAVIS, JOSEPH H., 1957. Multiple traumatic lesions of the infant skeleton. *Stanford med. Bull.*, **15**, 259-73.

KAPLAN, MORRIS, 1962. Deaths of young studied by city. *New York Times*.

52. KEMPE, C. HENRY, et al., 1962. The battered-child syndrome. *J. Am. med. Assn*, **181**, 17-24.
53. LEIKEN, S. L., et al., 1963. Clinical pathological conference: the battered child syndrome. *Clin. Proc. Children's Hosp., Wash., D.C.*, **19**, 301-06.
54. LESERMAN, SIDNEY, 1964. There's a murderer in my waiting room. *Med. Econ.*, **41**, 62-71.
55. MCCORT, J., et al., 1964. Visceral injuries in battered children. *Radiology*, **82**, 424-28.
56. MCHENRY, THOMAS, GIRDANY, BERTRAM R., and ELMER, ELIZABETH, 1963. Unsuspected trauma with multiple skeletal injuries during infancy and childhood. *Pediatrics*, **31**, 903-08.
57. MERRILL, EDGAR J., et al., 1962. *Protecting the battered child.* Denver, Col., Children's Division, American Humane Association.
58. MILLER, DONALD S., 1959. Fractures among children. *Minnesota Med.*, **42**, 1209-13; 1414-25.
59. MINTZ, A. A., 1964. Battered child syndrome. *Texas J. Med.*, **60**, 107-08.
60. MORRIS, MARIAN G., and GOULD, ROBERT W., 1963. Role reversal: a necessary concept in dealing with the 'battered child syndrome'. *Am. J. Orthopsychiat.*, **33**, 298-99.
61. MORRIS, MARIAN G., GOULD, ROBERT W., and MATTHEWS, PATRICIA J., 1964. Toward prevention of child abuse. *Children*, **11**, 55-60.
62. MYREN, RICHARD A., and SWANSON, LYNN D., 1962. *Police work with children.* Children's Bureau, Welfare Administration, U.S. Department of Health, Education and Welfare. U.S. Government Printing Office.
63. O'DOHERTY, N. J., 1964. Subdural haematoma in battered babies. *Developl Med. Child Neurol.*, **6**, 192-93.
64. OETTINGER, KATHERINE B., 1964. Protecting children from abuse. *Parents*, **39**, 12.
65. PFUNDT, T. R., 1964. The problem of the battered child. *Postgraduate Med.*, **35**, 426-31.
66. PLATOU, R. V., 1964. Battering. *Bull. Tulane med. Fac.*, **23**, 157-65.
67. POTTS, W. E., and FORBIS, O. L., 1962. Willful injury in childhood—a distinct syndrome. *Arkansas med. Soc.*, **59**, 266-70.
68. REIN, MARTIN. 1963. *Child protective services in Massachusetts.* Waltham, Florence Heller Graduate School for Advanced Studies in Social Welfare, Brandeis University.
69. REINHART, J. B., et al., 1964. The abused child: mandatory reporting legislation. *J. Am. med. Assn*, **188**, 358-62.
70. REZZA, EMILIO, and DE CARO, B., 1962. Fratture ossee multiple in lattante associate a distrofia, anemia e ritardo mentale. *Acta Paediatrica Latina*, **15**, 121-39 (with numerous references to European articles).
71. RICE, M. P., 1964. The battered child. *Henry Ford Hospital med. Bull.*, **12**, 401.
72. RIESE, HERTA, 1920. *Heal the hurt child.* Chicago, Univ. Press.
73. SCHACHTER, M., 1952. Contribution to the clinical and psychological study of mistreated children; physical and moral cruelty. *Giorn. Psichiat. Neuropatol. (Ferrara)*, **80**, 311-17.
74. SCHLEYER, F., and PIOCH, W., 1957. Fatal outcome by crush syndrom after continuous beatings of a child. *Monatsschrift Kinderheilkunde*, **105**, 392-94.
75. SCHLOESSER, PATRICIA T., 1964. The abused child. *Bull. Menninger Clinic*, **28**, 260-68.
76. SCHROTEL, S. R., 1961. Responsibilities of physicians in suspected csess of brutality. *Cinicinnati J. Med.*, **42**, 406-07.

77. SHAW, ANTHONY, 1963. How to help the battered child. *RISS* (National Magazine for residents, internes, and senior students published by *Medical Economics*), **6**, 71-104.
78. SHERRIFF, H., 1964. The abused child. *J. S. Carolina med. Assn*, **60**, 191-93.
79. SILVER, HENRY K., and KEMPE, C. HENRY, 1959. The problem of parental criminal neglect and severe physical abuse of children. Read at annual meeting of the American Pediatric Society, May 1959. *Am. J. Dis. Children*, **98**, 528.
80. SILVERMAN, F. N., 1953. The roentgen manifestations of unrecognized skeletal trauma in infants. *Am. J. Roentgenol., Rad. Ther. Nucl. Med.*, **69**, 413-27.
81. SILVERMAN, F. N., 1965. The battered child. *Manitoba med. Rev.*, **45**, 473.
82. SNEDEKER, LENDON, 1962. Traumatization of children. *New Eng. J. Med.*, **267**, 572.
83. SWANSON, LYNN D., 1961. Role of the police in the protection of children from neglect and abuse. *Fed. Probation*, **25**, 43-48.
84. TEN BENSEL, R. W., and RAILE, R. B., 1963. The battered child syndrome. *Minnesota Med.*, **46**, 977-82.
85. WOOLLEY, P. V., Jr., and EVANS, W. A., Jr., 1955. Significance of skeletal lesions in infants resembling those of traumatic origin. *J. Am. med. Assn*, **158**, 539-43.
86. WOOLLEY, P. V., Jr., 1963. The pediatrician and the young child subjected to repeated physical abuse. *J. Pediat.*, **62**, 628-30.
87. YOUNG, LEONTINE, 1964. *Wednesday's children: a study of child neglect and abuse*. New York, McGraw Hill.

Articles

88. The battered child syndrome. *Currents in public health* (Ross Laboratories), 1962.
89. Wilful injuries to children. 1962. (Abbott Laboratories). *What's new*.
90. *New York Times*, May 5, 1962; November 11, 1963; March 21, 1964; April 5, 1964; November 8, 1964.
91. The battered baby, 1966. *Brit. med. J.*, i, 601.

Editorials

92. 1961. *J. Am. med. Assn*, **176**, 942-43.
93. 1962. *J. Am. med. Assn*, **181**, 42.
94. The battered child syndrome. 1963. *J. Louisiana med. Soc.*, **115**, 322-24.
95. Physicians required to report child beatings. 1963. *Minnesota Med.*, **46**, 876.
96. The child abuse problem in Iowa. The extent of the problem, and a proposal for remedying it. *J. Iowa State med. Soc.*, **53**, 692-94.
97. More on the battered child. 1963. *New England J. Med.*, **269**, 1436.
98. The abused child, parents, and the law. 1964. *Rhode Island med. J.*, **47**, 89-90.
99. Assaulted children. 1964. *Lancet*, i, 543-44.
100. Child abuse and the physician's responsibility. 1964. *Postgraduate Med.*, **35**, 446.
101. *News Report*. 1961. *Med. Wld News*, **2**, 30.

XXII

THREE HISTORIC PAPERS

When the vexed question of the nature and classification of states of childhood psychosis is under discussion, three names are rarely omitted—those of de Sanctis, Heller and Kanner. All three have delimited a syndrome in the field.

The paper by de Sanctis, published in 1906, contains his first clear description of *Dementia Praecocissima*, a description elaborated later, in 1925, in his book 'Neuropsichiatria Infantile'. Heller described his first six cases of *Dementia Infantilis* in 1908; the paper published here is the result of his 22 years of additional experience and the study of 28 cases. Kanner's paper contains his first description of the syndrome called by him *Early Infantile Autism*, published in 1943 in a journal that has now ceased publication.

It is hoped that making these papers readily available will be a contribution to the study of childhood psychosis and a useful prelude to the chapters that follow.

1

ON SOME VARIETIES OF DEMENTIA PRAECOX*

Professor SANTE DE SANCTIS
University of Rome

Introductory Note by the Editor

This translation is of an historic paper by de Sanctis. In the course of assessing Kraepelin's description of Dementia Praecox, he delineates a syndrome, *Dementia Praecocissima* with which his name was subsequently always associated; this syndrome is invariably considered in any discussion of the nature of childhood psychosis.

De Sanctis in the first part of the introduction puts the case for continued re-assessment of Kraepelin's views. In the second part he considers the relationship between phrenasthenia (mental retardation) and dementia praecox (premature insanity) and in doing so identifies the first issue to be discussed later in his paper. In this part of the introduction he also explains how it has often been suggested, e.g. by Toulouse, that before puberty there exists only phrenasthenia and after it only psychosis. De Sanctis disagrees as he believes that dementia praecox exists in childhood; this he calls dementia praecocissima (very premature) and constitutes the second issue to be discussed later in his paper. In the third part of his introduction de Sanctis observes that dementia praecox might be thought to be misnamed, as it can appear in later life, and so he postulates that the process started early but the signs were delayed in appearing; this is the third issue to be discussed later in his paper. In the fourth part of his introduction, he points to the possibility that early signs of dementia praecox may exist and be neglected; this is the fourth issue discussed in his paper. In his conclusion, he expresses views on classification and includes some discussion of the etiology of dementia praecox.

This paper was reproduced with the kind cooperation of Professor Carlo de Sanctis, the son of the author. The translator has taken pains to retain the style of the author as published in a journal at the beginning of the twentieth century.

Introduction

I

Dementia praecox is always a subject of great topicality. Most alienists have accepted the essentials of Kraepelin's concept; the Americans (Edward Cowles, F. X. Dercum, Adolph Meyer, Sprague and Hill, Dunton, etc.)[1] have done so no less than the Germans and the Italians. It is true,

---

* Translated by Maria-Livia Osborn, Research Assistant, The Institute of Family Psychiatry, Ipswich, from the original Italian paper published in 1906 in *Rivista Sperimentale di Freniatria*, **32**, 141-65.

however, that the French are not yet resigned to suffer a German import of such scientific and practical importance. While others, as for instance J. Séglas and recently A. V. Parant, greatly restrict the Kraepelian concept; others like Regis and E. Maradon de Montyel (just to quote the most recent)[2] pronounce as indubitably false the concept of dementia praecox, adhering instead, in name, in prognosis and in aetiology, to the description given by Christian.[3] The English are no less cautious in accepting Kraepelin's ideas. This is demonstrated by the controversy generated by a work of Conolly Norman[4]. Nevertheless, French and English psychiatry too have been partly influenced by the nosographic and clinical views of the illustrious psychiatrist of Munich. Who could, in fact, deny that the views of Kraepelin do not continue to shake the whole of modern psychiatric thought?

Once more, interest has been focused on the simple kind of dementia praecox (dementia simplex)[5] recognized by some of Kraepelin's followers[6] and discussed at length by O. Diem in 1903[7] and G. Monod[8] this year (1906)[9].

The nosographic and symptomatologic relationships between dementia praecox and hallucinatory psychoses are also still a subject of study by those who are unwilling to expand the Kraepelinian concept too much, e.g. Ziehn and the school of L. Bianchi in Italy[10]; it is also a subject of controversial discussion between our young alienists (Angiolella and Vedrani). In all the clinics and in all the mental hospitals one talks about dementia praecox; there are passionate discussions about it in the German, American and French press, as well as in ours. In these last few years, it has been the favourite topic in national and regional congresses of English, German and French neurologists and alienists. In the forthcoming international medical congress in Lisbon, it will be the subject of papers by W. Weygandt, by W. Tschisch and by Tamas Maestre Pérez from Madrid.

I believe it would be a good thing to discuss, reassess and correct these views. By having too circumscribed clinical categories and giving too much importance to symptoms we have reached in one jump an oversimplification. We must start again to subdivide, to separate and to distinguish; we must re-do a piece of work which has already required much study and much acumen by German and French psychiatrists. The followers of Kraepelin may well dislike this, but it would do no harm if they, as well as the misoneists, would keep in mind the extraordinary caution with which the Teacher of Munich deals with psychiatric problems[11].

Kraepelin is not sure whether the morbid process is always the same in the various forms grouped under the term 'dementia praecox'; he insists that such grouping is temporary, admitting that there are still no viewpoints by which it would be possible to group the material satisfactorily. He declares himself ready to renounce the previously preferred term 'dementia praecox'[12].

Therefore, every conscientious contribution to the nosography of dementia praecox may have a value not to be despised. Observation of clinical cases in the institutions of which I am in charge, and in my private practice, gives me the opportunity to discuss some issues.

II

First of all, I was particularly interested in one question, that of the relationships between dementia praecox and phrenasthenia.

Shüle[13] talks of hebephrenic idiocy, grouping together under this term those cases of juvenile insanity which end in idiocy, and those which are complicated by it. He observes that the true hebephrenia does not always develop from idiocy and that sometimes hebephrenia culminates in idiocy (not dementia, please note!).

At first, Shüle's acute observation may seem to cause confusion, but to appreciate it, despite its insufficient precision, one must remember an opinion expressed by Morel[14]. He pointed out that in some cases dementia is only the last phase of a development in a foetal anomaly with which the adolescent has been born. Again it is a significant coincidence that it was Morel who used the term 'démence précoce' for the premature dementia, which sometimes develops at puberty in the children of alcoholics and of the insane.

Toulouse[15] reaffirmed the enlightened view of Morel, when he stated that puberty is the dividing line between congenital psychic weaknesses and those acquired, or insanities, so that dementia praecox by the time of puberty should be regarded, Toulouse states, as idiocy in an individual congenitally predisposed to it.

But for some time a number of psychiatrists have already affirmed without reticence that the mental conditions of the weak and the imbeciles (phrenasthenics) become worse at puberty.

This fact has not escaped Esquirol and those who have described primary dementia, hereditary insanity, hebephrenia, heboidophrenia, moral insanity and various psychic disturbances which accompany and follow puberty.

Finzi and Vedrani[16] pointed to the 'relative frequency' with which imbeciles and idiots present symptoms of dementia praecox at puberty, or earlier, and sometimes following puberty. Finzi had himself noted that a dementia praecocissima may constitute a form of phrenasthenia. Many years ago I[17] spoke of progressive phrenasthenias. This term referred to the fact which I have often observed that phrenasthenic children, both the cerebral palsied and aparalytics (excluding epileptics) presented, despite the appropriate medico-pedagogic treatment, with advancing age, a mental deterioration progressively more accentuated (educational arrests and regressions). Certainly this was happening more frequently among school children in institutions for mentally deficients and abnormals, than among those in the ordinary elementary schools; this fact was recently noted by A. Cramer[18].

I do not feel like insisting on the term and on the concept of progressive phrenasthenias. On the contrary, it seems superfluous to bring under discussion Toulouse's premise, that is to say, whether a mental weakening appearing at puberty is, by definition, of phrenasthenic nature[19].

If we are to avoid academic discussion, I believe that, on the one hand, the classic concept of phrenasthenia given by Esquirol must be respected, and on the other, we must not doubt the autonomy of a psychosis, which usually develops at puberty, and which today we term dementia praecox.

However, more recently, I have had occasion to observe another fact of undoubted interest; that among phrenasthenic children some are to be found with a type of mentality clearly vesanic* (dementia praecox mentality)[20]. I could not decide, then, if those cases were individual variants of psychopathology, or true dementia praecox, which, taking into account the age of the patients, I termed *dementia praecocissima*. However, the fact remained and was not made less important by the difficulty of interpretation.

Thus, two distinct questions arise:

1. If, how and when dementia praecox does appear in phrenasthenics?

2. If a prepubertal dementia praecox exists, that is to say, a dementia that because of the time at which it presents, deserves the term 'praecocissima'.†

III

Another question was suggested by a different set of observations. The authors who follow the views of Kraepelin, and Kraepelin himself, have admitted that dementia praecox is not always a pubertal or juvenile psychosis, as it may appear in paranoid form in those aged over 30, and even in those over 40 or 45[21]. I think that this belief about the aetiology of dementia praecox must be reassessed. I certainly have no wish to doubt the possibility of cases of apparently primary states of dementia in the fifth decennium of life; I just wish to discuss whether these states of dementia are to be regarded, without any doubt, as due to dementia praecox. Please, allow me a preliminary observation.

If we agree purely and simply as to the possibility of development of a catatonic or paranoid form at the end of the fourth and during the fifth decennium, we implicitly sanction the breaking up of the aetiological harmony in the group-unit of dementia praecox. Again, on what basis can the unit of form be kept, when it is admitted: that there can be recovery; that in the first attacks there may be no intellectual *deficit*; that the state of

---

* Vesania—an early term and concept meaning insanity. Translator's note.

† *Praecocissima*—very premature, as against *Praecox*, premature. Translator's note.

dementia constitutes nothing more than 'a result'[22]; that the form at times has a continuous course and at other times it so frequently remits as to appear even intermittent; and lastly that it can happen even in advanced age, that is to say at over 45 years?

Although repeating old criticisms, Maradon de Montyel rightly observes that it is not proper to call a psychosis 'dementia' with a recovery rate estimated by some to be 44 per cent; moreover, I add, when it is stated that in a number of cases intelligence remained unaffected[23]. Also it is, to say the least, useless to call a condition 'praecox' (premature) when it can appear so late in life. Therefore unity could be maintained on symptomatologic criteria only—criteria so opposed, as a taxinomic rule, by Kraepelin and his followers! Therefore, it seems to me that we must at least seriously discuss the fact, so easily admitted nowadays, of the late appearance of dementia praecox and find its causes, as far as it is possible.

IV

Another question, distinct from those mentioned above, and yet connected with them, concerns the childhood of dementia praecox patients. It is admitted that hebephrenia, as other forms of dementia praecox, may appear in subjects previously intelligent and completely normal; but I have been able to collect together some curious facts, which raise serious doubts about the claim for mental integrity of those who become cases of dementia praecox. These facts have at least caused one to ask whether in the childhood of these subjects there are often already revealing signs of their destiny. This problem could be connected with the aetiology of dementia praecox.

V

To sum up, I would like to discuss the following clinico-nosographic problems concerning dementia praecox.

1. Does a *subsequens or comitans dementia praecox* exist (which follows or accompanies phrenasthenia)?

2. Does a dementia *praecocissima* (of childhood) exist?

3. Does a *dementia praecox retardata* exist? (Later the reason will be clear why I prefer the qualifying adjective *retardata* (deferred) rather than 'late' which comes to mind first.)

4. Has dementia praecox in its *subsequens* or *comitans* forms, as well as in its *retardata* form, any premonitory signs in the evolutive ages of life?

In this brief preliminary note I make no claim at all to answer these questions conclusively, but my aim here is to summarize, very concisely, the results of my clinical experience on this subject and so to invite the alienists to collect together the necessary documents for the final resolutions of these problems.

1. *Dementia praecox subsequens* or *comitans*[24].

Provisionally I will thus call the dementia praecox, which usually appears in mentally defective subjects, that is the so-called phrenasthenics (idiots, imbeciles, retarded, mentally deficients, etc.). Perhaps not all alienists are as convinced as I am about the frequency of this form; and yet this fact can so easily be observed that it would not seem worth pausing over it, if various alienists were not so obstinate in confusing the true dementia praecox of the phrenasthenic, with periods of agitation common to idiots and imbeciles, or confusing it with psychopathologic states such as episodes of delirium, depression, etc. in the so-called degenerates. It is in deference to the precision which clinical forms must take, that I insist on this, which, so as to understand each other, I provisionally call *dementia praecox subsequens* or *comitans*. Actually, this variety is very common; in a few months and in a restricted field of observation, that is outside the asylum, six cases have come my way, all of which I have carefully studied and followed for a fairly long time. I now believe that in the prognosis of educable phrenasthenic children the possibility of *dementia praecox* must be taken into serious account.

Here are my conclusions about this clinical variety, from my personal experience:

(*a*) Dementia praecox *subsequens* or *comitans*, a fairly frequent variety, is more common in females than in males. Of my last six cases, four were females.

(*b*) In my six cases it first appeared between 12 and 20 years.

(*c*) The immediate apparent causes were: in one case a fever; in another a *surmenage* (?) (illtreatment), in two more or less intense emotions (fears, fright); in the other two, determining causes were elusive.

(*d*) Of the six cases, in one only the preceding phrenasthenic form was serious; in the other four it was fairly serious (mental retardation of a medium degree). One of the female patients had been able to learn— without special teaching—to read and write well and even to learn the basic elements of a foreign language (see typical case)—the other three subjects had all been able to go through, over the years, the first three years of elementary education. But in all, mental retardation had been ascertained since their infancy, by both their families and their doctors. Thus, on the basis of my experience, I can state that seriously ill phrenasthenics are less prone than the others to dementia praecox.

(*e*) All six cases were aparalytic phrenasthenics, but among the cases I have observed previously, in two the original mental retardation was accompanied by epileptic attacks.

(*f*) The symptoms which indicated dementia praecox in my six cases were, in order of frequency, as follows: strangeness of character and capriciousness; apathy; depressed mood; guilt; negativism; hallucinations; agitation. In only one of the six cases was there pronounced catatonia.

(g) In general, in phrenasthenics struck by dementia praecox it is evident that the intellectual decline starts at about 11 or 12 years, and sometimes later, and progresses, at least for some months or a few years, so that it is necessary to interrupt any pedagogic treatment. More serious cases—those who come to the attention of the alienist—take on the guises of the hebephrenic forms, or of the paranoid forms; but many cases, that thus go unobserved, must be classified as forms of simple dementia. Some of these cases, which in 1901 partly suggested to me the concept of educational regressions[25], were in fact placid intellectual declines. Reading again what Kahlbaum wrote about the heboid forms and some cases in the literature (Diem, Cramer, Monod) termed simple or arrested dementia, I found them to be similar in all aspects to some of my cases of educational regression[26].

It seems to me unnecessary to refer to all six of the most recent cases which I have observed. I will report one only as a sample of the clinical variety which I am describing.

Typical case: S. A., female, aged 17 years.

The family is not altogether free from mental disorders; but five sisters and two brothers of the patient enjoy good physical and mental health. A has had no pathological episodes in her infancy or in her childhood, but from early years has shown poor intelligence which was evident both at home and at school. She was dull, unable to concentrate, of poor memory and, despite perfect physical development, was considered by all to be feebleminded. However, her behaviour was always normal; she studied willingly, so much so that, with great effort, she was able to complete all the elementary school course and two years of the middle school, and to learn a little French.

But we must note that she was educated in private schools, run by religious orders, and that she had to repeat the same year several times. However, her first communion* marked the beginning of feelings of guilt and depression. Nevertheless she remained of perfectly good behaviour until she was 16. At this age, with an increasing feeling of guilt, A started to present clear changes of behaviour; there was less show of affection towards her parents, negativism, disobedience, odd ideas and, as her mother said: 'strange ideas'.

There were days when A would even refuse to eat, saying that she wanted to mortify the flesh. She spent the Spring and Summer of 1905 moderately well, but in August became very restless, odd and difficult to reach. In September, when I saw her for the first time and did not know her anamnesis, I diagnosed her as a case of common dementia praecox. On October 3rd she was admitted to my clinic and on the 26th of the same month she was transferred to a sanatorium, because she had become agitated, odd, with swings of mood, changing her mind every moment and obstinately refusing to eat and to leave her room.

The following is a brief description of the objective symptoms presented by A at my clinic and in the sanatorium between 10th of October and 20th November.

She was a well-developed, dark-haired, eurhythmic subject; height 162 cm; weight 51 kg with underdeveloped thyroid;[27] she presents, however, a definite anatomical and functional facial asymmetry, the right half of the face being more mobile than the left; physiological functions are regular, except for some days when

* In the Roman Catholic Church this is taken when the child is about 7 years old—Translator's note.

she has halitosis, constipation, and sleep disturbances. No alteration in muscular strength in active and passive movements, in reflexes or in sensation.

On the mental side one is struck mostly by her silly behaviour, motor and affective instability, and meaningless talk. At times the patient is very agitated, destructive, threatening suicide, wants to run away, but nevertheless laughs and grimaces. During calm periods, she laughs or weeps, or she retires into obstinate silence, or expresses absurd ideas, says meaningless words, assumes stereotyped attitudes and affected and grotesque poses. Some days her negativism is extreme; for several days she has refused all food, is closed in mutism, refusing even to micturate and so necessitating the use of a catheter several times.

In her speech I have noted frequent clang associations, rhyming, word mutilation, neologisms, echolalia, verbigeration and word-salad (Wortsalat); the same symptoms were reflected in her writings. The following is an example of her talk:

'And I am sure that all the Saints in Heaven will help me in the end to become a novice of the sacramentalists, and there should be no more locomotives, nor carriages, nor horses. But all should walk with their legs. One must never rest by day or by night, but I would wish that nobody got drunk, and was impolite, lazy and vagabond, but that all worked by their own effort, and that the vines should be all thrown into the fire, in short, all burned and also the corn, etc. . . . in short everybody should be the same, or all should eat the same like in an institution.' Another time, the patient said, with much laughter: 'Sel . . . selleri . . . Good selleri. I shall do it, you shall do it, they shall do it. The French is beautiful . . . ne pas, papa, Napoleon, tigers, cruel beasts . . . No, no, no.' In the above passage superficial and clang associations are many. Even more characteristic are the writings of A. Below is one of her letters:

'My dear D.M.,
   Please send me half an onion, because instead of being called 'Assunta', I am called 'Addolorata', therefore you will be so kind as to send me also the tears of Our Lady.'

To another letter written in very bad French to her parents, she added the following words as postscript:

'But only tell the priest of St. Mary to change the name of Lucifer, or to call him in a different way, as I am afraid of him.'

The patient expresses the most absurd ideas, her state is openly demented. On the whole, during three months I have observed her, I found in her all the mental symptoms of dementia praecox.

2. *Dementia Praecocissima*

The authors who have dealt with hebephrenia, with heboidophrenia, simple or primary dementia etc. have not admitted the possibility that these diseases could also present many years before puberty. Stecker, Kahlbaum, Fink, Clouston, Bevan-Lewis, Ball Mairet, Spitzka and Marro all denied such a possibility. Seppilli[28] found puberty psychoses uncommon even between the ages of 12 and 14 years. But it would be useful to note that the so-called moral insanity (occurring after a trauma, an illness, or emotional shock) was found even among children. Again, in Bertschinger's figures there are also cases of dementia praecox at 10 years of age. However, it can be said that as yet there is no literature on *dementia praecocissima*. Kraepelin limits his remarks to stating that some observations make it likely that perhaps some states of mental weakness appearing in early childhood should be regarded as hebephrenic manifestations; he compares some catatonic disorders of the idiots to those found in the terminal phases of dementia praecox, and quotes Masion's findings. Weygandt warns us that it is still an open question whether dementia praecox can be found before puberty.

In my paper, mentioned above, on 'Some types of mental deficiency', I said: 'For me there is no doubt that there are not infrequently mental deficiencies (phrenasthenias) in childhood, characterized, more or less, by the mental symptomatology of heboid and hebephrenic states ... there is no doubt as to whether we are in the presence of a separate clinical entity, or of a variety of phrenasthenia'. I can now confirm this, but I must enlarge on it. It seemed likely to me at that time, as I have already said, that the vesanic type was simply a type of mentality found in those of inferior intellect, since we must always carefully acknowledge causes of real intellectual *deficit* in infancy and in childhood, other than those producing phrenasthenia. My belief was reinforced also by the fact that children of the vesanic type of mentality could some times benefit from medico-pedagogic treatment, no less than phrenasthenic children of other mental types. However, I now have an objection; nobody could really exclude, because even phrenasthenics with vesanic mentality can improve, that they were not cases of true dementia praecox. From the recovery and educatability of the patients (therapeutic criterion) I made a wrong premise, thus suggesting that dementia praecox would be, always and in all its forms, incurable. Now, instead, I can state that some children regarded as phrenasthenic and presenting with frank vesanic mentality have not only improved, but have been cured. In this case, logic suggests that they were not phrenasthenic with vesanic mentality, but real cases of dementia praecox because, putting the symptomatology on one side, it is more logical to admit the cure of an attack of dementia praecox than that of a true phrenasthenia, which, to be precise, should not be regarded as an active pathologic process, but as the final result of a process.

Having said this, it is understood that I do not mean that all phrenasthenics with vesanic mentality are cases of dementia praecox. On the contrary, I would like to add that we must not confuse with dementia praecox other psychoses, which are commonly observed in children from 5 to 8 years of age, and which are usually cured. As examples, I will quote, because I have had occasion to observe them, states of hysterical dreaming, strange forms of delusion resembling paranoia in miniature, and hallucinatory psychoses. Also we must not confuse with dementia praecox other forms of dementia to be found in children; e.g. epileptic dementia, which is not at all rare. In conclusion, I do not diagnose dementia praecocissima unless the classic symptomatology of dementia praecox is present; I exclude it (admitting only a diagnosis of vesanic mentality type) when the child from early infancy has presented symptoms of dementia praecox and when, with vesanic mentality, he presents with such somatic phenomena (paresis, spasms, hypoplasia, etc.) to make us suspect prenatal or infantile cerebral palsy. I cannot, however, exclude cases of inherited syphilis from the diagnosis of dementia praecocissima. Indeed, it is strange that often my cases of dementia praecocissima have syphilitic parents and have the so-called ocular syphilitic stigmata. But, for the moment, I do not wish to go into details; enough that we can establish a form of dementia praecox in childhood, which I call *dementia praecocissima*, the prognosis of which is perhaps not always as grave as that of dementia praecox in adolescents and in adults, but which, like some heboid forms described by Kahlbaum, is sometimes cured.

A few months ago, while expanding my views to a German colleague, I learned from him that he too had come across dementia praecox in children, who were subsequently cured, and that Professor Binzwanger of Jena had also had a similar interesting case.

I. Typical Case: Flavio D., aged 10 years, male (observed in 1899).

Irascible father, impulsive but healthy. Paternal siblings excitable and of unconventional behaviour; mother 'chesty'; maternal grandfather alcoholic and brutal; maternal great-aunt insane.

F was born at full term by spontaneous delivery, teethed early, the first tooth appearing at four months and complete dentition by the first year. He started to walk at 3 years. Was late in developing speech and could pronounce words well only by the age of 5. He was always irritable even as a small child, but could attend school and profit a little by it; he has now completed the second year of elementary school. However, father notices that in the last two years the child's behaviour has become very strange and F is by now so changed that he cannot control him, he refuses to do whatever he is asked, and for this reason father has brought him to me.

Well-developed child, slightly pale, brachycephalic, large faced, flat nosed. Weight 26·500 kg, height 126 cm, some degenerative signs. Poor general nutritional state. Weak respiration; F has bronchitis frequently, but his heart is healthy, though prone to palpitations, especially at night. Appetite poor. Excessive perspiration at night, both in summer and in winter. Heavy sleeper, but with frequent night terrors. Moves about a lot in his sleep. Trophic state of muscles, normal. Quick superficial reflexes, normal patellas. Normal active and passive movements. When asked, can achieve all digital movements, but it takes time and patience to get him to perform them, as he is inattentive most of the time or indulges in playing about. Normal muscular strength. Vision: Right Visual Acuity $= \frac{1}{3}$; Left Visual Acuity $= \frac{1}{2}$. Distinguishes well green, red and yellow. Hyperaesthesia of the retina with reflex lacrimation. Localised trachoma of the tarsal conjunctivas. Tegmental sensation, normal; great tolerance to pain provoked by mechanical stimuli. Well-developed feeling of being satiated, but poor feeling of hunger. F's attention can be engaged quickly and held for a fair period, unless he is playing. Often he will contemplate an object at length and ask many questions about it. Fair memory; very good musical memory; father says F has a 'good ear' for music. Can add and subtract numbers up to 1,000; finds multiplications difficult. Can read fairly well, but writes very badly. Is afraid of the dark, but seems to have no fear of other things. Frequent and quick outbursts of rage; no erotic tendencies observable. No feeling of pity: F is cruel to animals; shows rather vivid organic emotivity, cries and laughs with extreme ease, but his feelings are blunted. He is unaffectionate. His spasmodic laugh is peculiar, in short bursts, but very easily provoked by a word or an event a bit lively. When I asked him why he laughs so noisily and at such length, he either does not answer or says 'who knows?' His mood is usually gay, but mostly changeable. His behaviour is silly; unmotivated actions, grotesque poses, grimaces, affected walk and greeting. Infantile curiosity. Tendency to solitude and to alcoholic drinks. Dislikes collective games, avoids company and prefers to do nothing and to grimace by himself. Well-developed mimicry; mimics other people's expressions and gestures. Dislikes cleanliness, is untidy and unstable. At school behaves aimlessly, but shows fair memory and when it seems that he has not understood at all what the teacher has explained, he surprisingly repeats what she has said or read out. At times he has a really fatuous expression: laughs, repeats several times any gesture or movement, moves about, twists, grimaces with his mouth and eyes; and all this without any reason on earth. Father adds that often at home F will repeat the same word for many minutes; sometimes this is accompanied by the repetition of head and hand movements (stereotypy with verbigeration). Some days displays extreme negativism, even to the point of refusing to eat.

More recently I have been able to gather more data of the utmost interest from this patient, whom I had not seen since 1899. F has changed a great deal during the last six years. For about two years his condition was as described above, and his father was desolate; but then, the father reports, F became more serious, he sent him to work and at last, now that he is 15, is earning five liras per week.

The patient's improvement is due to neither teaching nor drugs. It came about slowly during the 'prepubertal period', after his mental deficiency and insanity, as his father puts it, had lasted for about six years. I cannot guarantee that a cure will follow this improvement. It is more likely that F will remain with a degree of intellectual *deficit*.

The diagnosis of dementia praecocissima in the above case seems to me correct without any doubt, for the following reasons: (*i*) the illness did not manifest itself in the neonate or infant, when phrenasthenia commonly appears, but it presented only during childhood; (*ii*) it did not seem to have obvious causes and had no concomitant motor or sensory symptoms; (*iii*) it presented the common symptoms of dementia praecox; (*iv*) unlike phrenasthenia it ran a well-defined course, like a true pathological process. I have observed at least five similar cases, which I believe I could distinguish from cases of phrenasthenia with vesanic mentality; however, in none of them I observed any improvement of the mental deficiency syndrome, as in the case described above.

I would now like to report one of those cases which leaves us in doubt whether it is a case of dementia praecocissima or of vesanic mentality in phrenasthenia.

Doubtful case: G. M., aged 6 years, male (observed in 1899).

The paternal grandfather committed suicide for love when aged 55. Father is amoral, a liar, a sham, very sensual, of very unconventional behaviour, has never loved his son Guiseppe. A paternal great-aunt died in an asylum; a paternal great-uncle was regarded as half insane; the paternal uncles are of unconventional behaviour and are all over-sexed. Mother is feeble-minded, vain, a great lover of entertainments and pleasures, jealous of her husband. A sister is a healthy and rather beautiful girl, and therefore loved by the parents. G was delivered by forceps (full term). He suffered much during breast feeding, and later too was often insufficiently fed. Ill-treated, or at least neglected by his parents, he suffered many traumata as a young child. Always wetted his bed, and his aunt states that this habit is due to his mother, who would never see that he was made to micturate properly. Congenital syphilis is suspected. He is unable to learn, and therefore was always expelled from all the schools to which he gained admission. In the winter of 1899 he was admitted to my nursery school for mentally deficient poor children.

He is a normally developed child, dark haired, weight 17·600 kg, height 107 cm. Broad hands, short fingers, small nails; narrow forehead, dark straight hair with abnormal whorls; small ocular bulbs, dark irises; slightly asymmetrical face; abnormally implanted and shaped teeth.

G's general nutritional state is very poor; respiration is normal and the heart healthy. Nocturnal enuresis. Sleep, usually deep. G presents stenosis of the left nostril, caused by deviation of the nasal septum; cartilaginous growth in the same nostril, nasal catarrh.

Slow superficial reflexes, normal deep reflexes, normal pupillary reflexes. Trophic state of muscles normal. Slight hypotonia in lower limbs. Alternating strabismus. Movements (on request) of the face, tongue, neck, body and upper limbs cannot be assessed because of the mental state of the child; however, there seems to be no relevant anomaly in them. Motor ability is poorly developed. G needs help always and in everything. Manual muscular strength seems normal. G has tics and sucks his fingers. Vision and hearing are normal. Blunted sensibility (skin and mucose surfaces) to pain produced by mechanical stimuli. Voracity.

Attention is little developed, there is sluggishness and wandering. Poor memory. No ability in arithmetic at all. Very poor emotional feelings, no show of affection to parents, no empathy with other children. Usual mood hostile or expansive, always restless, silly behaviour. Extraordinary tendency to negativism. Paradoxical suggestibility (by contradiction). G presents attacks of absolute mutism lasting several days. Many times he has refused to micturate or to take food. Often, too, he has been caught eating furtively a piece of bread, which he had kept in his pocket. Wilfulness and negativism, these are the main traits of his character; at the nursery school, he is silent; solitary, but again, if at least excited, becomes impulsive. G has a stereotyped smile, which does not wane even when he rushes into impulsive actions.

To a superficial observer these would seem the stigmata of idiocy, but they are not, because at the end of the day, when he returns to his home, G comes out of his mutism and even relates what he has seen and heard at school. Therefore, it can be easily excluded that G's behaviour is a product of pathological timidity; G is not timid, rather he is insensitive and impulsive.

After three months, during which his state did not change, he left the nursery school and I was unable to have any more news about him.

In this case the diagnosis is doubtful, because observation of the course of the illness evades us, and we know nothing of the beginning of it. The alternating strabismus, too, and a slight spastic paraplegia make one think of many forms of arrested cerebral palsy. Certainly one notes in G at least a type of vesanic mentality.

3. *Dementia Praecox Retardata*

Cases of dementia praecox presenting at about 40 years of age, in the climacteric and even after the age of 50, are not to be accepted as such, without a detailed account. Diagnosis is often based exclusively on symptoms and especially on stereotypy, negativism, hallucinations and absurd delusions. It seems to me that the symptomatologic criterion is not enough. Moreover I am convinced that, at least in some cases, the diagnosis of dementia praecox is not even dependent on one of the classic symptoms of this psychosis, but rather is reached by exclusion. Thus, once amentia, manic-depressive psychosis, paranoia, undefined delusional states or presenile dementia have been excluded, what could a fanatical follower of Kraepelin diagnose when presented, for instance, with a woman of 45, who is not an alcoholic and has no past history of psychopathy, but presents with hallucinations, absurd hypochondriacal delusions, and instability of mood, and in whom the whole syndrome is frankly chronic? Patients like this are not at all rare.

Not long ago, I had occasion to observe a patient of about 52 years of age, who was in a sanatorium abroad because of continuous and very vivid hallucinations, agitation, and grandiose delusions, but with a perfect memory and presenting no direct signs of intellectual decline. Some years ago, Professor Kraepelin diagnosed her as a case of dementia praecox because she presented, and still presents, a stereotyped movement, which consists of beating the top of her head with her right hand, thus causing that part of her head to be bald.

Confronted with such cases, I don't see why one should not think of the diagnostic possibility of other psychoses. We must have no logoidolatry or logophobia.* Some syndromes would justify the term of paranoid dementia, if this form could be conceived by itself, i.e. outside the concept of dementia praecox, as postulated by Séglas[29]; others are frank persecution syndromes, like those described by Lasègue, and unfortunately nowadays a little neglected; others correspond to the more typical evolutive chronic delusion described by Magnan.

I would see nothing amiss if in some cases one would diagnose hallucinatory psychosis, as is the practice of Ziehen, Wernicke, Séglas[30], Bianchi, Morselli and others; or amentia or chronic confusion like it is done by the French; in yet other cases the diagnosis could be persecution delusion, in others perhaps (primary) dementia of middle age, and so on.

Of course, I am only putting forward hypotheses, because to create a clinical entity it is not sufficient to have found a characteristic syndrome, but it is necessary to relate to it a particular history, a given aetiology, and when possible, a pathogenesis. However, it seems to me that to have solved a great nosographic problem by creating the dementia praecox entity and grouping together a vast number of previously isolated syndromes, does not by any means solve all the nosographic problems posed by psychiatry. For example, it is possible to disagree with the extension given to the term 'sensory psychosis'† by some people of the Neopolitan school; one may have reserves on the presumed primary nature of hallucinations in cases of hallucinatory or sensory psychosis[31], but from the nosographic point of

---

* Love and hate of words—Translator's note.
† *Frenosi sensoria* in the original—Translator's note.

view it seems to me that dementia praecox does not have wings as ample as to cover all those cases (excluding, of course, periodic forms, manic-depressive psychosis, alcoholism, etc.) where the predominant symptoms are illusionary perception, multiple hallucinations and absurd delusions. We must not forget that Kraepelin[32] wrote: 'there is no reason to believe that it would be impossible to upset the whole medley of observations (on dementia praecox) in a large or a small number of well-defined morbid states and therefore to abandon the much contested collective term of *dementia praecox*, which has only a descriptive and provisional value'.

However, there is no doubt in the existence of psychoses with hallucinations, which develop in the fourth or fifth decennium of life, are very chronic, show all the signs of a mental deterioration and are nevertheless curable. Cases of so-called late recovery are well known (referred to as 'spätheilung' by the Germans; cases reported by Ventra, Riva, Algeri, Kreuser)[33].

Certainly a number of cases, diagnosed as dementia praecox in the fourth or fifth decennium, must be distinguished from true dementia praecox. Excluding hallucinations or certain compulsive movements which are easily taken for motor stereotypy, some sayings—a kind of verbal exorcism—and some delusional, but passing ideas, can these cases not be included with the hallucinatory psychoses, when they are not of psychasthenic character? On another occasion I have demonstrated that various forms of negativism can be found outside dementia praecox[34], and even neologisms (impossible as this seemed to the lamented Dr Finzi) can be observed in psychasthenics of vivid intelligence[35], just like clang associations, verbigeration and other symptoms of dementia praecox are found in other psychoses and even in pellagra (Lombroso, Finzi, Vedrani). It has been said that dementia praecox is characterized by an illness of the will (Kraepelin), or of perception (Weygandt), or by loss of harmony between intellectual, emotional and volitional activities and the thymuspsyche and the noöpsyche (Stransky). This, in theory; but in practice many patients with hallucinations act without motivation and in a silly and absurd way, related perhaps less to the hallucinatory content than to the disassociation of thought, perturbation and disorientation, which follow a true hallucination or which goes with the affective change, caused by the hallucination—these phenomena are an index of a pure and simple perturbation[36] of consciousness and not of a true intellectual *deficit*.

Nevertheless, it seems to me undeniable that there are cases where, because of the symptomatologic criterion, the diagnosis of deferred dementia praecox is imperative.

The following is the only case I have observed.

Typical case: A. M., aged 46 years, female, ill for the last three years.

The main symptoms were and still are: every kind of eccentricity, odd behaviour, like passing water on to the floor and smearing herself with menstrual blood; threatening suicide; unmotivated laughter; at times stiff poses, stereotyped movements, like scratching her breast.

The husband states that A was previously quite sane and completely normal and that she became ill suddenly, complaining of pains in her stomach and the uterus. Soon she showed no interest in her children or in her husband; she no longer kissed them, or asked about them; however she was not depressed, she would often laugh at the slightest provocation, leave the house and stay out longer than was her usual practice and always without plausible motives. After two months, even lay people regarded her as insane.

A is a woman of medium height, well fed, with healthy organs in her chest and abdomen. Her menses started at the age of 12 and are still regular. Her sleep is disturbed by strange and 'continuous' dreams; a particular dream is recurrent, but the patient cannot or will not tell its contents. No motor pathology present: reflexes of the mucosa, skin, muscles and tendons, normal; muscular strength in the hands (average from 5 measurings), on the right hands, 33 kg, on the left 29 kg. No tremors. No hypoaesthesia or abnormality of sensation.

One could say, a very common case. But, on the contrary, it was enough to suggest to me some considerations on the form which I have called *dementia praecox retardata*, because a stringent inquiry into the past history of the patient has revealed an anamnesis not at all free from symptoms, unlike the one previously gathered a bit hurriedly from the family. I could instead establish facts which, in my opinion, have special significance. They are as follows:

1. At puberty A often felt very unwell with headaches, irritability and capriciousness; presented at the same time bigotry and coquetry; pessimism. Once, because of these episodes, had to miss school for 22 consecutive days. No hysteria.

2. At the time of her marriage, whims and eccentricities, childish behaviour, feelings of guilt, changeable mood.

3. During the following years A was always of good behaviour, a good manager in the home, loving toward her children, but excessively avaricious, too meticulous in housekeeping, overreligious, diffident and too preoccupied with her own health: her own doctor of that period used to describe her as 'a bit hysterical'.

However, psychopathic episodes and hysteria can be excluded, but nevertheless mood disorders remain, which cannot be overlooked.

Thus, in our patient there seems to be late dementia praecox. But does it deserve the term 'late'? It is not unlikely that the intellectual *deficit* instead of appearing suddenly, was already manifest in adolescence and that, as it was only partial, it escaped attention. Perhaps it is a delayed dementia praecox, as if from adolescence onward it was slow in developing. Would it not, then, be more correct to talk of *dementia praecox retardata*? Here I would like to express my doubt that if a meticulous search of the patient's past history was undertaken in every case of late dementia praecox, perhaps it would still be possible to retain in the dementia praecox group the aetiologic criterion of an early age (of onset), which, to the disadvantage of clarity, is increasingly vanishing. Such a research in case histories, the importance of which is self evident, should be undertaken by someone with access to the rich material of the asylums. With my one case, I could do no better than to stimulate discussion in my colleagues.

Premonitory Signs

In conclusion a query, which is indeed linked to what I have said on *dementia retardata*: does *dementia praecox*, usually, show premonitory signs at a very early age? In my experience, I could answer: very often.

I have had at my disposal only very slight material, but I am nevertheless convinced that the records of patients suffering from dementia praecox are never, or very seldom, unblemished. Not only is their heredity usually contaminated (it is admitted that 75 per cent or more have an obvious hereditary disposition), but they themselves show changes of mood, or intellectual decline, or episodes of mania or of depression, etc. So much so that when I am presented with a case of a young subject suffering from hallucinations, confusion, or mania, and when the syndrome does not clearly indicate the exclusion of dementia praecox, I deem a totally unblemished family and individual history a valid criterion for exclusion of dementia praecox.

I already held these convictions, based exclusively on my own personal clinical experience, when I started to read again the chapter on dementia praecox in the seventh edition of Kraepelin. I was a bit surprised, but much gratified, to see Kraepelin concedes that there are frequent psychopathologic phenomena in the precedents of patients with dementia praecox even of late onset: timidity, oddity, bigotry, affected behaviour, irritability, weak moral fibre and intellectual weakness; he also refers to similar observations by Schroeder.

Conclusion

Nevertheless, looking over the literature on dementia praecox the difference between the cases described is striking. There is a category of patients, previously normal and intelligent, who develop dementia praecox through a period of stress at an age varying between 20 and 45 years; while another category comprises predestined individuals, who in adolescence and in the first flush of youth were already prone to melancholia, hallucinations and psychomotor excitement, or who in the silence of their tumultuous symptoms (simple dementia) tend to complete their parabola towards a precocious intellectual decline, as if they had drawn from nature a cerebral organization and structures without resistance. In this second category are found the phrenasthenics destined to dementia praecox.

Is it possible that this clinico-aetiologic classification is then rational? Let us examine the pathogenic hypotheses that have been advanced for the dementia praecox. Truly, not many of them are plausible: but autointoxication due to abnormal internal secretion of the sexual glands, advanced by Kraepelin, seems to have some foundation[37].

Kraepelin, however, interprets very widely the hypothetical relation between dementia praecox and sexual functions, as he assumes that there are autointoxications, capable of giving rise to the cerebral process of dementia praecox, whenever the sexual glands are active—at puberty, during menstruation, during pregnancy and at the climacteric. But, the modes of activities of the sexual glands are different in each of these events and it is difficult to understand how the physiological hurricane of puberty can leave the brain unharmed, and then pregnancy or the climacteric can be so injurious at an age when cerebral evolution has been accomplished, and in people who accomplished it normally (sound brains).

However, we must still ask: why should previously defective and normal personalities equally yield to such an autointoxication? Is the great and universally accepted frequency of already ill patients in dementia praecox a mere coincidence?

But let us turn to pathological anatomy. In the various forms of dementia praecox, together with the easily found brain anomalies of the insane and the melancholics (Kierman, 1877, and all the modern authors: Nissl, Deny, Voisin, Ballet, Hoch, Meyer, etc.) and with blood anomalies—by no means specific (Deny, Lhermitte and Camus, W. Prout, etc.)—have been found more distinct morphologic or structural modifications of the cerebral cortex, like hypoplasias, atrophies, deviations of development, specific localizations of the deeper cortical strata, particularly of the associative areas, and cellular atrophies and degenerations (Dunton, Alzheimer, Lugaro, Klippel and Lhermitte). Thus it seems to me difficult to explain some structural alterations and specific localizations, without admitting particular and strong predisposition of the brain in dementia praecox.

It is more rational to think that dementia praecox is a psychosis with unique pathogenesis and aetiology, which strikes the developing organism with varying force and at a different rate.

The neurasthenics too have always been divided into two categories; those in whom the illness has been caused by exhaustion—a kind of occasional neurasthenics—for whom the word neurasthenia was coined; and those predisposed or constitutionally prone to it (by some termed degenerate neurasthenics). But what a difference between the two categories! No likeness of symptoms can ever bring together those momentarily exhausted and those of weak constitution. It is nothing more than an analogy, like the one so abused by the French between exhaustion phenomena and hysterical phenomena. It is indeed because of taxonomic criteria, initiated by Kraepelin (course and prognosis criteria), that we should again limit the concept of neurasthenia and apply it only to constitutional hypobulics, to sentimentalists, to hypochondriacs, and to the more or less periodical pessimists. This is, in fact, the aim of the modern nosography of neurasthenia.

The same should be done for dementia praecox. The victim of dementia praecox can indeed become ill even late in life, as if he were paying his constitutional debt at a deferred date, but this does not exempt him from being predestined to it, and the signs of his destiny, if one looks carefully, can be found even in his childhood. How many times the first epileptic attack occurs late in life in those predestined to epilepsy by congenital cerebral disease! Signs of prenatal encephalitis, or porencephaly, or microgyria, are found at autopsy of epileptics who had their first attack when already 25 or 30 years old. But in these cases, before the onset of the attack, other signs indicated the congenital disease: slight motor anomalies, abnormality of behaviour, defective mentality, etc.

A true dementia praecox exploding in a constitutionally healthy and already completely developed and consolidated organism is unthinkable. Cases of dementia praecox of the fourth and fifth decennium of life in previously mentally stable and robust subjects, and cases of individuals later reported to have reacquired their lost intellectual patrimony, should all be re-assessed; the nosography of psychiatry would undoubtedly benefit by it.

Kraepelin himself cannot understand how a psychic organism, which up to adulthood has developed normally and vigorously, should, without apparent cause, suddenly arrest its development and often disintegrate. Not even the gravest hereditary predisposition, he adds, could explain this extraordinary fact. What then? . . . It is a question of nosography; the syndrome is not enough to define a group. Why not believe that in those cases we are dealing with a psychosis other than dementia praecox?

I believe that the admission of dementia praecox in psychiatry is invaluable, but on condition that dementia praecox should be understood to mean a psychosis tied to constitutional predisposition and to conditions of psychic development, and which is, from its onset and for its nature, a true dementia, and therefore always with a grave prognosis. It is not enough for the mental weakening to appear to be present, it must be real and therefore of long duration, like in amentia or in delusional forms; or in nervous exhaustion[38].

NOTES

1. COWLES, E., 1899. The progress in the clinical study of psychiatry, lecture to the American Psychiatric Association, 28th May. F. X. Dercum, lecture on the classification of mental illnesses, to the American Neurological Assn., June 1901, also in *J. Amer. med. Assn*, February, 1905. Also the very recent work of D'Orsay Hecht in *J. nerv. ment. Dis.*, 1905, No. 11, with bibliography.
2. In *J. Neurologie*, 1905, No. 1-2.

3. CHRISTIAN, 1899. De la Demence Precoce des Jeunes Gens. In *Annales Medicopsycholog*. The more recent French opinion about the vexed question was revealed in a discussion on vesanic dementias, to which participated Brisaud, Régis, Deny, Parant, Vallon, Garnier etc. See *Revue Neurologique*, August, 1904.
4. NORMAN, CONOLLY, 1904. Dementia praecox. *Brit. med. J.*, Oct. 15th, 972-76.
5. Not to be confused with *Dementia simplex* of Rieger, who by *Dementia simplex* meant only Kraepelin's *dementia praecox*.
6. WEYGANDT, 1902. *Atlas u. Grundriss der Psychiatrie*.
7. OTTO DIEM, 1903. Ein Klinischer Beitrag zur Kenntniss der Verblödungspsychosen—Die einfache demente Form der *Dementia praecox. Archiv. f. Psychiatrie u. Nervenheilk*, **37**, No. 1.
8. GUSTAVE MONOD, 1905. Les formes frustes de la démence précoce, Thèse de Paris, 1905.
9. Was Kahlbaum right in creating his heboidophrenia as a form distinct from the hebephrenia described by Hecker, and distinct from moral insanity and idiocy? Heboidophrenia, simple form of dementia praecox, primary dementia of Sommer and primary dementia of puberty as described or recognised by Wideroe, Sprague, Marro, Wille, Wernicke, etc. are they or are they not the same form? They are problems still awaiting a definitive solution.
10. For the relation between dementia praecox and sensory psychosis see the recent monograph by Frangnito, O., 1905. La Frenosi sensoria. *Annali di Nevrologia*, **13**, No. 3.
11. See the 7th German edition of the Treatise of Kraepelin. All my citations refer to this edition.
12. And it would really be better to give it up! Many confusions would so be avoided. In fact, what are the dementia praecox of Morel, that of Christian, that of Tschisch, compared with the dementia praecox of Kraepelin? But certainly we must not replace the term *dementia praecox* with *dementia simplex*, as suggested by Rieger; we would go from one misunderstanding to another.
13. SCHULE: *Clinical psychiatry*. Italian translation.
14. *Etudes des maladies mentales*. Paris. 1860.
15. TOULOUSE: Classification des maladies mentales. *Revue de Psychiatrie*, February 1900.
    See also S. de Sanctis: Sulla Classificazione delle psicopatie. *Riv. sper. di Freniatria* 1902. Atti del Congresso Freniatrico di Ancona, 1901.
16. FINZI and VEDRANI, 1899. Contributo alla dottrina della demenza precoce, *Riv. sper. di Freniatria*, No. 1-2.
17. de SANCTIS, S., 1902. Sui criteri e i metodi per la educabililtà dei deficienti. Paper presented at the psychiatric Congress in Ancona, 1901. *Riv. sper. di Freniatria*.
18. CRAMER, A., 1902. *Entwickelungsjahre und Gesetzgebung*.
19. BOURNVILLE (C. R. de Bicêtre, 1897) terms idiocies also the mental weakenings appearing at the beginning of puberty, at 13 or 14 years, following cerebral pathological processes. Esquirol terms it accidentally acquired idiocy. In these cases it would perhaps be better to talk of consecutive dementias (traumas or inflammatory processes of the meninges or of the brain, or tumours, etc.).
20. de SANCTIS, S., 1905. Su alcuni tipi di mentalità inferiore. Paper presented at the 5th International Congress of Psychology. See also the Annali della R. Clinica psichiatrica di Roma, 1905.

21. Case reported by A. PICK (Uber primäre Demenz bei Erwachsenen. *Prager medezin.* Wochensche. No. 32 1904). More famous is the case reported by Schroeder, where dementia praecox would have started at 59 years! (quoted by Kraepelin).
22. See TANZI, *Treatise of psychiatry*, p. 584. Also Kraepelin, who writes as follows: 'With the term *dementia praecox* it has been possible to group together provisionally a series of pathological pictures, having in common that they result in particular states of mental weakness'. If the state of dementia is not primary, that is to say if it is not visible from the first stages of the invasion of the illness, I cannot see why we must oppose Serbsky's concept of *dementia secundaria progressiva* (progressive secondary dementia).
23. See a paper by Pfersdorff on the prognosis of dementia praecox, presented at the meeting in Baden-Baden, 27th-28th May, 1905.
24. Professor Tamburini suggests that this form should be called *dementia praecox phrenasthenica*. See the discussion of my paper to the *R. Accademia di Roma*, 28th January, 1906.
25. See my above-mentioned paper to Psychiatric Congress in Ancona, 1901.
26. I say 'some'; and above I have said that the term 'educational regression' was suggested to me partially by the cases I am referring to, precisely because educational regressions can be caused not only by the placid or tumultuous decline of intelligence during puberty, but also by epileptic forms, by the environment, by early intoxications and by other unknown causes.
27. Note this detail. In another case of hebephrenia, which I have noted elsewhere, there was swelling of the thyroid glands and Bosedowian symptoms. However, further interpretation evades us. In the case described here, thyroid extract tablets produced no change.
28. SEPPILLI, 1886. Delle psicosi della pubertà. *Proc. 5th Congr. Societa Freniatrica Italiana.*
29. SÉGLAS, 1900. La demence paranoide in Annales medico-psychologiques. Sept. and Oct.
30. SÉGLAS, 1899. *Leçons cliniques.* Pg. 450 and following. See also Farnarier: *La psychose hallucinatoire aigue.* Thèse de Paris.
31. See the above mentioned work by O. Frangnito. *La Frenosi sensoria.*
32. IBID.
33. It is not new, nor out of place, to say that psychiatrists should retrace their steps and look again at the work of Maynert and Wernicke.
34. de SANCTIS, 1900. Psicopatologia delle idee de negazione. *Manicomio moderno* (Nocera-inferiore). **16**.
35. de SANCTIS, 1902. Intorno alla psicopatologia dei Neologismi. *Annali di Nevrologia*, **20**.
36. It does not seem right to me to affirm that hallucinations cannot disorientate and perturb the mind. If an hallucination is really such, it has a more or less permanent disintegrating power, as is seen even in people who are hallucinated, but not insane. Besides, it has been denied (Möbius) that dreams can cause more or less passing mental disturbances, saying that it is the insanity which provokes the dream and not vice versa. Instead my data (see 'I Sogni', Torino 1899 and Die Träume-Halle, 1901) and others collected in the literature confirm the opposite.
37. I have observed a typical case of dementia praecox, where periodically the thyroid would visibly swell, and also three cases of classic dementia praecox, where the thyroid was very poorly developed.
38. Of course the characteristics of the variety which I have here called dementia praecocissima could be partially different from those of the common dementia praecox.

2

ABOUT DEMENTIA INFANTILIS*

THEODOR HELLER

Introductory Remarks by the Translator

In recent years, psychotic states in young children have been frequently described in American literature. Their relationship to schizophrenia is still a matter of debate although the term 'childhood schizophrenia' has come into wide use. The basic articles by Howard Potter, Louise Despert, Leo Kanner, Loretta Bender, Margaret Mahler and other American contributors are well known to all interested in this subject, but earlier European literature on psychosis, schizophrenia and dementia praecox in childhood is hardly accessible to the American reader.

Occasionally authors in this country make use of the diagnostic term, 'Heller's syndrome', as a disease sui generis and different from infantile autism, pseudo-feeblemindedness or childhood schizophrenia. It seemed advisable to make available an English translation of one of the original papers by Theodor Heller which describes his 'syndrome' and tries to differentiate it from other psychotic or schizophrenia-like illnesses in childhood. Whether such a clinical differentiation is valid remains for the reader to decide.

The paper is here rendered in its entirety in as literal a translation as possible. Some overly long German sentences have been broken down into several parts. To avoid semantic confusion, a short glossary of German and English technical terms has been added. Heller's paper appeared originally in the 5th (Schluss-) Heft, 37. Band, pages 661-667. *Zeitschrift fuer Kinderforschung*, Berlin: Julius Springer Verlag, 1930. (It has been translated through their kind permission.) Theodor Heller was a collaborating editor of that journal.

At the Fifth Congress for Remedial Education at Cologne (1930) Professor Corberi of Milan submitted a discussion remark in Italian following the lectures by Professor H. W. Maier (Zuerich) and by Dr P. Seelig (Berlin) concerning schizophrenia-like conditions in childhood. Lack of time prevented a translation and reading of Professor Corberi's remarks at that meeting. These remarks deal primarily with dementia infantilis which had been observed and described by me for the first time. Professor Corberi compares dementia infantilis with the dementia praecocissima described by Sante de Sanctis. He concludes that these two symptom-complexes, which often are confused with each other and are erroneously taken to be identical, represent actually two different conditions. The

---

* Translated by the late Wilfred C. Hulse, M.D., Child Psychiatric Section, The Mount Sinai Hospital, New York, and reproduced by kind permission of Mrs Ilse C. Hulse and the Editor of *The Journal of Nervous and Mental Disease*, where it appeared in June 1954 (vol. 119).

assumption that dementia praecocissima is an early form of dementia praecox in childhood is also incorrect. It is not easy to gain a completely clear understanding from the available literature about Sante de Sanctis' concept of dementia praecocissima as he seems to include under this designation different types of psychoneuroses of early childhood, all resulting in idiotic regression. I have asked Professor Corberi who has published on this subject* a number of times to clarify by means of a detailed summary what Sante de Sanctis and his school understand by the term 'dementia praecocissima'. We will then be able to judge the validity of objections made by some German researchers who believe that in dementia praecocissima we are dealing primarily with post-encephalitic states, progressive forms of mental deficiency and similar cases. Yet such revisions and critiques have to be reserved for the medical author. I will restrict myself to giving in the following pages a picture of dementia infantilis to the extent to which my research and my experiences have enabled me to gain insight into this condition and its interrelated factors.

During the years 1905 and 1906 I was given to observe and to evaluate an unusually large number of feebleminded children. I was particularly impressed by a number of cases whose past histories were so similar that there could remain no doubt as to a close inner connection. These children came from different countries and from differing social strata. These were children who—without preceding illness—had become conspicuous in their third and fourth years through early symptoms which one might sum up (if such a designation is appropriate at this early age) as character changes which presented themselves primarily by changes of mood. These had been placid or lively children by nature until that time; now they became moody, negativistic, disobedient, often raging without reason, and whining; not rarely they started to destroy their toys of which they had made reasonable use before. Many showed definite anxiety states, occasionally of a hallucinatory character. With these stormy symptoms, or in rare cases more quietly and without affective blows, there developed a mental process of regression which led within a few months to a complete loss of speech and to complete idiocy. The language became impoverished by degrees, words were distorted, sentences could not be repeated any longer, and finally, the children stopped speaking altogether. The capacity to understand language was lost with the exception of some primitive remnants. During this regressive process, motoric degeneration became frequently evident. The children acquired tic-like movements; they grimaced, posed in peculiar positions. Their condition reminded one of the erethism of certain idiots. Many became incontinent, losing control of urine, sometimes also of faeces; it became necessary to feed them. During all this there

* Corberi, 1925. Una sindrome demenziale grave nell' età infantile. *Atti della Società Lombarda di Scienze Mediche e Biologiche*. **13**.—Fasc. VI. Milano.

Ibid., 1926. Sindromi di regressione mentale infanto-giovanile. *Rivista di Patologia nervosa e mentale*. **31**. Fasc. 1. Firenze. Gennaio-Febbraio.

remained a certain degree of attentiveness which was particularly evident in their ability to focus ('Blickrichtung').

Without exception, all parents maintained that the children had been intelligent before the onset of this condition. In a few cases, the information given by the parents suggested that some of these children had been very gifted. Of course, we had to be cautious in evaluating these statements, as it is well known that parents generally overestimate the intellectual achievements of their children, especially in retrospect. But there was no doubt that these children had once been able to speak and to understand the spoken word, that they had possessed the ability for independent action commensurate to their ages. In no way could they have been called very retarded or feebleminded, nor had their character development been particularly conspicuous.

The lowest mental level was reached within an average of nine months. No improvement was observed in any of the children after that. As a rule the children remained from then on in a state of extreme idiotic regression. Great motor restlessness, stereotypies and tic-like habits remained in the foreground. Throughout this, the children maintained their misleading intelligent facial expression. Particularly impressive was the clear look in their eyes and the apparent attention which these children frequently seemed to pay to whatever went on around them. They proved to be unresponsive to any approach through remedial education. Through careful therapeutic nursing some could be trained to eat by themselves and to keep clean.

As a rule the parents expected a recovery of the lost functions; they were cruelly disappointed as the low mental status persisted and as the child lapsed into complete idiotic regression.

In 1908 I published 6 cases in the Journal for Research and Treatment of Juvenile Feeblemindedness (*Zeitschrift fuer die Erforschung und Behandlung des jugendlichen Schwachsinns*. Jena, Gustav Fischer). I had illustrated this article with photographs of these children. During his stay at Vienna in 1907, Professor Weygandt had examined psychiatrically one of my cases. I had previously acquainted him with my observations and had suggested the designation dementia infantilis for these cases. Professor Weygandt was able to concur completely with my observations and also accepted the name dementia infantilis. This term was chosen merely to designate a state of mental deterioration occurring in childhood; it did not intend to indicate in a more precise manner the origin of this process nor to connect it with other symptom complexes of similar nature. Professor Weygandt published the results of these observations during the same year in the above-mentioned journal under the title 'Idiotie und Dementia praecox'. Through an oversight the paper fails to refer to my observations and communications.

Various authors have since described cases of dementia infantilis (Higier, Jancke, and others). More recently in 1921, Julius Zappert made dementia infantilis the topic for a presentation at the meeting of the

German Paediatric Association (*Deutsche Gesellschaft fuer Kinderheilkunde*) at Jena. His material comprised 13 cases, in all of whom he could consistently observe the following stages:

1. Normal mental and physical development during the first years of life;
2. Onset of the illness between the third and fourth years of life;
3. Psychic and intellectual changes demonstrated by ineffectiveness of educational and recreational (zerstreuender) influences; marked restlessness, excited and occasionally anxious behaviour, increasing dementia;
4. Appearance of speech disorders in the beginning and during the course of the illness;
5. Maintenance of motor functions and complete lack of focal symptoms from the central nervous system;
6. Final complete idiotic regression;
7. Non-imbecilic facial expression and looks ('Blick').

I have collected case material of 28 children with dementia infantilis. All of them had thorough medical examinations so that any confusion with other diseases may be completely ruled out. Special caution was taken to prevent the sneaking-in of encephalitis lethargica cases. Any case where doubts existed about the parental reports, even if they described a regressive process similar to dementia infantilis, was excluded. Likewise, cases were not included in the above number if no definite record could be established because of a preceding illness. In all cases, the catastrophic mental decline occurred in the same fashion, the past histories conformed in all important features, if one discounted the self-deceptive stories of parents reporting short-lived temporary improvements. I have nothing further of importance to add to my observations published in 1908.

The reports about the follow-up studies of children who have gone through a dementia infantilis are of interest. All of the children remained in complete idiotic regression, did not speak, did not understand anything or only very little. They were unable to keep themselves occupied, were restless and years later still showed tics and stereotyped movements similar to those which had developed during or immediately after the (acute state of the) illness. The majority had been referred to nursing homes or to mental institutions, as they could not be kept at home because of their restlessness. Malaria therapy was tried in one case but no success was noted after repeated attacks of fever. Some of the patients had by now reached adult age; despite their severe idiotic regression, they gave the superficial impression of much greater intelligence than the idiots with whom they were placed. Their looks and the expression in their eyes ('Blick') encouraged many of the unfortunate parents not to give up hope for recovery, even after years of a continuous low mental level. Again and again physicians and directors of institutions were approached by these parents and asked to initiate 'treatment' ('Kuren'). In one instance, parents had travelled from one therapist to the next having been told about someone's efforts to cure feeblemindedness. Finally, they began to consult quacks of different schools and vocations. After all these many trials and tribulations, having tried every possible thing, the condition of the patient had at the very end not improved in the slightest noticeable degree.

Professor Emil Redlich, to whom I was able to present several of these ill children, concerned himself with the question whether we might not possibly be dealing with an early form of dementia praecox. At first he thought that there seemed to exist a certain similarity between dementia infantilis and some forms of schizophrenia. Later he was amazed to find the nearly photographic likeness of the course the illness took. He then became convinced that dementia infantilis was a peculiar regressive process which did not belong to the group of schizophrenias, which was of an unknown nature, impossible to speculate about.

Professor Maier and Dr Seelig have pointed out in the above-mentioned lectures that cases belonging to the schizophrenias are extremely rare in childhood and might not exist at all. During a period of 35 years I have had the opportunity to examine and evaluate an extremely large number of abnormal children. In all this time I only once had the occasion to observe a case of schizophrenia in childhood, which has been established beyond any doubt. This is the case of S.S., born March 24, 1917. From her past record we learned the following: She is the second child of healthy Jewish parents. No cases of mental disorders or nervous diseases have occurred in this family. Her birth was normal and so was her development during the first years of life. She learned to walk and to speak at the normal time. She showed only feeding difficulties—she belonged to the group of poor eaters. There was no other educational unusualness: she was intelligent, liked picture books and story telling. She understood all she was told and asked reasonable questions. This her father was able to show by many convincing examples. She began to show peculiarities at the age of 5, laughing occasionally without reason, whispering to herself words which made no sense. Later she showed a preference for odd positions, appeared sometimes as though 'rooted to the spot', would get stuck occasionally in the middle of an action, for instance, raising her hand with a spoon without getting it into her mouth. It also happened that she would suddenly accelerate her steps and start to run. She ran away from her nurse during outdoor walks. She lost interest in games, became whining, negativistic, incontinent. At the age of 7, one could not induce her to get up; she stayed in bed and had to be spoon-fed, taking little nourishment, often for several days. She lost control over urine and faeces and remained lying in this dirty mess. On December 5, 1924, she was brought to Vienna and was admitted to my institution. She was first examined by Professor von Wagner-Jauregg, who stated that we were dealing with an early form of dementia praecox, a diagnosis which was confirmed in every way during the subsequent period. The child was first catatonic with outspoken flexibilitas cerea. Occasionally, this catatonic state was interrupted by a state of excitement. In this state, the child would run around, touch everything, throw things to the floor as if in a state of high spirits. Everything edible was consumed ravenously by S.; her voracity had no limits at times like this. She spoke Polish and German words in a disconnected way. She carried out orders; on occasions she even did some sewing or other little housework during such a period showing remarkable manual dexterity. Then suddenly and unexpectedly the catatonic state returned, the child sat in her little chair in frozen poses, she had to be fed and would use the toilet only when ordered and with adult help. But one had the impression that even in the catatonic state, S. observed whatever was going on around her. On occasions one could find proof of this: when once again, she moved freely about the room, she found without hesitation things in the closet which the nurse had put there while the child had been lying in bed, apparently completely withdrawn. Once while being left alone in bed in a frozen pose, she got up, ate within an extremely short time the nurse's supper that was left on the table in the bedroom and was found again motionless in bed by the returning nurse.

Step by step, the child's intelligence declined more and more. She stopped speaking, became unable to keep herself occupied in the simplest fashion, and was unable to understand the meaning and use of the tools and toys put at her disposal. The catatonia moved into the background more and more and was replaced by a state of silliness and idiotic regression. The child now sits idly in her little chair, laughs without cause, plays monotonously in the manner of idiots with little blocks or plates and displays a ravenous appetite which she tries to satisfy with garbage, left-overs and crumbs from the floor. Teaching attempts find the child without response and in complete apathy. She does not take notice of other children and shows no interest in their games and occupations. She lately gained a lot of weight. She is just approaching the onset of puberty.

No further explanation is needed to show that this early form (Fruehform) of schizophrenia is entirely different in its course from the cases of dementia infantilis which have been observed until now. Cases of encephalitis lethargica are also sharply differentiated from dementia infantilis. Children with encephalitis present a picture totally different from our cases. Besides, catastrophic declines of intelligence, which we have learned to recognize as absolutely typical for dementia infantilis, do not occur in patients with encephalitis. Complete idiotic regressions can probably be observed but rarely in encephalitis lethargica.

Physicians and educators depend on one another for the diagnosis and treatment of feebleminded juveniles; they depend on mutual help and mutual cooperation. This has been the way in which all progress has been achieved in orthopedagogics. Whenever the remedial educator (orthopedagogist) makes observations in his practice which can contribute to medical research, he should not hesitate to communicate such material. In the same manner, the physician should not miss any opportunity to acquaint the educator with facts, experiences and observations which can stimulate and enrich the practical fields of teaching and education. In the area of remedial education, the arts of medicine and pedagogy interlink with each other; they also overlap in part and it is just through this common cultivation of certain areas, that the best and most persistent successes have been achieved. Many areas in the science of infantile feeblemindedness are still very much in the dark. Enlightenment is needed for a better concept and a clearer understanding of the therapy and its limitations. This is how I should like to have understood the goals and purposes of my observations which the remedial educator offers to the physician.

GLOSSARY

Blows of affect	Affektstoesse
Catastrophic mental decline	geistiger Absturz
Frozen poses	starre Posen
High spirits	Uebermut
Idiotic regression—idiocy	Verbloedung
Mental deterioration	geistige Veroedung
Motoric degeneration	Entartung der Motorik
Remedial Education (Orthopedagogics)	Heilpaedagogik
Symptom complexes	Krankheitsbilder oder—erscheinungen
Therapeutic nursing	Pflegebehandlung

3

AUTISTIC DISTURBANCES OF AFFECTIVE CONTACT*

LEO KANNER
M.D.

Since 1938, there have come to our attention a number of children whose condition differs so markedly and uniquely from anything reported so far, that each case merits—and, I hope, will eventually receive—a detailed consideration of its fascinating peculiarities. In this place, the limitations necessarily imposed by space call for a condensed presentation of the case material. For the same reason, photographs have also been omitted. Since none of the children of this group has as yet attained an age beyond 11 years, this must be considered a preliminary report, to be enlarged upon as the patients grow older and further observation of their development is made.

Case 1. Donald T. was first seen in October, 1938, at the age of 5 years, 1 month. Before the family's arrival from their home town, the father sent a 33-page typewritten history that, though filled with much obsessive detail, gave an excellent account of Donald's background. Donald was born at full term on September 8, 1933. He weighed nearly 7 pounds at birth. He was breast fed, with supplementary feeding, until the end of the eighth month; there were frequent changes of formulas. 'Eating,' the report said, 'has always been a problem with him. He has never shown a normal appetite. Seeing children eating candy and ice cream has never been a temptation to him.' Dentition proceeded satisfactorily. He walked at 13 months.

At the age of 1 year 'he could hum and sing many tunes accurately'. Before he was 2 years old, he had 'an unusual memory for faces and names, knew the names of a great number of houses' in his home town. 'He was encouraged by the family in learning and reciting short poems, and even learned the Twenty-third Psalm and 25 questions and answers of the Presbyterian Catechism.' The parents observed that 'he was not learning to ask questions or to answer questions unless they pertained to rhymes or things of this nature, and often then he would ask no question except in single words'. His enunciation was clear. He became interested in pictures 'and very soon knew an inordinate number of the pictures in a set of *Compton's Encyclopedia*'. He knew the pictures of the presidents 'and knew most of the pictures of his ancestors and kinsfolk on both sides of the house'. He quickly learned the whole alphabet 'backward as well as forward' and to count to 100.

It was observed at an early time that he was happiest when left alone, almost never cried to go with his mother, did not seem to notice his father's home-comings, and was indifferent to visiting relatives. The father made a special point of

* Reprinted from *The Nervous Child*, 1943, 2, by kind permission of the author and the publishers.

mentioning that Donald even failed to pay the slightest attention to Santa Claus in full regalia.

> He seems to be self-satisfied. He has no apparent affection when petted. He does not observe the fact that anyone comes or goes, and never seems glad to see father or mother or any playmate. He seems almost to draw into his shell and live within himself. We once secured a most attractive little boy of the same age from an orphanage and brought him home to spend the summer with Donald, but Donald has never asked him a question nor answered a question and has never romped with him in play. He seldom comes to anyone when called but has to be picked up and carried or led wherever he ought to go.

In his second year, he 'developed a mania for spinning blocks and pans and other round objects'. At the same time, he had

> A dislike for self-propelling vehicles, such as Taylor-tots, tricycles, and swings. He is still fearful of tricycles and seems to have almost a horror of them when he is forced to ride, at which time he will try to hold on to the person assisting him. This summer (1937) we bought him a playground slide and on the first afternoon when other children were sliding on it he would not get about it, and when we put him up to slide down it he seemed horror-struck. The next morning when nobody was present, however, he walked out, climbed the ladder, and slid down, and he has slid on it frequently since, but slides only when no other child is present to join him in sliding. . . . He was always constantly happy and busy entertaining himself, but resented being urged to play with certain things.

When interfered with, he had temper tantrums, during which he was destructive. He was 'dreadfully fearful of being spanked or switched' but 'could not associate his misconduct with his punishment'.

In August, 1937, Donald was placed in a tuberculosis preventorium in order to provide for him 'a change of environment'. While there, he had a 'disinclination to play with children and do things children his age usually take an interest in'. He gained weight but developed the habit of shaking his head from side to side. He continued spinning objects and jumped up and down in ecstasy as he watched them spin. He displayed

> An abstraction of mind which made him perfectly oblivious to everything about him. He appears to be always thinking and thinking, and to get his attention almost requires one to break down a mental barrier between his inner consciousness and the outside world.

The father, whom Donald resembles physically, is a successful, meticulous hard-working lawyer who has had two 'breakdowns' under strain of work. He always took every ailment seriously, taking to his bed and following doctor's orders punctiliously even for the slightest cold. 'When he walks down the street he is so absorbed in thinking that he sees nothing and nobody and cannot remember anything about the walk.' The mother, a college graduate, is a calm, capable woman, to whom her husband feels vastly superior. A second child, a boy, was born to them on May 22, 1938.

Donald, when examined at the Harriet Lane Home in October, 1938, was found to be in good physical condition. During the initial observation and in a two-week study by Drs Eugenia S. Cameron and George Frankl at the Child Study Home of Maryland, the following picture was obtained:

There was a marked limitation of spontaneous activity. He wandered about smiling, making stereotyped movements with his fingers, crossing them about in the air. He shook his head from side to side, whispering or humming the same three-note tune. He spun with great pleasure anything he could seize upon to spin. He kept throwing things on the floor, seeming to delight in the sounds they made. He arranged beads, sticks, or blocks in groups of different series of colours. Whenever he finished one of these performances, he squealed and jumped up and down. Beyond this he showed no initiative, requiring constant instruction (from his mother) in any form of activity other than the limited ones in which he was absorbed.

Most of his actions were repetitions carried out in exactly the same way in which they had been performed originally. If he spun a block, he must always start with the same face uppermost. When he threaded buttons, he arranged them in a certain sequence that had no pattern to it but happened to be the order used by the father when he first had shown them to Donald.

There were also innumerable verbal rituals recurring all day long. When he desired to get down after his nap, he said, 'Boo (his word for his mother), say "Don, do you want to get down?"'

His mother would comply, and Don would say: 'Now say "All right"'.

The mother did, and Don got down. At mealtime, repeating something that had obviously been said to him often, he said to his mother, 'Say "Eat it or I won't give you tomatoes, but if you don't eat it I will give you tomatoes,"' or 'Say "If you drink to there, I'll laugh and I'll smile"'.

And his mother had to conform or else he squealed, cried, and strained every muscle in his neck in tension. This happened all day long about one thing or another. He seemed to have much pleasure in ejaculating words or phrases, such as 'Chrysanthemum'; 'Dahlia, dahlia, dahlia'; 'Business'; 'Trumpet vine'; 'The right one is on, the left one is off'; 'Through the dark clouds shining'. Irrelevant utterances such as these were his ordinary mode of speech. He always seemed to be parroting what he had heard said to him at one time or another. He used the personal pronouns for the persons he was quoting, even imitating the intonation. When he wanted his mother to pull his shoe off, he said: 'Pull off your shoe'. When he wanted a bath, he said: 'Do you want a bath?'

Words to him had a specifically literal, inflexible meaning. He seemed unable to generalize, to transfer an expression to another similar object or situation. If he did so occasionally, it was a substitution, which then 'stood' definitely for the original meaning. Thus he christened each of his water-colour bottles by the name of one of the Dionne quintuplets—Annette for blue, Cécile for red, etc. Then, going through a series of colour mixtures, he proceeded in this manner: 'Annette and Cécile make purple'.

The colloquial request to 'put that *down*' meant to him that he was to put the thing on the floor. He had a 'milk glass' and a 'water glass.' When he spit some milk into the 'water glass', the milk thereby became 'white water'.

The word 'yes' for a long time meant that he wanted his father to put him up on his shoulder. This had a definite origin. His father, trying to teach him to say 'yes' and 'no', once asked him, 'Do you want me to put you on my shoulder?'

Don expressed his agreement by repeating the question literally, echolalia-like. His father said, 'If you want me to, say "Yes"; if you don't want me to, say "No"'.

Don said 'yes' when asked. But thereafter 'yes' came to mean that he desired to be put up on his father's shoulder.

He paid no attention to persons around him. When taken into a room, he completely disregarded the people and instantly went for objects, preferably those that could be spun. Commands or actions that could not possibly be disregarded were resented as unwelcome intrusions. But he was never angry at the interfering *person*. He angrily shoved away the *hand* that was in his way or the *foot* that stepped on one of his blocks, at one time referring to the foot on the block as 'umbrella'. Once the obstacle was removed, he forgot the whole affair. He gave no heed to the presence of other children but went about his favourite pastimes, walking off from the children if they were so bold as to join him. If a child took a toy from him, he passively permitted it. He scrawled lines on the picture books the other children were colouring, retreating or putting his hands over his ears if they threatened him in anger. His mother was the only person with whom he had any contact at all, and even she spent all of her time developing ways of keeping him at play with her.

After his return home, the mother sent periodic reports about his development. He quickly learned to read fluently and to play simple tunes on the piano. He began, whenever his attention could be obtained, to respond to questions 'which require yes or no for an answer'. Though he occasionally began to speak of himself as 'I' and of the person addressed as 'you', he continued for quite some time the pattern of pronominal reversals. When, for instance, in February, 1939, he stumbled and nearly fell, he said of himself, '*You* did not fall down'.

He expressed puzzlement about the inconsistencies of spelling: 'bite' should be spelled 'bight' to correspond to the spelling of 'light'. He could spend hours writing on the blackboard. His play became more imaginative and varied, though still quite ritualistic.

He was brought back for a check-up in May, 1939. His attention and concentration were improved. He was in better contact with his environment, and there were some direct reactions to people and situations. He showed disappointment when thwarted, demanded bribes promised him, gave evidence of pleasure when praised. It was possible, at the Child Study Home, to obtain with constant insistence some conformity to daily routine and some degree of proper handling of objects. But he still went on writing letters with his fingers in the air, ejaculating words—'Semicolon'; 'Capital'; 'Twelve, twelve'; 'Slain, slain'; 'I could put a little comma or semicolon'—chewing on paper, putting food on his hair, throwing books into the toilet, putting a key down the water drain, climbing on to the table and bureau, having temper tantrums, giggling and whispering autistically. He got hold of an encyclopedia and learned about fifteen words in the index and kept repeating them over and over again. His mother was helped in trying to develop his interest and participation in ordinary life situations.

The following are abstracts from letters sent subsequently by Donald's mother:

September, 1939. He continues to eat and to wash and dress himself only at my insistence and with my help. He is becoming resourceful, builds things with his blocks, dramatizes stories, attempts to wash the car, waters the flowers with the hose, plays store with the grocery supply, tries to cut out pictures with the scissors. Numbers still have a great attraction for him. While his play is definitely improving, he has never asked questions about people and shows no interest in our conversation. . . .

October, 1939 [a school principal friend of the mother's had agreed to try Donald in the first grade of her school]. The first day was very trying for them but each succeeding day he has improved very much. Don is much more independent, wants to do many things for himself. He marches in line nicely, answers when called upon, and is more biddable and obedient. He never voluntarily relates any of his experiences at school and never objects to going. . . .

November, 1939. I visited his room this morning and was amazed to see how nicely he cooperated and responded. He was very quiet and calm and listened to what the teacher was saying about half the time. He does not squeal or run around but takes his place like the other children. The teacher began writing on the board. That immediately attracted his attention. She wrote:

>   BETTY MAY FEED A FISH.
>   DON MAY FEED A FISH.
>   JERRY MAY FEED A FISH.

In his turn he walked up and drew a circle around his name. Then he fed a goldfish. Next, each child was given his weekly reader, and he turned to the proper page as the teacher directed and read when called upon. He also answered a question about one of the pictures. Several times, when pleased, he jumped up and down and shook his head once while answering. . . .

March, 1940. The greatest improvement I notice is his awareness of things about him. He talks very much more and asks a good many questions. Not often does he voluntarily tell me of happenings at school, but if I ask leading questions, he answers them correctly. He really enters into the games with other children. One day he enlisted the family in one game he had just learned, telling each of us just exactly what to do. He feeds himself some better and is better able to do things for himself. . . .

March, 1941. He has improved greatly, but the basic difficulties are still evident. . . .

Donald was brought for another check-up in April, 1941. An invitation to enter the office was disregarded, but he had himself led willingly. Once inside, he did not even glance at the three physicians present (two of whom he well remembered from his previous visits) but immediately made for the desk and handled papers and books. Questions at first were met with the stereotyped reply, 'I don't know'. He then helped himself to pencil and paper and wrote and drew pages and pages full of letters of the alphabet and a few simple designs. He arranged the letters in two or three lines, reading them in vertical rather than horizontal succession, and was very pleased with the result. Occasionally he volunteered a statement or question: 'I am going to stay for two days at the Child Study Home'. Later he said, 'Where is my mother?'

'Why do you want her?' he was asked.

'I want to hug her around the neck.'

He used pronouns adequately and his sentences were grammatically correct.

The major part of his 'conversation' consisted of questions of an obsessive nature. He was inexhaustible in bringing up variations: 'How many days in a week, years in a century, hours in a day, hours in half a day, weeks in a century, centuries in half a millennium', etc., etc.; 'How many pints in a gallon, how many gallons to fill four gallons?' Sometimes he asked, 'How many hours in a minute, how many days in an hour?' etc. He looked thoughtful and always wanted an answer. At times he temporarily compromised by responding quickly to some other question or request but promptly returned to the same type of behaviour. Many of his replies were metaphorical or otherwise peculiar. When asked to subtract 4 from 10, he answered: 'I'll draw a hexagon'.

He was still extremely autistic. His relation to people had developed only in so far as he addressed them when he needed or wanted to know something. He never looked at the person while talking and did not use communicative gestures. Even this type of contact ceased the moment he was told or given what he had asked for.

A letter from the mother stated in October, 1942:

> Don is still indifferent to much that is around him. His interests change often, but always he is absorbed in some kind of silly, unrelated subject. His literal-mindedness is still very marked, he wants to spell words as they sound and to pronounce letters consistently. Recently I have been able to have Don do a few chores around the place to earn picture show money. He really enjoys the movies now but not with any idea of a connected story. He remembers them in the order in which he sees them. Another of his recent hobbies is with old issues of *Time* magazine. He found a copy of the first issue of March 3, 1923, and has attempted to make a list of the dates of publication of each issue since that time. So far he has gotten to April, 1934. He has figured the number of issues in a volume and similar nonsense.

Case 2. Frederick W. was referred on May 27, 1942, at the age of 6 years, with the physician's complaint that his 'adaptive behaviour in a social setting is characterized by attacking as well as withdrawing behaviour'. His mother stated:

> The child has always been self-sufficient. I could leave him alone and he'd entertain himself very happily, walking around, singing. I have never known him to cry in demanding attention. He was never interested in hide-and-seek, but he'd roll a ball back and forth, watch his father shave, hold the razor box and put the razor back in, put the lid on the soap box. He never was very good with cooperative play. He doesn't care to play with the ordinary things that other children play with, anything with wheels on. He is afraid of mechanical things; he runs from them. He used to be afraid of my egg beater, is perfectly petrified of my vacuum cleaner. Elevators are simply a terrifying experience to him. He is afraid of spinning tops.
>
> Until the last year, he mostly ignored other people. When we had guests, he just wouldn't pay any attention. He looked curiously at small children and then would go off all alone. He acted as if people weren't there at all, even with his grandparents. About a year ago, he began showing more interest in observing them, would even go up to them. But usually people are an interference. He'll push people away from him. If people come too close to him, he'll push them away. He doesn't want me to touch him or put my arm around him, but he'll come and touch me.
>
> To a certain extent, he likes to stick to the same thing. On one of the bookshelves we had three pieces in a certain arrangement. Whenever this was changed, he always rearranged it in the old pattern. He won't try new things, apparently. After watching for a long time, he does it all of a sudden. He wants to be sure he does it right.
>
> He had said at least two words ['Daddy' and 'Dora', the mother's first name] before he was 2 years old. From then on, between 2 and 3 years, he would say words that seemed to come as a surprise to himself. He'd say them once and never repeat them. One of the first words he said was 'overalls'. [The parents never expected him to answer any of their questions, were *once* surprised when he did give an answer—'Yes'.] At about 2½ years, he began to sing. He sang about 20 or 30 songs, including a little French lullaby. In his fourth year I tried to make him ask for things before he'd get them. He was stronger-willed than I was and held out longer, and he would not get it but he never gave in about it. Now he can count up to into the hundreds and can read numbers, but he is not interested in numbers as they apply to objects. He has great difficulty in learning the proper use of personal pronouns. When receiving a gift, he would say of himself: 'You say "Thank you" '.

He bowls, and when he sees the pins go down, he'll jump up and down in great glee.

Frederick was born May 23, 1936, in breech presentation. The mother had 'some kidney trouble' and an elective cesarean section was performed about two weeks before term. He was well after birth; feeding presented no problem. The mother recalled that he was never observed to assume an anticipatory posture when she prepared to pick him up. He sat up at 7 months, walked at about 18 months. He had occasional colds but no other illness. Attempts to have him attend nursery school were unsuccessful: 'he would either be retiring and hide in a corner or would push himself into the middle of a group and be very aggressive'.

The boy is an only child. The father, aged 44, a university graduate and a plant pathologist, has travelled a great deal in connection with his work. He is a patient, even-tempered man, mildly obsessive; as a child he did not talk 'until late' and was delicate, supposedly 'from lack of vitamin in diet allowed in Africa'. The mother, aged 40, a college graduate, successively a secretary to physicians, a purchasing agent, director of secretarial studies in a girls' school, and at one time a teacher of history, is described as healthy and even-tempered.

The paternal grandfather organized medical missions in Africa, studied tropical medicine in England, became an authority on manganese mining in Brazil, was at the same time dean of a medical school and director of an art museum in an American city, and is listed in *Who's Who* under two different names. He disappeared in 1911, his whereabouts remaining obscure for 25 years. It was then learned that he had gone to Europe and married a novelist, without obtaining a divorce from his first wife. The family considers him 'a very strong character of the genius type, who wanted to do as much good as he could'.

The paternal grandmother is described as 'a dyed-in-the-wool missionary if ever there was one, quite dominating and hard to get along with, at present pioneering in the South at a college for mountaineers'.

The father is the second of five children. The oldest is a well-known newspaper man and author of a best-seller. A married sister, 'high-strung and quite precocious', is a singer. Next comes a brother who writes for adventure magazines. The youngest, a painter, writer, and radio commentator, 'did not talk until he was about 6 years old', and the first words he is reported to have spoken were, 'When a lion can't talk he can whistle'.

The mother said of her own relatives, 'Mine are very ordinary people'. Her family is settled in a Wisconsin town, where her father is a banker; her mother is 'mildly interested' in church work, and her three sisters, all younger than herself, are average middle-class matrons.

Frederick was admitted to the Harriet Lane Home on May 27, 1942. He appeared to be well nourished. The circumference of his head was 21 inches, of his chest 22 inches, of his abdomen 21 inches. His occiput and frontal region were markedly prominent. There was a supernumerary nipple in the left axilla. Reflexes were sluggish but present. All other findings, including laboratory examinations and X-ray of his skull, were normal, except for large and ragged tonsils.

He was led into the psychiatrist's office by a nurse, who left the room immediately afterward. His facial expression was tense, somewhat apprehensive, and gave the impression of intelligence. He wandered aimlessly about for a few moments, showing no sign of awareness of the three adults present. He then sat down on the couch, ejaculating unintelligible sounds, and then abruptly lay down, wearing throughout a dreamy-like smile. When he responded to questions or commands at all, he did so by repeating them echolalia fashion. The most striking feature in his behaviour was the difference in his reactions to objects and to people. Objects absorbed him easily and he showed good attention and perseverance in playing with them. He seemed to regard people as unwelcome intruders to whom he paid as little attention as they would permit. When forced to respond, he did so briefly and returned to his absorption in things. When a hand was held out before him so that he could not possibly ignore it, he played with it briefly as if it were a detached object. He blew out a match with an expression of satisfaction with the achievement, but did not look up to the person who had lit the match. When a fourth person entered the room, he retreated for a minute or two behind the bookcase, saying, 'I don't want you', and waving him away, then resumed his play, paying no further attention to him or anyone else.

Test results (Grace Arthur performance scale) were difficult to evaluate because of his lack of cooperation. He did best with the Seguin form board (shortest time, 58 seconds). In the mare and foal completion test he seemed to be guided by form entirely, to the extent that it made no difference whether the pieces were right side up or not. He completed the triangle but not the rectangle. With all the form boards he showed good perseverance and concentration, working at them spontaneously and interestedly. Between tests, he wandered about the room examining various objects or fishing in the wastebasket without regard for the persons present. He made frequent sucking noises and occasionally kissed the dorsal surface of his hand. He became fascinated with the circle from the form board, rolling it on the desk and attempting, with occasional success, to catch it just before it rolled off.

Frederick was enrolled at the Devereux Schools on September 26, 1942.

Case 3. Richard M. was referred to the Johns Hopkins Hospital on February 5, 1941, at 3 years, 3 months of age, with the complaint of deafness because he did not talk and did not respond to questions. Following his admission, the interne made this observation:

> The child seems quite intelligent, playing with the toys in his bed and being adequately curious about instruments used in the examination. He seems quite self-sufficient in his play. It is difficult to tell definitely whether he hears, but it seems that he does. He will obey commands, such as 'Sit up' or 'Lie down', even when he does not see the speaker. He does not pay attention to conversation going on around him, and although he does make noises, he says no recognizable words.

His mother brought with her copious notes that indicated obsessive preoccupation with details and a tendency to read all sorts of peculiar interpretations into the child's performances. She watched (and recorded) every gesture and every 'look', trying to find their specific significance and finally deciding on a particular, sometimes very farfetched explanation. She thus accumulated an account that, though very elaborate and richly illustrated, on the whole revealed more of her own version of what had happened in each instance than it told of what had actually occurred.

Richard's father is a professor of forestry in a southern university. He is very much immersed in his work, almost entirely to the exclusion of social contacts. The mother is a college graduate. The maternal grandfather is a physician, and the rest of the family, in both branches, consists of intelligent professional people. Richard's brother, 31 months his junior, is described as a normal, well developed child.

Richard was born on November 17, 1937. Pregnancy and birth were normal. He sat up at 8 months and walked at 1 year. His mother began to 'train' him at the age of 3 weeks, giving him a suppository every morning 'so his bowels would move by the clock'. The mother, in comparing her two children, recalled that while her younger child showed an active anticipatory reaction to being picked up, Richard had not shown any physiognomic or postural sign of preparedness and had failed to adjust his body to being held by her or the nurse. Nutrition and physical growth proceeded satisfactorily. Following smallpox vaccination at 12 months, he had an attack of diarrhoea and fever, from which he recovered in somewhat less than a week.

In September, 1940, the mother, in commenting on Richard's failure to talk, remarked in her notes:

> I can't be sure just when he stopped the imitation of word sounds. It seems that he has gone backward mentally gradually for the last two years. We have thought it was because he did not disclose what was in his head, that it was there all right. Now that he is making so many sounds, it is disconcerting because it is now evident that he can't talk. Before, I thought he could if he only would. *He gave the impression of silent wisdom to me. . . .* One puzzling and discouraging thing is the great difficulty one has in getting his attention.

On physical examination, Richard was found to be healthy except for large tonsils and adenoids, which were removed on February 8, 1941. His head circumference was 54½ cm. His electroencephalogram was normal.

He had himself led willingly to the psychiatrist's office and engaged at once in active play with the toys, paying no attention to the persons in the room. Occasionally, he looked up at the walls, smiled and uttered short staccato forceful sounds—'Ee! Ee! Ee!' He complied with a spoken and gestural command of his mother to take off his slippers. When the command was changed to another, this time without gestures, he repeated the original request and again took off his slippers (which had been put on again). He performed well with the unrotated form board but not with the rotated form board.

Richard was again seen at the age of 4 years, 4 months. He had grown considerably and gained weight. When started for the examination room, he screamed and made a great fuss, but once he yielded he went along willingly. He immediately proceeded to turn the lights on and off. He showed no interest in the examiner or any other person but was attracted to a small box that he threw as if it were a ball.

At 4 years, 11 months, his first move in entering the office (or any other room) was to turn the lights on and off. He climbed on a chair, and from the chair to the desk in order to reach the switch of the wall lamp. He did not communicate his wishes but went into a rage until his mother guessed and procured what he wanted. He had no contact with people, whom he definitely regarded as an interference when they talked to him or otherwise tried to gain his attention.

The mother felt that she was no longer capable of handling him, and he was placed in a foster-home near Annapolis with a woman who had shown a remarkable talent for dealing with difficult children. Recently, this woman heard him say clearly his first intelligible words. They were, 'Good night'.

Case 4. Paul G. was referred in March, 1941, at the age of 5 years, for psychometric assessment of what was thought to be a severe intellectual defect. He had attended a private nursery school, where his incoherent speech, inability to conform, and reaction with temper outbursts to any interference created the impression of feeblemindedness.

Paul, an only child, had come to this country from England with his mother at nearly 2 years of age. The father, a mining engineer, believed to be in Australia now, had left his wife shortly before that time after several years of an unhappy marriage. The mother, supposedly a college graduate, a restless, unstable, excitable woman, gave a vague and blatantly conflicting history of the family background and the child's development. She spent much time emphasizing and illustrating her efforts to make Paul clever by teaching him to memorize poems and songs. At 3 years, he knew the words of not less than 37 songs and various and sundry nursery rhymes.

He was born normally. He vomited a great deal during his first year, and feeding formulas were changed frequently with little success. He ceased vomiting when he was started on solid food. He cut his teeth, held up his head, sat up, walked, and established bowel and bladder control at the usual age. He had measles, chickenpox, and pertussis without complications. His tonsils were removed when he was 3 years old. On physical examination, phimosis was found to be the only deviation from otherwise good health.

The following features emerged from observation on his visits to the clinic, during five weeks' residence in a boarding home, and during a few days' stay in the hospital.

Paul was a slender, well built, attractive child, whose face looked intelligent and animated. He had good manual dexterity. He rarely responded to any form of address, even to the calling of his name. At one time he picked up a block from the floor on request. Once he copied a circle immediately after it had been drawn before him. Sometimes an energetic 'Don't!' caused him to interrupt his activity of the moment. But usually, when spoken to, he went on with whatever he was doing as if nothing had been said. Yet one never had the feeling that he was willingly disobedient or contrary. He was obviously so remote that the remarks did not reach him. He was always vivaciously occupied with something and seemed to be highly satisfied, unless someone made a persistent attempt to interfere with his self-chosen actions. Then he first tried impatiently to get out of the way and, when this met with no success, screamed and kicked in a full-fledged tantrum.

There was a marked contrast between his relations to people and to objects. Upon entering the room, he instantly went after objects and used them correctly. He was not destructive and treated the objects with care and even affection. He picked up a pencil and scribbled on paper that he found on the table. He opened a box, took out a toy telephone, singing again and again: 'He wants the telephone', and went around the room with the mouthpiece and receiver in proper position. He got hold of a pair of scissors and patiently and skilfully cut a sheet of paper into small bits, singing the phrase 'Cutting paper', many times. He helped himself to a toy engine, ran around the room holding it up high and singing over and over again, 'The engine is flying'. While these utterances, made always with the same inflection, were clearly connected with his actions, he ejaculated others that could not be linked up with immediate situations. These are a few examples: 'The people in the hotel'; 'Did you hurt your leg?'; 'Candy is all gone, candy is empty'; 'You'll fall off the bicycle and bump your head'. However, some of those exclamations could be definitely traced to previous experiences. He was in the habit of saying almost every day ,'Don't throw the dog off the balcony'. His mother recalled that she had said those words to him about a toy dog while they were still in England. At the sight of a saucepan he would invariably exclaim, 'Peten-eater'. The mother remembered that this particular association had begun when he was 2 years old and she happened to drop a saucepan while reciting to him the nursery rhyme about 'Peter, Peter, pumpkin eater'. Reproductions of warnings of bodily injury constituted a major portion of his utterances.

None of these remarks was meant to have communicative value. There was, on his side, no affective tie to people. He behaved as if people as such did not matter or even exist. It made no difference whether one spoke to him in a friendly or a harsh way. He never looked up at people's faces. When he had any dealings with persons at all, he treated them, or rather parts of them, as if they were objects. He would use a hand to lead him. He would, in playing, butt his head against his mother as at other times he did against a pillow. He allowed his boarding mother's hands to dress him, paying not the slightest attention to *her*. When with other children, he ignored them and went after their toys.

His enunciation was clear and he had a good vocabulary. His sentence construction was satisfactory, with one significant exception. He never used the pronoun of the first person, nor did he refer to himself as Paul. All statements pertaining to himself were made in the second person, as literal repetitions of things that had been said to him before. He would express his desire for candy by saying. '*You* want candy'. He would pull his hand away from a hot radiator and say, '*You* get hurt'. Occasionally there were parrot-like repetitions of things said to him.

Formal testing could not be carried out, but he certainly could not be regarded as feebleminded in the ordinary sense. After hearing his boarding mother say grace three times, he repeated it without a flaw and has retained it since then. He could count and name colours. He learned quickly to identify his favourite victrola records from a large stack and knew how to mount and play them.

His boarding mother reported a number of observations that indicated compulsive behaviour. He often masturbated with complete abandon. He ran around in circles emitting phrases in an ecstatic-like fashion. He took a small blanket and kept shaking it, delightedly shouting, 'Ee! Ee!' He could continue in this manner for a long time and showed great irritation when he was interfered with. All these and many other things were not only repetitions but recurred day after day with almost photographic sameness.

Case 5. Barbara K. was referred in February, 1942, at 8 years, 3 months of age. Her father's written note stated:

First child, born normally October 30, 1933. She nursed very poorly and was put on bottle after about a week. She quit taking any kind of nourishment at 3 months. She was tube-fed five times daily up to 1 year of age. She began to eat then, though there was much difficulty until she was about 18 months old. Since then she has been a good eater, likes to experiment with food, tasting, and now fond of cooking.

Ordinary vocabulary at 2 years, but always slow at putting words into sentences. Phenomenal ability to spell, read, and a good writer, but still has difficulty with verbal expression. Written language has helped the verbal. Can't get arithmetic except as a memory feat.

Repetitious as a baby, and obsessive now: holds things in hands, takes things to bed with her, repeats phrases, gets stuck on an idea, game, etc., and rides it hard, then goes to something else. She used to talk using 'you' for herself and 'I' for her mother or me, as if she were saying things as we would in talking to her.

Very timid, fearful of various and changing things, wind, large animals, etc. Mostly passive, but passively stubborn at times. Inattentive to the point where one wonders if she hears. (She does!) No competitive spirit, no desire to please her teacher. If she knew more than any member in the class about something, she would give no hint of it, just keep quiet, maybe not even listen.

In camp last summer she was well liked, learned to swim, is graceful in water (had always appeared awkward in her motility before), overcame fear of ponies, played best with children of 5 years of age. At camp she slid into avitaminosis and malnutrition but offered almost no verbal complaints.

Barbara's father is a prominent psychiatrist. Her mother is a well-educated, kindly woman. A younger brother, born in 1937, is healthy, alert, and well developed.

Barbara 'shook hands' upon request (offering the left upon coming, the right upon leaving) by merely raising a limp hand in the approximate direction of the examiner's proffered hand; the motion definitely lacked the implication of greeting. During the entire interview there was no indication of any kind of affective contact. A pin prick resulted in withdrawal of her arm, a fearful glance at the pin (not the examiner), and utterance of the word 'Hurt!' not addressed to anyone in particular.

She showed no interest in test performances. The concept of test, of sharing an experience or situation, seemed foreign to her. She protruded her tongue and played with her hand as one would with a toy. Attracted by a pen on the desk stand, she said: 'Pen like yours at home'. Then, seeing a pencil, she inquired: 'May I take this home?'

When told that she might, she made no move to take it. The pencil was given to her, but she shoved it away, saying, 'It's not my pencil'.

She did the same thing repeatedly in regard to other objects. Several times she said, 'Let's see Mother' (who was in the waiting room).

She read excellently, finishing the 10-year Binet fire story in 33 seconds and with no errors, but was unable to reproduce from memory anything she had read. In the Binet pictures, she saw (or at least reported) no action or relatedness between the single items, which she had no difficulty enumerating. Her handwriting was legible. Her drawing (man, house, cat sitting on six legs, pumpkin, engine) was unimaginative and stereotyped. She used her right hand for writing, her left for everything else; she was left-footed and right-eyed.

She knew the days of the week. She began to name them: 'Saturday, Sunday, Monday', then said, 'You go to school' (meaning, 'on Monday'), then stopped as if the performance were completed.

Throughout all these procedures, in which—often after several repetitions of the question or command—she complied almost automatically, she scribbled words spontaneously: 'oranges'; 'lemons'; 'bananas'; 'grapes'; 'cherries'; 'apples'; 'apricots'; 'tangerine'; 'grapefruits'; 'watermelon juice'; the words sometimes ran into each other and were obviously not meant for others to read.

She frequently interrupted whatever 'conversation' there was with references to 'motor transports' and 'piggy-back', both of which—according to her father—had preoccupied her for quite some time. She said, for instance, 'I saw motor transports'; 'I saw piggy-back when I went to school'.

Her mother remarked, "Appendages fascinate her, like a smoke stack or a pendulum'. Her father had previously stated: 'Recent interest in sexual matters, hanging about when we take a bath, and obsessive interest in toilets'.

Barbara was placed at the Devereux Schools, where she is making some progress in learning to relate herself to people.

Case 6. Virginia S., born September 13, 1931, has resided at a state training school for the feebleminded since 1936, with the exception of one month in 1938, when she was paroled to a school for the deaf 'for educational opportunity'. Dr. Esther L. Richards, who saw her several times, clearly recognized that she was neither deaf nor feebleminded and wrote in May, 1941:

> Virginia stands out from other children [at the training school] because she is absolutely different from any of the others. She is neat and tidy, does not play with other children, and does not seem to be deaf from gross tests, but does not talk. The child will amuse herself by the hour putting picture puzzles together, sticking to them until they are done. I have seen her with a box filled with the parts of two puzzles gradually work out the pieces for each. All findings seem to be in the nature of a congenital abnormality which looks as if it were more of a personality abnormality than an organic defect.

Virginia, the younger of two siblings, was the daughter of a psychiatrist, who said of himself (in December, 1941): 'I have never liked children probably a reaction on my part to the restraint from movement (travel), the minor interruptions and commotions'.

Of Virginia's mother, her husband said: 'She is not by any means the mother type. Her attitude [toward a child] is more like toward a doll or pet than anything else'.

Virginia's brother, Philip, five years her senior, when referred to us because of severe stuttering at 15 years of age, burst out in tears when asked how things were at home and he sobbed: 'The only time my father has ever had anything to do with me was when he scolded me for doing something wrong'.

His mother did not contribute even that much. He felt that all his life he had lived in 'a frosty atmosphere' with two unapproachable strangers.

In August, 1938, the psychologist at the training school observed that Virginia could respond to sounds, the calling of her name, and the command, 'Look!'

> She pays no attention to what is said to her but quickly comprehends whatever is expected. Her performance reflects discrimination, care, and precision.

With the non-language items of the Binet and Merrill-Palmer tests, she achieved an IQ of 94. 'Without a doubt', commented the psychologist,

> Her intelligence is superior to this. . . . She is quiet, solemn, composed. Not once have I seen her smile. She retires within herself, segregating herself from others. She seems to be in a world of her own, oblivious to all but the centre of interest in the presiding situation. She is mostly self-sufficient and independent. When others encroach upon her integrity, she tolerates them with indifference. There was no manifestation of friendliness or interest in persons. On the other hand, she finds pleasure in dealing with things, about which she shows imagination and initiative. Typically, there is no display of affection. . . .

> *Psychologist's note, October, 1939.* Today Virginia was much more at home in the office. She remembered (after more than a year) where the toys were kept and helped herself. She could not be persuaded to participate in test procedures, would not wait for demonstrations when they were required. Quick, skilled moves. Trial and error plus insight. Very few futile moves. Immediate retesting reduced the time and error by more than half. There are times, more often than not, in which she is completely oblivious to all but her immediate focus of attention. . . .

> *January, 1940.* Mostly she is quiet, as she has always worked and played alone. She has not resisted authority or caused any special trouble. During group activities, she soon becomes restless, squirms, and wants to leave to satisfy her curiosity about something elsewhere. She does make some vocal sounds, crying out if repressed or opposed too much by another child. She hums to herself, and in December I heard her hum the perfect tune of a Christmas hymn while she was pasting paper chains.

> *June, 1940.* The school girls have said that Virginia says some words when at the cottage. They remember that she loves candy so much and says 'Chocolate', 'Marshmallow', also 'Mama' and 'Baby'.

When seen on October 11, 1942, Virginia was a tall, slender, very neatly dressed 11-year-old girl. She responded when called by getting up and coming nearer, without ever looking up to the person who called her. She just stood listlessly, looking into space. Occasionally, in answer to questions, she muttered, 'Mamma, baby'. When a group was formed around the piano, one child playing and the others singing, Virginia sat among the children, seemingly not even noticing what went on, and gave the impression of being self-absorbed. She did not seem to notice when the children stopped singing. When the group dispersed she did not change her position and appeared not to be aware of the change of scene. She had an intelligent physiognomy, though her eyes had a blank expression.

Case 7. Herbert B. was referred on February 5, 1941, at 3 years, 2 months of age. He was thought to be seriously retarded in intellectual development. There were no physical abnormalities except for undescended testicles. His electro-encephalogram was normal.

Herbert was born November 16, 1937, two weeks before term by elective cesarean section; his birth weight was 6¼ pounds. He vomited all food from birth through the third month. Then vomiting ceased almost abruptly and, except for occasional regurgitation, feeding proceeded satisfactorily. According to his mother, he was 'always slow and quiet'. For a time he was believed to be deaf because 'he did not register any change of expression when spoken to or when in the presence of other people; also, he made no attempt to speak or to form words'. He held up his head at 4 months and sat at 8 months, but did not try to walk until 2 years old, when suddenly 'he began to walk without any preliminary crawling or assistance by chairs'. He persistently refused to take fluid in any but an all-glass container. Once, while at a hospital he went three days without fluid because it was offered in tin cups. He was 'tremendously frightened by running water, gas burners, and many other things'. He became upset by any change of an accustomed pattern: 'if he notices change, he is very fussy and cries'. But he himself liked to pull blinds up and down, to tear cardboard boxes into small pieces and play with them for hours, and to close and open the wings of doors.

Herbert's parents separated shortly after his birth. The father, a psychiatrist, is described as 'a man of unusual intelligence, sensitive, restless, introspective, taking himself very seriously, not interested in people, mostly living within himself, at times alcoholic. The mother, a physician, speaks of herself as 'energetic and outgoing, fond of people and children but having little insight into their problems, finding it a great deal easier to accept people rather than try to understand them'. Herbert is the youngest of three children. The second is a normal, healthy boy. The oldest, Dorothy, born in June, 1934, after 36 hours of hard labour, seemed alert and responsive as an infant and said many words at 18 months, but toward the end of the second year she 'did not show much progression in her play relationships or in contacts with other people'. She wanted to be left alone, danced about in circles, made queer noises with her mouth, and *ignored persons completely* except for her mother, to whom she clung 'in panic and general agitation'. (Her father hated her ostensibly.) 'Her speech was very meagre and expression of ideas completely lacking. She had *difficulties with her pronouns* and would repeat "you" and "I" instead of using them for the proper persons.' She was first declared to be feebleminded, then schizophrenic, but after the parents separated (the children remaining with their mother), she 'blossomed out'. She now attends school, where she makes good progress; she talks well, has an IQ of 108, and—though sensitive and moderately apprehensive—is interested in people and gets along reasonably well with them.

Herbert, when examined on his first visit, showed a remarkably intelligent physiognomy and good motor coordination. Within certain limits, he displayed astounding purposefulness in the pursuit of self-selected goals. Among a group of blocks, he instantly recognized those that were glued to a board and those that were detachable. He could build a tower of blocks as skilfully and as high as any child of his age or even older. He could not be diverted from his self-chosen occupations. He was annoyed by any interference, shoving intruders away (without ever looking at them), or screaming when the shoving had no effect.

He was again seen at 4 years, 7 months, and again at 5 years, 2 months of age. He still did not speak. Both times he entered the office without paying the slightest attention to the people present. He went after the Seguin form board and instantly busied himself putting the figures into their proper spaces and taking them out again adroitly and quickly. When interfered with he whined impatiently. When one figure was stealthily removed, he immediately noticed its absence, became disturbed, but promptly forgot all about it when it was put back. At times, after he had finally quieted down following the upset caused by the removal of the form board, he jumped up and down on the couch with an ecstatic expression on his face. He did not respond to being called or to any other words addressed to him. He was completely absorbed in whatever he did. He never smiled. He sometimes uttered inarticulate sounds in a monotonous singsong manner. At one time he gently stroked his mother's leg and touched it with his lips. He very frequently brought blocks and other objects to his lips. There was an almost photographic likeness of his behaviour during the two visits, with the main exception that at 4 years he showed apprehension and shrank back when a match was lighted, while at 5 years he reacted by jumping up and down ecstatically.

Case 8. Alfred L. was brought by his mother in November, 1935, at 3½ years of age, with this complaint:

> He has gradually shown a marked tendency toward developing one special interest which will completely dominate his day's activities. He talks of little else while the interest exists, he frets when he is not able to indulge in it (by seeing it, coming in contact with it, drawing pictures of it), and it is difficult to get his attention because of his preoccupation. . . . There has also been the problem of an overattachment to the world of objects and failure to develop the usual amount of social awareness.

Alfred was born in May, 1932, three weeks before term. For the first two months, 'the feeding formula caused considerable concern but then he gained rapidly and became an unusually large and vigorous baby'. He sat up at 5 months and walked at 14.

> Language developed slowly; he seemed to have no interest in it. He seldom tells experience. He still confuses pronouns. He never asks questions in the form of questions (with the appropriate inflection). Since he talked, there has been a tendency to repeat over and over one word or statement. He almost never says a sentence without repeating it. Yesterday, when looking at a picture, he said many times, 'Some cows standing in the water'. We counted fifty repetitions, then he stopped after several more and then began over and over.

He had a good deal of 'worrying':

> He frets when the bread is put in the oven to be made into toast, and is afraid it will get burned and be hurt. He is upset when the sun sets. He is upset because the moon does not always appear in the sky at night. He prefers

to play alone; he will get down from a piece of apparatus as soon as another child approaches. He likes to work out some project with large boxes (make a trolley for instance) and does not want anyone to get on it or interfere.

When infantile thumb sucking was prevented by mechanical devices, he gave it up and instead put various objects into his mouth. On several occasions pebbles were found in his stools. Shortly before his second birthday, he swallowed cotton from an Easter rabbit, aspirating some of the cotton, so that tracheotomy became necessary. A few months later, he swallowed some kerosene 'with no ill effects'.

Alfred was an only child. His father, 30 years old at the time of his birth, 'does not get along well with people, is suspicious, easily hurt, easily roused to anger, has to be dragged out to visit friends, spends his spare time reading, gardening, and fishing'. He is a chemist and a law school graduate. The mother, of the same age, is a 'clinical psychologist', very obsessive and excitable. The paternal grandparents died early, the father was adopted by a minister. The maternal grandfather, a psychologist, was severely obsessive, had numerous tics, was given to 'repeated hand washing, protracted thinking along one line, fear of being alone, cardiac fears'. The grandmother, 'an excitable, explosive person, has done public speaking, published several books, is an incessant solitaire player, greatly worried over money matters'. A maternal uncle frequently ran away from home and school, joined the marines, and later 'made a splendid adjustment in commercial life'.

The mother left her husband two months after Alfred's birth. The child has lived with his mother and maternal grandparents. 'In the home is a nursery school and kindergarten (run by the mother), which creates some confusion for the child.' Alfred did not see his father until he was 3 years, 4 months old, when the mother decided that 'he should know his father' and 'took steps to have the father come to the home to see the child'.

Alfred, upon entering the office, paid no attention to the examiner. He immediately spotted a train in the toy cabinet, took it out, and connected and disconnected the cars in a slow, monotonous manner. He kept saying many times, 'More train—more train—more train'. He repeatedly 'counted' the car windows: 'One, two windows—one, two windows—one, two windows—four window, eight window, eight windows'. He could not in any way be distracted from the trains. A Binet test was attempted in a room in which there were no trains. It was possible with much difficulty to pierce from time to time through his preoccupations. He finally complied in most instances in a manner that clearly indicated that he wanted to get through with the particular intrusion; this was repeated with each individual item of the task. In the end he achieved an *IQ of 140*.

The mother did not bring him back after this first visit because of 'his continued distress when confronted with a member of the medical profession'. In August, 1938, she sent upon request a written report of his development. From this report, the following passages are quoted:

> He is called a lone wolf. He prefers to play alone and avoids groups of children at play. He does not pay much attention to adults except when demanding stories. He avoids competition. He reads simple stories to himself. He is very fearful of being hurt, talks a great deal about the use of the electric chair. He is thrown into a panic when anyone accidentally covers his face.

Alfred was again referred in June, 1941. His parents had decided to live together. Prior to that the boy had been in eleven different schools. He had been kept in bed often because of colds, bronchitis, chickenpox, streptococcus infection, impetigo, and a vaguely described condition which the mother—the assurances of various paediatricians to the contrary notwithstanding—insisted was 'rheumatic fever'. While in the hospital, he is said to have behaved 'like a manic patient'. (The mother liked to call herself a psychiatrist and to make 'psychiatric' diagnoses of the child. From the mother's report, which combined obsessive enumeration of detailed instances with 'explanations' trying to prove Alfred's 'normalcy', the following information was gathered.)

He had begun to play with children younger than himself, 'using them as puppets—that's all'. He had been stuffed with music, dramatics, and recitals, and had an excellent rote memory. He still was 'terribly engrossed' in his play, didn't want people around, just couldn't relax:

> He had many fears, almost always connected with mechanical noise (meat grinders, vacuum cleaners, street cars, trains, etc.). Usually he winds up with an obsessed interest in the things he was afraid of. Now he is afraid of the shrillness of a dog's barking.

Alfred was extremely tense during the entire interview, and very serious-minded, to such an extent that had it not been for his juvenile voice, he might have given the impression of a worried and preoccupied little old man. At the same time, he was very restless and showed considerable pressure of talk, which had nothing personal in it but consisted of obsessive questions about windows, shades, dark rooms, especially the X-ray room. He never smiled. No change of topic could get him away from the topic of light and darkness. But in between he answered the examiner's questions, which often had to be repeated several times, and to which he sometimes responded as the result of a bargain—'You answer my question, and I'll answer yours'. He was painstakingly specific in his definitions. A balloon 'is made out of lined rubber and has air in it and some have gas and sometimes they go up in the air and sometimes they can hold up and when they got a hole in it they'll bust up; if people squeeze they'll bust. Isn't it right?' A tiger 'is a thing, animal, striped, like a cat, can scratch, eats people up, wild, lives in the jungle sometimes and in the forests, mostly in the jungle. Isn't it right?' This question 'Isn't it right?' was definitely meant to be answered; there was a serious desire to be assured that the definition was sufficiently complete.

He was often confused about the meaning of words. When shown a picture and asked, 'What is this picture about?' he replied, 'People are moving *about*'.

He once stopped and asked, very much perplexed, why there was 'The Johns Hopkins Hospital' printed on the history sheets: 'Why do they have to say it?' This, to him, was a real problem of major importance, calling for a great deal of thought and discussion. Since the histories were taken at the hospital, why should it be necessary to have the name on every sheet, though the person writing on it knew where he was writing? The examiner, whom he remembered very well from his visit six years previously, was to him nothing more nor less than a person who was expected to answer his obsessive questions about darkness and light.

Case 9. Charles N. was brought by his mother on February 2, 1943, at $4\frac{1}{2}$ years of age, with the chief complaint, 'The thing that upsets me most is that I can't reach my baby'. She introduced her report by saying: 'I am trying hard not to govern my remarks by professional knowledge which has intruded in my own way of thinking by now'.

As a baby, the boy was inactive, 'slow and phlegmatic'. He would lie in the crib, just staring. He would act almost as if hypnotized. He seemed to concentrate on doing one thing at a time. Hypothyroidism was suspected, and he was given thyroid extract, without any change of the general condition.

His enjoyment and appreciation of music encouraged me to play records. When he was 1½ years old, he could discriminate between eighteen symphonies. He recognized the composer as soon as the first movement started. He would say 'Beethoven'. At about the same age, he began to spin toys and lids of bottles and jars by the hour. He had a lot of manual dexterity in ability to spin cylinders. He would watch it and get severely excited and jump up and down in ecstasy. Now he is interested in reflecting light from mirrors and catching reflections. When he is interested in a thing, you cannot change it. He would pay no attention to me and show no recognition of me if I enter the room. . . .

The most impressive thing is his detachment and his inaccessibility. He walks as if he is in a shadow, lives in a world of his own where he cannot be reached. No sense of relationship to persons. He went through a period of quoting another person; never offers anything himself. His entire conversation is a replica of whatever has been said to him. He used to speak of himself in the second person, now he uses the third person at times; he would say, 'He wants'—never 'I want'. . . .

He is destructive; the furniture in his room looks like it has hunks out of it. He will break a purple crayon into two parts and say, '*You* had a beautiful purple crayon and now it's two pieces. Look what *you* did'.

He developed an obsession about faeces, would hide it anywhere (for instance, in drawers), would tease me if I walked into the room: 'You soiled your pants, now you can't have your crayons!'

As a result, he is still not toilet trained. He never soils himself in the nursery school, always does it when he comes home. The same is true of wetting. He is proud of wetting, jumps up and down with ecstasy, says, 'Look at the big puddle *he* made'.

When he is with other people, he doesn't look up at them. Last July, we had a group of people. When Charles came in, it was just like a foal who'd been let out of an enclosure. He did not pay attention to them but their presence was felt. He will mimic a voice and he sings and some people would not notice any abnormality in the child. At school, he never envelops himself in a group, he is detached from the rest of the children, except when he is in the assembly; if there is music, he will go to the front row and sing.

He has a wonderful memory for words. Vocabulary is good, except for pronouns. He never initiates conversation, and conversation is limited, extensive only as far as objects go.

Charles was born normally, a planned and wanted child. He sat up at 6 months and walked at less than 15 months—'just stood up and walked one day—no preliminary creeping'. He has had none of the usual children's diseases.

Charles is the oldest of three children. The father, a high-school graduate and a clothing merchant, is described as a 'self-made, gentle, calm, and placid person'. The mother has 'a successful business record, theatrical booking office in New York, of remarkable equanimity'. The other two children were 28 and 14 months old at the time of Charles' visit to the Clinic. The maternal grandmother, 'very dynamic, forceful, hyperactive, almost hypomanic', has done some writing and composing. A maternal aunt, 'psychoneurotic, very brilliant, given to hysterics', has written poems and songs. Another aunt was referred to as 'the amazon of the family'. A maternal uncle, a psychiatrist, has considerable musical talent. The paternal relatives are described as 'ordinary simple people'.

Charles was a well developed, intelligent-looking boy, who was in good physical health. He wore glasses. When he entered the office, he paid not the slightest attention to the people present (three physicians, his mother, and his uncle). Without looking at anyone, he said, 'Give me a pencil!' and took a piece of paper from the desk and wrote something resembling a figure 2 (a large desk calendar prominently displayed a figure 2; the day was February 2). He had brought with him a copy of *Reader's Digest* and was fascinated by a picture of a baby. He said, 'Look at the funny baby', innumerable times, occasionally adding, 'Is he not funny? Is he not sweet?'

When the book was taken away from him, he struggled with the hand that held it, without looking at the *person* who had taken the book. When he was pricked with a pin, he said, 'What's this?' and answered his own question: 'It is a needle'.

He looked timidly at the pin, shrank from further pricks, but at no time did he seem to connect the pricking with the *person* who held the pin. When the *Reader's Digest* was taken from him and thrown on the floor and a foot placed over it, he tried to remove the foot as if it were another detached and interfering object, again with no concern for the *person* to whom the foot belonged. He once turned to his mother and excitedly said, 'Give it to you!'

When confronted with the Seguin form board, he was mainly interested in the names of the forms, before putting them into their appropriate holes. He often spun the forms around, jumping up and down excitedly while they were in motion. The whole performance was very repetitious. He never used language as a means of communicating with people. He remembered names, such as 'octagon', 'diamond', 'oblong block', but nevertheless kept asking, 'What is this?'

He did not respond to being called and did not look at his mother when she spoke to him. When the blocks were removed, he screamed, stamped his feet, and cried, 'I'll give it to you!' (meaning 'You give it to me'). He was very skilful in his movements.

Charles was placed at the Devereux Schools.

Case 10. John F. was first seen on February 13, 1940, at 2 years, 4 months of age.

The father said: 'The main thing that worries me is the difficulty in feeding. That is the essential thing, and secondly his slowness in development. During the first days of life he did not take the breast satisfactorily. After fifteen days he was changed from breast to bottle but did not take the bottle satisfactorily. There is a long story of trying to get food down. We have tried everything under the sun. He has been immature all along. At 20 months he first started to walk. He sucks his thumb and grinds his teeth quite frequently and rolls from side to side before sleeping. If we don't do what he wants, he will scream and yell.'

John was born September 19, 1937; his birth weight was 7½ pounds. There were frequent hospitalizations because of the feeding problem. No physical disorder was ever found, except that the anterior fontanelle did not close until he was 2½ years of age. He suffered from repeated colds and otitis media, which necessitated bilateral myringotomy.

John was an only child until February, 1943. The father, a psychiatrist, is 'a very calm, placid, emotionally stable person, who is the soothing element in the family'. The mother, a high-school graduate, worked as secretary in a pathology laboratory before marriage—'a hypomanic type of person; sees everything as a pathological specimen rather than well; throughout the pregnancy she was very apprehensive, afraid she would not live through the labour'. The paternal grandmother is 'obsessive about religion and washes her hands every few minutes'. The maternal grandfather was an accountant.

John was brought to the office by both parents. He wandered about the room constantly and aimlessly. Except for spontaneous scribbling, he never brought two objects into relation to each other. He did not respond to the simplest commands, except that his parents with much difficulty elicited bye-bye, pat-a-cake, and peek-a-boo gestures, performed clumsily. His typical attitude toward objects was to throw them on the floor.

Three months later, his vocabulary showed remarkable improvement, though his articulation was defective. Mild obsessive trends were reported, such as pushing aside the first spoonful of every dish. His excursions about the office were slightly more purposeful.

At the end of his fourth year, he was able to form a very limited kind of affective contact, and even that only with a very limited number of people. Once such a relationship had been established, it had to continue in exactly the same channels. He was capable of forming elaborate and grammatically correct sentences, but he used the pronoun of the second person when referring to himself. He used language not as a means of communication but mainly as a repetition of things he had heard, without alteration of the personal pronoun. There was very marked obsessiveness. Daily routine must be adhered to rigidly; any slightest change of the pattern called forth outbursts of panic. There was endless repetition of sentences. He had an excellent rote memory and could recite many prayers, nursery rhymes, and songs 'in different languages'; the mother did a great deal of stuffing in this respect and was very proud of these 'achievements': 'He can tell victrola records by their colour and if one side of the record is identified, he remembers what is on the other side'.

At $4\frac{1}{2}$ years, he began gradually to use pronouns adequately. Even though his direct interest was in objects only, he took great pains in attracting the attention of the examiner (Dr Hilde Bruch) and in gaining her praise. However, he never addressed her directly and spontaneously. He wanted to make sure of the sameness of the environment literally by keeping doors and windows closed. When his mother opened the door 'to pierce through his obsession', he became violent in closing it again and finally, when again interfered with, burst helplessly into tears, utterly frustrated.

He was extremely upset upon seeing anything broken or incomplete. He noticed two dolls to which he had paid no attention before. He saw that one of them had no hat and became very much agitated, wandering about the room to look for the hat. When the hat was retrieved from another room, he instantly lost all interest in the dolls.

At $5\frac{1}{2}$ years, he had good mastery of the use of pronouns. He had begun to feed himself satisfactorily. He saw a group photograph in the office and asked his father, 'When are they coming out of the picture and coming in here?'

He was very serious about this. His father said something about the pictures they have at home on the wall. This disturbed John somewhat. He corrected his father: 'We have them *near* the wall' ('on' apparently meaning to him 'above' or 'on top').

When he saw a penny, he said, 'Penny. That's where you play tenpins'. He had been given pennies when he knocked over tenpins while playing with his father at home.

He saw a dictionary and said to his father, 'That's where you left the money?'

Once his father had left some money in a dictionary and asked John to tell his mother about it.

His father whistled a tune and John instantly and correctly identified it as 'Mendelssohn's violin concerto'. Though he could speak of things as big or pretty, he was utterly incapable of making comparisons ('Which is the bigger line? Prettier face?' etc.).

In December, 1942, and January, 1943, he had two series of predominantly right-sided *convulsions*, with conjugate deviation of the eyes to the right and transient paresis of the right arm. Neurologic examination showed no abnormalities. His eyegrounds were normal. An electroencephalogram indicated 'focal disturbance in the left occipital region', but 'a good part of the record could not be read because of the continuous marked artefacts due to the child's lack of cooperation'.

Case 11. Elaine C. was brought by her parents on April 12, 1939, at the age of 7 years, 2 months, because of 'unusual development': 'She doesn't adjust. She stops at all abstractions. She doesn't understand other children's games, doesn't retain interest in stories read to her, wanders off and walks by herself, is especially fond of animals of all kinds, occasionally mimics them by walking on all fours and making strange noises'.

Elaine was born on February 3, 1932, at term. She appeared healthy, took feedings well, stood up at 7 months and walked at less than a year. She could say four words at the end of her first year but made no progress in linguistic development for the following four years. Deafness was suspected but ruled out. Because of a febrile illness at 13 months, her increasing difficulties were interpreted as possible postencephalitic behaviour disorder. Others blamed the mother, who was accused of inadequate handling of the child. Feeblemindedness was another diagnosis. For 18 months, she was given anterior pituitary and thyroid preparations. 'Some doctors', struck by Elaine's intelligent physiognomy, 'thought she was a normal child and said that she would outgrow this'.

At 2 years, she was sent to a nursery school, where 'she independently went her way, not doing what the others did. She, for instance, drank the water and ate the plant when they were being taught to handle flowers'. She developed an early interest in pictures of animals. Though generally restless, she could for hours concentrate on looking at such pictures, 'especially engravings'.

When she began to speak at about 5 years, she started out with complete though simple sentences that were 'mechanical phrases' not related to the situation of the moment or related to it in a peculiar metaphorical way. She had an excellent vocabulary, knew especially the names and 'classifications' of animals. She did not use pronouns correctly, but used plurals and tenses well. She 'could not use negatives but recognized their meaning when others used them'.

There were many peculiarities in her relation to situations:

> She can count by rote. She can set the table for numbers of people if the names are given her or enumerated in any way, but she cannot set the table 'for three'. If sent for a specific object in a certain place, she cannot bring it if it is somewhere else but still visible.

She was 'frightened' by noises and anything moving toward her. She was so afraid of the vacuum cleaner that she would not even go near the closet where it was kept, and when it was used, ran out into the garage, covering her ears with her hands.

Elaine was the older of two children. Her father, aged 36, studied law and the liberal arts in three universities (including the Sorbonne), was an advertising copy writer, 'one of those chronically thin persons, nervous energy readily expended'. He was at one time editor of a magazine. The mother, aged 32, a 'self-controlled, placid, logical person', had done editorial work for a magazine before marriage. The maternal grandfather was a newspaper editor, the grandmother was 'emotionally unstable'.

Elaine had been examined by a Boston psychologist at nearly 7 years of age. The report stated among other things:

> Her attitude toward the examiner remained vague and detached. Even when annoyed by restraint, she might vigorously push aside a table or restraining hand with a scream, but she made no personal appeal for help or sympathy.

At favourable moments she was competent in handling her crayons or assembling pieces to form pictures of animals. She could name a wide variety of pictures, including elephants, alligators, and dinosaurs. She used language in simple sentence structure, but rarely answered a direct question. As she plays, she repeats over and over phrases which are irrelevant to the immediate situation.

Physically the child was in good health. Her electroencephalogram was normal.
When examined in April, 1939, she shook hands with the physician upon request, without looking at him, then ran to the window and looked out. She automatically heeded the invitation to sit down. Her reaction to questions—after several repetitions—was an echolalia type reproduction of the whole question or, if it was too lengthy, of the end portion. She had no real contact with the persons in the office. Her expression was blank, though not unintelligent, and there were no communicative gestures. At one time, without changing her physiognomy, she said suddenly: 'Fishes don't cry'. After a time, she got up and left the room without asking or showing fear.

She was placed at the Child Study Home of Maryland, where she remained for three weeks and was studied by Drs Eugenia S. Cameron and George Frankl. While there, she soon learned the names of all the children, knew the colour of their eyes, the bed in which each slept, and many other details about them, but never entered into any relationship with them. When taken to the playgrounds, she was extremely upset and ran back to her room. She was very restless but when allowed to look at pictures, play alone with blocks, draw, or string beads, she could entertain herself contentedly for hours. Any noise, any interruption disturbed her. Once, when on the toilet seat, she heard a knocking in the pipes; for several days thereafter, even when put on a chamber pot in her own room, she did not move her bowels, anxiously listening for the noise. She frequently ejaculated stereotyped phrases, such as, 'Dinosaurs don't cry'; 'Crayfish, sharks, fish, and rocks'; 'Crayfish and forks live in children's tummies'; 'Butterflies live in children's stomachs, and in their panties, too'; 'Fish have sharp teeth and bite little children'; 'There is war in the sky'; 'Rocks and crags, I will kill' (grabbing her blanket and kicking it about the bed); 'Gargoyles bite children and drink oil'; 'I will crush old angle worm, he bites children' (gritting her teeth and spinning around in a circle, very excited); 'Gargoyles have milk bags'; 'Needle head. Pink wee-wee. Has a yellow leg. Cutting the dead deer. Poison deer. Poor Elaine. No tadpoles in the house. Men broke deer's leg' (while cutting the picture of a deer from a book); 'Tigers and cats'; 'Seals and salamanders'; 'Bears and foxes'.

A few excerpts from the observations follow:

> Her language always has the same quality. Her speech is never accompanied by facial expression or gestures. She does not look into one's face. Her voice is peculiarly unmodulated, somewhat hoarse; she utters her words in an abrupt manner.
>
> Her utterances are impersonal. She never uses the personal pronouns of the first and second persons correctly. She does not seem able to conceive the real meaning of these words.
>
> Her grammar is inflexible. She uses sentences just as she has heard them, without adapting them grammatically to the situation of the moment. When she says, 'Want me to draw a spider', she means, 'I want you to draw a spider'.
>
> She affirms by repeating a question literally, and she negates by not complying.
>
> Her speech is rarely communicative. She has no relation to children, has never talked to them, to be friendly with them, or to play with them. She

moves among them like a strange being, as one moves between the pieces of furniture of a room.

She insists on the repetition of the same routine always. Interruption of the routine is one of the most frequent occasions for her outbursts. Her own activities are simple and repetitious. She is able to spend hours in some form of daydreaming and seems to be very happy with it. She is inclined to rhythmical movements which always are masturbatory. She masturbates more in periods of excitement than during calm happiness. . . . Her movements are quick and skilful.

Elaine was placed in a private school in Pennsylvania. In a recent letter, the father reported 'rather amazing changes':

She is a tall, husky girl with clear eyes that have long since lost any trace of that animal wildness they periodically showed in the time you knew her. She speaks well on almost any subject, though with something of an odd intonation. Her conversation is still rambling talk, frequently with an amusing point, and it is only occasional, deliberate, and announced. She reads very well, but she reads fast, jumbling words, not pronouncing clearly, and not making proper emphases. Her range of information is really quite wide, and her memory almost infallible. It is obvious that Elaine is not 'normal'. Failure in anything leads to a feeling of defeat, of despair, and to a momentary fit of depression.

Discussion

The 11 children (eight boys and three girls) whose histories have been briefly presented offer, as is to be expected, individual differences in the degree of their disturbance, the manifestation of specific features, the family constellation, and the step-by-step development in the course of years. But even a quick review of the material makes the emergence of a number of essential common characteristics appear inevitable. These characteristics form a unique 'syndrome', not heretofore reported, which seems to be rare enough, yet is probably more frequent than is indicated by the paucity of observed cases. It is quite possible that some such children have been viewed as feebleminded or schizophrenic. In fact, several children of our group were introduced to us as idiots or imbeciles, one still resides in a state school for the feebleminded, and two had been previously considered as schizophrenic.

The outstanding, 'pathognomonic', fundamental disorder is the children's *inability to relate themselves* in the ordinary way to people and situations from the beginning of life. Their parents referred to them as having always been 'self-sufficient'; 'like in a shell'; 'happiest when left alone'; 'acting as if people weren't there'; 'perfectly oblivious to everything about him'; 'giving the impression of silent wisdom'; 'failing to develop the usual amount of social awareness'; 'acting almost as if hypnotized'. This is not, as in schizophrenic children or adults, a departure from an initially present relationship; it is not a 'withdrawal' from formerly existing participation. There is from the start an *extreme autistic aloneness* that, whenever possible, disregards, ignores, shuts out anything that comes to the child from the outside. Direct physical contact or such motion or noise as threatens to disrupt the aloneness is either treated 'as if it weren't there' or, if this is no longer sufficient, resented painfully as distressing interference.

According to Gesell, the average child at 4 months of age makes an anticipatory motor adjustment by facial tension and shrugging attitude of the shoulders when lifted from a table or placed on a table. Gesell commented:

> It is possible that a less definite evidence of such adjustment may be found as low down as the neonatal period. Although a habit must be conditioned by experience, the opportunity for experience is almost universal and the response is sufficiently objective to merit further observation and record.

This universal experience is supplied by the frequency with which an infant is picked up by his mother and other persons. It is therefore highly significant that almost all mothers of our patients recalled their astonishment at the children's *failure to assume at any time an anticipatory posture* preparatory to being picked up. One father recalled that his daughter (Barbara) did not for years change her physiognomy or position in the least when the parents, upon coming home after a few hours' absence, approached her crib talking to her and making ready to pick her up.

The average infant learns during the first few months to adjust his body to the posture of the person who holds him. Our children were not able to do so for two or three years. We had an opportunity to observe 38-month-old Herbert in such a situation. His mother informed him in appropriate terms that she was going to lift him up, extending her arms in his direction. There was no response. She proceeded to take him up, and he allowed her to do so, remaining completely passive as if he were a sack of flour. It was the mother who had to do all the adjusting. Herbert was at that time capable of sitting, standing, and walking.

Eight of the 11 children acquired the *ability to speak* either at the usual age or after some delay. Three (Richard, Herbert, Virginia) have so far remained 'mute'. In none of the eight 'speaking' children has language over a period of years served to convey meaning to others. They were, with the exception of John F., capable of clear articulation and phonation. Naming of objects presented no difficulty; even long and unusual words were learned and retained with remarkable facility. Almost all the parents reported, usually with much pride, that the children had learned at an early age to repeat an inordinate number of nursery rhymes, prayers, lists of animals, the roster of presidents, the alphabet forward and backward, even foreign-language (French) lullabies. Aside from the recital of sentences contained in the ready-made poems or other remembered pieces, it took a long time before they began to put words together. Other than that, 'language' consisted mainly of 'naming', of nouns identifying objects, adjectives indicating colours, and numbers indicating nothing specific.

Their *excellent rote memory*, coupled with the inability to use language in any other way, often led the parents to stuff them with more and more verses, zoologic and botanic names, titles and composers of victrola record pieces, and the like. Thus, from the start, language—which the children did not use for the purpose of communication—was deflected in a considerable measure to a self-sufficient, semantically and conversationally valueless or grossly distorted memory exercise. To a child 2 or 3 years old, all these words, numbers, and poems ('questions and answers of the Presbyterian Catechism'; 'Mendelssohn's violin concerto'; the 'Twenty-third Psalm'; a French lullaby; an encyclopaedia index page) could hardly have more meaning than sets of nonsense syllables to adults. It is difficult to know for certain whether the stuffing as such has contributed essentially to the course of the psychopathologic condition. But it is also difficult to imagine that it did not cut deeply into the development of language as a tool for receiving and imparting meaningful messages.

As far as the communicative functions of speech are concerned, there is no fundamental difference between the eight speaking and the three mute children. Richard was once overheard by his boarding mother to say distinctly, 'Good night'. Justified scepticism about this observation was later dispelled when this 'mute' child was seen in the office shaping his mouth in silent repetition of words when asked to say certain things. 'Mute' Virginia—so her cottage mates insisted—was heard repeatedly to say, 'Chocolate'; 'Marshmallow'; 'Mama'; 'Baby'.

When sentences are finally formed, they are for a long time mostly parrot-like repetitions of heard word combinations. They are sometimes echoed immediately, but they are just as often 'stored' by the child and uttered at a later date. One may, if one wishes, speak of *delayed echolalia*. Affirmation is indicated by literal repetition of a question. 'Yes' is a concept that it takes the children many years to acquire. They are incapable of using it as a general symbol of assent. Donald learned to say 'Yes' when his father told him that he would put him on his shoulders if he said 'Yes'. This word then came to 'mean' only the desire to be put on his father's shoulders. It took many months before he could detach the word 'yes' from this specific situation, and it took much longer before he was able to use it as a general term of affirmation.

The same type of *literalness* exists also with regard to prepositions. Alfred, when asked, 'What is this picture about?' replied: 'People are moving *about*'.

John F. corrected his father's statement about pictures on the wall; the pictures were '*near* the wall'. Donald T., requested to put something *down*, promptly put it on the floor. Apparently the meaning of a word becomes inflexible and cannot be used with any but the originally acquired connotation.

There is no difficulty with plurals and tenses. But the absence of spontaneous sentence formation and the echolalia type reproduction has, in every one of the eight speaking children, given rise to a peculiar grammatical phenomenon. *Personal pronouns are repeated just as heard*, with no change to suit the altered situation. The child, once told by his mother, 'Now I will give you your milk', expresses the desire for milk in exactly the same words. Consequently, he comes to speak of himself always as 'you', and of the person addressed as 'I'. Not only the words, but even the intonation is retained. If the mother's original remark has been made in form of a question, it is reproduced with the grammatical form and the inflection of a question. The repetition 'Are you ready for your dessert?' means that the child is ready for his dessert. There is a set, not-to-be-changed phrase for every specific occasion. The pronominal fixation remains until about the sixth year of life, when the child gradually learns to speak of himself in the first person, and of the individual addressed in the second person. In the transitional period, he sometimes still reverts to the earlier form or at times refers to himself in the third person.

The fact that the children echo things heard does not signify that they 'attend' when spoken to. It often takes numerous reiterations of a question or command before there is even so much as an echoed response. Not less than seven of the children were therefore considered as deaf or hard of hearing. There is an all-powerful need for being left undisturbed. Everything that is brought to the child from the outside, everything that changes his external or even internal environment, represents a dreaded intrusion.

Food is the earliest intrusion that is brought to the child from the outside. David Levy observed that affect-hungry children, when placed in foster-homes where they are well treated, at first demand excessive quantities of food. Hilde Bruch, in her studies of obese children, found that overeating often resulted when affectionate offerings from the parents were lacking or considered unsatisfactory. Our patients, reversely, anxious to keep the outside world away, indicated this by the refusal of food. Donald, Paul ('vomited a great deal during the first year'), Barbara ('had to be tube-fed until 1 year of age'), Herbert, Alfred, and John presented severe feeding difficulty from the beginning of life. Most of them, after an unsuccessful struggle, constantly interfered with, finally gave up the struggle and all of a sudden began eating satisfactorily.

Another intrusion comes from *loud noises and moving objects*, which are therefore reacted to with horror. Tricycles, swings, elevators, vacuum cleaners, running water, gas burners, mechanical toys, egg beaters, even the wind could on occasions bring about a major panic. One of the children was even afraid to go near the closet in which the vacuum cleaner was kept. Injections and examinations with stethoscope or otoscope created a grave emotional crisis. Yet it is not the noise or motion itself that is dreaded. The disturbance comes from the noise or motion that intrudes itself, or threatens to intrude itself, upon the child's aloneness. The child himself can happily make as great a noise as any that he dreads and move objects about to his heart's desire.

But the child's noises and motions and all of his performances are as *monotonously repetitious* as are his verbal utterances. There is a marked limitation in the variety of his spontaneous activities. The child's behaviour is governed by an *anxiously obsessive desire for the maintenance of sameness* that nobody but the child himself may disrupt on rare occasions. Changes of routine, of furniture arrangement, of a pattern, of the order in which everyday acts are carried out, can drive him to despair. When John's parents got ready to move to a new home, the child was frantic when he saw the moving men roll up the rug in his room. He was acutely upset until the moment when, in the new home, he saw his furniture arranged in the same manner as before. He looked pleased, all anxiety was suddenly gone, and he went around affectionately patting each piece. Once blocks, beads, sticks have been put together in a certain way, they are always regrouped in exactly the same way, even though there was no definite design. The children's memory was phenomenal in this respect. After the lapse of several days, a multitude of blocks could be rearranged in precisely the same unorganized pattern, with the same colour of each block turned up, with each picture or letter on the upper surface of each block facing in the same direction as before. The absence of a block or the presence of a supernumerary block was noticed immediately, and there was an imperative demand for the restoration of the missing piece. If someone removed a block, the child struggled to get it back, going into a panic tantrum until he regained it, and then promptly and with sudden calm after the storm returned to the design and replaced the block.

This insistence on sameness led several of the children to become greatly disturbed upon the sight of anything broken or incomplete. A great part of the day was spent in demanding not only the sameness of the wording of a request but also the sameness of the sequence of events. Donald would not leave his bed after his nap until after he had said, 'Boo, say "Don, do you want to get down?" ' and the mother had complied. But this was not all. The act was still not considered completed. Donald would continue, 'Now say "All right" '. Again the mother had to comply, or there was screaming until the performance was completed. All of this ritual was an indispensable part of the act of getting up after a nap. Every other activity had to be completed from beginning to end in the manner in which it had been started originally. It was impossible to return from a walk without having covered the same ground as had been covered before. The sight of a broken crossbar on a garage door on his regular daily tour so upset Charles that he kept talking and asking about it for weeks on end, even while spending a few days in a distant city. One of the children noticed a crack in the office ceiling and kept asking anxiously and repeatedly who had cracked the ceiling, not calmed by any answer given her. Another child, seeing one doll with a hat and another without a hat, could not be placated until the other hat was found and put on the doll's head. He then immediately lost interest in the two dolls; sameness and completeness had been restored, and all was well again.

The dread of change and incompleteness seems to be a major factor in the explanation of the monotonous repetitiousness and the resulting *limitation in the variety of spontaneous activity*. A situation, a performance, a sentence is not regarded as complete if it is not made up of exactly the same elements that were present at the time the child was first confronted with it. If the slightest ingredient is altered or removed, the total situation is no longer the same and therefore is not accepted as such, or it is resented with impatience or even with a reaction of profound frustration. The inability to experience wholes without full attention to the constituent parts is somewhat reminiscent of the plight of children with specific reading disability who do not respond to the modern system of configurational reading instruction but must be taught to build up words from their alphabetic elements. This is perhaps one of the reasons why those children of our group who were old enough to be instructed in reading immediately became excessively preoccupied with the 'spelling' of words, or why Donald, for example, was so disturbed over the fact that 'light' and 'bite', having the same phonetic quality, should be spelled differently.

Objects that do not change their appearance and position, that retain their sameness and never threaten to interfere with the child's aloneness, are readily accepted by the autistic child. He has a good *relation to objects*; he is interested in them, can play with them happily for hours. He can be very fond of them, or get angry at them if, for instance, he cannot fit them into a certain space. When with them, he has a gratifying sense of undisputed power and control. Donald and Charles began in the second year of life to exercise this power by spinning everything that could be possibly spun and jumping up and down in ecstasy when they watched the objects whirl about. Frederick 'jumped up and down in great glee' when he bowled and saw the pins go down. The children sensed and exercised the same power over their own bodies by rolling and other rhythmic movements. These actions and the accompanying ecstatic fervour strongly indicate the presence of *masturbatory orgastic gratification*.

The children's *relation to people* is altogether different. Every one of the children, upon entering the office, immediately went after blocks, toys, or other objects, without paying the least attention to the persons present. It would be wrong to say that they were not aware of the presence of persons. But the people, so long as they left the child alone, figured in about the same manner as did the desk, the bookshelf, or the filing cabinet. When the child was addressed, he was not bothered. He had the choice between not responding at all or, if a question was repeated too insistently, 'getting it over with' and continuing with whatever he had been doing. Comings and goings, even of the mother, did not seem to register. Conversation going on in the room elicited no interest. If the adults did not try to enter the child's domain, he would at times, while moving between them, gently touch a hand or a knee as on other occasions he patted the desk or the couch. But he never looked into anyone's face. If an adult forcibly intruded himself by taking a block away or stepping on an object that the child needed, the child struggled and became angry with the hand or the foot, which was dealt with per se and not as a part of a person. He never addressed a word or a look to the owner of the hand or foot. When the object was retrieved, the child's mood changed abruptly to one of placidity. When pricked, he showed fear of the *pin* but not of the person who pricked him.

The relation to the members of the household or to other children did not differ from that to the people at the office. Profound aloneness dominates all behaviour. The father or mother or both may have been away for an hour or a month; at their homecoming, there is no indication that the child has been even aware of their absence. After many outbursts of frustration, he gradually and reluctantly learns to compromise when he finds no way out, obeys certain orders, complies in matters of daily routine, but always strictly insists on the observance of his rituals. When there is company, he moves among the people 'like a stranger' or, as one mother put it, 'like a foal who had been let out of an enclosure'. When with other children, he does not play with them. He plays alone while they are around, maintaining no bodily, physiognomic, or verbal contact with them. He does not take part in competitive games. He just is there, and if sometimes he happens to stroll as far as the periphery of a group, he soon removes himself and remains alone. At the same time, he quickly becomes familiar with the names of all the children of the group, may know the colour of each child's hair, and other details about each child.

There is a far better relationship with pictures of people than with people themselves. Pictures, after all, cannot interfere. Charles was affectionately interested in the picture of a child in a magazine advertisement. He remarked repeatedly about the child's sweetness and beauty. Elaine was fascinated by pictures of animals but would not go near a live animal. John made no distinction between real and depicted people. When he saw a group photograph, he asked seriously when the people would step out of the picture and come into the room.

Even though most of these children were at one time or another looked upon as feebleminded, they are all unquestionably endowed with good *cognitive potentialities*. They all have strikingly intelligent physiognomies. Their faces at the same time give the impression of *serious-mindedness* and, in the presence of others, an anxious *tenseness*, probably because of the uneasy anticipation of possible interference. When alone with objects, there is often a placid smile and an expression of beatitude, sometimes accompanied by happy though monotonous humming and singing. The astounding vocabulary of the speaking children, the excellent memory for events of several years before, the phenomenal rote memory for poems and names, and the precise recollection of complex patterns and sequences, bespeak good intelligence in the sense in which this word is commonly used. Binet or similar testing could not be carried out because of limited accessibility. But all the children did well with the Seguin form board.

Physically, the children were essentially normal. Five had relatively large heads. Several of the children were somewhat clumsy in gait and gross motor performances, but all were very skilful in terms of finer muscle coordination. Electroencephalograms were normal in the case of all but John, whose anterior fontanelle did not close until he was $2\frac{1}{2}$ years old, and who at $5\frac{1}{4}$ years had two series of predominantly right-sided convulsions. Frederick had a supernumerary nipple in the left axilla; there were no other instances of congenital anomalies.

There is one other very interesting common denominator in the backgrounds of these children. *They all come of highly intelligent families.* Four fathers are psychiatrists, one is a brilliant lawyer, one a chemist and law school graduate employed in the government Patent Office, one a plant pathologist, one a professor of forestry, one an advertising copy writer who has a degree in law and has studied in three universities, one is a mining engineer, and one a successful business man. Nine of the 11 mothers are college graduates. Of the two who have only high-school education, one was secretary in a pathology laboratory, and the other ran a theatrical booking office in New York City before marriage. Among the others, there was a free-lance writer, a physician, a psychologist, a graduate nurse, and Frederick's mother was successively a purchasing agent, the director of secretarial studies in a girls' school, and a teacher of history. Among the grandparents and collaterals there are many physicians, scientists, writers, journalists, and students of art. All but three of the families are represented either in *Who's Who in America* or in *American Men of Science*, or in both.

Two of the children are Jewish, the others are all of Anglo-Saxon descent. Three are 'only' children, five are the first-born of two children in their respective families, one is the oldest of three children, one is the younger of two, and one the youngest of three.

Comment

The combination of extreme autism, obsessiveness, stereotypy, and echolalia brings the total picture into relationship with some of the basic schizophrenic phenomena. Some of the children have indeed been diagnosed as of this type at one time or another. But in spite of the remarkable similarities, the condition differs in many respects from all other known instances of childhood schizophrenia.

First of all, even in cases with the earliest recorded onset of schizophrenia, including those of de Sanctis' dementia praecocissima and of Heller's dementia infantilis, the first observable manifestations were preceded by at least two years of essentially average development; the histories specifically emphasize a more or less gradual *change* in the patients' behaviour. The children of our group have all shown their extreme aloneness from the very beginning of life, not responding to anything that comes to them from the outside world. This is most characteristically expressed in the recurrent report of failure of the child to assume an anticipatory posture upon being picked up, and of failure to adjust the body to that of the person holding him.

Second, our children are able to establish and maintain an excellent, purposeful, and 'intelligent' relation to objects that do not threaten to interfere with their aloneness, but are from the start anxiously and tensely impervious to people, with whom for a long time they do not have any kind of direct affective contact. If dealing with another person becomes inevitable, then a temporary relationship is formed with the person's hand or foot as a definitely detached object, but not with the person himself.

All of the children's activities and utterances are governed rigidly and consistently by the powerful desire for aloneness and sameness. Their world must seem to them to be made up of elements that, once they have been experienced in a certain setting or sequence, cannot be tolerated in any other setting or sequence; nor can the setting or sequence be tolerated without all the original ingredients in the identical spatial or chronologic order. Hence the obsessive repetitiousness. Hence the reproduction of sentences without altering the pronouns to suit the occasion. Hence, perhaps, also the development of a truly phenomenal memory that enables the child to recall and reproduce complex 'nonsense' patterns, no matter how unorganized they are, in exactly the same form as originally construed.

Five of our children have by now reached ages between 9 and 11 years. Except for Vivian S., who has been dumped in a school for the feeble-minded, they show a very interesting course. The basic desire for aloneness and sameness has remained essentially unchanged, but there has been a varying degree of emergence from solitude, an acceptance of at least some people as being within the child's sphere of consideration, and a sufficient increase in the number of experienced patterns to refute the earlier impression of extreme limitation of the child's ideational content. One might perhaps put it this way: While the schizophrenic tries to solve his problem by stepping out of a world of which he has been a part and with which he has been in touch, our children gradually *compromise* by extending cautious feelers into a world in which they have been total strangers from the beginning. Between the ages of 5 and 6 years, they gradually abandon the echolalia and learn spontaneously to use personal pronouns with adequate reference. Language becomes more communicative, at first in the sense of a question-and-answer exercise and then in the sense of greater spontaneity of sentence formation. Food is accepted without difficulty. Noises and motions are tolerated more than previously. The panic tantrums subside. The repetitiousness assumes the form of obsessive preoccupations. Contact with a limited number of people is established in a twofold way: people are included in the child's world to the extent to which they satisfy his needs, answer his obsessive questions, teach him how to read and to do things. Second, though people are still regarded as nuisances, their questions are answered and their commands are obeyed reluctantly, with the implication that it would be best to get these interferences over with, the sooner to be able to return to the still much desired aloneness. Between the ages of 6 and 8 years, the children begin to play in a group, still never *with* the other members of the play group, but at least on the periphery *alongside* the group. Reading skill is acquired quickly, but the children read monotonously, and a story or a moving picture is experienced in unrelated portions rather than in its coherent totality. All of this makes the family feel that, in spite of recognized 'difference' from other children, there is progress and improvement.

It is not easy to evaluate the fact that all of our patients have come of highly intelligent parents. This much is certain, that there is a great deal of obsessiveness in the family background. The very detailed diaries and reports and the frequent remembrance, after several years, that the children had learned to recite 25 questions and answers of the Presbyterian Catechism, to sing 37 nursery songs, or to discriminate between 18 symphonies, furnish a telling illustration of parental obsessiveness.

One other fact stands out prominently. In the whole group, there are very few really warmhearted fathers and mothers. For the most part, the parents, grandparents, and collaterals are persons strongly preoccupied with abstractions of a scientific, literary, or artistic nature, and limited in genuine interest in people. Even some of the happiest marriages are rather cold and formal affairs. Three of the marriages were dismal failures. The question arises whether or to what extent this fact has contributed to the condition of the children. The children's aloneness from the beginning of life makes it difficult to attribute the whole picture exclusively to the type of the early parental relations with our patients.

We must, then, assume that these children have come into the world with innate inability to form the usual, biologically provided affective contact with people, just as other children come into the world with innate physical or intellectual handicaps. If this assumption is correct, a further study of our children may help to furnish concrete criteria regarding the still diffuse notions about the constitutional components of emotional reactivity. For here we seem to have pure-culture examples of *inborn autistic disturbances of affective contact*.

XXIII

THE NATURE OF CHILDHOOD PSYCHOSIS

LAURETTA BENDER

M.D.

Director, Research Child Psychiatry, Children's Unit,
Creedmoor State Hospital, Queens Village, New York

The childhood psychoses have been a rich field for world-wide investigation for this century and even before. Still, in these 1960s there is little agreement as to what is meant by childhood psychosis, although recently there have been many papers trying to clarify this subject.

1

Definition

In England, K. Cameron[53] classified under the psychotic syndromes of childhood, the schizophrenic, manic or depressive, toxic exhaustive, epileptic, and others. M. Rutter[158, 159] who followed Cameron at Maudsley, believes that child psychoses are not a part of schizophrenia but are associated with a chronic brain syndrome in pre-puberty children and that a psychosis developing at or after puberty may be similar to schizophrenia in adults. M. Creak[61] speaks of childhood psychoses and schizophrenia as identical. Her contributions refer mostly to young children similar to those L. Kanner, United States, has described since 1943[108] as his specific syndrome of early infantile autism 'generically related to schizophrenia' and since 1957 Kanner, and Eisenberg[70], Kanner's associate and follower at Johns Hopkins, have identified it as one of the schizophrenias (Bleuler)[45]. This view has been accepted implicitly by some Americans (Ekstein, Bryant and Friedman)[73] and emphasized by others. Thus W. S. Langford[122] reported that the Committee for Child Psychiatry of Group for the Advancement of Psychiatry (GAP) in 1963 offered a classification of Child Psychotic Disorders under three age periods of childhood. In early childhood, early infantile autism (Kanner), symbiotic infantile psychosis (M. Mahler)[128] and other psychotic reactions such as atypical development (Rank)[148] could be recognized. In later childhood schizophreno-form and other psychotic reactions occurred. In the adolescent period, acute confusional states, schizophrenic reactions of the adult type and other psychotic reactions occurred.

At a regional meeting of the American Psychiatric Association on Diagnostic Classification in Child Psychiatry it was said[122] that psychotic reactions would be classified with brain damage whether of the schizophrenic form or not and that there was a tendency 'to feel that we ought to abandon the term childhood schizophrenia and refer to childhood psychoses' since there is a 'question as to whether the psychoses of early childhood bear any relationship to adult schizophrenic processes'.

M. Tramer, Switzerland[194] expressed his opinion that the nosological confusion and lack of definition concerning childhood schizophrenia is largely caused by 'certain notions in the United States giving rise to the problem as to whether childhood schizophrenia exists at all as a disease entity'. Tramer said that experience shows that in childhood there is a schizophrenic disease process of which heredity is a known main cause and which runs a course into adult schizophrenia. It is based on a primary endogenous process and a secondary one due to the patient having to cope with his problems in a human environment. He believes, however, that it is rare and presents a clinical picture similar to the adults. He protests the more frequent diagnoses made in the United States[28]. Tramer[192] reported a case of infantile schizophrenia which he examined at 12 years but whose mother wrote a diary of him starting at birth. It is of interest that the mother had influenza in the third month and the infant weighed only 2,540 grams at birth. His atypical development started at once, he was autistic in the third year and then became increasingly disturbed, lost his speech and regressed into a chronic course.

D. A. Van Krevelen (Netherlands)[197, 198, 199] recognizes Kanner's syndrome of early infantile autism as a specific syndrome of a psychotic nature but states that it is a pathological development arising from cerebral lesions in which the parent-child relationship is unimportant. He[199] emphasizes H. Asperger's (Austria)[4] report on the autistic psychopath in childhood who presents pictures of psychoses in childhood in families with histories of psychoses. Also early infantile autism and autistic psychopathy in later childhood occurred in the same family. Van Krevelen shows that children with early infantile autism have brain damage and consequently he believes that it is the result of early brain damage in cases of autistic psychopathy on an inherited basis. C. Burns, England[52], has reported a ten-year follow-up on five such cases and found that they had all made a 'schizoid adjustment'. Two, at least, had been diagnosed at some period in childhood as childhood schizophrenia. Berner and Spiel[42] also report on seven juvenile delinquents who presented a picture of infantile autism early and of autistic psychopathy of Asperger later.

This author believes that childhood psychoses should not be considered synonymous with childhood schizophrenia. Psychotic states associated with brain damage, with the convulsive states, with encephalitis, and with other stressful situations occur in childhood and are certainly psychoses. The question of manic-depressive psychoses and reactive depressions have been often discussed in the literature. But these subjects will be reported on elsewhere in this book.

This author feels that she must give her own definition, to clarify her point of view: Schizophrenia in childhood is the same process as schizophrenia in adulthood; it is a psychobiologic entity determined by an inherited predisposition, an early physiologic or organic crisis, and a failure in an adequate defence mechanism; schizophrenia persists for the lifetime of the individual but exhibits different clinical or behavioural or psychiatric features at different epochs in the individual's development and in relationship to compensating or decompensating defences which can be influenced by environmental factors (Bender)[21]. Thus we see the autistic and symbiotic features in infancy and early childhood[21], the psychosis of later childhood and the pseudo-neurotic (Hoch and Polatin)[100] and pseudo-psychopathic[22] features of adolescence. Many states of schizophrenia are not psychotic by virtue of latency, of remissions, of adequate neurotic defences or in response to treatment. The confirmation of the diagnosis in late adolescence or adulthood in several follow-up studies with co-workers is seen as confirming this definition[30, 32, 37].

2

Historical Notes

The history of childhood psychoses has been often told. Usually it is said to be a disease recognized only in the 20th century starting with the description of *dementia praecocissima* by de Sanctis[162] and described and investigated, particularly in the United States for the last 25 years (Bellak[12], Bradley[51], Despert[67], Ekstein et al.[73], Gianascol[86], Howells[101], Kanner[107], Kessler[116], Rubinstein[156]).

J. Louise Despert was one of the first in the United States[66] to describe diagnostic criteria and therapy in verifiable cases of childhood schizophrenia. In a 1965 book[67], *The emotionally disturbed child, then and now*, she maintains that careful perusal of historical documents from many countries does not reveal any evidence of schizophrenia in childhood before this century and that there is undoubtedly an increase in this illness, which she calls primarily an ego disease associated with a parallel weakening of the family structure with a correlated increase in the disturbances in the parent-child relationship.

Leo Kanner, who wrote the first American textbook in *Child psychiatry*[107] has repeatedly emphasized that Americans neglected the European history of child psychiatry while there was none in America before this century.

Kanner[112] refers to the following English and European reports of cases of psychoses or insanity in children before 1900. Gottfried Keller, Munich (1713); J. E. D. Esquirol, France (1830); J. B. F. DesCuret, France (1841); Emminghaus, Germany (1887); W. W. Ireland, England (1898); N. Manheimer, England (1899); H. Maudsley, England (1880); P. Moreau deTours, France (1888). In the twentieth century there was also, according to Kanner, A. Homburger, Germany (1926); S. de Sanctis, Italy (1925); J. Lutz, Switzerland (1937); T. Ziehen, Germany (1926); Heller, Germany (1908).

It is of considerable interest that the term *demence praecoce* was first used by B. B. Morel in 1860[138] for a 13-year-old boy, previously normal but whose mother and grandmother were insane, and who developed an acute psychosis which passed into a hebetude-like torpor 'the dire termination of hereditary madness' (quoted by P. Wender, 1963) and also that Kahlbaum[105] divided the paraphrenias into three age-based psychoses, neophrenia, hebephrenia and presbyphrenia.

E. A. Rubinstein[156] contested Kanner's statement that America offered nothing before 1900 and referred to case reports of psychotic or insane children with discussions by Benjamin Rush (1812); James MacDonald (1845); I. M. Kerlin (1878); and S. V. Clevenger (1883) who reviewed the literature, and Spitzka (1880) who stated that insanity occurs early in life due to hereditary transmission, and the causes were usually organic except for sudden fright. Harriett Alexander (Chicago)[1] besides blaming the acute diseases, especially the exanthemata of childhood, for psychotic states, was the first to discuss the psychological and developmental problems of childhood. She recognized a wide variety of neurotic and psychotic states in childhood. B. Sachs wrote two treatises[160,161] on mental illness in children, describing them as dementia praecox and manic depressive insanity similar to adults.

John Haslam (1809) reported by G. E. Vallient[196] recounted the case of a 5-year-old boy admitted to Bethlem Asylum in 1799 that would seem to fit the description of Kanner's early infantile autism.

A number of papers reporting cases of childhood schizophrenia were published in the 1920s (see Goldfarb and Dorsen)[90]; Hart, (1927); Kasanin and Kaufman (1929); A. A. Brill (1926). In 1930, more clinical discussions followed the work of Potter[145], including Despert[66]; W. Bromberg (1933); Bender[15,16]; Piotrowsky (1937). Lutz[127] in Switzerland published his first paper on childhood schizophrenia in 1937.

3
Review: Childhood Psychosis, United States, to 1956

Introduction

A significant contribution to the knowledge of childhood schizophrenia was made by R. Ekstein, K. Bryant, and S. W. Friedman, when they compiled and analysed the literature (especially for the United States) for the 10-year period 1946 to 1956, with a bibliography of 542 items in L. Bellak's *Schizophrenia: a review of the syndrome*[73]. They credit Bellak[12] with a similar review for the previous 10 years and include this work in their survey. This reviewer will summarize much of Ekstein, Bryant and Friedman's work before going on to consider the ten-year period since 1956.

Authors in the United States contributing to the literature are viewed as appearing on a spectrum from Kallmann[106], who has presented the evidence for the hereditary basis for schizophrenia; through Bender[21] and her theory of a maturational disorder; Kanner[111] and Rank[148] and their associates, who acknowledge a constitutional factor but stressed the importance of the personality and attitudes of the parents, the emotional quality of the parent-child relationship and the early environmental influences as having a noxious effect on the development of the schizophrenic child. The spectrum is further extended by Mahler[128] with her studies on the effect of the mother-child symbiosis on the development of ego identity with its special importance for schizophrenia in constitutionally vulnerable children; the psychoanalysts and ego psychologists exemplified by Beres[41], Gianascol[86], Hartman[95], Smolen[180], and their extensive researches into personality and ego function from a psychodynamic point of view, many of whom postulated some constitutional weakness also; and Despert[67] and Szurek[188] and Blau[44] who see childhood schizophrenia as an ego disorder with only psychogenic factors arising from the family climate and the suppressed neurotic problems of the parents.

The trend to establish the unique dynamic identity of schizophrenia as an illness of childhood, as distinguished from its manifestations peculiar to adults, and with definite diagnostic criteria, received its greatest impetus from the work of Kanner[108, 110], Bender[18] and Mahler[129, 131]. Their descriptions of early infantile autism, childhood schizophrenia, and symbiotic psychosis, have established clinical pictures and have provided us with the necessary criteria that have enabled us to begin to emerge from the nosologic confusion inherent in the problem of schizophrenia.

Childhood Schizophrenia: Lauretta Bender and Associates

Ekstein's formulation of Bender's contribution emphasized her clinical studies and research at Bellevue Hospital, New York City, for over 20 years (first reports of schizophrenic children)[15, 16] in which the concept of this disorder was developed on a biological basis. In early writing[18] childhood schizophrenia was conceived as a well-recognized syndrome with a characteristic behaviour disorder in every area of functioning of the personality based on a biological dysfunction akin to encephalopathy. In 1948[18] there was introduced the concept of plasticity as characterizing the schizophrenic disturbance, supported by Gesell's concept[85] in his book *Embryology of behaviour*. Thus childhood schizophrenia was seen as involving a maturational lag at the embryonic level characterized by a primitive plasticity in all areas from which subsequent behaviour develops. This disordered maturation was seen as genetically determined, in agreement with Kallmann[106] and activated by a physiological crisis such as birth, or any of the prenatal and perinatal accidents. Anxiety was seen as the core organismic response calling forth a variety of defence mechanisms.

Bender used Gesell's categories of embryological development as the areas of dysfunction in the schizophrenic infant or young child. These included the homeostatic mechanisms arising in the vaso-vegetative areas; respiratory patterns related to speech, language and ideation; sleep and wakefulness associated with changing states of consciousness; muscular tone responding to vestibular sensations; and tonic-neck reflex motor patterning. These functional areas are subject to abnormal maturation, when the genetically determined schizophrenic process leads to an embryonic plasticity or undifferentiated patterning in all experiences. This leads to the schizophrenic disorder in the infant and child from early in life.

The term dysmaturation was used by some of Bender's associates (Freedman[81], Caplan[54], and Helme[39]). All of these emphasized the importance of the biological process of maturation and the development of the personality resulting from the interaction of the organism with the environment for the understanding and etiology of childhood schizophrenia. The process of dysmaturation they consider the primary cause with its roots in the foetal development of the human organism. Secondary is the anxiety which every organism experiences when it undergoes a disturbance of its biological equilibrium. How the organism then attempts to counter the disorganizing effects of both the anxiety and the disturbed equilibrium constitutes what Bender and her associates describe as the tertiary symptoms that determine the great variety of clinical pictures presented by schizophrenic children.

Basic to Bender's work is the belief that genetic factors determine the infant's vulnerability to a schizophrenic type of maturational disorder when a biological crisis decompensates the stability. This is related to Kallmann's[106] conclusions 'that children with schizophrenia at an early age (before puberty) are distinguished by (*i*) a specific vulnerability factor in the enzymatic range, and (*ii*) by a general constitutional inability or low ability to control through compensatory activities this basic deficiency in the complex process of growth and maturation'. Kallmann's findings also indicate an early effect in schizophrenic children of the same genotype assumed to be responsible for the basic symptoms of adult schizophrenia. Bender believes that the decompensating factor, in many cases at least, is a pre- or perinatal damage or biological crisis of some nature. Therefore many schizophrenic children show evidence of biological defects or brain damage in addition to the three-phase disorder of schizophrenia itself.

Cultural as well as familial factors have concerned Bender and Grugett[38] seeking the social factors interacting with biological and hereditary substrata. Statistical data was acquired from large numbers of child patients studied from 1934-1951 at Bellevue Hospital in New York City, regarding their racial, religious, cultural, social and family relationships. There was a male/female ratio under seven of two/one, and from seven to eleven the males exceeded the females as much as five times. Similar ratios were found by Kallmann, who believed it was a true biological and not a cultural difference. It is also recorded by Eisenberg and Kanner[71].

There was no specific pattern of family life regarding emotional, social and economic climate of these children admitted freely (without selection) in a large city hospital. However, severe emotional illness and psychotic states of parents and grandparents pointed to clinical confirmation of possible genetic factors[31].

At Bellevue Hospital, Peck, Rabinovitch and Cramer[140] confirmed the viewpoint that there was no uniform pattern of family life dynamics and no typical pathological attitudes of mothers to account for child's illness on psychogenic basis. Freedman[81] also agreed with this. Rabinovitch[146] emphasized the primary disturbance inborn in the child and saw the mother's negative attitude as her response to rejection by the schizophrenic child unable to respond to her affection, distorting normal relationship between them.

Paul Schilder's Contributions

Paul Schilder[173] paid great attention to the biological features of schizophrenia. The tendency for schizophrenics to give in to postural changes; to turning on the longitudinal axis with divergence of the outstretched hands in response to the passive turning of the head; the automatic compliance to clinging[174] (see also Bowlby[49]); the ocular motor reflexes; and the negativism. These have also been referred to as 'soft neurological signs'[172] to distinguish them from neurological signs due to structural brain pathology.

The turning on the longitudinal axis with divergence of the outstretched hands spontaneously or in response to passive turning of the head in schizophrenic children, has been called the whirling test (Bender[18]) confirmed by Teicher[191], Silver[178], Rachman and Berger[147], Colbert and Koegler[59].

Schilder[173] had expressed the hope that psychoanalysis of children would bring to light the psychogenic factors or trauma in infancy that

2u

would be sufficient to account for the severity of the symptoms and the malignancy of the course of schizophrenia in contrast to a simple neurosis. Psychoanalysis, even in his own experience, had failed in adults to uncover such factors. He considered that psychoanalytic work with children, including that of Melanie Klein[117], had been disappointing in this regard.

Schilder's[171] concept of the body image as a continuously evolving, labile, never static construction from total perceptual experiences, determined by the total life experiences and reflecting the psychopathology in schizophrenia, has been widely accepted. It has contributed much to psychological thinking in schizophrenia, particularly of children (Bender[18, 30] and Keeler[40]).

Leo Kanner's Syndrome: Early Infantile Autism

When Leo Kanner first introduced the unique syndrome of early infantile autism in 1943[108], he was impressed with the innateness and specificity of the syndrome and stated that it seemed to be 'a pure culture example of inborn autistic disturbance of affective contact'.

The innateness was inferred from the observation that the condition was present from the beginning of life or as early as the first and second year and thereafter distorted the development of the child in a characteristic way. In this he was following Adolf Meyer's teaching that mental disorders were habit disorganization determined by constitutional weaknesses and life experience.

This specificity of the syndrome was based on two primary features[110]; (*i*) extreme autistic aloneness, and (*ii*) an anxious obsessive desire for the preservation of sameness in environment, daily routine and experiences. Four secondary features were also described: (*i*) a language disturbance[109] with mutism or non-communicative language with echolalia, bizarre language, thought disturbances, failure to use first person pronoun; (*ii*) a skilful relationship with non-human objects; (*iii*) an intelligent appearing facies often with some evidence of isolated areas of high cognitive ability while (*iv*) testing at a low level of intellectual functioning.

Early observations and repeated experience with the parents of these children led Kanner to conclude that there was a typical consistent pattern in the parents' personalities and in their characteristic attitudes toward their children, which seemed to underlie the dynamics of the children's psychopathological condition or at least to further emphasize the specific characteristics. Kanner[111] described the parents as characteristically cold and obsessional, sophisticated and intelligent, but adjusting to life and their relationships in the most impersonal and mechanical manner. They were often professional people, emotionally undemonstrative, and disdainful of any frivolities. It was stated that they reared their children in an emotionally refrigerated atmosphere and kept empathy and warmth out of their lives. He felt that the parents had escaped the psychotic proportions of their offspring and could be spoken of as successful autistic adults in whom there was a familial trend.

Although studies of the families of Kanner's series of children with early infantile autism did not reveal as high a genetic incidence of schizophrenia in other members of the family as reported by other workers (Kallmann, Bender), Kanner repeatedly referred to the probable genetic factor because of the characteristics of the parents and the evident constitutional or innate features in the children. Kanner has agreed that other etiological factors must be considered. It has been admitted that 10 per cent of the parents seen in the Johns Hopkins Clinic did not fit the stereotype, and those who do, have raised normal children and that similarly frigid parents are seen who do not have autistic offspring[71]. He has mentioned[110] that brain damage might be a factor in some cases, but he never documented this.

He did emphasize that the parents undoubtedly influenced the psychopathology in the child but he never implied or stated that early infantile autism was a strictly psychogenic condition, which has been widely assumed.

Since 1956, both Kanner[114] and Eisenberg[71] have offered the concept that early infantile autism is in itself a specific clinical syndrome belonging to the heterogeneous group of schizophrenias as defined by Bleuler[45]. Thus it is denied by them that there is a unitary disease of schizophrenia which may occur in childhood or even from the 'beginning of life' as early infantile autism. Thus also they see the possibility of multiple etiological factors but a specific syndrome reaction.

Follow-up studies of Kanner's original group of children with early infantile autism revealed that those children who had some degree of useful speech by five years had a 50 per cent chance at fair to good adjustment in a school setting by adolescence[71]. This represented a third of the total group. However, the adolescent autistic children who did not emerge from their illness subsequently functioned at a severely retarded level[70]. The later course of these patients has not been published.

As late as 1964[113] Kanner said, 'This concept of early infantile autism was diluted by some to deprive it of its specificity so that the term is used as a pseudo-diagnostic waste basket for a variety of unrelated conditions and a nothing-but psychodynamic etiology was decreed by some as the only valid explanation so that further curiosity was either stifled or scorned'.

A very extensive literature has developed following Kanner's concept. Some workers have started out quite close to Kanner's teachings that 'innate as well as experiential factors conjoin to produce a clinical picture'[71]. They ultimately come to the conclusion or to work with the idea that familial climate or parental, especially maternal, relationship with the child or psychogenic factors are most important.

On the other hand, a recent (1965) review by Menolascino[137] has indicated that the literature reveals the wide divergence in views on the cause of autistic reactions in childhood. Thirty-four children reported by him presented initial clinical pictures of autism but were found to be divisible into eight distinct etiological sub-groups.

Margaret Mahler's Symbiotic Psychosis

Margaret Mahler's concept of symbiotic psychosis syndrome has had three important consequences. (*i*) She has emphasized this particular syndrome in the early period of childhood schizophrenia in children who are 'constitutionally vulnerable and predisposed to the development of a psychosis . . . creating the vicious cycle of the pathogenic mother-child relationship'[132]. (*ii*) She has also used this clinical experience to evolve ideas about the development of the infant's personality from a psychoanalytic point of view. (*iii*) And of course she has worked out a therapeutic regime directed logically at both mother and child. It would seem that she has been misrepresented by such statements as the importance of her work is in the 'elucidation of the significance of the infant-mother symbiotic relationship for the genesis of childhood schizophrenia'[73].

In her most recent and widely read paper on this subject, Mahler[130] states that she believes that the clinical picture of childhood schizophrenia depends on the stage of maturity of the central nervous system and the integrating function of the ego and that a psychosis afflicts only constitutionally vulnerable infants. She claims that her main thesis is that 'the cardinal difficulty is an inability of the psychotic infant to use the external maternal ego for restructuralization of his own rapidly maturing, vulnerable ego'. The basic dynamic mechanisms are described by her as 'psychotic, delusional, autistic modes of adjustment which appear to aim at the restoration of omnipotent oneness with the symbiotic mother but also leads to panicky fear of fusion and dissolution of the self'.

Children with Atypical Development: Beata Rank and Co-workers

Rank[149] and her co-workers have studied a group of young psychotic children whom they refer to as children of atypical development. They have been impressed with the hereditary and constitutional role in the etiology and agree that they are referring to the same children that others call schizophrenic, though some may be brain damaged, etc. Follow-up studies[152] to the age of 22 on 125 of their first children with atypical development, did indeed show that 45 or 36 per cent were severely retarded, regressed or arrested; 7 per cent were minimally or moderately retarded; 43 or 34 per cent were brittle schizoid, eruptive schizoid or schizophrenic. Sixteen or 12·8 per cent were classified as normal or neurotic, responding to treatment.

Their studies[148], which are largely therapy-oriented, have placed the emphasis on psychodynamic factors inherent in the early parent-child relationship. Rank feels that it is more profitable to study the role of the post-natal psychological factors in the emergence of the disturbance which she calls ego fragmentation, since something can be done about this even though it may not be the basic etiological factor. She found, for example, that the majority of mothers of the atypical children she studied, were either psychotic and had to be hospitalized repeatedly, or were immature narcissistic, trying to maintain a fictitious image of themselves as woman, wife and mother, or the 'as if' mother of Helene Deutsch[68].

Emotional Deprivation

There has been a marked tendency in the United States to misconstrue the work of important contributors in the effort to emphasize psychogenic factors, especially the mother-child relationship. This is seen in the work of Mahler, though she has never failed to make her position clear. Kanner, too, as stated above, has denied that the refrigerator parents he has described, were the sole cause of early infantile autism.

There has been a similar misuse of Spitz's work. He has made important contributions in his studies of emotionally deprived infants and those who are separated from the mother. He has shown the effects of deprivation on the developing personality and has discussed hospitalism and anaclitic depressions[181]. He has related these experiences to mourning reactions, depression and melancholia. He has referred to them as 'psychoses'. He has never, however, implied or stated that there was any relationship to childhood schizophrenia. In his classification of psychogenic diseases of infancy[182] which he relates to a wrong kind of mother-child relationship or a deficiency in it, he does not include schizophrenia or autism. He uses this material to elaborate psychoanalytic concepts in personality development.

John Bowlby's (England) extensive and important studies on maternal deprivation and more recently on separation anxiety, and his psychoanalytic studies of the relationship of child and mother, have contributed very much indeed to our understanding of normal personality development and its deviations in relationship to various vicissitudes in the mother-child tie[47, 48, 49, 50]. His work re-emphasizes many important factors in the development of the child's personality. These include the infants' need for skin contact (Ribble)[153], their drive for clinging (Hermann[96], Schilder[174]) and the significance of the early smile response in the evolution of object relation (Spitz and Wolf[183]). There is also the relationship of birth trauma to anxiety (Rank[150], Greenacre[93]). He refers, too, to the contributions of ethnology in the understanding of personality development exemplified in Harlow's work with infant monkeys raised in various situations of separation from their mothers.

Bender[23] in a summarizing statement on emotional deprivation and its implication in child psychiatry emphasized that typically the emotionally deprived infant suffers lack of development of the personality and ego and super ego formation; such a child lacks the capacity to identify, to love, to hate, to feel guilt or anxiety. There is retardation in language and concept formation and consequently in mental development. The schizophrenic child is basically anxious with some defence mechanism. The withdrawn autistic schizophrenic child may partially resemble an emotionally deprived one but a child with a symbiotic psychosis is quite different. Of course, an emotionally deprived child may be also latently schizophrenic, perhaps abandoned by schizophrenic parents, or maybe also brain damaged, and thus the clinical picture may be confused.

Ego Psychology and Psychoanalysis

Ego psychology under the leadership of Heinz Hartman[95] has had many contributors to the study of the psychotic child whether thought of as schizophrenic or not. Hartman has made it clear that a predisposition exists in the child to make him vulnerable to a psychosis, nevertheless ego psychology helps in the understanding of what goes on in mother and child and in the relationship between them.

A constitutional defect in the perceptual apparatus is postulated which may cause the child to have a distorted view of reality and interfere in object representation and relationship and in self-representation. There is no effort to determine the why or the how of the postulated constitutional defect in the perceptual apparatus. But there is a very considerable literature which elaborates findings in the study of ego development in the psychotic child and the associated mother-child relationship, sometimes remembering the constitutional defect as the causative factor (Starr[184], Weil[203]), but often referring to the mother's failure to meet the child's needs as the cause of the psychosis (Geleerd[84]). This literature has been sympathetically developed to 1956 by Ekstein, Bryant and Friedman[73] who identify themselves with the ego psychology movement.

Difficulties in ego and object boundaries in schizophrenia as described by Federn[77], have come under study by the ego psychologists, as has also the body image concepts of Schilder, which undergo distortions in schizophrenia also and almost specifically in childhood (Bender[18, 30, 40]).

Some (Beres[41]) would like to withdraw the term schizophrenia and use terms describing variants of ego deviation in childhood disorders, in order to emphasize a primary interest in the vicissitudes of ego development and defences. Schizophrenia is seen as the result of ego regression and the schizophrenic process as the breakdown of those unique human qualities that constitute the ego.

Ekstein[73] and his co-workers refer to the children they have studied as borderline or schizophrenic-like and this implies that the problems lie entirely in the ego structure without a postulated constitutional defect. Recently (1964)[55] their work is known as 'therapeutic-action research'.

Fantasy of omnipotence, as a stage in normal development which is retained characteristically in young schizophrenic children, has also come under study (Geleerd[84], Weil[202, 203]). Introjections were also studied following the teachings of Melanie Klein[117] which has been taken up especially by Winnicott in England with his important contribution on transitional objects[204]. These two writers have spoken of psychotic phases in infantile development, a concept which is not, however, accepted by everyone. Jack Rapoport[151], an American student of Melanie Klein, observed introjected objects in schizophrenic children and led to a considerable literature on this subject in the United States (Furer[83], Jaffe[103]).

Most of the work done by the ego psychologists is in the framework of therapy. Theories and interpretations are elaborated which are observed under these rather special conditions with selective patients. This author finds some difficulty in the universal use of the term 'ego' since this has come to be thought of as though it were a structural reality by many who could never define it. It is hard to conceptualize what is meant by saying 'The schizophrenic process is the breakdown of those unique human qualities that constitute the ego'.

Mahler[129] has concluded that psychoanalytic methods had to be used to understand the dynamics of childhood schizophrenia. It must be recognized that autism is only a 'mechanism for serving the psychotic child's need for survival' to help the child 'to cope with, ward off the panic created by his symbiotic-parasitic needs and his dread of the dissolution of his identity through the pull and threat of symbiotic fusion with his mother'. She also recalled that as far as psychoanalytic ego-psychology was concerned Hartman had indicated a quarter of a century earlier that research in schizophrenia contributed to the understanding of the ego and its functions.

Szurek[188] and his co-workers accept the concept that childhood schizophrenia is wholly psychogenic and determined by post-natal influences, some of which are the suppressed unconscious drives and unresolved conflicts from the childhood of the parents.

4

Modern Perspectives in Childhood Psychosis, 1956-66

Organic Factors Emphasized in the United States

There have been a number of workers in the United States who have elaborated on organic or constitutional factors in the etiology of childhood schizophrenia and allied conditions. Clemens Benda[13] speaks of an inherited weakness of drives, a total organismic deficiency which could account for all the defects in the development in the total personality disorder of the young schizophrenic child. Later Benda[14] distinguishes between mental defect, autism and childhood psychosis. Mental defect is exemplified by a focal brain damage. Autism is the result of a specific 'inability to handle symbolic form and assume an abstract attitude or use speech and communication'. Schizophrenia he believes is a disease process probably associated with some kind of auto-toxic biochemical effects and possibly secondarily causing neuropathological changes in the brain; the psychotic child has a developmental disorder of integration which interferes with his contact with his environment. Heller's disease, he emphasizes, is a rare, progressive, deteriorating process.

Malamud[133] reported on six children who had been diagnosed childhood schizophrenia and on post-mortem examination found that they all had a familial deteriorating brain disease (two pairs of siblings with amaurotic familial idiocy, the others atypical). He claimed that the diagnosis of childhood schizophrenia is often inadequate or misleading, noting that in the cases he examined the role of organic factors were either ignored or underestimated. Of course, Malamud, as a neuropathologist sees only those cases selected by death, which are few. Malamud also does not recognize Heller's disease as a proven entity. Kanner[107] in his text book *Child psychiatry*, clearly distinguished between Heller's disease and early infantile autism.

Paul Yakovlev[208, 209] postulates inborn visceral metabolic and motility disorders which in turn disrupt the homeostasis, autonomic, locomotive and emotional life of the child, interfering with normal development. He suggests that this may result in organic pathology of the brain which in turn aggravates the condition.

Kurt Goldstein[91] argues for an inborn defect in the capacity to abstract in the 'abnormal child'. 'Early childhood psychoses' result from consequent defects in development and maturation and from inadequate behaviour in the environment (mother). He wishes to avoid the distinguishing 'autistic' and 'symbiotic' conditions because they may be no more than different reactions by which the abnormal organism has come to terms with the world.

Recent United States Books on Childhood Psychosis

During the 1960s several books have appeared on the subject of the childhood psychoses. The five most significant ones are the products of United States clinical and research psychology with its emphasis on methodology, research structure, data collecting and analysis, and hypothetical modes. To this author it sometimes seems as though the child and his problem, i.e. the psychosis, is lost in the process. However, current controversies are dealt with and important contributions are made.

William Goldfarb's book *Childhood schizophrenia*[87] is a report of five years research on 26 'schizophrenic' children 6-6 to 11-2 years in the Henry Ittleson Research Centre for Childhood Research, New York, a residential treatment centre for severely disordered young children. Children selected were those so disturbed or deviant in their behaviour and development that they could not attend the usual schools and who belonged to intact families. A psychiatric diagnosis was not considered important. The term childhood schizophrenia was used as a broad term to cover gross disorders in young children's behaviour and development. It is stated that 'it is not the usual precursor of the schizophrenia of later onset nor should the two be regarded as equivalent'.

Hypotheses were held for two classes of etiology which led to their studies of: (*i*) the role of the family in relational and interactional patterns affecting psychosexual experiences and motivation, and; (*ii*) the significance of foetal and early childhood trauma in the clinical expression of cerebral dysfunction.

The research curiosity was directed to the area of the 'cyclical reverberating interplay between causes and consequences in the theoretical model'. There is no research curiosity for the causes of the family pathology, the parental perplexity, or the considerable prenatal and paranatal disorders of the brain.

The 26 experimental children were compared with 26 matched normal children from a public school. The research consisted of extensive batteries of tests and appraisals providing physical, behavioural, and familial data. The schizophrenic children were found to be uniformly inferior to normal children in perceptual processes, in conceptual functions requiring abstraction and categorization, in speech and communicative ability and in psychomotor capacities. There was a suggested 'receptor intolerance' for distance receptor modalities such as visual and auditory in contrast to proximal sensory or touch experiences; probably the most original contribution of the study. Eighteen of the 26 schizophrenic children were organically impaired while none of the control children were so damaged. The mean Full IQ on the WISC of the schizophrenic children was 72·4 as compared to 108·8 for the controls.

It was postulated that the behaviour deficiencies found in childhood schizophrenics can be produced either by neurological defects in the child or by abnormal conditions in the rearing environment (failure on the part of the family to reinforce desirable modes of adaptive response in the child).

Thus Goldfarb sees in childhood two schizophrenic clusters which he designates as 'organic' and 'non-organic'. The 'non-organic' schizophrenic child is seen as the result of a 'particular type of paralysis of parental function termed "parental perplexity" '. The brain damage in the 'organic' children was confirmed by neurological evaluation by a paediatric neurologist (Taft)[190].

To a considerable extent this book has failed to show Goldfarb's contribution to the field of childhood psychosis. In a later paper[88] he again states that childhood schizophrenia is not an entity but indicates a child with ego manifestation of particular deficits to which we assign the label. He specifies four areas of deficits: (*i*) aberration in receptor behaviour by avoiding distance receptors, hearing and seeing, as instruments for monitoring executive acts; and thereby leading to disturbances in orientation in time, space, reality and self-awareness; (*ii*) a defect in abstracting and categorizing incoming stimuli or a primary cognitive defect; (*iii*) a hedonic aberration or lack of dynamic force behind integrative behaviour, or a deficient response to pleasure and pain; (*iv*) finally a failure in external psychosexual stimulation or reinforcement due to perplexed parents.

He finally concludes that the schizophrenic child merely seems to be equipped with a narrower repertoire of responses than the normal. He seems to derive his conclusions from the learning theory a United States school of psychology applied to a selected group of children, some of whom may have been only brain damaged.

Austin M. Des Lauriers' book *The experience of reality in childhood schizophrenia*[65] is derived from his experiences at the Children's Unit of the Topeka State Hospital. The book consists of two parts. The second reports on the therapy of seven youngsters, 13 to 16 years old, who were chronically withdrawn cases of childhood schizophrenia. The first part deals with theoretical considerations concerning the psychological experience of reality, its relation to schizophrenia, and the approach to and appraisal of psychotherapy. His approach is essentially derived from ego psychology, somewhat modified by earlier (1926-27) association with Bender and a Bellevue experience with schizophrenic children and Schilder's concept of body image. In childhood schizophrenia he saw 'a structural deficiency in personality development which left the child incapable of experiencing reality in a meaningful and goal-directed way . . . incapable of establishing stable reality relationships because he lacked whatever was necessary for reality experience to take place'.

He then sought for the conditions necessary in the development of the human being for the experience of reality and for the stable establishment of reality relationships. He found within the psychoanalytic framework a conceptual model of the experience of reality influenced by David Rapaport's work on ego psychology and some of Rapaport's ideas on the works of Schilder, Piaget, Werner, Hartman, Kris, Spitz and Federn.

Schizophrenia, for him, is evidently the same process throughout the total life period—childhood, adolescence and adulthood. Having defined it from the point of view of its intrinsic psychological causes, as a structural deficiency involving a severe diminution of narcissistic cathexis of body boundaries and preventing the possibility of reality experiences and reality relationships, he attempted a therapeutic approach to prove his theory. This is what the book is about and it is well done.

The Genain quadruplets, a case study and theoretical analogies of heredity and environment in schizophrenia (1963), edited by David Rosenthal[155] is a case study of a schizophrenic family—mother, father (and his mother) and identical quadruplet daughters, all schizophrenic in varying degrees, and an analysis of research data by 25 contributors, mostly research psychologists from the National Institute of Mental Health. This includes data on intellectual and physical development, electroencephalogram studies, handwriting, human figure drawings, and Rorschach protocols were most revealing in terms of showing schizophrenic features in the various members of the family and the degree of severity of each at any one time.

David Rosenthal, the editor, in his theoretical overview, offers three theories for the etiology of schizophrenia. (*i*) Monogenic—biochemical; (*ii*) Diathesis-stress; (*iii*) Life experience. The concept of multiple etiology is offered, meaning that some cases of schizophrenia are due to one etiology, and others to another. For this author it seems probable that all three etiologies (and others!) occur in all cases.

The significant contribution here is the case study, the story of Gertrude, the schizophrenic mother of the schizophrenic quadruplets, inexorably living out her life drama with a schizophrenic husband (also epileptic), and mother-in-law.

The evaluation of the four girls' psychoses accepts their genetically identical background as a constant. The most significant life experience factor for all four girls was thought to be that their mother did not regard them as individuals in their own right but rather as an extension of herself and the girls devoted themselves to living out their mother's mandate, thus sacrificing their own personalities. Each internalized a different aspect of the mother's personality according to the mother's 'set' (fantasies, projections, perceptions, and expectations) towards her. The 'favoured' daughter, Nora, was to be dependent upon her mother in a symbiotic relationship; the second, Myra, was to live out her mother's independent strivings; the third, Iris, was to repress her instinctual drives as her mother tried to do; and the fourth, Hester, was the embodiment of the 'bad' drives which the mother tried to deny. Hester had the smallest birth weight and developed the least satisfactorily. She first showed her schizophrenic illness at about three years by anxious masturbatory behaviour.

Each girl in her psychosis is seen as caricaturing the role her mother assigned to her. Each assignment (by the mother) was unconsciously and narcissistically made and represented an aspect of the mother's early emotional deprivation, conflicts, and anxiety-producing experiences. It was as though the mother had to fulfil herself in these daughters.

The personality patterns which emerged in this study help clarify hypotheses about the nature of the mother-child relationship in schizophrenia due to genetic factors as was established here. However, it still does not make clear what the schizophrenia is. Is it something genetically determined that makes the child vulnerable to the mother's unconscious mandates? Or does it only exist intrinsically in the relationship between mother and child? None of the structured research methods contribute to our understanding of the genetic factor.

This concept of the influence of the mother's 'set' derived from her own infantile conflicts has been advanced by S. Szurek[188] and Adelaide Johnson[104] and others[179]. A recent review of a psychodynamic approach to childhood schizophrenia is by Gianascol[86] from Szurek's staff at the Langley Porter Neuropsychiatric Service, San Francisco. He concludes that as a result of their studies 'highly significant and independent confirmation of our clinical hunches, gives further impetus to our study of parental psychopathology and the modes of family interaction through which the disorder (childhood schizophrenia) arises'. A recent sophisticated review[8] indicates that some United States authors emphasize the importance of certain family backgrounds and social learning variables in the histories of many schizophrenics.

Bernard Rimland's *Infantile autism—the syndrome and its implications for a neural theory of behaviour*[154] is a highly speculative book derived, admittedly by the author, a clinical psychologist, from the literature not only in psychology but also in genetics, neurology, neurophysiology, and biochemistry; some 500 items in all. He does not hesitate to assert that infantile autism is a unique condition in children of a certain kind of superior parent, that it is not related to schizophrenia, that there are no psychogenic factors but a biological one which results in an impairment between sensation and memory. Rimland then speculates that the reticular formation is the right site for the dysfunction in autism since the reticular formation might be 'the site linking sensory input with the prior content of the brain'. He further postulates that hyperoxia at the time of birth may cause the lesion in the reticular formation of children who become autistic. He compares this to blind children with retrolental fibroplasia, caused by hyperoxia in incubators in which these premature babies were placed, since conditions similar to autism have been described by some authors, especially Keeler[115]. Bender and Andermann[35] have shown that these are not cases of autism but of gross brain damage related to the conditions which led to early premature birth. Rimland continues to speculate on a theory of behaviour and intelligence and personality.

Samuel Beck's *Psychological processes in schizophrenic adaptation*[11] is a follow-up and elaboration on his *Six schizophrenias*[9]. His work is based on Rorschach studies on carefully selected and controlled populations of schizophrenics including childhood schizophrenics.

In his first book, Beck found that one of his six schizophrenias, the SG group, was for schizophrenic children only. He found that as children developed they patterned out of one group but into another. He stated that schizophrenia is a permanent character structure—once a schizophrenic—always a schizophrenic. However, there are latent patterns too, when a schizophrenic is not psychotic. He also stated that schizophrenia in children is not *ipso facto* a cause for pessimism; it dictates planning.

In his 1965 book, Beck reports on studies of schizophrenic children from the Michael Reese Hospital and from the Orthogenic School, both in Chicago. He saw two different patterns related to the severity of the illness in the Michael Reese Hospital children. However, later in development both patterns shifted; the sicker children unhappily progressed into the core, dream or sanctuary schizophrenias. He refers to 'fate and chance, i.e. environmental vicissitudes, together with whatever destiny in heredity makes for mental disorders so converged in their effects . . . to develop schizophrenia'. Some of both groups of children in later studies had improved into transition and some into neurotic patterns. As children they were in a fluid changing state which, as Beck points out, is recognized implicitly or explicitly in the writings of various students of childhood schizophrenia. He also has a good deal to say about the variety of psychological symptomatology and of ego inadequacies and about the nature of defences and the possibility that schizophrenia itself is a defence.

Beck[10] was more specific in a discussion of Bender's paper on pseudo-psychopathic schizophrenia in adolescence[22] in which it had been stated that 'schizophrenia has been viewed as a life-long process but a psychosis occurs only when more satisfactory defences fail' and a pseudo-psychopathic behaviour was often observed in adolescent boys who were known to have childhood schizophrenia before puberty. Beck said that this confirmed his thinking that schizophrenics continue indefinitely in some sort of schizophrenic adjustment. His schizophrenic children shifted from one schizophrenic pattern into another over the years but always remained in one of the patterns. They were never free of the latency for schizophrenia. 'Whether the schizophrenic is to become psychotic is a function of the ego's stamina and of the stresses to which the vicissitudes of life subject it.'

New York Contributions: Lauretta Bender and Associates

Bender and her associates and co-workers at Bellevue City Hospital and Creedmoor State Hospital, New York, have continued their clinical and research reports over the past ten years.

It is a part of Bender's definition of childhood schizophrenia that a pre- or perinatal defect, trauma or damage or a 'physiological crisis' is the stress that decompensates the genetically vulnerable child and produces a clinically recognizable picture of childhood schizophrenia[24, 26, 32]. Because such organic factors are so often present, it is particularly difficult to make a differential diagnosis with a non-schizophrenic brain damaged child[29]. Both may use autism as a withdrawal defence against the anxiety arising from disorganization or lack of organization. Some years may pass before the more typical longitudinal course of schizophrenia may prove itself[30, 32] or convulsions or other clear neurological patterns develop[25], such as a continuous course of low grade mental deficiency. These latter cases may be combinations of brain damage, mental deficiency and schizophrenia.

Faretra and Bender[75] confirmed Knoblock and Pasamanick[118], whose epidemiological studies led to the concept of a 'continuum of pregnancy casualties' in deviant developmental disorders of children. Faretra and Bender found that maternal bleeding and toxaemia during the pregnancy, and especially prematurity of the infant, occurred frequently enough to be considered significant in childhood schizophrenia. Zitrin et al.[210] at Bellevue Hospital found a significantly higher incidence of prematurity among the total cases of mental disorders in children and among schizophrenic children than controls.

Bender's[31] findings for familial incidence of schizophrenia in children diagnosed childhood schizophrenia agreed with Kallmann[106] with a high incidence in parents and siblings, indicating the highest vulnerability for pre-puberty boys.

The concept of plasticity as the specific characteristic of schizophrenic disorders in function and behaviour was first formulated by Bender in 1948[20]. In a summation[33] it was postulated that evolutionary processes in development of the human brain, mentality, and behaviour may represent causes for stress in the child in the process of maturation. Undetermined pleuripotential plastic states appear to be characteristic for those brain functions specifically human and last in evolutionary development and still evolving. Clinical experience has shown that in all maturational lags in children, primitive plastic phenomena of an embryonic nature is the characteristic dysfunction. Childhood schizophrenia is such a maturational lag with a pattern of behavioural disturbance in all areas of central nervous system functions, characteristically plastic at an embryonic level.

This explains the common underlying pattern of disturbance in schizophrenia, in the visceral or autonomic functions, in perception, mentation, language, in motor activity and emotional-social behaviour. It also may make understandable the great variety of clinical pictures and symptomatology which are presented by schizophrenic children. It accounts for the response to physiological and pharmacological therapies which have aimed at reducing the plastic patterning in homeostasis, in the tone of the vascular bed of viscera and in the motor system, in perception and the affective and social behaviour. It explains the schizophrenic tendency for regressions, remissions, and even accelerated, precocious, and creative capacities and the reverberating anxiety which is at the core of the schizophrenic experience.

Some therapeutic procedures have interesting implications for basic concepts. There is a theoretical interest in serotonin as possibly related to schizophrenia, and LSD-25 and some of its derivatives are serotonin inhibitors. Also, LSD-25 and derivatives are stimulants to the autonomic nervous system with specific effects on the tone of the vascular bed. They also have specific effects on perception, causing perceptual experiences to be more vivid. Their psychotomimetic properties might possibly break through autistic defences. With these features in mind an effort has been made to use some of these drugs (LSD-25, UML-491 (Sansert) and psilocybin (Sandoz) in a therapeutic programme[36, 76]. They have appeared to be effective in these areas with the continuous daily administration of the drug and also to have had a favourable influence on the clinical course.

Autonomic Nervous System and Childhood Psychosis

Studies on the autonomic nervous system were made by Faretra[76] with the Funkenstein test and these drugs. She showed that there was a considerable variability in the vital functions with an increasing potentiation toward normal findings. These recordings suggest evidence of plasticity in the patterning of these autonomic functions in the children, which tends to be corrected by the d-lysergic acid medication.

L. Rubin[157] included autistic and normal children in his studies of autonomic dysfunction in the psychoses leading to his theory that the psychoses are 'chronic disordered autonomic' states with an imbalance between the adrenergic-cholinergic mechanisms.

There have been several references in the literature to the frequent occurrence of coeliac syndrome in schizophrenic children (Graff and Handford[92], Bender[27]). This condition can best be understood as an immaturity of the intestinal system. The relationship between gut motility and serotonin has been documented by Sandler[165]. In turn serotonin has been implicated in the psychoses.

Schizophrenic Infants: Barbara Fish

Most important work has been done by Fish[78, 79, 80] in her studies of infants. Fish by examining at one month and following to $9\frac{1}{2}$ years a series of infants in a well baby clinic, found 'that it was possible to detect an infant who later became schizophrenic by applying Bender's criteria to a random sample of infants (and that this) provides direct corroboration of her concept that the schizophrenic child is distinguished at an early age from his non-schizophrenic peers by specific biologic signs of disordered maturation. Furthermore, later development illustrated the features predicted by Bender, namely (*i*) overall plastic patterning of development in all areas; (*ii*) immature homeostasis; (*iii*) early torporous state; (*iv*) molluscuous muscle tone; and (*v*) immature posture and motor activity'.

Fish and Alpert[79] made a study of the neurological development of infants born to schizophrenic mothers and were able to observe deviations in the state of consciousness, vestibular function, motility and muscle tonus, as early as the first day of life and continuing into the early months of infancy.

They observed immature vestibular responses to caloric stimulation in two infants by sustained tonic deviations to the side of the slow component rather than the expected nystagmus, and this tended to persist. Similar studies were made by Colbert *et al.*[59] on older children. They called attention to Lorente de No's[125] experimental studies indicating that the rapid component depends upon the functioning of the reticular formation, and it was suggested that the persistent tonic response in these deviate infants is related to dysfunction in the development of this system.

Biochemical Studies: Siva Sankar

Important work has been started on the biochemical aspects of schizophrenia in childhood by Siva Sankar and his associates[166, 167, 168]. Biogenic amines received some attention and justifiably so in view of their involvement in the actions of psychoactive drugs, and in phenylketonuria (Nadler and Hsia[139], Perry[142]). Elevated levels of serotonin have been reported in autistic children by Schain and Freedman[170]. Perry[141] (see also Sankar et al.[168]) reported the occurrence of N-methylmetanephrine in the urines of 3 out of 18 juvenile psychotics. However, Shaw and his colleagues[176, 177] could not find any significant differences between schizophrenic and non-schizophrenic children with respect to the effect of tryptophan loading on the urinary excretion of indoles nor with respect to the urinary aminoacid due to excretion patterns. Heeley[97] reported impaired metabolism of tryptophan (pyridoine-dependent systems) in 9 out of 16 children who showed deviant behaviour from a very early age, but not in children who regressed into psychotic behaviour at a later age.

A summary of these biochemical findings shows that in most of the tests, the autistic schizophrenic children stand on one end of the test results and the non-schizophrenic children on the other end. The non-autistic schizophrenic children are usually in between.

The schizophrenic (autistic) child compares to a chronologically younger non-schizophrenic patient. This observation gives biochemical support to the theory of 'maturational lag' in childhood schizophrenia. The involvement of biogenic amine uptake by the thrombocytes, differences in plasma electrolyte and complex lipids may indicate involvement of possibly a defect in adenosine triphosphate production and also a defect of neural functions of complex lipids, biogenic amines and of electrolytes. It is interesting to speculate that childhood schizophrenia (autism) may be a lipidosis.

That the permeability of the erythrocyte may be involved in childhood schizophrenia is indicated by the observation that the ratio of adenosine triphosphatase activities in the lysed blood and whole blood (B/A) is much higher in the schizophrenic children. Lipoprotein complexes (e.g. hematosides of RBC Stroma) are usually involved in permeability of cells. The differences in several enzymatic activities, especially lactic dehydrogenase and alkaline phosphatase, show that the autistic child is comparable to more primitive types of tissues (e.g. embryonic or cancer tissues) in the lag of development of biochemical and metabolic ingenuities, but not to the extent to indicate muscular, osseous or hepatic dysfunction. The interpretation of the data was in terms of biochemical parameters or as characteristic profiles of childhood schizophrenia rather than pointing to the biochemical etiology of the disease.

Psychological Studies

Bender as the author of the Visual Motor Gestalt Test[17] has found its use in studying schizophrenic children especially revealing of immaturity, fluidity, plasticity, and variability in the visual motor gestalt function[19] which continues into adulthood[30].

Wechsler and Jaros[201] have explored the possibility of a specific schizophrenic pattern in the intellectual function of children. The Wechsler Intelligence Scale for Children was used in the study of schizophrenic children of normal intelligence from Bellevue Hospital, from Creedmoor State Hospital, and from the League Day School of New York. It was found that by analysing the WISC subtests in terms of signs and test patterns it was possible to differentiate between schizophrenic and non-schizophrenic children in a considerable percentage of cases. A measure of variability was determined by combining any one of three signs such as the verbal score being 16 points more than performance score, with subtests that suggest a higher abstract ability in schizophrenics. This piece of work tends to confirm clinical impressions that when schizophrenic children have adequate intelligence they show great variability in different functions and at different times, they are often highly verbal and abstract in their thinking, which also suggests the characteristic of plasticity in schizophrenic children.

Language of Schizophrenic Children

The language of schizophrenic children has come in for a great dea of study since the earliest intensive clinical observations (Potter[145], Despert[66], Kanner[109], Bender[18], Goldfarb[89]). But there has been a marked upsurge of interest in this area during the 1960s. Cunningham and Dixon[64] observed an autistic boy over six months, analysing his speech quantitatively and qualitatively in terms of Piaget's (1959) classification. They found that it resembled the language of a 24-30-month-old child quantitatively, it was inferior as a means of communication. Ekstein[72] made a study on the acquisition of speech in the autistic child and found that echolalia serves the function of restitution, the restoration of the mother's voice, and the recognition of the ego offering an example of 'regression in the service of the ego'.

Wolff and Chess[207] analysed the language of 14 schizophrenic children under 8 years of age. They found that the most striking abnormality was stereotyped repetition appropriate to earlier levels of development or to previous experiences accompanied by a lack of expression of curiosity, or of spontaneity or awareness of changing situations. Cobrinik[57, 58] in two studies, found that verbal stereotypy in schizophrenic children should be considered in the larger framework of behavioural dissociation. It reveals the child's inability to derive meaning from speech and to use it for individual communicative purposes or of obtaining satisfaction from organizing experiences; they resort to emphasizing the concrete derivative aspects of speech.

Summary of United States Studies: Paul Hoch

Paul Hoch[99] in a summarizing paper on schizophrenia said, 'We consider schizophrenia basically to be an organic disorder. . . . Clinical and experimental evidence that what we call schizophrenia is a special form of integrative disorganization. This disorganization pattern is widespread and as characteristic as the so-called organic reaction types. Schizophrenia occurs in every culture and may be precipitated by different noxae in predisposed individuals. This predisposition is inherited. We could further speculate that a pre-eminently cortical impairment occurs in the so-called organic psychoses. On the other hand, a pre-eminently subcortical impairment occurs in schizophrenia or a disruption of normal relationship between cortex and subcortex'.

At this time Hoch did not mention schizophrenia in childhood but in 1950, when discussing Bender's paper 'The psychotic child' (Bender, 1952) before the New York Academy of Medicine, he said, 'Dr Bender in her studies confirms many deviations in schizophrenic children which are known in adult schizophrenics. As she follows her line of observation, it will ultimately be profitable in elucidating the etiology of this order.

'Schizophrenia, originally described as a disease, was later seen as a reaction of the individual to stress situations. Today it is understood by many as a biological deviation from the norm: that the homeostatic regulation of the individual is disturbed. Schizophrenia is not a mental disease, it is a disease of the whole individual. This is true for schizophrenic adults and it is true for schizophrenic children too.'

British Studies in Child Psychosis

The influence of Melanie Klein[117] on the understanding of childhood psychosis from her psychoanalytic studies in children is well known and has been referred to in the discussion on psychoanalysis. Her definition of a childhood psychosis as a failure to project the introjected bad parent is a classic. Her emphasis upon the greater anxiety in psychoses arising from the early developmental stages in the depressive and paranoid phases has had considerable influence in the understanding of psychoses and the justification for psychoanalytic intervention in early childhood.

Anna Freud's[82] contributions, especially resulting from her observations at the Hampstead Child-therapy Clinic set up in London during the war, have contributed to understanding of deviate development in children and therefore to the psychoses, but especially in terms of corrective therapy.

In Winnicott's many psychoanalytic contributions to childhood, only rather casual references to the psychoses are made. The definition of childhood schizophrenia as an 'environmental deficiency disease' has been ascribed to him and defended by him[205, 206]. However, he modifies this definition by saying that schizophrenia is a failure in the maturation process 'itself a matter of heredity' and also a failure in the facilitating environment. It has already been pointed out that his most important contribution was his delineation and elaboration of transitional objects and phenomena.

We have also discussed the important work of John Bowlby for over 25 years and with world wide influence from his 1941 *Maternal care and mental health*[47] to his latest papers on the relationship of the child and mother[49], separation anxiety[50] and ethology which have enhanced the psychoanalytic literature in the understanding of the development of the normal and the abnormal child[48].

M. Creak has contributed a number of important clinical studies[60, 61, 62, 63]. She was a member of the working party which formulated nine points distinguishing early childhood psychosis as the schizophrenia syndrome of childhood (1963). She summarised them as follows: (*i*) impairment of emotional relationships with people; (*ii*) unawareness of his own personal identity; (*iii*) pathological preoccupation with certain objects without regard to their accepted functions; (*iv*) resistance to change in environment and a desire to maintain sameness; (*v*) abnormal perceptual experiences; (*vi*) excessive and illogical anxiety; (*vii*) speech never acquired, lost or immature; (*viii*) distortion in motility pattern; (*ix*) a basic serious retardation with possible islets of higher mental functions of skill.

These criteria would seem to apply best to young schizophrenic children with Kanner's syndrome of autism. They would not adequately describe Mahler's symbiotic syndrome or the schizophrenic pre-puberty child widely recognized in the United States.

In Creak's[61] careful study of the type of psychotic children she has noted many organic factors. In 100 cases there were 12 cases with epilepsy, two died and proved to have neurolipidoses at autopsy, 17 recovered sufficiently to function adequately, 13 were chronically institutionalized for severe retardation and 40 functioned inadequately at home. Thus the course of the children followed up by Creak were similar to the children with atypical development treated at the J. J. Putnam Centre in the United States by Rank and her associates[152] and by Bender and her associates[30, 32]. While Creak[62] concludes that many of these psychotic children have minimal brain damage and she feels it is not known how this factor of 'organicity' produces the familiar clinical picture; Rutter in a series of recent articles[158, 159] argues that the psychotic child is not schizophrenic but suffers from a general or chronic organic damage of the brain in which psychogenic factors play only a secondary role.

Stroh[186] claims that there are probably multiple causative factors among which no one is indispensable; therefore the term schizophrenia should be avoided. Schain and Gannet[169] discuss 50 cases of infantile autism claiming a general similarity to previous descriptions of such cases, but finding convulsive seizures in the history of 42 per cent and recurrent seizures in 20 per cent so that he argued that the limbic system might be the site for the cerebral abnormality in these cases.

Stott, Glasgow[185] claims that infants damaged by prenatal or paranatal factors are more vulnerable to maternal deprivation. He refers to gestational stress to mothers in concentration camps during the war in England and Germany, to a variety of maternal illnesses such as rubella, and to infantile illnesses. He speaks of an 'unforthcomingness' personality defect and mental subnormality which may be blamed on maternal deprivation in these situations.

Rachman and Berger[147] (Maudsley Hospital) made a critical study of the whirling and postural behaviour in schizophrenic children. They reviewed the literature from Schilder[171] to Goldfarb[87]. They examined schizophrenic children and appropriate controls (matched intelligence) and confirmed that comparatively many schizophrenic children whirl and have poor postural control in contrast to the control subjects, and that the whirling is unrelated to intellectual level.

Hutt *et al.*[102] have made an important behavioural and electro-encephalographic study on autistic children. The characteristic behaviour of these children was observed and related to EEG records which showed low voltage with irregular activity and no established rhythm. The hypothesis was advanced that autistic children are in a chronically high state of physiological arousal.

In England we find an early interest in psychoanalytic mechanisms, a preoccupation with maternal deprivation and with early traumatic experiences especially during the war, but gradually the emphasis changed to a recognition of many organic factors. The interest has been centred on the young poorly developed child. Some have doubted the existence of true schizophrenia in childhood.

Childhood Psychosis in Western Europe

Kanner's early infantile autism has been well accepted in Europe as a recognizable syndrome. However, its relationship to schizophrenia of adult life has been questioned and there has been little acceptance of the idea that the etiology was psychogenic, arising from an unsatisfactory mother-child relationship. There has been an emphasis on constitutional or hereditary factors or on cerebral pathology (Van Krevelen[197, 199, 200], Holland; deWit[69], Holland; Tramer[194], Switzerland; Asperger[6], Austria; Schoenfelder[175], Germany.

Childhood schizophrenia is accepted by European paedopsychiatrists but only as an extension downward before puberty of the adult form of the illness, occurring rarely as a distinct change in personality after normal development (Stutte[187], Germany; Fanconi and Lutz[74]; Tramer[194], Switzerland; Gross[94], Bosch[46], Lempp[124], Germany). Asperger[6] also has stated that organic brain disorders with mental retardation can resemble infantile autism and childhood schizophrenia and that the anxiety engendered by such condition produces psychotic states.

Asperger's autistic psychopathy of childhood was first described by him in 1944[4] (see also 1950[5], 1961[7]) at the same time when the United States workers, Kanner and Bender, were describing early infantile autism and childhood schizophrenia. There has been considerable European discussion concerning the relationship between these conditions especially emphasized by Van Krevelen[198, 199]. But cases and follow-up reports have been made by Berner and Spiel[42], Germany; Burns[52], England; and Tramer[192], Switzerland. This author would see the 'autistic psychopath' as similar to her description of the pseudo-psychopathic schizophrenia of adolescents (Bender)[22].

Manghi[135] of Milan, Italy, found signs of cerebral lesions in psychotic children sufficiently often to justify the conclusions that psychotic behaviour is favoured or determined by encephalitic lesions and dysfunctions.

Anna Lisa Annell's work in Sweden is well known for extensive clinical treatment and follow-up reports[2, 3]. She takes childhood schizophrenia for granted finding that it continues into the adult life of the individual.

Childhood Psychoses in Eastern Europe

Bilikiewicz, Poland[43] in his textbook *Psychiatria Kliniczna* recognizes childhood schizophrenia as a rare form of adult schizophrenia and Heller's syndrome as also a form of schizophrenia.

In Russia also we are told (Lourie)[126] that childhood schizophrenia is seen as a part of adult schizophrenia. In general children's mental disorders are considered to have an organic basis. Sukhareva[189], considered the dean of Soviet child psychiatry, emphasizes heredity (enzymatic) and intrauterine noxious agents and traumas as most significant. As early as 1948 he recognized the effect of war conditions on increasing the incidence of emotional disturbances in children, except for epilepsy and schizophrenia.

Uschakow, Moscow[195] has written a good clinical description of 200 schizophrenic children 13 to 16 years, in which the onset was either acute between 11 to 13 years, or slow from early childhood, many cases resembling either Heller's or Kanner's syndromes.

Childhood Psychoses in Japan

Japanese child psychiatrists have been active in the area of child psychoses. Before the war they followed the mid-European, especially German teaching and emphasized the organic basis in all mental disorders (Makita)[134]. Since the war many have come to the United States to learn from child psychiatric centres, especially with Szurek in San Francisco,

Kanner in Baltimore, and Bender in New York, and Rank in Boston, so that all schools of thought are represented. Kuromaru[120, 121] 'Kyoto School' has studied especially the intrafamily relationship in autistic and schizophrenic children. He has found more distortions in family relationship in the non-organic schizophrenic children than the organic. He also emphasized a feature peculiar to Japan, which had to do with the intensely important role of the grandmother in the family dynamism.

Sakamoto, Osaka[163, 164] has reported on cases of both infantile autism and childhood schizophrenia and believes they run a similar chronic course in adulthood. He has written a paper emphasizing psychodynamics of schizophrenic children who are firesetters.

Israel

Marcus[136] discusses cases from Israel which he calls borderline states of childhood from the point of view of ego psychology. He argues for hereditary constitutional and emotional factors and refers to Hartman's concept of a constitutional ego weakness plus early emotional trauma. He finds that psychoanalytic theories help in understanding what happens to the personality.

India

An interesting report comes from E. Hoch[98] from India. She noted an increase of autism in the clinics in Luchnow, Delhi and Bombay where the preponderance of fathers came from the academic professions and the armed services and concludes that the emergence from an empathic symbiotic stage of culture into a more individualistic existence results in personality disturbance in the presence of organic brain disease, which she found present in a minimum of 38 per cent of cases. She also noted that illiterate peasants in the Himalayas, who breast feed their babies until they are four, brought retarded children to the clinics that appeared to be autistic.

REFERENCES

1. ALEXANDER, H. C. B., 1893, 1894. Insanity in children. *Alien. Neurol.*, **14**, 409; **15**, 27.
2. ANNELL, A., 1963. Follow-up study on psychotic children. *Acta Psychiat. Scand.*, **39**, 235.
3. ANNELL, A., 1963. Periodic catatonia in a seven year old. *Acta Paedopsychiat.*, **38**, 48.
4. ASPERGER, H., 1944. Die 'autischen Psychopathen' in Kindersalter. *Arch. Psychiat. Nervenkr.*, **117**, 76.
5. ASPERGER, H., 1950. Bild un sociale Wertigkeit der autischen Psychopathen. *Proc. II Internat. Cong. Orthopedog.*, Amsterdam.
6. ASPERGER, H., 1960. Behavior problems and mental retardation. In *Mental Retardation*, Proc. First Internat'l Med. Conf. Ed. Bowman, P. W. New York, Grune and Stratton.

REFERENCES

7. ASPERGER, H., 1961. Autischen Psychopathen. In *Heilpaedgogik*. Vol. 3. Vienna, Springer.
8. BAXTER, J., WILLIAM, J., and ZEROF, S., 1966. Child rearing attitudes and disciplinary fantasies of parents of schizophrenics and controls. *J. nerv. ment. Dis.*, **141**, 567.
9. BECK, S., 1954. *The six schizophrenias*. New York, American Orthopsychiatric Association.
10. BECK, S., 1959. Discussion of L. Bender, Pseudopsychopathic schizophrenia in adolescence. *Am. J. Orthopsychiat.*, **29**, 509.
11. BECK, S., 1965. *Psychological processes in the schizophrenic adaptation*. New York, Grune and Stratton.
12. BELLAK, L., 1948. *Dementia Praecox, A Review*. New York, Grune and Stratton.
13. BENDA, C., 1954. Psychopathology of childhood. In *Manual of child psychology*, 2nd Ed., Carmichael, L. New York, John Wiley.
14. BENDA, C., 1960. Childhood schizophrenia, autism, and Heller's disease. In *Mental retardation*, Proc. First Internat'l Med. Conf. Ed. Bowman, P. W. New York, Grune and Stratton.
15. BENDER, L., 1937. Art and therapy in mental disturbances in children. *J. nerv. ment. Dis.*, **86**, 249.
16. BENDER, L., 1937. Behavior problems in children of psychotic and criminal parents. *Genet. Psychol. Mono.*, **19**, 229.
17. BENDER, L., 1938. *A visual motor gestalt test and its clinical use*. New York, Am. Orthopsychiat. Assn.
18. BENDER, L., 1947. Childhood schizophrenia, a clinical study of 100 schizophrenic children. *Am. J. Orthopsychiat.*, **17**, 40.
19. BENDER, L., 1949. Psychological principles of the visual motor gestalt test. *Trans. N.Y. Acad. Sci.*, **11**, 164.
20. BENDER, L., 1950. Anxiety in disturbed children. In *Anxiety*. Ed. Hoch, P. New York, Grune and Stratton.
21. BENDER, L., 1956. Schizophrenia in childhood, its recognition, description and treatment. *Am. J. Orthopsychiat.*, **26**, 499.
22. BENDER, L., 1959. The concepts of pseudopsychopathic schizophrenia in adolescents. *Am. J. Orthopsychiat.*, **29**, 491.
23. BENDER, L., 1960. Emotional deprivation in infancy and its implication in child psychiatry. *A Crianca Portuguesa*, **19**, 83.
24. BENDER, L., 1960. Diagnostic and therapeutic aspects of childhood schizophrenia. In *Mental retardation*, Proc. First Internat'l Med. Conf. Ed. Bowman, P. W. New York, Grune and Stratton.
25. BENDER, L., 1961. Childhood schizophrenia and convulsive states. *Rec. Adv. biol. Psychiat.*, **3**, 96.
26. BENDER, L., 1961. Clinical research from in-patient services for children—1920-1957. *Psychiat. Quart.*, **35**, 88.
27. BENDER, L., 1961. Celiac syndrome in schizophrenia. Letter to the editor. *Psychiat. Quart.*, **35**, 586.
28. BENDER, L., 1961. Schizophrenie de l'enfant. *Méd. et Hyg.*, **19**, 508.
29. BENDER, L., 1962. Organicity in schizophrenic children (functioning at a defective level). *Proc. London Conf. Scient. Study of Mental Deficiency*, **2**, 411.
30. BENDER, L., 1963. The origin and evolution of the gestalt function, body image and delusional thought in schizophrenia. *Rec. Adv. biol. Psychiat.*, **5**, 38.
31. BENDER, L., 1963. Mental illness in childhood and heredity. *Eugen. Quart.*, **10**, 1.
32. BENDER, L., 1964. Twenty-five year view of therapeutic results. In *Evaluation of psychiatric treatment*. Eds, Hoch, P., and Zubin, J. New York, Grune and Stratton.

33. BENDER, L., 1966. The concept of plasticity in childhood schizophrenia. In *Psychopathology of schizophrenia.* Eds, Hoch, P., and Zubin, J. New York, Grune and Stratton.
34. BENDER, L., 1967. The visual motor gestalt test in six and seven year old normal and schizophrenic children. In *Psychopathology of mental development.* Eds, Zubin, J., and Jervis, G. A. New York, Grune and Stratton.
35. BENDER, L., and ANDERMANN, K., 1965. Brain damage in blind children with retrolental fibroplasia. *Arch. Neurol.*, **12**, 644.
36. BENDER, L., FARETRA, G., COBRINIK, L., and SANKAR, S., 1966. The treatment of childhood schizophrenia with LSD and UML. In *The biological treatment of mental illnesses.* Ed. Rinkel, M. New York, L. C. Page.
37. BENDER, L., FREEDMAN, A. M., GRUGETT, A. E., and HELME, W., 1952. Schizophrenia in childhood, a confirmation of the diagnosis. *Trans. Am. Neurol. Assn*, **77**, 67.
38. BENDER, L., and GRUGETT, A. E., 1956. A study of certain epidemiological problems in a group of children with childhood schizophrenia. *Am. J. Orthopsychiat.*, **26**, 131.
39. BENDER, L., and HELME, W. H., 1953. A quantitative test of theory and diagnostic indicators of childhood schizophrenia. *Arch. Neurol. Psychiat.*, **70**, 413.
40. BENDER, L., and KEELER, W. R., 1952. The body image of schizophrenic children following electroshock therapy. *Am. J. Orthopsychiat.*, **22**, 335.
41. BERES, D., 1956. Ego deviation and the concept of schizophrenia. *Psychoanal. Study Child*, **11**, 1964.
42. BERNER, P., and SPIEL, W., 1960. On a special group of autistic juvenile delinquents. *Acta Paedopsychiat.*, **27**, 193.
43. BILIKIEWICZ, T., 1960. *Psychiatria Kliniczna*, 2nd Ed. Warsaw, Panstwowy Zaklad Wydawnictw Lekarskich.
44. BLAU, A., 1962. Childhood schizophrenia. *J. Am. Acad. Child. Psychiat.*, **1**, 225.
45. BLEULER, E., 1911. *Dementia Precox, or the Group of Schizophrenias.* Zinkin, J. (Trans.). New York, Internat. Univ. Press.
46. BOSCH, A., 1962. *Der Fruehekindliche Autism.* Berlin, Springer.
47. BOWLBY, J., 1951. *Maternal care and mental health.* Geneva, W.H.O.
48. BOWLBY, J., 1957. Ethological approach to research in child development. *Brit. J. med. Psychol.*, **30**, 230.
49. BOWLBY, J., 1958. The nature of the child's tie to its mother. *Internat. J. Psychoanal.*, **39**, 1.
50. BOWLBY, J., 1960. Separation anxiety; a critical review of the literature. *J. Child Psychol. Psychiat.*, **1**, 251.
51. BRADLEY, C., 1941. *Schizophrenia in childhood.* New York, Macmillan.
52. BURNS, C., 1964. Autopathy, follow-up of cases. *Acta Paedopsychiat.*, **31**, 357.
53. CAMERON, K., 1958. Symptom classification in child psychiatry. *Revue de Psychiat. Infant.*, **25**, 241.
54. CAPLAN, H., 1956. The role of deviant maturation in pathogenesis of anxiety. *Am. J. Orthopsychiat.*, **26**, 94.
55. CARUTH, E. and MEYERS, M., Eds, 1964. Project on childhood psychosis. *Reiss-Davis Clinic Bull.*, **1**, 4.
56. COBRINIK, L., 1966. An exploratory study of speech in severely disturbed schizophrenic children. *Psychiat. Quart.*, **40**. In Press.
57. COBRINIK, L., and FARETRA, G., 1966. Verbal stereotypy in childhood emotional disorders. *Rec. Adv. biol. Psychiat.*, **8**.
58. COBRINIK, L., and POPPER, L., 1961. Developmental aspects of thought disturbances in schizophrenic children. A Rorschach study. *Am. J. Orthopsychiat.*, **31**, 170.

59. COLBERT, E. G., KOEGLER, R., and MARKHAM, C., 1959. Vestibular dysfunction in childhood schizophrenia. *Arch. Gen. Psychiat.*, **1**, 600.
60. CREAK, E. M., 1962. Juvenile psychoses and mental deficiency. *Proc. London Conf. on Scient. Study of Mental Deficiency*, **2**, 389.
61. CREAK, E. M., 1963. Childhood psychoses; a review of 100 cases. *Brit. J. Psychiat.*, **109**, 84.
62. CREAK, E. M., 1963. Schizophrenia in early childhood. *Acta Paedopsychiat.*, **30**, 42.
63. CREAK, E. M., 1964. The problem of the mentally handicapped child. *Acta Paedopsychiat.*, **31**, 325.
64. CUNNINGHAM, M. A., and DIXON, C., 1961. A study in language of an autistic child. *J. Child Psychol. Psychiat.*, **2**, 193.
65. DES LAURIERS, A. M., 1962. *The experience of reality in childhood schizophrenia.* New York, Inter. Univ. Press.
66. DESPERT, J. L., 1938. Schizophrenia in children. *Psychiat. Quart.*, **12**, 366.
67. DESPERT, J. L., 1965. *The emotionally disturbed child, then and now.* New York, Vantage Press.
68. DEUTSCH, H., 1942. Some forms of emotional disturbances and their relationship to schizophrenia. *Psychoanalyt. Quart.*, **11**, 301.
69. DEWIT, J., 1964. Some critical remarks on 'maternal deprivation.' *Acta Paedopsychiat.*, **31**, 340.
70. EISENBERG, L., 1956. The autistic child in adolescence. *Am. J. Psychiat.*, **112**, 607.
71. EISENBERG, L., and KANNER, L., 1957. Early infantile autism, 1943-1955. *Am. psychol. Assn Psychiat. Research Reports*, **7**, 55.
72. EKSTEIN, R., 1964. On the acquisition of speech in the autistic child. *Reiss-Davis Clinic Bull.*, **1**, 1963.
73. EKSTEIN, R., BRYANT, K., and FRIEDMAN, S. W., 1958. Childhood schizophrenia and allied conditions. In *Schizophrenia: a review of a syndrome.* Ed. Bellak, L. New York, Logos Press.
74. FANCONI, G., and LUTZ, J., 1958. Psychologie und Psychopathologie im Kindesalter. In *Lehrbach der Paediatrie*, vol. 5. Basel, Benno Schwabe.
75. FARETRA, G., and BENDER, L., 1962. Pregnancy and birth histories of children with psychiatric problems. *Proc. III World Cong. Psychiat.*, **2**, 1329.
76. FARETRA, G., and BENDER, L., 1965. Autonomic nervous system responses in hospitalized children treated with LSD and UML. *Rec. Adv. biol. Psychiat.*, **7**, 1.
77. FEDERN, P., 1952. *Ego psychology and the psychoses.* New York, Basic Books.
78. FISH, B., 1959. Longitudinal observations of biological deviations in a schizophrenic infant. *Am. J. Psychiat.*, **116**, 25.
79. FISH, B., and ALPERT, M., 1963. Patterns of neurological development in infants born of schizophrenic mothers. *Rec. Adv. biol. Psychiat.*, **5**, 24.
80. FISH, B., WILE, R., SHAPIRO, T., and HALPERN, F., 1966. The prediction of schizophrenia in infancy; a ten year follow-up. In *Psychopathology of schizophrenia.* Eds. Hoch, P., and Zubin, J. New York, Grune and Stratton.
81. FREEDMAN, A. M., 1954. Maturation and its relation to the dynamics of childhood schizophrenia. *Am. J. Orthopsychiat.*, **24**, 487.
82. FREUD, A., 1965. *Normality and pathology in childhood.* New York, Internat. Univ. Press.
83. FURER, M., HOROWITZ, M., TEC, L., and TOOLAN, J. V., 1957. Internalized objects in children. *Am. J. Orthopsychiat.*, **27**, 88.
84. GELEERD, E. R., 1946. A contribution to the problem of psychosis in childhood. *Psychoanal. Study Child*, **2**, 271.
85. GESELL, A., 1945. *Embryology of behavior.* New York, Harper and Bros.

86. GIANASCOL, A. J., 1963. Psychodynamic approach to childhood schizophrenia, a review. *J. nerv. ment. Dis.*, **137**, 336.
87. GOLDFARB, W., 1961. *Childhood schizophrenia.* Cambridge, Mass., Harvard Univ. Press.
88. GOLDFARB, W., 1964. An investigation in childhood schizophrenia. *Arch. Gen. Psychiat.*, **11**, 620.
89. GOLDFARB, W., BRAUNSTEIN, P., and LORGE, I., 1956. A study of speech patterns in a group of schizophrenic children. *Am. J. Orthopsychiat.*, **26**, 544.
90. GOLDFARB, W., and DORSEN, M. M., 1956. *Annotated bibliography of childhood schizophrenia.* New York, Basic Books.
91. GOLDSTEIN, K., 1959. Abnormal mental conditions in infancy. *J. nerv. ment. Dis.*, **128**, 538.
92. GRAFF, H., and HANDFORD, A., 1961. Celiac syndrome in the case histories of five schizophrenics. *Psychiat. Quart.*, **35**, 306.
93. GREENACRE, P., 1941. The predisposition to anxiety. *Psychoanal. Quart.*, **10**, 66, 610. Reprinted in Greenacre, P. (1952) *Growth and personality.* New York, W. W. Norton.
94. GROSS, H. P., and SCHALLENGE, H., 1965. Autistic behaviour and its causes in childhood. *Ztsch. Kinderheilkunde*, **92**, 343.
95. HARTMAN, H., 1953. Contribution to the meta-psychology of schizophrenia. *Psychoanal. Study Child*, **8**, 177.
96. HERMANN, I., 1936. Sich-Anklammern-auf-Suche-Gehen. *Int. Z. Psychoanal.*, **22**, 349.
97. HEELEY, A. F., and ROBERTS, G. E., 1965. Tryptophane metabolism in psychotic children. *Dev. Med. & Child Neurol.*, **7**, 46.
98. HOCH, E., 1964. Indian children in a psychiatric playground. *Transcultural Res.*, **1**, 40.
99. HOCH, P., 1966. Schizophrenia. In *The psychopathology of schizophrenia.* Eds, Hoch, P., and Zubin, J. New York, Grune and Stratton.
100. HOCH, P., and POLATIN, J., 1949. Pseudoneurotic forms of schizophrenia. *Psychiat. Quart.*, **23**, 448.
101. HOWELLS, J. G., 1962. Trends in British child psychiatry. *J. Am. Acad. Child Psychiat.*, **1**, 591.
102. HUTT, S. J., HUTT, C., LEE, D., and OUNSTED, C., 1965. A behavioral and EEG study of autistic children. *J. Psychiat. Res.*, **3**, 181.
103. JAFFE, S. L., 1966. Hallucinations in children at a state hospital. *Psychiat. Quart.*, **40**, 88.
104. JOHNSON, A. M., and SZUREK, S. A., 1952. The genesis of antisocial acting-out in children and adults. *Psychoanal. Quart.*, **21**, 323.
105. KAHLBAUM, K., 1863. *Die gruppierungen der psychischen krankheiten und die einteilung der seelen storungen.* Danzig.
106. KALLMANN, F. J., and ROTH, B., 1956. Genetic aspects of preadolescent schizophrenia. *Am. J. Psychiat.*, **112**, 599.
107. KANNER, L., 1935. *Child psychiatry*, 3rd ed. 1957. Springfield Ill., C. C. Thomas.
108. KANNER, L., 1942-43. Autistic disturbance in affective contact. *Nerv. Child*, **2**, 217.
109. KANNER, L., 1946. Irrelevant and metaphorical language in early infantile autism. *Am. J. Psychiat.*, **103**, 242.
110. KANNER, L., 1949. Problems of nosology and psychodynamics of early infantile autism. *Am. J. Orthopsychiat.*, **19**, 416.
111. KANNER, L., 1954. Childhood schizophrenia. *Am. J. Orthopsychiat.*, **24**, 526.
112. KANNER, L., 1962. Emotionally disturbed children—an historical review. *Child Dev.*, **33**, 97.

113. KANNER, L., 1964. Foreword to B. Rimland. *Infantile Autism.* New York, Appleton-Century Crafts.
114. KANNER, L., 1965. Infantile autism and the schizophrenias. Read at a panel meeting of the Am. Psychiat. Assoc. May 4, 1965, New York City, for Stanley R. Dean Research Award.
115. KEELER, W. R., 1958. Autistic patterns and defective communication in blind children with retrolental fibroplasia. In *Psychopathology of communication.* Eds, Hoch, P., and Zubin, J. New York, Grune and Stratton.
116. KESSLER, J. W., 1966. *Psychopathology of childhood.* Chap. II. Englewood Cliffs, N. J., Prentice-Hall.
117. KLEIN, M., 1937. *The psycho-analysis of children.* Strachey, A. Trans. London, Hogarth.
118. KNOBLOCK, H., and PASAMANICK, B., 1960. Complications of pregnancy and mental deficiency. In *Mental retardation,* Proc. First Internat'l Med. Conf. Ed. Bowman, P. W. New York, Grune and Stratton.
119. KOEGLER, R. K., and COLBERT, E. G., 1959. Childhood schizophrenia. *J. Am. med. Assn,* **171,** 1045.
120. KUROMARU, S., 1964. A study of Japanese families of autistic and schizophrenic children. *Abstr. Am. Psychiat. Assn,* p. 187.
121. KUROMARU, S., OKADA, S., and TAKAHASI, I., 1964. An aspect of family structure in childhood schizophrenia. *Jap. J. Child Psychiat.,* **5,** 100.
122. LANGFORD, W. S., 1964. Reflection on classification in child psychiatry as related to the activities of the Committee on Child Psychiatry of the Group for the Advancement of Psychiatry. In *Diagnostic classification in child psychiatry,* Eds, Jenkins, G. L., and Cole, J. A.P.A. Psychiat. Res. Report.
123. LEBOWITZ, M., COLBERT, E. G., and PALMER, J. O., 1961. Schizophrenia in children. *J. Dis. Child.,* **102,** 55.
124. LEMPP, R., 1964. The significance of early brain damage in children with childhood neurosis. *Acta Paedopsychiat.,* 152.
125. LORENTE DE NO, R., 1933. Vestibular-ocular reflex arc. *Arch. Neur. Psychiat.,* **30,** 245.
126. LOURIE, R., 1963. Child psychiatry in the U.S.S.R. *J. Am. Acad. Child Psychiat.,* **2,** 569.
127. LUTZ, J., 1937. Ueber die Schizophrenie im Kindesalter. *Schweiz. Arch. Neurol. Psychiat.,* **39,** 335; **40,** 141.
128. MAHLER, M., 1952. On child psychoses and schizophrenia. Autistic and symbiotic infantile psychoses. *Psychoanal. Study Child,* **7,** 286.
129. MAHLER, M. S., 1964. Foreword. *Childhood Psychoses. The Reiss-Davis Clinic Bull.,* **1,** 54.
130. MAHLER, M. S., 1965. On early infantile psychoses, the symbiotic and autistic syndromes. *J. Acad. Child Psychiat.,* **4,** 554.
131. MAHLER, M. S., FURER, M., and SETTLAGE, C. F., 1959. Severe emotional disturbances in childhood. In *American handbook of psychiatry.* Ed. Arieti, S. New York, Basic Books.
132. MAHLER, M. S., and GOSLINER, B. J., 1955. On symbiotic child psychosis. *Psychoanal. Study Child,* **10,** 215.
133. MALAMUD, N., 1959. Heller's disease and childhood schizophrenia. *Am. J. Psychiat.,* **116,** 215.
134. MAKITA, K., 1965. The present situation of child psychiatry in Japan. *Acta Paedopsychiat.,* **32,** 223.
135. MANGHI, E., 1963. Segni di lesione cerebrale in un gruppo di bambini con comportamento psicotico (schizofrenico). *II Congresso Europeo di Pedopsichiatria,* p. 1.

136. MARCUS, J., 1963. Borderline states in childhood. *J. Child Psychol. Psychiat.*, **4**, 207.
137. MENOLASCINO, F. J., 1965. Autistic reactions in early childhood: differential diagnostic considerations. *J. Child Psychol. Psychiat.*, **6**, 203.
138. MOREL, B. B., 1860. *Traite des Maladies Mentales*. Paris.
139. NADLER, H. L., and HSIA, D. Y., 1961. Epinephrine metabolism in phenylketonuria. *Proc. Soc. expl biol. Med.*, **107**.
140. PECK, H. B., RABINOVITCH, R. D., and CRAMER, J. B., 1949. A treatment program for parents of schizophrenic children. *Am. J. Orthopsychiat.*, **19**, 592.
141. PERRY, T. L., 1962. Urinary excretion of amines in phenylketonuria and mongolism. *Science*, **136**, 879.
142. PERRY, T. L., 1963. N-methylmetanephrine: excretion by juvenile psychotics. *Science*, **139**, 587.
143. POLLACK, M., and KRIEGER, H. P., 1958. Oculomotor and postural patterns in schizophrenic children. *Arch. Neur. Psychiat.*, **79**, 720.
144. POLLIN, W., STABENAU, J. B., MOSHER, L., and TUPIN, J., 1966. Life history of differences in identical twins discordant for schizophrenia. *Am. J. Orthopsychiat.*, **36**, 492.
145. POTTER, H. W., 1933. Schizophrenia in children. *Am. J. Psychiat.*, **12**, 1253.
146. RABINOVITCH, R. D., 1951. Observations on the differential study of severely disturbed children. *Am. J. Orthopsychiat.*, **22**, 230.
147. RACHMAN, S., and BERGER, M., 1963. Whirling and postural control in schizophrenic children. *J. Child Psychol. Psychiat.*, **4**, 137.
148. RANK, B., 1955. Intensive study and treatment of preschool children who show marked personality deviations or 'atypical development', and their parents. In *Emotional problems of early childhood*. Ed. Caplan, G. New York, Basic Books.
149. RANK, B., and MACNAUGHTON, D., 1950. A clinical contribution to early ego development. *Psychoanal. Study Child*, **5**, 53.
150. RANK, O., 1924. *The trauma of birth*. London, Kegan Paul. (English Trans., 1929.)
151. RAPOPORT, J., 1944. Phantasy objects in children. *Psychoanalyt. Rev.*, **31**, 316.
152. REISER, D. E., and BROWN, J. L., 1964. Patterns of later development in children with infantile psychosis. *J. Am. Acad. Child Psychiat.*, **3**, 650.
153. RIBBLE, M. A., 1943. *The rights of infants*. New York, Columbia Univ. Press.
154. RIMLAND, B., 1964. *Infantile autism*. New York, Appleton-Century Crafts.
155. ROSENTHAL, DAVID (Ed.). *The Genain quadruplets*. New York, Basic Books.
156. RUBINSTEIN, E. A., 1948. Childhood mental disease in America; a review of literature before 1900. *Am. J. Orthopsychiat.*, **18**, 314.
157. RUBIN, L. S., 1961. Patterns of pupillary dilatation and construction in psychotic adults and autistic children. *J. nerv. ment. Dis.*, **133**, 2.
158. RUTTER, M., 1965. Classification and categorization in child psychiatry. *J. Child Psychol. Psychiat.*, **6**, 71.
159. RUTTER, M., 1965. The influence of organic and emotional factors on the origin, nature and outcome of childhood psychosis. *Dev. Med. Child. Neurol.*, **17**, 518.
160. SACHS, B., and HAUSMAN, L., 1926. *Nervous and mental disorders from birth through adolescence*. New York, Hoeber.
161. SACHS, B., 1895. *A treatise on the nervous diseases of children for physicians and students*. New York, Wood.
162. DE SANCTIS, S., 1908. Dementia praecocissima des frueheren Kindesalter. *Folia Neuro-Biologica*, **2**, 9.

163. SAKAMOTO, M., 1960. Symptoms of childhood schizophrenia. *Anniversary issue—Prof. Yuzo Naka's 61st birthday*. Osaka City Univ. Med. School.
164. SAKAMOTO, M., 1960. A dynamic psychopathology of fire setting in schizophrenic children. *Osaka City Med. J.*, **6**, 59.
165. SANDLER, M., 1961. Brain function and the 5-hydroxyindoles. *Cerebral Palsy Bull.*, **3**, 456.
166. SANKAR, D. V. S., 1965. Effects of psychoactive drugs on particulate norepinephrine levels, plasma glucose and 17-hydroxycortico-steroids and urinary excretion of biogenic amines and their metabolites. *Fed. Proc.*, **24**, 195.
167. SANKAR, D. V. S., CATES, N., BROER, P., and SANKAR, B., 1963. Biochemical parameters in childhood schizophrenia (autism) and growth. *Rec. Adv. biol. Psychiat.*, **5**, 76.
168. SANKAR, D. V. S., GOLD, E., PHIPPS, E., and SANKAR, B., 1962. General metabolic studies on schizophrenic children. *Ann. N.Y. Acad. Sci.*, **96**, 392.
169. SCHAIN, R. J., and GANNET, H., 1960. Infantile autism. *J. Pediat.*, **57**, 560.
170. SCHAIN, R. J., and FREEDMAN, D. X., 1961. Studies on 5-hydroxy indole metabolism in autistic and other mentally retarded children. *J. Pediat.*, **58**, 315.
171. SCHILDER, P., 1935. *Image and appearance of the human body*. New York, Internat. Univ. Press. 1950. English Trans.
172. SCHILDER, P., 1964. *Contributions to developmental neuropsychiatry*. Ed. Bender, L. New York, Internat. Univ. Press.
173. SCHILDER, P., 1936. The psychology of schizophrenia. *Psychoanal. Rev.*, **26**, 380.
174. SCHILDER, P., 1939. Relation between clinging and equilibrium. *Internat. J. Psychoanal.*, **20**, 58.
175. SCHOENFELDER, T., 1964. Ueber fruehkindliche Antriebsstoerungen. *Acta Paedopsychiat.*, **31**, 112.
176. SHAW, C. R., and SUTTON, H. E., 1960. Metabolic studies in childhood schizophrenia: amino and excretion patterns. *Arch. Gen. Psychiat.*, **3**, 519.
177. SHAW, C. R., LUCAS, J., and RABINOVITCH, R. D., 1959. Metabolic studies in childhood schizophrenia; effects of tryptophan loading on indole excretion. *Arch. Gen. Psychiat.*, **1**, 366.
178. SILVER, A., 1952. Postural and righting responses in childhood schizophrenia. *Psychiat. Quart.*, **29**, 272.
179. SINGER, M. T., and WYNNE, M. D., 1963. Differentiating characteristics of parents of child schizophrenics. *Am. J. Psychiat.*, **120**, 234.
180. SMOLEN, E. M., 1965. Some thoughts on schizophrenia in childhood. *J. Am. Acad. Child Psychiat.*, **4**, 443.
181. SPITZ, R., 1946. Anaclitic depression. *Psychoanal. Study Child*, **2**, 313.
182. SPITZ, R., 1951. Psychogenic disease in infancy. *Psychoanal. Study Child*, **6**, 255.
183. SPITZ, R., and WOLF, K. M., 1946. The smiling response, a contribution to the ontogenesis of social relations. *Genet. Psychol. Monogr.*, **34**, 57.
184. STARR, P. H., 1954. Psychoses in children; their origin and structure. *Psychoanal. Quart.*, **23**, 544.
185. STOTT, D. H., 1962. Abnormal mothering as a cause of mental subnormality. *J. Child Psychol. Psychiat.*, **3**, 79.
186. STROH, G., 1960. On the diagnosis of childhood psychosis. *J. Child Psychol. Psychiat.*, **1**, 238.
187. STUTTE, H., 1957. Die prognose der Schizophrenien des Kindes und Jugendalters. *Proc. 2nd Internat. Cong. Psychiat.*, **1**, 328.

188. SZUREK, S. A., 1956. Psychotic episodes and psychotic maldevelopment. *Am. J. Orthopsychiat.*, **26**, 519.
189. SUKHAREVA, G. E., 1947-48. Psychological disturbances in children during war. *Am. Rev. Sov. Med.*, **5**, 32.
190. TAFT, L. T., and GOLDFARB, W., 1964. Prenatal and perinatal factors in childhood schizophrenia. *Dev. Med. Child Neurol.*, **6**, 32.
191. TEICHER, J. D., 1941. Preliminary survey of motility in children. *J. nerv. ment. Dis.*, **99**, 277.
192. TRAMER, M., 1931. Die Entwicklungslinie eines psychotischen Kindes. *Schw. Arch. f. Neur. u. Psychiat.*, **27**, 383. Also translated, Brunch, H., and Cottington, F. 1942. *Nervous Child*, **1**, 232.
193. TRAMER, M., 1961. Schizoid psychopathy or schizophrenia. *Acta Paedopsychiat.*, **29**, 136.
194. TRAMER, M., 1962. Childhood schizophrenia as a problem of nosology. *Acta Paedopsychiat.*, **29**, 337.
195. USCHAKOW, G. K., 1965. Symptomotologie der initial Periode der im Kindes —oder Jugendalter beginnenden Schizophrenie. *Psychiatrie, Leipzig*, **17**, 41.
196. VALLIENT, G. E., 1962. John Haslam on early infantile autism. *Am. J. Psychiat.*, **119**, 376.
197. VAN KREVELEN, D. A., 1960. Autismus infantum. *Acta Paedopsychiat.*, **27**, 97.
198. VAN KREVELEN, D. A., 1962. The psychopathology of autistic psychopathy. *Acta Paedopsychiat.*, **29**, 22.
199. VAN KREVELEN, D. A., 1963. On the relationship between early infantile autism and autistic psychopathy. *Acta Paedopsychiat.*, **30**, 303.
200. VAN KREVELEN, D. A., 1964. Autism and iatrogenic disorder. *Acta Paedopsychiat.*, **31**, 129.
201. WECHSLER, D., and JAROS, E., 1965. Schizophrenic patterns on the WISC. *J. clin. Psychol.*, **3**, 288.
202. WEIL, A. P., 1953. Clinical data and dynamic considerations in certain cases of childhood schizophrenia. *Am. J. Orthopsychiat.*, **23**, 518.
203. WEIL, A. P., 1953. Certain severe disturbances of ego development in childhood. *Psychoanalyt. Study Child*, **8**, 271.
204. WINNICOTT, D. W., 1953. Transitional objects and transitional phenomena. *Int. J. Psychoanal.*, **34**. Also in *Collected Papers*, 1958. New York, Basic Books.
205. WINNICOTT, D. W., 1954. Psychotic illness in relation to environmental failure. In *Collected papers thru Pediatrics to Psychoanalysis*. New York, Basic Books.
206. WINNICOTT, D. W., 1965. *The maturational process and the facilitating environment* (Papers 1957-63). New York, Internat. Univ. Press.
207. WOLFF, S., and CHESS, S., 1965. An analysis of the language of 14 schizophrenic children. *J. Child Psychol. Psychiat.*, **6**, 29.
208. YAKOVLEV, P. I., WEINBERGER, M., and CHIPMAN, C. E., 1958. Heller's syndrome as a pattern of schizophrenic behavior disturbance in early childhood. *Am. J. Ment. Defic.*, **53**, 318.
209. YAKOVLEV, P. I., 1948. Motility, behavior and the brain. *J. nerv. ment. Dis.*, **107**, 313.
210. ZITRIN, A., FERBER, P., and COHEN, D., 1964. Pre- and paranatal factors in mental disorders in children. *J. nerv. ment. Dis.*, **139**, 357.

XXIV

THERAPEUTIC MANAGEMENT OF SCHIZOPHRENIC CHILDREN

WILLIAM GOLDFARB
M.D., Ph.D.

Director, Henry Ittleson Center for Child Research, Riverdale, New York

1
Introduction

The discussion to follow will consider the therapeutic management of schizophrenic children. Such discussion would seem to be entirely reasonable at the present time, inasmuch as the current climate surrounding psychiatric management of childhood schizophrenia is strongly optimistic. The intention to treat is distinctly dominant, as is evidenced in the very rapid growth of specialized clinical services for schizophrenic children, including residential, day and outpatient programmes, as well as of specialized non-clinical services, including schools, camps, and recreational programmes. The psychiatric and educational communities have thus responded boldly to the pressure for services for these extremely disturbed children and their families.

However, in the main, the impetus has been based more on therapeutic conviction than on secure knowledge. Certainly, information regarding childhood schizophrenia is not completely clear and unqualified: and the burgeoning of facilities for psychotic children has occurred in spite of the fact that the epidemiology of childhood psychosis is not established; evaluations of therapeutic methods have been rare and, at best, inconclusive; and—most important of all—the diagnosis is too broadly encompassing and etiological factors are not firmly established.

As one soon observes in clinical practice, a major hindrance to the formulation of a specific therapy is the fact that the classification of childhood psychosis is assigned to a great diversity of children. Indeed, various workers have classified the children by different names such as childhood schizophrenia,* e.g.[2, 3, 5, 6, 7, 11, 19] autistic psychosis[13], symbiotic psychosis[15, 16], atypical disorder[20], borderline psychosis[9] and chronic brain syndrome[14]. To a degree, the variations in nosology reflect the diversity noted among the children in quantitative and qualitative aspects of ego expression, in growth, and in the contributions of biological and psychosocial factors to the disorders of the children. The different subdivisions of psychosis suggested by these observers also reflect differing guidelines or criteria for diagnosis. Some observers have stressed phenomenology[2]; some have stressed onset history[7]; and some have stressed etiologic subgroupings[15].

Also, it must be understood that each of the treatment modalities used in the treatment of childhood psychosis had been designed originally for non-psychotic children. For example, milieu therapy evolved out of older designs for substitute care of dependent children and individual psycho-therapy had originally been developed for milder reactive behaviour disorders. Certainly, the original rationalizations of these treatment forms were not based on the special characteristics of psychotic children.

Fortunately the situation is not entirely ambiguous inasmuch as various workers in the past two decades have had genuine experience in comprehensive management of schizophrenic children. This intimate contact with the children as they have coped with the demands of reality has increased empirical and practical understanding of their treatment requirements. The warm human engagement with the children throughout the day under circumstances permitting detailed observation of social and relational responses has also stimulated systematic research.

Can one proceed from the diagnosis of childhood schizophrenia to the specification of a precise and universally applicable plan of treatment? The question can only be answered in the negative. Terms like 'psychosis', 'childhood schizophrenia' or 'autism' are so broad that in themselves they do not automatically imply a tight precise pattern of personality traits, symptoms, history, pathogenic influence and cause. It follows that a specific and universally applicable therapy for childhood psychosis comparable to the penicillin treatment of pneumococcal pneumonia is not possible. In actual clinical practice, the classification of a child as 'psychotic' or 'schizophrenic' ordinarily carries little weight in the devising of an individualized therapeutic plan for that child. To formulate a coherent and relevant plan for each individual child, the therapeutic team is more disposed to assay in the greatest detail his adaptive strengths and weaknesses and the contribution of biological and psychosocial factors and then to weigh the environmental accommodations necessary to assist in the normalization of his ego structure. There is also likely to be reference to

* We shall use this diagnostic designation in the present report.

group as well as individual therapeutic processes, to interpersonal as well as intrapsychic phenomena, to somatic as well as to social kinds of influence. Suffice it to say that although it is difficult to talk of a single therapeutic technique, it is surprisingly feasible to discuss a rationale or a point of view for the orderly treatment of psychotic children. In what follows, therefore, an attempt will be made to define such a rationale and to suggest objectives and format for the treatment of these children.

Therapeutic conviction in itself is highly desirable. Psychotic children are so aberrant and abrasive in behaviour, their emotional requirements are so monumental and their progress in treatment is ordinarily so slow, that they offer limited emotional returns to the adults who care for them. Belief in the capacity of such children to change and an initial desire to assist the children toward greater fulfilment does assist the teacher, therapist, or child-caring person to sustain an enduring commitment to burdensome aspects of interaction with the children throughout a long treatment period.

The desire to heal, however, is not in itself a sufficient basis for the treatment of psychotic children. A conscious, deliberate and clearly articulated treatment point of view which permeates all aspects of the therapeutic climate is essential and, indeed, is what distinguishes professional skill from the mere desire to heal. A coherent rationale for treatment has an organizing and coordinating function. Thus, it enables the evolution of an overall climate of value to all the varieties of children found among psychotic children; and it offers a basis for an individualized therapeutic plan for each child. A rationalized and unified approach to treatment makes it possible to relate the different varieties of treatment service available for schizophrenic children (for example, day, residential and outpatient) and the different varieties of treatment technique (for example, milieu, individual and drug). Finally it facilitates the coordination of the surprising number of people and disciplines to which the schizophrenic child is inevitably exposed in any serious programme of comprehensive treatment. Coordination is necessary because the teacher, child-care worker, and psychotherapist each possesses his own skills and modes of expression. It is possible, however, for each discipline to buttress the efforts of the others, provided they all hold to common therapeutic objectives.

An explicit rationale is also essential to avoid the hazards which may be expected when adults in the treatment installation react intuitively to the children. Too often such intuitive reactions euphemistically described as 'common sense', represent the naïve point of view of adults lacking an explicit framework for responding to the children. Indeed these intuitive responses may frequently represent the adult workers' own biases without reference to the children's needs and, of even greater risk, may block the discovery of what is really happening to the child in treatment. In this kind of unreflective circumstance, harmful relationships may become fixed and unchanging.

2
Corrective Socialization

If there is not a specific treatment technique, is there a treatment point of view which might be regarded as specifically appropriate for the rehabilitation of schizophrenic children? Here proposed is such a reconstructive approach which has evolved as a result of recent systematic investigations including detailed life process observations. The approach has been termed 'corrective socialization'. In brief it presumes that (i) the central finding in childhood schizophrenia consists of primary deficiencies in self directive or self regulative functions organizing personality. For purposes of discussion we shall call this aspect of personality the 'ego'. (ii) The key to treatment is the correction of these primary deficiencies in ego, and (iii) the major instrument for correcting these deficiencies are processes of social experience and human interaction.

To illuminate the rationale of corrective socialization as a therapeutic approach strategically suited to the needs of schizophrenic children, the discussion to follow will consider answers to a number of questions:

1. Who are the children classified as schizophrenic? More precisely what are the diagnostic criteria for the classification of childhood schizophrenia? How homogeneous are the children classified as schizophrenic?

2. What are the key adaptive deficiencies of schizophrenic children?

3. What part do intrinsic organismic factors in the child and extrinsic environmental factors play in the manifestations of adaptive failure which characterizes schizophrenic children?

4. What are the specific objectives and formal qualities of a social environment which would tend to overcome the deficiencies of schizophrenic children?

Diagnosis of Childhood Schizophrenia

Criteria for the diagnosis of childhood schizophrenia are first presented since it is useful first to define the kinds of children who are diagnosed as schizophrenic and the range of disorders subsumed by the diagnosis. A recent set of nine diagnostic criteria reflect those commonly employed by child psychiatrists[5]. These nine criteria include the following:

1. Gross and sustained impairment of emotional relationships.

2. Apparent unawareness of personal identity to a degree inappropriate to his age.

3. Pathological preoccupation with particular objects or certain characteristics of them, without regard to their accepted functions.

4. Sustained resistance to change in the environment.

5. Abnormal perceptual experience in the absence of discernible organic abnormality.

6. Acute excessive anxiety, frequently precipitated by change.
7. Impaired speech and language.
8. Distortion in motility.
9. Serious intellectual retardation with islets of normal or better intellectual skill.

These criteria would seem to be a sufficient basis for the designation of a homogeneous class of children. In actual fact, however, each of these criteria is very broad in definition. For example, the term 'impaired emotional relationships' refers on the one hand to children who have no attachments or internalized image of the human person at all and also to those who desire to possess and ingest important persons and to struggle against any kind of physical separation from them. Or impaired speech includes total mutism as well as children who speak but show many kinds of deviation from culturally expected signals. Or intellectual retardation may be severe in the case of some schizophrenic children, while other children may be very superior in intelligence while demonstrating special islands of symbolic impairment. It turns out, therefore, that while all schizophrenic children deviate conspicuously from normal in human relationship, perception, cognition and motor response, there is great diversity among the children in all their symptoms and characteristics. The important conclusion to be drawn is the necessity for a highly individualized treatment programme suited to the unique needs of individual children regardless of those characteristics held in common by all.

Adaptive Deficiencies of Schizophrenic Children

Nevertheless is there a central disturbance which is manifested by all schizophrenic children and which thus implies a common therapeutic approach for all? It can be stated unequivocally that in all cases of childhood schizophrenia the children suffer from a failure in self regulation and self direction; and the key to their maladaptive responses is a pervasive state of deficiency in ego equipment as they interact with their environment. If specific ego functions are studied, it can be shown that although they show normal thresholds of sensory acuity (vision, audition, touch), they demonstrate incapacities in the patterning of sensory stimuli into configurations (perception) and in their ability to categorize perceptions on the basis of common traits (conceptualization)[11]. Their difficulties in generalizing the essential attributes in new situations is expressed in disorientation to time, place and person. Situations remain unfamiliar, devoid of meaning and cut off from previous experience. Most disturbing to them are their disordered body concepts so that they are unable to attain a clearly differentiated, unified and stable body representation.

An important aspect of the schizophrenic child's deficiencies in adaptive response is the absence of necessary tools for monitoring and organizing behaviour. Of significance in this regard is their tendency to avoid auditory and visual input. This tendency to exclude distance stimuli seriously limits the ability to anticipate and to cope discriminatively with the outer environment.

In addition, schizophrenic children tend to be highly limited in range of pleasurable and painful response. This hedonic restriction deprives the children of the most salient motivations for coordinating and directing behaviour. It also narrows the children's potentiality for learning since the environmental possibilities for influencing learning are reduced.

The defect in goal directed action is accompanied by deficiencies in the inner awareness of self which accompanies effective action. In every case the schizophrenic child does not perceive his responsibility for initiating and carrying through successful action. He therefore does not have the basis for distinguishing self from non-self, nor does he attain feelings of continuity of self-feelings he must achieve to experience constancy and permanence in himself and in the non-self. The most dramatic examples of failures in self awareness are represented in disordered, fragmented and unstable body concepts.

Because of his deficiencies in self awareness and his inability to give meaning to new experiences by connecting them with previous learnings, the schizophrenic child is constantly confused. Feelings of ambiguity and puzzlement overwhelm him and are the basis for fears of cataclysmic proportion.

The fact to be stressed is that the major categories of ego impairment, that is, in purposeful behaviour, in the monitoring and directing of purposeful response and in the consciousness of self as a responsible, intact and initiating agent of action, are at the basis of what distresses schizophrenic children most. They do not orient themselves and attend to reality, give it meaning and adapt successfully to its requirements. There is a great deal of evidence that these children struggle to overcome the frightening strangeness and meaninglessness of a reality which does not assume the aspects of predictability and form. They also demand repeatedly of the therapist or the therapeutic environment that steps be taken to diminish the vagueness and uncertainty of experience. They communicate this demand through signs of puzzlement and panic. In turn the human environment is called on to relieve them of their sense of mystification by expanding each child's repertoire for coping with reality as he trades information with it.

The notion of specific functional constituents of ego has been stressed since 'ego' is an abstraction while the specific functions for dealing with reality are immediately observable and, therefore, definable. It is impractical, therefore, to set the goal of curing the questionable entity 'childhood schizophrenia' while one can approach the improvement of specified ego functions with optimism. One investigation employing tests of many functions has suggested that all schizophrenic children show defects in three major areas of self regulation, that is perceptual integration, self awareness (identity) and in communication[11]. Adaptive impairment, therefore, in a schizophrenic child requires improvement in each of these areas. Thus, the child must learn to attend to visual and auditory stimuli, particularly as connected with the human person. He must achieve clearly articulated concepts of his body, of himself as distinguished from others, and of temporal and spatial character of reality. And he must learn to communicate with others as a basis for relating to others and for defining reality. In our clinical experience it is reasonable to expect improvement in each of these three aspects of ego provided a suitable corrective environment is organized.

Causal Factors

A knowledge of causal factors in each case of childhood schizophrenia should assist the specification of a preferred regimen. The proposed theory of etiology is one which postulates that a variety of factors, distal (e.g. hereditary, brain damage) as well as immediate (psychosocial), and extrinsic (environmental) as well as intrinsic (cerebral), operate to a varying extent and with varying degree of combination in each schizophrenic child to produce his characteristic deficits. When the ego impairments and expressions are interpreted as adaptational manœuvres in which intrinsic predispositions and extrinsic pressures of the environment play a part, a specific treatment plan for each child is facilitated.

Thus when the schizophrenic child is physiologically intact, we have been impressed by a dramatic paralysis of parental function characterized by parental responses of extreme passivity, marked uncertainty, lack of spontaneity, and absence of empathy with the child, which add up to make a perplexed parent. Such parents are characterized by a lack of perception of the child's needs, bewilderment and inactivity in the face of the child's socially unacceptable or bizarre behaviour, and a nearly total absence of control of the child[12, 17]. A therapeutic climate is characterized by adult responses that are polar opposite of those manifested by the perplexed parent.

Environmental failure is also apparent when the family is unable to meet the special challenge of children with primary and intrinsic incapacities such as those caused by brain damage. The brain injury in itself does not explain the uniquely disordered functional manifestations of the children whom we term schizophrenic. The original incapacities of brain-damaged children, which are frequently apparent at birth, are, in such cases, exaggerated by the familial responses they provoke. The children strive to order reality and to survive, always adapting to external pressures and the pressures of larger psychosocial systems such as the family, and yet are always caught within the bounds set by their own limitations. Because the familial requirements and conduct are beyond their restricted functional capacities, their adaptive efforts miscarry. They are left bewildered, frightened, and even more circumscribed in their engagement with reality than they need be. While corrective socialization cannot cure the intrinsic cerebral defect in these children, it can do much to counteract the inappropriate adjustments which they have made to living.

Treatment Objectives

The preferred working conviction, therefore, is that, notwithstanding theories of ultimate cause and regardless of the child's own central areas of vulnerability, the environment has failed in every case to facilitate normal development. Somehow, each schizophrenic child has missed the social experiences he has required to develop into a whole person. In contrast, a therapeutic environment strives to cement the gaps in ego structure which previous experience had either failed to correct by errors of omission or aggravated by errors of commission. In accord with our analysis of the major adaptive defects of schizophrenic children, objectives in their treatment include:

1. The stimulation and enhancement of all ego functions, including perceptual, conceptual, psychomotor and communicative. Here, we also refer to the child's affective and social behaviour.

2. The stimulation and enhancement of self awareness processes, essential in the attainment of a clearly articulated self identity.

3. The stimulation and enhancement of control processes, involving an adequate and essential attention to visual and auditory processes, the cultivation of pleasurable responses and the attainment of suitable pain reactions.

The Therapeutic Environment

These therapeutic objectives determine the major constituents of a therapeutic environment for schizophrenic children. If, as we have maintained, the schizophrenic child suffers primarily from deficits in essential behavioural functions, treatment must offer him ego building experiences. In these experiences, temporal, spatial and human influences are employed to improve the child's self regulative abilities, to reduce the anxieties stemming from deficiencies in self awareness and to increase the range of gratification in his encounters with people and nature at large.

To do so, the child must be provided with many opportunities for active response and learning throughout the day. Careful programming of a day rich in experiences increases the child's skills. Of equal significance, in pursuing these experiences the child can become aware of himself as an actor, can improve his initiative and experience success and pride.

The optimal environment for assisting a schizophrenic child in his construction of reality is one which is readily perceived by the child. The first source of therapeutic influence is thus a clearly articulated environment which, on the one hand, is sensitive to those specific ego deficits which each schizophrenic child lacks and, on the other hand, responds in an affirmative and energetic fashion to enlarge the child's adaptive equipment.

The child-caring adults should try to create a world which by its very structure consistently contradicts the child's own aberrant inclinations. Thus the adults may actively and assertively establish constructive standards of response in all aspects of child routine such as schooling, eating, sleeping and all other features of child care. Though mutuality and tolerance of the children's adaptive expressions are essential, the adults decide those features of child behaviour which will be approved and which disapproved.

Clear and precise delineation of the boundaries of time, space and role behaviour are also essential. Although they must of course be comprehensible to the child, such structural definition of the temporal, spatial and role expectations of the environment is a powerful force for 'normalizing' the children's behaviour. By careful programming, the child is taught appropriate times for sleeping, eating, schooling, recreation and the many other activities of childhood. He is taught the appropriate locales for these activities. Gradually the child learns to distinguish the varying roles adults play in his life. This kind of environmental definition gives the children the feedback of external response necessary to assist them to organize existent capacities and to achieve more mature levels of response.

The atmosphere that evolves actively stresses impulse control, assists the children to wait for gratifications and to tolerate reasonable restraints and limitations. It also intrudes on unreal and wishful fantasy and contradicts the bizarre as far as feasible. Such a climate is obviously not permissive but neither is it unkind. It merely presumes that in the creative act of growing every child must have an environmentally defined framework within which he can assay the effects of his actions and develop discriminative awareness of himself in action.

What is also important to recognize, is that the well-structured environment presents many opportunities for augmenting the schizophrenic child's construction of reality and his self awareness. An example of a typical adult-child encounter within a requisite environmental framework is the following anecdote.

>When the counsellor came on duty in the morning she found Sarah sitting in barefooted dejection on her bed. Her long black hair was in matted disarray; hanging limply about her neck and face. Her pyjama top was open leaving her partially exposed. The buttons of her pyjamas having been torn off by her were strewn about the floor as were facial tissues from her incessant nose blowing.
>
>On seeing her counsellor Sarah moaned in pain that she had something in her mind. 'There's a disk in my head', she went on. 'It hurts me, please cut open my head and take the disk out. Get me some medicine. I need some medicine to clean up my mind.' The counsellor commented positively that there was no disk in Sarah's head, that her discomfort was probably a headache, and something everyone felt every so often.
>
>'Sarah', she said, 'pick up the tissues and throw them in the waste basket. You know we don't throw them on the floor, and also pick up the buttons. I'm surprised

at you! We'll have to save them and you'll sew them back on this afternoon. While you're doing that I'll get you the aspirin.'

When the counsellor returned Sarah took the two aspirins and forgetting the disk in her head went on to her nose.

'Emily', she said. 'I'm tired of my nose, my nose hurts, my mouth hurts, Emily my whole life hurts.'

'I know, Sarah', Emily replied, 'you have a cold; everyone feels uncomfortable with a cold, but your cold will get better. Your nose won't hurt and your mouth won't feel dry. Go get a drink of water, your mouth will feel better, and then get your clothes and start dressing.'

Sarah got her drink of water, and walking to the clothes closet she suddenly clutched her genitals with one hand, and while groping for clothing with the other, she began moaning.

'My vagina hurts,' she said. 'I can feel it, it feels like its bubbling. Oh, I'm afraid it's going to bubble over.'

The counsellor overhearing this asked Sarah if she had as yet urinated since awakening. 'Did you make since you've been up? You probably have to urinate and that's why you feel discomfort.'

Sarah admitted that she had not urinated, but then went on in soliloquy to say over and over, 'I have to urinate, but I can't. I'm afraid to, my vagina hurts.'

The counsellor patiently instructed Sarah to go to the toilet, sit down, and urinate. 'It will not hurt. When you're finished you will feel better. Come back immediately and start dressing.'

Sarah followed the counsellor's instructions explicitly. On returning she seemed more at ease.

'You were right, Emily', she said, 'I did have to urinate.'

She began dressing industriously for a few minutes and then paused, calling for Emily. 'Emily', she asked philosophically, 'what price do we pay for living—for dying? Is there a future? Is there danger in the future . . . ?'

'Sarah', Emily replied sharply, 'this is nonsense for a little girl to be talking, and I want you to stop it. At 7.30 in the morning I don't know about the price of living and dying or the future. I know it's time to get dressed, to get washed, to make your bed. I also know that you're late and the other girls are ahead of you, and you're going to hold us up for breakfast. So stop your questions now and start your routines.'

'Emily', Sarah replied, 'I like you', and moved off to complete her routines.

In this anecdote it is to be noted that the child-caring adult actively engages with Sarah in an effort to reduce the child's fears stemming from her disordered self-awareness. The adult is empathically sensitive to what is disturbing Sarah and responds immediately and intuitively to the child's expressions which signal confusion regarding reality. Most important, in meeting Sarah's need to schematize her body experiences and thereby to give them meaning, the child-caring person becomes important to the child and an object for the child's affection. It is to be noted, however, that this kind of maturing encounter occurs within the structural expectations of an adult environment which requires, for example, that Sarah dress herself, show a requisite degree of neatness, and join the other children in the day's programme of activities at the scheduled time. Bizarre manifestations and autistic expression in Sarah are intruded on and set right. The adult by her communications gives the child a language for describing and explaining her body sensations. This language is comprehensible and acceptable to others; and in addition to defining Sarah's reality it helps Sarah to achieve a degree of emotional mutuality with other people.

Some of the more general features of the therapeutic design follow directly from what we know of schizophrenic children as a whole. Inasmuch as schizophrenic children are highly diversified in the specific constituents of ego, however, any environment which aims to correct their adaptive deficits must achieve a high level of individualization in its programme of care. Although a basic climate relates its structure, its mores and rules to the common requirements of schizophrenic children, there is a fundamental need for individualization of environmental response to meet the unique needs of each child. It can, for example, be stated unequivocally that every phase of the environment should be alerted to the part that communication plays in facilitating behaviour and relational response and in defining the child's reality. Similarly, all the children need assistance in improving their communicative proficiency. The mute, autistic child needs to be offered response contingencies which reinforce in sequence interest in humans, then in the human voice, in vocalization, in the production of words, in symbolization and finally in the elaboration of complex linguistic structures. But the bright, overideational child with flat, toneless vocalization is encouraged to achieve appropriate affective expression as an aspect of the reversal of his social isolation.

Apart from its individualization of response, the effectiveness of the therapeutic environment is determined by the immediacy of its presence and its responsiveness to all the behavioural manœuvres of the child. Attention is paid to each relational episode in which the schizophrenic child participates at the moment of the social encounter.

Similarly, in a corrective environment, every schizophrenic symptom is viewed as an accommodative effort by the child. Unless an effort is made to understand the adaptive objective of the schizophrenic child's strivings, the response contingencies essential to facilitate ego growth are unclear. Under these circumstances treatment efforts lead to blunders which may even be harmful to the child. Clinical experience has confirmed, for example, that at the moment when panic over his sense of mystification is at its peak the schizophrenic child is asking for an environmental response which will diminish his confusion. If this demand is not met he becomes still more frightened and prefers to exclude the environment. Most significantly, the adult who fails to give the child the explanations he needs to assist him in giving form to reality recedes in importance as a facilitating agent for the child.

Professional Coordination

Representatives of many disciplines have been enlisted in the organized effort to overcome the disabilities of schizophrenic children, including psychiatrists, neurologists and other medical specialists, child-care workers, teachers, case workers, psychologists and remedial specialists. In addition, many varieties of therapeutic procedure have been employed—psychotherapy, environmental design, education, and chemotherapy. Psychiatric direction of the therapeutic programme is suited to the effective coordination of the many disciplines and procedures involved and assures attention to the biological, social and psychological features of childhood schizophrenia.

The therapeutic point of view embodied in the concept of corrective socialization is most obviously represented in the technique of milieu therapy. Milieu therapy exploits the opportunities for ego corrective influence offered by countless encounters with the schizophrenic child in the course of child care and education. However, it must be understood that milieu therapy is consonant with all the specialized procedures of psychiatry including drug treatment and individual psychotherapy. Both chemotherapy and individual psychotherapy are useful for overcoming the child's confusions and adaptive deficiencies and for improving his construction of reality. They will, therefore, be considered briefly in terms of their specialized objectives and especially in terms of their integration into a broad programme of corrective socialization.

Chemotherapy

The objectives of chemotherapy are best considered in the light of the broad goals of treatment. The approach of corrective socialization assumes that all the characteristic symptoms and phenomena of childhood schizophrenia have an adaptational significance. They represent ultimate outcomes of transactions between the child with his intrinsic predispositions and his environment. The approach of corrective socialization also assumes that learning and human interaction are the primary agents for modifying the functional deficits of schizophrenic children. Within this basic framework for treatment, drugs are utilized as adjuvant agents for the purpose of enhancing the impact of social processes on the children.

While they may alter a child's accessibility to stimulation and influence, drugs do not in themselves undo the complex skein of learned responses or create entirely new behavioural characteristics. The latter can only emerge out of real life experience. Merely making a child manageable is not equivalent to cure or genuine improvement. In addition, in circumstances where there are adequate and sufficient therapeutic personnel, and where detailed human attention is provided for the child's communications and requirements, most of the children are, in fact, manageable without drugs. Custodial installations lacking in personnel and programme are likely to depend on drugs alone to reduce the problems of managing the children. When these children in custodial environments are transferred to therapeutic settings, it is frequently possible to reduce very sharply the drugs they have been receiving and to manage the children very simply by careful concern with their individual needs. Obviously the employment of drugs in child psychiatry must be accompanied by a continuing search for the psychological and social factors contributing to the deficiencies of each schizophrenic child and the reversal of their disturbing influence.

Nevertheless, drugs do have a clear and certain job to perform. They do, in fact, affect some varieties of symptomatic behaviour in schizophrenic children which interfere with their environmental engagement. Thus, for example, they are useful in reducing their anxiety, their excessive sensory sensitivity, their distractibility, their deficient impulse control and their hyperactivity. These deviations in overall adaptive characteristics hinder schizophrenic children as they strive to develop improved relationships and understanding of reality. By affecting these overall qualities of ego, pharmacotherapy can make selected children more receptive to psychotherapy and social influence. It may be of assistance, therefore, in facilitating the child's adjustment to his peers, his tolerance for the special requirements and educative experience of the classroom, and his accessibility to psychotherapeutic methods which depend on communicative attention and insight. Pharmacotherapy is thus a reasonable component of a comprehensive programme of psychiatric treatment.

Precautions need to be mentioned briefly. Drugs need to be selected which aim at the relief of clearly defined symptoms which interfere with learning, social adjustment and psychotherapy. Individualization of dosage programme is usually essential, since the effective range varies from child to child. They should be reduced or eliminated as soon as possible. Precautions against toxicity must be taken. Assuming rational choice of drug and attention to effective dosage and toxicity, a great deal of success can be achieved in using drugs to support treatment and social influence.

A review which has been made of about 10 years of clinical experience in one treatment installation for schizophrenic children between 6 and 12 years of age has shown that the major target symptoms for which chemotherapy has been employed include: apathy, anxiety, hypersensitivity, hyperactivity, distractibility and disturbance in impulse control. The drugs employed most often for the relief of these symptoms may be summarized as follows:*

		Target Symptoms
1.	Trifluo-perazine (Stelazine)	apathy
		hypoactivity
		withdrawal
		anxiety
2.	Chlorpromazine (Thorazine)	anxiety
		hyperactivity
		impulse disturbance

* More complete summaries of chemotherapy for children and its evaluation may be found elsewhere. [8,10,18]

		Target Symptoms
3.	Diphenhydramine (Benadryl)	anxiety hyperactivity impulse disturbance
4.	Dextro-amphetamine (Dexedrine)	hyperactivity impulse disturbance

Milieu Therapy

For purposes of discussion, it is desirable to offer definitions which differentiate individual therapy from milieu therapy. Milieu therapy is the deliberate and planned design of a total environment in accord with a clear therapeutic objective for each child. The constituents of the milieu are all aspects of the atmosphere, except for psychotherapy and pharmacotherapy. Among them are the daily activities arranged for the children including eating, going to sleep and waking, schooling, recreation, dress; and the many varieties of interaction among the children, between the children and adults, and among the adults themselves.

Individual Therapy

Individual psychotherapy refers rather to an intimate human interchange between adult therapist and child in which the encounter is guided by a systematic theory of human behaviour. Fundamental to such a theory are the psychoanalytic propositions that human responses are motivated and purposeful, that behaviour is adaptational and best explained within the context of continuing interaction of the person and his environment, and that motivations may be unconscious or outside the individual's conscious awareness. Intrapsychic conflicts arise when conscious and unconscious goals are contradictory. To understand the meaning of a child's responses requires the interpretation of unconscious motivations. Such meaning is inferred on the basis of the convergence of data gathered in play therapy, verbal interview and direct life observation.

There has been a great deal of discussion of the comparative merits of individual psychotherapy and milieu therapy. Some treatment installations use milieu therapy alone; others emphasize both milieu therapy and individual therapy; others view the residential or day hospital programme merely as a background to support the child's accessibility to individual psychotherapy. Actual clinical experience in applying milieu therapy and individual therapy alone, and in conjunction with each other* would support the position that both therapeutic modalities are essential in a comprehensive programme of treatment for the schizophrenic child.

* At the Ittleson Center, milieu therapy under the direction of a psychoanalytically trained psychiatrist, was employed as a sole technique in the residence for two years; and then individual therapy was added to the programme. The coordination of the two treatment forms has been an active concern of the professional staff for the past 11 years.

For some of the children, the significance of the social climate is of primary value. For others, the experience of individual psychotherapy is most meaningful to the child. The optimal programme is one in which the two facets of treatment contribute to each other.

By their mutual and reciprocating influence, too, the two forms of treatment take on a special character. Because observations of each child by child-care workers and teachers are made over the entire day, the individual therapist is in an unusual position to know precisely and in detail each child's external reality. The link between individual and group processes, and the relationship between reality and the child's fantasies are readily inferred. The climate as designed by the adults defines the child's external world, and the introspective explorations of individual therapy probe intrapsychic processes in the child and bring to view how the child is experiencing and interpreting his milieu. This kind of information regarding the child's private interpretations of his environmental situation is only attainable within the individual therapeutic relationship, and is of inestimable value for designing a climate which is meaningful for each child. Often, the individual therapist who is most sensitive to the manifestations and details of adaptation can assist the adults involved in the design of the milieu to respond to the child in a manner which will have most constructive effect on the building of the child's ego.

The psychotherapist is equipped to deal with motivational and conflictual aspects of ego organization which arise. While child-care workers and teachers are busily engaged in defining reality for the child, the therapist may strategically and skilfully deal with the child's affective responses to that reality, his adaptive style and those of his defences which miscarry.

In a therapeutic milieu which recognizes the essential role of the milieu, individual therapy thus has an irreplaceable role in deepening the professional understanding of the psychodynamic and adaptive significance of the child's symptoms and behaviour. In addition, where conflicts may be hindering the child in his efforts to cope with reality, the therapist serves the function of exposing and resolving the conflicts. Serious conflicts and emotional defences similar to those noted in childhood neurosis do arise in the development of schizophrenic children and they can best be dealt with within the framework of individual therapy by qualified therapists.

It is important to grasp, however, that intrapsychic conflict is a more basic adaptive problem in children suffering from the usual range of reactive behaviour disorders and neurotic reactions than in schizophrenic children. The pivotal problem in the schizophrenic child is his structural defect in ego, that is, his deficiency in the functions necessary for self regulation in the course of his interaction with his environment. Conflicts and the defensive accommodations they provoke do arise in schizophrenic children, but these conflictual manifestations are not as important as the primary deficits in purposeful function. Therefore, in individual therapy of schizophrenic children, no less than in milieu therapy, the therapist's objective is to assist them to orient themselves to a shifting, ambiguous world.

The corrective implication of individual therapy is recognized by most workers who have described specialized forms of individual therapy for schizophrenic children. Thus, for example, Mahler[16] recommends a 'corrective symbiotic' experience. The child is helped to relive the regressive, symbiotic phase of development directly with the mother and then gradually to replace the old relationship with a new, less demanding relationship with the mother. Alpert[1] also describes a 'corrective object relationship' in which the therapist and teacher serve as suitable objects to compensate for early maternal failures. Des Lauriers[6], too, implies a direct corrective approach wherein the schizophrenic child is provided with actual experiences for the purpose of improving his awareness of his body and psychological identity. They all, therefore, recognize the fundamental therapeutic necessity for positive nutrition and stimulation of the defective ego.

Impairments in ego functions such as perceptual attention, human interest and attachment, organization of reality, communication, responsiveness to rewards and punishments must be overcome by socializing experiences. The assumption is made that the schizophrenic child has missed essential ego-nurturing experiences and that experiences for stimulating and reinforcing adaptive functions must be given to him in individual as well as milieu therapy. This point is stressed because there is some degree of professional confusion represented in the notion that the ultimate therapeutic manœuvre is analytic interpretation to the schizophrenic child who presumably will be able to utilize his capacity for logical reasoning to alter his behaviour. An interesting example of this confusion is the report of Caruth and Ekstein[4] on the use of the metaphor with borderline and schizophrenic children. Although the authors develop at length the use of this relational tool to maintain contact with the patients and note its value in enhancing empathic communication, they nevertheless state, 'It is but a preliminary approximation to the final therapeutic act, which ultimately will consist of a classical interpretation at the level of secondary process'. This is an arbitrary therapeutic requirement. Talking to a child at his level of understanding and emotional tolerance is not merely preparation for the final therapeutic act. If the therapist interests a non-communicating and emotionally isolated child in communication and in human relationship, then the therapist's responses are the primary therapeutic acts. Efforts to improve a schizophrenic child's insight via analytic interpretation may have little significance for him because of intrinsic limitations in receptor and communicative capacity and, even more, perhaps, because he primarily needs new environmental and adult response to achieve a higher level of integrative response.

Family Treatment

In evolving a corrective therapeutic programme based on social processes, attention is inevitably given to therapeutic objectives with the family of the schizophrenic child. Some treatment centres are so pessimistic about the possibilities for change in the families of schizophrenic children that they are inclined to exclude the family from therapeutic considerations. Under these circumstances, the family is kept isolated from the treatment programme. The parents and siblings remain unchanged and their emotional reactions to the treatment of the schizophrenic child remain unexplored. However, other treatment centres are impressed by the necessity for altering the pattern of family interaction if the child's gains in treatment are to be sustained on his return home after a period of comprehensive treatment.

Although it is easier to exclude the family from treatment, there is much to be gained from a family oriented programme of treatment. This kind of a programme entails treatment of the parents and siblings as individuals; but in recent years treatment of the family as a group has also been promising. Therapy of the family as a unit brings into sharp focus the style of family behaviour and the relationship between patterns of psychosocial behaviour in the family and the adaptive responses of the psychotic child. Failures in family communication and the challenge such failures have on the schizophrenic child's ego are illuminated. Focused efforts can then be made to correct the communicative and relational errors in the family.

Albert had been treated in residence for four years with clinical improvement. He became less wooden and less withdrawn. His speech became more expressive. He gave up his bizarre body mannerisms, such as flapping. His Wechsler IQ improved 35 points. He was achieving in school beyond the average for his age.

To achieve these results, the therapeutic programme in residence had combined a number of constituent therapeutic techniques. Thus a great deal of consideration had been given to all of his daily experiences in his group of peers, in the many aspects of child care and in school. Similarly, he had been in intensive individual therapy for the four years of his stay in the residence; and each of the family members including father, mother and younger sister had been in individual psychotherapy.

In arriving at a plan for his discharge from the residence and his return to the community, the professional staff felt there would be advantage in offering Albert the normalizing experiences of school and community with which he was now prepared to cope. There remained a considerable uncertainty regarding the dynamics of his family organization, the various psychological roles of the individual family members and particularly of the role of the child patient in the family, and the style of communication within the family. Individual treatment of the parents and children had permitted each singly or in clusters to present contradictory information, to lie, to distort reality and to exercise a massive pattern of denial. It was obvious that a new therapeutic format was necessary if the patterns of psychosocial response in the family were to come to view for purposes of therapeutic modification. It was decided that this would be most feasible in conjoint family therapy where the interactional characteristics, the defensive distortions and the communicative ambiguities would appear in the public light of mutual examination. Individual treatment sessions would also be employed as indicated.

During the first year of family treatment, the most sustained theme was the management of sexual expression in the family. This was occasioned by the parents' complaints regarding Albert's uncontrollable sexual behaviour. He masturbated to excess, even in the company of others at home and in the classroom. He would peer under girls' skirts, touch their breasts, would announce to the class if a girl was wearing a brassiere, and approach girls with comments such as 'I'd like to make babies with you!' The parents were paralysed and inert in response to Albert's sexual behaviour, and asked what could be done. Albert, on the other hand, complained he did not have a clear idea of what was appropriate sexual behaviour. In fact, he attributed his confusion regarding sexual control to his parents' very inconsistent behaviour. He wondered if it was proper for a father to 'goose' him and for his mother to barge into his bedroom unannounced to see if he was masturbating.

In a typical family interchange, the father's evasiveness and denial of his own responsibility for stimulating the children sexually emerged in bold relief. Albert, who is ordinarily unexpressive and wooden, appealed to the psychiatrist. 'Is it right for a father to goose his son?' When the father denied behaving as his son had described, Albert was supported by his sister. The father tried to intimidate the children, attacked their 'foolishness' and said uncomfortably that the goosing was infrequent and had only occurred recently. The children were frightened and tearful as they exposed the father. Albert's sister affirmed 'Every time we pass him he pinches us in the back and he's done it for as long as we can remember.' The father became furious and shouted 'If I can't act natural with my kids, maybe they'd be better off if I'd leave home'. His inclination to intimidate the children by leaving them was linked to his repetitive threat to Albert since his son's discharge from the residence that he would 'put' him away again and was dealt with.

In similar sessions, discussions of the parents' behaviour were initiated by the children. They talked of their parents' exhibitionism and lack of respect for privacy. They described the parents' inappropriate nudity and complained that both parents would come into the bathroom unannounced when they were bathing and toileting. With great hesitation, they complained of the father's excessive use of punishments which combined elements of cruelty and erotic arousal. For example, the father would punish the children by strapping their bare buttocks.

The contradictions and inconsistencies in the parental behaviour were considered at length. Along with their apparent disapproval of Albert's masturbation and sexual preoccupation, they had been stimulating him to be sexually uncontrolled. The contribution of these inconsistencies to Albert's sexual confusion was stressed. At the same time, in regular individual sessions with Albert, his role in the sexual confusion of the family was examined. The realistic consequences of his uncontrolled sexual behaviour was examined with him since he was unaware of how his behaviour had isolated him from his peers and might even result in another placement away from home. He was also confronted with his defensive tendency to use 'illness' and 'confusion' as rationalizations for his inadequate controls.

This therapeutic approach had definite and positive consequences. Albert's aberrant behaviour ceased. Masturbation continued but was not exercised in public. The diminution in mutual sexual arousal at home resulted in diminished anxiety in Albert. In general, he showed greater impulse control and his learning and peer relationships improved. Most important of all Albert and his family showed improved clarity and forthrightness in their communication with each other.

The present discussion has emphasized that the main deficiencies in schizophrenic children represent failures in adaptive functions involved in their engagement with reality. It has further maintained that their ability to organize reality in a meaningful fashion is determined in part by the response of the environment. The milieu is therefore viewed as the essential and minimal therapeutic resource nourishing and correcting the fragmented egos of the children. This rehabilitative ego-building role is shared by the specialized forms of individual and family therapy for schizophrenic children. So far it has been suggested that a corrective environment must react decisively at the moment of the child's actions; and that the environmental response must aim at the facilitation of growth in specified ego functions which are impaired.

3

Community Planning

Preferred Size of Treatment Unit

It must also be recognized that the irreplaceable and primary therapeutic agent for the schizophrenic child needs to be the human person. Learning machines are available and programmed schedules of reinforcement can be employed to improve specified classes of functional response such as language. However, the ultimate goal in treatment includes the development and consolidation of normal patterns of human attachment and relatedness. To attain this goal, the schizophrenic child requires the intimate socializing impact of the human being himself. Human availability and responsiveness are feasible only when the number of children under care is small relative to the number of professional adults.* The optimal atmosphere is one in which the children and adults all know each other intimately.

Duration of Treatment

Practical experience in the management of schizophrenic children has also confirmed that a corrective human influence must be exercised for very prolonged periods of time. Perceptible improvement in ego functions is achieved by a gradual process of growth.

Variety of Services

In addition, a recent study of the professional requirements of these children from birth through a post-discharge period from the residential centre of 5-10 years has clearly confirmed that the residential placement is only one episode in their clinical histories. All had contact with clinical agencies long before the residential placement. In addition, it has become

---

* Although absolute standards do not exist, the Ittleson Center for Child Research provides 20 to 24 children with 3 psychiatrists on a half-time basis, a psychiatric supervisor, 4 teachers, 10 to 11 child-care workers, a child-care supervisor, 2 to 3 caseworkers, and a large group of maintenance and other ancillary personnel.

increasingly clear that after discharge there is a need for psychiatric and other specialized assistance by the children throughout their childhood, and by their families. For example, prior to placement in the psychiatric residence of the Ittleson Center for Child Research at the age of 6 years, a schizophrenic girl and her family had already had the following professional consultations for her problems at different times and in sequence: paediatrician, psychiatrist, psychologist, family agency, therapeutic nursery, child guidance and brief hospital inpatient psychiatric service. After $4\frac{1}{2}$ years of treatment in the specialized treatment residence of the Ittleson Center she was improved, but the family situation was so unsettled she required foster care. She was thus sent to an institution for dependent children. After two years she was discharged to her family but required special class placement. When her mother suddenly became acutely depressed, psychiatric treatment was arranged for the mother. Another example of multiple service needs is that of a schizophrenic boy placed at the age of 6 in the Ittleson Center. Before placement, and beginning at 2 years of age, he had been studied by paediatricians for slow development, by psychologists, by a speech pathology clinic and by the inpatient children's service of the city psychiatric hospital. He was treated for four years at the Ittleson Center with marked improvement. He was discharged to his home at 10 years of age, with arrangement for outpatient treatment. He quickly gave evidence of coping poorly with the pressures of the normal school environment and of the family itself which had not altered significantly in its psychosocial characteristics. He became withdrawn and suicidal. He was then brought back to the Ittleson Center day hospital programme with quick return to his level of adjustment at the time of discharge from the residence. After two years in the day centre, he was able to return to an advanced educational programme in a public high school but has remained in individual treatment on an outpatient basis. In addition, the entire family has been involved in conjoint family therapy.

These brief follow-up summaries of two children indicate their changing clinical needs throughout childhood. They have required a very broad range of specialized psychiatric services, including outpatient, day and residence services, and cooperative relationships with community resources, such as the schools. Such longitudinal studies of clinical need provide evidence that the preferred community programme for schizophrenic children is one which makes all these services available to the child. In addition, a rounded programme enveloping all the special services as constituents would permit coordination of services for each child. It would also facilitate the attainment of skill in the differential use of professional services for the children at varying points in their historic development. This kind of community programme would accept psychiatric responsibility for the schizophrenic child when the child's severe ego disabilities first became manifest. Thereafter, guided by the child's requirements of any given time, the community programme would foster an easy shift from one professional service and level of professional responsibility to another.

REFERENCES

1. ALPERT, A., 1963. A special therapeutic technique for prelatency children with a history of deficiency in maternal care. *Am. J. Orthopsychiat.*, **33**, 161-82.
2. BENDER, L., 1947. Childhood schizophrenia. Clinical study of one hundred schizophrenic children. *Am. J. Orthopsychiat.*, **17**, 40-56.
3. BRADLEY, C., 1941. *Schizophrenia in childhood.* New York, MacMillan.
4. CARUTH, E., and EKSTEIN, R., 1966. Interpretation within the metaphor. *J. Child Psychiat.*, **5**, 35-46.
5. CREAK, M., 1961. Schizophrenic syndrome in childhood; progress report of a working party. *Cerebr. Palsy Bull.*, **3**, 501.
6. DES LAURIERS, A. M., 1962. *The experience of reality in childhood schizophrenia.* New York, Internat. Univ. Press.
7. DESPERT, L. J., 1938. Schizophrenia in children. *Psychiat. Quart.*, **12**, 366-71.
8. EISENBERG, L., 1964. Role of drugs in treating disturbed children. *Children*, **11**, 167-73.
9. EKSTEIN, R., and WALLERSTEIN, J., 1954. Observations on the psychology of borderline and psychotic children. *Psychoanalytic study of the child*, vol. 9. New York, Internat. Univ. Press.
10. FISH, B., 1960 Drug therapy in psychiatry: psychological aspects. *Comprehensive Psychiat.*, **1**, 55-61.
11. GOLDFARB, W., 1961. *Childhood schizophrenia.* Cambridge, Mass., Harvard University Press for the Commonwealth Fund.
12. GOLDFARB, W., SIBULKIN, L., BEHRENS, M., and JAHODA, H., 1958. Parental perplexity and childhood confusion. In *New frontiers in child guidance.* Ed. Esman, A. H. New York, Internat. Univ. Press.
13. KANNER, L., 1944. Early infantile autism. *J. Pediatr.*, **25**, 211-17.
14. KNOBLOCH, H., and PASAMANICK, B., 1962. Etiologic factors in 'early infantile autism' and childhood schizophrenia. Address to International Congress of Paediatrics, Lisbon, Portugal.
15. MAHLER, M. S., 1958. Autism and symbiosis. Two extreme disturbances of identity. *Inter. J. Psychoanal.*, **39**, 1-7.
16. MAHLER, M. S., and FUHRER, M., 1960. Observation on research regarding the 'symbiotic syndrome' of infantile psychosis. *Psychoan. Quart.*, **29**, 317-27.
17. MEYERS, D. I., and GOLDFARB, W., 1961. Studies of perplexity in mothers of schizophrenic children. *Am. J. Orthopsychiat.*, **31**, 551-64.
18. NICHTERN, S., 1962. Chemotherapy in child psychiatry. In *Child psychiatry and the general practitioner.* Eds, Krakowski, A. J., and Santara, D. A. Springfield, Ill., Thomas.
19. POTTER, H. W., 1933. Schizophrenia in children. *Am. J. Psychiat.*, **12**, 1253-70.
20. RANK, B., 1949. Adaptation of the psychoanalytic technique for the treatment of young children with atypical development. *Am. J. Orthopsychiat.*, **19**, 130-39.

XXV

ACUTE ORGANIC PSYCHOSES OF CHILDHOOD*

AETIOLOGY AND SYMPTOMATOLOGY

G. BOLLEA

Professor of Child Neuropsychiatry, University of Rome, Italy

1
Introduction

By 'acute organic psychoses' is meant all psychopathological manifestations, reversible or irreversible, which have a causal connection with a somatic illness, whether this involves extracerebral organs and systems firstly, and then the brain, or whether it is localized only or mostly in the nervous system. Thus 'symptomatic psychoses' and 'organic psychoses' are considered synonymous by the author.

The literature on acute organic psychoses of childhood and adolescence is strangely scarce and confused both on phenomenology and on nosography. Psychiatrists have paid very little attention to this field and paediatricians, for their part, have given little consideration to these syndromes as most of them have a rapidly reversible symptomatology. Paediatricians hold that these syndromes have little importance (with the exception of the comatose states) in relation to the general picture of the illness which causes them. Again, many authors do not consider that febrile delirium, which as we shall see is one of the less severe forms, should be included among organic psychoses. Bleuler[2] stated that children react with delirium very easily, and therefore this disturbance is of no great significance. Often, too, it is very difficult to make a differential diagnosis between symptomatic psychoses and syndromes purely reactive to physical acute or sub-acute illnesses, because in the infant and in the child it is more difficult than in the adult to separate physical from psychological factors.

* Translated by Maria-Livia Osborn, Research Assistant, The Institute of Family Psychiatry, Ipswich and East Suffolk Hospital, Ipswich.

Thus, to define this area better, a lengthy and fuller observation is needed in order to arrive at a more specific description of symptomatology, and therefore to a more precise diagnosis. It is important to follow every case of acute organic psychosis for a long time, clinically and by laboratory tests, even after a complete recovery.

Above all it must be remembered that in the literature there are scientific statements, valid in themselves, but which are handed down from one author to another as axioms; these statements should be assessed more critically. (*i*) The validity of Bonhoeffer's[3] principle, also for childhood and adolescence, i.e. that the psychopathological manifestation of exogenous origin should be the same whatever the nature of the illness and the causal factor. (*ii*) The almost invariable absence of symptomatic psychic disturbances below the age of 3 years, when instead the exogenous reaction is represented exclusively by convulsions. (*iii*) The almost invariable complete reversibility of the psychopathological picture, except in those cases tending to dementia.

Kraepelin[6], and many other authors of his time, tried without success to establish specific psychopathological forms for each disease. However, Bonhoeffer's attempt to establish a uniformity of features of the exogenous reaction and its independence from the causal disease has gone too far in the opposite direction, i.e. there has been no incentive to collect ample clinical material and analyse more accurately the correlation between psychopathology, aetiology, pathogenesis and pathological anatomy. Instead the classic and fundamental symptoms of the exogenous reaction (disorder of consciousness, drowsiness or agitation, hallucinatory delirium) have been the starting point for the conclusion that any syndrome approximating this phenomenology has an organic nature.

However, in the formative years, especially in infancy and childhood, the brain, depending on its degree of maturity is particularly sensitive and vulnerable. Therefore Bonhoeffer's[3] principle of exogenous reaction should be substituted by that of chronogenous reaction, i.e. a phenomenological reaction linked to the chronological factor in which the noxa acted.

Moreover, we must always remember that in childhood and adolescence not only in every disease, but in every group of diseases, the organic attack tends to select the same specific area (perivenous encephalitis, diffuse alterations of the circulation, especially venous, encephalitis of the basal nuclei, enzymatic intracellular blocks, leuko-encephalitis, localized oedemas with or without Nissl's acute cellular degeneration) which must perforce partially influence the acute psychopathological picture and in particular the eventual outcome. The latter, of course, is also influenced by the premorbid personality and by the familial environment.

In considering the almost inevitable absence of symptomatic psychic disturbances below the age of 3 years, when convulsions are the only reaction, it must be remembered that the convulsion is often the culminant point of an altered psychic state, which at this age presents a less pronounced symptomatology in the shape of apathy, inertia and detachment from the environment, or contortions and agitation without aim. 'He does not look at me', 'he doesn't see me', 'he does not recognize me', and 'he has a pain somewhere' are perhaps the anxious maternal correlations of a confusional state with which agitation may be associated. Loose words, which the child often utters without any link with reality or with his needs, are also an indication of changes in his psyche. But often the convulsion is sudden, or so close to the beginning of the noxa, that this period of psychic change is not easily noticed by the parents.

It must be added that in every severe form of hydric and electrolytic disquilibrium there is a picture of psychic disturbance of the confusional type, as it will be specified later, that is to say a change in awareness of the environment.

However, it is difficult to establish at what age an exogenous reaction can occur. The child should be:

1. Old enough to be orientated in time and space and capable of recognizing the objects around him.

2. Capable of communicating this ability, or better still it should be possible to interpret clinically any change in this ability. Theoretically this should already be possible at 12 months, but in practice a diagnosis is only possible some months later. In fact, cases of drug poisoning (especially atropine) between 15 to 20 months have been described.

Four points about the complete reversibility of phenomena must be kept in mind:

1. The frequency with which electroencephalographic alterations are observed after acute illness.

2. The problem, discussed at length in contemporary scientific literature, of the characterological consequences of a micro-pathology often related to a symptomatic psychosis of the neonatal stage and infancy, which had previously been underevaluated. This is the so-called 'psycho-organic infantile syndrome'; the classic syndrome presents the following symptoms: lack of learning, lack of retentive memory, lack of ability to conceptualize and to reproduce shapes (hence dyslexia, dysgraphia, difficulty in learning geometry), lack of concentration, retardation of thought, frequent fluctuations of disturbed behaviour.

3. The increasing frequency of sub-acute encephalopathies with a history of symptoms of acute organic psychosis, even if in these cases a history of convulsions is more frequent.

4. The frequency with which a symptomatic psychosis, that often is relapsing, may indicate an initial dysmetabolic state (Hartnup disease, prolinoemia, etc.).

Prognostically, therefore, four groups of acute organic psychoses may be considered:

(*a*) Forms which are reversible within a few days or several months.
(*b*) Irreversible forms, which result in:

(i) mental retardation, of varying degree.
(ii) mental regression up to dementia.
(iii) convulsive syndrome.
(iv) leuko-encephalitis, etc.

(c) Partially reversible forms: infantile psycho-organic syndrome (brain damage); grave behaviour disorders.

(d) Relapsing and atypical forms:

(i) Benign.
(ii) Malignant, which become, after various crises, true psychoses (symptomatic schizophrenia).

After these preliminary considerations, it would be useful to discuss the acute organic psychoses, firstly, from the aetiopathogenic point of view and, secondly, from the symptomatologic and nosographic point of view.

2

Aetiology

Introduction

As has already been stated, no distinction is made here between acute symptomatic psychoses and acute organic psychoses. Some authors would consider the first to be caused by diseases or by toxic, metabolic, endocrine, extracerebral changes, which are only secondary causes of brain lesions; and the others to be caused primarily by cerebral diseases (cranial trauma, tumors, meningeal encephalitis, chemical intoxications, etc.) This distinction, apparently clear and simple, is often impossible in clinical practice when considering the acute phase.

The pathogenesis of symptomatic psychoses is very controversial, it is, however, always due to several factors. The cerebral disorder may be of a functional nature, acting directly or indirectly on the cerebral metabolism, or strictly of an organic nature due to a lesion of the cellular substratum. A strong disquilibrium of the hydric balance, e.g. caused by toxic infection, may produce an acute Nissl's cellular degeneration of the nervous cells which, depending on age, may be rapidly reversible, or may develop into cellular death; an infectious disease may cause a cerebral oedema, a secondary perivenous encephalitis, or a very acute toxic haemorrhagic encephalitis. In these cases, it is difficult to establish the moment of onset of the psychic disorder and hence the difficulty of classification.

Even more difficult is the distinction between the two forms in many chemical intoxications, when the agent can act concurrently on several organs and systems, including the nervous system. In these cases the psychosymptomatology may be caused, in the acute phase, either by a direct action, or by a secondary autointoxication of other extracerebral lesions.

Another reason for keeping together the two acute forms is that the fundamental symptom for both is a dimming or, even more usual, a disorder of consciousness of varying severity. Incoherence of thought is here secondary, unlike in the acute states of endogenous and functional psychic disorders. The primacy of disorder of consciousness is very distinct in childhood and is the characteristic element of every form of acute organic psychosis, from the slightest to the gravest.

'Acute organic psychoses' will thus be the term used here, and in discussing their pathogenesis the following groups will be considered: (1) Those with cerebral causes: (*a*) vascular, (*b*) infectious, (*c*) tumours or hypertensions, (*d*) traumatic, (*e*) related to epilepsy. (2) Those with extra-cerebral causes: (*a*) para- and post-infective encephalitis, (*b*) disorders of metabolism, endocrine disorders and auto-intoxications, (*c*) hetero-intoxications: (*i*) accidental; (*ii*) by poisonous substances and drugs, (*d*) avitaminosis. (3) Those with physical agents: (*a*) sun or heat stroke, (*b*) accidental hypothermia, (*c*) electric trauma, (*d*) radiation and burns. (4) Those with unknown causes.

In order to orientate the reader, the most frequent causes of acute organic psychoses will be briefly reviewed. It seems unnecessary to refer in detail here to the specific symptoms of illness, or to the neurological signs that may be present, as these are discussed later. Instead a brief description is given, for some psychoses, of the most frequent psychopathological pictures to be found in childhood.

Cerebral Causes

Vascular disorders (*i*) *Cerebral embolism:* This is rare in childhood and usually follows the migration of thrombi in congenital cardiopathy, or of microthrombi in endocarditis. The onset is sudden with torpor and sometimes convulsions.

(*ii*) *Cerebral haemorrhage:* This is rare in childhood. Sometimes presents in the Sturge-Weber syndrome and in the course of some systemic diseases, like leukaemia, haemophilia and Werlhof's disease. Usually the establishment of the disorder of consciousness is rapid, sometimes preceded by a brief period of excitement, and soon followed by coma.

(*iii*) *Cerebral thrombosis:* This is extremely rare in childhood, except the form affecting the dura mater. The onset of the disorder of consciousness is usually sudden, sometimes preceded by a brief period of confusion, and soon developing into coma.

(*iv*) *Migraine:* This is rare before puberty. In the prodromal period sometimes hallucinatory twilight states are present and, in ophthalmic migraine, visual hallucinations. Associated with it there might be dysphoria, which only exceptionally develops into a state of psycho-motor excitement. Seldom, states equivalent to migraine are present with disorders of the twilight type and with acute anxiety.

Infections. In childhood, the younger the child the graver and of earlier presentation is the entity of the disorder of consciousness, which tends to develop into coma quite rapidly. The most frequent are tubercular meningitis, meningococcic meningitis, most types of encephalitis, rabies and chorea minor.

(*i*) *Tubercular meningitis:* In the prodromal phase, mood changes are often observed, or apathy and sadness. Then, when the disease has developed, drowsiness and torpor alternate with periods of motor excitement and, sometimes, with confusional delirium.

(*ii*) *Meningococcal meningitis:* In the initial period there is torpor, with alternating states of restlessness, sometimes reaching the point of confusional excitement.

(*iii*) *Herpetic encephalitis:* The disorder is generally limited to a stage of torpor, which may, sometimes, progress into coma.

(*iv*) *Encephalitis caused by neurotropic viruses:* Here we have states of clouding, sometimes alternating with restlessness.

(*v*) *Rabies:* In rabies acute anxiety with agitation is present. Sometimes, especially in infancy and childhood, there are forms where depression is common.

(*vi*) *Chorea:* At the beginning there is often a period of depression and anxiety, then emotional lability, disorders of memory and concentration, and, very seldom, a slight clouding of consciousness.

Tumours or hypertensions. When the acute psychotic disorder is tied to intercranial tumours and to hypertensions in general, it is impossible to distinguish a characteristic psychopathology, because the disorders usually take on the guise of torpor, apathy and slow mentation, tied to the hypertension. Some of the symptomatology may be dictated by the site of the lesion. In *tumours of the 3rd ventricle and of the hypothalamus* sleep disorders are often present, they may be followed by coma. In the initial phases of *cerebral stem damage* a confusional state and torpor can be observed. *Tumours of the temporal lobe* are often associated with psycho-motor disorders and confusional states, whilst in occipital tumours psychosensory disorders are often frequent. Lastly, in *tumours of the frontal lobe* disorders of mood and of memory are prevalent, such as fatuous euphoria.

Particular mention must be made of psychological disorders related to the presence of a haematoma. The onset of the symptomatology is often acute and consists of disorders of alertness deteriorating into coma; in chronic forms, in addition to the neurological symptoms, are often observed changes of mood, inattention, instability and sleep disorders. This symptomatology is in many respects analogous to that found in forms of cerebral abscess with slow development.

Lastly, mention must be made of cranio-pharyngioma, which fairly often, in its slow development, may show a characteristic symptomatology displaying slow mentation, depression and insomnia.

Traumata. In addition to the general lesion due to the functional disorder of the traumatized brain, psychological disorders may be present, consisting, in the first instance, of loss of consciousness and coma. In a few cases, the only symptom of cerebral damage may be a twilight state which may present with confusion and slowness of thought, or, in the 'lucid' form, characterized by vivacity reaching hypomania. It must be noted that control of consciousness is reacquired fairly soon, even if amnesia of the traumatic event still persists.

Epilepsy. Sometimes in the phase *preceding the fit*, the patient may present a state of acute anxiety, experienced as terror and perplexity. On the other hand, in childhood, experiences of depersonalization and déjà-vu are rare. The *fit* may sometimes show the characteristics of a periodic psychosis, with coma, confusional states, dysthimia, delirium and hallucinations. In the phase *following a grand mal fit* disorders of alertness are prevalent, there might be a twilight state simple or complicated by psychomotor automatism. In *petit mal*, the phase following the fit may deteriorate to the point of lucid delirium, hallucinosis and oneirism.

Lastly, it is to be remembered the psychological disorder which sometimes follows the pharmacological control of the fits (Landort's syndrome), represented by compulsive and aggressive behaviour.

Extra-cerebral Causes

Encephalitis during and following infectious diseases. The most common of these diseases are: influenza, typhus, scarlet fever, measles, chicken-pox, small-pox, mumps, pertussis, enterovirosis, infections related to vaccinations, leukocytosis, tuberculosis, brucellosis, acute rheumarthritis, malaria, acute yellow atrophy of the liver, blood diseases (haemolytic syndromes, thalassemia, etc.), pneumonia, diphtheria and erysipelas.

Due to the sensitivity typical to childhood, toxic and infectious diseases are the most common causes of acute organic psychoses, which, because of their common characteristics, present in fairly similar forms, even if they have a different aetiology. Some of the most characteristic are: *influenza*, which might present symptomatology varying from a twilight state to a confusional agitated state; *typhoid fever*, presenting a confusional state in which torpor is predominant; *salmonella* infections where, although seldom, stuporose states may be present.

Even in exanthemas, the younger the child the greater can be the psychotic reaction, especially in proportion to the gravity of the febrile state. This psychosymptomatology is not specific and can include both states of torpor and somnolence, and confusional delirium.

Particular mention must be made of disorders appertaining to post-vaccinal encephalitis, which appear 5-15 days after vaccination or revaccination and are characterized mostly by a state of torpor. Only in those cases where the symptomatology is that of grave haemorrhagic encephalitis, is a confusional state with delirium present; this may be accompanied by convulsions and by various pareses (somnolent-paretic syndrome).

Disorders of metabolism—Endocrine disorders—Auto-intoxications. The most common of these disorders are: diabetes, hypoglycaemia, porphyria, nutritional deficiencies, hypertoxic gastroenteritis, continual vomiting, anorexia nervosa, coeliac disease, uraemia, hyper- or hypo-thyrosis, hyper- or hypoparathyrosis, hyper- or hypoadrenalinaemia, hyper- or hypopituitarism, hyper- or hypogonadism, cardiopathies, nephropathies, hepatopathies (acute yellow atrophy of the liver, infective haepatitis), blood diseases (leukaemia, haemolytic syndromes, thalassaemia, haemorrhagic diathesis, hypochromic anaemia, polycythaemia).

In other pathological states, where the *hydroelectrolytic balance* is altered, psychological disorders might be present, characterized mostly by changes of consciousness, which give rise to various manifestations ranging from a shrinking of the field of consciousness with torpor, to symptoms of confusional sub-excitement. These forms may be observed in *acute hypertoxic enteritis, in periodical vomiting* and, in general, in all those pathological conditions which cause *acute disorder of the hydroelectrolytic balance.*

In some forms of *anorexia nervosa*, acute psychotic symptoms related to the general debility may sometimes be superimposed on the specific psychopathology. In metabolic diseases, and in particular in *diabetes*, acute psychotic symptoms can be observed, though rarely, which precede the onset of coma. These psychological disorders are represented by confusional delirium and psycho-motor agitation, followed by a progressive deterioration which rapidly develops into torpor and coma.

Conversely, hypoglycaemic conditions, whatever the cause, are characterized by the presence of neuro-vegetative symptoms, with anxiety and agitation of sudden onset, often ending in convulsions, with automatic activity, probably due to temporal lobe excitation.

In *true uraemia*, psychotic disorders may have the two fundamental characteristics of acute onset with a symptomatology of confusion and delirium, or of sub-acute onset, where the delirium and confusion is preceded by torpor, with grave dysphoric reactions and also pseudo-dissociation of thoughts.

In *haepatic disorders*, acute psychotic manifestations may be present, although rarely; these are preceded by a period of torpor or apathy, which is followed, sometimes rapidly, by reactions typified by cataleptic poses. Oneiric states with torpor and stupor, at times with psychomotor agitation and confusion, are present in chronic hepatic conditions; these are not always related to the general state, and often are not correlated with the specific liver disease.

In *porphyria*, side by side with the characteristic neurological symptoms and physical abdominal symptoms, acute psychotic episodes may arise, sometimes recurrent and characterized either by a picture of hallucinations and delirium with excitement, or by episodes of dysphoria with twilight.

In *congenital myxoedema*, within the basic psychological disorders (torpor, apathy, mental deficiency) acute confusional episodes may sometimes present.

Hetero-intoxications. The most common intoxications are due to: alcohol, barbiturates, lead, mercury, petroleum derivatives, bromides, carbon tetrachloride, carbon disulphide, carbon monoxide, atropine, ferrous salts, scopolamine, chloride, amphetamine, arsenic, opium and its derivatives, antibiotics, cortisone, ACTH, isoniazid, ergot, poisonous fungi, botulism, cocaine, morphia and heroin, hashish, LSD, hydantoinate, psycho-pharmacological drugs, salicylic acid and its derivatives, helminthiasis, anticryptogamics, camphor, antihistamine drugs, vermifuges, insect stings, poisonous snake bites.

Acute intoxication due to the intake of *alcohol* has fairly typical characteristics in the child, as the phase of inebriation and excitement is very brief, and passes almost at once into the phase of coma.

Barbiturate intoxication depends on the mode of intake and absorption of the substance. Psychotic symptomatology may start with a brief period of restlessness and anxiety, which is often followed by a progressively diminished alertness, culminating in coma.

Some subjects have an allergy to calomel; this condition is infrequently found nowadays, but when present it manifests acrodynia, anorexia and behaviour disorders with marked elements of general uneasiness, agitation and some confusion.

CO poisoning depends on the degree of gas saturation in the blood; from an initial phase characterized by general unwellness, frontal headache, nausea and torpor, it progresses to a graver phase where somnolence increases to the point of coma.

Lead poisoning, in the acute phase, causes an acute cerebromeningeal oedema (acute lead encephalopathy) and presents either simple torpor, or a confusional state, or psychosensory disorders associated to a state of irresistible somnolence.

Atropine poisoning is diagnosed from reddening and dryness of the mucous membranes, dilation of the pupils, from initial periods of excitement and uncoordinated movements, as if the patient were trying to grab an imaginary object; this period is soon followed by a state of drowsiness, sometimes accompanied by hallucinatory phenomena.

Intoxication by poisonous fungi generally begins with a state of excitement and hallucinations, followed by mental confusion culminating in torpor and coma.

Generally, drug poisoning is diagnosed by symptomatology of the exogenous reaction type. During therapy with *cortisone* or with *ACTH*, transitory mood changes are sometimes observed, both towards euphoria and towards depression with excitement.

Of the drugs, those of particular interest at the present time are hashish and *LSD*, because of the alarmingly widespread use they have among adolescents. The symptomatology of acute *hashish* intoxication is characterized by vivid perceptive distortions, by the production of vivid thoughts with an euphoric and self-appreciative content, and by changes in the perception of the rhythm of time. The symptomatology of acute *LSD* intoxication includes obvious changes in time and space conceptions, and abnormal behaviour typified by thought and affective disorders, sometimes accompanied by fearful anxiety and perceptual visual hallucinosis.

Hydantoinate, because of intolerance, may initially cause ataxia and diarrhoea, but seldom causes psychological changes. Prolonged treatment with it may produce spatio-temporal disorientation, which may reach the point of confusional state with hallucinations.

Camphor produces clouding of consciousness followed by convulsions in sensitive subjects.

Avitaminosis. In this group, the most common disorders causing psychological symptoms are pellagra, beriberi, scurvy and Hartnup disease. During *pellagra*, when the disease is in an advanced stage, acute confusional symptoms may be present. In *Hartnup disease*, in addition to nystagmus and cerebral ataxia, the initial period may present, during the cycles of re-exacerbation of symptoms, emotional instability and slight confusional states. However, in this disease, the psychological disorders are due more to the lack of nicotinic acid, which disturbs the tryptophan metabolism.

Physical Agents

These include heat stroke, exposure, electric trauma, radiation and burns.

The younger the child, the more sensitive he is to thermal factors—warmth and cold—because his thermo-regulating mechanisms are still imperfect.

Sun stroke and *heat stroke* present a psychosymptomatology dominated by disorders of the oneiric and delusional type, sometimes associated to phosphenes, to a general feeling of unwellness, vertigo and nausea.

In *exposure* (accidental hypothermia) the psychosymptomatology is usually distinguished at the onset by a phase of hyperexcitability followed by an oneiric-confusional phase, which tends to develop into coma.

In *electric trauma* the psychosymptomatology is dominated by disorders of the oneiric and delusional type, often accompanied or alternated with states of excitement with twitching of the muscles, myoclonia and convulsions.

In an acute *radiation* disease, psychological disorders are manifested by a confusional state, usually followed by coma.

3
Symptomatology

Symptomatological manifestations will be discussed in this section and consideration must be given to the symptomatological framework proposed by various authors; they are often not only based on a different terminology, but have also a different conceptual approach. This depends on:

(*i*) The difference in approach to the problem by paediatricians and by psychiatrists.

(*ii*) The difference in historical approach by the German, French and Anglo-Saxon schools, which, however, have given little consideration to the problem on the basis of the clinical material in childhood, but rather have applied to childhood the characteristics of acute organic psychoses in adults.

(*iii*) A different meaning, or extension of meaning, given to some terms (acute delirium, febrile delirium, amentia, confusional state, coma, etc.).

It would take too long to compare these meanings, their semantic justifications and their grouping by syndromes. In general, it can be said that many, especially in the paediatric field, consider two groups only: febrile delirium and coma, even if subsequently they divide the coma into a state of clouding, slight coma or stupor, and deep coma. Others add hallucinations, others talk of a state of hallucinosis or oneiric delusional state. Others still, especially psychiatrists, group together various forms under the term 'amential state' or 'confusional state', without, however, stressing the considerable differences which may exist between the adult and the child.

As it is necessary to go more deeply into this phenomenological analysis, a classification of disorders is proposed here, which could include all the multiform symptomatology of acute organic psychoses. As has already been said, experience shows that, in almost all cases, disorders of consciousness are particularly significant. The delusional element and psycho-sensory changes are always secondary, even if, in some cases, they may become uppermost.

In some forms (group V-VI) of the classification adopted here, acute psychosis presents a picture, which completely covers the slight state of disorientation, always present at the beginning of symptomatology. It must be also stressed again that in almost all cases it is only possible to diagnose a 'state' and not a 'syndrome', because of the difficulty to gather under single syndrome entities a symptomatology which often includes many elements (disorientation, delirium, agitation, etc.) with a different degree of importance from case to case, from day to day, or even from hour to hour.

At present, research does not allow us to show clinically specific syndromes of acute psychosis. Moreover, there is no direct correlation between the gravity of the basic disease, gravity of anatomic-pathologic lesion and psychopathological picture. With the exception of epilepsy and of some pictures of cerebral tumours, there is no significant correlation between the psychopathological picture and the eventual topographic localization of the anatomical lesion. Nor is there a single modality of clinical beginning in respect to the same pathological cause, so numerous are the variables concurring in the pathogenesis of the psychopathological picture (gravity of the cause, easy electrolytic disquilibrium, age, personality structure, anatomic-pathologic basis, onset, gravity, type, intensity of oedema, etc.).

Moreover, we must always remember that the younger the child, the less specific, but more violent is the psychotic reaction, and that, conversely, the nearest the patient is to adulthood, the more coloured is the psychotic disorder by his basic character traits.

The pathogenic mechanisms directly responsible for the psychopathology are cerebral oedema and intracellular electrolytic disquilibrium, or, in general, a cellular dismetabolism more or less acute, which in most cases causes, on the isto-pathological level, the picture of acute Nissl disease. Oedema and acute Nissl disease can be caused by (*a*) vascular changes (perivenus encephalitis, thrombophlebitis, haemorrhagic encephalitis, etc.) (*b*) inflammations, from intermediate toxic products of the metabolism directly related to the basic disorder.

In addition to the data specifically related to the basic organic aetiological disorder, the biochemistry almost always presents an hydric disquilibrium (rapid and alarming in early childhood) and an electrolytic disquilibrium especially for chlorine and potassium.

Leukocytosis is frequent, with relative lymphopenia; disorders of serum and cerebrospinal fluid with hyperazotemia are almost invariably present.

There are no specific laboratory investigations. Those undertaken are the same as those needed for the study of various cerebral and extracerebral causes. Here, therefore, are presented only those electroencephalographic pictures, which in some cases may be indicative of the gravity of the clinical case. It is impossible to talk of specific electroencephalographic pictures, but rather of pictures indicating an unspecific cerebral disorder. Thus are observed slowing of basal rhythms and changes of the blocking reaction. As for the slow waves, these may sometimes appear in a hypersynchronic form during hyperpnoea, sometimes in the posterior regions and coinciding with opening of the eyes. Sometimes the slow waves express themselves through a slow disrhythmia, which does not represent a true disorganization of the tracing as the alpha rhythm is not altogether suppressed. The various changes are in direct proportion to the presence of confusional disorders.

The symptomatology of acute organic psychoses will now be considered according to the classification in Table 1.

TABLE 1

Classification of acute organic psychoses

I	Disorders of consciousness	State of drowsiness Confusional state Oneiric state or oneirism Acute febrile delirium Stuporose state Comatose state or coma Twilight state
II	Disorders of ego awareness	Episodes of depersonalization
III	Psycho-sensory disorders	Illusions and hallucinations Hallucinosis state
IV	Thought disorders	Acute delusional syndrome
V	Affective disorders	Acute anxiety state Reactive depression Hypomania
VI	Psycho-motor disorders	Catalepsy
VII	Behaviour disorders	Aggressive outbursts of destructiveness Temporary perversion of instincts Perverse mood

Disorders of Consciousness

General. Consciousness is considered as a function controlling the spatio-temporal organization of life experience and therefore capable of transforming exterior reality into interior reality and capable of communicating it by meaningful signs and symbols (gestures, actions, words). This function is dependent on many variables, i.e. the threshold and frequency of external stimuli, the speed of transmission, etc. These variables are correlated with other variables of a physical and chemical nature. Consciousness is, therefore, a relay controller between the tactile and sensory stimuli system, and the perceptive and representational relating system, or between some perceptive sectors and some representational sectors.

As Lhermitte[8] suggested, the following can be considered schematically: a consciousness of the outside world, which changes in confusional states, from clouding of consciousness to coma; a body consciousness which changes when there is unawareness of physical illness, and an ego consciousness which changes in states of depersonalization and in temporary crises. However, in studying the structure of states of changed awareness of the environment, we must consider also the degree, the lucidity and the field of consciousness. There might be quantitative disorders and hence only a lowered or heightened threshold of consciousness, or qualitative disorders with a distorted understanding or distorted perception of stimuli, or a restriction of the field of operations which causes a poor 'reception' of exterior reality.

This phenomenological analysis can be useful in establishing a finer correlation between the clinical picture of psychopathology and the level and extent of organic change. We already know that, in general, the complex of those nervous structures responsible for a constant state of consciousness can be involved in lesions and functional disorders at three levels:

(a) in confusional states, usually at cortical level and in the Flechsig's oval bundle (Bini[1], Massenti[9]).

(b) at the level of the superior parts of the stem in the mid brain, and, in more serious cases, in the thalamus, when there is intermittent loss of consciousness without neuro-vegetative disorders, as there are in stuporose or sub-comatose states.

(c) at the level of the inferior part of the brain stem, in coma (with serious neuro-vegatative disorders). In both (b) and (c) there are serious functional disorders or lesions in the activating ascending reticular system.

Drowsiness or clouding of consciousness. This may be a moderate disorder of consciousness, or the premonitory sign of a confusional state, or of coma.

The patient is apathetic, inert, detached, or irritable and agitated; there is perseveration in his behaviour, aimless and continuous movement, and he appears rather indifferent, but not frightened. He cannot concentrate and relate facts; he answers only if pressed, giving contradictory answers, which may not show a true disorientation in time and space. However, the mode of contact with the environment, the erratic behaviour without aim and rather incoherent, the difficulty of concentration in intellectual work, the lack of appreciation of his condition and of his existential situation, show that there is a definite disorder of alertness.

Case History

Carla, T., female, 12 years old.

It seems that her psycho-motor development was slow. Enuresis up to 5 years. Usual childhood exanthemas. Was kept in the first grade for two years at school, and then completed the five elementary grades with great effort. First menstruation at 11 years 6 months. Excessive eater. Evident obesity (60 Kg) evenly distributed. Ten days ago she started a slimming treatment by drugs, the name of which she does not remember, but which she has taken in greater doses than prescribed. For the last seven days she has been listless, weak, drowsy, she sings monotonously, touches everything she sees but with no interest, does not speak, answers by monosyllables, cannot obey simple instructions, as if forgetting them immediately. Was hospitalized urgently by her family.

On examination she is uncooperative, moves continuously and is aimlessly busy. Is not very disorientated in space and time, but had difficulty in remembering being taken to hospital and what has happened, is not agitated, is unaware of being ill, beats rhythmically and monotonously her abdomen, cannot concentrate, talks to herself with short phrases, often incoherently.

All laboratory tests were negative, except the EEG and the sedimentation rate.

After six days the patient is lucid, orientated in time and space, answers to the point. Remembers with a certain vagueness the preceding days and can reconstruct only partially what has happened.

Confusional State. A confusional state can be primary or secondary: it is primary when it dominates the clinical picture and is not preceded by an obvious infectious and toxic cause, or by trauma. As such, it is very rare in childhood, indeed some authors exclude it completely in this age group, but it may be sometimes observed in the mentally retarded, in particular in pre-adolescents, but even in these cases an autotoxic aetiology cannot be excluded.

Almost invariably the confusional state is secondary, or at least symptomatic of an infectious and toxic state, or of other accountable causes, which have been discussed already, whether these directly cause brain lesions (encephalitis, meningo-encephalitis), or whether they act through other pathogenic mechanisms. The clinical picture is very much the same throughout childhood, even if in approaching puberty there is an increase of mixed forms with frequent psychosensory disorders of interpretation.

The main pathological elements in the clinical picture are changes in concentration, conceptual thought and orientation.

The patient's mind is clouded, he is semi-conscious, disinterested in his environment, almost always impatient, irritable and agitated. He goes from one thing to another, busies himself in an aimless fashion and tears up his sheets. He appears anxious, and at times terrified. In some cases agitation can be the dominating factor, aggravating the state of prostration and dehydration. Continuous 'boasting' may accompany it, but this is also incoherent, compulsive and related to odd recollections of the past (especially of school days), to oneiric elements, or to momentary auditive impressions connected by assonance or analogy. There is great difficulty in concentrating, which in older children makes even the smallest intellectual effort difficult; the patient, however, tries hard to overcome his confusion and to answer even simple questions, but his answers are slow, and often incoherent. He makes an obvious vain effort to get his perception right, but instead he becomes lost in details.

There are obvious disorders of fixative memory and clear disorientation in time and space. The patient does not know where he is and believes he is at school or at home; seeing the white-clad doctor he becomes uncertain and keeps looking about. Sometimes he knows that he is in hospital, but cannot remember the street or the town where he lives, nor how long he has been in hospital. He may not recognize his parents, his siblings or other members of the family. He is aware of his lack of comprehension, but it does not cause him anxiety, on the contrary, he tries to coordinate his few memories by chatting, or he rapidly changes the subject of the conversation.

This state may be accompanied by other groups of symptoms caused by disorders of perception (illusions, hallucinations), or disorders of interpretation (delusional thoughts, oneirism).

At times these symptoms dominate the clinical picture and for this reason each of them will be described by itself.

Oneiric Confusional State or Oneirism. Lafon[7] says 'Oneirism is to dreaming what mental confusion is to sleeping'.

On a foundation of confusional disorder of consciousness, described above, a delusional manifestation is frequently set up which is characterized by a succession of visual illusions and hallucinations, following each other without any order, or rapidly linked in scenes with different themes (school, play, siblings, etc.). The patient lives these scenes intensely, sometimes pleasurably, but almost always with anxiety, dread and fear. Imagination, illusion, hallucination and reality are not distinct, but mingle in surging and unconnected scenes which usually provoke in the child an incubus, a feeling of impending danger, which he cannot express, hence his anxious and frightened aspect.

In its most grave form this frequently happens in toxic states, while in less serious forms it is characteristic of the febrile bouts of childhood and is easily confused with a syndrome which most authors call 'infantile acute febrile delirium'. In these cases oneirism is prevalently nocturnal.

When these episodes of oneiric confusion are brief (from a few hours to one or two days), have a sudden onset and a sudden end, and are recurrent, the first consideration must be the possible presence of epilepsy.

Case History

Anthony, S., male, 12 years old.

Third child in family, normal delivery, normal psycho-physical development. When 5 and 6 years old was treated for 'lymphatism'. Frequent winter bronchitis up to 8-9 years. Very good at school, where he is in the first year of secondary education. Following mumps, his progress was fairly regular in the first few days. After a week the patient's temperature is almost normal, but he is very restless, anxious and complains continuously. In the following 24 hours the restlessness increases, he is confused and talks nonsense. His parents request hospitalization.

On admission the patient is confused, disorientated in time and space, does not recognize his parents; he complains continuously, wants to get up, tears up his shirt, cannot answer to the point and keeps repeating his name and surname.

He talks continuously and incoherently about school, without any logic. Has periods when he is absent, detached and lies with his eyes closed, murmuring stereotyped words and sentences.

In the evening, and even more so at night, he is very agitated, has visual and auditory hallucinations, and complains of frightening visions and dreams: he sees his teacher threatening him, hears strange voices, now sweet, now menacing; with broken words he manages to relate the theme of his visions—'school, car, bed, knife, innocent, kill, suffer', etc.

On the third day of admission the restlessness is greatly decreased, he starts to look less frightened, and ceases to complain of fearful dreams and hallucinations. Mental confusion still persists: it is impossible to get his attention or an adequate reply, except 'yes' and 'no' when invited to eat. After seven days he starts to recognize his parents and the place where he is; he eats fairly regularly. He still has a period of agitation towards the evening fearing nightmares, especially in the hypnogogic period; 'Because I cannot control my thought and have a succession of frightening visions'. 'Why frightening?' 'Frightening, frightening.' The contents of these visions cannot be discussed as he obstinately refuses to do it. This evening anxiety lasts for some months. Seen again after two months, he had complete amnesia of the period he was ill.

Acute and Febrile Delirium. In the adult, acute delirium is a very grave organic syndrome which even today shows a high mortality rate. The symptomatology is rather uniform: severe dehydration, toxic faces, dry and cracked lips, very furred blackish tongue, severe vascular fragility, fever progressing in bouts and resistent to the usual antipyretics, sitophobia, psycho-motor agitation, deep disorganization of consciousness.

In childhood, on the other hand, we talk of 'acute, but febrile delirium'. By this term we understand, more than a syndrome, a very frequent symptom, to which paediatricians attach little importance, a symptom which tends to recur in the same individual, usually up to the end of childhood, whenever his body temperature increases considerably. When the temperature is at its highest and during its fall, especially if there is a crisis, the child has an almost complete disorder of ideation; he says words without any connection or logical sense, or repeats again and again themes of his daily life seen in a distorted form; he is slightly restless, rocks his inert head on the pillow, looks at his parents absently, as if he did not know them. Or he has an anxious and frightened appearance, as if he saw something frightening.

It is better to describe febrile delirium together with the disorders of consciousness because, even if there is thought disorder more or less manifest according to age, a disorder of consciousness in a determining form is always present.

It is difficult to say whether there is just a clouding of consciousness, common in hyperthermia, or a narrowing of consciousness of a twilight type, or a fluctuation of consciousness of an oneiric type. Disorientation, therefore, is usually slight and after the episode there is a fragmentary recollection of what has happened. Delirium lasts minutes or several hours, then disappears when the temperature comes down, or a few hours after it. If the symptomatology is more marked, then we have the clinical picture which we have described as 'oneiric confusional state'.

The simple febrile delirium tends to recur whenever there is a high fever, has a good prognosis and usually disappears when the child is 10 or 11 years old. Its pathogenesis is perhaps associated with a particular individual sensitivity to the toxic picture of simple hyperthermia, but when febrile delirium continues after the fever has abated, or presents the same picture as the oneiric confusional state, then the prognosis is less favourable and the pathogenesis is similar to that of other confusional states.

However, almost invariably the two pictures are described by various authors under the common heading of 'febrile delirium'.*

The author thinks it is better to keep the two pictures separate and, even accepting the term 'acute febrile delirium', despite it being a picture quite different from the homonymous syndrome of adult psychiatry, he regards it as limited to those cases in which delirium is present in the febrile period only, tends to recur in each period of acute hyperthermia and has always a good prognosis. All cases presenting delirium lasting longer than the febrile period, with a more distinct change of consciousness and signs of oneirism, must be considered separately, as they need a different treatment and may have a less favourable prognosis.

Stuporose State. Here the disorganization of consciousness is graver. The contact with the outside world is greatly altered, even if it presents in flashes. The patient is drowsy and does not answer unless strongly stimulated. He does not eat, and often refuses food and drink. There is loss of sphincter control, and diminished tendon and corneal reflexes, but there are no cardio-respiratory disorders, nor difficulty in deglutation. The stuporose state is more frequently found in grave encephalitis, especially if convulsions are also present. In some subjects with an hereditary predisposition to endogenous psychoses, this state may present even when the causal factor is not very grave clinically.

Case History

Mario, T., male, 5 years old.

Second child in family. Nothing notable in his pathological anamnesis except recurring tonsilitis in winter. When 4 years old, catarrhal otitis in right ear. Five days ago hit the left side of his forehead against the washbasin. After 24 hours a headache developed, which increased in the following days. After 48 hours, there was fever (37·5-39°C); the tonsils were very inflamed (positive swab for streptococcus viridans); vomiting.

The patient scratches his nose rhythmically, rocks his head to one side, recognizes his parents with difficulty and more by their voices than by sight, is restless and anxious.

After four days he has a cluster of left tonic-clonic convulsions with loss of consciousness lasting for one hour. He partially regains consciousness after some hours. Since then patient is occasionally enuretic for eight days.

At times he answers, but only after persistent urging and then incoherently. He has long periods when he is completely lost; turns his eyes aimlessly; his aspect is not anxious, on the contrary he does not even ask for food, as if lost. Then he gradually passes to a state of great psychomotor agitation; tears up the sheets and gets out of bed.

* In some textbooks, all forms of acute organic psychosis are grouped under the term 'delirium' (Kanner[5]) which has replaced the ancient Hippocratic term 'phrenitis', by which for centuries were described all psychic disorders, symptomatic of acute organic central affections. Here the term 'delirium' is used only in its phenomenologic meaning of fairly grave disorder of the rational schemata; the ego is no longer able to compare one scheme to another and therefore cannot correct them.

Laboratory tests and blood chemistry, normal; EEG, frequency potential theta—delta waves 2-4 c.s. Acute diffuse pain. After eight days the pain, always rather intense, became localized to the right hemisphere, especially in the middle-posterior-central position.

After six days the stuporose state starts to regress. There are no more convulsions. Sphincter control returns; for some days he is confused with clear disorientation, especially in time. On the fifteenth day, everything is back to normal. The patient has no recollection at all of the whole period of his illness. The EEG is back to normal at the end of the third month.

Coma. Here the disintegration of consciousness is complete. There is total suppression of cerebral functions. Coma can vary in depth, can have a sudden onset or be the last stage of a worsening psychic disorder which in a few hours or in a few days will bring the patient from simple drowsiness to an almost complete loss of relational life, that is to say to coma. (In many textbooks of paediatrics, three stages of coma are considered: (*i*) clouding and drowsiness stage; (*ii*) slight coma stage; (*iii*) deep coma stage.) The patient is no longer in touch with his environment and perception is lost. A very painful stimulation is needed to obtain a reaction (a muscular reaction, a fleeting mydriasis, a change of expression, etc.). The child lies still with a vacant look, his eyes half closed; the corneal reflex is very weak or absent.

Characteristic of coma is the presence, in addition to the grave disorder of consciousness, of rather serious neuro-vegetative disorders, which always worsen the prognosis. Neurological disorders are neither constant nor specific and consist almost invariably of diffuse hypotonia, decrease or loss of tendon reflexes with possible bilateral Babinski's reflex. Of course, here are excluded those cases where neurological examination points instead to a particular cerebral lesion (cranial trauma, circulation disorders, certain post-vaccination, or post-exanthematic encephalites, etc.).

Neuro-vegetative disorders consist essentially of:

(*i*) Changes in the respiratory rhythm: shallow, rapid, inefficient respiration, or Kussmaul's breathing, or Cheyne-Stokes respiration; this disorder produces anoxia which in turn aggravates the comatose state.

(*ii*) An increase of perspiration aggravating the hydric disquilibrium which is almost invariably present.

In addition there is hyperthermia, tachycardia, arterial hypotension, difficulty in, or loss of deglutation. The general aspect is typical to the dehydrated child: dry tongue, deep-set eyes with dark lines, sharpened features, flabby skin, a lost and anguished aspect.

Twilight State (or state of narrowing of consciousness).* This is a shrinking of the field of action of consciousness. The psychic world of the child is suddenly restricted to one sector of thinking and feeling. It is a

---

* The sub-title 'narrowing of consciousness', has been added because many authors by 'twilight state' mean the 'Dammerige Bewusstsein' of Jaspers[4], which is a form of destructuration of consciousness, of change of consciousness, more than narrowing of it, as is meant here.

closed circle within which his psychic activity is like normal, even if there is a degree of clouding of consciousness. The child acts and moves like an automaton (somnambulism), he can carry out apparently coordinate actions, but has poor perception of external stimuli, he cannot fix them, and hence will have total or partial amnesia of them. Echolalia and echopraxia can be observed.

In childhood this state is usually associated with epilepsy both as a psychic disorder during a crisis and as a post-crisis situation. Many epileptic fugues happen during the twilight stage; the child acts coherently as if in a state of second consciousness: he might go to the home of relations, or to the station and catch a train. Then suddenly after hours or days, he realizes that he is in a different place.

Antisocial behaviour may also take place (stealing, arson, etc.) which, however, before pre-puberty is never as violent as in the adult. This is an experience of total depersonalization; the patient lives a complete doubling of his person with an actor ego and a spectator ego.

This twilight state, however, can also be present in acute toxic states and during convalescence of other acute organic psychoses. Even in the latter case it can last several days, causing great concern to the parents because of the strange and perplexing temperament assumed by the patient, who is enclosed in his own small world; his replies are unsure, incoherent and given with great detachment.

Disorders of Ego Awareness

Depersonalization. This phenomenon is much more common in childhood than it is generally admitted. Cases of depersonalization in 5-year-old children have been reported.

To avoid the innumerable discussions about its definition, depersonalization is here regarded as a non-specific symptom which may present in many psychiatric syndromes. On the phenomenological level, following Wernicke's classification, three forms of depersonalization can be considered: (*i*) Auto-psychic, with a feeling of strangeness about the true ego. (*ii*) Somato-psychic, with disorders of corporal awareness, which may reach the point where the body scheme is changed. (*iii*) Allopsychic, with a feeling of strangeness of the perceptive world (derealization).

Before the age of 10, the somato-psychic form is the most common. The child feels his body changed, separated from himself, from his ego, or realizes a body deformed as whole, which he compares with his past body; this causes fearful anguish because he feels that the situation cannot be changed.

During puberty the auto-psychic form is prevalent instead. The youth has the sensation, almost painful, of losing his personality, he no longer has a feeling of ego unity, he feels strange to himself, a spectator of his ego, which he no longer can control: 'What is happening to my person?'

The allopsychic form is never found in toxic-infectious or post-traumatic forms, but it is relatively more frequent in temporal epilepsy.

Depersonalization is common in psychic disorders caused by physical agents, where it can often present as autoscopy.

Case History

Eris, D., male, 8 years 8 months old.

Born by normal delivery. Normal physical development. Psycho-motor development normal. Early sphincters control: at 12 months, following rigid training by mother. Frequent tonsillitis up to 8 years, when he underwent tonsillectomy. Between age 5 and 8: measles, pertussis and paradenolymphytis. Mother very demanding in the educational field. Very good school progress, but from the beginning of school attendance has shown various tics. At 8 years 6 months, an episode of electric shock; loss of consciousness for a few seconds, he fell and lost faeces. Since then, once or twice a day he has sudden periods of anxiety and is in a daze for some hours. During these periods he is in a true state of depersonalization: he feels that he is no longer himself and that his arms and legs are enormous; he sees himself enormous and deformed. Other times he has the sensation of not existing and feels 'changed inside' and people too 'are no longer the same'.

EEG, dysrhythmia, with alpha well represented among potentials of inferior frequency: the voltage is low. With hyperpnoea synchronization slow and diffuse (3 c/s).

This symptomatology disappears after eight days. After three years the patient reports no disorders and the EEG too is perfectly normal.

Psychosensory Disorders

Illusions and Hallucinations. These are very common in acute organic psychoses, although never as an isolated picture, but always accompanied by a clouding of consciousness or a confusional state. These are mainly present in febrile delirium and in oneiric confusional state (already described). Any object in the room may cause an illusion; the stains on the wall become phantoms; the movement of a curtain, that of an intruder; the table is the teacher's desk, etc.

Hallucinations, mostly visual, are simple and very distinct: animals, lights, mountain scenes, devils, cars, or sounds and voices of school mates and of teachers. Often, in younger children, we can perceive the presence and type of hallucinations from their behaviour: they cover their ears, speak to the wall, make defensive movements, stare fixedly at a point in the room, etc.

Often the hallucinations persist even when the confusional state has improved and, in febrile delirium, after the temperature has returned to normal. In these cases, they present during the state of drowsiness, almost as a hypnogogic hallucination. Only occasionally, they are frightening, but usually they cause anxiety because of the recollection of certain happenings of daily life which they provoke. It is the picture of oneiric confusional state, already described.

Hallucinosis. The state of hallucinosis differs from the confusional state and from delirium with hallucinations, because with it there is no disorder of consciousness. Orientation is good and the sensorium clear, and hallucinations are almost always auditory. It is very rare in childhood, usually never present during the acute stage, but rather during the convalescence of infectious diseases, especially toxic. It is found more commonly in patients of low intellect. It is very difficult to find clinical evidence of it. The patient is anxious, fearful, has a neurotic and hypochondriacal symptomatology; it is difficult to relate this picture, understandable in a convalescent, to a psycho-sensory disorder which is not spontaneously reported by the patient, especially if he is of low intellect.

During the convalescence of every debilitating acute toxic-infectious disease we must be alert to the possible presence of psychosensory disorders. These, even if not always true to type, as in states of hallucinosis, are certainly much more frequent than we are led to believe by the literature on the subject.

The typical alcoholic hallucinosis of adults has no corresponding disorder in childhood, whilst cases have been described of hallucinosis in atropine intoxication and during convalescence of cerebral rheumatism which had been treated with large doses of salycilates.

Thought Disorders

Acute Delirium Syndrome. This is the most puzzling of the symptomatic psychoses. It is distinguished both from the acute febrile delirium, because in this we have a disorganization of thought of short duration on a background of changed consciousness, and from the confusional state, because there is no disorder of consciousness. The patient is lucid and orientated in time and space. In addition to experiencing delirium, the child must have reached a certain psychic maturity, hence this syndrome is very rare before the age of 6 or 7 years, and rare before 11 years. Prepuberty is the most favourable age of presentation. It is more frequent in those of poor intelligence, with poor cultural heritage and poor critical faculties. The author has observed it after acute articular rheumatism, after grave choreas and after isolations. It appears at the end of the illness and during the first few days of convalescence in an acute or sub-acute form and can last for a few weeks or many months. Usually it disappears when the child's school and social life returns to normal.

The deliriums are many, absurd and at times fantastic: of being poisoned, of grandeur, religious and often hypochondriac. There is fear that food is drugged or poisoned; one patient will become a great hairdresser, the greatest; the little shepherd will be the new Jesus, who will convert the world; another, 10 years old, alleges that unknown to all, he is married with four children to keep. Psychosensory disorders are frequent; unknown voices issuing orders, or fearful visions (e.g. ghosts coming out of the wardrobe), or erotic visions, or visions of wicked gypsies, or of

Christ pointing the way to be followed. It is impossible to challenge the delirium: the child, unlike the adult, does not attempt to prove their reality, but folds up within himself, shrugs his shoulders or gets angry.

In childhood the pathogenesis of this form is difficult to solve, as we do not have the help of the pre-morbid personality. Many assert that the physical illness unleashes an endogenous illness, hence we are not dealing with an organic psychosis; others, conversely, basing their assumption on the absence of an obvious pre-morbid personality and on the fact that the syndrome often presents in encephalopathics of low intellect, tend to maintain that there is a causal relation with the organic illness. Laboratory tests are either silent or of no significance. Even the EEG can be perfectly normal, or of a non-developing type, or may present slow rhythms, which are common in all acute organic psychoses and during their convalescence.

In some cases the course is significant; the syndrome progresses in waves, and the psychotic understructure of the personality slowly emerges. In others, instead, the delirium syndrome, after some weeks or months, becomes less pronounced and then disappears; the home, school and social behaviour becomes adequate, the child has little recollection of the thought disorder and is left only with a feeling of tiredness, boredom and irritation. Unfortunately there are no catamnestic studies of these syndromes, whilst in adult psychiatry Kraepelin[6] asserted that 3 per cent of his cases of schizophrenia had undergone a bout of delirium in childhood; he does not specify whether they happened after an infectious disease or for other causes. The problem, thus, is left open, but it seems important to bring it anew to the attention of the clinical psychiatrist.

Affective Disorders

These forms of acute anxiety, depression and hypomania must not be confused with feelings of anxiety, of general unwellness, of anguish, of true sadness, of instability, of motor restlessness, which very often precede an infective or febrile disease. These phenomena are perhaps due to disorders of coenaesthesia very common in children. Here, instead, by affective disorders it is meant a pathological state of the affect rather long lasting, for days or for weeks, which presents immediately after the climax of the organic or cerebral affection, or at the beginning of convalescence. They are often observed in cerebral traumata, in auto-toxic forms and after chorea. Sometimes the depressive form is very long lasting with an atypical neurotic and hypochondriac picture which compels a differential diagnosis from a schizophrenia beginning.

The chronological link with the organic or central disease is clear, even if it is not always easy to explain the pathogenic link, as, after all, is true for other disorders already reviewed here. Many authors maintain that the premorbid personality is of great importance and that the disease is only a further expression of it. Even if, in some cases, this hypothesis is accepted, it would be wrong to generalize. Moreover, as a rule, the cerebral lesion is the direct cause of the psychic picture. Some forms of anxiety, or better, of anxious confusion, are reminiscent of the 'sham rage', which is experimentally provoked in animals by stimulation of the thalamus, and the euphoric, hypomanic state is very reminiscent of the organic frontal syndrome.

Psycho-motor Disorders

Catalepsy. This psychopathological reaction is seldom observed and then only in pre-puberty; it is relatively more frequent in those with a degree of mental retardation. On a background of confusional state, there is psycho-motor arrest with hypertonia, or a plastic muscular resistance. Often there is only an obvious initial motor difficulty; every movement must be passively started, then the patient can continue doing it, even if with difficulty and slowly. This form is always accompanied by a fairly organized delirium syndrome, which usually becomes more obvious when the cataleptic symptom starts to disappear. Initially, there is difficulty in differential diagnosis with acute schizophrenic syndrome, but the diagnosis is made clear by the anamnesis, which usually reveals an acute aetiology and a normal pre-morbid personality, and by the course of the disease which usually concludes with rapid and permanent recovery.

Case History

Ugo, T., *male, 12 years old.*

Third and last child in the family. Mother died when the boy was 5. He lives on a mountain farm in great isolation. Father is a farm worker. Father says that because he was 'not very intelligent' he has not been sent to school regularly. He was listless, closed within himself, nature loving, wandering alone in the woods and on the mountain. Since his brothers left for boarding school, he has had few occasions to speak to other people. Since the age of 9, he has been assistant shepherd and has been tending a herd of 30 sheep.

After a sunstroke with headache, vomit, restlessness and fever, he was brought to the town. His temperature reached 38°C and he was confused, restless and deliriant. After two days the fever abated, but the psychosymptomatology became worse, hence his hospitalization was requested. The boy appears disorientated in time and space, he believes himself in his mountain hut, talks very little and only after stimulation: 'Jesus, the people must be saved'. He looks dumbfounded; motor initiative is blocked, he tends to remain in an assumed position, although there is a certain purposefulness in his actions, which are always undertaken slowly and with great effort, after much verbal prompting and initial help in the movement. *Flexibilitas cerea* of the upper limbs, very variable in the same day.

After a few days the picture changes. Catalepsy decreases, the patient talks more and some hints of delirium of a religious theme are clear—he must save the soul; Jesus was a shepherd like himself; he will become the new Jesus; everybody must be good, nobody must hurt the sheep; we must pray; the sun is God; the sun is the master of mankind.

Initially the neurological examination is negative, except for the changes in muscular tone already described. For ten days there is slight hyperazotemia and slight leukocytosis with lymphopenia. All other analyses of blood, urine and cerebrospinal fluid were normal. EEG showed a clear and diffuse prevalence of slow alpha rhythm with a considerable disorganization of outline. During the fourth week of the illness, the outline became normal.

The patient is orientated, he now answers to the point with a language indicative of his initial mental debility. The WISC indicates an IQ of 65, but with better results in the performance test (75) than in the verbal tests. He remembers hardly anything of the whole period of the illness. His recollections stop at the moment when he was taken from his hut to the town.

Behaviour Disorders

Aggressive Outbursts of Destructiveness. The state of hyperkinesis, of overactivity and motor agitation often observed in confusional states, and which can be interpreted as a liberation of archaic psychomotor automatisms, can change during, or soon after convalescence to a state of aggressive destructiveness: the child's nature changes completely, he is aggressive, throws all kinds of things (plates, knives, stools) at members of his family and other people, he kicks, spits, throws about chairs and stools, breaks things, climbs up the windows, throws heavy objects on to the street. This is not a continuous state, but happens in outbursts. His behaviour appears normal, only a bit dysphoric, asthenic and bored—understandable symptomatology in convalescence; then suddenly, often for a slight reproach or a little denial, the outburst is unleashed and lasts for a few minutes or for some hours. The child does not respond to reasoning or to punishment, and afterwards has a confused recollection of the episode.

These destructive episodes are classic in epileptic twilight states, but the author has often seen them in traumata of the brain stem, especially under the age of 6-7 years, when they may last for several months. In addition to this specific traumatic aetiology, it appears that these episodes are more frequent when the disorder of consciousness has been severe, that is to say, after stuporose states and comas.

Case History

Fabio, A., male, 4 years 10 months old.

No pathology in the anamnesis up to the age of 4. At 4, he was knocked down by a car, resulting in a fracture at the base of the skull with otorrhagia, tetraplegia and coma. After 12 hours, general convulsion, repeated after seven days. Remained in coma for 35 days.

At about the 10th-15th day, the tetraplegia regressed, but he recommenced to walk and talk only at the end of the second month. At the same time post-traumatic diabetes insipidus appeared.

At the end of the third month, motility, speech and state of consciousness had returned to normal. Testing shows a normal intelligence. Continuous and violent aggression against people and things became manifest. The child would break everything and would throw down without reason anything he could lay his hands on. He would throw plates and knives at his nanny, his parents or his siblings.

Nothing could stop him, neither gentleness nor punishment. He moved continuously, running about, shouting and changing toys all the time. Often enuretic and encopretic. Sometimes he would play with his own faeces. Only towards evening he would calm down and his night sleep was normal. During this state, the EEG showed a left occipital focus.

After two months the picture was considerably changed and the aggressive destructive state changed to outbursts of aggressive destruction, which became increasingly infrequent and ceased almost completely after about a year.

4
Conclusion

For the sake of completion only, I will conclude with a few remarks on treatment.

First of all therapy must be specific to the causal agent or disease, when these are known. Moreover, symptomatic treatment is necessary, which must tend to re-establish the humoral equilibrium, almost always changed in these subjects: the electrolytic equilibrium must be re-established as soon as possible and, at the same time inflammation, oedema, toxicity and avitaminosis must be counteracted with cortisone derivatives, liver extracts, hypertonic glucose solutions, etc. Particular attention must be paid to conditions involving the cardiac circulation with special caution because of the neurotropic effects of some analeptic and some stimulant drugs commonly in use (coramine, cardiazol, etc.).

It must always be remembered that at times the state of agitation may induce secondary disorders of metabolism (hyperazotemia, hyperglycemia, etc.) which in turn may aggravate the toxic psychotic state. In those cases where excitement is a predominant factor, it is useful to sedate the patient using psychopharmacological drugs, such as promazine, butobarbitone, etc. In cases of very severe agitation electro-shock therapy may be useful.

Lastly, it must not be forgotten the importance of environmental stimuli in conditioning and giving negative stimulation in these psychopathological states. It is however, necessary that the patient should be kept in a calm and serene environment, sufficiently ventilated and at a constant temperature. The patient's possible self-destructive impulses must not be neglected, hence during recovery he must be under constant visual observation.

REFERENCES

1. BINI, L. and BAZZI, T., 1959. *Trattato di Psichiatria*. Milano, F. Vallardi.
2. BLEULER, E., 1955. *Lehrbuch der Psychiatrie*. IX Ed. Berlin, Springer Verlag.
3. BONHOEFFER, K., 1930. Ueber die neurologischen und psychischen Folgerscheinungen der Schwefel Kohlenstoff Vergiftung.
4. JASPER, K., 1959. *Allgemeine Psychopatologie*. Berlin, Springer Verlag.
5. KANNER, L., 1935. *Child Psychiatry*. Oxford, Blackwell Scientific Publications.
6. KRAEPELIN, E., 1919. *Allgemeine Psychopatologie*. Berlin, Springer Verlag.

7. LAFON R., 1963. *Vocabulaire de Psychopédagogie et de Psychiatrie de l'Enfant.* Paris, P.U.F.
8. LHERMITTE, J., 1963. In Lafon, R. *Vocabulaire de Psychopédagogie et de Psychiatrie de l'Enfant.* Paris, P.U.F.
9. MASSENTI, C., 1946. Studio istopatologico dell'ipotalamo nelle psicosi di tipo reazione esogeno. *Riv. Sperim. di Freniatria,* 72.

XXVI

THE CHILD AT SCHOOL

John C. Glidewell
Ph.D.

*Professor of Educational Psychology,
The University of Chicago, Chicago, Illinois, U.S.A.*

The child at school grows and develops in a well-defined social system in the classroom. Finding or being assigned a position in the social structure of the classroom is associated with the process of learning the alternate modes of behaviour available and the consequences of adopting each mode —a process of socialization. Socialization at school produces some stress for all children; it produces behaviour problems in a few children; it occasions psychiatric illness in still fewer children.

The findings from empirical research continue to clarify the nature of the socialization process at school, the manifestations of distress at school, the antecedents of the appearance of behaviour problems at school, and the processes and effects of preventive and therapeutic mental health programmes for school children. The following sections contain an attempt to summarize the relevant data and to review the more recent research activities. Given the conditions of international information dispersion and the preoccupations of the reviewer, almost all of the information comes from work in the United States, England, and Germany. Corrections and extensions of scope are anticipated with enthusiasm.

1
The Psycho-social Context of Life at School

The Development of Classroom Social Structure

Reliable data from many sources have shown the speed with which the social structure of a classroom develops. Within a few weeks—perhaps within a few hours—of the first meeting of an elementary school classroom, the individuals in it had found, or were allocated, a readily observable position along at least three dimensions of social structure: interpersonal attraction, perceived competence, and social power. The rapid development of such differentiated positions has been noted by such trained observers as Moreno[96] in 1934, Bonney[14] in 1942; and Lippitt and Gold in 1959[82]. It has been perceived by teachers as shown by such work as that of Laughlin[76] in 1954, Bower[16] and Boyd[18] in 1960. It has been perceived by the children themselves, as indicated by sociometric and near-sociometric studies by a large number of investigators such as Moreno[96] in 1934; Jennings[66] in 1937; Bonney in 1942[14] and 1943[15]; Force[40] in 1954; Lippitt and Gold[82] in 1959.

Research along the same lines gives a clear picture of a quite stable social structure in elementary school classrooms in a wide variety of social and economic settings. The stability extends over a school year, from one year to the next, and over several school years. As early as 1926, Beth Wellman[143] observed the constancy of playmates and workmates over a period of five months. Later Moreno[96] in 1934; Jennings[66] in 1937; Newstetter[98] in 1938; Criswell[29] in 1939; and Hunt and Solomon[64] in 1942 found a persistence of social structure over several weeks or several years. Bonney's correlational studies in 1942 and 1943 showed that positions in the classroom social structure at the beginning of the year were positively correlated with those at the end of the year and those of the subsequent year (the coefficients ranged from 0·68 to 0·94). Lippitt and Gold[82] examined stability over one year separately for interpersonal attraction, perceived competence, and social power. The findings indicated an average correlation between positions at the beginning and the end of the year at about 0·70 for social power and about 0·80 for both attraction and competence. Such correlations have been found in many studies over a number of years in many different social settings in the United States. They have indicated a core of stable social structure in the typical classroom in that culture. The stability should not be interpreted as rigidity. Based upon the data cited, on the dimension of interpersonal attraction, one could predict that the pupils of a classroom would remain in the same one-tenth of their class from one year to the next and be correct about one time out of two.

In summary it is clear that the social structure of an elementary school classroom develops quickly—within a few weeks at most—and remains relatively stable throughout the school year.

The Components of Social Structure in the Classroom

The components of the classroom social system are mutually attracted pairs and sub-groups, plus a few continuing isolates, as demonstrated by Moreno[96] in 1934; Jennings[66] in 1937; Criswell[29] in 1939; and Bonney[15] in 1943. The stable sub-groups tend to be composed of children—usually of the same social class and sex—who have similar values and personality traits, who are often in contact with one another, and who are in close proximity in the classroom and in the neighbourhood as shown by Seagoe[116] in 1933; Kuhlen and Lee[74] in 1943; and Austin and Thompson[4] in 1948, as well as Moreno, Jennings and Bonney. A centralized hierarchy, as distinguished from a diffuse structure, seems to provide greater stability, to produce more accurate self-perception of status, but it provides a less emotionally supportive 'social climate' as shown by the work of Schmuck[113] in 1962 and 1963[114].

In general, most children hold an accurate perception of the classroom social structure and their own position in it. Potashin[102] demonstrated this awareness in an economically privileged community; Goslin[50] obtained similar findings in a middle-class community: Lippitt[83] and his associates produced similar data in studying delinquent boys.

Dimensions of Social Structure in the Classroom

Three dimensions of social structure have emerged from the researches of the last 30 years: interpersonal attraction, perceived competence, and social power. Interpersonal attraction is the most widely studied. In the most simple form it means that each child is more attracted to some of his classmates than others and that some children are more widely liked than are other children. Perceived competence represents the views of the children about the competence of their peers at the tasks required at school. Perceived competence is task-specific, it differs from the classroom to the playground. Nonetheless it tends to be generalized by children. Some children are seen as *generally* more competent than others. Social power is the ability to influence other children—the ability of a child to get others to do what he wants them to do. Although the three dimensions are conceptually distinct dimensions of social structure, they are empirically related. Attraction and power appear to be the most closely related in elementary school classrooms (r about 0·60); attraction and competence, next most closely related (r about 0·40) and power and competence, least (r about 0·30). (See the review by Glidewell[43].) An important implication of these empirical relationships is that elementary school children are more influenced in their behaviour by the peers they like than they are influenced by peers they perceive to be competent.

Teacher Power and Its Use

A large number of investigations have indicated systematic effects of the degree of dispersion and the manner of employment of the social power and emotional acceptance of the teacher. Intervention of any sort at any point in the system has been demonstrated to produce effects in all the related parts and, sometimes, throughout the classroom social system. The manner of intervention of a teacher into the affairs of any individual pupil influences not only the response of the individual pupil, but also (*a*) the behaviour of many watching pupils, (*b*) the perception by the peer group of the fairness of the teacher, and (c) the perception by the peer group of the target pupil's power and competence—in sum, the whole social organization and work pattern of the classroom. The dynamics of these teacher-classroom relationships were particularly well analysed and demonstrated in the work of Thelen[134-35] in the late 1940s and early 1950s, of Flanders[39] in 1951 and subsequently, of Rehage[104] in 1951, of Levitt[78] in 1955, of Leeds[77] in 1956, of Perkins[101] in 1957, of Birth and Prillwitz[11] in 1959, Tausch[130-33] in 1958, 1960, and 1962, of Gnagey[48] in 1960, of Kounin, Gump, and Ryan[73] in 1961, and Minuchin[94] in 1964.

Of particular significance are two recent studies. Bronfenbrenner[21] and his colleagues in 1965 found that a child's report of his teacher's behaviour toward him showed a closer relationship to his own value reports than did his report of his parents' behaviour. Schmuck and Van Egmond[115] in 1965 also found that parental attitudes toward school and achievement were less important in affecting academic work than the child's relationship with his teacher. Both studies were conducted in the classroom. Had they been conducted at home, the findings may have been different, but both studies, independently, have shown the salience of the teacher in the classroom social system.

The particular effects of the teacher's dispersion of his power and emotional acceptance have included: (*i*) increased pupil-to-pupil interaction, (*ii*) reduced interpersonal conflicts and anxieties, (*iii*) increased mutual esteem and self-esteem, (*iv*) wider dispersion and flexibility of peer power, (*v*) greater tolerance for divergent opinions in the initial phases of problem-solving, (*vi*) greater convergence of opinion in the later phases of problem-solving, (*vii*) increased self-initiated work, and (*viii*) increased independence of opinion. Such dispersion alone has not, however, produced any regular improvement in academic achievement.

Stress at School

Schooling is a socialization process. With all its variations from culture to culture, socialization is a conformity-inducing process. Schooling is a special socialization process and it induces special sorts of conformity. It demands that a child adapt himself readily to many new situations and apply himself to the mastery of new skills with great regularity and intensity. The classroom social system demands, also, that he approach other children positively and respond to them in accord with their expectations. Depending upon the temperament of the child, schooling produces more or less conflict between the urges of the child and demands of the teacher and the peer group. Even the most temperamentally well-suited child, however, experiences some conflict between the urges he feels and the psycho-social demands he perceives, and, accordingly, he experiences some 'stress'.

Isolation in the classroom has been a matter of considerable interest and a subject of considerable research. The findings have been consistent: isolation is associated with intra-personal stress, anxiety, low self-esteem, poor interpersonal skills, and psychiatric illness. The findings have been consistent in such studies as those of Gronlund[53] in 1959, Mensh and Glidewell[90] in 1958, Smith[121] in 1958, Bower[16] in 1960, and Horowitz[62] in 1962. Of less interest has been the 'invisible child'. Painter[100] has reported that, in the practice of child psychiatry, some quite healthy children have been referred to him as emotionally ill. Their only symptom was that they seemed to be unaware of the social expectations of their peers. Unlike the isolates, who are usually painfully aware of the rejection of their peers, these 'invisible' children were simply unconcerned about the social pressures from their peers or unaware of them. Hudgins and Loftis[63] in 1966 have commented upon the 'invisible child' who was not rejected by other children and was not an isolate in the usual sense. He simply was not noticed by other children or by adults. Further, he did not seem to need to be noticed. Stringer and Glidewell[127] in 1966 have made similar comments. Trained observers in the classroom had great difficulty because a few children simply went unnoticed during the observation period. Gronlund[53] in 1959 and Northway[99] in 1944 observed that there were some healthy, self-sufficient or socially uninterested children who seemed to be unaware of the classroom social structure or their position in it. The nature of the personality and social adaptation of such 'invisible children' is not clear from the data, but it is clear that they cannot be categorized as isolates and they cannot be assumed to be psychiatrically ill.

Still less interest has been shown in the development of small 'contra-cultures' of pairs and sub-groups in the classroom. Such contra-cultures set values upon, approve of, and award status for behaviour which have characteristics opposite from those approved by most pupils and the teacher. The experiment of Kerstetter and Sargent[70] in 1940, the work of Kerr[69] in 1945 and of Shoobs[120] in 1947 have shown the nature of such contra-cultures in the classroom and their resistance to change. Again, such contra-cultures must be distinguished from children who are isolates, because the anti-social nature of their behaviour does not necessarily indicate psychiatric illness, as aggravating to teachers and parents as it may be.

Stringer[125-26] has produced data indicating that elementary school children do not show a steady rate of achievement year by year. By far the largest proportion of children show a cyclical trend in achievement rates, usually annual in frequency of the cycle. If a child shows a rapid rate of achievement one year, he is likely to show a slow rate of achievement the next. In schools in which pupils are subjected to considerable pressure for achievement, the rapid rate may continue for two years before the cycle reverses and a slow rate appears. Accordingly, in studying the relationships between achievement and behaviour problems, a pupil's rate of achievement must be judged in the context of his usual cyclical pattern. Stringer has identified some deviant low patterns of achievement, which become remarkably stable during the first few years of school and remain relatively fixed for the next six or eight years. Groups of pupils showing such deviant low patterns (cycles) tend to have a high proportion of disturbed children. Knowledge of such patterns can be used to some advantage for screening for behaviour problems, but such screening still produces a considerable rate of missed cases and false positives.

The data available are not yet specific enough, but there are some clear inferences that life at school is particularly stressful to a child who, by temperament, is bright enough, but is slow to approach new situations or withdraws from them, is irregular in his work habits, is slow in adapting to changes in his environment, has a low frustration tolerance, is frequently negative in his mood. Such children seem to be very similar to those designated by Birch, Thomas, and Chess[10, 26, 137] as the 'difficult' children, who have shown such temperament since the first few months after birth. Such children very frequently develop behaviour problems at school, but, given the consistency of school demands and some tolerance for and support during the delay in adapting to change, such children do adapt to school, even with zest and enthusiasm. In a few cases, damage to the central nervous system or some physical defect has been involved, but generally the behaviour problem arises out of an interaction between the temperament of the child and the socialization demands of the school. Fortunately, most children show regular, positive approaches to school and adapt readily to the socialization demands. The exact prevalence of the problems has not been the subject of very careful study, and the data are unsatisfactory, but in the United States (and on the Isle of Wight) something like six to ten per cent of children in school manifest such behaviour problems to the point of needing professional assistance; perhaps two per cent require intensive clinical treatment.

Summary

Within a few weeks—perhaps within a few hours—of the first meeting of an elementary school classroom, the individuals in it find, or are allocated, a readily observable position along at least three dimensions of social structure: interpersonal attraction, perceived competence, and social power. The quickly-formed structure remains stable throughout the school year and remains to some extent the same during following years. The classroom social system is composed of mutually attracted pairs and sub-groups plus a few isolates. The sub-groups are usually made up of children of the same sex and social class who have similar values and personality traits and are often in contact with one another. Most children are aware of their position in the classroom social structure. The teacher has great influence over the classroom social system; and the dispersion of the teacher's power and emotional acceptance has induced such changes as (*i*) increased pupil-to-pupil interaction, (ii) reduced interpersonal conflict and anxieties, and (iii) increased mutual and self esteem. Depending upon the temperament of the child, socialization in school produces more or less conflict between the felt urges of the child and the perceived demands of the school. Life at school is particularly stressful for the child who, by temperament, is slow to approach new situations or withdraw from them, is irregular in his work habits, is slow in adapting to changes in his environment, and is frequently negative in mood. While behaviour problems are most frequent among such children, given consistency in school demands, tolerance for delay in adapting to change, and support during frustration, such children do adopt to school, even with zest and enthusiasm.

2

Manifestations of Distress at School

The Search for Syndromes

In spite of extensive efforts to validate assessments of mental health and illness at school, the specification of conceptually and empirically distinct emotional problems of school children has been unsatisfactory. Studies in the U.S.A. by Ackerson[1] in 1931, in Leicester by Cumming[30] in 1944, in Minneapolis by Griffiths[52] in 1952, in St. Louis County[109] in 1954-59, in Buffalo by Lapouse and Monk[75] in 1958, in the County of Buckinghamshire by Shepherd, Oppenheim, and Mitchell[119] in 1966, on the Isle of Wight by Rutter and Graham[108] in 1966, and reviews by Rutter[107] in England in 1965 and the Group for Advancement of Psychiatry[55] in the U.S.A. in 1966—all these studies entailed the analyses of the appearance and course of symptoms of emotional problems, but none of them yielded empirically delineated problem entities. All the studies cited involved a sample of school children, most of whom presented no serious problems. Perhaps the prevalence of true symptoms of illness is too low to permit analyses which will do what is generally desired, that is: (i) clearly distinguish one kind of problem from another, (ii) assess the degree of severity of the problem, (iii) identify the significant points in the course of development of the problem, (iv) yield some possible inferences about the nature of the forces which brought on the problem, and (v) yield some testable inferences about the kind of treatment appropriate to the management or elimination of the problem.

Analyses of the manifestations of distress in more seriously disturbed children has shown more progress. For example, Lorr and Jenkins[84] in 1953, extending the work of Hewitt and Jenkins[60] in 1946 and Jenkins and Glickman[65] in 1946, analysed data from clinical case records and found five replicable factors: (i) socialized delinquency, (ii) internal conflict, (iii) unsocialized aggressiveness, (iv) schizoid personality and (v) brain injury. Rutter[107] in 1965 reviewed a number of research findings and confirmed the distinction of anti-social behaviour from the other disorders. He also suggested that developmental disorders could be empirically differentiated from both anti-social and neurotic disorders—in the clinic but not necessarily at school. He added a distinguishable hyperkinetic syndrome. Another review by the Group for the Advancement of Psychiatry[55] yielded a detailed classification. When similar information on general, non-clinical samples of children is analysed, no such clear-cut factors emerge—except for anti-social behaviour. (See for example the analyses of Glidewell[44] in 1966.)

When teachers are asked to report the behaviour problems of children in school, they do give rather clear indications of what they consider to constitute manifestations of distress at school. For example, in some of the St. Louis County[109] studies, factor analyses of behaviour problems (reported by some 60 teachers on six samples each of 200 elementary school children) showed that the teacher perceptions could be accounted for by four factors: (*i*) lack of emotional control, (*ii*) defects of interpersonal skills, (*iii*) anti-social behaviour, and (*iv*) slow academic achievement. There was also a possible fifth factor—hyperactivity—but it was not so clearly a separate entity, being often involved in lack of emotional control and in defects of interpersonal skills.

These findings converge with those of the investigators who were stimulated by Wickman's[145] contrast (in 1928) of the views of teachers and clinicians of the significance of the behaviour problems of children. For example, Stouffer[123] in 1952 and Beilin[9] in 1959 questioned Wickman's methods and findings and produced evidence that teachers then tended to agree rather well with clinicians about the significance of specified behaviour problems. Their data also indicated that the teachers were concerned about particular problems of the same sort: emotional control, interpersonal skills, pro-social behaviour, and achievement.

Identification of Emotional Problems

To say that teachers and clinicians agree about the significance of behaviour problems is not to say that either of them see the problems as psychiatric illnesses. Agreement between teachers and clinicians about whether particular children were mentally ill has been rather irregular in the United States. Ullmann[140] in 1952 in Maryland, Glidewell[45] and his associates in 1957 in Missouri, and Bower[16] in 1960 in California found rather substantial agreement (about 80 per cent) between teachers and mental health specialists, but each worked with samples selected in rather different ways. Goldfarb[49] in 1963 in Maryland found less agreement (about 60 per cent). The indications are that, to teachers, distress at school is clearly not the same thing as mental illness. The problems to which they are sensitive appear to be more accurately considered to be evidences of ineffective socialization: Labile emotional control, interpersonal ineptness, anti-social behaviour, and lagging achievement. Connected with, or underlying, such problems may be some neurology defect or some psychiatric pathology such as an incipient schizophrenia, but teachers rarely undertake such judgments. The findings available do show that pupils identified by teachers as presenting severe behaviour problems represent a sub-population with a high risk of neuropsychiatric illness, but the sub-populations requires further diagnostic study.

Findings such as those of Mitchell and Shepherd[95], Rutter[107] and Glidewell[44] also confirm that children behave differently at school from the way they behave at home. Not only teachers' judgments but also mothers' reports, peer reports (sociometric), achievement records, and psychological tests have been studied as psychiatric screening instruments. Mitchell and Shepherd[95] in 1966 reported findings from Buckinghamshire County indicating adequate screening requires data from both home and school, used jointly. The St. Louis County[109] Studies in the 1950's, the studies by Smith[121] in 1958, the studies by Stringer[127] in the 1960s, and a variety of other works have produced roughly comparable results. Given a prevalence of eight per cent of school children needing professional attention (but not intensive treatment), and adjusting the screening method to select 10 per cent of the children, the children selected by screening will include about half those children actually in need of attention. Of the children selected about 40 per cent will actually require attention. Such screening results appear quite unsatisfactory. Consider, however, the low cost of such screening as compared to psychiatric diagnosis, and consider that at least a brief diagnostic study of 10 per cent of children might someday be possible. Finding half the cases by diagnosis of one-tenth the children appeals to one's optimism. Actually, even a quite accurate screening which identified all the children in need of professional attention, is still impractical. Such a case load would completely swamp the resources available even in the most privileged communities. Currently, in practice, referral has been to a large extent based upon the judgment of mothers and teachers. The most appropriate screening development would be the training of mothers and teachers to become more competent referral agents, and the supplementation of their judgments by other data, like achievement records, structured interviews, and peer reports.

Prevalence and Incidence

A wide variety of surveys based upon teacher reports and ratings have been undertaken. (See for example, those of Griffiths[52], Bower[16], Glidewell[46], Rutter and Graham[108], Mitchell and Shepherd[95]. There is a remarkable convergence of findings that six to ten per cent of school children are in need of some professional attention. The nature of the problems which occasion this need, however, is altogether unclear. It has been proposed by some anthropologists and at least one psychiatrist (Gruenberg[56]) that about ten per cent of the members of any social system

Table 1

Prevalence of Behaviour Symptoms in School Children

	St. Louis County—Boys and Girls 8 yrs of age			Buckinghamshire County—Boys only 5–11 yrs of age			Buffalo, N.Y.—Boys and Girls 6–12 yrs of age		
	567	211	778	2,732	344	3,076			482
	Adjusted*	Maladjusted*	Total	Adjusted	Maladjusted	Total	Adjusted	Maladjusted	Total
Nervousness	29	42	33						
Eating Trouble	29	30	29						36
Daydreaming	17	28	21						
Temper Tantrums	17	24	19						
Unusual Fears	17	22	18	05	11				43
Withdrawn with Children	04	15	07	10	17				
Acting out with Children	06	16	09						
Wetting	14	16	14	01	05				17
Overactivity	11	22	14						49
Lying	12	17	13						
Frequent Crying	11	16	13						
Speech Trouble	08	10	09						
Thumbsucking	08	09	09	03	07				10
Trouble Sleeping	06	15	08						
Stomach Trouble	08	09	08						
Withdrawn with Adults	01	02	01						
Acting out with Adults	06	07	06						
Destructiveness	04	12	07						
Fuss about School	03	08	05						
Sex Trouble	01	03	02						
Stealing	01	04	02	01	04				
Disinterested in School				06	12				
Nightmares									28
Temper Loss									48
Restlessness									30
Stuttering									04
Nail Biting									17
Nose Picking									26
Teeth Grinding									14

* Corrected for sex and social class differences.

will find it difficult to meet the demands of the system—no matter what the system or the demands. The question remains. Which of the deviants are ill?

In the St. Louis County[109] Studies, the nature of the problem has been somewhat better defined—from the point of view of the teacher. The most prevalent problems were problems of emotional control They included temper tantrums, day dreaming, unusual fears, and frequent crying. They appeared in about 20 per cent of school children. About one-fourth of the problems were considered serious enough to require professional attention. The next most prevalent problem was some defect in interpersonal skills, appearing in about 15 per cent of school children. About one-third of these problems were considered serious enough to require professional attention. Anti-social behaviour was found in only five per cent of school children, but the problem was considered serious enough to require professional attention four-fifths of the time.

These data, along with much other data, re-emphasize the need to make more clear distinctions between deviancy and psychiatric illness. There would be a real tragedy in the shifting of the responsibility or socialization from the parents and teachers to the psychiatrist. No matter how much value a society may set upon originality and creativity, the socialization process remains fundamentally a conformity-producing process. Psychiatric illness is but one of the factors which can induce anti-social behaviour; it can also induce pro-social behaviour.

It is informative, however, to look at the prevalence of particular symptoms in an unselected school population. The findings from St. Louis County[109], Buckinghamshire County, and Buffalo, N.Y. are available as examples. The data are shown in Table 1.

3
Antecedents of Distress at School

Constitution and Temperament

Recently a number of scientists have become interested again in the interaction between nature and nurture in the development of psychiatric disorders in childhood. The longitudinal studies of Birch, Thomas, and Chess[26, 137] in New York in 1966 represent an excellent example of this reawakened interest. Since 1956 they have followed a sample of 136 children, representing 96 per cent of an original sample retained over a ten-year period. Data have been collected by interviews with parents and teachers, by direct observation of the children at home and at school, and by standardized tests. Psychiatric evaluation and periodic clinical follow-up examination have been completed on each case of behaviour disturbance. In most of the children the consistency of the expressions of temperament at different ages was striking. Significant changes occurred in a few children. More important, both the constancies and the changes could be explained, in the concepts of the investigators, by the interaction between the temperament of the child and the demands of his environment.

Analyses over the first five years of life indicated that the temperamental constancies and changes could be differentiated by five variables: (*i*) regularity of biological functions, (*ii*) adaptability in new situations, (*iii*) positiveness of approach, (*iv*) mood, and (*v*) intensity of reactions. The most prevalent combination of these factors involved regularity of life style, positive approach to new stimuli, easy adaptation to change, a preponderance of positive mood, and reactions of mild to moderate intensity. Such children are easy to socialize and they show few problems in school. Generally, parents, paediatricians, psychiatrists, and pedagogues like them.

The diametrically opposite combination is the least prevalent. As indicated in the foregoing section, life at school is particularly difficult for children who respond to new stimuli negatively or by withdrawal, who are slow in adapting to changes in their environment, who show frequent negative moods, and who react with great intensity. The temperament of the child is not in itself a problem. The social system of the school can sometimes provide a consistent set of demands, tolerance for slow adaptation to change, and personal support during intense negative moods, and the difficult child adapts to the school. Teachers who understand that their role is one influence—but not an all-determining one—on the child, often find such children predictable, dependable, independent in their opinions, and zestful in their responses to the learning demands at school.

Socialization at school is still, however, primarily a conformity-inducing process, and the intense, negative, slow to adapt child presents more behaviour problems than other children. The New York studies[26, 137] have identified mild to severe behaviour problems of some form—of both long and short duration—during the five years of follow-up in 42 of the 136 children. The environmental demands which produced stress to the point of symptom formation were not the same for all children. The intense, negative, slow-to-adapt children showed a higher incidence of behaviour problems—typically in response to impatient, inconsistent, and punitive demands from adults. The moderate, positive, adaptable children showed a lower incidence of behaviour problems. When they did present problems it was in response to conflicting demands between the home and some external agent—often a school.

Intellectual Resources

A number of investigators have found relationships between intelligence test scores and the position of the child in the social structure of the classroom. Examples of such studies over the last twenty years include those of Bonney[14, 15] in 1942 and 1943, Young and Cooper[147] in 1944, Potashin[102] in 1946, Shoobs[120] in 1947, Grossman and Wrighter[54] in 1948,

Laughlin[76] in 1954, Deitrich[33] in 1964, and Sells and Roff[118] in 1967. The correlations range between 0·00 and 0·45; they average about 0·20.

The relationship between intelligence and achievement is exceedingly well known. Except when the general level of intelligence of the sample is high enough to make non-intellectual factors more salient—or when distress interferes with intellectual functioning—the correlation between intellect and achievement varies around 0·40.

Other work has demonstrated that the utilization of intelligence increases with both the interpersonal attraction and the social power of the child in the classroom. Especially cogent are the findings of Van Egmond[141] in 1960, Schmuck[113] in 1962 and 1963[114], and Schmuck and Van Egmond[115] in 1965.

Family Dynamics

Family influences have been sometimes confused with temperament, but it is clear that the child begins school with certain resources and vulnerabilities which have developed from the interaction of his temperament and the child-rearing practices of his parents. The literature in this area is extensive. Some recent reviews include those of Caldwell[24] on child-rearing practices during infancy, Yarrow[146] on separation from parents, Becker[8] on parental discipline, Kohlberg[71] on the development of morals, and Clausen[27] on family structure. The weight of the current evidence leans toward the reduction in the importance once given to parental behaviour during infancy and an increase in the importance given to parental behaviour during childhood, including the school years.

One pervasive concept used to interpret the mediation between family influences and school influences has been the concept of self esteem. Conceiving family influences to be salient in the preschool development of self esteem, one can show connections between self esteem, position in the classroom social structure, and the utilization of intelligence in the achievement tasks at school. Baron[6] found in 1951 that girls high in peer status in their classrooms felt a clear sense of efficiency in coping with environmental demands. Girls of low classroom status, however, often felt inadequate to meet what they perceived as excessive environmental demands. Coopersmith[28] in 1959 found high self esteem to be associated with high interpersonal attraction for peers. He also found that pupils with low self esteem tended to show greater anxiety. The connection with anxiety and other manifestations of distress has been confirmed by McCandless, Castameda, and Palermo[85] in 1956, Trent[138] in 1957, Douglas[35] in 1959, Horowitz[62] in 1962, and Feldhusen and Thurston[38] in 1964.

While these studies have not established that self esteem is a concept comprehensive enough to mediate all the connections between family dynamics and school dynamics, they do indicate that the concept will cover many of the connections. The recent studies of Stringer[127] and her colleagues showed that self esteem accounted for more of the mediating variance than any of a number of other family-based personal resources, such as interpersonal skills, competence, responsibility, productivity, and enjoyment.

Behind the development of self esteem is the interplay between the temperament of the child and style of child-rearing of the parents. The many analyses of the impact of child-rearing styles show at least some convergences, as indicated in any of several reviews of such works as those of Bowlby[17] in 1951, Baldwin[5] in 1955, Miller and Swanson[92-93] in 1958 and 1960, Heckhausen and Kemmler[57-58] in 1957 and 1959, Sears, Maccoby, and Levin[117] in 1957, and Whiting and Child[144] in 1953.

Parental control has been a focus of attention for all the investigations. Control to the point of dominance tends to produce problems in children of almost any temperament; parental submission to their children is likewise troublesome. (See especially Baumert[7], Sears *et al.*[117], Bronfenbrenner[22], and Swanson[129].) Taken alone, the extent of control exercised by the parents has not explained the variability in behaviour problems. Taken jointly with variations along the love-hostility dimension, somewhat more explanation is possible, as shown by Miller and Swanson[93], Bronfenbrenner[22] and Sears[117] and his colleagues. Parental sense of responsibility for the behaviour of their children tends to be associated with a sense of potency to influence the behaviour, according to the work of Gildea[42] and her colleagues. No single combination of these dimensions of parenthood is associated with behaviour problems in children, but the rates at which such problems appear does vary significantly from one combination to another. The parent who sees himself as one of many influences upon his child's behaviour, who is more dominant than submissive, who expresses more affection than hostility, who feels more potent than impotent, and who acts more responsible for his children than irresponsible—such a parent has been found to have fewer children with behaviour problems at school than parents characterized by any other combination of these variables. Much unexplained residual variations in childhood behaviour problems remain—at home and at school.

Socio-cultural Background

Mechanic[86] has pointed out, in a series of provocative papers that data about illness represent two kinds of phenomena: (*i*) the condition of the person, and (*ii*) his reaction to his condition.

The behaviour of both the individual and that of his associates is influenced by both kinds of phenomena. As Mechanic[86] and others have demonstrated, the cultural background of the individual influences his reaction to his condition—to a small but significant extent.

Ethnic Factors. Zbarowski[148] reported in 1952 that, during interviews in a New York City hospital, Jewish and Italian adult patients related that their mothers showed great concerns about possible illness or injury.

They also showed alarm at small symptoms of disorders such as coughs and sneezes. Such great concerns were not so often characteristic of the parents of 'old Americans' and Irish patients. One possible outcome of such health concerns may have appeared in the fact that Jewish families in Anderson's study in 1958[2] showed the lowest infant mortality rate of all groups studied, including native white population, after controls for family size and income. As shown in one of Mechanic's[87] investigations, however, cultural factors account for only a small part of the variations in concern about or response to illness.

Sex Roles. The socialization of males and females is different in all cultures. The social expectation for one's sex are powerful forces in school as elsewhere. Mechanic[88–89] found in 1964 and 1965 that age-sex roles influenced the fear of getting hurt and attention to pain more than maternal attitudes or maternal illness behaviour. Schmuck and Van Egmond[115] in 1965 found that for girls the utilization of intelligence was reduced by loss of social acceptance, whereas, for boys, it was more reduced by loss of social power. Generally, boys have poorer relations with teachers than girls do. Boys are more often seen by teachers as having mental health problems. Girls are more apt to respond to social pressure by conformity and are more apt to approach teachers with pleas for help. The sex and social class interaction on withdrawal (see the following) in relations with other children reflect the variations in sex roles from one social class to another. Such findings are typical of such investigations as those of Gildea *et al.*[42], Lippitt and Gold[82], Bower[16], Boesch[13], and Ullmann[140].

Socio-economic Factors. Along another dimension, Koos[72] found in 1954 that the lower classes were less likely than the (relatively) upper classes to view themselves as ill when they had particular symptoms, and less likely to seek medical help. Saunders[112] in 1954 found that deprived Spanish-speaking families were more likely to rely on folk medicine and family care than were 'Anglos' in Southwest U.S.A. These findings would lead one to expect that lower-class mothers would report fewer behaviour symptoms to an interviewer and would less often seek professional help in dealing with symptoms. The former expectation was supported by the St. Louis County data[109]. For those children perceived by their teachers as 'maladjusted' at school, but not for others, the lower-class mothers reported fewer symptoms. The latter expectation was also supported by Turner's[139] analysis of the data from the St. Louis County[109] studies. She found that the lower classes were indeed less often in contact with mental health resources, but that the making of contact by the mother and child was more closely related to the severity of the child's problems (as seen by the teacher) than it was related to social class.

Still another study in St. Louis County, reported by Glidewell[44] in 1966, showed a significant interaction between sex and social class in their associations with tendencies to withdrawal in interpersonal relations with other children. Apparently the tendency to withdraw in social interaction was so uncommon among lower-class boys (three per cent) that, in that sample, *all* lower-class boys (versus two-fifths of middle-class boys) who tended to withdraw were seen by teachers as disturbed. Among lower-class girls the prevalence of withdrawal was more typical of that of most children (eight per cent), but the symptom still alerted the teacher. Two-thirds of the lower-class girls (versus only one-fourth of middle-class girls) who presented the symptom were seen by the teacher as disturbed.

One study provided an analysis of social class differences in the incidence of new symptoms among white elementary school children (ages 8-11). While the lower-class boys showed a significantly lower prevalence of withdrawal than middle-class boys, they showed no lower incidence. The conclusion is that episodes of withdrawal appeared almost as often among lower-class boys as among middle-class boys, but they did not last as long. The data suggest that the socialization forces acting on lower-class white boys in the U.S.A. move them away from passivity and toward assertiveness. For middle-class white boys, on the other hand, the pressure acts in both directions—in conflict. The middle-class male, as suggested by Green[51], is expected to be both well-mannered and aggressive and is allocated considerable social power. The lower-class male is expected to be less well-mannered and more aggressive but he is allocated little social power outside his own social class.

Anti-social behaviour has generally been found more prevalent in the lower-classes, but, as stated previously, such sociologically influenced anti-social behaviour may reflect good rather than poor psychiatric health. The data available indicate that it is not the assertive anti-social behaviour but the withdrawn passive behaviour which requires psychiatric attention in the lower classes.

Community Contra-cultures

The cultural gap between the urban slum Negro and the school in the U.S.A. has been most difficult to close. The work of Rainwater[103] presents a good example of the data available. It seems certain that the slum develops community and family roles, values, and concerns which are markedly different from those of the school—usually reflecting the values of the middle-classes. (See the reports of Davis[32], Deutsch[34], Miller[91] and Riessman[105].)

Swallow[128] in 1967 studied the nursery school behaviour of 58 children of slum Negro mothers. She interpreted her data to indicate that the younger, more assertive mothers, either by modelling or by direct tuition, induced their girls to put on whatever performance the situation demanded for the attainment of desired rewards—in nursery school or elsewhere. The older, more stoic mothers induced their daughters to accept their disadvantaged position more stoicly and even stubbornly to avoid any 'proper' performance for rewards. Boys were of less interest to and less influenced by their mothers than girls. Eyeferth's[37] study in 1959 showed the differences in sex identifications in mulatto children of Negro occupation soldiers in West Germany.

Smith and Geoffrey[122] in 1965 reported their very careful, coordinated observations of a classroom in a slum school. Their notes showed a parade of dramatic events, often violent, which were sensational to the middle-class eye, but were more commonplace to the slum children. More critical than the dramatic events was the pervasive sense of defencelessness of the children—defencelessness against almost all the demands from the world around them. Perhaps in desperation, each child sought alliances with other children, close identification with an 'in-group', full involvement in the 'here and now', and a pawn-like resignation toward the future. It is in such a context that the significance of the social-class and sex interaction effects on the withdrawal of the lower-class male becomes clear. The withdrawal is not just deviance. It is a disturbance of the developmental process, and it may leave the slum Negro boy—especially at adolescence—significantly deprived of both self-esteem and interpersonal skills.

4
Prevention of Behaviour Problems at School

General

The most common approaches to prevention of behaviour problems in children appear to be mental-health education for parents, mental-health training for teachers, preschool screening examinations, mental-health consultation for teachers and administrators, crisis intervention, and modifications of the social systems of the school.

Parent Education

Convinced that behaviour problems in children were fundamentally based in the nature of the parent-child relationship, many leaders of the various mental-health movements have invested their efforts in parent education programmes. The assumption was most problems are, at least in part, amenable to resolution by information and intelligence. The assumption has a long and honourable history. Professional practitioners have undertaken to provide parents with information about the nature of child development and the nature of the processes of parent-child interaction in everyday life. Brim[20] has published an excellent survey of the development of parent education up to about 1960.

One of the first difficulties encountered by such programmes arose out of some role confusions in the relationship between psychiatrists and laymen. The planners of parent education programmes have usually designed the approach to allow the practitioner to provide general information and to avoid giving any specific advice about dealing with the problems of particular children. At the same time, the practitioner was often confronted in public by parents who made urgent requests for advice about particular children otherwise unknown to the practitioner. To refuse to give any help seemed to be a violation of role responsibilities, but to offer specific advice in such a setting was too hazardous to be responsible.

Some programme planners decided not to use professional practitioners at all. They were much influenced by the popularity of group discussion techniques and the research such as that of Lewin's[79] showing the effects of groups discussion techniques on attitude change during the 1950s. In accord with this trend, a number of programmes were developed and offered as discussions among laymen, led by laymen, trained in discussion leadership only. The Mental Health Association of St. Louis, Missouri and of Austin, Texas, have developed, maintained, and conducted research upon such programmes for a number of years.

The discussions were focused upon parent-child relationships and interactions. They were conducted at meetings of school-related organizations, which requested the services of the Mental Health Association in presenting and leading the discussions. Typically, a film or skit was used to initiate the meeting and stimulate the discussion. The leader was a layman—usually middle or upper-middle class—especially trained by the association in methods of leading group discussions. He was not trained, as he explicitly announced to his group, in any field of mental health. The discussion leader was trained to encourage widespread participation, the acceptance of a wide variety of viewpoints, and the feeling of individual autonomy in deciding how to rear one's children.

Preliminary research by Glidewell, as reported by Gildea[41] suggested that, based upon observed performance, the successful layman discussion leader was the one who generally interacted vigorously with the group but was not upset by long pauses or periods of low activity. He was also slow to intervene into disagreements within the group or to intervene only to clarify the issue or orient the discussion. He did not demand interaction or contribution by the members, but he readily reinforced that interaction which did appear. He appeared to be less fearful of failure to achieve a 'good' group discussion. His behaviour reflected a primary concern about accurate orientation to the goals of the discussion and to the current contributions to the discussion.

Initially the success of the programmes was defined simply as the continued requests for them. The failures—the discontinuation of the requests—were analysed by Brashear[19] and later by Gildea[41]. Negro groups and lower-class groups were difficult to involve, and, at times, openly hostile toward the method. Captive groups—those groups who agreed to but did not spontaneously request the programme—rejected the method more often than those who took the initiative in requesting the programme.

Armstrong[3] investigated the interrelations among several factors involved in programme evaluation and found two clusters of relationships. The reported satisfaction of the discussion leader and the client group's programme chairman are associated with each other and with the physical setting in the first cluster. This cluster is, however, surprisingly unrelated to the second. The second cluster indicates that smaller middle-class groups repeatedly ask for mental-health education programmes and that the larger lower-class groups do not repeat their requests. Whether or not programmes are repeatedly requested is, however, almost unrelated to their satisfaction with the programme—in both social classes.

The tentative interpretation is that the middle classes, being committed to working for future rewards and to great faith in education as a way of improving life, keep trying to solve their problems by education—even in face of variable outcomes. On the other hand, the lower classes, seeking immediate rewards and having less faith in education as a way of improving life, discontinue their efforts when faced by variable outcomes.

Two experimental evaluations of such educational programmes have been mounted in the U.S.A. In the Austin, Texas, experiment, as reported by Hereford[59], laymen-led parent education showed significant effects on 648 parents (mostly mothers). The effects included changed attitudes toward acceptance of child behaviour, understanding of child behaviour, and trust of children. The programmes also increased the parents' concern about their own adequacy as parents. The children of the parents in the experimental groups (as compared with the children of parents in control groups) showed increases in interpersonal attractiveness to their peers at school. Against teachers' rating, however, the children showed no improvement.

In the St. Louis County Studies[109] the parents in the experimental groups showed relatively little attitude change as compared to the controls. Their children, however, in the eyes of their mothers, showed some improvement—immediately (during the first year) in the middle classes, subsequently (during the second year) in the lower classes. As in the Austin experiment, however, the evaluation of the programme against teachers' ratings was not favourable.

Judged against the background of Bronfenbrenner's[23] review of changes in child-rearing practices through time and across social classes, and Kaufman's[68] analyses of biographies, the data available suggest that parent education methods do have impact in the form of small amounts of change in parent behaviour accumulating over time, first in the middle classes and then, by diffusion more than education, in the lower classes, with a constant lag between the two social classes through time. More perspective on the data—and more experimental data—are needed before the preventive effectiveness of these changes can be satisfactorily determined.

Teacher Training

One of the most frequent laments of professional practitioners is that teachers are not more skilful in the management of children with behaviour problems. Almost as frequently, teachers express regret that they have so little success in teaching the few 'problem' children who seem a part of almost every classroom. In an analysis of the development of school mental-health services, Glidewell and Stringer[47] found one source of frustration in the differences between the focus of responsibility in the health institution and the educational institution. The classic clinical orientation is that the practitioner—the healing agent—must focus his attention and responsibility on the health of the individual patient. The classical educational orientation is that the practitioner—the socialization agent—must focus his attention and responsibility on finding some accommodation between the individual child and the society into which he is being socialized. In the course of teacher training the clinician tends to demand of the teacher more attention and responsibility to the individual than is feasible in the school. The teacher tends to demand of the clinician more attention and responsibility to the classroom and the community than is feasible in the clinic. Similar distinctions have been reported by Lindemann[81] of the Wellesley group, by Neubauer and Beller[97] and by Sarason[111] of the Yale group.

A second difficulty in teacher training appears to be rooted in the traditional clinical assumption that the significant problems lie within the individual and that the modification of his environment will lead only to new manifestations of the problems in a different form. In contrast, the traditional educational assumption has been that the manifest problem lies in the socialization process. Reduction of the problem, to the educator, means modification of the approach of some of the agents of the society. Most often, for the educator, the critical agent is the parent; less often the teacher. Although it was drawn from work with late adolescents, Sanford's[110] interpretation of his research on the educational process includes a discerning analysis of the conflict. He found essentially that professional educators must necessarily create tensions and conflicts in students because of their responsibility to confront the students with ideas and feelings which are deviant from those to which he is committed. He also found that professional educators can—by modifying their organization, roles, or policies—improve the institutional management of tensions in the students. Counsellors in the school, Sanford proposed, were more appropriately used for one-to-one individual support for students who were sufficiently vulnerable that the necessary institution-generated tensions became too disabling for learning. Clinicians were more appropriately used when the student must be temporarily removed from the school and relieved of the student role.

A third frustration seemed to arise out of differing assumptions about effective approaches to behaviour change. Glidewell and Stringer[47] found that the teacher regularly employs and is regularly rewarded for appeals to the intellect. Most children respond readily. The clinician is seldom rewarded for appeals to the intellect. Most of his patients are patently unresponsive to such appeals. He does regularly employ appeals to motivation and emotion. His experience has included repeated rewards for such appeals. The teacher and the clinician have accumulated a considerable consistent experience; each has been rewarded for his own approach; each has a clearly different approach. It is not so clear to the teacher that it has been with just those children who do not respond to appeals to the intellect that she has needed help. It is not so clear to the clinician that only very few of the children in a classroom do not respond to appeals to the intellect —almost all the children in the clinic do not. Accordingly, the teacher-training process has been subject to considerable frustration for both the teachers and the clinicians who undertake to train them in the field of mental health. The programmes do continue, however, no doubt based upon the faith in the educational process and the willingness of the middle-class teacher and clinicians to delay rewards.

Preschool Check-up

In the early 1950s the Wellesley group undertook to mount a comprehensive preschool psychiatric check-up. Their findings were that the practice made possible the identification of behaviour problems one to four years earlier than had been possible in the past without such checks. They also found that identification was tension-inducing as well as informative. Some teachers and parents were not very sympathetic with the early identification, and the service ran into the typical difficulties associated with therapeutic clinical services in schools—difficulties to be discussed in the following section.

Stringer and Glidewell[127] in the early 1960s, undertook a somewhat different attempt to accomplish the same results. All the mothers of children entering kindergarten were requested to come to the school for an interview with a psychiatric social worker. The interview was to be accomplished as a part of a research project on child development. No offer of assistance or advice to the mother was made. An offer was made, however, for future conferences on the initiative of the mother, if she wished to discuss further any of her relationships with any of her children. About 40 per cent of the mothers took advantage of the opportunity for the additional conferences. In the course of this programme the clinicians found very few of the typical concerns about stigma, parental inadequacy, or premature intervention into a problem the child will grow out of. The tentative interpretation is that the mothers were not asked to take the patient role, as they have by implication, in other such programmes. Data are not yet available on the preventive effectiveness of this two-year-old programme.

Mental-Health Consultation in Schools

Gerald Caplan[25] at Harvard has been the initiator of a new and well-defined practice of mental-health consultation with teachers. The consultant may be from any one of the several disciplines—psychiatry, psychology, social work, nursing, education. He is made available to the teacher in the school at specified times. He develops his role in the school gradually, but regularly insists that he is not in the school to see children. He will consult with any teacher about her difficulties with any child who is hard to teach, but he does not take any direct action with the child. As the role develops according to Caplan's prescriptions, the consultant and his consultee discuss the child—who is the client even though not seen by the consultant. Attention is focused upon the relationship between the teacher and the pupil. The teacher is encouraged to examine his role, how he performs it with the particular child, and the implications of his role performance for the behaviour of the child. A considerable literature has developed around this technique; case histories in detail have been reported; and further literature is developing. No experimental research upon the outcomes of the consultation has been completed as yet.

Hollister[61] at North Carolina, Visotsky[142] in Chicago and Stringer[125] in St. Louis have developed other approaches to mental health consultation in the schools, particularly consultation with administrators about school policies. Again case histories are available but no experimental research.

System Intervention in Schools

Glidewell in St. Louis and Lighthall[80] in Chicago have begun to develop a more clearly-defined approach to preventive intervention at the system level. The two will collaborate upon the development of training and research in system intervention in the autumn of 1967. Such a programme of intervention may include—in addition to the clarification of the role to school personnel—regular observation, data collection, and analyses of psycho-social phenomena at school; reporting to the members of the school social systems the outcomes of observations, data collections, or analyses; confrontations of appropriate persons with stress-inducing information; provision of consultation in support of persons coping with stress-inducing information; development of temporary social systems or sub-systems for dealing with stressful situations at school; development of new methods of tension management and conflict resolution in the social systems at school. The approach, like Caplan's, is adult-orientated, but, unlike Caplan's it is not individual-orientated. The focus is upon the system. The approach is altogether speculative; experience is yet to be evaluated.

5

Clinical Services in the School

General

Until recently most of the attention to the child in the school has been some adaption of clinical services either within the school or as an adjunct to the school. The traditional child guidance services became available to schools—in limited amounts—in the 1930s and have been available since. Some larger school systems, like that in New York City, have maintained their own clinical services. Others have used the services made available by private practitioners or by health agencies—voluntary and official.

Referral and Relief.

Research on school mental health services has indicated that teachers regularly seek relief from the real stresses generated by the behaviour of severely ill children in their classrooms. It is very widely observed that the initial response to newly available clinical services it to seek some relief—realistically or unrealistically—from the stresses produced by neurotic, psychotic, damaged, or strongly anti-social children. Even though the number of such children is exceedingly small, the need for relief from their disturbances of the classroom is quite clear and strong. The existence and strength of this force has been often demonstrated, for example by Lindemann[81] in 1957, Gildea[41] in 1959 and Stringer[124] in 1962. At the same time, data from the same studies showed that teachers tend to refer only about one-third of the children who they believe to be in need of professional attention. Interviews with such teachers indicate that they know that most children (in St. Louis County, 80 per cent; in Buckinghamshire, 60 per cent) do lose their symptoms within a year or two. They also know that referral to the clinic will bring on some stigma in the school and the neighbourhood. In addition, their experience with the children they have referred had led to expectations that they will get little feedback from the clinic and that the few clinical suggestions for classroom management they do receive will seem to them to be unrealistic. To a teacher, it seems wise not to refer children until it is clear that they are not going to get better. Such reactions have been reported at the Thayer Conference[31] of the Division of School Psychologists of the American Psychological Association, in the report of the survey of the work of the Bureau of Child Guidance of the New York Public Schools[12], and at the Tri-state Conference on School Psychology[36] in 1962. Lighthall[80] has published a provocative review entitled, 'School Psychology: An Alien Guild'.

Social Class Mediation

Studies of social class as a mediating force in psychiatric services in the school indicate that the current services get only little response from and give less attention to lower-class families. (See, for example, the work of Kahn *et al.*[67], in 1951; Roach *et al.*[106] in 1958 and Glidewell[44] in 1966.) It would appear that parents and children of the lower classes do not participate readily in verbal interchanges about motivation and emotionality so typical of psychiatric services. The more concrete forms of therapy would appear to show more promise. This is particularly a problem in working with children from highly developed contracultures in the community served by the school.

The Educational Institution and the Health Institution

Clinical services for school children move along with greatest facility when the child is sufficiently ill to be removed from the school at least temporarily and treated within the health institution of the community. Such differences as inattention to the individual, focus of responsibility, and approaches to behaviour change remain intact as differences. Neither institution places pressure upon the other to conform to its own values and norms. The child can differentiate the two environments and he develops differentiated expectations. It is clear that it is the child who is the patient; not the teacher. As long as the child remains clearly injured or ill, he can be relieved of his usual responsibilities for achievement in school, and he can concentrate upon getting well so that he can return to his usual responsibilities. Probably less than one per cent of pupils can be treated in this way.

The remaining pupils who need clinical services must be treated while they remain in school, and the school and the clinic must develop some form of collaboration to cope with the conflicts of values and norms between the two institutions.

6

Summary

The social structure of an elementary school classroom develops quickly and remains relatively stable through a school year. The positions of the children in the structure can be differentiated by at least three dimensions: interpersonal attraction, perceived competence, and social power. The classroom social structure is composed of mutually attracted pairs and subgroups of children of similar personal and social characteristics. Most children hold an accurate perception of their position in the classroom social structure. The teacher holds great social power in the classroom and by contracting or extending his power and acceptance he can influence the pupil-to-pupil interaction, interpersonal conflict and intrapersonal anxiety, and the mutual and self esteem of the pupils. The stress of socialization in the classroom tends to be greater for pupils who by temperament are slow in approach to others, irregular in work habits, slow in adapting to new situations, and frequently negative in mood. Approximately six to ten per cent of children in school manifest some sort of behaviour problems justifying some professional attention; about two per cent require intensive treatment.

Unselected samples of school children show no clear syndromes of symptoms except the anti-social syndrome. The symptoms of children who have come to the attention of clinicians do show some discernible syndromes, but there is little consensus on classification. Most reviewers distinguish anti-social syndromes from developmental from neurotic from psychotic from injury to the central nervous system. Children behave differently at school and at home. The prevalence of specific behaviour problems has been studied on several samples of children, but generalization of the prevalence is still tenuous.

Behaviour problems appear to develop out of the interaction of several antecedents, principally, temperament, cultural background, family dynamics, intellectual resources and the extent and manner of the teacher's exercise of his power and acceptance of pupils at school. The fewest behaviour problems appear in children of the parent who sees himself as one of many influences upon his child, is more dominant than submissive, feels more potent than impotent, acts more responsible than irresponsible. Studies of the interaction of such parental personality, child temperament, and classroom management have been slow in developing, and much unexplained variance in behaviour problems remains.

The prevention of behaviour problems at school has been attempted with some small success—in the middle classes—by parent education in child development. Mental-health training for teachers continues to be a widespread practice, but the conflicts between the values and assumptions of the community health institution and the community educational institution make its impact unclear. Some form of preschool screening—preferably one in which the parent and child are not required to take the patient role—holds some promise but remains largely untested. Mental-health consultation in the school has been widely developed but not yet experimentally evaluated. System intervention and the therapeutic use of the public school classroom is still highly speculative, but the data available indicate that such an approach may have the greatest preventive potential. Clinical services within the school have been plagued with inter-institutional conflicts, but clinical treatment of children who are clearly seen as ill or injured and who are removed from school for treatment has been more nearly conflict-free.

REFERENCES

1. ACKERSON, L., 1958. *Children's behaviour problems.* Chicago, Univ. Press.
2. ANDERSON, O., 1958. Infant mortality and social and cultural factors: historical trends and current patterns. In *Patients, physicians, and illness.* Ed. Jaco, E. G. New York, Free Press.
3. ARMSTRONG, J., 1958. *Program evaluation research.* St. Louis, Miss., Mental Health Assn of St. Louis.
4. AUSTIN, M. C., and THOMPSON, G. G., 1948. Children's friendships: a study of the bases on which children select and reject their best friends. *J. educ. Psychol.*, **39**, 101.
5. BALDWIN, A. L., 1955. *Behavior and development in childhood.* New York, Dryden Press.
6. BARON, D., 1951. Personal-social characteristics and classroom social status: a sociometric study of fifth and sixth grade girls. *Sociometry*, **14**, 32.

7. BAUMERT, G., 1952. *The youth of post-war years: living conditions and reaction modes.* Darmstadt. Eduard Roether Verlag.
8. BECKER, W. C., 1964. Consequences of different kinds of parental discipline. In *Review of child development research*, vol. I, Eds, Hoffman, M. L., and Hoffman, L. W. New York, Russell Sage Foundation.
9. BEILIN, H., 1959. Teachers' and clinicians' attitudes toward the behavior problems of children: a reappraisal. *Child develop.*, **30**, 9.
10. BIRCH, H. D., THOMAS, A., and CHESS, S., 1966. Implications for concepts of behavior disorders of children of renewal of interest in early individual differences. A paper read at the annual meetings of the Amer. Psychol. Assoc., New York.
11. BIRTH, K., and PRILLWITZ, G., 1959. Leadership types and group behaviour in school children. *Z. Psychol.*, **163**, 230.
12. Board of Education, 1955. *Bureau of child guidance of the New York public schools: a survey.* New York, The Board of Educ.
13. BOESCH, E., 1962. *Authority and achievement behavior in Thailand.* Frankfurt, Berlin, Alfred Metzner Verlag.
14. BONNEY, M. E., 1942. A study of social status on the second grade level. *J. genet. Psychol.*, **60**, 271.
15. BONNEY, M. E., 1943. The relative stability of social, intellectual, and academic status in grades II to IV, and the inter-relationships between these various forms of growth. *J. educ. Psychol.*, **34**, 88.
16. BOWER, E. M., 1960. *Early identification of emotionally handicapped children in school.* Springfield, Ill., Charles Thomas.
17. BOWLBY, J., 1951. *Maternal care and mental health.* Monograph Series No. 2. Geneva, W.H.O.
18. BOYD, G. R., 1960. Classroom adjustment of the underchosen child. Unpublished report. Troy, Ala., Troy State College.
19. BRASHEAR, E. L., KENNEY, E. T., BUCHMUELLER, A. D., and GILDEA, M. C.-L., 1954. A community program of mental health education using group discussion methods. *Amer. J. Orthopsychiat.*, **24**, 554.
20. BRIM, O. G., Jr., 1959. *Education for child rearing.* New York, Russell Sage Foundation.
21. BRONFENBRENNER, J., DEVEREAU, E. C., Jr., SUCI, G. J., and RODGERS, R. R., 1965. Adults and peers as sources of conformity and autonomy. Unpublished manuscript. Ithaca, N.Y. Cornell Univ., Dept. of Child Develop. & Fam. Rels.
22. BRONFENBRENNER, J., 1961. Toward a theoretical model for the analysis of parent-child relationships in a social context. In *Parental attitudes and child behavior.* Ed. Glidewell, J. C. Springfield, Ill., Charles Thomas.
23. BRONFENBRENNER, J., 1958. Socialization and social class through time and space. In *Readings in social psychology.* Eds, Maccoby, E. E., Newcomb, T. M., and Hartley, E. L. New York, Henry Holt.
24. CALDWELL, B. M., 1964. The effects of infant care. In *Review of child development research.* Vol. I. Eds, Hoffman, M. L., and Hoffman, L. N. New York, Russell Sage Foundation.
25. CAPLAN, G., 1959. *Concepts of mental health and consultation.* Washington, D.C., Children's Bureau, Dept. of H.E.W.
26. CHESS, S., THOMAS, A., and BIRCH, H. G., 1959. Characteristics of the individual child's behavioral responses to the environment. *Amer. J. Orthopsychiat.*, **29**, 791.
27. CLAUSEN, J. A., 1966. Family structure, socialization and personality. In *Review of child development research*, vol. II, Eds, Hoffman, L. W., and Hoffman, M. L. New York, Russell Sage Foundation.

28. COOPERSMITH, S., 1959. A method for determining types of self-esteem. *J. abnorm. soc. Psychol.*, **59**, 87.
29. CRISWELL, J., 1939. Social structure revealed in a sociometric retest. *Sociometry*, **11**, 69.
30. CUMMING, J. D., 1944. The incidence of emotional problems in school children. *British J. educ. Psychol.*, **14**.
31. CUTTS, N. E. (Ed.), 1955. *School psychologists at midcentury*. Washington, D.C., Amer. Psychol. Assn.
32. DAVIS, A., 1948. *Social class influences of children's learning*. Cambridge, Mass., Harvard Univ. Press.
33. DEITRICH, F. R., 1964. Comparison of sociometric patterns of sixth grade pupils in two school systems: ability grouping compared with heterogeneous grouping. *J. educ. Res.*, **57**, 507.
34. DEUTSCH, M., 1963. The disadvantaged child and the learning process. In *Education in depressed areas*. Ed. Passov, A. H. New York, Teachers Coll. Press, Columbia Univ.
35. DOUGLAS, V., 1959. The development of two families of defense. *Dissert. Abstr.*, **20**, 1438.
36. EISERER, P. E. LIEBERFRUEND, S., and WHITE, M. A., 1962. *Proc. 12: State conference on school psychology*. Unpublished report.
37. EYEFERTH, K., 1959. A study of negro mulatto children in West Germany. *Vita humana*, **2**, 102.
38. FELDHUSEN, J. F., and THURSTON, J. R., 1964. Personality and adjustment of high and low anxious children. *J. educ. Res.*, **56**, 265.
39. FLANDERS, N. A., 1951. Personal-social anxiety as a factor in experimental learning situations. *J. educ. Res.*, **45**, 100.
40. FORCE, D. G., Jr., 1954. A comparison of physically handicapped children and normal children in the same elementary school classes with reference to social status and self-perceived status. *Dissert. Abstr.*, **14**, 1046.
41. GILDEA, M. C.-L. 1959. *Community mental health*. Springfield, Ill., Charles Thomas.
42. GILDEA, M. C.-L., GLIDEWELL, J. C., and KANTOR, M. K., 1961. Maternal attitudes and general adjustment in school children. In *Parental attitudes and child behavior*. Ed. Glidewell, J. C. Springfield, Ill., Charles Thomas.
43. GLIDEWELL, J. C., KANTOR, M. B., SMITH, L. M., and STRINGER, L. A., 1966. Socialization and social structure in the classroom. In *Review of child development research*, vol. II. Eds, Hoffman, L. M., and Hoffman, M. L. New York, Russell Sage Foundation.
44. GLIDEWELL, J. C., 1966. *Studies of mothers' reports of behavior symptoms in their children*. Report IX. Symposium of definition and measurement of mental health. Fort Worth, Texas, Institute of Behavioral Research, Texas Christian Univ.
45. GLIDEWELL, J. C., MENSH, I. N., and GILDEA, M. C.-L., 1957. Behavior symptoms in children and degree of sickness. *Amer. J. Psychiat.*, **114**, 47.
46. GLIDEWELL, J. C., DOMKE, H. R., and KANTOR, M. B., 1959. Behavior symptoms in children and adjustment in public school. *Human Organiz.*, **18**, 123.
47. GLIDEWELL, J. C., and STRINGER, L. A., 1967. The Educational Institution and the Health Institution. In *Behavioral science frontiers in education*. Eds, Hollister, W. G., and Bower, E. M. New York, John Wiley.
48. GNAGEY, W. J., 1960. Effect on classmates of a deviant student's power and response to a teacher-exerted control technique. *J. educ. Psychol.*, **51**, 1.
49. GOLDFARB, A., 1963. Teacher ratings in psychiatric case finding. *Amer. J. Public Hlth*, **53**, 1919.

50. GOSLIN, D. A., 1962. Accuracy of self perception and social acceptance. *Sociometry*, **25**, 283.
51. GREEN, A. W., 1946. The middle class male child and neurosis. *Amer. Sociol. Rev.*, **11**, 31.
52. GRIFFITHS, W., 1952. *Behavior difficulties in children as judged by parents, teachers and children themselves.* Minneapolis, Minn. Univ. Press.
53. GRONLUND, W. E., 1959. Applying sociometric results to educational problems. In *Sociometry in the classroom.* Ed. Gronlund, N. E. Part III. New York, Harper.
54. GROSSMAN, B., and WRIGHTER, J., 1948. The relationship between selection, rejection and intelligence, social status, and personality amongst sixth grade children. *Sociometry*, **11**, 346.
55. Group for Advancement of Psychiatry, 1966. *Psychopathological disorders in childhood: theoretical considerations and a proposed classification.* New York, Publications Office, Group for the Advn. of Psychiat.
56. GRUENBERG, E. A., 1960. Personal communication.
57. HECKHAUSEN, H., and KEMMLER, L., 1957. Conditions for the formation of child independence. *Z. expl angew. Psychol.*, **4**, 603.
58. HECKHAUSEN, H., and KEMMLER, L., 1959. Mothers' views on training problems. *Psychol. Rundschau.*, **10**, 83.
59. HEREFORD, C. F., 1963. *Changing parental attitudes through group discussion.* Austin, Texas, Univ. Texas Press.
60. HEWITT, L. E., and JENKINS, R. L., 1946. *Fundamental patterns of maladjustment: the dynamics of their origin.* Springfield, The State of Illinois.
61. HOLLISTER, W. G., 1966. Personal communication.
62. HOROWITZ, F. D., 1962. The relationship of anxiety, self concept and sociometric status among 4th, 5th and 6th grade children. *J. abnorm. soc. Psychol.*, **65**, 212.
63. HUDGINS, B. B., and LOFTIS, L., 1966. The invisible child in the arithmetic class: a study of teacher-pupil interaction. *J. genetic Psychol.*, **108**, 143-52.
64. HUNT, J. McV., and SOLOMON, R. A., 1942. The stability and some correlates of group status in a summer camp group of young boys. *Amer. J. Psychol.*, **55**, 33.
65. JENKINS, R. L., and GLICKMAN, S., 1946. Common syndromes in child psychiatry. *Amer. J. Orthopsychiat.*, **16**, 244.
66. JENNINGS, H. H., 1937. Structure of leadership-development and sphere of influence. *Sociometry*, **1**, 99.
67. KAHN, J., BUCHMUELLER, A. D., and GILDEA, M. C.-L., 1951. Group therapy for parents of behavior problem children in public schools: failure of the method in a negro school. *Amer. J. Psychiat.*, **108**, 351.
68. KAUFMAN, I., 1963. Researches into the role of parents in the light of 200 biographies. Unpublished Ph.D. Dissertation. Bonn.
69. KERR, M. A., 1945. A study of social acceptability. *Element. Sch. J.*, **45**, 257.
70. KERSTETTER, L. M., and SARGENT, J., 1940. Re-assignment therapy in the classroom as a preventive measure in juvenile delinquency. *Sociometry*, **3**, 293.
71. KOHLBERG, L., 1964. Development of moral character and moral ideology. In *Review of child development research*, vol. I. Eds, Hoffman, M. L., and Hoffman, L. W. New York, Russell Sage Foundation.
72. KOOS, E., 1954. *The health of Regionville.* New York, Columbia Univ. Press.
73. KOUNIN, M. S., GUMP, P. V., and RYAN, J. J., 1961. The ripple effect in discipline. *Element. Sch. J.*, **59**, 158.
74. KUHLEN, R. G., and LEE, B. J., 1943. Personality characteristics and social acceptability in adolescence. *J. educ. Psychol.*, **34**, 321.

REFERENCES

75. LAPOUSE, R., and MONK, M. A., 1958. An epidemiologic study of behavior characteristics in children. *Amer. J. Public Hlth.*, **48**, 1134.
76. LAUGHLIN, F., 1954. *The peer status of sixth and seventh grade children.* New York, Bureau of Publications, Columbia Univ. Teachers College.
77. LEEDS, C. H., 1956. Teacher attitudes and temperament as a measure of teacher-pupil rapport. *J. appl. Psychol.*, **40**.
78. LEVITT, E. E., 1955. Effect of a 'casual' teacher training program on authoritarianism and responsibility in grade school children. *Psychol. Rep.*, **1**, 449.
79. LEWIN, K., 1947. Frontiers in group dynamics. *Hum. Relat.*, **1**, 5.
80. LIGHTHALL, F. F., 1963. School psychology: an alien guild. *Elem. School J.*, **63**, 361.
81. LINDEMANN, E., 1957. Mental health in the classroom: the Wellesley experience. A paper read at the annual meetings of the Amer. Psychol. Assn, New York.
82. LIPPITT, R., and GOLD, M., 1959. Classroom social structure as a mental health problem. *J. soc. Issues*, **15**, 40.
83. LIPPITT, R., POLANSKY, N., and ROSEN, S., 1952. The dynamics of power: a field study of social influence in groups of children. *Hum. Relat.*, **5**, 37.
84. LORR, M., and JENKINS, R. L., 1953. Patterns of maladjustment in children. *J. Clin. Psychol.*, **9**, 16.
85. McCANDLESS, B. R., CASTAMEDA, A., and PALERMO, D. S., 1956. Anxiety in children and social status. *Child Development*, **27**, 385.
86. MECHANIC, D., and VOLKART, E. H., 1961. Stress, illness behavior and the sick role. *Amer. sociol. Rev.*, **26**, 51.
87. MECHANIC, D., 1962. The concept of illness behavior. *J. chron. Dis.*, **15**, 189.
88. MECHANIC, D., 1964. The influence of mothers on their children's health attitudes and behavior. *Pediatrics*, **33**, 444.
89. MECHANIC, D., 1965. Perception of parental responses to illness. *J. Hlth hum. Beh.*, **6**, 253.
90. MENSH, I. N., and GLIDEWELL, J. C., 1958. Children's perceptions of relationships among their family and friends. *J. exper. Educ.*, **27**, 65.
91. MILLER, W., 1965. Focal concerns of lower class culture. In *Poverty in America*. Eds, Ferman, L. A., Kornblum, J. L., and Haber, A. Ann Arbor, Mich., Univ. Mich. Press.
92. MILLER, D. R., and SWANSON, G. E., 1958. *The changing American parent.* New York, John Wiley.
93. MILLER, D. R., and SWANSON, G. E., 1960. *Inner conflict and defence.* New York, Henry Holt.
94. MINUCHIN, P., 1964. Children's sex role concepts as a function of school and home. Paper read at American Orth. Assn, Chicago, Illinois.
95. MITCHELL, S., and SHEPHERD, M., 1966. A comparative study of children's behaviour at home and at school. *Brit. J. educ. Psychol.*, **36**, 248.
96. MORENO, J. L., 1934. *Who shall survive?* Washington, D.C., Nervous and Mental Disease Pub. Co., No. 58.
97. NEUBAUER, P. B., and BELLER, E. K., 1958. Differential contribution of educator and clinician in diagnosis. In *Orthopsychiatry and the school.* Ed. Krugman, M. New York, Amer. Orthopsychiat. Assn.
98. NEWSTETTER, W. I., FELDSTEIN, M. J., and NEWCOMB, T. M., 1938. *Group adjustment.* Cleveland, Ohio, Western Reserve Univ. Press.
99. NORTHWAY, M. L., 1944. Outsiders: a study of the personality patterns of children least acceptable to their age mates. *Sociometry*, **7**, 10.
100. PAINTER, P., 1962. Personal communication.
101. PERKINS, H. V., 1957. A study of selected factors influencing perceptions of and changes in children's self-concepts. *Dissert. Abstr.*, **17**, 567.

102. POTASHIN, R. A., 1946. A sociometric study of children's friendships. *Sociometry*, **9**, 48.
103. RAINWATER, L., and YANCEY, W. L., 1967. *The Moynihan report and the politics of controversy*. Cambridge, Mass., Mass. Inst. Techn. Press.
104. REHAGE, K. J., 1951. A comparison of pupil-teacher planning and teacher directed procedures in eighth grade social studies classes. *J. educ. Res.*, **45**, 111.
105. RIESSMAN, F., 1962. *The culturally deprived child*. New York, Harper and Row.
106. ROACH, J. L., GURRSLIN, O., and HUNT, R. G., 1958. Some social-psychological characteristics of a child guidance clinic case load. *J. consult. Psychol.*, **22**, 183.
107. RUTTER, M., 1965. Classification and categorization in child psychiatry. *J. clin. Psychol. Psychiat.*, **6**, 71.
108. RUTTER, M., and GRAHAM, P., 1966. Psychiatric disorder in 10 and 11 year old children. *Proc. Royal Soc. Med.*, **59**, 382.
109. St. Louis County Health Dept., 1965. General research report. Clayton, Mo., The Health Dept.
110. SANFORD, N. A., 1966. *Self and society*. New York, Atherton Press.
111. SARASON, S., 1966. *Psychology in a community setting*. New York, John Wiley.
112. SAUNDERS, L., 1954. *Cultural differences in medical care*. New York, Russell Sage Foundation.
113. SCHMUCK, R. A., 1962. Sociometric status and utilization of academic abilities. *Merrill-Palmer Quart.*, **8**, 165.
114. SCHMUCK, R. A., 1963. Some relationships of peer liking patterns in the classroom to pupil attitudes and achievement. *School Rev.*, **71**, 337.
115. SCHMUCK, R. A., and VAN EGMOND, E., 1965. Sex differences in the relationship of interpersonal perceptions to academic performance. *Psychol. in the Schools*, **2**, 32.
116. SEAGOE, M. V., 1933. Factors influencing the selection of associates. *J. educ. Res.*, **27**, 32.
117. SEARS, R. R., MACCOBY, E., and LEVIN, H., 1957. *Patterns of child rearing*. Evanston, Ill., Row, Peterson.
118. SELLS, S. B., and ROFF, M., 1967. *Peer acceptance-rejection and personality development*, Fort Worth, Texas. Institute of Behavioral Research, Texas Christian Univ.
119. SHEPHERD, M., OPPENHEIM, A. N., and MITCHELL, S., 1966. Childhood behavior disorders and the child guidance clinic: an epidemiological study. *J. Child. Psychol. Psychiat.*, **7**, 39.
120. SHOOBS, N. E., 1900. Sociometry in the classroom. *Sociometry*, **10**, 154.
121. SMITH, L. M., 1958. The concurrent validity of sex personality and adjustment tests for children. *Psychol. Monogr.*, **77**, No. 457.
122. SMITH, L. M., and GEOFFREY, W., 1965. *Toward a model of teacher decision-making in an urban classroom*, St. Louis, Mo. Final report, project S-048, Grad. Institute of Educ., Washington University.
123. STOUFFER, G. A. W., JR., 1952. Behavior problems of children as viewed by teachers and mental hygienists. *Ment. Hyg.*, **36**, 271.
124. STRINGER, L. A., 1962. The development of a school mental health service in a local health dept. A paper presented at the 8th Annual Symposium on School Health, Univ. of Kansas Medical School, Kansas City, Kansas.
125. STRINGER, L. A., 1963. The role of the school and the community, in mental health programs. *J. sch. Hlth*, **33**, 385.
126. STRINGER, L. A., MCMAHAN, A., and GLIDEWELL, J. C., 1962. *A normative study of academic progress in elementary school children*. Clayton, Mo., St. Louis County Health Dept.

127. STRINGER, L. A., and GLIDEWELL, J. C., 1967. *Early detection of emotional problems in children.* Final report. Clayton, Mo., St. Louis County Health Dept.
128. SWALLOW, C., 1967. Patterns of mothering A.D.C. children. Unpublished Masters Thesis, Washington University, St. Louis, Missouri.
129. SWANSON, G. E., 1961. Determinants of the individuals defenses against inner conflict: review and reformulation. In *Parental attitudes and child behavior.* Ed. Glidewell, J. C. Springfield, Ill., Charles Thomas.
130. TAUSCH, A. M., 1958. Experimental studies on the behaviour of teachers toward children in difficult training situations. *Z. expl Angew. Psychol.*, 5, 127.
131. TAUSCH, A. M., 1958. Special training situations in practical school instruction; frequency, cause and type of solution by teachers: an empirical study. *Z. expl angew. Psychol.*, 5, 657.
132. TAUSCH, A. M., 1960. The effect of the kind of verbal prohibitions. *Z. Psychol.*, 164, 215.
133. TAUSCH, A. M., 1962. Various non-autocratic behavior forms in their effect upon children in conflict situations. *Z. expl angew. Psychol.*, 9, 339.
134. THELEN, H. A., 1950. Educational dynamics: theory and research. *J. soc. Issues*, 6, 5.
135. THELEN, H. A., (Ed.), 1951. Experimental research toward a theory of instruction. *J. educ. Res.*, 45, 89.
136. THELEN, H. A., 1961. Teachability grouping: a research study of the rationale, methods, and results of 'teacher-facilitative' grouping. Unpublished report. Chicago, Ill., Univ. Chicago Dept. of Educ.
137. THOMAS, A., CHESS, S., BIRCH, H. G., and HERTZIG, M. E., 1960. A longitudinal study of primary reaction patterns in children. *Comp. Psychiat.*, 1, 103.
138. TRENT, R. D., 1957. The relationship of anxiety to popularity and rejection among institutionalized delinquent boys. *Child Develpm.*, 28, 379.
139. TURNER, V., 1900. Effects of sex, social class, and extent of maladjustment on approaches to mental health resources. Unpublished report. Clayton, Mo., St. Louis County Health Department.
140. ULLMANN, C. A., 1952. *Identification of maladjusted school children.* Washington, Public Health Monograph No. 7, U.S. Public Health Service.
141. VAN EGMOND, E., 1960. Social interrelationship skills and effective utilization of intelligence in the classroom. Unpublished doctoral dissertation (prefinal draft), Univ. of Michigan.
142. VISOTSKY, H. M., 1963. Personal communication.
143. WELLMAN, B., 1926. The school child's choice of companions. *J. educ. Res.*, 14, 126.
144. WHITING, J. W. M., and CHILD, I. L., 1953. *Child training and personality.* New Haven, Conn., Yale Univ. Press.
145. WICKMAN, E. V., 1928. *Children's behavior and teachers' attitudes.* New York, Commonwealth Fund.
146. YARROW, L. J., 1964. Separation from parents during early childhood. In *Review of child development research*, vol. I. Eds, Hoffman, M. L., and Hoffman, L. W. New York, Russell Sage Foundation.
147. YOUNG, L. L., and COOPER, D. H., 1944. Some factors associated with popularity. *J. educ. Psychol.*, 35, 513.
148. ZBAROWSKI, M., 1952. Cultural components in responses to pain. *J. soc. Issues*, 8, 16.

XXVII

RESIDENTIAL CARE OF CHILDREN

Sven Ahnsjö

M.D.

Professor in Child Psychiatry, Karolinska Institute, Stockholm, Sweden

1

Introduction

Institutions and their Development

The great importance of the complete family for the development of a child's personality is indisputable. Furthermore, a normal family situation seems to be the best way of satisfying the child's need for security during his years of development. Although all efforts aiming at the welfare of children are directed towards the realization of a family upbringing, there has always been, and always will be, a need of institutional care.

The general course of development of institutional care of children and adolescents, as well as of adults, has been characterized by the fact that at first charity organizations, often ecclesiastical, but also lay, were responsible for it. This was before the State and other public institutions gradually took over firstly most of the controlling powers, and subsequently the full responsibility for institutional care and its expansion.

It has also been characteristic of the development that it has moved away from collective care of undifferentiated groups towards differentiation by categories. In the first place a distinction was made between children and adults, and then between the healthy and those who are handicapped in various ways, the mentally ill and those who are physically disabled. Recently, the aim has been to gradually supply care away from the institution, and to provide care by foster parents or in private families, supplemented, where necessary, by control and supervision on the part of the authorities.

When the need arises to confine adults to an institution, the protection of the community from the individual has always played an important part, whereas in the case of children or adolescents the need to help, protect, care and educate them has always been more prominent. Emergency situations of many kinds create the need of institutions even for healthy children of all ages. Various categories of physically or mentally ill children necessitate special facilities for observation and treatment, which often can be adequately provided only by an institution.

Institutions: A Necessary Evil

As far as adults are concerned, modern care trends aim towards rehabilitation and readjustment to society, and consequently to a minimum of institutional care. In the case of children and adolescents, institutional life has such obvious disadvantages that our efforts must be directed towards the reduction of institutional care to a minimum. This implies, however, that other child-care practices must be intensified, especially foster care, which in many countries is efficiently developed, but which requires, in addition, the development of allied facilities and controls. Even if we consider institutions a necessary evil, we must see to it that their defects are eliminated as much as possible.

Fundamental requirements for Child-care Institutions

'The small-group principle'

Regardless of the character of the clientele, a fundamental principle must be to create a homelike atmosphere within an institution, as far as this is feasible. Generally, large institutions do not lend themselves to this. In all circumstances conditions must be provided within the institution for assuring the 'small-group principle' to the greatest possible extent.

This implies that the planners of modern institutions should endeavour to create small care units. Experience in numerous branches of care, has shown that each unit should be limited to six or seven children. To arrive at these small groups, the large institution should be divided up, so that the care units consist in all cases of no more than eight to ten beds.

Each department should have several single bedrooms, especially where there are adolescents, and, as a general rule, it is to be recommended that no more than four children should share a room. A single room should measure 7×8 m, a two-beds room 10×12 m, a three-beds room 14×16 m and a four-beds room 18×18 m: that is to say an area of 4×5 m per child. The children should have individual space at their disposal in the bedrooms and should be also allowed to occupy them in the daytime.

In general, each department should comprise a dayroom and a dining-room, as well as space for play and for spare-time occupations. Access to a kitchen, or a kitchenette has an excellent therapeutic value.

Surveys on sanitary equipment have shown that it is valuable to provide a bath tub for every seventh child, a wash basin for every third child, and a w.c. for every fifth child. The toilets and the wash basins should be screened off and adapted to the ages of the children. For older children, a toilet could be equipped with an ordinary wash basin and a shower, besides the w.c. Such a toilet unit should be available for each group of three children. Instead of a bathroom, a Finnish steam-bath (sauna) may be installed.

Here it is also important to point out the need for a room for the personnel on duty, since they no longer need to live within the institution.

The site of the institution. Institutions for temporary care, as well as those intended for permanent care, should be so situated as to allow members of the children's family to visit them, and the children to take home leave. If it becomes necessary to have one special institution for a large district, and if travelling to and from the institution is difficult and expensive, it is important to facilitate contact with the children's families in other ways, for instance, through telephone conversations, correspondence, free travelling, etc.

Internal life of the institutions. The internal life of the institutions depends on the personnel, their number and quality. If a home-like atmosphere is to be attained by individual attention to the children, a numerous staff is unfortunately necessary. A small number of employees necessarily results in the adoption of unfavourable rules, many regulations, and heavy demands as to order and discipline, all of which produce the unpleasant institutional system, that we are striving to avoid in order to attain acceptable child care. A sufficient number of employees therefore constitutes the basic prerequisite for adequate work. According to circumstances, estimates should be made on the basis of one child, or a maximum of three children per employee. The direction of the institution must, in addition, be so qualified that they can provide for the training of personnel, inasmuch as untrained staff must take on nursing duties, which is apparently the rule even in highly developed countries.

The training of nursing personnel must be aimed at making them so acquainted with mental hygiene that each employee, man or woman, is conscious of the necessity to endeavour to compensate the children for what they are lacking by being in an institution. It is necessary to understand all the problems confronting the children, especially on the day of admission, when the child, as a rule, is anguished, coming from a situation laden with conflict to a strange and hence perhaps even more frightening environment, which the child may wrongly interpret as representing punishment. By introducing the child to his new environment in the right way and answering his questions, false conceptions and anxiety may be changed into affection and a feeling of security, with the effect that the child will easily adjust. Often the situation may be simplified, if children and members of their family are allowed to familiarize themselves with the institution before the child's final admission; this can be done through early visits by family members or home visits by the children, where this is possible. The training of nursing personnel should also aim at conveying knowledge of group dynamics, involving interrelations between children, and interplay between children and adults. It is necessary to endeavour to satisfy the children's need for contact, especially when it becomes acute, as at bedtime. It is then desirable that the child's particular nurse should be present, or that the communication between children and personnel should be intensified by other means. Monotony easily permeates institutional life, and it is essential that the entire nursing staff should know by what methods monotony can, and should, be broken. The personnel should seize every opportunity to create variation and let the children experience changes of rhythm, brought about by breaks in the daily routine. The available premises should be utilized with a view to creating coziness, a good atmosphere and, occasionally, festivity. Make the kitchen contribute to a home-like atmosphere, and allow the children to decorate their rooms according to their own ideas and keep their personal belongings there. Use meals as occasions for conversation, if this is possible. All this, and much more, not least anything that can radically contribute to break the sterility of institutional life, as home leaves, excursions, journeys and the like, should also be part of the institution's activities.

What has just been said, as a principle, does not in the least imply that children in institutions should be spoilt, or that they should be allowed to do as they please. On the contrary, they should also encounter resistance and experience disappointment, in other words meet the same situations that occur in an ordinary home. The essential thing is to create a basis for security and affection, which will permit a normal development of emotions and reactions to be borne and tolerated by both the children and the personnel. It is quite proper to make claims on children, but they must be commensurate to the degree of maturity of the child, to his development and to the other aspects of the situation.

Another important principle in institutional care is that personnel in charge of children include males and females. The need of male personnel is as essential in institutions for young children, or teenage girls, as in boys' homes, as essential in institutions for temporary, or permanent care, as in institutions for observation and treatment.

Finally it is indispensable to provide suitable toys, games and books for different ages and in sufficient quantities; the need should be stressed also for spacious premises for hobby activities, gymnastics and swimming, as well as for playgrounds with equipment for outdoor games.

2

Institutional Care on Social Indications

On the occasion of childbirth, illness and even death within an ordinary family, the children may usually expect help from relatives, friends and acquaintances. When this is not possible, the children will find themselves in a socially exceptional situation which calls for institutional care. The children concerned are usually physically healthy and mentally normal. The situation is in principle the same, where an unmarried mother has no home or, for other reasons, cannot herself take care of her child.

The institutional care needed in such cases is of a temporary nature and should cease as soon as other facilities become available such as either return to the parental home, or, if this is not feasible, placement in another family.

The type of institution that can be envisaged in such cases is in the first place, homes for mothers, infant homes, and homes for children and adolescents up to the age of 20 years. It is desirable that homes of this type should be centrally situated within the respective receiving areas, so that, for instance, school children may be able to continue to attend their usual school. Siblings should not be split between different homes or departments, and differentiation according to sex, or age, should be avoided as far as possible. For adolescents from 15 to 20 years it is, however, necessary to provide separate homes for boys and girls.

Each community should have a plan for institutional care and the responsibility for direction and supervision should be delegated to local authorities. Further a higher social authority should be in charge of the central supervision, and should follow and stimulate the development of institutional care.

Institutions should not accommodate more than 20 children. In addition to the physicians responsible for the care of the children's physical health, the homes should offer facilities for consultations with child psychiatrists, child psychologists and social workers, so that the home can be used for periods of observation. It should thus be possible to undertake there the surveys that should serve as a guide for the future placement of children. A child psychiatric team can, of course, serve several homes within a region.

Because it has proved difficult to provide private homes for certain categories of children, in particular adolescents, special homes of the small-home type have been recommended; they are located in villas, terraced houses, or rented flats, and the care is provided by a married couple—a form of qualified family care.

3

Institutional Care for Physically Handicapped Children and Adolescents

In a civilized society, physically handicapped children and adolescents should have the same right to education and vocational training as normal children. As far as possible, they should, however, also attend normal schools, preferably with normal children, or, if this is not possible, be placed in special classes, or subdivisions of classes. Due to the fact that normal schools are now, as distinguished from what was done earlier, built and equipped with the needs of these children in mind, especially the needs of children with motor disorders, with the help, *inter alia*, of an extended school transport system it is possible to provide an increasing number of handicapped children with educational facilities in their local school. For certain categories, like the blind, the deaf, and children with severe motor disorders, who can generally be accepted in a limited number only, we are, however, faced with the necessity of gathering them in institutions, where the specialized teachers must also be centred. In those schools where facilities exist for the education of these categories of handicapped children, facilities must, however, be provided for them to live in hostels or private homes in the immediate vicinity of the school. It is important that all these categories of handicapped should be connected with a regional hospital and with the treatment centre for handicapped children of the children's department of such a hospital.

Institutions for the Blind

These institutions are intended for preschool training, schooling and vocational training. They should include observation centres, and *inter alia*, be responsible for providing the parents with information and advice, to enable them to start the necessary systematic training at the nursery school age. The advisory department for preschool education should be connected with these institutions, and preschool supervisors should be responsible for the management within a certain region, the size of which may, however, vary. Preschool children may spend periods from three to six months, or more, at the institution, and for part of this time the mother should be present.

Adolescents who are blind, or have defective vision, should receive education within the usual vocational school system, but special vocational schools for the blind are also necessary to provide training leading to the widest possible choice of profession.

Institutions for the Deaf

For the deaf early training in hearing and speech is necessary, as well as an even earlier home training. This can be supervised by the preschools for deaf children. The pupils of these schools may live in boarding schools, or, when possible, in their parental homes, or in certain cases, with foster parents. For the deaf several types of educational institutions are generally needed later, as well as special vocational and technical schools with their separate hostels.

Institutions for Children and Adolescents with Motor Disorders

In the case of children with severe motor disorders it is also impossible to avoid institutional care. Here, too, the institutions should provide, as for other categories of handicapped children, educational facilities for different levels of development, and the school should comprise, as for other categories of handicapped, a junior, an intermediate and a senior stage. The institutions should not cover too large an area, and should have close contact with a hospital and its various specialists. In any case, children with severe motor disorders should have gone through the hospitals for observation, exploration and decision, to the same extent as non-institutional children with a corresponding handicap.

Institutions for persons with motor disorders must be constructed in a manner adjusted to the clientele. The premises should offer facilities not only for long term care of children of different ages, but also for short term care (observation, appraisal, and treatment) with parents staying at the institution at the same time. Not only spastic children are among the patients, but also children with skeletal malformations, with operated hydrocephalus, or with spina bifida, who must receive treatment at a very early age with a view to motor training, sensorial training, and prosthesis training. This implies that the group is, and will remain, very difficult to tend and treat, and that its care will hence necessitate a numerous personnel. In addition to the nursing and the teaching personnel, physiotherapists, speech therapists, and occupational therapists constitute an important professional groups within the institution.

4

Institutional Care for Mentally Ill Children and Adolescents

Child and Youth Psychiatric Hospital Departments

The mental hygiene movement which developed in the 1920s, and the subsequent interest in juvenile delinquency with its continuous increase, had the effect that several countries initiated mental care for children and young people through so-called Child Guidance Clinics. Here, parents and authorities could obtain advice on educational problems from specialized physicians, psychologists, educators and social workers.

This practice has developed considerably in several countries, and the experience gained has led to a demand for the expansion of psychiatric services for children and adolescents. The need in each public health region for well-equipped child and youth psychiatric departments under qualified medical direction has become increasingly evident.

These child and youth psychiatric hospital institutions are intended for observation and treatment of those children who cannot be adequately observed and treated within the clinics of the child and youth mental welfare system, or at their branch establishments for out-patient care, namely the child guidance bureaux. These child and youth psychiatric departments within the hospital grounds should be built and planned as units independent of other hospital departments and have access to their own playgrounds. The number of beds should be limited. Each section should comprise of no more than six to eight children, and the youth sections should by some means or other be separated from the child sections. The total number of beds may vary, but should not, as a rule, exceed 32. Each section should have sizeable floor space, and should be provided with a separate kitchen, with a dining room and a playroom, and, as a rule, with rooms for various occupations, so that handicraft and recreation rooms should not be entirely located outside the departments. A child and youth psychiatric hospital department should also include classrooms, even though the education will be individual to a great extent.

Rooms for physicians, psychologists, child psychiatric social workers, and other assistants should generally be arranged in such a manner, as to be easily adapted also to the advisory activity of the child and youth mental care. Adjoining the department a day observation centre will generally be built for long term observation and for special treatment. These observation centres should, in their design, mainly correspond to kindergartens or afternoon homes for school children. Especially in the larger cities, thanks to such centres and in spite of daily observation and treatment, children and adolescents can spend their evenings and nights in their own homes, which in many cases is an advantage for all concerned. In the evenings, the premises may be utilized for different forms of group therapy for parents, as well as for the patients of the child and youth departments.

The child and youth psychiatric hospital departments are so planned and constructed as to facilitate also close cooperation with allied specialities, especially paediatrics and adult psychiatry and so that the services offered by the hospital can be utilized conveniently. A major advantage is that, in the evening, the patients will have access to the gymnasium and the rehabilitation facilities of the hospital, among other those for play, the swimming-pool, etc.

Treatment Homes Connected with Child and Youth Psychiatric Departments

The child and youth psychiatric hospital departments described above, as has been said, are intended to provide such observation and treatment as cannot be supplied by child guidance bureaux. The period of hospital care should not be extended beyond the time necessary for the use of all hospital facilities needed by the patient's state of health. Thus, if the child has undergone the necessary observation for a medical decision, and if his state of health no longer necessitates hospital treatment, he shall not be treated in a hospital department of this type any further. The natural and desirable course is that the boy, or girl should be cared for in the parental home and that the treatment should be continued at Child Guidance Clinics. Unfortunately, return to the former environment is not always possible, even though efforts may have been made during the child's hospital stay to prepare the parents for such a possibility. Neither is it always suitable or possible to arrange for care in another family, a solution which is always aimed at in the first instance, where the parental home for one reason or another cannot be expected to provide continual care and treatment. In such situations it may become necessary to arrange for care and treatment in an institution, in order to promote the proper personality development of the child concerned. It is therefore desirable to attach subdivisions to the child and youth mental welfare organization, two types of treatment homes for certain special purposes.

1. *Treatment homes for children from disturbed environments, neurotic children, etc.* This type of treatment home is intended for children and adolescents who, after investigation in a hospital department, or in a Child Guidance Clinic, need continued observation, or additional specialized care and treatment during a limited period, usually of no more than a year, and often much less, before they can be returned to the parental home for continuous care, or placed in another family. The disorders met here are generally of a neurotic nature, responding to environmental therapy and psychological treatment; other cases include patients with symptoms of brain injury, who after hospital treatment, need a period of stabilization and rehabilitation with continued medication and psychotherapy. The patients are school children, often in need of personal tuition before they are ready for ordinary schooling, and adolescents who will gradually be trained for employment, sometimes after occupational therapy and training by other organizations.

Treatment homes of this type have already been in operation for several years and have proved adequate for their purpose. The number of such homes is still far too limited, but new units are being planned on an expanding scale. At least two homes of this nature are estimated to be needed for each child psychiatric hospital department.

Treatment homes of this type should consist of small institutions for a maximum of about ten children, and should occupy detached buildings with spacious grounds for the children's outdoor games. They should fit naturally into built up areas. The equipment should correspond to that of an ordinary home environment.

2. *Treatment homes for children with character disorders.* This type of treatment home is intended for children and adolescents of normal, or somewhat feeble intelligence, whose difficulties are, in the majority of cases, connected with early character disorders, for which institutional care is necessary for different reasons, and where the treatment period is expected to be relatively long. We are here dealing with a border area of the so-called reformatory schools discussed below, with their more acute anti-social or delinquent clientele. The treatment homes are intended for a clientele mainly younger than that of the reformatory schools.

Like the homes for neurotic children damaged by an adverse environment, these treatment homes should have a close connection with the child psychiatric hospital departments, but should nevertheless be situated outside urban agglomerations, on a site where there are ample facilities for outdoor life in wood and field.

For homes of this type, the estimated number of beds is 18 to 20, broken up, if possible, into smaller units with five to seven children each. Today, preference is given to units with a very small number of children, no more than seven or eight per home, and the aim is to establish more numerous homes, where the children will be distributed according to sex and age.

Institutions for Psychotic Children and Adolescents (Mental Hospitals)

The type of child and youth psychiatric institution provided by mental hospitals for children and adolescents has not existed hitherto. Usually psychotic children have had to be admitted to mental hospitals for adults, where, in general, they have enjoyed considerable personal attention from physicians as well as from the nursing staff. The available treatment facilities have also been utilized to the greatest possible extent. However, so far, treatment facilities especially adapted to this category of patients hardly exist in any country. The children have thus been admitted to the ordinary departments, and have been mixed with other patients in a mental hospital. Where the morbid symptoms have been of a more severe character, it has been necessary to keep the children in departments for agitated patients. Psychotic children often become very disturbed and trying, because of their illness. Therefore, they frequently constitute an irritating factor for elderly patients, or patients who for other reasons are especially sensitive and irritable.

The care of the mentally diseased cannot be said to ever have had suitable treatment facilities for adolescents, either during or immediately after puberty. It is true that, like the children, they have enjoyed personal attention, and have received such treatment as the hospitals have been able to provide within their facilities. It has, however, been necessary to give the children care and treatment together with other categories of patients, at times in departments with patients with severe or protracted illnesses. For adolescents with schizophrenic symptoms the contact with severely ill patients with similar symptoms, must be very unfavourable from the psychological point of view. Considering the great plasticity of behaviour of these age groups, there is considerable risk of aggravating the symptoms of the illness in so unfavourable an environment. Moreover, many adolescents have had a disturbing effect on older patients on account of their liveliness. Only when the adolescents have grown somewhat older, they have been able to fit fairly well into the environment in the mental hospitals.

Mental hospitals for children and adolescents should be intended for children of 10 to 20 years, who have been stricken by mental illness of a psychotic character and for whom the care provided at the child and youth psychiatric hospital departments has not given satisfactory results. Such mental hospitals should be well-equipped with ample differentiation of facilities, and should be capable of providing different treatment and rehabilitation facilities, including schooling, and vocational training. It is considered appropriate to build such mental hospitals for 40 to 50 patients, distributed among four or five departments.

Mental Nursing-homes for Children and Adolescents

This type of home corresponds to the above-mentioned treatment home, and should be a home-like institution for younger children and for older children and adolescents, provided they do not need mental hospital treatment and care. Children of this category are now staying in a number of different institutions, sometimes after a period of observation and treatment in child and youth psychiatric departments.

In the first instance it was intended to establish these homes in conjunction with mental hospitals for children and adolescents. Usually the children concerned are chronically ill, so that the nursing period will sometimes be relatively long. It can often be expected that they will stay for several consecutive years, in some cases during their entire period of growth, until they reach the age at which they can be transferred to the institutional care for mentally ill adults. Because of this it is important that these children should not be placed at such a distance from their own homes, that visits by their parents, and contact with the parental home in general, becomes difficult. Child psychiatrists, too, have welcomed such nursing-homes, and in future they should be attached to the child and youth psychiatric hospital departments. This applies especially to the homes for the younger children.

Homes of this type should, like the treatment homes, consist of small units so situated as to allow easy access to the open country, to its fauna and flora, and yet they should not be located in a place so isolated that communication with the mental hospital, or the child and youth psychiatric department on which they are dependent becomes difficult.

Institutional Care and Schools for the Intellectually Retarded

The intellectually retarded constitute a very large group in the community. The frequency figures for all grades, from IQ 70 and below is estimated, for different ages, at one to three per cent.

Within the modern care of the retarded, efforts are made to coordinate all measures of care and attention on which this category of mentally handicapped are dependent.

In many countries special legislation exists, which determines the structure of the public help, support, etc. which should be provided.

Usually, a division is made between the institutions for care and the educational schools, often with a widely differentiated system of institutions within each sector.

For each given area, a central board should be responsible for the development of the organization under the supervision of a medical, or educational public authority. This central board, or its delegates, should also be entrusted with the control of admission and discharge.

Institutions for Care (Nursing-homes)

The nursing-homes are intended to provide care for the severely mentally retarded, to stimulate and activate them through exercises, training and occupation.

It is important to separate nursing-homes for retarded children and work-homes for adults, as well as from the schools for the mentally retarded. If, for some reason, this is not feasible, it is essential that the nursing-home for children should have a separate entrance, and sufficient ground for the children to be outdoors without constraint, together with visitors, and without having to meet adult patients.

It is very important to have institutions for the care of children of different ages, and to have facilities in the homes for nursing certain categories of sick children as well as infants. It is essential, in view of the present development within the domain of metabolic disorders, that the nursing institutions should be so located that a close contact can be maintained with the hospital specialists in the child field such as paediatricians, child psychiatrists, and child surgeons.

It is evident that children in this category, who can receive care in their parental home, or in another family, should also have the above advantages. In this case, the parental home should receive a public care allowance and the central board should engage personnel (experts, such as work therapists, physiotherapists, speech therapists, and social workers) for ambulatory assistance. This personnel should be attached to institutions where the children concerned can also receive temporary care, when needed.

The nursing-homes should also be differentiated into two or more groups according to age and depending on the total number of children cared for. Apart from infant homes, children under seven years should constitute one group, those from 7 to 12 another, and children of 12 to 16 years yet another group. No differentiation according to sex should be necessary, but for the older age groups separate sanitary facilities for boys and girls should be available.

Certain mentally retarded children are, because of their violence, destructiveness or uncleanliness, unsuitable for ordinary nursing-homes. As their number may not justify the setting up of a special department within the institution, several regional districts, or areas, should jointly establish special nursing departments, or hospitals. However, not to make visiting by the children and by members of their family too difficult, this arrangement should be avoided whenever possible.

For the slightly older adolescents, facilities are needed within the institution for work in sheltered workshops where their abilities can be utilized in different ways.

Schools for the Mentally Retarded

Within the normal educational system, the mentally retarded with an intelligence quotient below about 70 (Terman-Merrill) usually do not receive tuition. They are instead referred to special boarding-schools, or special schools, if they are what is called 'educable', generally within the IQ limits of 45 to 70 (or even 40 to 75).

The present trend is for such children, as well as various types of physically handicapped children, to receive their education, as far as possible, within the framework of the normal school, in special classes for the mentally retarded. The compulsory school attendance is usually extended for these children and may continue up to the time when they are 21, or even 23 years old.

The boarding schools generally comprise three types of homes: preschool homes, school homes and vocational homes. In preference, the education of the mentally retarded should be provided by day schools, or there should be places for day school pupils in conjunction with homes for preschool children, school homes or vocational homes, and the children should thus preferably live with families. Another possibility is to arrange for weekly boarding and lodging in school homes and vocational homes, possibly in ordinary private residences within the school district.

Institutions of an exclusive boarding school type, should, however, exist in a sufficient number for the educational requirements within each area. Among the mentally retarded there are, of course, also children with motor disorders, or with other handicaps (epileptic, crippled, deaf or blind). As these children cannot receive adequate care in boarding schools, it is important that facilities for their care should be provided by institutions serving larger areas within the framework of the welfare system for the retarded.

Complications of a different character, such as defiance with tantrums, inclination to escape, or other disturbed or anti-social behaviour, necessitate other types of special institution. For these, too, several areas should cooperate in order to make possible an adequate differentiation of the clientele. Under certain conditions it may be necessary to set up institutions with a very wide catchment area, maybe even nation-wide institutions, for a special clientele.

Educational institutions for the mentally retarded should have facilities for differentiating the clientele. Usually a division into preschool pupils, younger school pupils, older school pupils and vocational school pupils is recommended. Boys and girls are usually placed in separate school homes and vocational homes. Here, however, the circumstances may allow variations.

It is very important for these pupils that due attention should be paid to their need for social training; meaningful spare-time activities should be provided during hours when no teaching is taking place. Contact should thus be maintained with local organizations, and cooperation should be established with athletic, temperance and other associations, whose members should also be encouraged to visit the institutions.

Further, it is necessary to pay attention to vocational and occupational training. All pupils who have aptitudes must be given opportunities. For the pupils who can and should be discharged, it is also essential that this is facilitated through discharging them to boarding homes for temporary or prolonged placement. These homes should then be situated so that there is access to work in 'sheltered' factories or some form of semi-sheltered factory within the industry.

The central board, mentioned at the beginning of this chapter, which is also intended to be responsible for the schools, has a task involving great responsibility for the destiny of the pupils even after the termination of their education and vocational training.

Like the reformatory school clientele, the school clientele is dependent on the cooperation between the institutions and the regional hospitals and their specialists. The school physician of the boarding schools should be responsible for this cooperation, unless the institutions themselves employ the specialists needed to meet their requirements.

5

Institutional Care for Children with Epileptic Symptoms

The necessity of special institutions for the care of children with epileptic symptoms can be seriously questioned. The symptom concerned, fits, are not decisive in themselves but require investigation. Such an investigation should, in principle, be undertaken, in the case of children, in a paediatric department with access to neurological and child psychiatric expert advice. The majority of cases can be freed from attacks through medication, and uncomplicated cases should be treated as healthy. Should there be complications, such as mental retardation, the patient should receive adequate treatment and appropriate placement. Children who have attacks resistant to treatment which occur too frequently for them to be cared for in their parental home, or who need long-term observation are few. Where special institutions should be established for them, a large receiving area is required. This, again, would often cause the children to live a long distance away from their own home. In view of this, it would be better, and possible, where a need for special units exists, to attach them to already existing institutions for children with motor disorders, or otherwise handicapped children, within the smaller areas where such establishments are situated.

Usually, it is the behaviour disorders of these children that necessitate special observation facilities. Investigations should then take place at child psychiatric departments in conjunction with child neurological units. In certain cases mental hospitals for children and adolescents, or mental nursing homes, may offer a more adequate form of care for these children; in other cases, other institutions may be more suitable, such as the treatment homes for children with character disorders.

6

Residential Care of Juvenile Delinquents

The concept of juvenile delinquency is undoubtedly interpreted in various ways in different parts of the world. Usually, however, a strict legal-administrative definition is used, and children from 7 or 8 years to 18 years who have been committed to institutions, either through a court decision or by order of an appropriate authority, are included in this category. They have usually manifested such disorders as aggression and destructiveness, in most cases combined with recalcitrance at school. In the older children there may be also abuse of alcohol, spirit or drugs, running away from home, promiscuity and venereal disease. The majority of this clientele are recidivists as far as institutional detention is concerned. These children and adolescents have thus frequently been subjected to other measures by society, such as observation and treatment in child psychiatric departments and treatment homes, changes of school, attempts at placement with foster parents, etc.

The need for detention and institutional care is in general three or four times greater for boys than for girls.

For this clientele institutional care has, in principle, been aiming on the one hand, at removing the individual from a possible 'delinquent sub-culture', and, on the other, at giving him the treatment necessary to make him capable of social behaviour. The latter has often implied different forms of so-called medico-educational treatment, the former has consisted of placing the person concerned as far from his own home as possible.

Gradually, there has been a shift from individual care of admitted children to group treatment of them and their families, and subsequently to treatment including the whole family. Experiments have even been made with admission of entire families to a special family cottage within an institution. In this case (the children's village of Ska, Sweden) the institution concerned has been next to a treatment home for children and adolescents with character disorders, although it is not attached to any child and youth psychiatric department. It should be regarded as the next step from a residential treatment home for children, where modern methods of treatment are tested in practice. To make family treatment possible, these institutions, although they may be situated at a certain distance from the cities, should be near enough for transport facilities to be available, so that parents can visit the children and the latter can go citme on leave. This is, of course, possible only in the vicinity of larger hoies.

Outside larger cities it is, however, necessary to have a relatively wide receiving area for this clientele; this is often an obstacle to the desirable family treatment. The need of differentiation according to sex as well as to age, and further of a differentiation according to the nature of the clientele, has the effect that the organization to be created must usually include a considerable area. However, in principle it is desirable that several, and smaller institutions should be established. The clientele should not risk total loss of contact with their original environment.

It is also important that the institutions should not be situated in a spot so isolated that it becomes difficult to keep in touch with advisory personnel of different kinds, such as child and youth psychiatrists, psychologists, etc. Even though this type of institution is not intended for children with acute mental illness, who should instead be admitted to child and youth psychiatric departments or to mental hospitals for children and adolescents, there will always be need for medico-psychological treatment. This is particularly the case in this type of institution where 'closed door' type institutional care is necessary.

School Homes

These homes are intended to provide care and treatment for the special group of delinquent children who do not fit into other institutions, such as mental hospitals or institutions for the mentally retarded, but who have been admitted to institutional care by the authorities, and who, because of their age or other reasons, are still subject to compulsory education. This implies that the clientele of school homes will usually include boys and girls under 16 years. The lower age limit in institutions of this type should usually be about 11 or 12 years. Besides the sex-specific differentiation, other differentiation facilities are also needed, and it is desirable to be able to separate the youngest children, children with weak intelligence and more mentally abnormal children from the other clientele, and to place the categories mentioned in more specialized school homes. Should this not be possible, the imparting of education should be differentiated. This is particularly necessary as there are generally more children in the age group of 14-16 years than in the group of 11-13 years, and the clientele will thus be largely dependent on the facilities for practical work and vocational guidance, as well as education. Cooperation with the ordinary school system is often highly valuable for the solution of the school problems of older children. A considerable number of pupils must, however, be exempted from school attendance at the age of 15, and instead enter vocational education and occupational training in the vocational schools.

In order to obtain purposeful tuition, this clientele need not only education in special classes, but frequently entirely individual tuition, too. The teachers should have adequate qualifications, and these can hardly be demanded, unless favourable employment conditions are offered, with opportunities for further training, fellowships etc. Furthermore, buildings, educational materials and other equipment should be of the same standard in these school homes as in the special classes of the ordinary schools. Of special importance is access to audio-visual facilities, such as tape recorders, slide projectors, film projectors etc. In order to obtain results the teaching must be varied and concrete. The central, as well as the local educational supervision must, like the social and the medical supervision, have a stable organization.

Vocational Schools

For the senior clientele (children of 15 to 18 years and, occasionally, adolescents up to 21 years) a larger number of different institutions are required as well as more differentiation facilities within the institution.

Even though the pupils are distributed as much as possible among the different schools according to their degree of intelligence, to the possible type of their character disorder, and/or according to other criteria, the clientele will nevertheless be heterogeneous with regard to occupational conditions. Usually, the pupils lack all vocational training and any stable connection with the labour market. It should, therefore, be of great importance to provide the pupils with such working habits and knowledge, through instruction and training, as to facilitate their social adjustment. Each school must be equipped to undertake this phase of the educational treatment.

Generally, boys' schools of different categories are better equipped for differentiation, work training and vocational instruction. Metal engineering and repair work are considered to be specially suitable branches with a view to vocational orientation.

Broadly speaking, that part of the treatment of the pupils which is covered by the term vocational instruction and work training should include a therapy-related occupation without vocational orientation as well as vocational guidance and aptitude testing, in addition to special work training and a certain amount of occupational education. It is important that the institutions maintain continuous contact with organizations dealing with vocational guidance and the labour market, and that cooperation is established with the employment agencies in the locality where the institution is situated.

In principle, each school should be oriented towards one or two vocational branches capable of furnishing an overall work-training, and leading to different sectors of employment, In the case of vocational schools for boys it is appropriate to have mechanical workshops (for metal engineering, forging, welding and repair work and, possibly, motor engineering) and carpentry (building carpentry and interior fittings, cabinet-making and factory woodwork). The vocational schools for girls may include housekeeping (including household management of institutions, restaurants etc.) and sewing, with basic training for milliners, furriers and the clothing industry, but certain mechanical jobs are also suitable.

It is important to endeavour to place the pupils, as early as possible, with local craftsmen or in local industries for work training and for aptitude testing within certain trades or professions.

The vocational instruction in the institutions should be combined, as much as possible, with production, which, however, necessitates qualified teachers and suitable premises and machines. A realistic production and work training programme demands groups of 12-16 pupils, which are not always easy to handle.

However, the advantages are so great that production possibilities should be sought. One of the advantages is that the premium system for application can be replaced by a wage system, or even by piecework rates based on a group arrangement.

Spare-time Activity

For school homes as well as vocational schools it is essential to organize spare-time activities in a satisfactory manner. Access to suitable literature and a daily routine permitting variety in respect of physical work, instruction, play and sports, as well as rest, are equally important. Cooperation with organizations of different kinds can be very valuable in creating contacts between the pupils and the community. This requires instructors and leaders qualified for their task, as well as premises, gymnasiums and sports grounds.

Special Detention Departments

Institutions for anti-social children and adolescents are often charged with the treatment of juvenile delinquents who would otherwise be committed to prison. This and the degree of disturbance of the clientele, which is often considerable, have brought about a demand for care combined with detention in such institutions.

It is, however, contrary to all modern principles that children and adolescents should be detained or even subjected to custody in institutions which, in practice, resemble prisons.

If closed institutional departments exist, they must have, or be given, a positive mission in educational work. The positive part should then be less dependent on the merely technical arrangements for preventing escape than on the facilities to offer to the pupils care in a small group, with opportunity for intensive contact with and influence by the personnel. The quiet atmosphere in such small units may by itself exercise a favourable influence on mentally disturbed pupils. In schools of this nature there should therefore be facilities for such care in special departments, as a phase of treatment of the clientele.

Closed institutional care should be resorted to only after careful consideration, and mainly as a disciplinary measure in cases where this type of treatment is considered necessary; for example to prevent escapes, acts of violence or the like, or in order to facilitate a necessary investigation.

The stay in a special department should not exceed two months, if there are no special reasons for extension, and in all cases a psychiatrist should participate in the appraisal.

Treatment in a closed department must be combined with a particular occupation, with workshops within, or adjoining, the department, and the time spent there should be meaningful. Such special departments should be well staffed with personnel.

Aftercare

In order to avoid a period of treatment longer than is absolutely necessary, each institution should arrange for treatment facilities outside the school. To begin with, the pupils may be tested, perhaps by a transfer to special discharge sections with limited staff. A discharge section could be advantageously located in an area outside the school, for example in rented flats. It should, like other school departments, have a full-time staff. Through the services of the school, a pupil should also have the opportunity to become a boarder in a private family, where he will receive care, education and supervision. The pupil may also be tried out in special residential homes with full board in a home-like atmosphere, once he has obtained work.

Special personnel, attached to the institutions, should be responsible for aftercare arrangements, and also for maintaining contact with the pupil's parental home, or with the authorities of his own home, in case the pupil must return there or if another solution must be found.

7

The Future Development of Institutional Care

As living conditions and the general standard of the community improve, the need for institutional care for normal children and adolescents will become increasingly less. Thus, institutional care will become more and more utilized for the observation and treatment of the physically and mentally handicapped. The demands made on the personnel directing the institutions, as well as on the staff that will tend, observe and treat the clientele, are likely to increase continuously.

For large groups of handicapped the educational problems have been so predominant that it has been natural to focus on education and to establish schools for such categories as the blind, the deaf and the mentally retarded, as well as to aim treatment towards the development of their capabilities. Of course, these needs continue to exist, but developments in medicine, psychology and sociology have gradually increased the demands for precise diagnosis and for various forms of treatment for all groups of physically and mentally ill children and adolescents, whether developmentally abnormal, disabled or with character disorders.

In the majority of countries, child and youth psychiatry, with its teamwork by physicians, psychologists, social workers and educators, is becoming an increasingly necessary instrument of observation and treatment.

The shortage of qualified psychiatrists, clinical psychologists, child psychiatric social workers and educators with special training makes the rational institutional care of children and adolescents impossible practically everywhere. Adequate development depends on the increase of these groups of cooperating specialists and on the provision of the appropriate instruction and training required by each speciality.

At the child and youth psychiatric hospital departments, and the related treatment homes and advisory bureaux, these categories of personnel can obtain their practical tuition. Once such an organization has been built up, all institutions situated within the corresponding receiving-area, can successfully come to benefit by the work of those qualified, cooperating specialists. For institutions of various kinds, this means that they will escape from the isolation that often characterizes them, and will instead derive constant stimulation from a qualified centre for child and youth psychiatry. In large cities, where it is more difficult to realize such a combination of skills, each institution or group of institutions should have its own complete team consisting of a chief physician, assistant physicians, clinical psychologists etc. The risk of isolation here will not be as great as within less densely populated receiving-areas.

Contact between the child and youth psychiatric team and institutions of various kinds also makes it possible to provide continuous training, and, not least, advanced training, for the institutions' nursing staff through courses and conferences, where the problems of institutionalized children and adolescents can be discussed by experts.

REFERENCES

1. AHNSJO, S., 1958. Child psychiatry in Sweden. *Acta Paedopsychiat.*, **25**, 131-36.
2. AHNSJO, S., 1963. A treatment home in conjunction with a child and youth psychiatric department. *Acta Paedopsychiat.*, **30**, 88-94.
3. ANNELL, ANNA LISA, 1965. Child psychiatry in Sweden. *Acta Paedopsychiat.*, **32**, 90-94.
4. GRUNEWALD, K. R., 1963. Child psychiatry in Sweden. *Acta Paedopsychiat.*, **30**, 190-93.

5. GRUNEWALD, K. R., 1963. Föräldrarföreningar för handikappade barn (parent-teacher associations for handicapped children). *Barnavård och Ungdomsskydd*, 6.
6. HELLGREN, KARIN, 1964. Barnpsykiatrisk verksamhet bland handikappade (child psychiatric practice among the handicapped). *Svensk Läkartidning*, 12.
7. HOFFSTEN, BIRGITTA, VON, 1949. Jag är rädd för anstalter. (Fear of institutions.) *Vi*, 8.
8. ISRAEL, J., 1963. *Socialpsykologi*. Stockholm.
9. JONSSON, G., and KÄLVESTEN, ANNA-LISA, 1964. 222 stockholmspojkar (222 Stockholm boys). Stockholm.
10. KLACKENBERG, G., 1956. Studies in maternal deprivation in an infant's home. *Acta Paediat.*, 45.
11. REINIUS, E., 1952. Hur skall barnhemmen bäst möta sina ändrade funktioner? (How should the children's homes perform their altered functions in the best manner possible?) *Barnavård och Ungodms skydd*, 2.
12. SIMONSEN, KAREN, 1947. *Examination of children from children's homes and day-nurseries*. Kopenhemn.
13. SLAVSON, S.-R., 1954. *Re-educating the delinquent*. New York.

Statens (The State of Sweden) offentliga utredningar (The Swedish Government Official Reports):

Psykisk barna- och ungdomsvard (Child and youth mental care). S.O.U. 1957: 40, Inrikesdepartementet.

Behandlingshem och mentalsjukhem för barn och ungdomar (Treatment home and mental nursing-homes for children and adolescents). S.O.U. 1958: 20, Inrikesdepartementet.

Verksamhet vid ungdomsvårdsskolorna (Reformatory schools practice). S.O.U. 1959: 25, Socialdepartementet.

Barn på anstalt (Children in institutions). S.O.U. 1965: 55, Socialdepartementet.

Yrkesutbildningen (Occupational education). S.O.U. 1966: 3, Ecklesiastikdepartementet.

XXVIII

THE STRATEGY OF FOLLOW-UP STUDIES, WITH SPECIAL REFERENCE TO CHILDREN *

LEE N. ROBINS
Ph.D.
Professor of Sociology in Psychiatry

AND

PATRICIA L. O'NEAL
M.D.
Associate Professor in Psychiatry

1

Uses for the Follow-up Study

Natural Histories and the Evaluation of Therapy

A follow-up study compares measures on the same population at two or more points in time. It is a useful technique in child psychiatry in two ways: it permits observing and recording the fate of symptoms over a period of time and the emergence of new symptoms, and it permits evaluating the effect of treatment when outcomes of treated and untreated groups are compared. The phenomenon initially observed and followed may be a disease, a set of symptoms, or a pattern of behaviour. In psychiatry we sometimes deal with clearly defined entities or diseases but often with a symptom or with an item of behaviour which is judged abnormal but cannot be given the status of a symptom. This is particularly so in the case of child psychiatry, where the classification of functional disorders is even less satisfactory than it is for the remainder of psychiatry.

The first type of follow-up study, the observation of the outcome of a

* Support for this work has come from U.S. Public Health Grants MH-07126, MH-5398, and MH-7081.

symptom or syndrome, should ideally allow observation, description and recording of the *unmodified* course of an illness or item of behaviour. But society seldom fails to intervene when illness or maladaptive behaviour occurs. That intervention may be by educators, social workers, or the judiciary more often than by the physician. Given this perspective, the follow-up study concerned with natural history differs from the study concerned with therapy only in emphasis. The natural history study of the development, course, and outcome of an illness must necessarily take into account the possible effects that various kinds of deliberate intervention may have had. These effects can be taken into account by studying a group large enough to allow for the probable occurrence of various kinds of manipulation and the influence of various kinds of environmental factors.

Follow-up studies offer more, however, than learning the outcome of a disease or a therapy. One can also learn something about the incidence of various illnesses and symptoms in a given population, ages of onset, the setting in which various behaviours first appear, fluctuations in these behaviours, and settings in which behaviours diminish or disappear. A physician will readily recognize the practical value of these kinds of information.

Can Follow-up Studies Reveal Causes?

We have discussed the value of follow-up studies as providing base line data about outcome and as providing a test of treatment success. They are valuable for these purposes because they permit making predictions about outcome. Thinking about prediction has been closely tied in with thinking about causes. Can follow-up studies of children tell us what causes adult psychiatric illness?

To argue that certain events contribute to the occurrence of illness, i.e. are 'causes', you have to be able to show that when these events occur among well persons, more of them are thereafter found to be sick than when the events do not occur. This is not proof, of course, but it is the best one can do in the absence of an experimental demonstration. Some workers, recognizing that retrospective studies have trouble in establishing temporal connections between events and the onset of illness, have thought that follow-up studies would solve these problems. It is our opinion that while follow-up studies, like cross-sectional studies, suggest *hypotheses* about causes when certain events and illnesses are found to occur in the lives of the same persons, they can rarely offer direct evidence that these events *preceded* the illness. Let us suppose that a follow-up study is done with child patients and child control subjects. The patients *are* patients because they already have symptoms. We are obviously, then, not in a position to witness the onset of their illnesses. Indeed, except for being closer to the starting point, and therefore better able to get accurate information, we are in no better position to know whether certain events preceded the symptoms or followed them than we would have been if we had first seen the patient as an adult and obtained a history from him. In either case we would be getting a *retrospective* history. But what about the control subjects? Since they are *well* as children, will we be able to explain the illness of those who are found to be ill at follow-up? There are two sets of events that might explain their illness: events occurring before the beginning of the study, and events occurring in the interval between intake and follow-up. For events occurring in this interval, we have the same problem as with the patients. When we find control subjects who are sick at follow-up and who have suffered possibly causal events in the interval since intake, we cannot be sure that the events preceded the onset of symptoms. For both patients and such control subjects, we can only develop causal hypotheses based on the observation that more subjects who experienced such events became sick than did those who did not. But even in building hypotheses, we will need to be cautious about assuming the order of occurrence, since personality changes associated with psychiatric illness commonly create personal difficulies such as job loss, disruption of relationships, and geographical moves. Follow-up studies have a real advantage over cross-sectional studies, however, in relating events *present at intake* to the outcome of control subjects. If the control subjects, well at intake, who have had family patterns, class status, or presumably traumaic experiences similar to those of patients are found at outcome to be psychiatrically ill, we do have *both* a correlation between environment and psychiatric illness *and* the certainty that the events presumed noxious *predated* the illness. This is much better evidence for a causal connection than is mere correlation. We will still be a long way from *proving* cause or knowing the mechanisms through which these events cause illness.

Follow-up studies of children then are particularly suitable for developing and testing causal hypotheses that relate events occurring early in life to illnesses that are most likely to develop between intake and follow-up, that is, illnesses that begin *neither* in early childhood nor late in life.

2

Issues in the Overall Design of Follow-up Studies

The Study Population

The ideal study population obviously varies with the problem one is trying to solve. Yet there are at least two basic criteria that must be met: (*i*) obtaining an adequate sample of the group to which you want to extrapolate your findings and (*ii*) providing a reasonable control or comparison group.

The Study Group. Researchers are too often satisfied with their study group merely because they have selected an unbiased sample of a specific population. But a study group is valuable only to the degree that findings about it can be extrapolated to *other* populations. One studies the outcomes of patients seen over a given interval, e.g. between 1960 and 1965, not for their intrinsic interest, but in order to predict how patients seen in later years or in other places can be expected to turn out. But the composition of patient populations differs with time and locale. In designing a follow-up study, one has to keep in mind the fact that the population to which the findings will be applied in the future may differ in many ways from the population studied. It one wants a base line estimate of recovery rates against which to evaluate new treatments, it is of no help to know that '60 per cent of all patients previously seen were well after 10 years' unless the patients previously studied by chance had the same characteristics as patients now receiving the new treatment. But if base line statistics are presented, not for the total group of patients, but for specifically-defined sub-samples, e.g. for boys 6-10 referred by the school for poor academic success or girls 14-16 referred by the juvenile court for promiscuity, they are much more useful. If recovery rates for such sub-samples are available, one can extrapolate from them to expected recovery rates for new populations with different parameters. An expected rate of recovery in the new population can be computed by weighting the recovery rates for the sub-groups in the original study to match their proportions in the new patient group. To allow this weighting procedure, the earlier study must obviously have contained the whole spectrum of patient types found in the new population, even though they need not have been represented in the *same proportions*. But even if some kinds of cases did not appear in the original study, the types which *did* appear will provide estimates for the same kinds of cases in the new populat on.

It is important that the study from which base line findings come have had *enough* cases in the more important sex, age, and comp'aint categories to permit making stable estimates of their outcome. With a 100 cases of boys under 12 referred for theft, for instance, a 60 per cent recovery rate without treatment tells you that the chances are 95 out of 100 that if you studied another untreated group with these characteristics, their recovery rate should be somewhere between 50 per cent and 70 per cent. In a treated group, then, more than 70 per cent would have to recover to argue that treatment had made any difference. If the recovery rate had been based on only 30 cases, 60 per cent of whom had recovered, a recovery rate as high as 77 per cent in another group could be expected by chance alone. Treatment would have to produce even better results than this if we are to believe it has been effective. Since we are interested in predicting outcome for sub-samples with specific age and sex characteristics, so that we will be able to make predictions for future populations, it is wise to select cases to follow in such a way that there will be *enough* cases in the various cross-classifications to provide a stable estimate of their outcome. We suggest, then, what survey researchers call a *stratified* sample rather than a simple random sample or a consecutive series. A stratified sample sets quotas for various sub-populations. Subjects may still be randomly selected within the quota limitations.

Stratification makes sense, however, only if one has some prior knowledge about which variables are likely to influence outcome. Such knowledge comes from prior follow-up studies and from clinical observation. We found in our own follow-up study (Robins)[10] that recovery is more common in boys than in girls, and in children referred for 'nervousness' than in children referred for antisocial behaviour. But we also know that clinic populations usually provide many more boys than girls and that a higher proportion of boys than of girls are referred for anti-social behaviour (Tuckman)[14]. To stratify on sex and presenting complaint, then, it might be necessary to follow *every* anti-social girl available, while anti-social boys could be sampled at a much lower rate to provide roughly equal numbers of anti-social boys and girls.

The Control Group. The need for a control group has now been well accepted for any study that concerns the effects of intervention. Claims for the success of drug therapy, for instance, are treated sceptically if there is no 'placebo' group for comparison, unless the illness is well known to have a very poor prognosis. It is less widely accepted that natural history studies also require control groups, perhaps because we are less sceptical about predictions of poor outcome in the absence of treatment than we are about claims for the success of treatment. Nonetheless, we cannot argue that children with certain symptoms, if untreated, have a poor prognosis, unless we can compare their outcome with that of similar children without symptoms. Children free of psychiatric symptoms may develop psychiatric illness as adults. To argue that childhood symptoms are ominous, the adult illness rate for children with these symptoms must be higher than the rate for children without them (i.e. the control subjects).

The particular kind of control group needed depends, of course, on what point the follow-up study is trying to make. To show that intervention should be considered for children with a particular complaint, one needs to compare the outcomes of untreated children with this complaint to the outcomes of children who are well. But to show that children with one kind of complaint need care more than do children with another, one obviously needs to compare outcomes of two untreated complaint groups—one with complaint A and one with complaint B. On the other hand, to show that a particular *treatment* is valuable, one must compare experimental and control groups with the *same* complaint, but the experimental group must have received the treatment while the control group has not.

It is simple to decide whether study and control groups should be alike or different with respect to their chief complaint. But it is not simple to decide in what other ways they need to be alike. For better or worse, the follow-up study takes the laboratory experiment as its model. When the problem to be explored is the effect of treatment, the parallel to the laboratory situation is obvious. The two groups to be compared should be alike with respect not only to their presenting problem, but also in all respects that might influence outcome. They should differ *only* in whether or not they received treatment. The goal is straightforward, but its achievement is difficult. In laboratory experiments, the experimenter can randomly assign subjects to the treated and untreated groups. He assumes that randomization will cancel out the effects of background variables he cannot control. But when children to be followed come from treated and untreated populations in the real world, presence or absence of treatment is never random, but depends on the practitioner's decision and on the family's and the child's acceptance of treatment. The practitioner recommends treatment for children he believes likely to be successful candidates. He may well consider children who are less seriously ill the better candidates. Obviously, if the initial prognosis for the treated group is better than for the untreated, a better outcome following treatment should not be attributed only to the effect of the treatment. The fact that the family and child must be *receptive* to treatment, if the child is to receive it, may also muddy the design. The family's and child's very belief that therapy is valuable may make the therapy more effective. But more importantly, it is well known that positive attitudes toward psychiatric intervention are more common in the well-to-do and the well-educated. We do not yet know to what extent these socio-economic variables may themselves affect outcome. Perhaps children from comfortably-off homes would have had a better prognosis even *without* treatment.

In view of the fact that the decision to give and to accept treatment may predict outcome, it may well be the case that comparable treated and untreated groups are available to research only when the demand for treatment is vastly greater than the supply. If there are insufficient facilities for treating all the persons considered likely to benefit and desiring treatment, cases on the waiting list who never come to treatment can provide a control group whose families were originally as eager for treatment as were the families of treated cases and who were judged by the practitioner to be as good candidates for therapy. Such waiting lists can provide nearly ideal control subjects.

For natural history follow-up studies aimed at comparing outcomes of children with symptoms and children without, the question of what kind of design would approximate a laboratory experiment is not so easily answered. In the classical experiment, one evaluates the effect of the experimental variable, 'other things being equal'. The use of this phrase 'other things being equal' is based on the assumption that the experimenter has himself *created* the experimental condition whose outcome is being tested. The 'other things' which are equal, therefore, do not contain any of the *causes* of the experimental condition. But the occurrence of symptoms is a 'natural' experiment, to which the researcher has made no contribution. To know whether the presence of a complaint in childhood is associated with particular kinds of outcomes, one wou'd like to isolate the effect of the complaint from the effect of background variables. Unfortunately, the background variables on which it is important to match controls and patients may very well have played a role in the appearance of the patient's illness. For instance, a child may steal because his parent does. If we try to match parents' behaviour as one background variable, the control subjects who do not steal despite having a parent who does will not be 'normal' controls, but children unusually resistant to the parent's example. If they turn out better than the patients, we will not know whether this means that stealing has a bad prognosis or that being able to resist the parental example has a particularly good prognosis. In any case, it may be hard to find enough such exceptional control subjects.

Yet if factors like family patterns are *not* used as criteria for selecting the control group, the study is open to the criticism that the apparent differences in outcome are attributable not to the patient's behaviour problems but to the level of pathology in his family situation. The dilemma here resides in the fact that family patterns which may have contributed to the occurrence of the child's behaviour problems have many additional effects as well. The criminal parent who may have contributed to his child's delinquency will also have damaged the child's reputation in the community. Consequently the community will *expect* the child to be 'no good like his father', an expectation which may well have important consequences for the child's chances of remission.

Faced with this real dilemma in trying to segregate the child's pathology and its causes from background variables that may independently influence his adult adjustment, the researcher can only compromise the experimental model. The most reasonable compromise appears to be a decision to match patients and control subjects only on those characteristics which in the general population are at least as often associated with an absence of pathology as with its presence. This compromise restricts the closeness of the match between controls and patients. Control subjects may easily be found to match patients with respect to class and family type if the match for class is limited to categories as broad as 'guardian is a blue-collar worker' and if the match for family type is limited to categories as broad as 'broken home'. But if the class status of the family is more narrowly defined in terms of how much of the time the family has been dependent on social agencies and if the family type is defined in terms of the *reason* for the break (e.g. desertion), enough well children may not be found to serve as controls.

The fact that there is no perfect solution to the problem of selecting control subjects for natural history studies does not mean that control subjects are not valuable nor that rough attempts to equate backgrounds of patients and control subjects are not much better than no attempts. It *does* mean that when the outcome for patients is found to differ from the outcome for control subjects, one must consider the possibility that uncontrolled background differences may largely account for the finding.

Prospective or post facto *Follow-Ups?*

The defining characteristic of the follow-up study is that it requires information about the same group of people collected at two or more points in time. The researcher has an option as to whether he personally collects the materials from the subjects at either or both points in time. Indeed, follow-up studies have varied from one extreme, sometimes called panel studies, in which the researcher sees the subjects repeatedly from the beginning to the end of the follow-up period (e.g. Chess[2], Macfarlane[5] to the opposite extreme, known as record linkage studies, where the researcher does not control the collection of data at all, but locates subjects in two or more rosters collected at different time periods for other purposes (Christiansen[8], Roff[11], Nameche[3]). There have of course also been examples of intermediate types, such as the Cambridge-Somerville Youth Study (McCords)[6], in which subjects were seen intensively during the initial period, but their outcomes evaluated through police records without personal contact, and our study of child guidance clinic patients (Robins)[10] in which records provided initial information, but personal interviews (as well as records) were used to obtain outcome information.

If the purposes of the follow-up study require collecting childhood materials *directly*, the researcher has no alternative to a prospective study. He must take his measures in childhood and wait patiently for his subjects to age enough to make it profitable to restudy them. If, however, the predictors of outcome in which he is interested have been collected in connection with the child's normal progress through life—e.g. in school records or neonatal hospital records—or in connection with the child's coming to psychiatric attention, the researcher can choose between a prospective study, in which he selects children and waits for them to age, and a *post facto* study. If he chooses the *post facto* study, he can select subjects for whom childhood information was collected sufficiently long ago so that the follow-up period has already elapsed. He can then immediately conduct interviews with them as adults or obtain adult record information about them. To decide which kind of follow-up study to do, the researcher must weigh the time saved by using the latter method against the loss of an opportunity to design the intake research instrument that would have been possible with a prospective study.

We would argue in favour of the second or *post facto* follow-up whenever it is feasible, not only because it has been successful for us, but because we believe the advantages of being able to design the research intake interview are somewhat illusory. Studies of psychiatric outcome for children require a longer follow-up period to reach a decisive answer than is necessary for most other kinds of studies. There is the danger, in planning a research project that extends over the 20 years or so required to get the child past most of the age of risk for diseases like schizophrenia or alcoholism, that one may change one's tastes or one's locale and so give up the project or leave it to others to carry on. If others must finish it, they are no better off than the first researcher would have been using existing records, since the original collection of data was not designed with the special interests of the 'clean-up' team in mind. But even if the first researcher has sufficient perseverance to stay with his task to the end, new knowledge obtained by others (and himself) before he reaches the time for follow-up will probably have changed the state of the field enough so that he will wish he had asked different questions originally, or had at least scored answers in a different way.

And yet each researcher who starts with existing records regrets that they are not better. Is this an insoluble dilemma? Perhaps, but records *could* be much more useful for research than they usually are.

The kinds of data that would permit testing most of the current theories about factors related to the outcome of psychiatrically ill children are not so esoteric that any practitioner could not record them if he knew what was needed. If a few rules for recording at intake were adhered to, children seen now in hospitals, in clinics, and in private practice could well be used in 20 years by the practitioner himself or by someone else for research into the antecedents of adult problems. The list below contains the minimum data that should be collected. To do so, the doctor should use an intake form to insure collecting equivalent information for each patient.

A. Identifying data for use in later location of the patient and his records:
   1. Date and place of birth.
   2. Complete name, signed by the patient (or his parent if he is below school age), so that we need not rely on the intake interviewer's guesses at spellings. (In our previous study, we wasted great amounts of time searching for a Mr Newman who was really Mr Neumann and a Robert White was really *James* Robert White.)
   3. Names of all members of his household, their ages, and their relationship to the patient.
   4. Source of referral.

B. Description of the problem behaviour:
   1. The presenting complaint:
      (*a*) Its nature.
      (*b*) Its frequency.
      (*c*) The date of its first occurrence.
   2. Other complaints (described as above).
   3. Observations of behaviour by the psychiatrist or social worker.
   4. Behaviour problems elicited by direct questioning, but *not* complained of.

The description of the presenting complaints should be concrete, rather than interpretative. That is, 'he hits children at school' is preferable to 'he is aggressive'. 'He refuses to go anywhere with relatives or family friends unless accompanied by his mother' is preferable to 'he is overdependent'. Such concrete descriptions of behaviour will allow future researchers to categorize behaviour as seems most profitable at the later time rather than having to depend on categorizations by therapists using divergent definitions or using conceptual schemes that may seem less relevant in later years. Examining the 30-year-old clinic records used for our study, we found that concrete descriptions of behaviour reported by the social worker were extremely useful, and sounded completely contemporary, while the psychiatrist's evaluations sounded quaint and were quite untranslatable into modern terminology. 'Insecurity', 'affectionless character', 'inhibition of emotional expression', and other terms in current use, may in later years be just as perplexing to the researcher and as lacking in concrete referents as we found the psychiatrist's 30-year-old descriptions such as 'his whole understanding of life is on the basis of presenting to him dogmatic experiences that demand a stereotyped reaction from which there is no latitude of deviation' or 'her output of energy is moderate, but only in a restricted way is it expended in a well-synthesized manner'.

Making a careful distinction between complaints offered and answers to direct questions by the psychiatrist is particularly important if one hopes to assemble for follow-up studies materials collected at different times and by different psychiatrists. It is easy to elevate the reported rates of such common childhood behaviour as masturbation or lying by asking each child referred whether he has ever done these things. Since psychiatrists differ in the degree of probing for such behaviour and the levels at which they consider such behaviour to constitute symptoms, complaints volunteered by the referring agency are probably better predictive tools than is behaviour probed for. At least the behaviour complained of has occurred often enough or has been serious enough to mobilize people in the child's environment to take action.

We have argued here for more careful and consistent reporting of identifying data and complaint histories for children treated. While current recording techniques may be below desirable standards, at least *some* information is always available. But the same cannot be said for children referred but not treated. When a child is *not* treated, identifying data and a description of his complaint are seldom preserved. Yet such children would constitute the ideal control group for later evaluation of the success of treatment. It would be invaluable to have the information listed above recorded for *all* patients referred, with the addition, in the case of the untreated, of the reason treatment was not initiated and facilities to which the child was subsequently referred.

It may be utopian to hope that physicians will voluntarily set and adhere to minimum standards of record-keeping in order eventually to contribute their patients and unaccepted referrals to follow-up studies. Perhaps the answer lies in the area-wide registers of psychiatric patients which have recently been set up (Bahn)[1]. The register provides forms which must be filled out for each new patient admitted to a psychiatric facility. These registers in the United States have not yet successfully enrolled private physicians in their enterprise, nor have they requested records for untreated patients, but they promise to be excellent sources for choosing child patients for follow-up, and will also steer the researchers to those psychiatric facilities the child has used in later years.

Records, Interviews or Both?

The decision about whether records or interviews or a combination of the two are to be used at the intake point and again at the follow-up point will depend on the adequacy of and the freedom of access to existing records, the willingness and ability of subjects to be interviewed, and the validity of the responses given in interview. If the study population is made up of severely mentally deficient or brain-damaged children, records at both intake and follow-up will probably be as useful as interviews. If children are very young at intake, interviews can obviously be conducted only with relatives. On the other hand, if the prevalence of psychiatric disease is the outcome which one wishes to predict, interviews are essential at the endpoint, since we now well know that the treated cases which appear in records represent only a small proportion of the psychiatrically ill.

But setting aside situations in which the necessity for records or interviews is self-evident, there are advantages to both that are less commonly recognized.

Psychiatrists who are accustomed to asking for and obtaining intimate information from patients may tend to undervalue records as an important adjunct to evaluating the adult outcome of children. It is important to remember that at follow-up, the relationship with the subject has been initiated by the *doctor*. The subject is *not* asking for help and is not convinced that his contribution of the absolute truth is essential to his improvement or his continued well-being. It is perhaps remarkable that despite the fact that they have nothing obvious to gain by being interviewed, the vast majority of subjects agree to cooperate and answer the most personal questions honestly. But not *all* subjects will be found for interview at follow-up; not all those found will agree to cooperate; and of those who cooperate, not all will answer completely honestly. The use of records permits reducing the bias in the sample resulting from the non-response of some subjects and the lack of candour of others. We found in our previous follow-up study that concealment of discreditable behaviour was most common when the behaviour had been discontinued years before (Robins)[10]. It is then the most improved subjects, and therefore in some ways the most interesting, who are likely to be misidentified by using interviews alone. Another advantage of records is in elucidating answers given in interview. A subject in our current study reported that two years earlier he had had a 'nervous breakdown' with hospitalization subsequent to discovering his wife's infidelity. Only on reading the hospital record did it become clear that the wife's 'infidelity' was part of the subject's paranoid delusional system. His delusions were so well organized that they could not be detected in an interview. In this case, the record was essential to making a correct diagnosis. Another subject, when asked whether he had ever been in a hospital or sanatorium as a result of any psychiatric problem, denied psychiatric hospitalization. Yet records showed that he had been treated in a Federal hospital for narcotics addiction. We thought at first that he had attempted to conceal this in his interview, but on reviewing the interview protocol, we noted that he had named the location of the hospital in answering our question 'Have you ever lived out of St Louis?' and later in the interview admitted addiction to narcotics. He obviously had not considered drug addiction a psychiatric problem, nor the hospital to which he had been sent as a prisoner a psychiatric hospital. Records are, then, very helpful in avoiding errors resulting from the interviewer's and subject's failure to share common definitions of terms.

If it appears that the goals of the study could be met with data that records contain, it may seem unnecessary to interview. That is, if outcome is to be judged by educational level, mortality, hospitalization, or incarceration, the relevant information could theoretically be found in school records, death records, hospital records, and police records. The fly in the ointment, however, is that failure to locate a record does not necessarily mean it does not exist. In the study now in progress, for instance, we have sought subjects in the records of the school system and the Armed Forces, among others. A sizeable minority of those for whom we had found no such record reported in interview attending secondary school or serving in the Armed Forces. With information from the interview specifying which school and dates attended, which branch of the Service and dates of enlistment, we have often been able to locate a misplaced record or a record on which the identifying data did not quite agree with ours. (Boys often push their year of birth back two or three years if they want to enlist before they are of legal age.)

We are convinced that the most accurate estimate of outcome is obtained when *both* interviews and records are secured and when the researcher attempts to reconcile interview and record information. Each helps to illumine the other.

Adults or Children as Index Cases?

Post facto follow-up studies of children can use as the basis for the selection of subjects either a characteristic of the subjects as *children* or a characteristic of the subjects as *adults*. That is, one can either ask a question such as 'How do child guidance clinic patients turn out?' or alternatively 'What were schizophrenics like as children?' It has been more common to select cases on the basis of a childhood characteristic (as in our study, and in studies by the Gluecks[4], Terman[13], Skeels[12], Macfarlane[5], and the McCords[6]), but a few studies have started with adults and then located them as children in rosters of schools or children's clinics. The use of adult status as the basis for the selection of index cases is the more efficient method for studying childhood predictors of *rare* phenomena or of events occurring late in life. If one seeks childhood predictors of schizophrenia or suicide, even a population of disturbed children, such as our child guidance clinic population, will produce very few cases by age 45. But one can identify *adult* cases (in mental hospitals for schizophrenia, or from coroners' reports for suicides) and interview their relatives to learn where to look for records concerning their childhoods. From the school, birth, or clinic records that include the patient, an appropriate control subject can be chosen. Further information about the childhoods of both patients and controls can be sought in school records, juvenile police records, hospital and clinic admissions. Information about the kinds of families from which they came can be obtained by seeking similar records for their siblings and seeking records concerning their parents in social agency, hospital, and police records dating from their childhoods. These records can also be supplemented by retrospective interviews with relatives.

3
Tactics for Solving Problems Inherent in Follow-up Studies

Many methodological problems met in executing a follow-up study are not at all different from those met in the course of a cross-sectional study. Both kinds of studies present problems of sampling, interview design, interviewer training, maximizing cooperation, developing analytical codes for data reduction, planning statistical treatment. Many texts (see, for instance, Riley)[9] have dealt much more adequately with these problems than this brief chapter can. But there are methodological problems that are specific to the follow-up study. These have to do with treating the time intervals represented by the intake and follow-up periods, criteria for inclusion and omission of subjects, and methods for locating subjects, maximizing recovery rates, and avoiding contamination between data coming from the two time periods.

The Inequality of Time Intervals

The follow-up study concerns itself with three time periods: the history before intake; the 'current status' at follow-up; and the interval history between intake and the 'current status'. Ideally these periods should have the same duration for each subject. In practice, the time periods may vary widely between subjects. The length of the pre-intake period varies with the age of the subject at intake. Children who come to treatment before age 6 have had no opportunity to show many of the symptoms found in older children—school retardation, sexual deviance, poor work performance, to mention the most obvious. Subjects who vary in age at intake will also vary in age at follow-up, and consequently will have had varying numbers of years at risk for divorce, or job achievement, or other indices of adjustment that are restricted to adults. They will also vary in the proportion of the age of risk they have passed through in the development of various psychiatric illnesses. An equal interval of elapsed time between intake and follow-up is the easiest for the researcher to achieve. He can designate the year of intake and the year of follow-up. But even here he is hampered by the fact that the higher the proportion of the original cases he tries to recover, the greater the gap will be between the date of locating the first subject and the last. Subjects who are easy to find tend to be interviewed first, and therefore to have the shortest interval between intake and follow-up.

Epidemiologists have developed actuarial techniques for taking into account differences in years at risk which are applicable to follow-up studies. But the statistical elegance of age-specific rates cannot compensate for the instability of findings based on very few cases. When the original population varies markedly in age at intake and years between intake and follow-up, the cases in the higher age ranges at follow-up are inevitably sparse.

Some of the ways in which we attempted to minimize time inequalities in our previous study may illustrate possibilities for reducing this problem.

1. We restricted the period of referral to a few years. Some studies have followed patients seen over the whole history of a clinic—often as much as a 15 or 20 year period. At follow-up some of the recent patients are still children, while patients seen early are middle-aged. When the age difference is so great, outcomes are not comparable.

2. We supplemented the childhood history available at intake with juvenile records of treatment, school records, and juvenile police and juvenile court records. While this kind of supplementation does not provide the intense survey of symptomatology throughout childhood that would have been available had all patients come to the clinic in their late teens, at least it told us whether the younger patients ever developed serious antisocial behaviour in childhood. What we tried to do, in effect, was to raise the intake age to 18 for all the subjects, regardless of when they actually appeared in the clinic.

3. We made the follow-up interval sufficiently long (30 years) so that the subjects had been adult for many years. A reasonably stable adjustment could, then, be expected to exist at follow-up. Since changes are most rapid in youth, the longer the follow-up interval, the less difference do initial age discrepancies make.

4. We defined 'current status' as a 10-year period. The duration of 'the present' must be limited in some way. One day or one year is not sufficient because many of the criteria useful for assessing current adult adjustment imply an adjustment over time. Current job adjustment, for instance, includes the ideas of amount of unemployment and number of job

changes, both of which are meaningful only over time. The use of a fixed length of time to define 'the present' means that at least in this one of the three time periods every subject can have the same number of years at risk.

The methods we used minimized differences in the length of the intake period and gave 'current status' a uniform duration in approximately the same age ranges. These methods reduced the problem of varying time periods, but did not solve them. In a study now in progress, we have been able further to reduce the time variation by limiting the sample to men born within a five-year period, and by shortening the follow-up interviewing period to one year. We have also found it advisable to define the 'current status' as a 5-year rather than a 10-year period because many agencies destroy records after 5 years' inactivity.

Criteria for Inclusion of Subjects

Subjects can be included in a follow-up study only when data for both time periods can be obtained. If childhood information is inadequate or if subjects die before they reach adulthood, obviously their childhood patterns cannot be related to their adult patterns. It is a mistake, however, to omit subjects for whom it is merely *inconvenient* to collect adult data—those who have died recently, who are out of town, or who are hard to find at home. We found in our previous study that early death, absence from home, and geographical mobility were all strikingly related to psychiatric status. Alcoholics and sociopaths have elevated mortality rates, seldom remain in their home towns, are much more likely than other subjects to be incarcerated at follow-up, and if free are seldom found at home in the evening. Similarly, in our current study of Negro men, the ones hard to locate are found to lead very atypical existences. Some of them literally have *no* home address, but sleep occasionally at relatives' homes, sometimes at their girl friend's apartment, sometimes at a male friend's home. Moynihan[7] has noted the temporary disappearance of the young Negro male from census statistics and his reappearance at a later age. The young Negro male is only an extreme example of the fact that accessibility to interview and style of life adjustment are closely associated. Omitting subjects who are dead or difficult to locate obviously biases results. Investigating outcomes only for those readily found exaggerates both the rate of stable adjustment in a population and the rate of institutionalization. For this reason, follow-up studies that are to produce reliable results are expensive. We estimate that it cost approximately as much to locate the 76th to 90th per cent of our sample as to locate the whole first 75 per cent.

Methods of Locating Subjects to Maximize Recovery Rates

There are several generalizations which can be made about conditions under which subjects are hard or easy to locate.

1. The longer the elapsed time between the original contact and the time of follow-up, the greater will be the difficulty in locating the subjects.

2. The less stable the subjects, in terms of work habits and residence, the harder location is. Instability is not entirely a negative factor, though. Highly unstable people often leave in their wake a rich variety of public records. It is often possible to trace their progress from crime to crime or in the files of public agencies.

3. Men are easier to find than women because men do not routinely change their name and they register for the draft.

4. The more information one has about a given subject the easier it is to find him. This includes knowing complete identifying data, relatives' names, occupation, interests, and the part of the city in which he is likely to spend his leisure time.

Among the various public and private records that have provided us clues to the location of subjects are records of social agencies, the police, hospitals, driver's licence rosters, credit ratings, Armed Services and veterans' records, marriage and death records, lists of registered voters, unemployment compensation records, and lists of taxpayers.

In the course of our studies, we have learned many techniques for simplifying the process of locating subjects. It is hard to judge how many of these have general utility. But there seem to be certain broad principles.

If one plans to use both records and interviews, locating subjects for interview should *follow* the search for records. In the process of checking adult records, one will accumulate occupational histories, previous addresses, names of relatives, and learn whether there are errors in or additions to the original identifying data, such as middle names, aliases, etc. All such data assist in location.

In checking records, we often discover the name of one or more relatives. When we are unable to locate a subject it seems logical to ask help from his relative before resorting to other measures. Beware! Some relatives, particularly mothers, not only refuse to give any information but also alert the subject so that when he is located he will refuse to be interviewed. Other relatives, of course, are extremely helpful.

When using records, either for the location of a subject or to obtain follow-up information, there is always the chance that a pertinent record will be missed or that it will be found but cannot be identified as belonging to the subject. One learns that the order in which records are pursued has a good deal to do with avoiding such problems. In our study, police records have been generally the best place to start. The reasons are as follows: first, a large percentage of the population appears in the police files, since even the upright may have a traffic offence. Second, the police record race, place of birth, date of birth, address, occupation, and frequently height, weight and physical disabilities, as well as the offence, permitting positive identification based on childhood information, and providing much new information that will be helpful in identifying the subject in other files. Third, the police make out a new card for each contact, so that the address and occupation can be *dated*. Agencies that keep running files frequently record new contacts without bothering to recheck addresses or birth dates so that changes in address are not noted and original errors in birth dates remain uncorrected.

Once a complete set of identifying data has been obtained from a source such as the police, identification becomes possible in much less adequate files. A name and an early address alone may be sufficient to positively identify the subject in, for instance, the files of a credit bureau. And that file may, in turn, yield the subject's current address.

Old addresses are also useful for locating subjects by methods other than record search. Sometimes relatives with whom the subject once lived are still at the old address. If not, the neighbours often know where the subject has moved. Finally, the old address provides a clue to choosing among addresses found in the current City Directory or telephone book for subjects with common names. The address closest to the old address is the best choice, for city dwellers who move usually stay in the same neighbourhoods.

Maximizing Cooperation

The exact procedure to be followed in order to obtain the highest rate of interviews undoubtedly varies with the kind of population being studied. Pilot studies provide an opportunity to experiment with ways of obtaining cooperation from subjects. Especially if the subject was seen first as a child and is now being seen at follow-up as an adult, he probably will not know the investigators and may not even remember having been seen in a clinic or hospital. He will have to be convinced not only that the research is valuable, but that he has been correctly identified as a potential subject. It has been our experience that the best procedure is to write a letter which explains the general purpose of the study and says that the subject can expect to hear later from the investigator. This letter should be short, general, and avoid emphasis on the psychiatric nature of the study or on the nature of the original problem. Offering a rationale for the study which does not distinguish between patients and control subjects is best, so that a subject does not identify himself as belonging to one group or the other. The letter may invite the subject to call for an appointment if he wishes, but should not specify when the interviewer will visit him. Setting a definite time for the visit gives the subject an opportunity to avoid being seen and thus to become one of the most time-consuming problems in follow-up studies—the subject who neither cooperates nor refuses outright. While not alerting him to the time of the planned visit avoids *this* problem, it may mean that the interviewer does not find the subject at home or free at the time of the first visit, and a number of visits may be necessary.

Offering to pay a subject for his time is a controversial issue in research. Middle-class subjects may be insulted and suspicious of the motives of the researcher if payment is offered. On the other hand, in the study now in progress with a predominantly lower-class male population, the offer of payment seems to be responsible for a surprisingly high rate of cooperation and a tremendous saving in time and funds. As a result of offering in our letter a higher rate to subjects who volunteer to come to our office for the interview than to those we interview at home, we find that half of the subjects interviewed have volunteered. Less than 2 per cent of those personally asked for an interview have refused. The advantages are not only those of low refusal rates and having to spend little time in fruitless efforts to see subjects at home, but also in providing in the office a more private interviewing situation than most slum homes afford. We have also been startled by the high level of honesty with which subjects have reported the one kind of activity we have checked against record reports—narcotics use. It is possible that accepting payment has created a moral obligation to provide all the facts requested. At least payment does not seem to have interfered with achieving candid answers.

Avoiding Contamination of Intake and Follow-Up Data

In follow-up studies, as in an experiment, it is necessary to protect against the evaluation of the outcome's being influenced by the experimenter's knowledge about the pre-existing characteristics of the subject. Unlike an experiment, it is *also* necessary in a *post facto* follow-up study to protect against a knowledge of the outcome's having an influence on the evaluation of the pre-existing state. That is, a coder analysing outcome may be biased by knowing what the subject was like as a child; and the coder knowing outcome, may equally well exaggerate in the childhood record phenomena that might have allowed the prediction of the outcome. Preventing contamination in both directions is facilitated by *not* allowing the interviewer to know whether he is interviewing a patient or a control subject, and keeping this information from the coder as well. It is also helpful to have different persons score childhood and adult protocols. Despite the best of intentions, however, it is hard to keep the early and late data separate. It is often necessary to include some questions about childhood in the follow-up interview (to make sure, for instance, that school records obtained are complete), and in any case, subjects frequently reminisce about their childhood in interview. Where 'double-blind' methods fail, the best safeguard seems to be scoring the data in a factual way that allows as little scope as possible to the coder's overall evaluations. The degree of inadequacy of the childhood home, for instance, is more adequately scored by enumerating the ways in which it was inadequate (family on welfare, father deserted, mother cited for neglect, child underweight, clothes dirty at intake, etc.) than by the coder's overall judgment which places the home on a 7-point scale. Computers are particularly useful for recoding scores on a large set of criteria into a scale score. Such analysis techniques also produce better predictive tools than do pre-arranged scales because criteria can be dropped when they are found not to predict outcome.

We have discussed here some of the basic problems in follow-up studies, and some of the ways we have tried to mitigate these problems. To discuss methods further would involve us in the details of bookkeeping necessary to cumulate and reconcile information from various records and from interviews, in the details of designing interview schedules to allow standardization combined with flexibility, and in the design of codes and an analysis plan. Such topics would be of interest only to people personally involved in doing follow-up studies.

Enough has been said, without elaborating these other technical problems, to show that carrying out a follow-up study requires considerable planning, financial resources, and effort. It has been fashionable recently, at least in the United States, to include an evaluation plan in every demonstration project that attempts to improve the treatment of children. These evaluations have not, in general, answered the important question: Are the methods used more effective than previously available methods? They have instead offered information on how many cases were seen, how many visits per case, the cost per visit, and how many children were discharged as 'well', 'improved' or 'unimproved'. They have generally failed to develop criteria for improvement that would permit comparisons between one treatment technique and another; they have failed to present evidence that the levels of improvement achieved would not have occurred over the same time interval without therapy or using older methods; and they have failed to specify which kinds of syndromes responded to treatment. When we consider the vast amounts of money and effort that are being poured into the treatment process, it would seem that the investment of the time, effort, and expertise needed to evaluate treatment by carefully designed follow-up studies is not excessive. But a casual evaluation may well be worse than none at all, since it may falsely confirm us in our habits or falsely overthrow our confidence in perfectly adequate techniques.

REFERENCES

1. BAHN, ANITA K., GARDNER, E. A., ALLTOP, L., KNATTERUD, G. L., and SOLOMON, M., 1966. Admission and prevalence rates for psychiatric facilities in four register areas. *Am. J. Public Health*, **52**, 2033-51.
2. CHESS, STELLA, THOMAS, A., RUTTER, M., and BIRCH, H. G., 1963. Interaction of temperament and environment in the production of behavioral disturbances in children. *Amer. J. Psychiat.*, **120**, 142-47.
3. CHRISTIANSEN, H. T., 1958. The method of record linkage applied to family data. *Marriage and Family Living*, **20**, 38-43.
4. GLUECK, S., and GLUECK, ELEANOR, 1940. *Juvenile delinquents grown up*. New York, The Commonwealth Fund.
5. MACFARLANE, JEAN W., 1964. Perspectives on personality consistency and change from the guidance study. *Vita Humana*, **7**, 115-26.
6. McCORD, W., and McCORD, JEAN, 1959. *Origins of crime*. New York, Columbia Univ. Press.
7. MOYNIHAN, D. P., 1965. *The negro family: the case for national action*. U.S. Department of Labor.

8. NAMECHE, G., WARING, MARY, and RICKS, D., 1964. Early indicators of outcome in schizophrenia. *J. Nerv. Ment. Dis.*, **139**, 232-40.
9. RILEY, MATHILDA W., 1963. *Sociological research: a case approach.* New York, Harcourt, Brace and World.
10. ROBINS, LEE, 1966. *Deviant children grown up: a sociological and psychiatric study of sociopathic personality.* Baltimore, Williams and Wilkins.
11. ROFF, M., 1956. Preservice personality problems and subsequent adjustment to military service: gross outcome in relation to acceptance-rejection at induction and military service. *U.S. Air Force School of Aviation Medicine. Report No.* 55-138.
12. SKEELS, H. M., and SKODAK, MARIE, 1965. Techniques for a high-yield follow-up study in the field. *Public Health Reports*, **80**, 249-57.
13. TERMAN, L. M., and ODEN, MELITA H., 1959. *The gifted group at mid-life, genetic studies of genius V.* Stanford, Cal., Stanford Univ. Press.
14. TUCKMAN, J., and REGAN, R. A., 1966. Problems referred to children's outpatient psychiatric clinics. *J. Hlth Human Behav.*, **7**, 54-58.

AUTHOR INDEX

This index covers volumes 1, 2 and 3 of the Modern Perspectives in Psychiatry series, the figures in bold type denoting the volume of entry.

Abe, S. **2**: 52, 86
Abelson, R. **1**: 140, 149
Abercrombie, M. L. J. **1**: 212, 219, 232
Aberle, D. F. **3**: 141, 150
Abood, L. G. **2**: 279, 285
Abraham, K. **1**: 485, 487, 493
Abramovitz, A. **1**: 128, 149; **2**: 565, 574
Abramson, H. A. **2**: 614
Abramyan, L. A. **2**: 428, 445
Abt, L. G. **2**: 386
Acheson, R. M. **3**: 21, 56
Ackerman, N. W. **1**: 368; **3**: 125, 150, 357, 359, 368
Ackerson, L. **1**: 370, 398; **3**: 739, 757
Adams, C. W. M. **2**: 84
Adams, H. B. **2**: 250, 252, 254
Adams, J. M. **3**: 60
Adams, R. B. **2**: 113, 127
Adams, R. D. **2**: 121, 122, 123, 127
Adams, S. **1**: 398
Addis, T. **2**: 103
Adelson, L. **3**: 585
Adey, W. R. **2**: 262
Adler, A. **2**: 150
Adrian, E. D. **2**: xix, 342, 348
Aftanas, M. **2**: 236, 263
Afterman, J. **3**: 155
Agadzhanian, N. A. **2**: 251
Agnew, H. W. **2**: 216, 218
Agranoff, B. W. **2**: 99, 103, 104
Agudov, V. V. **2**: 428, 445
Ahlenstiel, H. **2**: 271, 285
Ahnsjö, S. **3**: 764, 783
Ahrens, R. **1**: 89, 101
Aichhorn, A. **1**: 242, 247; **3**: 5
Ainslie, J. D. **2**: 619
Ainsworth, M. D. **1**: 19, 243, 247; **3**: 121, 283, 290, 545
Ainsworth, R. **2**: 262
Ajmone-Marsan, C. **2**: 286
Ajuriaguerra, U. **3**: 201, 202, 218
Akert, K. **2**: 217, 218
Åkesson, H. O. **1**: 43, 55
Akimoto, H. **3**: 369
Akmurin, I. A. **2**: 436

Alanen, Y. O. **2**: 410, 411, 417, 421, 422
Albee, G. W. **2**: 355, 386
Albrecht, R. M. **1**: 369
Albright, F. **2**: 46
Albright, G. A. **2**: 258
Albright, R. J. **2**: 263
Alcaraz, M. **2**: 189
Aldestein, A. M. **1**: 368
Aldridge, V. J. **2**: 192, **3**: 417
Alexander, D. **2**: 44
Alexander, F. **1**: 312, 334; **2**: 448, 477, 479; **3**: 473, 474
Alexander, H. C. B. **3**: 652, 676
Alexander, H. M. **2**: 252
Alexander, W. P. **1**: 195, 572, 584
Algeri, **3**: 603
Allee, W. C. **1**: 33, 36
Allen, A. **3**: 585
Allen, I. M. **1**: 344, 349
Allen, J. M. **2**: 85
Allen, L. **1**: 168, 400; **3**: 79
Allison R. S. **2**: 124, 127
Allport, G. **1**: 119, 146
Alltop, L. **3**: 803
Almy, T. P. **3**: 525
Alon, M. **3**: 336, 337, 334
Alperin, M. **2**: 255
Alpert, A. **1**: 245, 247; **3**: 700, 705
Alpert, M. **3**: 669, 679
Altman, J. **2**: 88, 101, 103, 104
Altman, J. W. **2**: 251
Altshuler, K. D. **2**: 449, 479
Alzheimer, A. **3**: 606
Amatruda, C. S. **1**: 233, 566, 585; **3**: 318, 470
Ambrose, G. J. **2**: 181, 187
Ambrose, J. A. **1**: 90, 101
Amen, E. A. **1**: 97, 101
Ames, L. B. **1**: 100, 101
Ancona, L. **3**: 141, 150
Andermann, K. **3**: 666, 678
Anders, J. M. **2**: 46
Anderson, **1**: 389
Anderson A. N. **3**: 123
Anderson, E. W. **2**: 285; **3**: 34, 56

Anderson, G. **3**: 56
Anderson, G. W. **3**: 23, 56
Anderson, J. E. **2**: 251
Anderson, L. R. **3**: 585
Anderson, N. **3**: 152
Anderson, O. **3**: 747, 757
Anderson, P. J. **2**: 84
Anderson, W. J. R. **3**: 27, 56
Andics, M. von **1**: 413, 426
Andrew, R. J. **1**: 28, 36
Andrews, J. P. **3**: 585
Andrews, T. G. **2**: 386
Andry, R. **1**: 374
Andry, R. G. **3**: 145, 150, 281, 290
Anell, B. **3**: 469
Angevine, J. B. (Jr.) **2**: 114, 129
Angiolella **3**: 591
Annell, A. L. **3**: 675, 676, 783
Annigoni, P. **2**: 143
Ann Josephine, Sister **2**: 45
Anthony, A. **3**: 315, 320
Anthony, E. J. **1**: 214, 232, 579, 584
Anthony, J. **1**: 238, 247, 412, 426, 487, 493
Antin, R. **2**: 422
Apley J. **1**: 310, 326, 334
Appelbaum, A. **2**: 482, 485
Appell, G. **3**: 98, 121, 122
Appleby, L. **2**: 418
Arajarvi, T. **3**: 525
Archer, G. T. **3**: 528
Arduini, A. **2**: 251
Aresin, N. **3**: 29, 56
Argyle, M. **1**: 374, 395, 398
Arieti, S. **2**: 420; **3**: 681
Aristotle, **2**: 139, 147
Armitage, S. **1**: 148
Armitage, S. G. **3**: 52, 56
Armstrong, J. **3**: 750, 757
Arnhoff, F. N. **2**: 251
Asch, H. **3**: 527
Aschaffenberg, G. **2**: 415, **3**: 13
Aserinsky, E. **2**: 199, 216
Ash, P. **2**: 365, 386
Ashcroft, G. W. **2**: 219, 220
Ashley, D. J. B. **2**: 44
Ashley, F. W. **2**: 615
Ashworth, P. L. **2**: 409, 421

805

AUTHOR INDEX

Askevold, F. **3**: 525
Aslanov, A. **2**: 555, 556
Asperger, H. **3**: 650, 651, 674, 675, 676, 677
Astington, E. **1**: 575, 584
Astrup, C. **2**: 391, 415
Atkinson, **3**: 293
Aubin, H. **2**: 702, 710
Aubry, J. **3**: 139, 150
Auerback, A. **2**: 415, 418, 480, 481, 483, 485, 486
Augburg, T. **2**: 262
Aukee, M. **3**: 525
Austin, M. C. **3**: 735, 757
Ausubel, D. B. **3**: 492
Ax, A. **2**: 293, 296, 309, 310
Ayats, H. **2**: 710
Ayllon, T. **1**: 139, 143, 146; **2**: 570, 573
Azima, H. **2**: 251
Azrin, A. H. **1**: 146
Azrin, N. **1**: 147

Babich, F. R. **2**: 104, 106
Babott, J. **3**: 58
Bach, G. R. **3**: 141, 150
Bachrach, A. J. **2**: 573
Bachrach, A. L. **1**: 146
Backett, E. M. **1**: 361, 368
Bacon, C. L. **2**: 481
Bacon, F. **1**: 9
Bacon, H. K. **3**: 146, 150
Badarraco, G. **3**: 201, 202, 218
Baer, D. M. **1**: 114, 136, 140, 142, 146, 147
Bagot, J. **1**: 375, 398
Bahn, A. K. **3**: 794, 803
Baikie, A. G. **2**: 46, 47, **3**: 60
Bailey, M. A. **2**: 221
Bailey, P. **2**: 448, 479
Bain, K. **3**: 585
Baird, D. **3**: 27, 56
Bakan, P. **2**: 257
Baker, A. **2**: 728
Baker, A. A. **2**: 614
Bakwin, H. **1**: 358, 368; **2**: 251; **3**: 9, 585
Bakwin, R. **1**: 358, 368
Baldridge, B. J. **2**: 216
Baldwin, A. L. **1**: 375, 398; **3**: 746, 757
Baldwin, M. **2**: 286
Balint, E. M. **1**: 368
Balint, M. **1**: 309, 311, 334; **2**: 457, 458, 477, 479, 686, 694; **3**: 121, 210, 218
Ballet, **3**: 606
Ball Mairet, **3**: 597
Bally, C. **2**: 217, 218
Balser, R. **1**: 413, 426
Banay, R. S. **1**: 383, 398
Bandura, A. **1**: 140, 146; **2**: 376, 386
Banks, R. **2**: 216

Bannister, D. **2**: 366, 367, 386
Banta, T. J. **3**: 151
Barber, T. X. **2**: 177, 179, 181, 187
Barbizet, J. **2**: 113, 127, 216
Barbour, R. F. **2**: 216
Barchilon, J. **2**: 614
Bargen, J. A. **3**: 527
Barik, H. **2**: 104
Barka, T. **2**: 84
Barker, J. C. **2**: 573
Barker, W. F. **3**: 528
Barmack, J. E. **2**: 218
Barmeyer, G. H. **3**: 585
Barnard, C. W. **2**: 251
Barnett, J. A. **1**: 382, 398
Barnett, P. E. **2**: 106
Barnett, S. A. **3**: 28, 56, 57
Baron, A. **2**: 251
Baron, D. **3**: 745, 757
Barondes, S. H. **2**: 98, 104
Barr, K. L. **1**: 51, 55
Barr, M. L. **1**: 51, 55; **2**: 20, 21, 44, 45, 47, 48
Barrett, B. H. **1**: 136, 146
Barrett, P. E. H. **2**: 216
Barron, A. **3**: 240, 250
Barron, A. J. **3**: 586
Barron, S. H. **3**: 154, 512, 525, 528
Barry, H. A. A. **3**: 146, 150
Barta, R. A. (Jr.) **3**: 585
Bartels, M. **3**: 85, 86, 97
Barth, T. **2**: 252
Bartlett, E. M. **1**: 192
Bartlett, F. C. **3**: 553, 568
Bartlett, J. E. A. **2**: 251, 272, 286
Barton, J. **3**: 57
Barton Hall, M. **1**: 487, 493
Barton Hall, S. **1**: 334
Basamania, B. **2**: 415
Basowitz, H. **1**: 482, 493
Bassin, F. V. **2**: 594
Bastiaans, J. **1**: 313, 335
Basu, G. K. **2**: 264
Batchelor, I. R. C. **1**: 412, 426
Bateson, G. **2**: 396, 399, 404, 410, 417, 418, 466, 479; **3**: 296
Batipps, D. M. **2**: 47
Batten, **3**: 9
Baumert, G. **3**: 746, 758
Baune, H. **1**: 368
Baxter, J. **3**: 677
Bayley, N. **3**: 121, 123
Bazett, C. **2**: 315, 348
Bazzi, T. **3**: 731
Beach, F. A. **2**: 128
Beard, G. **2**: 520
Beard, R. **1**: 82
Bearsley, R. K. **3**: 369, 370, 371
Beatman, F. L. **2**: 418, 420
Beavers, W. R. **2**: 411, 422

Bechterev, V. M. **1**: 104; **2**: 578, 582, 593
Beck, S. J. **2**: 418; **3**: 666, 667, 677
Becker, E. **2**: 412, 423
Becker, W. C. **3**: 145, 150, 154, 745, 758
Beckett, P. G. S. **2**: 16, 19, 298, 310, 410, 421; **3**: 153
Beckman, M. **2**: 143
Beecher, H. K. **2**: 603, 614, 616, 619
Beers, C. **3**: 6
Beh, H. C. **2**: 216
Béhague, P. **3**: 414, 416
Behrens, M. **3**: 705
Beilin, H. **3**: 740, 758
Beiser, H. R. **3**: 65, 79
Belenkov, N. U. **2**: 544, 555
Bell, **3**: 171
Bell, J. **2**: 4, 7, 17
Bell, N. W. **2**: 420; **3**: 146, 151, 152, 154
Bellak, R. **3**: 368
Bellak, L. **1**: 577, 584; **2**: 477, 480, 482, 695; **3**: 651, 653, 677, 679
Beller, E. K. **3**: 752, 761
Belleville, R. E. **2**: 216
Bellugi, U. **3**: 551, 553, 554, 568
Beloff, J. **2**: 146, 187
Belval, P. C. **2**: 104
Bena, E. **2**: 216
Benda, C. **3**: 661, 677
Bender, L. **1**: 93, 101, 236, 239, 247, 357, 368, 383, 384, 398, 408, 426, 473, 492, 493, 582, 584; **2**: 412, 423; **3**: 147, 610, 649, 651, 652, 653, 654, 655, 656, 657, 659, 660, 664, 666, 667, 668, 669, 671, 672, 675, 676, 677, 678, 679, 705
Bendix, R. **3**: 309, 319
Bene, E. **1**: 579, 584
Benedict, R. **3**: 295, 296, 312, 317, 353, 357, 362, 368
Beniest-Noirot, E. **3**: 129, 151
Ben Israel, N. **3**: 328, 344
Benjamin, F. B. **2**: 258
Benjamin, J. D. **1**: 244, 247; **2**: 449, 459, 480; **3**: 121
Bennett, A. M. H. **2**: 251
Bennett, E. L. **2**: 88, 103, 104
Bensch, C. **2**: 217
Benson, P. F. **1**: 320, 335
Bentinck, C. **2**: 252
Bentler, P. M. **1**: 128, 129, 146
Benton, A. L. **1**: 455, 472, 583, 584
Ber, R. **3**: 469
Bereday, G. **1**: 184, 190
Berenda, C. W. **2**: 355, 386
Beres, D. **3**: 653, 660, 678
Berg, H. M. **3**: 492

AUTHOR INDEX

Berg, I. A. **2**: 390
Berg, J. M. **1**: 57, 496, 502, 503, 516, 518, 520; **3**: 469
Berg, R. M. **3**: 472, 492
Bergemann, E. **2**: 45
Bergen, J. R. **1**: 494
Berger, M. **3**: 655, 674, 682
Berger, R. J. **2**: 201, 216, 220, 291, 292, 309; **3**: 391
Bergmann, P. **1**: 236, 247; **2**: 476, 480; **3**: 121
Bergmann, T. **2**: 480, **3**: 121
Bergstrand, C. G. **1**: 404, 405, 409, 426
Beringer, K. **2**: 426, 445
Berko, J. **3**: 553, 568
Berko, M. J. **1**: 219, 232
Berks, J. E. **3**: 529
Berlyne, D. E. **1**: 80, 82, 89, 101
Berman, P. W. **1**: 455, 472, 573, 585
Bernard, V. **2**: 679; **3**: 337, 344
Berner, P. **3**: 651, 675, 678
Bernfeld, S. **1**: 412, 426
Bernhard, W. **2**: 52
Bernhardt, K. G. **2**: 335, 371, 386
Bernhardt, K. S. **3**: 142, 151
Bernheim, H. **2**: 149, 150, 187
Bernstein, B. **3**: 537, 545
Bernstein, N. **2**: 436, 445
Beron, L. **3**: 146, 151
Berry, H. K. **1**: 507, 520
Bert, J. **2**: 217
Bertalanffy, L. von **3**: 96
Bertram, E. G. **1**: 51, 55; **2**: 44
Bertram, M. L. **2**: 21, 44, 45
Bertrand, C. **2**: 348
Bertrand, I. **2**: 45
Bertschinger, **3**: 597
Berze, J. **2**: 426, 445
Beteleva, T. G. **2**: 251
Bettelheim, B. **1**: 492, 493
Bettley, F. R. **2**: 181, 188,
Betz, B. J. **1**: 492, 493
Beutler, E. **2**: 45
Bevan-Lewis, **3**: 597
Bevers, T. G. **3**: 554, 568
Bexton, W. H. **2**: 251, 255, 260, 286, 299, 310
Bianchi, L. **3**: 591, 602
Biase, D. V. **2**: 264
Biber, B. **3**: 328, 333, 337, 344
Bibring, E. **1**: 410, 426
Bibring, G. L. **3**: 83, 84, 96
Bice, H. V. **1**: 472
Bickford, R. C. **2**: 112, 127
Bidwell **1**: 471, 472
Biel, J. H. **2**: 285
Biersdorf, K. R. **1**: 577, 584
Bijou, S. W. **1**: 114, 135, 141, 143, 146, 150
Bilikiewicz, T. **3**: 675, 678

Billing, L. **3**: 526
Binet, A. **1**: 97, 101, 185, 190, 570; **3**: 5
Bingham, J. **1**: 182, 190
Bingley, T. **1**: 464, 472
Bini, L. **3**: 719, 731
Binswanger, L. **2**: 517
Binzwanger, O. **3**: 599
Bion, W. R. **2**: 477, 480
Birch, H. G. **1**: 381, 398, 399; **3**: 74, 79, 474, 493, 738, 743, 758, 763, 803,
Birch, J. W. **1**: 217, 233
Birch, L. B. **1**: 171, 190, 233
Birdwhistell, R. L, **3**: 143, 151
Birman, B. N. **2**: 582, 594
Birnbach, S. B. **1**: 360, 368
Birth, K. **3**: 736, 758
Bishop, A. **2**: 45
Bishop, O. N. **2**: 45
Bizan, I. U. P. **2**: 251
Blachy, P. H. **2**: 251
Black, A. A. **2**: 614
Black, J. A. **1**: 436, 450
Black, S. **2**: 146, 153, 154, 155, 159, 162, 163, 164, 166, 167, 168, 169, 174, 175, 176, 178, 179, 182, 184, 185, 186, 188, 190, 191
Blacker, C. P. **1**: 255, 283
Blacker, K. H. **2**: 312
Blakemore, C. B. **2**: 573
Blank, C. E. **1**: 511, 520; **2**: 45
Blau, A. **3**: 653, 678
Bleuler, E. **2**: 4, 17, 265, 415, 426, 445; **3**: 649, 657, 678, 706, 731
Bleuler, M. **2**: 309
Bliss, E. L. **2**: 204, 216, 310; **3**: 97
Block J. **2**: 419; **3**: 142, 151
Block, J. **2**: 419
Blodgett, H. C. **1**: 165, 168
Blom, G. E. **3**: 525
Blomfield, J. M. **1**: 43, 55, 437, 450; **3**: 35, 57
Bloom, A. A. **3**: 526
Blum, R. **2**: 282, 286, 287
Blumberg, S. **2**: 422
Blundell, J. **2**: 176, 189
Boardman, H. E. **3**: 585
Boardman, W. **1**: 116, 146
Boatman, M. J. **2**: 465, 466, 480
Bocquet, F. **3**: 150
Bodian, D. **2**: 64, 84
Boesch, E. **3**: 747, 758
Bogen, J. E. **2**: 111, 127
Bogoch, S. **2**: 16, 17, 102, 103, 104
Boisen, A. T. **2**: 365, 386
Boismont, Brierre de **2**: 265
Boles, G. **1**: 226, 233
Bolland, J. **2**: 476, 480; **3**: 121, 249, 250

Bollea, G. **3**: 706
Bond, J. **2**: 47
Bonhoeffer, K. **2**: 427, 443, 445; **3**: 707, 731
Bonnard, A. **3**: 222
Bonney, M. E. **3**: 734, 735, 744, 758
Bonnier, P. **2**: 130, 132, 140, 145
Booher, J. **2**: 84
Böök, J. A. **1**: 43, 47, 55; **2**: 11, 17
Boonin, N. **2**: 680, 695
Borda, R. P. **2**: 190
Bordeaux, J. **2**: 190
Bordeleau, J. M. **2**: 635, 701, 710
Boring, E. G. **2**: 251
Borisova, **2**: 548
Borland, E. M. **2**: 216
Bornstein, B. **3**: 426, 453
Bornstein, M. B. **2**: 78, 84
Borrus, J. C. **3**: 58
Borton, H. **3**: 370
Bosch, A. **3**: 674, 678
Boss, M. **2**: 488, 510, 511, 517
Boston, M. **1**: 19
Bostroem, A. **2**: 441, 445
Boszormenyi-Nagy, I. **2**: 409, 420, 421, 480, 483, 485
Botkin, S.P. **2**: 435
Bourne, G. H. **2**: 44
Bourne, H. **1**: 518, 520; **3**: 532, 533, 545
Bournville, D.-M. **3**: 608
Bovet, L. **1**: 370, 398
Bowen, M. **1**: 112, 147; **2**: 394, 395, 396, 397, 398, 401, 414, 415, 464, 480
Bower, E. M. **3**: 734, 737, 740, 741, 747, 758
Bowlby, J. **1**: 15, 19, 36, 214, 215, 233, 243, 244, 247, 334, 485, 494; **2**: 449, 452, 457, 477, 480; **3**: 9, 82, 96, 121, 138, 151, 175, 209, 210, 218, 265, 266, 281, 282, 284, 290, 300, 301, 317, 340, 344, 545, 655, 659, 673, 678, 746, 758
Bowman, P. W. **3**: 676, 677, 681
Boyd, E. **2**: 46
Boyd, G. R. **3**: 734, 758
Boyd, H. **1**: 35, 36
Boyd, M. M. **2**: 216
Bracchi, F. **2**: 191
Brachet, J. **2**: 105
Bracken, H. van **2**: 387
Bradburn, N. M. **3**: 141, 151
Braden, I. **2**: 256
Bradford Hill, A. **3**: 21, 57
Bradley, C. **1**: 112, 147; **3**: 651, 678, 705
Bradley, P. B. **2**: 309, 635

AUTHOR INDEX

Brady, J. 1: 135, 136, 142, 147
Braid, J. 2: 149, 188
Brain, R. 2: 108, 124, 127, 129, 328, 330, 334
Braine, M. D. S. 1: 78, 82, 96, 101; 3: 470, 552, 568
Bram, F. M. 3: 317
Brandon, M. W. G. 1: 498, 501, 507, 508, 520
Brandon, S. 1: 384, 398
Brashear, E. L. 3: 750, 758
Brattgard, S-O. 2: 104
Brauchi, J. T. 2: 286
Braun, E. J. 3: 585
Braun, J. G. 3: 585
Braunstein, P. 1: 494; 3: 680
Bray, P. 2: 45
Brazelton, T. B. 3: 121
Brazier, M. A. B. 2: 84, 85
Breese, F. H. 1: 398
Breg, W. R. 2: 47
Breland, O. P. 3: 151
Bremer, F. 2: 251
Brengleman, J. C. 1: 399
Brenman, M. 2: 477, 482
Brennemann, J. 3: 10
Brenner, R. F. 1: 447, 448, 450
Bressler, B. 2: 252; 3: 525
Breuer, J. 2: 150, 156, 189, 490; 3: 293, 317
Briffault, R. 3: 126, 151
Briggs, J. H. 1: 57; 2: 46
Briggs, M. H. 2: 104
Briggs, S. M. 1: 521
Brill, A. A. 3: 652
Brilluen, L. 2: 440
Brim, O. G. (Jr.) 3: 749, 758
Brink, J. J. 2: 103
Brion, M. 2: 728
Brion, S. 2: 114, 127
Brisaud, 3: 608
Brittain, P. P. 2: 46
Broadbent, D. 1: 145, 147; 3: 566, 567, 568
Broberger, O. 3: 525
Broca, P. 2: 323, 331, 348
Brockway, A. L. 3: 414, 416
Brodey, W. M. 2: 397, 415, 416
Brodie, B. B. 2: 276, 286
Brodie, F. H. 1: 220, 234
Brodmann, 2: 66
Brodskii, V. Ya. 2: 104, 107
Brody, E. B. 2: 416
Brody, M. W. 2: 573
Brody, S. 3: 121
Broer, P. 3: 683
Bromberg, W. 1: 398; 3: 652
Bronfenbrenner, J. 3: 746, 751, 758
Bronfenbrenner, U. 3: 306, 317
Bronner, A. 1: 400
Brooke, E. 2: 695
Brophy, A. L. 2: 355, 386

Brosin, H. W. 2: 480
Brotemarkle, R. A. 2: 354, 386
Brower, D. 2: 386
Brown, C. H. 3: 525, 528
Brown, F. 1: 412, 426
Brown, G. 2: 315
Brown, G. W. 2: 412, 423, 679, 695
Brown, J. L. 3: 682
Brown, R. 3: 547, 551, 553, 554, 568
Brown, R. H. 1: 151; 2: 251
Brown, W. 3: 473, 493
Brownfield, C. A. 2: 251
Bruce, D. 3: 553, 554, 568
Bruce, H. M. 3: 29, 57
Bruch, H. 1: 313, 334; 3: 151, 642
Bruhn, G. C. 1: 426
Bruner, J. S. 2: 243, 251, 299, 310
Brunngraber, E. G. 2: 104
Brunton, M. 2: 46
Bryant, H. D. 3: 585
Bryant, K. 3: 649, 653, 660, 679
Bryson, S. 2: 251
Bubash, S. 2: 104, 106
Buch, M. K. B. 2: 171, 189
Buchmueller, A. D. 3: 758, 760
Buck, C. 2: 106
Buckton, K. A. 2: 47
Buckton, K. E. 3: 60
Bühler, K. 1: 61, 88, 101, 388; 3: 5
Bull, J. P. 2: 614
Bullard, D. M. 2: 423
Bullis, G. E. 1: 88, 102
Bunge, M. B. 2: 76, 84
Bunge, R. P. 2: 76, 84
Bunzel, B. 1: 408, 413, 426
Bur, G. E. 1: 50, 56; 2: 48
Burch, N. R. 2: 270, 286
Burch, P. R. J. 2: 15, 17
Burchard, J. 2: 570, 573
Burchinal, L. G. 3: 141, 151
Burgum, M. 3: 146, 151
Burkinshaw, J. 3: 24, 57
Burlingham, D. 2: 254, 481; 3: 141, 152, 221, 236, 237, 240, 241, 244, 250, 251, 265
Burney, C. 2: 252
Burnham, D. L. 2: 457, 458, 477, 480
Burns, C. 3: 650, 675, 678
Burns, C. L. C. 2: 191
Burns, D. B. 2: 181, 544, 550 555
Burns, N. M. 2: 252, 254
Burnstein, A. 1: 180, 191
Burt, C. L. 1: 80, 82, 174, 180, 185, 186, 187, 190, 253, 375, 398, 497, 520; 2: 383; 3: 545

Burton, A. 2: 420, 482
Burton, R. V. 3: 316, 318
Busemann, 3: 4
Butfield, E. 3: 562, 568
Butler, R. A. 2: 252
Butler, R. N. 2: 617
Butler, S. 2: 110, 127
Byers, L. W. 2: 15, 18

Cadilhac, J. 2: 216
Caffey, J. 3: 585
Cahan, A. 2: 46
Cairns, H. 2: 216
Cajal, S. 2: 67, 68, 71, 84
Caldwell, B. M. 3: 319, 482, 492, 745, 758
Caldwell, D. 2: 304, 311
Callagan, J. E. 2: 262
Callaway, E. 2: 298, 310, 312
Cambareri, J. D. 2: 252
Cameron, A. H. 1: 55, 520
Cameron, D. E. 2: 96, 104, 252
Cameron, E. 2: 327
Cameron, H. 1: 252, 283; 3: 9
Cameron, J. L. 1: 36, 247; 2: 308, 312, 481
Cameron, K. 1: 19, 112, 226, 233, 289, 305, 396, 398; 3: 649, 678
Cameron, T. 3: 545
Cammock, D. W. 1: 272, 283
Campbell, B. J. 1: 149
Campbell, D. 2: 573
Campbell, D. T. 2: 360, 386
Campbell, J. D. 1: 412, 426
Campbell, P. 2: 573
Camus, 3: 606
Candland, D. 2: 261, 262
Cannon, W. B. 2: 186, 191
Cantor, A. 2: 619
Cantor, G. N. 1: 96, 101
Caplan, G. 2: 477, 480, 676, 679, 694; 3: 341, 344, 525, 682, 753, 754, 758
Caplan, H. 2: 654, 678
Cappon, D, 2: 216
Caputo, D. V. 2: 411, 422; 3: 146, 151
Caravaggio, 2: 143
Carey, F. M. 2: 96, 105
Carey, N. 1: 174, 190
Carlander, O. 3: 469
Carmichael, H. T. 2: 476, 480
Carmichael, L. 3: 139, 151, 569, 677
Carney, R. E. 2: 104
Carothers, J. C. 2: 700, 701, 704, 710
Carpenter, M. B. 2: 86
Carpenter, R. G. 3: 526
Carr, 1: 224
Carr, D. H. 2: 34, 45, 48
Carr-Saunders, A. M. 1: 370, 398

Carrera, R. N. 2: 250, 254
Carretier, L. 3: 123
Carroll, H. A. 1: 195, 209
Carstairs, G. M. 2: 410, 421, 423, 702, 710
Carter, C. O. 1: 54, 55
Carter, F. F. 2: 355, 386
Carter, M. P. 1: 380, 400
Caruth, E. 3: 678, 700, 705
Case, H. W. 1: 114, 147
Casey, M. D. 2: 45
Castameda, A. 3: 745, 761
Castelnuovo-Tedesco, P. 3: 492, 525
Castiglione, Comtesse de 2: 142
Castiglioni, 2: 603
Castle, T. L. van de 2: 355, 386
Castro, R. 2: 699, 710
Catcheside, D. G. 1: 55
Cates, N. 3: 683
Cattell, R. B. 1: 185; 2: 375, 386
Catzel, P. 3: 469
Caudill, W. 2: 477, 480; 3: 351, 352, 357, 368, 369
Cavallin, H. 3: 145, 151
Caveny, E. L. 2: 365, 386
Cesa Bianthi, M. 3: 150
Cézanne, P. 2: 143, 726, 728
Chalmers, D. 2: 181, 191
Chamberlain, T. J. 2: 93, 97, 104
Chambers, E. G. 1: 351, 368
Chambers, R. 2: 252
Chambers, W. W. 2: 307, 312
Champney, H. 1: 375, 399
Chance, M. R A. 1: 25, 26, 27, 34, 36
Chang, J. 2: 104
Chapin, 3: 9
Chapman, A. H. 1: 327, 334; 3: 473, 492
Chapman, J. 2: 289, 309, 414, 423, 424; 3: 566, 568, 569
Charcot, J. M. 2: xxi, 149, 150, 188, 490
Charles, D. C. 1: 498, 520
Charny, I. W. 2: 252
Chase, W. P. 1: 88, 101
Chaslin, J. 2: 426, 445
Chaudhary, N. A. 1: 334; 3: 525
Chaudhry, M. R. 1: 470, 472
Chazan, M. 1: 131, 133, 134, 147
Cheek, F. E. 2: 411, 412, 422, 423; 3: 147, 151
Chekhova, A. N. 2: 435, 445
Chernukin, P. 1: 374, 399
Cherry, C. 1: 114, 147
Chertok, L. 2: 577, 582, 594
Chess, S. 1: 399, 409, 426; 3: 61, 62, 63, 64, 69, 70, 71, 77, 79, 474, 493, 671, 684,

738, 743, 758, 763, 792, 803
Chesser, E. 3: 585
Chidester, L. 1: 368
Child, I. L. 3: 146, 150, 156, 313, 320, 746, 763
Childs, B. 2: 45
Chinn, W. L. 3: 146, 151
Chipman, C. 1: 495; 3: 684
Chisholm, B. 2: 694
Chomsky, N. 3: 82, 96, 548, 568
Chow, K. L. 2: 258
Christian, 3: 591, 608
Christiansen, H. T. 3: 792, 803
Chu, E. H. Y. 1: 55; 2: 45
Clancy, J. 2: 573
Claparède, E. 2: 138, 145
Claridge, G. 2: 375, 381, 387
Clark, B. 2: 252
Clark, L. D. 2: 216
Clark, M. L. 2: 619
Clarke, A. D. B. 1: 216, 233, 334, 497, 517, 520; 3: 279, 290, 535, 545
Clarke, A. M. 1: 216, 233, 334, 497, 517, 520; 3: 279, 290, 535, 545
Clarke, C. M. 1: 57
Clarkson, P. 1: 368
Class, N. E. 3: 585
Clausen, J. A. 3: 745, 758
Cleghorn, R. A. 2: 258; 3: 528
Clein, L. 1: 154, 168
Clendinnen, B. G. 3: 53, 57
Cleveland, S. E. 2: 252
Clevenger, S. V. 3: 652
Clokie, H. 3: 34, 57
Close, H. G. 2: 45, 47
Clouston, T. S. 3: 597
Cloward, R. A. 1: 379, 399
Cobb, P. W. 1: 368
Cobb, S. 2: 322; 3: 530
Cobliner, W. G. 3: 176, 177, 199
Cobrinik, L. 3: 671, 678
Coburn, F. E. 2: 695
Coca, A. F. 2: 182, 188
Cochrane, W. A. 1: 507, 520
Coffey, V. 1: 516, 520; 3: 21, 22, 23, 57
Cohen—of Birkenhead, 1: 471, 472
Cohen, A. K. 1: 379, 399; 3: 146, 151
Cohen, B. D. 2: 219, 252, 296, 298, 302, 303, 309, 310, 311, 312
Cohen, D. 3: 684
Cohen, G. J. 3: 470
Cohen, H. D. 2: 98, 104
Cohen, J. 3: 407, 416
Cohen, K. 2: 180, 189
Cohen, M. 2: 311
Cohen, M. B. 2: 480

Cohen, M. R. 1: 6, 8, 19
Cohen, N. 2: 263; 3: 525
Cohen, R. A. 2: 476, 480
Cohen, S. I. 2: 252, 253, 260
Cohen, W. 2: 252
Cohen, Y. A. 2: 702, 710; 3: 316, 318
Colbert, E. G. 3: 655, 669, 679, 681
Cole, J. 3: 681
Coleman, R. W. 3: 121
Coleridge, E. H. 2: 286
Coleridge, S. T. 2: 268, 286
Coles, R. 3: 585
Collier, G. 2: 258
Collins, G. H. 2: 113, 127
Collins, L. F. 1: 17, 19, 106, 112
Collins, M. 1: 572, 584
Collins, W. 2: 258
Collins, W. F. 2: 259
Collumb, H. 2: 704, 710
Colonna, A. B. 3: 231, 238, 252
Compayre, 3: 5
Condillac, E. 2: 223
Condrau, G. 2: 488, 492, 517
Conlon, M. F. 3: 155
Connell, J. R. (Jr.) 3: 585
Connell, P. H. 1: 403, 413, 426, 535, 561
Connery, H. J. 2: 258
Conrad, J. 1: 373, 399
Conrad, K. 2: 365, 386, 426, 427, 433, 440, 445
Conway, C. G. 2: 573
Cook, L. 2: 96, 104
Cook, N. G. 1: 412, 413, 427
Cook, W. M. 1: 96, 101
Coolidge, J. C. 1: 151
Cooper, D. H. 3: 744, 763
Cooper, G. D. 2: 250, 252
Cooper, M. 3: 470
Cooper, M. M. 3: 525
Cooper, R. 2: 192; 3: 417
Cooper, R. D. 2: 421
Cooper, R. M. 1: 381
Coopersmith, S. 3: 745, 759
Coors, D. 2: 161, 188
Coppen, A. 1: 49, 55, 57, 513, 520, 521; 2: 45
Corberi, 3: 610, 611
Corinth, L. 2: 143
Corlett, K. 1: 501, 510, 520
Cornelison, A. 2: 401, 416, 417, 483
Cornelison, F. S. (Jr.) 2: 287, 309
Cornell, J. B. 3: 369
Corner, B. 3: 410
Corning, W. C. 2: 95, 104
Costa, E. 2: 286
Costello, C. G. 1: 118, 150; 2: 208, 216
Costero, I. 2: 74, 77, 78, 85
Cotte, S. 1: 408, 427
Cotter, L. H. 2: 47

AUTHOR INDEX

Coué, E. **2**: 149, 188
Court Brown, W. M. **2**: 45, 46, 47; **3**: 60
Courtney, J. **2**: 252, 253
Courtois, G. **2**: 544, 556
Cowie, V. **1**: 38, 43, 49, 54, 55, 57, 501, 506, 507, 513, 520, 521; **2**: 45
Cowles, E. **3**: 590, 607
Cox, C. **1**: 199, 201, 209
Cox, W. B. **3**: 585
Coyne, L. **2**: 480, 485
Crager, R. L. **1**: 573, 585
Craig, J. M. **1**: 502, 521
Crain, **2**: 76
Cramer, A. **3**: 593, 596, 608
Cramer, F. J. **2**: 251, 427, 445
Cramer, J. B. **3**: 655, 682
Cramer-Azima, F. J. **2**: 251
Crammer, J. L. **2**: 216
Crane, A. R. **3**: 145, 151
Cravens, R. B. **2**: 355, 388
Creak, E. M. **1**: 237, 247, 473, 475, 478, 480, 482, 483, 489, 494, 537, 561; **3**: 558, 568, 649, 673, 679, 705
Cressy, D. R. **1**: 374, 401, 402
Crick, F. H. C. **1**: 52, 57
Criswell, J. **3**: 734, 759
Critchley, M. **2**: 130, 134, 145, 211, 212, 216, 330
Crohn, B. B. **3**: 525
Crombie, D. L. **1**: 269, 283
Crome, L. **1**: 497, 509, 511, 514, 517, 518, 520
Cronbach, L. J. **2**: 252, 369, 386
Crosby, N. D. **1**: 116, 117
Cross, K. W. **1**: 269, 283
Crosse, V. M. **1**: 55, 520
Crowcroft, A. **3**: 531, 545
Crue, B. L. **2**: 85
Cruickshank, W. M. **1**: 472
Cruikshank, R. M. **1**: 99, 101
Cullen, J. H. **2**: 146, 188
Culver, C. M. **2**: 253
Cumming, E. **3**: 541, 545
Cumming, J. **2**: 418; **3**: 541, 545, 739, 759
Cunningham, C. **2**: 253
Cunningham, J. M. **1**: 257, 283
Cunningham, M. A. **3**: 671, 679
Curran, D. **1**: 384
Curry, R. L. **1**: 574, 584
Curtis, G. C. **3**: 585
Curtis, J. L. **3**: 151
Cushing, M. G. **3**: 526
Cutts, N. E. **3**: 759
Czermak, J. M. **2**: 147, 188
Czerny, **3**: 9

Dahlgren, K. G. **1**: 413, 426
Dale, H. **2**: 342
Dally, P. J. **1**: 334
Dalton, K. **1**: 399

Daly, R. L. **2**: 221
Danielli, J. **2**: 44
Daniels, G. E. **3**: 526, 529
Daniels, R. S. **2**: 220
D'Annunzio, G. **2**: 137
Darin de Lorenzo, A. J. **2**: 84
Darwin, C. R. **1**: 3, 20, 36; **2**: 147, 150, 188
Das, G. D. **2**: 88, 103, 104
Davenport, B. F. **2**: 370, 386
Davenport, R. K. **2**: 216
David, H. P. **2**: 355, 386, 387
David, L. **3**: 585
David, M. **3**: 98, 121, 122
Davidovsky, I. V. **2**: 428, 443, 445, 446
Davidson, A. B. **2**: 104
Davidson, M. **3**: 526
Davidson, R. G. **2**: 45
Davidson, W. M. **1**: 51, 55; **2**: 45
Davies, A. **3**: 546
Davies, D. L. **1**: 261, 283
Davies, R. L. **2**: 728
Davis, **1**: 174
Davis, A. **3**: 306, 307, 318, 748, 759
Davis, D. R. **2**: 410, 412, 421
Davis, D. V. **2**: 104
Davis, J. H. **3**: 586
Davis, J. M. **2**: 252, 253
Davis, K. **2**: 253
Davis, L. W. **2**: 188
Davis, R. **2**: 253
Davis, R. E. **2**: 103, 104
Davison, G. C. **2**: 377, 386, 564, 572, 573
Dawson, G. D. **2**: 174, 188; **3**: 397, 416
Day, J. **2**: 416, 487
Day, R. W. **2**: 45
de Almeida, J. C. **2**: 46
Deal, W. B. **2**: 218
De Caro, B. **3**: 587
Deckert, G. H. **2**: 273, 286
Deecke, L. **3**: 416
DeFrancis, V. **3**: 585, 586
de Grazia, S. **2**: 614
de Groot, M. J. W. **2**: 365, 388
Deiters, **2**: 79
Deitrich, F. R. **3**: 745, 759
Delacroix, F. V. E. **2**: 143
de la Fresnay, J. F. **2**: 128
Delage, J. **1**: 474, 494
de la Haba, G. **2**: 105
De Lasylo, **3**: 153
Delay, J. **2**: 114, 127, 410, 421, 620, 635, 636
De Lee, J. B. **2**: 190
Delhanty, J. D. A. **1**: 56
Delhougne, F. **2**: 178, 188
Dell, M. B. **3**: 414, 416
Delorme, F. **2**: 205, 218
Delsordo, J. D. **3**: 586
De Martino, R. **3**: 371
Dembicki, E. L. **3**: 52, 60

Dembo, D. **2**: 298, 310
Dement, W. C. **2**: 200, 201, 204, 216, 217, 218, 220, 221, 270, 286, 481; **3**: 453
Denber, H. **2**: 635
Dencker, S. J. **1**: 455, 472
Deniker, P. **2**: 421, 620, 635
Denis-Prinzhorn, M. **1**: 99, 102
Denker, R. **1**: 154, 168
Dennis, C. **3**: 526
Dennis, M. G. **2**: 253
Dennis, W. **1**: 90, 102; **2**: 253
Dennison, W. M. **2**: 46
Denny, M. **1**: 148
Deny, **3**: 606, 608
Dercum, F. X. **3**: 590
Der Heydt, V. von **3**: 122
Derouesne, C. **2**: 114, 127
Desai, M.M. **2**: 357, 386
de Sanctis, S. **1**: 473, 495; **3**: 3, 8, 589, 590, 608, 609, 610, 611, 646, 651, 652, 682
Descartes, R. **2**: 489, 500
DesCuret, J. B. F. **3**: 652
de Sonza, A. **2**: 48
Despert, J. L. **1**: 485, 494; **3**: 610, 651, 652, 653, 671, 679, 705
Deutsch, F. **3**: 527
Deutsch, H. **1**: 239; **3**: 83, 88, 96, 659, 679
Deutsch, M. **3**: 748, 759
Devault, M. **2**: 257, 311
Devereau, E. C. (Jr.) **3**: 758
Devereux, G. **2**: 701, 710
Devine, J. V. **2**: 106
Devore, I. **3**: 131, 132, 151
DeVos, G. **3**: 357, 369, 371
De Waelhens, A. **2**: 496
Dewey, J. **3**: 6
Dewhurst, K. **2**: 137, 145
de Wit, J. **3**: 674, 679
Dews, P. B. **1**: 135, 147
Dewson, J. H. **2**: 204, 217
Deyking, E. **2**: 412, 423
Diamond, M. C. **2**: 88, 104, 105
Diamond, S. **3**: 97
Diatkine, R. **3**: 201, 202, 212, 218, 219
Dick, A. P. **3**: 526
Dickens, C. **2**: 142
Dickey, M. **2**: 355, 386
Diem, O. **3**: 591, 596, 608
Diezel, P. H. **1**: 508, 520
Dilthey, **2**: 490; **3**: 295
DiMascio, A. **1**: 366, 368
Dingman, H. F. **2**: 48
Dingman, W. **2**: 97, 105
Dinitz, S. **3**: 27, 59
Dire, J. **2**: 46
Dispensa, J. **3**: 52, 57
Distler, L. **3**: 142, 154
Dittmann, A. T. **2**: 480
Dixon, C. **3**: 671, 679

AUTHOR INDEX

Doane, B. K. **2:** 253, 255, 260
Dobie, S. I. **2:** 252, 311
Dock, W. **3:** 526
Dodge, H. W. (Jr.) **2:** 127
Dodson, **1:** 388
Doering, C. R. **2:** 365, 386, 615, 619
Dohan, L. J. **2:** 616
Doi, L. T. **3:** 352, 357, 369
Doi, T. **3:** 369, 370
Doll, E. A. **1:** 231, 233
Doll, R. **3:** 57
Dollard, J. **1:** 170, 377, 399; **3:** 307, 318
Domino, E. F. **2:** 304, 307, 311, 312
Domke, H. R. **3:** 759
Donaldson, G. A. **3:** 526
Donaldson, J. **2:** 253
Donaldson, R. M. (Jr.) **3:** 527
Dongier, S. **2:** 555
Donoghue, J. D. **3:** 370
Donoso, C. M. **2:** 176, 189
Donovan, D. **3:** 586
Doob, L. W. **1:** 399
Dorcus, R. M. **2:** 161, 171, 177, 188
Doronin, G. P. **2:** 251
Dorsen, M. M. **3:** 652, 680
Douglas, H. **2:** 318
Douglas, J. W. B. **1:** 43, 55, 437, 450; **3:** 35, 37, 57, 534, 545
Douglas, V. **3:** 745, 759
Doupe, J. **2:** 179, 186, 188
Doust, J. W. **2:** 158, 189
Douyon, E. **2:** 705, 711
Dower, J. **3:** 526
Down, L. **3:** 3
Draguns, J. M. **1:** 97, 102
Dreese, M. **2:** 386
Drever, J. **1:** 572, 584
Drew, G. C. **1:** 365, 367, 368
Dreyfus-Brisac, C. **2:** 217
Driesch, H. **2:** 490
Drillien, C. M. **1:** 241, 247; **3:** 27, 34, 39, 43, 45, 47, 50, 55, 57
Driscoll, K. **1:** 56
Driver, M. **1:** 461, 472
Droz, M. B. **2:** 56, 84, 105
Dublin, C. C. **3:** 470
Dublin, L. I. **1:** 413, 426
DuBois, C. **3:** 318
Duke, D. I. **3:** 58
Dukes, W. F. **1:** 99, 102
Dumermuth, G. **2:** 45
Dumont, S. **2:** 176, 190
Dunbar, H. F. **1:** 314, 334, 355, 356, 357, 358, 366, 368; **2:** 178, 180, 189; **3:** 474
Duncan, A. G. **2:** 5, 17
Duncan, G. M. **3:** 586
Dunham, H. W. **2:** 412, 423
Dunlap, K. **2:** 568, 573
Dunn, H. G. **2:** 45

Dunsdon, M. I. **1:** 217, 233
Dunsdon, M. L. **1:** 460, 472
Dunsworth, A. D. **1:** 147
Dunton, W. R. **3:** 590, 606
Duran-Reynals, M. L. **2:** 614
Dürer, A. **2:** 143
Durfee, R. A. **2:** 355, 386
Durkheim, E. **1:** 413 426; **3:** 295, 315
Durrell, D. D. **1:** 581, 584
Du Toit, D. **2:** 257
Dwyer, T. F. **3:** 96
Dyer, W. G. **3:** 141, 151
Dysinger, R. H. **2:** 397, 415
Dzugaeva, C. **2:** 555

Earle, C. J. C. **1:** 473, 494
East, N. **1:** 383, 385, 399
Eaton, J. C. **3:** 57
Eaton, J. W. **2:** 700, 711
Eayrs, J. T. **3:** 53, 57
Eccles, J. C. **2:** 61, 84, 109, 127, 311, 348, 349
Eccleston, D. **2:** 219, 220
Echlin, F. A. **2:** 544, 555
Eckstein, R. **1:** 492, 494
Economo, C. von **2:** 66, 193, 217
Eddy, F. D. **3:** 526
Edgcumbe, R. **3:** 253
Edholm, O. G. **2:** 179, 188
Edisen, C. B. **2:** 618
Edmondson, M. S. **3:** 139, 155, 307, 320
Edstrom, J. E. **2:** 92, 105
Edwards, J. H. **1:** 49, 55, 497, 520; **3:** 27, 32, 57
Eels, K. **3:** 546
Egerton, N. **2:** 253
Egyhàzi, E. **2:** 52, 84, 92, 105
Ehrenpreis, T. **1:** 320, 334; **3:** 507, 508, 526
Eichmann, E. **3:** 29, 57
Eickhorn, O. J. **2:** 355, 386
Eilbert, L. R. **2:** 253
Eilenberg, M. D. **1:** 383, 399
Einstein, A. **2:** 187
Eisenberg, L. **1:** 130, 131, 134, 147, 237, 247, 481, 494; **3:** 147, 151, 649, 655, 657, 679, 705
Eisenson, J. **1:** 583, 584; **3:** 559, 568
Eisenstein, S. **2:** 479
Eiserer, P. E. **3:** 759
Eissen, S. B. **2:** 614
Eitinger, H. **2:** 703, 711
Ekbom, K. A. **2:** 136, 145
Ekdhal, M. **2:** 120, 129
Ekman, P. **2:** 614
Ekstein, R. **3:** 649, 651, 653, 660, 671, 679, 700, 705
Elder, E. H. **3:** 90, 96
Elder, K. A. **3:** 142, 151
Elkes, J. E. **2:** 288, 301, 309
Ellenberger, H. **2:** 699, 711
Ellingson, R. J. **2:** 189

Ellis, H. **2:** 280
Ellis, J. R. **1:** 56
Ellis, N. **1:** 82, 83, 135, 147
Ellison, E. A. **2:** 411, 422; **3:** 146, 151
Elmer, E. **3:** 586, 587
Elwood, D. L. **3:** 565, 569
Embree, J. **3:** 370
Emch, M. **1:** 389, 399
Emery, A. E. H. **2:** 46
Emminghaus, H. **3:** 2, 376, 390, 652
Emminghaus, M. **2:** 427, 446
Emmons, W. H. **2:** 199, 221
Engel, G. L. **1:** 319, 334; **2:** 477, 481; **3:** 496, 499, 510, 514, 519, 525, 526
Engelhardt, D. M. **2:** 615
Engelmann, T. G. **2:** 219
English, A. C. **1:** 563, 575, 585
English, H. B. **1:** 563, 575, 585
English, O. S. **1:** 313, 335; **2:** 476, 481; **3:** 139 151
Erickson, M. **1:** 147; **2:** 173, 177, 189, 418
Ericsson, N. O. **3:** 526
Erikson, E. H. **1:** 246, 247, 373, 376, 399; **2:** 450, 451, 452, 454, 455, 456, 457, 458, 460, 461, 463, 467, 468, 469, 470, 471, 478, 481; **3:** 122, 190, 199, 298, 302, 303, 304, 312, 314, 315, 318, 526, 545
Erikson, J. A. **3:** 492
Eron, L. D. **2:** 390; **3:** 138, 141, 147, 151
Ervin, F. R. **2:** 129
Ervin, S. M. **3:** 551, 553, 568
Erwin, D. T. **3:** 586
Erwin, W. J. **2:** 573
Escalona, S. **1:** 236, 247; **2:** 449, 481; **3:** 93, 96, 121, 122
Esdaile, J. **2:** 151, 189
Esecover, H. **2:** 614
Esman, A. H. **3:** 705
Esquirol, J. E. D. **2:** 265, 286, 715; **3:** 592, 652
Essen-Möller, E. **2:** 6, 17
Esterson, A. **2:** 421, 483
Evans, A. S. **2:** 412, 423
Evans, J. **2:** 328, 349
Evans, J. I. **2:** 206, 209, 217, 219, 220
Evans, K. A. **1:** 54, 55
Evans, W. A. (Jr.) **3:** 588
Evarts, E. V. **2:** 217, 266, 286
Everett, I. R. **1:** 79, 83
Ey, H. **2:** 426, 427, 428, 441, 446
Eyeferth, K. **3:** 748, 759
Eysenck, H. J. **1:** 16, 19, 41, 56, 104, 106, 107, 108, 109, 110, 111, 119, 121, 128, 142, 147, 152, 153, 154,

Eysenck, H. J.—cont. 157, 160, 161, 164, 168, 186, 190, 382, 399, 561, 576, 585; 2: 189, 353, 354, 357, 362, 364, 368, 373, 375, 376, 377, 378, 380, 381, 383, 449, 481, 558, 570, 573, 574; 3: 569
Eysenck, S. B. G. 1: 108; 2: 373, 375, 387
Ezriel, H. 2: 477, 481

Fabian, A. A. 1: 357, 368, 492, 494
Fabian, M. 2: 483
Fabre, I. M. 2: 147, 148, 189
Fabricius, B. 1: 35, 36
Faigin, H. 3: 329, 341, 344
Fain, M. 3: 214, 218
Fairbairn, W. R. D. 1: 244, 247; 2: 457, 481
Fairbanks, V. F. 2: 45
Fairburn, A. C. 3: 586
Fairweather, D. V. I. 1: 378, 399, 472
Fanconi, G. 3: 674, 679
Fantz, R. L. 1: 89, 102
Farber, E. 1: 129
Farber, S. M. 2: 47
Farberow, N. L. 1: 410, 427; 2: 419
Faretra, G. 3: 667, 669, 678, 679
Faris, M. D. 2: 485
Faris, R. E. L. 2: 412, 423
Farmer, E. 1: 351, 368
Farnarier, 3: 609
Farndale, J. 2: 695
Farquhar, H. G. 1: 325, 334
Farrow, J. T. 2: 107
Faubion, R. W. 2: 253
Faulk, M. E. (Jr.) 2: 314, 349
Faure, J. 2: 217
Favez-Boutonier, J. 3: 139, 152
Fechner, G. T. 2: 223
Federn, P. 2: 306, 312, 523, 529; 3: 543, 545, 660, 664, 679
Feighley, C. A. 2: 311
Feinberg, I. 2: 284, 285, 286
Feinstein, H. N. 3: 586
Feldhusen, J. F. 3: 745, 759
Feldman, M. P. 2: 568, 573
Feldman, P. E. 2: 614
Feldstein, M. J. 3: 761
Fellows, E. V. 2: 104
Fenger, G. 1: 269
Fenichel, O. 2: 614; 3: 144, 152, 419, 420, 453
Ferber, P. 3: 684
Ferenczi, S. 3: 210, 218
Ferguson, W. M. 3: 586
Ferguson-Smith, M. A. 1: 50, 56, 513, 520, 521; 2: 46
Ferman, L. A. 3: 761
Fernandes, X. 2: 711

Fernandez-Guardiola, A. 2: 189
Ferreira, A. J. 2: 410, 421
Ferster, C. B. 1: 114, 136, 137, 138, 139, 140, 143, 147
Fessard, A. 2: 128
Field, J. G. 1: 382, 399; 2: 127
Field, M. J. 2: 701, 704, 711
Fields, S. J. 2: 390
Fields, W. S. 2: 85
Filante, W. 2: 263
Finch, S. M. 3: 145, 152, 511, 515, 520, 521, 526, 528
Fink, 3: 597
Finley, C. B. 2: 651, 673
Finley, J. R. 1: 151
Finzi, 3: 592, 603, 608
Fischer, G. 3: 612
Fischgold, H. 2: 217, 218, 221
Fish, B. 1: 479, 494; 2: 458, 459, 481; 3: 669, 679, 705
Fish, L. 1: 515, 521
Fisher, C. 2: 3, 201, 217, 220, 449, 478, 481; 3: 453
Fisher, C. M. 2: 114, 121, 122, 127, 129
Fisher, H. K. 2: 614
Fisher, R. A. 2: 12, 17
Fisher, S. 2: 397, 416
Fisher, S. H. 3: 586
Fisher, V. 2: 218
Fisher, V. E. 2: 173, 189
Fisk, F. 2: 423
Fiske, D. W. 2: 246, 253, 259
Fixsen, C. 3: 156
Fjerdingstad, E. J. 2: 95, 97, 105, 106, 107
Flaherty, B. E. 2: 252, 255, 257, 259, 260
Flamm, H. 3: 23, 57
Flanagan, B. 1: 136, 147
Flanders, N. A. 3: 736, 759
Flato, C. 3: 586
Fleck, S. 2: 401, 402, 416, 417, 483; 3: 370
Fleming, E. E. 1: 585
Flenning, F. 2: 312
Flexner, J, B. 2: 98, 99, 105
Flexner, L. B. 2: 98, 99, 105
Flood, C. A. 3: 525, 526, 529
Floyer, E. B. 1: 460, 472
Flugel, F. 2: 464, 635
Flugel, J. C. 1: 182, 190; 3: 146, 152
Flye, J. 2: 236, 263
Fode, K. L. 2: 618
Fodor, J. A. 3: 554, 568
Folch-Pi, J. 2: 309
Foley, J. M. 2: 257, 299, 310
Folkart, L. 3: 253
Fölling, A. 1: 45, 504, 520; 3: 4
Fonberg, E. 2: 573
Fonda, C. P. 2: 365, 389
Fondeur, M. 3: 156

Fonkalsrud, E. W. 3: 528
Fontana, V. J. 3: 586
Forbis, O. L. 3: 587
Force, D. G. (Jr.) 3: 734, 759
Ford, C. E. 1: 55, 57; 2: 46
Ford, F. R. 1: 452, 472
Forea, I. 2: 47
Forgus, R. H. 1: 381
Forrer, G. R. 2: 614
Forrest, H. 2: 46
Forssman, H. 2: 46
Foss, B. 3: 97, 121, 122, 152, 252
Foudraine, J. 2: 412, 422
Foulds, G. 2: 614
Foulds, G. A. 2: 365, 387
Foulkes, D. 2: 217
Foulkes, S. H. 2: 477, 481
Foulkes, W. D. 2: 213, 217
Fowler, H. B. 2: 653, 673
Fox, B. 2: 390, 614
Fox, R. H. 2: 179, 188
Fox, S. S. 2: 253
Fozzard, J. A. F. 3: 60
Fracarol, La C. 2: 106
Fraccaro, M. 1: 55, 2: 46
Fraiberg, S. 3: 426, 453
Framo, J. L. 2: 421, 480, 483, 485
Frances, J. M. 1: 57
Frangnito, O. 3: 609
Frank, J. D. 2: 614, 615, 618; 3: 63, 79
Frank, T. 1: 494
Frankl, L. 3: 222, 223, 242, 244, 245, 250
Frankl, V. 2: 573
Franklin, A. W. 1: 435, 450; 3: 546, 569, 570
Franks, C. M. 1: 382, 399; 2: 357, 376, 387, 388, 570, 573
Fraser, G. R. 1: 508, 520
Fraser, H. F. 2: 216
Fraser, L. H. 2: 46
Frazer, J. G. 2: 653, 673
Frazier, S. H. 3: 586
Frederick II, 3: 158, 199
Fredericson, E. 2: 253
Freedman, A. 3: 470
Freedman, A. M. 1: 518, 520; 3: 654, 655, 678, 679
Freedman, D. X. 2: 276, 286, 306, 312, 416; 3: 670, 683
Freedman, N. 2: 615
Freedman, S. J. 2: 253, 254, 300, 311
Freeman, H. 1: 158, 168, 494; 2: 695
Freeman, J. 2: 182, 189; 3: 545
Freeman, J. A. 2: 84
Freeman, T. 1: 32, 36, 238, 247; 2: 308, 312, 458, 481; 3: 152
Fremming, K. 2: 10, 17
French, T. M. 2: 477, 479
Freud, A. 1: 241, 247, 252,

AUTHOR INDEX

305, 535; **2:** 254, 449, 452, 457, 458, 476, 480, 481, **3:** 6, 121, 122, 141, 152, 199, 200, 201, 208, 215, 216, 218, 221, 222, 225, 230, 232, 233, 234, 235, 236, 238, 244, 250, 251, 252, 265, 545, 672, 679
Freud, S. **1:** 82, 182, 237, 238, 242, 247, 251, 283, 358, 368, 411, 426; **2:** xix, xx, xxi, xxii, xxiv, xxv, 149, 150 156, 171, 173, 189, 200, 202, 209, 217, 266, 267, 448, 450, 452, 453, 454, 460, 461, 467, 468, 482, 488, 490, 498, 500, 501, 502, 505, 509, 511, 513, 514, 515, 517, 522, 523, 525, 526, 571, 625; **3:** 5, 6, 62, 63, 66, 79, 144, 177, 182, 200, 201, 202, 203, 210, 211, 213, 214, 218, 222, 246, 293, 294, 295, 298, 299, 301, 302, 313, 314, 317, 318, 418, 419, 421, 426, 441, 446, 453, 526, 537, 540, 544, 545
Freud, W. E. **3:** 232, 151
Freund, K. **1:** 164, 168; **2:** 568, 573
Freyberger, H. **2:** 479
Fried, J. **2:** 703, 711
Friedhoff, A. J. **2:** 277, 286
Friedjung, J. K. **3:** 445, 453
Friedlander, K. **1:** 370, 373, 399; **3:** 222
Friedlander, M. **2:** 143, 145
Friedman, A. S. **2:** 421
Friedman, M. **2:** 162, 163, 186, 188; **3:** 586
Friedman, M. H. F. **3:** 526
Friedman, N. **2:** 614
Friedman, S. **1:** 401
Friedman, S. W. **3:** 649, 653, 660, 679
Friedmann, **2:** 430; **3:** 245, 251
Fries, M. **3:** 423, 453
Froehlich, C. P. **2:** 357, 388
Frohman, C. E. **2:** 16, 19, 219, 293, 298, 309, 310
Fromm, E. **3:** 297, 318, 371
Fromm-Reichmann, F. **2:** 411, 419, 422; **3:** 303
Frost, J. D. **2:** 190
Fry, D. B. **3:** 554, 555, 570
Fry, L. **2:** 190
Fry, W. F. **2:** 418, 419, 420
Fujimori, M. **2:** 220
Fuller, E. M. **1:** 359, 368
Fulton, J. F. **2:** xxiii, 128
Furer, M. **3:** 661, 679, 681, 705
Furhman, A. **2:** 259
Furneaux, B. **3:** 558, 559, 568

Furst, S. **3:** 252

Gaarder, K. **2:** 312
Gabriel, L. **2:** 491, 517
Gabrilove, L. J. **3:** 525
Gaddum, **2:** 276
Gage, R. P. **3:** 528
Gaito, J. **2:** 85, 90, 105, 255
Gaitonde, M. R. **2:** 702, 711
Gakkell, L. B. **2:** 583, 594
Galambos, R. **2:** 111, 127
Galdston, R. **3:** 571, 586
Galen, **1:** 106; **2:** 596
Galigher, D. L. **2:** 617
Galkin, V. S. **2:** 254
Gallinek, A. **2:** 217
Galloway, T. McL. **3:** 57
Galton, F. **1:** 171, 173, 176, 184, 190, 199, 253; **2:** 3, 266, 271, 286
Gannet, H. **3:** 673, 683
Gannushkin, N. **2:** 444, 446
Gantt, H. **2:** 615
Gantt, W. H. **1:** 119, 129, 147, 390, 399
Garattini, S. **2:** 635
Gardner, E. A. **3:** 803
Gardner, J. E. **3:** 470
Gardner, L. I. **1:** 46, 57
Gardner, L. P. **3:** 141, 142, 152
Gardner, N. H. **2:** 411, 422
Garetz, F. K. **2:** 615
Garlock, J. H. **3:** 525, 526
Garner, A. M. **3:** 156, 527, 530
Garnier, **3:** 608
Garrison, F. H. **2:** 613, 615
Garrod, **3:** 9
Garrod, A. E. **1:** 39, 45, 504, 520
Garry, R. C. **3:** 31, 57
Gartner, M. A. (Jr.) **2:** 615
Gastaut, H. **2:** 217, 538, 555; **3:** 393, 414, 416
Gauthier, M. **1:** 47, 56, 521
Gavrilova, N. **2:** 539, 543, 547, 554, 555, 556
Gavron, H. **3:** 143, 152
Gazzaniga, M. S. **2:** 111, 127
Gedda, L. **1:** 41, 56
Geleerd, E. R. **1:** 238, 247; **3:** 660, 679
Gellerman, L. W. **1:** 91, 102
Gellhorn, E. **2:** 254
Genn, M. N. **1:** 369
Gennep, A. L. van **3:** 315, 316, 318
Geoffrey, W. **3:** 749, 762
Georgi, F. **1:** 482, 494
Gerard, D. L. **2:** 411, 422; **3:** 146, 152
Gerard, M. **3:** 527
Gerard, R. W. **2:** 104, 128, 266, 286
Gerson, M. **3:** 333, 337, 339, 345

Gerver, D. **3:** 565, 568
Geschwind, N. **3:** 561, 569
Gesell, A. L. **1:** 61, 88, 90, 98, 102, 218, 224, 225, 233, 564, 566, 585; **3:** 5, 292, 318, 341, 426, 453, 456, 470, 542, 640, 654, 679
Gesenius, H. **3:** 29, 30, 57
Getzels, J. W. **1:** 187, 190
Gewirtz, J. L. **1:** 140, 147, 150; **3:** 340, 345
Ghent, L. **1:** 93, 97, 102
Ghetti, V. **2:** 635
Gianascol, A. J. **3:** 651, 653, 665, 680
Gianelli, F. **1:** 521
Giarman, N. H. **2:** 276, 286, 306, 312
Gibbens, T. C. N. **1:** 370, 384, 399
Gibbons, D. C. **1:** 373, 376, 399
Gibbs, N. K. **1:** 510, 520
Gibbs, P. K. **3:** 306, 319
Gibby, R. G. **2:** 250, 252, 254
Gibney, F. **3:** 370
Gibson, E. J. **1:** 98, 103
Gibson, R. **2:** 457, 482
Gibson, R. W. **2:** 477, 480
Gidro-Frank, L. **2:** 171, 189
Giffin, M. E. **2:** 483
Gifford, S. **2:** 290, 309
Gilan, J. **3:** 337, 338, 345
Gilbaud, G. **2:** 221
Gilbert, C. W. **2:** 46
Gildea, M. C.-L. **3:** 746, 747, 750, 755, 758, 759, 760
Gilder, R. (Jr.) **1:** 369
Giliarovsky, V. A. **2:** 581, 594
Gill, C. **3:** 83
Gill, M. M. **2:** 449, 477, 482
Gill, T. D. **3:** 586
Gillespie, R. D. **1:** 252, 283, 487, 494
Gillies, S. **1:** 479, 495
Gillin, J. **2:** 706, 711
Gilloran, J. L. **3:** 139, 152
Ginsberg, **3:** 135, 152
Girard, C., **2:** 45
Girdany, B. R. **3:** 587
Gittins, J. **1:** 397, 399
Gjessing, R. **1:** 482, 494; **2:** 15, 17
Gladstone, A. I. **2:** 477, 480
Gladstone, I. **3:** 369
Glanzmann, E. **3:** 527
Glasco, L. **3:** 308
Glaser, E. M. **2:** 615
Glasky, A. J. **2:** 94, 105
Glasner, S. **2:** 421
Glasser, R. **2:** 253
Glasser, W. **1:** 393, 399
Glazer, N. **3:** 309
Gleser, G. **3:** 416
Glickman, S. **3:** 739, 760
Glickman, S. E. **2:** 105

Glidewell, J. C. **3**: 733, 735, 737, 740, 741, 747, 750, 752, 753, 754, 755, 758, 759, 761, 762, 763
Gliedman, L. H. **2**: 615
Glivenko, E. **2**: 539, 556
Glover, E. **2**: 363, 388, 449, 482, 615
Glozer, E. **1**: 494
Gluck, E. **3**: 5
Gluck, P. **1**: 359, 368
Gluckholn, C. **3**: 136
Glueck, E. T. **1**: 44, 56, 325, 334, 374, 375, 383, 399; **3**: 145, 152, 796, 803
Glueck, S. **1**: 44, 56, 325, 334, 374, 375, 383, 399; **3**: 145, 152, 796, 803
Glynn, J. D. **2**: 574
Gnagey, W. J. **3**: 736, 759
Goerer, G. **3**: 370
Goff, P. **3**: 528
Golan, S. **3**: 336, 341, 342, 343, 345
Gold, E. **3**: 683
Gold, M. **3**: 734, 747, 761
Goldberg, E. M. **2**: 412, 423, **3**: 145, 153
Goldberg, J. **2**: 263
Goldberg, L. R. **2**: 368, 388
Goldberg, M. A. **1**: 207, 208, 209
Goldberger, A. **3**: 244, 250
Goldberger, L. **2**: 225, 254, 255, 300, 311
Goldblatt, D. **2**: 85
Goldenweiser, A. A. **3**: 293, 294
Goldfarb, A. **3**: 740, 759
Goldfarb, W. **1**: 215, 233, 479, 494; **2**: 412, 423; **3**: 9, 279, 290, 545, 550, 568, 652, 662, 663, 671, 674, 680, 684, 685, 705
Goldfischer, S. **2**: 84
Goldfrank, **2**: 221
Goldfried, M. R. **2**: 254
Goldgraber, M. D. **3**: 527
Goldiamond, I. **1**: 143, 147
Goldie, L. **1**: 463, 472; **2**: 189
Goldman-Eisler, F. **3**: 548, 568
Goldstein, A. P. **2**: 605, 615
Goldstein, G. **3**: 528
Goldstein, J. **3**: 251
Goldstein, K. **1**: 240, 247; **3**: 549, 662, 680
Gollin, E. S. **1**: 97, 102
Gomirato, G. **2**: 105
Gonzales-Licea, A. **3**: 527
Goodacre, I. **1**: 451
Gooddy, W. **2**: 126, 127
Goode, W. J. **3**: 308, 318
Goodenough, D. R. **2**: 200, 217, 220
Goodman, J. **2**: 309

Goodnow, J. J. **2**: 218, 221, 295, 310
Goodwin, M. S. **3**: 124
Goolker, P. **2**: 365, 388
Gorbov, F. D. **2**: 254
Gordon, H. **2**: 180, 189
Gordon, H. L. **2**: 704, 711
Gordon, I. E. **1**: 574, 585
Gordon, J. E. **1**: 362, 368, 426
Gordon, L. V. **1**: 585
Gordon, M. **3**: 309
Gorer, G. **3**: 139, 152, 296
Gorman, J. G. **2**: 46
Gorton, B. E. **2**: 174, 189
Goslin, D. A. **3**: 735, 760
Gosliner, B. J. **3**: 681
Gottesman, I. I. **2**: 14, 18
Gottlieb, J. S. **2**: 16, 19, 219, 252, 288, 298, 309, 310, 311, 312; **3**: 53, 60
Gottschalk, L. A. **2**: 480, 481, 483, 485, 486
Gough, D. **1**: 435, 450
Gould, R. W. **3**: 587
Gowing, J. **2**: 263
Grab, B. **1**: 369
Grace, W. J. **3**: 527
Grad, J. C. **1**: 212, 234; **2**: 412, 423, 679, 695
Graff, H. **3**: 669, 680
Graham, F. K. **1**: 455, 472, 573, 585
Graham, M. A. **2**: 48
Graham, P. **3**: 739, 741, 762
Graham, R. W. **2**: 262
Grant, E. C. **2**: 20, 26, 34, 36
Grant, J. D. **1**: 373, 376, 377, 394, 395, 399, 400, 402
Grant, M. Q. **1**: 372, 376, 377, 394, 395, 399, 400, 402
Graveline, D. E. **2**: 251
Gray, E. G. **2**: 72, 84
Gray, J. A. **2**: 574
Gray, S. W. **3**: 141, 152
Graybiel, A. **2**: 252
Grayson, M. J. **3**: 526
Grebe, H. **3**: 33, 57
Green, A. **2**: 421
Green, A. W. **3**: 748, 760
Green, J. M. **1**: 463, 472
Green, L. **2**: 104
Green, M. **3**: 527, 528, 529
Greenacre, P. **1**: 240, 241, 248, 386, 400; **3**: 122, 659, 680
Greenberg, G. **2**: 260
Greenberg, I. M. **2**: 254
Greenberg, M. **3**: 20, 57
Greenblatt, M. **2**: 253, 254, 286, 300, 311
Greenfield, N. S. **2**: 480, 482, 483
Greengard, J. **3**: 586
Greenwood, A. **2**: 254
Greenwood, M. **1**: 368

Gregg, N. M. **1**: 502, 504, 514, 520; **3**: 20, 57
Gregory, E. **3**: 283, 290
Greifenstein, F. **2**: 257, 302, 311
Greiner, T. **2**: 615
Greiner, T. H. **2**: 270, 286
Grekker, R. A. **2**: 536, 556
Gresham, S. C. **2**: 218
Grewel, F. **3**: 561, 568
Griesinger, W. **2**: 426, 446
Griffin, G. A. **2**: 482
Griffin, M. E. **2**: 421; **3**: 153
Griffiths, D. L. **3**: 586
Griffiths, N. L. **1**: 581, 585
Griffiths, R. **1**: 224, 225, 233, 567, 585
Griffiths, W. **3**: 739, 741, 760
Grime, G. **1**: 368
Grimes, F. V. **2**: 615
Grimm, E. R. **3**: 83, 96
Grinker, I. G. **1**: 493
Grisell, J. L. **2**: 219, 296, 298, 309, 310
Grissom, R. J. **2**: 254, 261
Grivel, F. **2**: 221
Groen, J. **1**: 319, 334; **3**: 527
Gronlund, N. E. **3**: 760
Gronlund, W. E. **3**: 737, 760
Grønsetti, E. **3**: 141, 152
Gross, C. G. **2**: 96, 105
Gross, H. P. **3**: 674, 680
Gross, J. **2**: 217, 481
Gross, R. E. **3**: 527
Grossman, B. **3**: 744, 760
Grothe, M. **2**: 618
Grotjahn, M. **2**: 479
Grove, E. F. **2**: 182, 188
Gruenberg, E. A. **3**: 741, 760
Gruenberg, G. M. **1**: 150
Grugett, A. E. **3**: 655, 678
Gruhle, M. **2**: 426, 445
Grumbach, M. M. **2**: 45
Grunberg, F. **1**: 384, 400, 470, 472
Grunebaum, H. V. **2**: 254, 300, 311; **3**: 146, 152
Grunebaum, M. G. **3**: 545
Grunewald, K. R. **3**: 783, 784
Grunhut, M. **1**: 385, 400
Guilford, J. P. **1**: 184, 185, 186, 190
Gulick, W. L. **2**: 261, 262
Gulliford, R. **1**: 499, 520
Gump, P. V. **3**: 736, 760
Gumpert, G. **2**: 615
Gunderson, E. E. K. **2**: 254
Guntrip, H. **2**: 457, 482
Gurevitz, S. **1**: 493
Gurrslin, O. **3**: 762
Gutelius, M. F. **3**: 470
Guthrie, D. **1**: 95, 102
Guthrie, E. R. **2**: 560, 574
Guthrie, W. K. **3**: 9
Gutsch, A. **2**: 254
Guze, S. B. **2**: 48

AUTHOR INDEX

Guzman-Flores, C. 2: 189
Gwinn, J. L. 3: 586

Haber, A. 3: 761
Haber, M. M. 2: 263
Hackett, P. 2: 262
Hadfield, J. A. 2: 180, 189
Haffner, C. 1: 535
Haffner, H. 3: 528
Hagans, J. A. 2: 615, 619
Haggard, H. W. 2: 615
Hagman, C. 1: 125, 126, 129, 147
Hahn, P. 1: 151
Haldane, J. B. S. 2: 4, 7, 8, 18
Hale, F. 3: 20, 57
Haley, J. 2: 404, 417, 418, 419, 420, 479, 615
Haley, T. J. 2: 85
Hall, B. H. 2: 482, 483
Hall, C. S. 2: 218
Hall, S. 3: 6
Hallgren, B. 1: 44, 45, 56; 2: 4, 6, 11, 12, 18
Halliday, A. M. 2: 176, 189
Hallowell, A. J. 2: 700, 711
Halpern, F. 2: 481, 3: 679
Halpern, H. 3: 545
Halpern, H. 3: 545
Hamashi, I. 2: 142
Hambert, G. 2: 16, 18, 46
Hambling, J. 3: 251
Hamerton, J. L. 1: 50, 56, 514, 521
Hamilton, D. M. 2: 411, 422; 3: 146, 151
Hamilton, H. C. 3: 52, 58
Hamilton, M. 2: 615, 618
Hamilton, M. W. 3: 56
Hammack, J. T. 1: 149; 2: 221
Hammer, E. F. 1: 579, 585
Hampe, W. W. 2: 481
Hampson, J. G. 2: 47
Hampson, J. L. 2: 47
Hancock, C. 3: 586
Hancock, R. L. 2: 68, 84
Handford, A. 3: 669, 680
Handlon, M. W. 3: 156, 530
Handmaker, S. D. 1: 521; 2: 46
Handy, L. M. 1: 40, 57
Hanhart, E. 2: 11, 18
Hankoff, L. D. 2: 615, 700, 711
Hanna, T. D. 2: 254, 255
Hanselmann, 3: 4
Hansen, E. 1: 460, 472
Hansen, K. 2: 178, 188
Harden, D. G. 2: 45
Harding, G. F. 2: 355, 388
Harding W. G. 1: 504, 520
Hare, E. H. 2: 412, 423
Hargreaves, 3: 11
Hargreaves, G. R. 2: 615

Harlow, F. L. 3: 284, 290, 291
Harlow, H. F. 1: 35, 36; 2: 255, 299, 310, 449, 457, 482; 3: 122, 210, 219, 300, 314, 315, 318, 659
Harlow, M. K. 3: 318
Harms, E. 2: 220
Harms, I. 1: 437, 450, 517, 521
Harnden, D. G. 1: 55, 513, 520, 521; 2: 45, 46, 47
Harned, B. K. 3: 52, 58
Harper, E. O. 3: 527
Harper, F. V. 3: 586
Harper, P. 2: 574
Harrington, J. A. 1: 384, 400, 456, 472
Harris, A. 2: 255
Harris, D. B. 3: 141, 152
Harris, H. 1: 45, 56
Harrison, P. 2: 259
Hart, B. 2: xxi; 3: 652
Hartey, A. L. 2: 95, 105
Hartland, D. 2: 588
Hartley, E. L. 3: 317, 320, 758
Hartman, A. A. 3: 145, 152
Hartman, B. O. 2: 257
Hartmann, E. L. 2: 449, 482
Hartmann, H. 1: 237, 242, 248; 2: 449, 454, 482; 3: 122, 201, 213, 219, 233, 302, 306, 318, 545, 653, 660, 661, 664, 676, 680
Hartshorne, H. 1: 374, 400
Harvey, E. N. 2: 219
Hasek, J. 2: 263
Haslam, J. 3: 652
Hasselman, M. 2: 204, 218, 294, 309
Hathaway, S. R. 2: 355, 388
Haughton, E. 1: 146
Hauschka, T. S. 2: 48
Hauser, G. A. 2: 46
Hausman, L. 3: 682
Hauty, G. T. 2: 255
Havighurst, R. J. 3: 306, 318, 330, 546
Havlena, J. 3: 52, 60
Hawkins, D. R. 2: 218
Hawkins, J. R. 2: 619
Haworth, M. R. 1: 575, 576, 578, 585
Haworth, M. W. 3: 250, 251
Hayashi, A. 2: 220
Hayden, M. 2: 416
Head, H. 2: 130, 131, 145, 316, 348; 3: 561, 568
Healy, W. 1: 252, 375, 380, 400; 3: 5
Heard, W. G. 1: 151
Hearnshaw, L. S. 1: 334
Heath, H. 2: 614
Heath, R. C. 2: 301, 311
Heath, R. G. 2: 15, 18, 310, 312

Heatherington, R. R. 1: 334
Hebb, D. O. 1: 186, 190, 201' 209; 2: 89, 99, 105, 128, 224, 241, 243, 255, 258, 266, 286
Hécaen, H. 2: 330, 348
Hechter, O. 2: 105
Heckhausen, H. 3: 746, 760
Hediger, H. 3: 82, 90, 96
Hediger, N. 1: 30, 36
Heeley, A. F. 3: 670, 680
Heersema, P. 2: 419
Hegel, G. W. F. 2: 162, 491
Heidegger, M. 2: 489, 490, 492, 493, 494, 495, 496, 497, 516, 517, 579, 594
Heider, G. 2: 481
Heilig, R. 2: 178, 180, 189
Heimann, P. 2: 483
Heimer, C. 3: 470
Heims, L. 1: 400, 494
Heinicke, C. M. 2: 477, 482; 3: 145, 152, 283, 290
Heins, H. L. 3: 60
Held, R. 2: 218, 254, 255
Heller, T. 1: 478, 494; 3: 4, 13, 589, 610, 646, 652, 675
Hellgren, K. 3: 784
Hellman, I. 1: 561; 3: 122, 241, 243, 244, 245, 250, 251
Hellmann, K. 3: 51, 52, 58
Hellmer, L. A. 3: 154
Helme, W. H. 3: 654, 678
Helmholtz, 2: 223
Helmholtz, H. F. 3: 494, 527
Helvey, W. M. 2: 258
Hemphill, R. E. 2: 16, 18
Hendelman, W. J. 2: 85
Henderson, D. K. 1: 252, 283
Hendler, E. 2: 252
Henning, G. B. 2: 262
Henriques, F. 3: 139, 152
Henry, C. E. 1: 112
Henry, J. 2: 397, 416; 3: 312, 318
Henry, J. P. 2: 255
Herblin, W. F. 2: 107
Hereford, C. F. 3: 751, 760
Hermann, I. 3: 659, 680
Hermann, J. 3: 528
Hermann, R. S. 2: 386
Hermelin, B. 1: 230, 234; 3: 553, 557, 558, 569
Hernandez-Peon, R. 1: 25, 36, 2: 174, 176, 189, 255, 305, 306, 312, 538, 556
Herndon, C. N. 1: 507, 521
Herndon, R. M. 2: 72, 84
Heron, W. 2: 251, 253, 255, 260, 261, 286, 299, 310
Herrick, J. 1: 494
Herrick, V. E. 3: 546
Herrmann, R. S. 2: 258
Hersov, L. 1: 131, 133, 134, 148
Hertig, A. T. 3: 47, 58

3 G

816 AUTHOR INDEX

Hertzig, M. **1**: 399; **3**: 79, 763
Herzog, **1**: 451
Hess, J. H. **3**: 145, 152, 511, 515, 526
Hess, R. **3**: 393, 416
Hess, W. R. **2**: 193, 218, 314
Hetzer, H. **1**: 95, 102
Hewitt, D. **3**: 59
Hewitt, L. E. **1**: 400; **3**: 739, 760
Heyer, G. R. **2**: 178, 189
Heyman, H. **1**: 368
Higier, **3**: 612
Hijmans, J. **3**: 527
Hild, W. **2**: 73, 74, 75, 78, 80, 84
Hildreth, G. H. **1**: 581, 585
Hilgard, E. R. **1**: 104, 105, 148, 165, 168; **2**: 173, 189, 241, 255
Hilgard, J. R. **2**: 412, 423
Hill, **3**: 590
Hill, D. **1**: 400, 454, 461, 472, 478, 494
Hill, J. C. **2**: 255
Hill, J. D. N. **3**: 416
Hill, K. T. **2**: 255
Hill, L. B. **2**: 411, 422
Hill, O. W. **3**: 283, 290
Hill, R. **3**: 141, 152
Hilliard, L. T. **1**: 217, 233; **3**: 546
Hiltman, H. **2**: 357, 388
Himwich, H. E. **2**: 312
Hinde, R. A. **3**: 131, 152, 283, 291
Hindley, C. B. **1**: 148, 224, 233
Hinkle, L. E. **2**: 218
Hinsie, L. **2**: 574
Hinsie, S. E. **2**: 265, 388
Hinton, J. M. **2**: 218
Hippocrates, **2**: xix, 596
Hirao, T. **2**: 251
Hirsch, M. W. **2**: 614
Hirsch, S. **3**: 492
Hirsch, S. I. **2**: 416, 487
His, W. **3**: 51, 58
Hitler, **3**: 29
Hjelholt, G. **3**: 142, 152
Hoagland, H. **1**: 482, 494
Hobart, G. A. **2**: 219
Hobbs, G. E. **1**: 51, 55; **2**: 45
Hobhouse, **3**: 135, 152
Hobson, J. A. **2**: 221
Hoch, A. **3**: 606
Hoch, E. **2**: 704, 711; **3**: 676, 680
Hoch, P. H. **1**: 574, 585; **2**: 388, 635, 712; **3**: 290, 470, 651, 672, 677, 678, 679, 680
Hoche, **2**: 427, 443, 446
Hodes, R. **2**: 218, 255
Hodges, R. **1**: 179, 191
Hoedemaker, F. S. **2**: 218, 219
Hoff, H. **2**: 178, 180, 189

Hoffer, A. **2**: 15, 18, 281, 301, 311
Hoffer, W. **3**: 222
Hoffman, J. **2**: 261, 271, 286
Hoffman, L. M. **3**: 759
Hoffman, L. N. **3**: 758
Hoffman, L. W. **3**: 139, 152, 492, 758, 760, 763
Hoffman, M. L. **3**: 492, 758, 759, 760, 763
Hoffman, W. A. **3**: 525
Hoffmann, H. **2**: 6, 18
Hoffsten, B. von, **3**: 784
Hofling, C. K. **2**: 598, 615
Hofmann, **2**: 278
Hogben, **2**: 3
Hogne, **2**: 74
Holden, M. **2**: 217
Holden, M. S. **1**: 494
Holder, A. **3**: 246, 252
Holland, J. G. **1**: 135, 148; **2**: 106
Hollingshead, A. B. **2**: 411, 412, 422; **3**: 146, 155
Hollingsworth, L. **1**: 195, 196, 209
Hollister, L. E. **2**: 288, 309
Hollister, W. G. **3**: 754, 760
Holman, P. **3**: 281, 290
Holmberg, A. R. **2**: 700, 711
Holmes, F. B. **1**: 122, 124, 126, 130, 148, 154, 168
Holmes, G. **2**: 130, 131, 145, 316, 348
Holmes, M. B. **1**: 244, 248
Holmes, O. W. **2**: 615
Holowach, J. **3**: 527
Holt, E. B. **3**: 301, 302, 314, 318
Holt, K. S. **1**: 460, 472
Holt, R. R. **2**: 225, 254, 255, 300, 311, 449, 478, 482
Holtzman, W. H. **2**: 485
Holzberg, J. **2**: 417
Holzel, A. **1**: 334, 461
Homburger, A. **3**: 8, 376, 390, 652
Honigfeld, G. **2**: 615
Honisett, J. **3**: 43, 58
Honzik, H. C. **1**: 151, 165
Honzik, M. P. **1**: 168, 400; **3**: 79
Hood, H. B. **1**: 79, 83
Hopkins, J. **3**: 649
Hopkins, P. **3**: 251
Hopkins, T. R. **2**: 264
Hopwood, J. S. **2**: 211, 218
Horigan, F. D. **3**: 346
Horn, G. **2**: 176, 189
Horn, R. **1**: 283
Hornbeck, R. T. **3**: 52, 57
Horney, K. **3**: 297, 318
Horowitz, F. D. **3**: 679, 737, 745, 760
Horsley, S. **1**: 396, 400
Horwitz, L. **2**: 482, 485
Hoskins, R. G. **2**: 16, 18

Hoskovec, J. **2**: 216
Houde, R. W. **2**: 617
Housden, L. G. **3**: 586
Houston, W. R. **2**: 616
Hout, H. V. D. **2**: 357, 388
Hovey, G. T. **3**: 529
Howard, R. A. **2**: 255
Howe, L. P. **2**: 695
Howells, J. G. **1**: 251, 283, 535, 561, 577, 585; **2**: 391, 397, 415, 416, 423, 637, 673, 674, 684, 695; **3**: 125, 135, 140, 147, 153, 154, 254, 290, 356, 370, 546, 651, 680
Howes, D. H. **3**: 561, 569
Hsia, D.Y-Y. **1**: 53, 56
Hsia, H. Y. **3**: 670, 682
Hsu, T. C. **1**: 55
Hubel, D. H. **2**: 334
Hudgins, B. B. **3**: 737, 760
Hudgins, C. V. **2**: 178, 190
Hudson-Smith, S. **1**: 349
Huff, W. **2**: 85
Hugelin, A. **2**: 176, 190
Hughes, J. P. W. **3**: 57
Hull, C. L. **1**: 148, 159, 163, 165, 168; **2**: 295, 310, 376, 574, 616; **3**: 62
Hull, J. **2**: 256
Hume, P. B. **2**: 477, 482, 679
Humphrey, J. H. **2**: 188
Humphrey, M. **1**: 451
Humphries, O. **2**: 616
Hungerford, D. A. **1**: 55; **2**: 47
Hunt, A. C. **3**: 586
Hunt, A. D. (Jr.) **3**: 527
Hunt, E. B. **2**: 388
Hunt, H. F. **2**: 575
Hunt, J. McV. **3**: 734, 760
Hunt, R. G. **3**: 762
Hunt, W. A. **2**: 365, 386, 388
Hunter, J. **2**: 140
Hunter, W. F. **2**: 48
Huntington, D. S. **3**: 96
Hurlock, R. **1**: 180, 191
Hurst, A. **2**: xxi
Hurst, P. L. **1**: 502, 521
Hurwitz, E. **3**: 329, 332, 345
Hurwitz, I. **3**: 545
Husband, R. W. **2**: 188
Huschka, M. **1**: 182, 191
Husserl, E. **2**: 492, 517
Hutchinson, E. O. **3**: 43, 58
Hutchinson, J. H. **1**: 507, 521
Hutchinson, R. **1**: 252, 283
Hutt, C. **3**: 680
Hutt, S. J. **3**: 674, 680
Huxley, A. **2**: 280
Hyde, D. M. **1**: 79, 83
Hydén, H. **2**: 52, 55, 80, 84, 85, 87, 89, 90, 92, 93, 103, 105, 106, 110, 128

Iazdovski, V. I. **2**: 254
Ikeda, K. **2**: 519, 529

AUTHOR INDEX

Ilan, E. **3**: 341, 345
Ilg, F. L. **1**: 88, 102
Illingworth, R. S. **1**: 224, 233, 437, 450, 460, 472
Illsley, R. **1**: 378, 399, 455, 456, 472
Ilse, D. R. **1**: 31, 37
Imagawa, D. T. **3**: 60
Imber, S. D. **2**: 615
Ingalls, T. H. **3**: 22, 58
Ingleby, Viscount **1**: 392
Inglis, J. **2**: 301, 311
Ingram, A. J. **1**: 225, 226, 227, 233
Ingram, T. T. S. **3**: 45, 55, 57
Ingvar, D. H. **2**: 544, 556
Inhelder, B. **1**: 59, 72, 74, 75, 76, 78, 82, 83, 84, 100, 102; **3**: 97, 413
Inhorn, S. L. **1**: 56
Ipsen, J. **1**: 426
Ireland, W. W. **1**: 251, 283; **3**: 2, 652
Irvine, E. E. **3**: 338, 345
Irwin, O. C. **3**: 549, 569
Isaacs, S. **1**: 143
Isakower, O. **2**: 285, 286
Ishihara, T. **2**: 48
Israel, J. **3**: 784
Isserlin, **3**: 4
Itani, J. **3**: 132, 153
Itard, J. M. G. **1**: 231, 233
Ivanov, N. V. **2**: 577, 594
Ivanov-Smolensky, A. G. **2**: 437, 446, 531, 532, 533, 535, 536, 537, 556, 583, 594

Jackman, R. J. **3**: 527
Jackson, A. D. M. **1**: 515, 521
Jackson, C. W. **2**: 300, 311
Jackson, C. W. (Jr.) **2**: 256, 258
Jackson, D. D. **2**: 8, 18, 395, 404, 410, 417, 418, 419, 420, 464, 479, 480, 482; **3**: 370, 527
Jackson, J. H. **2**: 266, 323, 327, 335, 348, 427, 428, 432, 433, 446
Jackson, L. **1**: 577, 585
Jackson, M. **3**: 527
Jackson, P. W. **1**: 187, 190; **3**: 142, 153
Jackson, S. **1**: 369
Jaco, E. G. **3**: 757
Jacobi, **3**: 9
Jacobs, P. A. **1**: 55; **2**: 45, 46, 47
Jacobson, A. **2**: 106, 210, 211, 218, 219, 520, 529
Jacobson, A. L. **2**: 97, 104, 106
Jacobson, E. **2**: 449, 482, 562, 563, 574
Jacobson, T. S. **2**: 45

Jacobziner, H. **1**: 404, 409, 426; **3**: 586
Jacubczak, L. **1**: 114, 148
Jaensch, E. R. **1**: 179, 191
Jaffe, S. L. **3**: 661, 680
Jagiello, G. M. **1**: 56, 521
Jahoda, H. **3**: 705
James, **3**: 408
James, B. **2**: 574
James, M. **1**: 244, 248
James, W. **2**: 256, 346
Jameson, G. K. **1**: 335
Jancke, **3**: 612
Janet, P. **2**: 265, 490
Jankovic, B. D. **2**: 106
Janszen, H. H. **2**: 287, 309
Jaques, E. **2**: 477, 482
Jaramillo, R. A. **2**: 220
Jaros, E. **3**: 671, 684
Jarvik, M. E. **2**: 98, 104, 614
Jasper, H. **2**: 112, 128, 268, 286, 287, 316, 317, 319, 327, 345, 349, 538, 543, 556
Jasper, H. H. **2**: 128
Jaspers, K. **2**: 427, 430, 442, 446, 496, 497, 518, 616; **3**: 376, 390, 724, 731
Jay, P. **3**: 131, 153
Jefferson, G. **2**: 218
Jeffress, L. A. **2**: 128
Jekels, L. **3**: 419, 446, 454
Jendrassik, E. **2**: 180, 190
Jenkins, C. D. **3**: 456, 470
Jenkins, G. L. **3**: 681
Jenkins, J. J. **1**: 184, 191; **3**: 552, 569
Jenkins, R. L. **3**: 739, 760, 761
Jenkins, W. O. **1**: 141, 148
Jennings, H. H. **3**: 734, 735, 760
Jephcott, A. P. **1**: 380, 400
Jersild, A. T. **1**: 122, 124, 126, 129, 130, 132, 148
Jervis, G. A. **3**: 678
Jesperson, **3**: 549
Jessner, L. **2**: 480; **3**: 121, 454
Jessop, W. J. E. **3**: 21, 22, 23, 57
Jessop, W. J. N. **1**: 516, 520
Jewett, R. E. **2**: 98, 106
Joffe, W. G. **3**: 247, 248, 249, 251, 252, 253
John, E. **1**: 124; **2**: 95, 104
Johnson, A. M. **1**: 374, 386, 400; **2**: 411, 421, 462, 483; **3**: 153, 586, 665, 680
Johnson, M. M. **3**: 142, 146, 153
Johnson, R. T. **2**: 218
Johnson, T. **2**: 106
Johnson, V. E. **2**: 450, 483
Johnston, A. M. **1**: 361, 368
Johnston, A. W. **1**: 513, 521; **2**: 46

Johnstone, M. A. **2**: 62, 85
Jones, A. **2**: 242, 256
Jones, C. M. **3**: 530
Jones, D. C. **2**: 47
Jones, E. **2**: xxi; **3**: 79, 441, 450, 454
Jones, H. E. **1**: 119, 148; **2**: 263
Jones, H. G. **1**: 3, 19, 114, 116, 117, 148, 164, 168, 386, 400; **2**: 574
Jones, H. H. **3**: 586
Jones, K. W. **2**: 46
Jones, M. **2**: 675, 691, 695
Jones, M. B. **2**: 619
Jones, M. C. **1**: 113, 115, 124, 127, 128, 129, 130, 148
Jones, R. T. **2**: 306, 312
Jonsson, G. **3**: 784
Jordan, K. **3**: 494
Jores, A. **2**: 479
Joseph, M. C. **2**: 46
Josselyn, I. M. **3**: 142, 153, 154, 527, 528
Jost, A. **2**: 46
Jouvet, D. **2**: 201, 218, 221
Jouvet, M. **1**: 36; **2**: 174, 189, 202, 205, 216, 218, 221, 255, 556
Jung, C. **1**: 237, 248; **2**: xxii, xxv, 4, 18, 150, 271, 520; **3**: 145, 153

Kaffman, M. **3**: 338, 342, 345
Kafka, G. **2**: 189
Kagan, J. **3**: 66, 79, 141, 153
Kahlbaum, K. **2**: 425, 439, 446; **3**: 596, 597, 608, 652, 680
Kahn, E. **2**: 6, 11, 18, 218
Kahn, J. H. **1**: 242, 248, 291, 305; **2**: 144, 695; **3**: 755, 760
Kahn, M. W. **2**: 355, 388
Kaijser, K. **2**: 46
Kaila, E. **1**: 89, 102
Kales, A. **2**: 218, 219
Kalhorn, J. **1**: 398
Kallmann, F. J. **1**: 42, 56, 380, 481, 494; **2**: 5, 13, 14, 18; **3**: 653, 654, 655, 657, 668, 680
Kälvesten, A-L. **3**: 784
Kandinsky, V. **2**: 436, 446
Kann, J. **3**: 83, 96
Kanner, L. **1**: 44, 167, 168, 182, 183, 191, 235, 248, 252, 267, 283, 404, 408, 426, 473, 481; **2**: 412, 423; **3**: 1, 292, 318, 367, 370, 456, 462, 470, 541, 589, 610, 617, 649, 650, 651, 652, 653, 655, 656, 657, 659, 662, 671, 673, 674, 675, 676, 679, 680, 681, 705, 723, 731

Kansky, E. W. 2: 256
Kant, I. 2: 162, 490, 496, 500
Kantor, M. 2: 712
Kantor, M. B. 3: 759
Kantor, M. K. 3: 759
Kaplan, B. 3: 123
Kaplan, M. 3: 586
Kaplan, S. 1: 495
Kardiner, A. 3: 298, 304, 318
Karlins, M. 2: 261
Karmel, M. 3: 80, 88, 96
Karpman, B. 1: 370, 400
Karush, A. 3: 526, 529
Kasanin, J. 2: 411, 422; 3: 146, 153, 652
Kasinoff, B. H. 2: 221
Kast, L. 3: 8
Kasten, F. H. 2: 50, 84, 85
Kato, 2: 520; 3: 370
Katz, D. 3: 5, 153
Katz, J. 3: 251
Katy, R. 3: 142, 153
Kauffman, R. 2: 271, 285
Kaufman, I. 1: 400, 413, 426, 479, 494; 3: 652, 751, 760
Kaufman, M. R. 2: 614
Kawenoka, M. 3: 252, 253
Kay, E. 2: 417
Kay, J. H. 2: 253
Keddie, K. M. G. 2: 220
Kedrov, B. 2: 446
Keeler, W. R. 2: 656, 666, 678, 681
Keena, J. C. 3: 56
Keir, G. 1: 252, 283
Keith-Lee, P. 2: 105
Kellaway, P. 2: 190
Keller, G. 3: 652
Keller, W. K. 2: 188
Kelley, R. 2: 311
Kellmer-Pringle, M. L. 3: 545, 550, 569
Kelly, 1: 185
Kelly, E. L. 2: 256
Kelly, M. 2: 616
Kemmler, L. 3: 746, 760
Kempe, C. H. 3: 587, 588
Kendric, D. C. 1: 158, 168
Kennedy, A. 2: 178, 190
Kennedy, H. E. 3: 252, 253
Kennedy, J. L. 2: 198, 219, 221
Kenney, E. T. 3: 758
Kent, E. 1: 40, 56
Kenyon, F. E. 1: 406, 412, 426
Kerbikov, O. V. 2: 427, 446
Kerlin, I. M. 3: 652
Kerlinger, F. N. 3: 370
Kerr, M. A. 3: 737, 760
Kerstetter, L. M. 3: 737, 760
Kesaree, N. 2: 46
Kesner, R. 3: 52, 60
Kessell, W. I. N. 2: 415, 651, 674
Kessler, J. W. 3: 651, 681

Kety, S. S. 2: 15, 18, 107, 277, 286, 616
Kidd, C. B. 2: 46
Kidd, P. J. 2: 179, 188
Kierkegaard, S. 2: 491, 492, 495, 518
Kierman, 3: 606
Kiev, A. 2: 616, 617
Kim, K. 2: 410, 421
Kimble, D. P. 2: 106
Kimble, G. 1: 104, 105, 119, 148; 2: 295, 310
Kimble, J. P. 3: 565, 569
Kinch, J. W. 1: 376, 400
King, G. F. 1: 135, 136, 142, 148; 2: 365, 388
King, J. A. 2: 256
King, S. R. 2: 619
Kinsbourne, M. 3: 564, 569
Kinsey, J. L. 2: 256
Kirk, H. D. 1: 451
Kirman, B. H. 1: 56, 217, 233, 459, 496, 501, 502, 503, 506, 510, 516, 518, 520, 521; 3: 24, 57, 546
Kirschbaum, R. M. 1: 84
Kirscher, A. 2: 147, 148, 190
Kirsner, J. B. 3: 527, 529
Kiruma, D. 2: 252
Kish, G. B. 2: 251
Kissen, D. M. 2: 185, 190
Kitamura, S. 2: 256
Kitto, G. B. 2: 104
Klackenberg, G. 3: 784
Klapman, Y. W. 2: 579, 594
Klebanoff, L. B. 1: 479, 494
Klebanov, D. 3: 27, 58
Klein, E. 1: 131, 148
Klein, G. S. 2: 449, 450, 478, 483
Klein, M. 1: 252, 359, 369, 485, 487, 492, 494; 2: 449, 452, 456, 457, 458, 483, 3: 175, 200, 211, 212, 213, 214, 217, 219, 441, 443, 454, 540, 543, 544, 546, 656, 661, 672, 681
Kleine, W. 2: 219
Kleist, 2: 440
Kleitman, N. 2: 193, 199, 200, 216, 217, 219, 270, 286
Klett, C. J. 2: 389
Kline, N. S. 2: 635
Klinefelter, J. F. (Jr.) 2: 46
Klinger, P. D. 2: 103
Klippel, M. 3: 606
Klopfer, B. 2: 616
Klotz, R. 3: 33, 58
Kluckhohn, C. 3: 139, 153, 302, 313
Kluckhohn, F. 3: 305, 318, 371
Kluckhohn, R. 3: 315, 320
Klüver, H. 3: 82, 96
Knapp, P. H. 2: 477, 483
Knatterud, G. L. 3: 803
Knight, D. A. 2: 616

Knight, E. 2: 422; 3: 153
Knight, R. P. 2: 558, 571, 574
Knobloch, H. 1: 437, 438, 450, 500, 521; 3: 27, 58, 59, 667, 681, 705
Knowles, J. B. 2: 616
Knox, E. G. 1: 378, 400
Knox, R. S. 2: 46
Knox, W. E. 1: 53, 56
Koch, J. P. 3: 527
Koch, S. 3: 97
Koegler, R. 3: 655, 679, 681
Koella, W. P. 1: 494
Koenig, H. 2: 62, 85
Koepf, G. F. 2: 48
Koffka, K. 2: 490
Kogan, A. B. 2: 538, 544, 556
Kogan, K. L. 1: 573, 585
Kohlberg, L. 3: 745, 760
Kohler, W. 2: 490
Kohlmeyer, W. A. 2: 707, 711
Kokoschka, O. 2: 143
Kokubun, O. 2: 258, 260
Kolb, D. A. 2: 575
Kolb, L. C. 2: 616
Kolin, E. A. 2: 264
Kollar, E. J. 2: 219
Kondo, A. 2: 520, 530; 3: 370
Konorsky, J. 2: 128
Koos, E. 2: 747, 760
Kora, T. 2: 519
Koranyi, E. K. 2: 204, 219
Korchin, S. J. 1: 493
Korn, S. 3: 79
Kornblum, J. L. 3: 761
Kornetsky, C. 2: 616
Kornfeld, D. S. 2: 256
Kornhuber, H. H. 3: 409, 416
Kornitzer, M. 1: 441, 444, 446, 450
Korolkova, T. 2: 539, 556
Korsakoff, S. S. 2: 427, 436, 440, 446
Kothe, B. 2: 435, 446
Kounin, J. 2: 617
Kounin, M. S. 3: 736, 760
Kovach, K. 2: 263
Kraepelin, E. 1: 473, 487, 494; 2: xix, 4, 5, 18, 219, 415, 425, 428, 432, 440, 444, 446, 701, 711; 3: 3, 12, 388, 390, 590, 591, 593, 594, 597, 602, 603, 605, 606, 607, 608, 609, 707, 728, 731
Kraepelin, K. 2: 427
Krafft-Ebing, R. von, 2: 180, 190, 432, 446
Krakowski, A. J. 3: 705
Krall, V. 1: 359, 369
Kramer, M. 2: 216
Kranz, H. 1: 40, 56, 380
Krasner, L. 1: 135, 148; 2: 376, 388, 390, 570, 573, 575, 616,

AUTHOR INDEX

Krasnich, S. A. **2**: 594
Kravitz, H. **2**: 219
Krech, D. **2**: 88, 104, 105
Kreindler, A. **3**: 562, 570
Kreitman, N. **2**: 365, 366, 368, 388
Kretschmer, E. **2**: 444
Kreuser, **3**: 603
Krieger, H. P. **3**: 682
Kris, E. **2**: 449, 482; **3**: 121, 122, 201, 213, 219, 302, 306, 318, 664
Kris, E. B. **3**: 53, 58
Kris, M. **3**: 66, 79, 328, 345
Kristiansen, K. **2**: 544, 556
Kroeber, A. L. **3**: 293, 294, 298, 302
Kroger, W. S. **2**: 165, 178, 181, 190
Kronfeld, A. S. **2**: 427, 428, 446
Kruger, **2**: 490
Krugman, M. **3**: 761
Krupp, I. M. **2**: 15, 18
Kruse, H. D. **3**: 11
Krutetski, V. A. **1**: 174, 187, 191
Kubie, L. **2**: 245, 256
Kubie, L. S. **2**: 270, 286, 306, 312, 478, 483
Kubzansky, P. E. **2**: 256, 257, 260, 298, 310
Kuehl, F. A. **2**: 15, 18
Kuffler, St W. **2**: 85
Kugler, M. M. **3**: 526
Kuhlen, R. G. **3**: 735, 760
Kummer, H. **1**: 33, 37
Kuninobu, L. **2**: 262
Kunkle, E. G. **1**: 369
Kurauchi, K. **2**: 529
Kurland, A. A. **2**: 616
Kurland, D. **2**: 614
Kurlents, S. **2**: 258
Kuromaru, S. **3**: 676, 681
Kurtz, K. **1**: 120, 148
Kurtz, S. M. **2**: 84
Küstner, H. **2**: 182, 191
Kuznetsov, A. G. **2**: 251
Kuznetsov, O. N. **2**: 256
Kuznetsova, G. **2**: 539, 556

LaBarre, W. **2**: 616
Lafon, R. **3**: 721, 732
Lagercrantz, R. **3**: 526, 527, 528
Lagercrantz, S. **3**: 469
Laing, R. D. **2**: 410, 421, 464, 466, 483; **3**: 544, 546
Lairy, G. C. **3**: 393, 414, 416
Lajtha, A. **2**: 100, 106
Lajtha, L. G. **2**: 46
Lambercier, M. **1**: 99, 102
Lambo, T. A. **2**: 707, 711
Lamy, **3**: 21
Landauer, W. **3**: 20, 58
Landis, C. **1**: 148; **2**: 364, 388, 574

Landreth, C. **1**: 128, 148
Lang, A. **3**: 293, 318
Lang, P. **1**: 127, 149; **2**: 377, 388, 564, 572, 574, 575
Lang, T. **1**: 51, 56
Lange, **3**: 408
Lange, B. **1**: 269
Lange, J. **1**: 380
Lange, P. W. **2**: 93, 106, 427, 446
Langfeldt, G. **2**: 391, 392, 415
Langford, W. S. **1**: 360, 361, 369; **3**: 145, 153, 512, 516, 528, 649, 681
Langs, R. J. **2**: 617
Lanzkowsky, P. **3**: 470
Lapham, L. W. **2**: 62, 85
Lapouse, R. **3**: 739, 761
Laptev, **2**: 537, 556
Larson, W. **2**: 45
Larsson, T. **1**: 43, 56
Lasagna, L. **2**: 616, 619
Lasègue, E. C. **3**: 602
Lashley, K. S. **2**: 111, 128
Laties, V. G. **2**: 616
Latil, J. **3**: 122
Laubscher, B. J. F. **2**: 701, 702, 711
Laufer, M. **3**: 231, 232, 251, 252, 470
Laughlin, F. **3**: 734, 745, 761
Laulicht, J. H. **3**: 151
Laurence, K. M. **1**: 501, 521
Lauriers, A. M. des, **1**: 492, 494; **3**: 664, 679, 700, 705
Lauwerys, J. **1**: 184, 190
Laverty, S. C. **2**: 573
Lavery, L. **1**: 245, 248
Lavin, N. I. **2**: 573
Lawson, D. **1**: 222, 224, 233
Lawson, J. S. **2**: 424; **3**: 565, 569
Lawson, R. **1**: 145, 149
Lay, W. **1**: 173, 191
Layman, E. M. **3**: 470
Layne, R. S. **2**: 312
Layng, J. **1**: 283; **3**: 153, 290
Lazar, E. **3**: 10
Lazarus, A. **1**: 127, 128, 149; **2**: 560, 565, 567, 570, 571, 574, 575
Lazowick, L. M. **3**: 141, 153
Lazowik, A. D. **1**: 127, 149; **2**: 377, 388, 564, 572, 574
Lea, J. **3**: 559, 569
Leach, B. E. **2**: 15, 18, 311
Learned, J. **1**: 100, 101
Lebedev, V. I. **2**: 256
Lebedinskii, M. S. **2**: 593, 594
Lebedinsky, A. V. **2**: 256
Leblond, C. P. **2**: 62, 84, 86, 105
Lebovici, S. **3**: 122, 200, 202, 219
Lebowitz, M. **3**: 681
LeCron, L. M. **2**: 190

Lederman, I. I. **2**: 421
Lee, A. R. **2**: 421
Lee, B. J. **3**: 735, 760
Lee, D. **3**: 680
Lee, E. S. **2**: 711
Leeds, C. H. **3**: 736, 761
Lees, H. **2**: 219, 307, 309, 312
Le Gassicke, J. **2**: 219
Lehmann, D. **2**: 218
Lehmann, H. E. **2**: 616
Lehmann, T. G. **2**: 204, 219
Lehner, G. F. J. **2**: 357, 388
Lehtinen, L. E. **1**: 16, 19, 472, 517, 521
Leiberman, D. M. **2**: 386
Leiberman, J. **1**: 366, 368
Leibowitz, H. **1**: 99, 103
Leiderman, H. **2**: 260
Leiderman, P. H. **2**: 256, 257, 260, 261, 262, 310, 311
Leighton, A. **2**: 701, 711
Leighton, D. **3**: 136, 153
Leiken, S. L. **3**: 587
Leitch, M. **3**: 122
Lejeune, J. **1**: 47, 55, 56, 502, 512, 521
Lemere, F. **2**: 575
Lempp, R. **3**: 674, 681
Lenhard, L. W. **2**: 49
Lenihan, E. A. **1**: 84
Lenin, V. I. **2**: 578
Lenneberg, E. H. **3**: 97, 568
Lennenberg, E. **3**: 528
Lennox, B. **2**: 46, 48
Lennox, W. G. **1**: 384, 461, 472; **2**: 616
Lenz, **3**: 50, 51
Lenzo, J. E. **2**: 219, 309
Leon, C. A. **2**: 706, 711
Leon, H. V. **2**: 251
Leonhard, K. **2**: 219, 440, 446, 594
Lepore, M. **3**: 526
Leriche, **2**: 134
Leserman, S. **3**: 587
Lesèvre, N. **3**: 414, 416
Leslie, A. **2**: 616
Lesser, G. **1**: 140, 149
Lesser, R. E. **2**: 219
Lester, B. K. **2**: 287, 309
Letemendia, F. J. J. **1**: 384, 400, 456, 472
Levan, A. **1**: 46, 55, 57; **2**: 49
Levi, W. E. **3**: 492
Levi-Montalcini, R. **2**: 72, 85, 91
Levi-Strauss, C. **2**: 717, 728
Levin, H. **1**: 401, 580, 585; **3**: 141, 143, 153, 155, 320, 746, 762
Levin, M. **2**: 219
Levin, P. **3**: 528
Levine, A. **2**: 614
Levine, M. **3**: 171, 529
Levine, S. **2**: 264
Levinsky, S. V. **2**: 256

AUTHOR INDEX

Levinson, J. **2:** 45
Levitt, E. E. **1:** 152, 153, 154, 168; **3:** 736, 761
Levitt, G. E. **2:** 364, 388
Levitt, M. **3:** 139, 146, 155
Levy, D. M. **1:** 255, 283; **3:** 123, 303, 319, 642
Levy, E. Z. **2:** 259, 260
Levy, K. **3:** 244, 252
Levy, L. **2:** 252
Levy, L. H. **2:** 355, 388
Levy, R. **3:** 528
Levy, S. **1:** 383, 400
Lew, W. **2:** 103
Lewin, G. **3:** 327, 329, 340, 341, 343, 345
Lewin, K. K. **2:** 717; **3:** 5, 123, 542, 546, 761
Lewin, K. W. **3:** 586
Lewin, L. **2:** 635
Lewin, W. **2:** 113, 116, 120, 129
Lewinson, P. M. **3:** 565, 569
Lewis, A. **1:** 400, 486, 495; **2:** 120, 128
Lewis, B. M. **2:** 48
Lewis, C. M. **3:** 525
Lewis, E. D. **3:** 546
Lewis, E. O. **1:** 500, 521
Lewis, H. **1:** 379, 400, 428, 436, 443, 450, 451; **3:** 265, 281, 291
Lewis, J. H. **2:** 178, 190
Lewis, M. M. **1:** 95, 102; **3:** 546
Lewis, W. C. **2:** 480, 482, 483
Lewty, W. **2:** 260
Lezine, I. **3:** 123
Lhermitte, J. **2:** xxi, 130, 145; **3:** 606, 718, 732
Liberman, R. **2:** 616
Liberson, W. T. **3:** 414, 416
Libich, S. S. **2:** 585, 593, 594
Lichtenstein, E. D. **2:** 219
Lichtenstein, H. **3:** 302
Lichtenstein, P. **1:** 129
Lickorish, J. R. **1:** 562, 577, 585; **2:** 674; **3:** 153
Liddell, H. **1:** 119, 121, 149
Lidell, **1:** 389
Lidz, R. W. **2:** 401, 410, 416, 465; **3:** 370
Lidz, T. **2:** 402, 403, 416, 417, 464, 483; **3:** 363, 364, 366, 370
Liébeault, A. A. **2:** 149, 190
Lieberfruend, S. **3:** 759
Liebermann, M. **2:** 143
Lief, H. I. **2:** 618
Lief, N. R. **2:** 618
Lief, V. F. **2:** 618
Lifton, R. J. **1:** 389, 400; **2:** 219
Lighthall, F. F. **3:** 754, 755, 761
Lilienfeld, A. M. **1:** 401, 472
Lilienfeld, M. D. **3:** 528

Lillie, R. D. **2:** 85
Lilly, J. C. **2:** 224, 256, 257, 299, 310
Limentani, D. **2:** 411, 422
Lin, T. Y. **2:** 701, 711
Lind, D. L. **1:** 136, 142, 147
Lindemann, E. **1:** 426; **2:** 257; **3:** 528, 752, 755, 761
Lindemann, H. **2:** 257
Lindquist, E. F. **1:** 6, 19
Lindsley, D. B. **1:** 112; **2:** 257
Lindsley, D. F. **2:** 262
Lindsley, O. R. **1:** 114, 135, 136, 141, 143, 146, 149, 150
Lindsten, J. **2:** 35, 46, 47
Ling, B. C. **1:** 91, 102
Linn, E. L. **2:** 616
Linnaeus, C. **2:** 140
Linton, H. B. **2:** 617
Linton, R. **2:** 698, 711; **3:** 298, 304, 312, 318, 319
Lippitt, R. **3:** 734, 735, 747, 761
Lippmann, R. **1:** 133, 134, 149
Lippton, **3:** 329
Lipset, S. M. **3:** 309, 319
Lipton, E. L. **3:** 472, 473, 474, 475, 492
Lisle, A. (Jr.) **3:** 528
Litin, E. M. **2:** 483; **3:** 586
Little, W. J. **1:** 516, 521
Little, W. R. **1:** 400
Littner, N. **2:** 527
Livanov, M. N. **2:** 537, 538, 539, 543, 547, 554, 556
Livingston, R. B. **2:** 174, 190
Locke, J. **2:** 161, 162, 223
Lockman, R. F. **2:** 355, 356, 389
Lodahl, R. M. **2:** 257
Loeb, D. G. **1:** 327, 334; **3:** 492
Loewenstein, R. M. **1:** 242, 248; **2:** 449, 482; **3:** 122, 201, 213, 251, 306, 318
Loftis, L. **3:** 737, 760
Löfving, B. **1:** 455, 472
Logan, G. B. **1:** 352, 354, 369
Logan, H. H. **3:** 494, 528
Logan, R. F. L. **3:** 145, 153
Logan, W. P. D. **1:** 515, 521; **3:** 30, 58
Lombroso, C. **3:** 603
London, I. D. **2:** 357, 388
Long, E. R. **1:** 141, 149
Loomis, A. L. **2:** 219
Lorente de Nó **2:** 67, 109, 128; **3:** 669, 681
Lorenz, K. **1:** 34, 37; **2:** 483; **3:** 82
Lorge, I. **3:** 570, 680
Lorr, M. **2:** 371, 389; **3:** 739, 761
Lossen, H. **2:** 357, 389
Lourie, R. **3:** 675, 681

Lourie, R. S. **3:** 455, 470
Lovaas, O. I. **1:** 114, 140, 142, 149
Lovell, C. **1:** 370, 401
Lovell, K. **1:** 79, 83
Lovibond, S. H. **1:** 116, 117, 141, 149, 163, 168; **2:** 378, 389, 574
Lovinger, E. **1:** 148
Low, M. D. **2:** 169, 190
Lowry, **2:** 52
Loy, R. M. **1:** 515, 521; **3:** 58
Lu, Y. C. **2:** 410, 421
Lubin, A. **2:** 219, 221, 295, 310
Luborsky, L. **2:** 483, 616, 619
Luby, E. D. **2:** 204, 219, 288, 293, 304, 309, 311, 312
Lucas, C. J. **2:** 616
Lucas, J. **3:** 683
Lucas, L. **1:** 481, 495
Ludowyk, E. **3:** 240
Ludowyk, G. E. **3:** 252
Lugaro, **2:** 426; **3:** 606
Lumsden, C. E. **2:** 77, 85
Lundstrom, R. **3:** 20, 26, 58
Luria, A. R. **1:** 92, 95, 96, 102; **3:** 537, 546, 553, 557, 569
Lurie, L. A. **1:** 487, 495
Lurie, M. L. **1:** 487, 495
Lurie, O. R. **3:** 153
Luse, **2:** 58
Lussier, A. **3:** 239, 244, 250, 252
Luttges, M. **2:** 106
Lutz, J. **3:** 652, 674, 679, 681
Luxenburger, H. **2:** 10, 18
Lyketsos, G. C. **2:** 411, 422
Lyle, J. G. **1:** 212, 213, 230, 231, 233, 500, 521
Lynn, D. **3:** 141, 153
Lynn, R. **1:** 574, 585
Lyon, M. F. **2:** 22, 25, 27, 47
Lyons, A. S. **3:** 526, 528

McAndrew, H. **2:** 257
McBride, J. A. **2:** 47; **3:** 51
McBride, K. E. **3:** 561, 570
McCallum, H. M. **3:** 57
McCallum, W. C. **2:** 192; **3:** 417
MacCalman, D. R. **3:** 139, 153
McCandless, B. R. **3:** 745, 761
McCarthy, D. **3:** 549, 569
McClemont, W. F. **2:** 16, 19, 46
McCollum, A. T. **2:** 484
McConnell, J. **2:** 95, 106
McConnell, J. V. **2:** 151, 190
McConnon, K. **3:** 550, 569
McCord, J. **1:** 375, 379, 383, 384, 401; **2:** 422; **3:** 146, 154, 792, 796, 803
McCord, W. **1:** 375, 379, 383,

AUTHOR INDEX

384, 401; **2:** 412, 422; **3:** 154, 792, 796, 803
McCort, J. **3:** 587
McCourt, W. F. **2:** 253
McCraven, V. C. **3:** 311, 320
McCraven, V. G. **3:** 310
McCulloch, W. **2:** 123, 128
McDermott, J. F. **3:** 528
McDonald, A. D. **1:** 516, 521; **3:** 36, 37, 58
Macdonald, E. K. **1:** 445, 450
McDonald, I. M. **2:** 695
MacDonald, J. **3:** 652
Macdonald, N. **2:** 190
McEwen, B. S. **2:** 54, 87, 106
McFarland, R. A. **2:** 257
MacFarlane, J. W. **1:** 123, 134, 149, 154, 155, 168, 381, 400; **3:** 66, 67, 79, 792, 796, 803
McGaugh, J. **2:** 106
McGhie, A. **1:** 36, 247; **2:** 207, 208, 219, 289, 308, 309, 312, 414, 423, 424, 481; **3:** 566, 568, 569
McGie, H. **3:** 545
McGill, T. E. **2:** 261, 262
MacGillivray, R. C. **3:** 33, 58
McGirr, E. M. **1:** 507, 521
McGovern, V. J. **3:** 528
McGregor, D. **2:** 106
MacGregor, F. M. C. **3:** 136, 154
MacGregor, T. N. **2:** 46
McGuigan, J. F. **2:** 617
McHenry, T. **3:** 587
McHugh, L. **2:** 253
McKay, J. R. **3:** 528
McKee, A. F. **3:** 22, 60
Mackeith, R. **1:** 311, 334, 369; **3:** 250
McKellar, P. **1:** 170, 176, 178, 191
McKenna, F. **2:** 251
Mackenzie, D. Y. **1:** 502, 505, 521
McKenzie, R. E. **2:** 257
McKeown, T. **2:** 27, 31, 32, 58, 59
McKerracher, D. G. **2:** 686, 695
McKerracher, D. W. **3:** 44, 58
McKie, R. **2:** 257
McKittrick, L. S. **3:** 529
McLaughlin, M. M. **3:** 199
Maclean, N. **2:** 45, 46, 47
McLean, P. D. **2:** 267, 286
McMahan, A. **3:** 762
MacMahon, T. **3:** 27, 58
McMenemey, W. H. **1:** 54, 56
Macmillan, D. **2:** 695
McNair, D. M. **2:** 389
MacNaughton, D. **3:** 682
MacQueen, I. A. G. **1:** 353, 369
MacSorley, K. **2:** 6, 18
McWhinnie, A. M. **1:** 451

Maccoby, E. E. **1:** 401; **3:** 306, 317, 319, 320, 746, 758, 762
Maceroy, E. E. **3:** 143, 155
Machover, K. **1:** 579, 585
Mackler, D. **2:** 619
Maddi, S. R. **2:** 246, 253, 259
Magnan, V. **2:** 425, 446; **3:** 602
Magnuson, K. **2:** 253
Magonet, A. P. **2:** 181, 190
Magoun, H. W. **2:** 193, 219, 267, 286
Mahatoo, W. **2:** 253
Maher, B. A. **2:** 357, 389
Maher-Loughnan, G. P. **2:** 181, 190
Mahler, M. S. **1:** 242, 248, 483, 492, 495; **2:** 459, 483; **3:** 327, 610, 650, 653, 658, 659, 661, 673, 681, 700, 705
Maier, H. W. **3:** 610, 614
Maier, M. R. F. **1:** 377, 388, 401
Main, T. F. **2:** 477, 483
Major, R. H. **2:** 617
Majorov, F. P. **2:** 583, 594
Makarenko, **3:** 139, 140, 154
Makino, S. **1:** 55; **2:** 48
Makita, K. **3:** 347, 370, 371, 375, 681
Makulkin, R. F. **2:** 544, 556
Malamud, N. **3:** 662, 681
Malinowski, B. **2:** 603; **3:** 127, 134, 154, 293, 294, 296, 319
Malitz, S. **2:** 614
Malleson, N. **2:** 574
Malm, J. R. **2:** 256
Malmo, R. **2:** 348
Malmo, R. B. **2:** 293, 309
Malzberg, B. **2:** 5, 6, 18, 703, 711
Mancall, E. L. **2:** 114, 129
Mandelbaum, D. G. **2:** 257
Mandell, A. J. **2:** 204, 219
Mandell, M. P. **2:** 219
Mandler, G. **3:** 123
Manghi, E. **3:** 675, 681
Manheimer, N. **3:** 2, 652
Mann, D. **2:** 615
Mannheim, H. **1:** 380, 401
Manning, M. **1:** 349
Manor, R. **3:** 332, 345
Manson, M. M. **3:** 21, 22, 23, 26, 54, 58
Manson, M. N. **1:** 515, 521
Mantle, D. J. **2:** 45, 46, 47
Marbe, K. **1:** 351, 369
Marcel, G. **2:** 495, 496, 518
Marchbanks, G. **3:** 567, 569
Marcus, **1:** 361, 369; **3:** 676, 682
Marcuse, F. L. **1:** 577, 584
Margerison, J. **1:** 463, 464, 472
Margetts, E. **2:** 701, 711
Margolin, S. **3:** 516, 528

Margolis, R. **2:** 615
Markham, C. **3:** 679
Marks, C. S. **2:** 263
Marks, I. M. **2:** 390
Marmer, M. J. **2:** 190
Marmor, J. **3:** 319
Maron, L. **2:** 220
Marquhart, D. I. **1:** 377, 401
Marquis, D. G. **2:** 173, 189
Marrazzi, A. S. **2:** 275, 287
Marro, **3:** 597, 608
Marrs, M. **1:** 518, 520
Marshall, A. G. **3:** 43, 58
Martens, S. **2:** 311
Martin, F. M. **2:** 678, 695
Martin, W. E. **3:** 319
Marton, T. **2:** 262
Maruseva, A. M. **2:** 538, 556
Masion, **3:** 598
Masland, R. P. **3:** 528
Masling, J. **2:** 617
Mason, A. A. **2:** 152, 153, 176, 180, 181, 182, 184, 189, 190
Mason, M. K. **2:** 257
Massenti, C. **3:** 719, 732
Masserman, J. H. **1:** 129, 390, 401; **2:** 417, 418, 419, 420, 486, 574, 614, 695, 696
Massey, J. R. **2:** 85
Masters, W. H. **2:** 450, 483
Masterson, J. **1:** 413, 426
Matthews, J. **1:** 217, 233
Matthews, P. J. **3:** 587
Maudsley, H. **1:** 251, 283; **2:** 435, 436, 446; **3:** 2, 11, 15, 652
Maxwell, A. E. **1:** 6, 14, 19, 112
May, F. **1:** 149
May, M. A. **1:** 374, 400
May, R. **1:** 125; **2:** 511, 518
Mayer, G. W. **3:** 563
Mayer-Gross, W. **2:** 7, 18; **3:** 8, 569, 546
Mayimilian, C. **2:** 47
Maynert, **3:** 609
Mays, J. B. **1:** 378, 379, 401; **3:** 546
Mead, G. H. **3:** 546
Mead, M. **3:** 136, 137, 138, 154, 155, 209, 257, 291, 296
Meares, A. **2:** 165, 181, 190
Mechanic, D. **3:** 746, 747, 761
Mednick, S. A. **1:** 187, 191
Meduna, L. J. von **2:** xxii
Meeker, J. A. (Jr.) **3:** 528
Meerloo, J. A. M. **1:** 411, 413, 426; **2:** 617
Meers, D. **3:** 246, 252
Mefford, R. B. **3:** 565, 569
Mehlman, B. **2:** 365, 389
Meiks, L. T. **3:** 527, 528, 529
Meili, R. **2:** 357, 389

AUTHOR INDEX

Mekeel, 3: 302
Mele, H. 2: 177, 191
Mellbin, G. 2: 47
Mellins, R. G. 3: 456, 470
Mellman, W. J. 2: 47
Melville, M. M. 2: 46
Mendell, D. 2: 397, 416
Mendeloff, A. I. 3: 528
Mendelson, J. 2: 257, 261, 262, 311
Mendelson, J. H. 2: 256, 257, 260, 299, 310
Mendelson, M. 3: 474, 492
Mengel, C. E. 3: 470
Menkes, J. H. 1: 502: 521
Menninger, K. A. 1: 369
Menolascino, F. J. 3: 657, 682
Mensh, I. N. 3: 737, 759, 761
Menzel, E. W. 2: 216
Menzies, I. E. P. 2: 695
Merleau-Ponty, M. 2: 133, 145, 496, 518
Merrell, D. 1: 148
Merrill, E. J. 3: 587
Merrill, M. A. 1: 96, 103, 570, 586
Mesmer, F. A. 2: 147, 149, 190
Messinger, E. C. 1: 53, 56
Messinger, J. 3: 333, 338, 339, 345
Metfessel, M. 1: 370, 401
Métraux, R. 3: 139, 154
Metz, B. 2: 218, 221, 309
Metzner, R. 1: 120, 121, 129, 145, 149, 157, 168; 2: 376, 389
Meyer, A. 1: 252; 2: 7; 3: 6, 8, 10, 11, 12, 590, 606, 656
Meyer, E. 1: 91, 102
Meyer, J. S. 2: 257, 302, 311
Meyer, M. de 1: 136, 137, 138, 143, 147
Meyers, D. I. 3: 705
Meyers, M. 3: 678
Meyerson, L. 1: 227, 233
Mezaros, A. F. 2: 617
Miale, I. L. 2: 72, 85
Miasnikov, V. I. 2: 254, 257
Michael, J. 1: 139, 146
Michelangelo, 2: 143
Michener, W. M. 3: 528
Middlekamp, J. N. 3: 528
Mihailovic, L. J. 2: 91, 106
Mikuriya, I. 2: 530
Milcu, St M. 2: 47
Mill, J. S. 1: 9, 19, 200
Millar, T. P. 3: 471, 492
Millen, J. W. 1: 514, 515, 521; 3: 47, 52, 58, 60
Miller, 2: 376
Miller, A. 2: 216
Miller, D. 3: 304, 306, 319, 746, 761
Miller, D. S. 3: 587
Miller, G. 2: 263
Miller, G. A. 3: 565, 569

Miller, J. 2: 636
Miller, J. G. 2: 273, 287
Miller, J. R. 2: 45
Miller, L. 3: 154, 321, 338, 345
Miller, N. 1: 120, 121, 149, 399
Miller, N. E. 2: 106
Miller, O. J. 1: 521; 2: 47
Miller, S. C. 2: 257, 449, 478, 484, 486
Miller, W. 3: 748, 761
Miller, W. R. 2: 188
Millican, F. K. 3: 455, 470
Millichap, J. G. 1: 464, 472
Mills, E. S. 1: 585
Milner, B. 2: 112, 118, 119, 128
Mintz, A. 2: 357, 389
Mintz, A. A. 3: 587
Mintz, T. 1: 188, 191
Minuchin, P. 3: 736, 761
Mirsky, A. E. 2: 105
Mirsky, I. A. 3: 474, 493, 499, 528
Misiak, H. 2: 357, 389
Mitchell, B. 1: 79, 83
Mitchell, J. M. 2: 47
Mitchell, S. 3: 739, 741, 761, 762
Mitchell, S. A. 2: 220
Mitchell, S. W. 2: 198, 199, 219, 280
Mittwoch, U. 1: 507, 521
Miura, T. 3: 371
Mjassischev, V. N. 2: 590, 593, 594
Mnukhina, R. S. 2: 538, 556
Möbius, 3: 609
Model, E. 3: 253
Modell, A. 2: 285, 287
Modell, W. 2: 617
Modlin, H. C. 2: 485
Mohr, G. J. 3: 145, 154, 528
Mohr, J. P. 2: 573
Moll, A. 2: 582, 587, 594
Moloney, J. C. 2: 700, 711; 3: 357, 371
Monakhov, K. K. 2: 531
Monashkin, I. 2: 422
Monck, E. M. 2: 423
Money, J. 2: 34, 44, 47
Money-Kyrle, R. E. 2: 483
Moniz, E. 2: xxiii
Monk, M. A. 3: 739, 761
Monod, G. 3: 591, 596, 608
Monroe, L. J. 2: 208, 219
Montagu, A. 3: 312
Montgomery, J. 2: 616
Montyel, M. de 3: 591, 594
Moon, L. E. 2: 257
Mooney, R. L. 1: 585
Moore, B. W. 2: 106
Moore, K. L. 2: 44, 47
Moore, N. 2: 572, 574
Moore, R. C. 2: 257
Moore, T. 3: 279, 280, 291

Moorhead, P. S. 2: 47
Moran, E. 3: 565, 569
Moreau de Tours, J. 2: 265, 625, 3: 2, 652
Morel, B. A. 1: 496, 521; 2: 425, 446
Morel, B. B. 3: 592, 608, 652, 682
Morell, J. 2: 538, 556
Morello, M. 2: 257
Moreno, J. L. 2: 419, 594, 614, 616; 3: 734, 735, 761
Morgan, 2: 150
Morgan, C. G. 2: 128
Morgan, C. P. 2: 111, 127
Morgan, R. F. 2: 257
Morgenbesser, S. 2: 284, 287
Morgensen A. 1: 269
Morishima, A. 2: 45
Morison, R. A. H. 2: 617
Morita, S. 2: 519-530
Morlock, H. C. 2: 221
Morlock, J. V. 2: 221
Morningstar, M. E. 2: 260
Morozov, V. M. 2: 434, 446
Morozova, T. V. 2: 553, 556
Morrell, F. 2: 110, 128
Morris, D. 1: 28, 32, 37
Morris, G. O. 2: 219, 400, 416
Morris, J. McL. 2: 47
Morris, M. G. 3: 587
Morrisbey, J. 2: 388
Morrison, D. F. 2: 221
Morselli, E. 3: 602
Morselli, H. 1: 413, 426
Morton, A. 3: 585
Morton, W. D. 2: 105
Moruzzi. G. 2: 193, 219, 305, 311
Moses, L. 3: 526, 529
Mosher, L. 3: 682
Mosier, H. D. 2: 47, 48
Mosley, A. L. 2: 257
Moss, A. 3: 123
Moss, A. A. 2: 190
Moss, H. A. 3: 79
Mosteller, F. 2: 616
Motherby, G. 2: 599, 617
Motobayashi, F. 2: 257
Mott, F. W. 2: 9, 18
Moule, P. D. 3: 528
Mourgue, R. 2: 266, 287
Mowrer, O. H. 1: 110, 113, 116, 117, 119, 120, 121, 150, 162, 169, 399; 2: 376
Mowrer, W. 1: 113, 116, 150
Moyer, J. H. 2: 573
Moynihan, D. P. 3: 309, 799, 803
Moynihan, F. J. 586
Mueller, D. D. 3: 141, 146, 154
Muggia, A. 3: 493
Mukherjee, B. B. 2: 48
Muldal, S. 2: 46, 48
Mulder, D. W. 2: 127

AUTHOR INDEX

Mullan, S. 2: 335, 336, 338, 349
Muller, B. P. 2: 617
Müller, M. 2: 491, 518
Muller-Heyemann, D. 2: 582, 594
Mullin, C. S. 2: 257, 258
Mullins, J. F. 2: 180, 190
Mulry, R. C. 2: 618
Multari, G. 1: 97, 102
Munch, E. 2: 143
Munday, L. 1: 215, 234
Munn, N. L. 1: 150
Munnichs, J. M. A. 2: 258
Munro, T. A. 2: 11, 18
Murakami, H. 3: 371
Murawski, B. J. 2: 290, 309
Murdock, G. P. 3: 134, 154
Murphree, H. E. 2: 256
Murphy, C. W. 2: 258
Murphy, D. B. 2: 258, 260
Murphy, D. P. 3: 33, 58
Murphy, H. B. M. 2: 703, 711, 712
Murphy, I. C. 1: 382, 402
Murphy, J. B. 2: 219
Murphy, L. B. 1: 216, 234; 3: 66, 78, 79
Murray, H. A. 3: 302
Murray, J. H. 2: 617
Murray, J. M. 1: 200, 209; 2: 617
Murray, M. R. 2: 73, 75, 78, 80, 84, 85
Murray, N. 2: 190
Murtaugh, T. 2: 264
Mushatt, C. 2: 483; 3: 528
Mussen, P. 3: 142, 154
Myer, A. 1: 252
Myers, R. E. 2: 111, 128
Myers, R. L. 2: 251
Myers, T. I. 2: 258, 260, 299, 311
Myklebust, H. R. 3: 555, 569
Mylle, M. 2: 48
Mylnaryk, P. 3: 529
Myren, R. A. 3: 587

Nadler, H. L. 3: 670, 682
Naegels, K. D. 3: 141, 150
Naess, S. 3: 281, 291
Nagatsuka, Y. 2: 258
Nagayasu, A. 3: 371
Nagel, E. 1: 6, 8, 19
Nagera, H. 3: 231, 232, 234, 235, 236, 238, 246, 251, 252, 253
Nagler, S. 3: 327, 329, 333, 337, 341, 342, 343, 345
Naito, Y. 3: 371
Nakai, J. 2: 79, 80, 85
Nakamura, M. 3: 370
Nameche, G. 3: 792, 804
Napier, M. B. 1: 412, 426
Narbutowich, I. O. 2: 583, 594
Nardini, J. E. 2: 258

Nash, E. H. (Jr.) 2: 615
Nash, J. 3: 139, 146, 154
Nathan, P. 2: 115, 116, 128, 259
Nauta, W. J. H. 2: 219
Neale, D. H. 1: 138, 139, 150
Nechaeva, N. V. 2: 104, 107
Nefedov, Y. G. 2: 256
Nelson, E. 1: 369
Nelson, E. H. 2: 379, 390
Nelson, R. C. 3: 20, 60
Nelson, W. E. 3: 529
Nemetz, S. J. 2: 483
Netal, A. 1: 398
Netchine, S. 3: 393, 414, 416
Neubauer, P. B. 3: 344, 345, 346, 752, 761
Neugarten, 3: 330
Neumeyer, M. H. 1: 381, 382, 401
Neurath, L. 3: 252, 253
Neustadt, J. O. 2: 619
Neville, E. M. 1: 193, 209
Newbold, G. 2: 181, 187
Newcomb, T. M. 3: 317, 320, 758, 761
Newhall, S. M. 1: 213, 234
Newman, A. F. 2: 262
Newman, L. M. 3: 251
Newman, M. F. 2: 423
Newson, E. 3: 143, 154, 538, 546
Newson, J. 3: 143, 154, 538, 546
Newstetter, W. I. 3: 734, 761
Newton, I. 1: 8
Newton, N. 3: 83, 85, 97
Nicholls, J. G. 2: 85
Nicholson, M. A. 2: 252
Nicholson, N. C. 2: 177, 190
Nichtern, S. 3: 705
Nicolay, R. C. 3: 145, 152
Nielson, J. 2: 48
Nietzsche, F. 2: 495
Nightingale, F. 2: 719
Niner, R. 2: 253
Nissen, H. W. 2: 128, 258; 3: 90, 97
Nissen, Th. 2: 105, 106, 107
Nissl, F. 3: 8, 606, 707
Nitowsky, H. M. 2: 45
Niven, J. S. F. 2: 188
Nobel, K. 2: 217
Nodine, J. H. 2: 573
Nomura, A. 2: 519, 530
Norby, D. E. 2: 48
Norman, C. 3: 591, 608
Norman, E. 1: 237, 248, 477, 495
Norman, P. 2: 45
Norris, F. H. 2: 129
Norris, M. 1: 220, 234
Northway, M. L. 3: 737, 761
Norton, N. 2: 416
Norton, S. 2: 106
Nouillhat, F. 1: 479, 495
Novick, J. 3: 220

Novikova, L. A. 2: 251
Nowak, J. 3: 29, 58
Nowell, P. C. 2: 47
Ntsekhe, 1: 380, 400
Nursten, J. P. 1: 242, 248, 305
Nye, F. L. 3: 281, 291
Nye, I. 1: 374

Obermeyer, M. E. 2: 185, 190
Oblinger, B. 1: 146
O'Brien, J. R. 1: 617
Occomy, W. G. 2: 104
Oceguera-Navarro, C. 2: 96, 107
Ochs, S. 2: 57, 85, 110, 128
Ockey, C. H. 2: 48
O'Connell, D. N. 1: 97, 103
O'Connor, C. M. 2: 128, 217, 221
O'Connor, J. F. 3: 526, 529
O'Connor, N. 1: 19, 188, 191, 216, 230, 234, 320, 335; 3: 281, 291, 553, 557, 558, 569
Odegaard, O. 2: 703, 712
Oden, M. H. 3: 804
O'Doherty, N. J. 3: 587
Oettinger, K. B. 3: 587
Ogden, D. A. 1: 382, 401
Ogilvie, E. 1: 79, 83
Ogle, D. C. 2: 258
O'Gorman, G. 1: 473, 495; 2: 412, 423; 3: 147, 154, 402, 407
Ohlin, L. E. 1: 379, 399
Ohno, S. 2: 21, 23, 48
Ojemann, R. G. 2: 112, 113, 128
Okada, S. 3: 681
Okonogi, K. 3: 347, 371
Okuma, T. 2: 220
Oldfield, R. C. 3: 547, 548, 561, 569
Olin, B. M. 2: 614
Olley, P. 2: 216, 220
Olsen, T. 1: 412, 426
Olsson, T. 2: 145
Oltean, M. 2: 422
Olton, J. E. 1: 401
Omwake, E. 2: 484
O'Neal, P. 1: 378, 401; 3: 785
Opler, M. 2: 711, 712; 3: 292, 310, 319, 320, 371
Oppé, T. E. 2: 216
Oppenheim, A. N. 3: 739, 762
Orlando, R. 1: 135, 143, 150
Orlansky, H. 3: 301, 319
Ormiston, D. W. 2: 258
Ormond, R. E. 2: 15, 18
Orne, M. T. 2: 171, 190, 258
Orshansky, I. G. 2: 427
Orwell, G. 2: 258
Osborn, M. L. 3: 288, 291
Oseretskovsky, D. 2: 430
Osmond, M. 2: 15, 18, 281
Osmund, H. 2: 311

AUTHOR INDEX

Øster, J. 1: 43, 56
Osterrieth, P. A. 1: 93, 102
Ostow, M. 2: 477, 484
Ostrovsky, E. S. 3: 139, 145, 154
Oswald, I. 1: 164, 169; 2: 193, 195, 199, 206, 209, 214, 215, 216, 217, 219, 220, 291, 292, 309
Ottaway, J. H. 1: 506, 521
Otto, U. 1: 404, 405, 409, 426
Ounsted, C. 1: 451, 478, 495; 3: 680
Ovchinnikov, I. F. 2: 432, 446
Overzier, C. 2: 46, 48
Owens, H. F. 2: 312
Ozeretskovsky, D. 2: 446

Page, J. 2: 357, 389
Pai, M. N. 2: 212, 220
Paillas, N. 2: 176, 190
Paine, R. S. 1: 506, 521
Painter, C. 3: 80, 90, 97
Painter, P. 3: 737, 761
Palade, G. E. 2: 56, 85
Palay, S. L. 2: 53, 56, 72, 85
Palermo, D. S. 3: 745, 761
Palmer, J. O. 3: 681
Palmer, W. L. 3: 527, 529
Pampiglione, G. 3: 393, 414, 416
Paolino, R. M. 2: 106
Papez, J. W. 2: 267, 287
Pappas, N. 1: 147
Paracelsus, 3: 3
Parant, A. V. 3: 591, 608
Pare, C. M. B. 1: 51, 56, 506, 509, 520, 521
Parhad, L. 2: 701, 702, 712
Park, E. A. 3: 8
Park, W. W. 2: 48
Parker, J. 2: 262
Parker, R. A. 1: 445, 450
Parloff, M. B. 2: 484, 617
Parmelee, A. H. 2: 220
Parr, G. 1: 454; 3: 416
Parson, C. 1: 79, 83
Parsons, A. 2: 603, 704, 712
Parsons, O. A. 2: 262
Parsons, T. 2: 477, 484, 617, 705; 3: 145, 154
Parten, M. 1: 213, 234
Pasamanick, B. 1: 241, 248, 384, 401, 437, 438, 450, 456, 472, 500, 521; 3: 27, 58, 59, 667, 681, 705
Pasqualini, R. Q. 1: 50, 56; 2: 48
Passerini, D. 2: 191
Passin, H. 3: 371
Passouant, P. 2: 216
Passov, A. H. 3: 759
Patau, K. 1: 49, 56
Patch, R. W. 3: 309
Paterson, A. S. 2: 161, 191

Paton, S. 3: 8
Patrick, J. R. 1: 401
Patterson, D. G. 1: 184, 191
Patterson, T. L. 2: 178, 191
Patterson, V. 2: 419
Patti, F. A. 2: 173, 180, 191
Paul, G. L. 2: 377, 389, 564, 571, 574
Paulley, J. W. 1: 308, 335; 3: 529
Paulsen, C. A. 2: 48
Pavenstedt, E. 2: 480; 3: 121, 123, 352, 357, 454
Pavlov, I. P. 1: 104, 105, 2: xxii, xxiv, xxv, 150, 161, 191, 223, 321, 342, 376, 435, 446, 531, 532, 534, 547, 555, 556, 574, 578, 582, 590, 594; 3: 62, 385, 390
Payne, R. B. 2: 255
Payne, R. W. 2: 370, 389; 3: 564, 569
Payne, W. W. 1: 520
Payson, H. E. 2: 619
Pear, T. H. 1: 174
Pearse, A. G. E. 2: 85
Pearson, C. B. 2: 3, 389
Peck, H. B. 3: 655, 682
Peck, L. 1: 179, 191
Peel, E. A. 1: 79, 83
Peimer, I. A. 2: 538, 556
Pelliteri, O. 3: 57
Pelzel, J. 3: 371
Pemberton, J. 2: 415, 650, 674
Penfield, W. 2: 112, 128, 268, 313, 314, 315, 316, 317, 318, 319, 320, 324, 327, 328, 330, 331, 335, 336, 337, 345, 348, 349,
Penmeld, W. 2: 287
Pennington, L. A. 2: 390
Pennybacker, J. 2: 114, 129
Penrose, L. S. 1: 39, 40, 47, 48, 50, 56, 437, 450, 498, 499, 501, 502, 506, 511, 520, 521; 2: 3, 5, 6, 8, 9, 10, 11, 16, 17, 18, 19, 3: 546
Pentti, R. 3: 525
Pérez, T. M. 3: 591
Perier, 2: 76
Perkins, H. V. 3: 736, 761
Perlin, S. 2: 617
Perot, P. 2: 337, 338, 349
Perry, T. L. 3: 670, 682
Persinger, G. W. 2: 618
Persky, H. 1: 493; 2: 264
Peters, J. 2: 258
Petersen, D. R. 3: 145, 154
Peterson, D. 1: 106, 113
Peterson, E. 2: 75, 80, 84, 262
Peterson, G. M. 2: 92, 106
Peterson, H. G. (Jr.) 3: 586
Petrie, A. 2: 258; 3: 526
Petrilowitsch, H. 2: 444, 446

Pfeffer, A. Z. 2: 476, 484
Pfersdorff, 3: 609
Pfundt, T. R. 3: 587
Phaire, T. 1: 252, 284
Philbrook, R. 3: 58
Phillipson, H. 2: 421
Philpott, W. M. 2: 574
Phipps, E. 3: 683
Piaget, J. 1: 12, 19, 58-84, 87, 88, 90, 91, 93, 94, 95, 98, 99, 100, 102, 188, 213, 214, 218, 221, 224, 228, 229, 234, 237, 376, 401; 2: 243, 448, 452, 484, 726; 3: 5, 92, 96, 97, 176, 177, 292, 315, 319, 413, 415, 542, 550, 557, 569, 664, 671
Piaget, P. H. 2: 450
Picasso, P. 2: 143
Pick, A. 3: 609
Pigon, A. 2: 84, 105
Pincas, A. 3: 561, 570
Pincus, G. 2: 16, 18
Pinel, P. 2: xx, 725
Pinkerton, P. 1: 306, 323, 327, 330, 335
Pinsard, N. 3: 393, 416
Pinsky, R. H. 2: 619
Pinsley, R. H. 3: 527
Pintler, M. H. 3: 155
Pioch, W. 3: 587
Piotrowsky, 3: 652
Pippard, J. S. 1: 384
Pirch, J. H. 2: 106
Pirquet, C. von 2: 192
Pitt, D. B. 1: 515, 521
Pitts, F. N. 2: 48
Plato, 3: 28, 136
Platonov, K. I. 2: 578, 585, 594
Platou, R. V. 3: 587
Platt, J. W. 1: 320, 335
Plaut, A. 3: 527
Plesset, I. R. 1: 40, 57
Pleydell, M. J. 3: 22, 26, 59
Ploss, H. 3: 85, 86, 97
Plotnikoff, N. 2: 106
Plunkett, E. R. 2: 45, 48
Plunkett, G. B. 2: 220
Podolsky, E. 2: 211, 220
Poenaru, S. 2: 47
Polani, P. E. 1: 47, 57, 521; 2: 46, 48
Polansky, N. 2: 617, 3: 761
Polatin, J. 3: 651, 680
Polezhaev, E. F. 2: 538, 556
Pollack, M. 2: 254, 3: 684
Pollard, J. C. 2: 256, 258
Pollard, P. C. 2: 300, 311
Pollard, T. D. 2: 85
Pollin, W. 2: 414, 421, 424, 617; 3: 682
Pollitt, E. 2: 47
Polyakov, K. L. 2: 537, 538, 556
Pomerat, C. M. 2: 62, 73, 74, 77, 78, 80, 82, 85

AUTHOR INDEX

Ponce, O. V. **2**: 706, 712
Pond, D. A. **1**: 240, 248, 384, 400, 401, 437, 450, 452, 453, 454, 455, 456, 458, 461, 463, 470, 471, 472
Poo, L. J. **2**: 103
Popper, K. A. **2**: 379, 389
Popper, L. **3**: 678
Porritt, A. **1**: 256
Porta, J. **2**: 422
Potashin, R. A. **3**: 735, 744, 762
Potter, H. W. **3**: 610, 652, 671, 682, 705
Potts, W. E. **3**: 587
Powers, E. **1**: 401
Pozsonyi, J. **2**: 45
Prader, A. **1**: 50, 57
Prados, M. **2**: 327
Pratt, C. W. M. **3**: 60
Pratt, Y. H. **2**: 582, 594
Prausnitz, C. **2**: 182, 191
Prausnitz Giles, C. **2**: 185, 191
Prechtl, H. F. R. **1**: 383, 401, **3**: 95, 97
Prell, D. B. **1**: 41, 56
Premack, R. **2**: 258
Prentice, N. M. **3**: 545
Preston, G. H. **2**: 411, 422
Preyer, W. **2**: 147, 150, 191; **3**: 5
Price, J. S. **3**: 283, 290
Price, L. **2**: 264
Price, W. H. **2**: 16, 19
Priest, J. H. **2**: 48
Priest, R. G. **2**: 215, 220
Priest, R. J. **3**: 529
Prillwitz, G. **3**: 736, 758
Prince, M. **2**: 266
Prioleau, W. H. **2**: 259
Pritchard, M. **1**: 51, 57; **2**: 48
Prout, C. T. **2**: 411, 422; **3**: 146, 154, 156
Prout, W. **3**: 606
Provence, S. A. **2**: 484; **3**: 121, 251, 319, 329, 529
Prugh, D. G. **1**: 80, 84, 127, 150, 319, 335; **3**: 145, 154, 494, 529
Prysiazniuk, A. **2**: 263
Puck, T. T. **1**: 55; **2**: 48
Pugh, **2**: 159
Pugh, H. **3**: 553, 554, 568
Puner, H. W. **2**: 191
Puryear, H. B. **2**: 218
Pushkar, D. **2**: 263
Puskina, **2**: 548, 550
Putnam, J. J. **1**: 369
Putnam, M. C. **1**: 495; **3**: 123
Pygott, F. **1**: 383, 401

Quartermain, D. **2**: 106
Quastel, D. M. J. **1**: 495
Quastel, J. H. **1**: 482, 495
Quay, H. C. **3**: 154

Quibell, E. P. **1**: 225, 226, 227, 234

Rabin, A. I. **1**: 575, 576, 578, 585; **3**: 340, 343, 344, 345
Rabinovitch, R. D. **3**: 655, 682, 683
Raboch, J. **2**: 48
Racamier, P. C. **3**: 123
Rachford, **3**: 9
Rachman, S. J. **1**: 104, 118, 131, 137, 149, 150, 151, 166, 169, 561; **2**: 376, 377, 378, 387, 389, 564, 565, 569, 572, 573, 574, 575; **3**: 655, 674, 682
Radcliffe-Brown, A. R. **3**: 296
Radke, M. J. **3**: 142, 154
Radouco-Thomas, C. **2**: 635
Rafferty, J. E. **1**: 585
Rafi, A. A. **2**: 575
Raiborn, C. W. **2**: 85
Raiborn, C. W. (Jr.) **2**: 85
Raile, R. B. **3**: 588
Raimy, V. C. **2**: 371, 389
Raines, J. **2**: 569, 575
Rainwater, L. **3**: 748, 762
Rajam, P. C. **2**: 104
Ramet, J. **2**: 618
Ramón, Y. **2**: 84
Randt, C. T. **2**: 259
Rank, B. **1**: 236, 248, 487, 495; **3**: 13, 123, 650, 653, 658, 673, 676, 682, 705
Rank, O. **3**: 659, 682
Rapaport, D. **2**: 245, 259, 267, 287, 449, 452, 454, 484; **3**: 92, 97, 123, 340, 343, 345, 357, 664
Raphael, T. **2**: 48
Rapoport, J. **3**: 661, 682
Rashkis, H. A. **2**: 617
Raskin, H. F. **3**: 527
Rasmussen, J. E. **2**: 258, 259
Rasmussen, T. **2**: 317, 320, 349
Rathod, N. H. **2**: 617
Raven, J. C. **1**: 203, 570, 573, 578, 585
Ravenette, A. T. **1**: 191; **2**: 390
Rawson, A. J. **1**: 357, 358, 369
Rawson, I. **3**: 123
Raymond, A. **2**: 365, 386
Raymond, M. J. **2**: 575
Rayner, R. **1**: 118, 151
Read, G. D. **2**: 172
Rebuck, J. W. **3**: 529
Rechtschaffen, A. **2**: 205, 220
Reckless, W. C. **1**: 370, 401
Record, R. G. **3**: 27, 31, 32, 35, 36, 58, 59
Reding, G. R. **2**: 213, 220
Redl, F. **3**: 337, 345
Redlich, E. **3**: 614
Redlich, F. C. **2**: 416

Redlo, M. **3**: 470
Reed, G. F. **2**: 259
Reed, P. A. **3**: 529
Rees, **3**: 11
Regan, R. A. **3**: 804
Regis, H. **2**: 555; **3**: 591, 608
Rehage, K. J. **3**: 736, 762
Rehin, G. F. **2**: 678, 695
Reichard, S. **1**: 413, 427; **2**: 411, 422; **3**: 146, 154
Reifenstein, E. C. (Jr.) **2**: 46
Rein, M. **3**: 587
Reinhart, J. B. **3**: 587
Reinius, E. **3**: 784
Reischauer, E. O. **3**: 371
Reiser, D. E. **3**: 682
Reiser, M. F. **3**: 493
Reissman, F. **3**: 748
Reitman, E. E. **2**: 252
Rembrandt, **2**: 143
Rémond, A. **3**: 414, 416
Remstad, R. **3**: 142, 155
Renfrew, C. E. **3**: 556, 570
Revans, R. W. **2**: 695
Reynolds, D. J. **2**: 564, 572, 574
Reynolds, V. **1**: 26, 37
Reznikoff, M. **2**: 617
Rezza, E. **3**: 587
Rheingold, H. **1**: 139, 150; **3**: 97, 123, 128, 151, 153, 155
Rhine, S. **2**: 107
Rhodin, J. **2**: 69, 86
Ribble, M. A. **2**: 241, 259; **3**: 163, 167, 170, 179, 185, 199, 300, 319, 423, 454, 659, 682
Ribot, **2**: 436, 446
Ricci, J. **2**: 417
Rice, M. P. **3**: 587
Rice, R. G. **3**: 59
Richards, M. E. **3**: 146, 155
Richards, T. W. **2**: 617
Richardson, M. W. **2**: 191
Richmond, F. **3**: 27, 34, 57
Richmond, J. **3**: 508, 529
Richmond, J. B. **3**: 300, 319
Richmond, J. P. **3**: 492
Richter, D. **1**: 508, 521; **2**: 100: **3**: 11
Ricks, D. **2**: 422, **3**: 804
Ricoeur, P. **2**: 496, 518
Riddoch, G. **2**: 134, 145, 330
Rieger, **3**: 608
Riese, H. **3**: 587
Riesen A. H. **2**: 259, 310
Riseman, D. **1**: 244, 248
Riessman, F. **3**: 762
Riley, M. W. **3**: 797, 804
Rimland, B. **3**: 666, 682
Rin, H. **2**: 706, 712
Rinkel, M. **1**: 366, 368; **2**: 614, 635; **3**: 678
Rioch, D. M. **2**: 420
Rioch, J. **1**: 368
Riskin, J. **2**: 420

Ritchie Russell, W. 1: 218, 234
Ritson, E. B. 2: 219
Ritvo, S. 2: 464, 484; 3: 123
Riva, 3: 603
Rivers, W. H. R. 1: 175, 191; 2: 617, 618
Riviere, J. 2: 483
Rix, A. 3: 528
Roach, J. L. 3: 755, 762
Robbins, L. C. 3: 62, 63, 79
Robbins, L. L. 2: 471, 484, 486
Robert, A. 3: 414, 416
Roberts, C. L. 2: 258
Roberts, G. E. 3: 680
Roberts, J. M. 2: 615, 618
Roberts, L. 1: 342, 349; 2: 318, 328, 331, 349
Roberts, R. B. 2: 105, 110, 128
Robertson, J. 1: 210; 2: 59, 477, 484; 3: 123, 241, 242, 252
Robertson, J. B. S. 1: 138, 150
Robertson, J. S. 3: 25, 26, 59
Robertson, M. H. 2: 250, 259
Robertson Smith, D. 2: 45
Robin, A. A. 1: 382, 401
Robins, L. N. 1: 378, 401; 3: 785, 789, 792, 795, 804
Robinson, A. 1: 55; 2: 48
Robinson, B. 2: 255
Robinson, J. 2: 259
Roche, M. 3: 416
Rochford, G. 3: 552, 561, 562, 563, 564, 566, 570
Rodgers, R. R. 3: 758
Rodin, E. A. 2: 309
Roe, A. 2: 371, 389
Roff, M. 3: 745, 762, 792, 804
Roffwarg, H. P. 2: 220
Roger, A. 2: 555
Rogers, C. R. 2: 618
Rogers, M. E. 1: 401, 456, 472
Rogers, W. J. B. 1: 534
Rogler, L. H. 2: 411, 412, 422; 3: 146, 155
Rohrer, J. H. 2: 259; 3: 139, 155, 307, 320
Roigaard-Petersen, E. J. 2: 107
Roigaard-Petersen, H. H. 2: 105, 106
Roitbakh, A. I. 2: 538, 556
Romano, J. 3: 529
Rome, H. P. 2: 127
Rook, A. 2: 188
Rook, W. T. 2: 389
Rosanoff, A. J. 1: 40, 57
Rosanoff, I. A. 1: 40, 57, 380
Rosanski, J. 2: 287
Rose, F. C. 2: 114, 128
Rosen, B. C. 3: 305, 320
Rosen, H. 2: 287, 312

Rosen, I. 2: 710
Rosen, J. N. 2: 457, 458, 484
Rosen, S. 3: 761
Rosenbaum, G. 2: 252, 302, 305, 311, 312
Rosenbaum, G. P. 2: 410, 421
Rosenberg, S. 2: 548, 569, 570
Rosenblatt, B. 3: 243, 246, 252, 253
Rosenblatt, F. 2: 96, 97, 107
Rosenblatt, J. S. 3: 81, 97
Rosenblith, W. A. 2: 312
Rosenblueth, A. 2: 186, 191
Rosenbluth, D. 1: 19
Rosenfeld, E. 3: 343, 345
Rosenfeld, H. 2: 457, 458, 484
Rosenfeld, S. K. 3: 238, 239, 252
Rosenthal, D. 1: 152, 169; 2: 414, 424, 618; 3: 664, 665, 682
Rosenthal, M. J. 3: 371
Rosenthal, R. 2: 607, 614, 618
Rosenthal, V. 2: 219
Rosenthal, V. G. 2: 177, 191
Rosenzweig, L. 1: 585
Rosenzweig, M. R. 2: 88, 104, 105
Rosenzweig, N. 2: 267, 287
Rosenzweig, S. 1: 585; 2: 354, 389
Roshnov, V. E. 2: 583, 594
Rosman, B. 2: 417
Ross, D. C. 3: 73, 74, 79
Ross, J. 1: 150
Ross, J. B. 3: 199
Ross, J. P. 2: 220
Ross, R. B. 2: 107
Ross, S. 2: 355, 356, 389
Rossenkötter, L. 2: 212, 220
Rossi, A. M. 2: 222, 259
Rot, M. 3: 327, 345
Roth, B. 1: 42, 56, 481, 494; 2: 14, 18, 3: 680
Roth, C. 1: 140, 147
Roth, H. P. 3: 474, 493
Roth, M. 2: 7, 18; 3: 546, 569
Rothlin, E. 2: 635
Rothman, T. 2: 309
Rothney, J. W. M. 3: 142, 155
Rothschild, G. H. 2: 104
Rotter, J. B. 1: 578, 585
Rouart, 2: 427, 428, 446
Rounds, D. E. 2: 85
Rousch, E. S. 2: 177, 191
Roussy, 2: xxi
Rowe, J. 1: 446, 450
Rowell, T. E. 3: 129, 155
Rowland, G. L. 2: 482
Rowley, J. 2: 46
Roy, J. R. 2: 46
Rubel, A. J. 2: 706, 712
Rubenstein, B. O. 3: 139, 146, 155

Rubin, L. S. 3: 669, 682
Rubin, S. 1: 401
Rubinfine, D. L. 3: 123
Rubinstein, E. A. 2: 484, 617; 3: 651, 652, 682
Rubinstein, I. 2: 218
Rubinstein, L. 2: 252
Rubinstein, L. J. 2: 85
Rubright, W. C. 2: 220
Ruckebusch, Y. 2: 221
Rudhe, U. 3: 526
Rüdi, K. 1: 57
Rüdin, 2: 6
Rue, R. 3: 470
Ruesch, J. 2: 677, 695
Ruff, G. E. 2: 259, 260
Rumke, H. C. 2: 365, 389
Rundle, A. 1: 49, 57, 513, 521
Ruseev, V. V. 2: 544, 556
Rush, B. 3: 652
Russell, C. 1: 36, 37
Russell, D. S. 2: 85
Russell, I. S. 2: 110, 128
Russell, S. M. 2: 207, 208, 209, 219
Russell, W. M. S. 1: 26, 36, 37; 3: 131, 155
Russell, W. R. 2: 115, 116, 117, 120, 125, 128
Rutter, M. 3: 70, 79, 266, 291, 474, 493, 559, 570, 649, 673, 682, 739, 741, 762, 803
Ryan, J. J. 3: 736, 760
Rychlak, J. K. 2: 355, 389
Ryckoff, I. M. 2: 416, 487
Ryde, D. H. 2: 191

Sabbot, I. M. 2: 219
Sabshin, M. 2: 614, 618
Sachepizckii, R. A. 2: 593, 594
Sachs, B. 3: 4, 652, 682
Sachs, D. M. 3: 250
Sachs, H. 3: 454
Sadger, I. 3: 454
Sage, P. 2: 422, 3: 153
Sainsbury, P. 1: 413, 427, 495; 2: 412, 423, 679, 695
Sainsbury, R. 2: 388
Sakamoto, M. 3: 676, 683
Sakel, M. 2: xxii
Sakurai, T. 2: 529
Salimbene, 3: 158, 199
Salmon, P. 2: 386
Salter, A. 2: 575, 562
Salzberger, F. 1: 431, 432, 450
Salzinger, K. 1: 135, 136, 137, 138, 141, 142, 150
Sampson, H. 2: 221
Samson, W. 2: 263
Samuels, A. S. 2: 618
Sandberg, A. A. 2: 48
Sanderson, R. E. 2: 573

Sanderson, W. T. **3**: 129, 155
Sandler, A-M. **3**: 237, 252
Sandler, F. **3**: 56
Sandler, J. **1**: 243, 248; **2**: 476, 480; **3**: 121, 220, 245, 246, 247, 248, 249, 250, 251, 252, 253
Sandler, L. **3**: 123
Sandler, M. **3**: 669, 683
Sands, D. E. **1**: 305
Sands, H. H. **1**: 84
Sanford, N. **2**: 281, 282, 287; **3**: 752, 762
Sanford, S. **2**: 418
Sankar, B. **3**: 683
Sankar, D. V. S. **3**: 683
Sankar, S. **3**: 670, 678
Santara, D. A. **3**: 705
Santostefano, S. **2**: 355, 388
Sapir, E. **3**: 297, 302, 317
Sarason, S. **3**: 752, 762
Sarbin, T. R. **2**: 178, 190
Sargant, W. W. **1**: 492, 495
Sargent, H. D. **2**: 449, 471, 474, 483, 484, 485
Sargent, J. **3**: 737, 760
Sartre, J. P. **2**: 495, 496, 518
Sasaki, Y. **2**: 529
Satake, M. **2**: 52, 86
Satir, V. **2**: 420
Sato, I. **2**: 260
Satterfield, J. H. **2**: 174, 191
Saucier, J.-Frs. **2**: 699, 711
Saunders, J. **1**: 222, 234
Saunders, L. **3**: 747, 762
Saunders, M. G. **2**: 234, 263, 311
Saver, W. G. **3**: 528
Sawrey, W. L. **3**: 141, 153
Sayers, B. **1**: 114, 147
Scantlebury, R. E. **2**: 178, 191
Scarr, H. A. **3**: 369
Schachter, M. **1**: 408, 427; **3**: 587
Schadé, J. P. **2**: 217, 218
Schaefer, E. **3**: 121
Schaefer, K. E. **2**: 260
Schaefer, S. **3**: 123
Schafer, R. **2**: 449, 450, 457, 485; **3**: 357
Schafer, S. **2**: 417
Schaff, G. **2**: 218, 309
Schaffer, H. R. **1**: 80, 84, 86, 102, 214, 220, 221, 234, 244, 248; **3**: 281, 291
Schain, R. J. **3**: 670, 673, 683
Schallenge, H. **3**: 680
Schapiro, A. F. **2**: 618
Scheflen, A. E. **2**: 476, 485
Scheibe, K. E. **2**: 258
Scheibel, A. B. **2**: 260
Scheibel, M. E. **2**: 260
Scheier, I. H. **2**: 386
Scheiner, A. P. **2**: 49
Schelling, F. von **2**: 491, 496
Scher, J. M. **2**: 418, 574
Scherback, A. **2**: 427

Scherrer, H. **1**: 36; **2**: 174, 189, 255, 556
Schilder, P. **1**: 242, 248, 359, 368, 369, 408, 426; **2**: 130, 145, 426, 446; **3**: 207, 219, 655, 656, 659, 660, 664, 674, 683
Schilling, M. **2**: 264
Schlagenhauf, G. **2**: 486
Schlesinger, B. E. **1**: 320, 335
Schleyer, F. **3**: 587
Schloesser, P. T. **3**: 587
Schludermann, E. **2**: 263
Schmid, W. **2**: 48
Schmideberg, M. **1**: 182, 191, 393, 401; **2**: 618
Schmidt, H. O. **2**: 365, 389
Schmikel, R. D. **2**: 47
Schmitt, F. O. **2**: 110, 128; **3**: 96
Schmuck, R. A. **3**: 735, 736, 745, 747, 762
Schneck, J. M. **2**: 287
Schneider, J. **1**: 57
Schneider, K. **2**: 427, 444, 446
Schneidman, E. **2**: 419
Schneirla, T. C. **3**: 81, 90, 97
Schnurmann, A. **3**: 253
Schoenfelder, T. **3**: 674, 683
Scholtz, B. W. **3**: 470
Schonell, F. E. **1**: 585
Schonell, F. J. **1**: 581, 585
School, H. **1**: 494
Schröder, **3**: 1, 605
Schroedinger, E. **2**: 187, 191
Schrotel, S. R. **3**: 587
Schuell, H. **3**: 561, 570
Schuessler, K. F. **1**: 401
Schulman, I. **1**: 393, 401
Schultz, D. P. **2**: 246, 258, 260
Schulz, H. R. **2**: 220
Schulzinger, M. S. **1**: 363, 369
Schumer, F. **2**: 390
Schur, M. **2**: 123, 251
Schutte, W. **2**: 263
Schwartz, B. A. **2**: 207, 217, 218, 221
Schwartz, M. S. **2**: 477, 486, 619
Schwartz, O. **2**: 189
Schwartz, R. D. **3**: 343, 346
Schwartz, S. S. **2**: 428, 446
Schwenter, D. **2**: 147, 191
Schwitzgebel, R. **2**: 575
Scott, C. **1**: 369
Scott, E. M. **3**: 83, 97
Scott, H. D. **2**: 191
Scott, J. **2**: 218
Scott, J. K. **3**: 44, 59
Scott, L. W. **2**: 48
Scott, P. **1**: 412, 426, 487, 493
Scott, P. D. **1**: 370

Scott, R. D. **2**: 409, 421
Scott, R. W. **2**: 47
Scott, T. H. **2**: 251, 253, 255, 260, 299, 310
Scott, W. C. M. **1**: 485, 495; **2**: 457, 485
Scoville, W. B. **2**: 112, 128
Scrivener, J. **2**: 388
Seagoe, M. V. **3**: 735, 762
Seakins, J. W. T. **1**: 54, 57
Searles, H. F. **2**: 411, 422, 457, 458, 464, 466, 485
Sears, P. S. **3**: 155
Sears, R. R., **1**: 375, 399, 401; **3**: 141, 143, 153, 155, 301, 320, 746, 762
Seay, B. **3**: 284, 290, 291
Sechehaye, M. **2**: 457, 458, 485; **3**: 303
Seelig, P. **3**: 610, 614
Seeman, W. **2**: 365, 389
Segal, H. **2**: 456, 485
Segal, M. **3**: 334, 335, 336, 345
Segall, L. J. **2**: 45
Séglas, J. **2**: 591, 602, 609
Seguin, C. A. **2**: 703, 712
Selesnick, S. T. **2**: 479
Sells, S. B. **3**: 745, 762
Semmes, J. **2**: 258
Senden, M. von, **1**: 86, 102
Senf, R. **2**: 310
Senn, M. J. **3**: 302, 320
Sens, C. **3**: 123
Seplin, C. D. **3**: 141, 155
Seppilli, **3**: 597, 609
Serbsky, **3**: 609
Sergovich, F. R. **2**: 48
Serkov, F. I. **2**: 544, 556
Seror, **3**: 21
Sersen, E. A. **2**: 135, 145
Seth, G. **1**: 95, 102
Settlage, C. F. **2**: 481; **3**: 681
Seward, G. **3**: 319
Sewell, W. H. **3**: 309, 320
Shaddick, C. W. **1**: 504, 520
Shaffer, J. W. **2**: 35, 48
Shagam, A. N. **2**: 593, 594
Shakow, D. **2**: 289, 309, 355, 389, 476, 480, 485
Shanks, B. L. **2**: 218
Shapiro, A. **2**: 217, 220
Shapiro, A. K. **2**: 596, 618, 619
Shapiro, D. **2**: 260
Shapiro, E. M. **2**: 190
Shapiro, M. D. **1**: 141, 150, 170, 191; **2**: 379, 389, 390
Shapiro, T. **2**: 481; **3**: 679
Sharkey, P. C. **2**: 85
Sharp, V. H. **2**: 410, 421
Shatsky, J. **2**: 265
Shaver, E. L. **2**: 45
Shaw, A. **3**: 588
Shaw, C. R. **1**: 370, 401; **3**: 683
Shaw, L. **1**: 363, 369

AUTHOR INDEX

Shaw, M. W. **2**: 48
Shcherback, A. **2**: 446
Sheehan, J. **1**: 114, 150
Sheer, D. **2**: 252
Sheldon, W. H. **1**: 402; **3**: 5
Shelley, H. M. **2**: 702, 712
Shepheard, E. **3**: 245, 251
Shepherd, M. **1**: 150; **3**: 739, 741, 761, 762
Sherfey, M. J. **2**: 450, 485
Sheridan, M. D. **1**: 224, 234, 438, 450, 582, 585
Sherman, S. **2**: 420
Sherriff, H. **3**: 588
Sherrill, H. H. **1**: 369
Sherrington, C. S. **2**: 60, 315, 343, 349
Sherwood, S. L. **1**: 464, 472
Shevky, E. **3**: 308, 320
Shields, J. **1**: 40, 41, 57, 106, 113; **2**: 14, 18, 19
Shimoda, M. **2**: 519, 520
Shinagawa, F. **3**: 349, 371
Shmavonian, B. M. **2**: 252, 253, 262
Shneidman, E. S. **1**: 410, 427, 578, 586
Shoben, E. J. **1**: 375, 402
Shoemaker, D. J. **3**: 154
Sholl, D. A. **2**: 53, 68, 86
Shoobs, N. E. **3**: 737, 744, 762
Shorvon, H. J. **1**: 112, 113
Shottstaedt, W. W. **2**: 619
Shüle, **3**: 592, 608
Shurley, J. T. **2**: 226, 257, 260, 262, 299, 310
Sibulkin, L. **3**: 705
Sichel, H. S. **1**: 363, 369
Sidman, M. **1**: 144, 145, 150
Sidman, R. L. **2**: 72, 85
Siegel, C. D. **3**: 528
Siegel, J. **2**: 411, 422; **3**: 146, 152
Siegman, A. W. **3**: 145, 155
Sigal, J. **3**: 253
Silberer, H. **1**: 178, 191
Silver, A. **3**: 655, 683
Silver, H. K. **3**: 588
Silverman, A. J. **2**: 252, 253, 260
Silverman, F. N. **3**: 588
Simmel, E. **3**: 424, 425, 443, 454
Simmel, M. L. **2**: 134, 135, 145
Simmons, L. W. **2**: 694, 695
Simon, B. **1**: 174, 188, 191; **2**: 357, 390
Simon, C. W. **2**: 199, 221
Simon, G. B. **1**: 479, 495
Simon, J. **1**: 191
Simon, L. N. **2**: 94, 105
Simon, T. **1**: 185, 570
Simonds, C. **3**: 585
Simons, D. G. **2**: 260

Simonsen, K. **3**: 784
Simpkiss, M. J. **1**: 520
Simpson, L. **1**: 178, 191
Simpson, M. **3**: 141, 155
Simson, T. P. **2**: 435, 446
Sinclair-Gieben, A. H. **2**: 181, 191
Singer, J. L. **3**: 310, 311, 319, 320
Singer, M. B. **3**: 238, 253
Singer, M. T. **2**: 400, 416, 417, 464, 465, 485, 487; **3**: 683
Singh, R. P. **2**: 48
Sinha, A. K. **2**: 48
Sipová, L. **2**: 48
Sivadon, P. **2**: 713, 728
Sjögren, T. **1**: 56; **2**: 4, 6, 11, 12, 18
Skaar, A. **3**: 56
Skachkov, Y. V. **2**: 436, 446
Skeels, H. M. **1**: 432, 437, 443, 450, 517, 521; **3**: 796, 804
Skinner, B. F. **1**: 104, 105, 114, 135, 143, 150; **2**: 376; **3**: 62, 320, 551, 570
Skodak, M. **1**: 432, 443, 450; **3**: 804
Slater, E. **1**: 41, 57, 125, 150, 380, 402, 492, 495; **2**: 7, 14, 18, 19, 48, **3**: 546, 569
Slavina, **1**: 189
Slavson, S. K. **2**: 594
Slavson, S.-R. **3**: 784
Slochower, M. Z. **1**: 93, 102
Sluchevsky, I. **2**: 426, 446
Small, L. **2**: 355, 390
Smarr, E. R. **2**: 617
Smart, J. **2**: 62, 86
Smetterling, **3**: 332
Smid, A. C. **1**: 352, 354, 369
Smirnoff, D. **2**: 180, 191
Smirnov, G. D. **2**: 128
Smith, A. **2**: 115, 116, 128
Smith, A. J. **1**: 502, 506, 521
Smith, C. M. **2**: 695
Smith, D. **1**: 319
Smith, D. R. **1**: 51, 55
Smith, D. W. **1**: 56; **2**: 49
Smith, G. R. **2**: 181, 550, 555
Smith, J. M. **2**: 191
Smith, L. M. **3**: 737, 741, 749, 759, 762
Smith, M. **2**: 208, 216
Smith, N. J. **3**: 585
Smith, R. J. **3**: 369, 370, 371
Smith, R. W. **2**: 251
Smith, S. **2**: 258, 260
Smith, W. R. **2**: 261
Smolen, E. M. **3**: 653, 683
Smythe, H. **3**: 371
Smythies, J. R. **2**: 15, 18, 131, 276, 287
Snape, W. J. **3**: 526
Snedeker, L. **3**: 588
Snell, H. K. **2**: 211, 218

Snezhnevsky, A. V. **2**: 425
Snider, R. S. **2**: 85
Snyder, F. **2**: 221
Sobel, D. E. **3**: 53, 59
Soddy, K. **3**: 150, 152, 153, 154
Soffer, A. **2**: 260
Sohler, D. T. **2**: 417
Sokoloff, B. **3**: 470
Sokoloff, L. **2**: 107
Solnit, A. J. **2**: 484; **3**: 123, 251, 319, 529
Solomon, H. C. **1**: 114, 143, 150
Solomon, M. H. **2**: 423; **3**: 803
Solomon, P. **2**: 222, 224, 225, 251, 252, 253, 254, 255, 256, 257, 258, 259, 260, 261, 262, 310, 311
Solomon, R. **1**: 158, 169
Solomon, R. A. **3**: 734, 760
Solyom, L. **2**: 104
Sommer, K. H. **3**: 29, 56
Sommer, R. **3**: 608
Sommers, S. C. **3**: 529
Sontag, L. W. **3**: 28, 36, 59, 83, 97
Sorsby, A. **3**: 24, 57
Spaulding, P. J. **1**: 220, 234
Spearman, C. **1**: 185, 198, 209
Specht, **2**: 442, 446
Speck, R. V. **2**: 410, 421
Spector, W. G. **2**: 185, 191
Speltz, E. **1**: 225, 233
Spence, J. **1**: 252
Spencer, J. A. **3**: 529
Spencer-Booth, Y. **3**: 283, 291
Speranski, A. D. **2**: 254
Sperling, M. **1**: 313, 335; **3**: 418, 454, 511, 512, 516, 518, 529
Sperling, O. E. **3**: 443, 447, 454
Sperry, B. M. **3**: 545
Sperry, R. W. **2**: 91, 107, 111, 127
Spiegel, J. P. **2**: 408, 420
Spiel, W. **3**: 651, 675, 678
Spielberger, C. D. **3**: 551, 570
Spiers, B. W. **1**: 222, 234; **3**: 51
Spiker, C. C. **1**: 135, 151
Spinanger, J. **1**: 507, 520
Spinoza, B. **2**: 496
Spiro, H. M. **3**: 493, 525
Spiro, M. E. **2**: 703, 712; **3**: 325, 328, 330, 331, 332, 339, 340, 341, 346
Spitz, R. A. **1**: 89, 103, 485, 487, 495; **2**: 261, 299, 310, 449, 452, 454, 456, 457, 458, 459, 464, 485, 486; **3**: 9, 122, 123, 161, 168, 169, 170, 171, 172, 173, 174,

175, 176, 199, 202, 203, 204, 205, 206, 207, 208, 209, 219, 265, 291, 299, 300, 301, 313, 319, 320, 329, 423, 454, 545, 659, 664, 683
Spitzka, E. C. **3**: 597, 652
Spock, B. **3**: 63, 79, 194, 199, 306, 320
Spooner, C. E. **2**: 287
Sporn, M. B. **2**: 97, 105
Spradlin, J. E. **1**: 114, 135, 136, 137, 141, 143, 151,
Sprague, J. M. **2**: 307, 312; **3**: 590, 608
Spranger, **2**: 490
Sprimon, V. V. **2**: 584, 594
Sprince, M. P. **3**: 238, 239, 244, 245, 252, 253
Spurlock, J. **3**: 154, 512, 525, 527, 528
Staats, A. W. **1**: 135, 137, 138, 151
Staats, C. K. **1**: 137, 138, 151
Stabenau, J. R. **2**: 410, 421, 424
Stabenau, J. B. **3**: 682
Stafford, J. W. **2**: 615
Stafford-Clark, D. **2**: 149, 191; **3**: 28, 59
Stainbrook, E. **2**: 701, 702, 712
Stalnaker, J. M. **2**: 191
Stampfl, T. **2**: 575
Standler, C. B. **3**: 319
Stanescu, V. **2**: 47
Stanley, J. C. **1**: 141, 148
Stanton, A. H. **2**: 477, 486, 619
Staples, F. **2**: 575
Staples, R. **1**: 89, 103
Star, S. A. **2**: 365, 390
Stare, F. A. **2**: 254
Starr, A. **2**: 251
Starr, P. H. **3**: 660, 683
Staub, E. M. **1**: 84
Staudt, V. **2**: 357, 389
Stecker, **3**: 597
Stein, L. **1**: 261, 283, 561
Stein, M. H. **1**: 46, 57
Stein, M. I. **2**: 420
Stein, S. N. **2**: 480
Stein, Z. **1**: 499, 500, 521; **3**: 546
Steinbrook, R. M. **2**: 619
Steinhilber, R. **3**: 156
Steinschneider, A. **3**: 492
Steinschriber, L. **2**: 217
Stekel, W. **1**: 390
Stellar, E. **2**: 105, 307, 312
Stelzner, H. **1**: 394, 402
Stemmer, C. J. **3**: 95, 97
Stengel, E. **1**: 411, 412, 413, 427
Stephen, E. **1**: 210, 224, 225, 234, 472
Stephens, J. H. **2**: 391, 415

Stephens, W. N. **3**: 141, 155
Stephenson, C. W. **2**: 171, 191
Stern, E. **2**: 357, 390
Stern, L. O. **3**: 529
Stern, M. **2**: 255
Stern, R. M. **2**: 261
Stern, S. **3**: 337, 346
Stern, W. **1**: 70; **2**: 490; **3**: 5
Stettler-Von Albertini, B. **1**: 93, 102
Stevens, M. **1**: 369
Stevenson, H. W. **1**: 166, 169; **2**: 255
Stevenson, I. **1**: 151; **2**: 575
Stevenson, S. S. **3**: 31, 59
Stewart, A. **3**: 34, 59
Stewart, A. M. **3**: 27, 36, 59
Stewart, H. **2**: 181, 191
Stewart, J. S. S. **2**: 46
Stickler, G. B. **3**: 528
Stikar, J. **2**: 216
Stockard, C. R. **3**: 20, 59
Stockert, F. G. von, **2**: 133, 145
Stoll, **2**: 278
Stolz, L. M. **3**: 141, 155
Stone, A. R. **2**: 615
Stone, F. H. **1**: 235, 240, 248, 436, 450
Stone, L. J. **2**: 261
Storch, A. **2**: 426, 446
Stott, D. H. **1**: 379, 384, 402; **3**: 19, 35, 37, 42, 44, 50, 55, 59, 280, 291, 674, 683
Stouffer, G. A. W. (Jr.) **3**: 740, 762
Strang, L. B. **1**: 502, 506, 521
Stransky, E. **2**: 426, 446; **3**: 603
Straumit, A. Y. **2**: 593, 594
Strauss, A. A. **1**: 16, 19, 472, 517, 521
Strean, H. S. **3**: 146, 152, 155
Street, D. F. **1**: 383, 401
Street, D. R. K. **2**: 45
Streitfield, H. S. **3**: 474, 493
Strelchuk, I. V. **2**: 583, 588, 594
Streltsova, N. **2**: 444, 446
Strickler, C. B. **2**: 161, 191
Stringer, J. C. **3**: 752
Stringer, L. A. **3**: 737, 738, 741, 745, 752, 753, 754, 755, 759, 762, 763
Strodtbeck, F. **3**: 305, 318
Stroh, G. **3**: 673, 683
Strong, E. K. **3**: 141, 155
Strong, J. A. **2**: 16, 19, 46, 47
Stross, J. **3**: 222
Strother, C. **2**: 371, 390
Strupp, H. H. **2**: 483, 605, 616, 619
Stubbs, J. T. **2**: 261
Stukat, K. **2**: 619
Sturrock, J. B. **2**: 259
Stutsman, R. **1**: 567, 586

Stutte, H. **3**: 674, 683
Suci, G. J. **3**: 758
Suedfeld, P. **2**: 254, 261
Sugimoto, S. **2**: 257
Sukhareva, G. E. **2**: 435, 446; **3**: 675, 684
Sullivan, **1**: 451
Sullivan, C. **1**: 376, 402
Sullivan, H. S. **2**: 571; **3**: 189, 199, 297, 302, 303, 314, 320
Sullivan, T. M. **2**: 16, 19
Sully, J. **1**: 253; **3**: 5
Sumbajev, I. S. **2**: 585, 595
Summerfield, A. **2**: 357, 390
Sundberg, N. D. **2**: 355, 360, 390
Sunley, R. **3**: 139, 155
Surwillo, W. W. **2**: 293, 309
Susser, M. **1**: 499, 500, 521; **2**: 695; **3**: 546
Sutherland, E. H. **1**: 372, 402
Suttie, I. D. **1**: 172, 191, 244, 248
Sutton, H. E **3**: 683
Suzuki, J. **2**: 218; **3**: 371
Svechnikov, G. **2**: 428, 446
Sved, S. **2**: 104
Svien, H. J. **2**: 127
Swallow, C. **3**: 748, 763
Swanson, G. **3**: 304, 306
Swanson, G. E. **3**: 319, 761, 763, 746
Swanson, L. D. **3**: 587, 588
Swaroop, S. **1**: 369
Swartz, J. **2**: 261
Sweet, W. H. **2**: 113, 129
Sykes, E. G. **3**: 42, 59
Sylvester, P. E. **1**: 516, 517, 521
Symonds, C. **1**: 488, 490
Symonds, C. P. **2**: 114, 128, 199, 221
Symonds, P. M. **1**: 577, 586
Szasz, T. S. **2**: 365, 390
Szeminska, A. **1**: 59, 84
Szilard, L. **2**: 107, 187, 191
Szurek, S. A. **1**: 400, **2**: 465, 466, 480, 483; **3**: 13, 157, 199, 653, 661, 665, 675, 680, 684
Szyrynski, V. **1**: 579, 586

Taboroff, L. **3**: 473, 493
Taft, L. T. **3**: 663, 684
Takagi, R. **3**: 371
Takahashi, L. Y. **3**: 470
Takahasi, I. **3**: 681
Takuma, T. **3**: 371
Talbot, E. **2**: 486
Talbot, M. **1**: 133, 134, 151
Talland, G. A. **2**: 120, 129
Talmon-Garber, Y. **3**: 333, 346
Tamburini, **3**: 609
Tanner, J. M. **1**: 287, 305; **3**: 97, 413

Tanzi, 3: 609
Tarasov, G. K. 2: 593, 595
Tarsh, M. J. 1: 518
Tart, C. T. 2: 619
Tasch, R. J. 3: 142, 155
Tausch, A. M. 3: 736, 763
Tausig, T. 1: 147
Taussig, H. B. 3: 51, 59
Tay, 3: 4
Taylor, A. C. 2: 86
Taylor, A. I. 2: 46
Taylor, A. J. W. 2: 261
Taylor, A. M. 2: 220
Taylor, C. D. 1: 91, 103
Taylor, I. G. 3: 558, 559, 570
Taylor, W. S. 2: 355, 390
Tchistovitch, L. A. 2: 538, 556
Tec, L. 3: 679
Teicher, J. D. 3: 655, 684
Teitelbaum, H. A. 2: 615
Ten Bensel, R. W. 3: 588
Tepas, D. I. 2: 221
Teplitz, Z. 2: 219
Terman, L. M. 1: 96, 103, 185, 195, 199, 200, 201, 209, 570, 586; 3: 796, 804
Termansen, P. E. 2: 697
Terry, D. 2: 416, 417
Tessman, E. 1: 151
Tevetoglu, F. 3: 470
Thacore, V. R. 2: 220
Thaler, M. 3: 493
Thaler, V. H. 2: 260
Thalhammer, O. 3: 24, 25, 59
Thaver, F. 3: 371
Theis, S. 1: 434, 444, 450
Thelen, H. A. 3: 736, 763
Therman, E. 1: 56
Thistlethwaite, D. 1: 165, 169
Thom, D. 3: 6
Thomas, A. 1: 399; 3: 62, 68, 69, 70, 79, 204, 219, 474, 493, 738, 743, 758, 763, 803
Thomas, E. S. 2: 218
Thomas, M. 1: 578
Thomas, R. 3: 232, 240, 253
Thompson, B. 1: 445, 450
Thompson, C. B. 1: 398
Thompson, G. G. 3: 139, 155, 735, 757
Thompson, M. 3: 97
Thompson, R. U. 2: 190
Thompson, W. R. 2: 261; 3: 28, 59
Thomson, A. M. 3: 27, 56
Thomson, G. 1: 185
Thorek, P. 3: 529
Thorndike, E. L. 3: 570
Thornton, D. R. 1: 147
Thorpe, J. G. 2: 573, 614
Thorpe, W. H. 3: 82, 97
Thrasher, F. M. 3: 145, 155
Thrasher, G. 2: 218
Thuline, H. C. 2: 48

Thurber, E. 3: 154
Thursfield, 3: 9
Thurston, D. L. 3: 527
Thurston, J. R. 3: 745, 759
Thurstone, L. L. 1: 185, 186, 187, 191, 375, 402
Tibbets, R. W. 2: 619
Ticho, G. 2: 483
Ticho, T. 2: 483
Tietze, T. 2: 411, 422; 3: 146, 155
Tiira, E. 2: 261
Tiller, P. O. 3: 141, 155
Tiller, P. R. 2: 254
Tillman, C. 1: 413, 427; 2: 411, 422; 3: 146, 154
Tillman, W. A. 1: 369
Tilton, J. 1: 148
Timkin, K. R. 2: 422
Tinbergen, N. 1: 29, 37; 2: 486
Tinnan, L. M. 2: 253
Titchener, J. L. 3: 529
Tizard, B. 1: 463, 464, 472
Tizard, J. P. M. 1: 212, 213, 216, 217, 231, 234, 459, 461, 472, 500, 522
Tjio, J. H. 1: 46, 55, 57; 2: 49
Tobach, E. 3: 97
Tobey, H. P. 2: 250
Todd, E. M. 2: 85
Todd, J. 2: 137, 145
Tokarsky, V. M. 2: 578, 584, 595
Tolman, E. C. 1: 151, 165
Tonescu, V. 2: 47
Tong, J. E. 1: 382, 402
Toolan, J. M. 1: 405, 409, 427
Toolan, J. V. 3: 679
Toomey, L. C. 2: 617
Tooth, G. 2: 700, 701, 712
Tooth, G. C. 2: 695
Topping, G. 2: 423
Tough, I. M. 3: 47, 60
Toulouse, 3: 590, 592, 593, 608
Tourney, G. 2: 310
Towers, J. 2: 388
Towne, R. D. 3: 155
Townes, P. L. 2: 49
Tramer, M. 1: 478, 495; 3: 650, 674, 675, 684
Tranel, N. 2: 261
Trapp, G. P. 2: 390
Trasler, G. 1: 387, 402
Travis, R. C. 2: 198, 219, 221
Treacy, A. M. 2: 46
Tredgold, R. F. 1: 509, 522; 3: 546
Treisman, A. 3: 548, 559, 566, 570
Treisman, M. 2: 220
Trent, R. D. 3: 745, 763
Trethowan, W. H. 3: 145, 155
Trieschman, A. 3: 151

Troffer, S. A. 2: 619
Troll, W. 1: 56
Trosman, H. 2: 221
Trotter, W. 2: 47
Troussau, A. 1: 306; 3: 387
Trouton, D. S. 2: 619
True, R. M. 2: 171, 191
Truelove, S. C. 1: 334; 3: 525
Truex, R. C. 2: 86
Trumbull, R. 2: 260
Tschisch, W. 3: 591, 608
Tseng, S. C. 3: 141, 152
Tsirkov, V. D. 2: 544, 555
Tsuagn, M-T. 2: 6, 19
Tucker, D. F. 3: 58
Tuckman, J. 3: 789, 804
Tudor, R. B. 3: 472, 493
Tudor-Hart, B. H. 1: 95, 102
Tuke, W. 2: xx
Tupin, J. P. 2: 486
Tupin, J. T. 2: 421, 424; 3: 682
Turkevitz, G. T. 3: 97
Turle, G. C. 1: 305
Turnbull, R. B. 3: 528
Turnbull, R. C. 2: 5, 17
Turner, B. 2: 142
Turner, H. H. 2: 49
Turner, V. 3: 747, 763
Turpin, R. 1: 47, 56, 521
Twain, M. 2: 450
Tyler, D. B. 2: 221, 294, 309
Tyler, R. 3: 546
Tyler, V. 2: 570, 573
Tymms, V. 1: 520

Uhlenruth, E. H. 2: 619
Uhr, L. 2: 192, 258, 300, 311, 636
Ukhtomsky, A. A. 2: 437, 447
Ulett, G. A. 3: 416
Ullman, M. 2: 180, 192
Ullmann, C. A. 2: 740, 747, 763
Ullmann, L. P. 3: 376, 388, 390, 570, 573, 575
Ulvedal, F. 2: 261
Underwood, J. E. A. 1: 256
Ungar, G. 2: 96, 107
Ushakov, G. K. 3: 375, 390, 675, 684
Utina, I. A. 2: 107
Uzman, L. 2: 86

Vahia, N. 2: 702, 712
Valatx, J. L. 2: 221
Valder, L. O. 3: 151
Valenstein, A. F. 3: 96
Valero, A. 3: 469
Vallient, G. E. 3: 652, 684
Vallon, 3: 608
Vallotton, 2: 143
Van Alstyne, D. 3: 550, 570
Vance, F. L. 2: 355, 390
Vandenheuval, W. J. A. 2: 15, 18
Vanderhoof, E. 2: 573

AUTHOR INDEX

Van der Sar, A. **3**: 456, 470
Van der Valk, J. **1**: 313, 334, 335; **3**: 527
Van Egmond, E. **3**: 736, 745, 747, 762, 763
Van Hooff, J. A. R. A. M. **1**: 28, 37
Van Houten, J. **3**: 155
Van Krevelen, D. A. **3**: 650, 674, 675, 684
Van Meter, W. G. **2**: 307, 312
Van Winkle, E. **2**: 277, 286
Van Wulfften-Palthe, P. M. **2**: 261
Vaughan, G. **1**: 350
Vaughan, W. T. (Jr.) **1**: 426
Vedenov, N. F. **2**: 436
Vedrani, **3**: 591, 592, 603, 608
Veeder, **3**: 9
Velvovskii, I. Z. **2**: 593, 595
Ventra, **3**: 603
Vernon, H. M. **1**: 369
Vernon, J. **2**: 224, 254, 261, 262, 271, 286
Vernon, M. D. **1**: 85, 103; **3**: 546
Vernon, P. E. **1**: 80, 84, 184, 185, 191
Verplank, W. S. **1**: 135, 151
Viasemskii, I. V. **2**: 578, 595
Victor, M. **2**: 113, 114, 118, 119, 120, 127, 129
Vidal, G. **1**: 50, 56; **2**: 48
Viek, C. **3**: 382, 390
Viek, P. **1**: 121, 150
Vigotsky, L. S. **1**: 188
Vikan-Kline, L. **2**: 618
Villablanca, J. **2**: 262
Vimont, P. **2**: 218
Vincent, N. M. **3**: 52, 60
Vink-Bang, **1**: 94, 102
Vinogradov, M. I. **2**: 538, 556
Vinogradova, O. S. **3**: 553, 569
Vish, I. M. **2**: 595
Visotsky, H. M. **3**: 754, 763
Vispos, R. H. **2**: 251
Voas, R. B. **1**: 114, 150
Voegtlin, W. L. **2**: 575
Vogel, E. F. **3**: 151, 152, 154, 357, 371
Vogel, G. **2**: 217
Vogel, S. H. **3**: 357, 371
Vogt, O. **2**: 582, 595
Voisin, **3**: 606
Völgyesi, F. A. **2**: 147, 148, 192, 582, 584, 595, 619
Volkart, E. H. **3**: 761
Volsky, T. C. **2**: 355, 390
von der Heydt, V. **3**: 145, 155
von Felsinger, J. M. **2**: 616, 619
von Marées, **2**: 143
von Mehring, O. **2**: 619
von Pirquet, C. **2**: 182, 184, 192; **3**: 10

von Wagner-Jauregg, J. **3**: 614
Vorobjeva, V. A. **2**: 538, 556
Voth, H. M. **2**: 485
Waal, N. **1**: 492, 495
Waelder, J. **3**: 441, 454
Waelhens, A. de **2**: 518
Waelsch, **2**. 100
Wagatsuma, H. **3**: 357, 369, 371
Wagener, T. **2**: 217
Wagner, H. P. **1**: 56
Wahl, C. W. **2**: 411, 422; **3**: 146, 155, 156, 371
Wainrib, B. **2**: 104
Waldeyer, **2**: 53
Waldfogel, S. **1**: 130, 131, 134, 151
Walk, R. D. **1**: 98, 103
Walker, A. E. **2**: 112, 129, 317, 349
Walker, H. T. **2**: 44
Walker, W. M. **2**: 22, 60
Wall, A. J. **3**: 528
Wallace, C. D. **2**: 218
Wallach, H. **1**: 97, 103
Wallerstein, J. **3**: 705
Wallerstein, R. S. **2**: 449, 471, 473, 482, 484, 485, 486
Wallgren, A. **3**: 529
Wallinga, J. V. **2**: 365, 390
Wallis, H. **2**: 49
Walter, R. J. **3**: 525
Walter, W. G. **2**: 155, 166, 168, 169, 176, 188, 192; **3**: 391, 393, 397, 399, 407, 408, 416, 417
Walters, A. A. **1**: 372, 402
Walters, C. **2**: 262
Walters, G. **1**: 120, 148
Walters, R. H. **1**: 140, 146, 148; **2**: 262
Walton, D. **1**: 115, 151; **2**: 575
Walton, E. **3**: 146, 156
Wapner, S. **2**: 145; **3**: 123
Wardwell, E. **1**: 580, 585
Waring, M. **2**: 412, 422; **3**: 804
Warkany, J. **1**: 515, 522; **3**: 20, 60
Warren, A. H. **1**: 151
Warren, I. A. **3**: 529
Warren, R. **3**: 529
Warren. S. **3**: 529
Warren, W. **1**: 285, 305, 559, 561
Warrington. E. **3**: 564, 569
Wasserman, R. **3**: 526
Waszink, H. M. **3**: 456, 470
Watkins, P. **2**: 156, 192
Watson, J. **2**: 421; **3**: 153
Watson, J. B. **1**: 113, 118, 119, 151; **2**: 150
Watson, J. D. **1**: 52, 57
Watson, R. I. **3**: 83, 97

Watson, W. H. **2**: 702, 712
Watt, F. **2**: 253
Watterson, D. **1**: 400; **2**: 262
Watts, A. W. **3**: 372
Watzlawick, P. **2**: 420
Weakland, J. H. **2**: 404, 417, 418, 420, 479
Webb, J. W. **3**: 59
Webb, W. B. **2**: 216, 218
Webber, C. S. **3**: 492
Wechsler, D. **1**: 359, 369, 498, 522, 568, 586; **3**: 671, 684
Wedell, K. **1**: 219, 227, 234
Wedge, B. M. **2**: 680, 695, 700, 712
Weeks, A. **1**: 394, 402,
Wegman, T. G. **2**: 49
Weigl, E. **3**: 562, 570
Weil, A. P. **1**: 238, 239, 248; **3**: 660, 684
Weil, R. J. **2**: 700, 711
Weinberg, W. **2**: 12, 19
Weinberger, M. **1**: 495; **3**: 684
Weiner, A. **3**: 156
Weiner, H. **3**: 475, 493
Weiner, M. F. **2**: 422
Weinstein, **1**: 451
Weinstein, E. **2**: 135, 144, 145
Weinstock, H. I. **3**: 511, 529
Weisenberg, T. **3**: 561, 570
Weisman, A. D. **2**: 262
Weiss, E. **1**: 313, 335
Weiss, H. R. **2**: 207, 221
Weiss, P. **2**: 57, 86
Weitzenhoffer, A. M. **2**: 192
Weitzner, E. **3**: 253
Welch, B. E. **2**: 257, 261
Welch, G. **2**: 234, 263, 311
Wellman, B. **3**: 734, 763
Wenar, C. **3**: 62, 63, 79, 145, 156, 527, 530
Wende, S. **2**: 212, 220, 262
Wendell, B. **3**: 320
Wender, P. **3**: 652
Wendt, H. **3**: 156
Wenner, W. H. **2**: 220
Werboff, J. **3**: 52, 53, 60
Werkman, L. S. **1**: 481, 495
Werner, **2**: 243, **3**: 664
Werner, H. **2**: 145
Werner, M. **2**: 421
Wernicke, C. **2**: 331, 349, 426, 447; **3**: 602, 608, 609
Wertheimer, M. **2**: 490
West, C. D. **2**: 216
West, D. J. **1**: 381, 402
West, J. **3**: 318
West, J. W. **2**: 292, 309
West, L. J. **2**: 254, 260, 261, 265, 286, 287
Westerman, R. A. **2**: 107
Westermarck, E. A. **3**: 126, 156
Westheimer, I. J. **2**: 477, 482; **3**: 145, 152, 283, 290

3 H

AUTHOR INDEX

Wetterstrand, L. 2: 582, 595
Wexler, D. 2: 256, 257, 260, 261, 262, 299, 311
Weybrew, B. B. 2: 262
Weygandt, W. 3: 13, 591, 598, 603, 608, 612
Whatley, E. 1: 225, 226, 234
Whatmore, P. B. 2: 16, 19
Wheaton, J. L. 2: 262
Wheeler, 3: 135, 152
Wheelis, A. B. 3: 314, 320
Whetnall, E. 3: 554, 555, 570
Whipple, H. E. 2: 107
Whitaker, C. 2: 418, 419
White, B. 2: 255
White, B. V. 3: 530
White, J. G. 1: 114, 115, 151
White, M. A. 2: 411, 422; 3: 146, 154, 156, 759
White, R. B. 2: 448, 477, 486
White, R. W. 2: 467, 486; 3: 44, 60, 493
White, W. H. 3: 494, 530
Whitehorn, J. C. 2: 619
Whiting J. W. M. 3: 156, 313, 315, 316, 318, 320, 746, 763
Whitlow, G. C. 2: 615
Whitman, R. M. 2: 216
Whitty, C. W. M. 2: 113, 120, 129
Wickes, I. G. 2: 221
Wickman, E. V. 3: 740, 763
Wideroe, 3: 608
Wigan, E. R. 2: 174, 175, 176, 188
Wild, C. 2: 417
Wilde, O. 2: 132
Wilde, Lady 2: 142
Wilder, J. 2: 364, 390, 575
Wile, R. 2: 481; 3: 679
Wilgosh, L. 2: 263
Wilkens, B. 2: 614
Wilkens, H. 3: 528
Wilking, V. N. 1: 369
Wilkins, L. T. 1: 371, 372, 402
Wilkinson, E. M. 3: 45, 50, 55, 57
Wilkinson, J. 2: 256
Wilkinson R. T. 2: 202, 204, 221, 293, 309
Wille, 3: 608
Willer, L. 1: 494
Williams, B. 2: 253
Williams, C. D. 1: 115, 151
Williams, C. E. 1: 502, 520 522
Williams, E. B. 3: 564, 565, 570
Williams, G. W. 2: 177, 192
Williams, H. L. 2: 202, 218, 219, 221, 295, 310
Williams, J. 2: 47; 3: 677
Williams, M. 1: 586; 2: 114, 129; 3: 308, 320, 547, 552,

561, 562, 563, 566, 567, 569, 570
Williams, P. 1: 372, 402
Williams, R. L. 2: 216
Willmer, E. N. 2: 85
Willmott, P. 3: 136, 156
Willoughby, R. R. 2: 575
Willows, D. 2: 263
Wills, D. M. 3: 237, 238, 252, 253.
Wilmer, H. A. 2: 418
Wilson, D. C. 2: 651, 673
Wilson, E. 2: 182, 192
Wilson, E. B. 2: 88, 107
Wilson, H. 1: 379, 402
Wilson, M. G. 3: 22, 60
Wilson, R. 1: 378, 402
Wilson, R. A. 2: 45
Wilson, R. H. L. 2: 47
Winch, R. 3: 141, 156
Windle, C. 2: 258
Wing, J. K. 2: 423, 679, 695
Wingfield, A. 3: 548, 561, 569
Winner, A. 1: 435, 450
Winnicott, D. W. 1: 241, 243, 244, 248, 252, 333, 335, 393, 402, 442, 450, 523, 531; 2: 449, 452, 457, 458, 464, 477, 486; 3: 124, 139, 142, 156, 214, 219, 544, 661, 672, 684
Winnik, H. Z. 3: 333, 346
Winocur, G. 2: 263
Winograd, M. 3: 344, 346
Winokur, G. 3: 416
Winsor, C. B. 3: 334, 346
Winter, A. L. 2: 192; 3: 417
Winters, W. D. 2: 275, 287
Withers, E. 1: 225, 233
Witmer, 1: 451
Witmer, H. 1: 401
Witmer, L. 2: 354
Wittenborn, J. R. 1: 438, 443, 444, 449, 450
Wittenhorn, J. R. 2: 371, 390
Wittersheim, G 2: 221
Wittkower, E. D. 2: 697, 705, 711, 712; 3: 528
Wittson, C. L. 2: 386, 388
Witty, P. 1: 209
Wohlgemuth, A. 2: 575
Wohlwill, J. F. 1: 59, 84
Wolberg, L. R. 2: 192
Wolf, K. M. 1: 89, 103; 3: 265, 291, 352, 357, 659, 683
Wolf, S. 2: 615, 619; 3: 527, 530, 671, 684
Wolf, W. 2: 619
Wolfe, S. 2: 421
Wolfe, T. 1: 368
Wolfenstein, M. 3: 154, 155
Wolff, H. D. 2: 251
Wolff, H. G. 2: 218; 3: 474, 493, 527
Wolff, O. H. 1: 55, 520
Woff, P. H. 2: 449, 450, 486, 487; 3: 80, 82, 92, 97

Wolpe, J. 1: 113, 118, 119, 121, 127, 128, 129, 130, 131, 142, 151, 153, 157, 159, 162, 164, 169; 2: 376, 377, 390, 557, 560, 567, 575
Wolpert, E. A. 2: 201, 217, 221
Wolpin, M. 2: 569, 575
Wolstenholme, G. E. W. 2: 128, 217, 221
Wong, R. J. 3: 586
Wood, H. O. 3: 31, 57
Woodmansey, A. 2: 617
Woods, G. E. 1: 218, 234
Woods, H. M. 1: 368
Woodward, J. 1: 119, 151
Woodward, M. 1: 58, 79, 84, 214, 215, 224, 231, 234, 374, 402, 500, 517, 522
Woolf, L. I. 1: 502, 505, 507, 510, 515, 520, 521, 522
Woollam, D. H. M. 1: 514, 521; 3: 47, 60
Woolley, D. W. 2: 276, 287
Woolley, P. V. 2: 46
Woolley, P. V. (Jr.) 3: 588
Wooster, H. 2: 255
Wootton, B. 1: 374, 402
Worcester, J. 3: 59
Word, T. J. 3: 60
Worster-Drought, C. 1: 336, 349, 458
Wortis, H. 3: 456, 462, 470
Wortis, J. 2: 253, 260, 262
Wretmark, G. 2: 474, 493
Wright, D. 1: 494
Wright, D. G. 2: 362, 390
Wright, S. W. 2: 45
Wrighter, J. 3: 744, 760
Wulff, M. 3: 426, 454
Wynn, M. 3: 141, 156
Wynn-Williams, D. 1: 349
Wynne. L. 1: 158, 169
Wynne, L. C. 2: 395, 398, 399, 400, 401, 410, 414, 416, 464, 465, 466, 485, 487; 3: 363, 372
Wynne, M. D. 3: 683

Yakovlev, P. I. 1: 478, 495; 3: 662, 684
Yalom, I. 3: 527
Yancey, W. L. 3: 762
Yap, P. M. 2: 704, 706, 712
Yardley, J. 3: 527
Yarnis, H. 3: 525
Yarrow, L. J. 3: 124, 281, 291, 745, 763
Yates, A. J. 1: 114, 121, 151; 2: 377, 390, 576; 3: 565, 566, 567, 570
Yeh, M. 2: 45
Yelen, D. 2: 311
Yerkes, R. M. 1: 388; 3: 90, 97
Yinger, J. M. 3: 312

Yonebayashi, T. **3**: 705, 712
Yorke, C. **3**: 223
Yoshizumi, T. **2**: 48
Young, A. J. **2**: 617
Young, J. P. **3**: 492
Young, L. **3**: 588
Young, L. L. **3**: 744, 763
Young, M. **3**: 136, 156
Yudin, M. **2**: 444, 447
Yudkin, S. **1**: 311, 335
Yudovitch, F. I. **1**: 95, 102; **3**: 546
Yunis, J. J. **2**: 44, 47

Zak, S. E. **2**: 428
Zappella, M. **1**: 222; **3**: 469
Zappert, J. **3**: 612
Zbarowski, M. **3**: 746, 763
Zeigler, H. P. **1**: 99, 103
Zemlich, M. S. **3**: 83, 97
Zerof, S. **3**: 677
Ziegler, N. A. **2**: 49
Ziehen, T. **3**: 3, 8, 591, 602, 652
Ziferstein, I. **2**: 681, 695, 696
Zilboorg, G. **1**: 408, 427; **3**: 156
Zilkha, K. **2**: 48
Zimberg, S. **2**: 256
Zimmerman, R. **3**: 122
Zingg, R. M. **2**: 262
Zipf, G. K. **3**: 548, 570
Ziskind, E. **2**: 262, 263

Zitrin, A. **3**: 684
Zoob, I. **2**: 264
Zubek, J. P. **2**: 233, 234, 236, 253, 256, 263, 299, 300, 311
Zubin, J. **1**: 574, 585; **2**: 364, 371, 388, 390, 575, 712; **3**: 290, 470, 677, 678, 679, 680
Züblin, W. **1**: 57
Zuch, J. **2**: 217, 481
Zuckerman, M. **2**: 263, 264, 411, 422
Zuckerman, S. B. **2**: 357, 390; **3**: 132, 156
Zurabashvili, A. D. **2**: 426, 428, 447
Zweizig, J. R. **2**: 218

SUBJECT INDEX

This index covers volumes 1, 2 and 3 of the Modern Perspectives in Psychiatry series, the figures in bold type denoting the volume of entry.

Abdominal pain, **1**: 324
Ability
  wastage, **3**: 533
Abortion, **3**: 21, 35, 37
  spontaneous, **3**: 36, 51
  stress, **3**: 29
  threatened, **3**: 43, 45
Accident-proneness, **1**: 350
  emotional stress, **1**: 362
  family, **1**: 361
  incidence, **1**: 352
  personality, **1**: 356, 360
  predisposing factors, **1**: 357
  prevention, **1**: 365
  psychological factors, **1**: 355
  recognition, **1**: 363
  suicide attempts, **1**: 359
  treatment, **1**: 364
Accidents
  monotony, **2**: 272
  sensory deprivation, **2**: 247
Acetylcholinesterase, **2**: 88
Acrocephalosyndactyly, **3**: 33
Acting out
  existential interpretation, **2**: 512
Acute organic psychoses in childhood, **3**: 706-731
  aetiology, **3**: 709-715
  affective disorders, **3**: 728
  behaviour disorders, **3**: 730
  classification, **3**: 716-718
  coma, **3**: 724
  confusional states, **3**: 720
  definition, **3**: 706
  delirium, **3**: 722
  depersonalization, **3**: 725
  disorders of consciousness, **3**: 718
  drowsiness, **3**: 719
  hallucinations, **3**: 726
  hallucinosis, **3**: 726
  illusions, **3**: 726
  oneirism, **3**: 721
  psychomotor disorders, **3**: 729
  psychosensory disorders, **3**: 726
  stuporose state, **3**: 723
  symptomatology, **3**: 716-731

  thought disorders, **3**: 729
  twilight state, **3**: 724
Adaption
  of children, **3**: 72
Adaptive maturity
  peptic ulcers, **3**: 485
  promotion of, **3**: 488
Addiction
  drugs (*see* Drug addiction)
  pica and, **3**: 467
Adolescents, **1**: 285
  anorexia nervosa, **1**: 292
  anxiety, **1**: 290
  behaviour disturbances, **1**: 290, 293
  compulsions, **3**: 381
  conduct disorders, **1**: 293
  delinquency, **1**: 293, 386; **3**: 778
  delusions, **3**: 381
  depression, **1**: 290
  homosexuality, **1**: 294; **3**: 239
  hostels, **1**: 265
  hysterical conversion states, **1**: 292
  independence, **1**: 286
  in-patient units, **1**: 265, 297, 301
  institutional care, **3**: 767
  kibbutz, **3**: 336-339
  mentally ill, **3**: 770
  neurosis, **1**: 291; **3**: 379
  night hospitals, **1**: 265
  obsessional neurosis, **1**: 292
  personality development, **2**: 468
  personality disorders, **1**: 293
  physical development, **1**: 287
  physically handicapped, **3**: 768
  prognosis, **1**: 303
  psychiatric ill-health, **1**: 288
  psychoanalytic treatment, **3**: 227
  psychological characteristics, **1**: 285
  psychological development, **1**: 286
  psychosexual development, **3**: 243
  psychosomatic disorders, **1**: 296
  psychotic disorders, **1**: 294
  schizophrenia, **2**: 408, 412, 413, 434, 439; **3**: 378
  sexuality, **1**: 286
  treatment, **1**: 296, 298, 300, 302

836 SUBJECT INDEX

Adolescents—cont.
  vocational guidance, **1**: 581
Adopted children, **3**: 82
Adoption, **1**: 428
  applicants, **1**: 439, 449
  assessment of child, **1**: 436
  committee, **1**: 447
  consent, **1**: 434
  direct placings, **1**: 430
  follow-up, **1**: 443
  laws and regulations, **1**: 429
  legal aspects, **1**: 428, 441
  problems, **1**: 434, 440
  registered agencies, **1**: 429
  research, **1**: 445
  social aspects, **1**: 431
  social work, **1**: 447
  statistics, **1**: 428
  supply and demand, **1**: 431
  third-party placings, **1**: 430
Adrenochrome, **2**: 15, 281
Aerobic respiration, **2**: 54
Affect
  sleep deprivation, **2**: 291
Affectionless character, **1**: 244
Affective changes
  sensory deprivation, **2**: 227
Affective contact
  autistic disturbances, **3**: 617-648
Affective disorders
  in children, **3**: 728
Affective psychoses
  schizophrenia and, **2**: 5
Age
  vulnerability, **2**: 653
Age-regression
  Babinsky reflex, **2**: 171
  handwriting test, **2**: 171
  psychological, **2**: 170-171
  Rorschach studies, **2**: 171
Aggression
  chromosomes abnormality, **2**: 39
  kibbutz, **3**: 329, 338;
  organic psychosis, **3** 730
Agnosia, **2**: 124
  visual object, **2**: 124
Alcohol
  intoxication in children, **3**: 714
  prenatal effect, **3**: 52
  as teratogen, **3**: 52
Alcoholism
  amnesia, **2**: 119, 120
  avoidance conditioning, **2**: 568
  group hypnotherapy, **2**: 578, 592
Allergy
  hypnosis, **2**: 182-186
  inhibition, **2**: 183-186
Alpert's syndrome, **1**: 511
Alzheimer-Pick disease, **2**: 14
Amaurotic family idiocy, **3**: 4

Ambivalence, **1**: 27
  alternating expression, **1**: 27
  displacement activities, **1**: 28
  facial expression, **1**: 28
  redirection, **1**: 29
  simultaneous expression, **1**: 27
Amenorrhea
  hypnosis, **2**: 178
Amentia
  psychogenic, **3**: 532
Amines
  hypermethylation, **2**: 276, 277
  increase due to hallucinogens, **2**: 277
Aminoaciduria, **1**: 506
Amnesia, **2**: 111, 112, 153
  current events, **2**: 117
  head injury, **2**: 115, 125
  hippocampal excision, **2**: 112
  hypnotic, **2**: 153-156, 161
  Korsakoff's syndrome, **2**: 120
  pavor nocturnus, **3**: 442, 445
  post traumatic, **2**: 115, 126
  psychogenic, **2**: 122, 123
  retrograde, **2**: 116, 125, 126
  sleep walking, **2**: 211; **3**: 431, 432, 435
  tabula rasa, **2**: 161, 223
  temporal lobe lesions, **2**: 112
  transient global, **2**: 124
Amnesic indifference, **2**: 124
Amok, **2**: 705
Amphetamines, **2**: 280
Amphetaminic shock, **2**: 624
Amphetaminic sub-narcosis, **2**: 625
Anaclitic depression, **3**: 299, 300, 315, 659
  separation from mother, **3**: 174
  in ulcerative colitis, **3**: 516
Anaesthesia
  hallucinations, **2**: 273
  hypnotic, **2**: 172, 173, 176
  paranoid ideation, **3**: 88
Anarthria, **2**: 333
Androgen deficiency, **2**: 40
Anencephaly, **3**: 23
  emotional stress in pregnancy, **3**: 30, 31
  influence of season, **3**: 32
  maternal factors, **3**: 23, 26, 27, 30, 31, 32, 33
  social conditions, **3**: 26, 27
Animal behaviour (*see also* Ethology)
  Harlow's experiments, **1**: 35; **2**: 249, 299, 449, 457; **3**: 314, 315
  psychoanalysis, **2**: 450
  psychotogens, **2**: 277
Animal experiments
  stress in pregnancy, **3**: 28
Animal studies
  mother-infant at birth, **3**: 90
  parental care, **3**: 128
  perinatal mortality, **3**: 90

SUBJECT INDEX

separation, **1**: 35; **2**: 249, 299, 449, 457; **3**: 210, 283, 284, 300, 314, 315, 659
Anniversary reactions, **2**: 653
Anorexia, **1**: 114, 292, 324; **2**: 649
  psychotic symptoms, **3**: 713
Anosodiaphoria, **2**: 144
Anosognosia, **2**: 144
Anterospective longitudinal studies
  child development, **3**: 66
Anthropoids
  care of young, **3**: 131
Anthropology, **2**: 493
  cultural, **3**: 295, 296
  family, **3**: 133-136
  fathering, **3**: 133, 136
  marriage, **3**: 135
  parenting, **3**: 136
  philosophical, **2**: 493
  psychoanalysis, **3**: 295, 296
Anxiety, **2**: 558
  accident-proneness, **1**: 358
  acquired drive, **1**: 120
  adolescents, **1**: 290
  aetiology, **1**: 119
  attacks, **1**: 245
  conditioned inhibition, **2**: 559
  confinement, **1**: 121
  determinants of strength, **1**: 120
  existential analysis, **2**: 492, 493, 513
  experimental extinction, **2**: 568
  free-floating, **2**: 559
  hierarchies, **2**: 562
  in infants, **3**: 166, 206
  learning therapies, **2**: 557
  normal and abnormal, **1**: 122, 476
  peptic ulcers in children, **3**: 471, 487
  phobia (q.v.)
  placebo, **2**: 603
  predisposition, **1**: 240
  prevention, **1**: 125
  primitive societies, **2**: 704
  prototype, **3**: 206
  questionnaires, **2**: 561
  reinforcement, **2**: 559
  role of, **3**: 77
  sensory deprivation, **2**: 228
  treatment, **1**: 126, 129
Aphasia, **1**: 336, 343, 583; **2**: 118, 124, 329, 331
  brain injury, **2**: 329
  cortical excision, **2**: 321
  development of speech, **3**: 559
  electrical interference, **2**: 325, 326
  language imprinting, **2**: 329
  post-operative, **2**: 333
Apperception, **2**: 490
Apractognosia, **2**: 330
Apraxia, **2**: 124
Archetypes, **3**: 145
Architecture

child psychiatric clinics, **1**: 259
  psychiatric hospital, **2**: 719
Arousal
  cortical, **2**: 275
  level, **2**: 269, 270
Arteriosclerosis, **2**: 441
  cerebral, **2**: 119, 120
Association techniques, **1**: 576
Asthma, **1**: 317, 329
  deprived child, **3**: 167
  hypnosis, **2**: 181, 182
  mother-child relationship, **3**: 473
  reciprocal inhibition, **2**: 572
Astrocytes, **2**: 62
Ataxia
  intrapsychic, **2**: 426, 437
Attachment behaviour, **3**: 82
Attention, **2**: 330, 334, 344, 346
  absence, **2**: 176
  infant, **3**: 167
  inhibition, **2**: 334
Autism, early infantile, **1**: 136, 235, 475; **2**: 400, 412; **3**: 589, 617-648, 650, 652, 653, 661, 662, 666, 674
  aloneness, **3**: 639, 656
  cognitive ability, **3**: 656
  cognitive potentialities, **3**: 645
  development, **3**: 647
  echolalia, **3**: 641, 656
  families, **3**: 646
  follow-up of Kanner's cases, **3**: 657
  food, **3**: 642
  intellectual functioning, **3**: 656
  Kanner's case histories, **3**: 617-639
  language, **3**: 656
  loud noises, **3**: 642
  masturbation, **3**: 644
  memory, **3**: 640
  moving objects, **3**: 642
  objects relation, **3**: 644, 656
  parents, **3**: 656
  physical aspects, **3**: 646
  relation to people, **3**: 644
  sameness, **3**: 643, 656
  schizophrenia and, **3**: 646
  speech, **3**: 640
  speech training, **1**: 138
  spontaneous activity limitations, **3**: 644
Autistic thinking, **2**: 4
Autoerotism, **3**: 235
  infant, **3**: 167
  kibbutz, **3**: 329
Autohypnosis, **2**: 148, 181
Autointoxications, **3**: 713
Automatism, **2**: 437
Autonomic nervous system
  childhood psychosis, **3**: 669
Autoradiography, **2**: 51
Autoscopy, **2**: 139, 271
Autosomes, **2**: 24

SUBJECT INDEX

Aversion therapy, **1**: 163; **2**: 567 (*see also* Behaviour therapy)
Avitaminosis
   psychological disorders, **3**: 715
Axon, **2**: 51, 57
   cytologic features, **2**: 81
   hillock, **2**: 53, 57

Babinsky reflex, **2**: 171
Baby's body
   inspection by mother, **3**: 91
Baby's cry
   at birth, **3**: 89
   quality of, **3**: 94
Backward children
   separation from parents, **3**: 280
Barbiturate intoxication, **3**: 714
Battered child
   definition, **3**: 572
   description, **3**: 572
   parents, **3**: 573
Behaviour
   adaptive, **1**: 58, 81, 110
   aggressive, **1**: 543, 545
   anti-social, **1**: 245, 293, 523 (*see also* Delinquency)
   aspects, **1**: 24
   assertive, **2**: 562
   biochemistry, **2**: 93
   development, **1**: 60
   deviant, at school, **3**: 741
   disorders (*see* Behaviour disorders)
   facial expressions, **1**: 28
   flight (q.v.)
   heredity, **1**: 40, 41
   human, **1**: 23
   modification, **1**: 104 (*see also* Behaviour therapy)
   motivation, **1**: 32
   neurotic, **2**: 558
   non-social, **1**: 21
   organization, **1**: 30
   patterns, **1**: 61
   premental, **3**: 163
   problems, **1**: 106, 535
   problems prevention, at school, **3**: 749
   in schizophrenia, **1**: 135
   secondary circular reactions, **1**: 62
   sequence, **1**: 23
   social, **1**: 21, 30
   study, **1**: 21
   symbolic, **1**: 67
   temper tantrums, **1**: 115, 544
   temperamental individuality, **3**: 68
   territory, **1**: 30
   theory, **1**: 104
   therapy (*see* Behaviour therapy)
   units of, **1**: 21
   ward, **2**: 693
   withdrawn, **1**: 546

Behaviour disorders
   in adolescents, **1**: 290, 293
   genesis, **3**: 61
   kibbutz's children, **3**: 342
   organic psychoses, in children, **3**: 730
   prenatal influences, **3**: 28, 42-45
Behaviour therapy, **1**: 154, 555; **2**: 557
   assertive responses, **2**: 561, 569
   avoidance conditioning, **2**: 567
   clinical psychologist, **2**: 376
   desensitization *in vivo*, **2**: 564, 567
   efficacy, **2**: 570
   evaluation, **2**: 570
   experimental extinction, **2**: 376, 568
   experiments, **1**: 127; **2**: 377
   imaginal desensitization, **2**: 565
   neurotic behaviour, **2**: 558
   non-adversive electrical stimuli, **2**: 565
   non-specific therapeutic effects, **2**: 570, 571
   operant conditioning, **2**: 569
   patient's response to therapist, **2**: 566
   reciprocal inhibition, **1**: 114, 128; **2**: 560
   relaxation responses, **2**: 562
   schizophrenia, **2**: 570
   sexual responses, **2**: 567
   symptom substitution, **2**: 571
Behaviourist psychologists, **2**: 150
Biochemical lesions
   mental disorders, **2**: 627
Biochemistry (*see also* Metabolism)
   genetics, **1**: 45
   memory, **2**: 87
   psychosis, **1**: 482; **2**: 14, 17, 626
   sensory deprivation, **2**: 235
Bioelectrical phenomena, **2**: 50
Birth cry, **3**: 89
Birth mark, **3**: 19
Birth order
   malformations, **3**: 27
   mongolism, **3**: 27
Black patch psychosis, **2**: 248
Blacker Report, **1**: 255
Blind children
   cerebral responsiveness, **3**: 407
   development, **3**: 227, 236-238
   failure of development, **3**: 237
   hearing, **3**: 237
   institutional care, **3**: 769
   lack of external stimulation, **3**: 236
   nursery group, **3**: 224
   studies on, **3**: 236-238
Blindness
   colour, **1**: 177
   corporeal awareness, **1**: 218; **2**: 133
   hypnotic, **2**: 176, 177
   partial, intelligence tests, **1**: 572
   space-form, **2**: 34
   word-blindness, **1**: 137, 344
Bodily sensations, **2**: 131

SUBJECT INDEX 839

Body-concept, **2**: 136
  draw-a-man test, **2**: 138
  location in outer space, **2**: 138
Body image, **1**: 177, 218; **2**: 130 (*see also* Corporeal awareness)
  child, **3**: 185
  disruption, **2**: 289
  drug intoxication, **2**: 141
  sensory deprivation, **2**: 228
  Sernyl reactions, **2**: 302
Body-mind relationship, **2**: 490
Body-scheme, **2**: 130
  awareness, **2**: 330
Borderline children, **3**: 228, 238
Boston Habit Clinic, **3**: 6
Bowel pathology
  carcinoma, **3**: 496, 506, 508
  ulcerative colitis, **3**: 495
Brain
  biochemical plasticity, **2**: 87
  biochemistry and learning, **2**: 93
  changes due to experiences, **2**: 88
  cytology, **2**: 50
  damage (*see* Brain damage)
  function, **2**: 50
  mechanisms, **2**: 322
  protein formation, **2**: 100
  RNA synthesis, **2**: 90
Brain damage, **1**: 452 (*see also* Neurological impairment)
  assessment, **1**: 453, 573
  cerebral palsy, **1**: 219, 222, 225, 460
  clinical lesion, **2**: 323
  dreaming, **2**: 200
  environment, **1**: 456
  epilepsy (q.v.)
  infantile autism, **3**: 650
  infection during pregnancy, **1**: 515; **3**: 24-26
  intelligence test, **1**: 573
  memory impairment, **2**: 113, 114, 118
  perinatal factors, **1**: 516
  previous personality, **1**: 455
  schizophrenia, **2**: 414
  social effects, **1**: 490
  temperament, **3**: 74
  toxoplasmosis, **3**: 24, 25
  treatment, **1**: 458
  tumours, **2**: 81, 82, 328
Brain washing, **2**: 224, 240
Breast feeding, **3**: 86, 160
  cultural aspects, **3**: 298, 304
  kibbutz, **3**: 323
British Social Adjustment Guides, **3**: 42, 43
Broca's area, **2**: 326
Broken home
  influence on child, **3**: 389
Bruxism, **2**: 213
Buccal smear, **2**: 20, 30, 31, 37
Buddhism, **2**: 519, 521, 527

Camphor, **3**: 715
Cannabinols, **2**: 274, 281, 282
Carbon monoxide poison, **1**: 519; **3**: 714
  amnesia, **2**: 116, 120
Cardiac infarction
  body image, **2**: 141
Care
  parental (*see* Parental care)
Case conference, **1**: 263, 264
Castration anxiety, **2**: 461, 462
  Koro, **2**: 706
  sleep disorders, **3**: 429, 436, 448, 452
Catalepsy, **2**: 177
  in children, **3**: 729
Catatonia, **2**: 147, 148, 150, 151, 154, 157, 158, 177, 277
  oneiroid, **2**: 438
  schizophrenic, **2**: 425, 431, 433, 435, 438, 439
Catharsis, **2**: 604
Cellular membranes, **2**: 59
Cellular patterns
  cerebral cortex, **2**: 66
Central nervous system
  malformations, **3**: 27, 29, 31
  pre-natal damage, **3**: 23, 24, 25
Centrioles, **2**: 57
Cerebellar cortex
  cytology, **2**: 69
Cerebellum, **2**: 314
Cerebral anoxia
  amnesia, **2**: 116, 119, 120
Cerebral arteriosclerosis, **2**: 119, 120
Cerebral atrophy
  somnolence, **2**: 212
Cerebral cortex, **2**: 88, 89
  cellular patterns, **2**: 66
  cortical excision, **2**: 321, 324
  electrical interference, **2**: 325
  electrical stimulation, **2**: 324
  frontal lobes, **2**: 326
  interpretive, **2**: 330, 335, 338, 339
  perception, **2**: 335
  planned initiative, **2**: 326
  programming, **2**: 326, 340, 348
  sensory and motor areas, **2**: 315-321
  speech areas, **2**: 325, 330, 336, 339
  trans-cortical connections, **2**: 317, 333
  uncommitted, **2**: 326, 338, 340, 348
Cerebral embolism, **3**: 710
Cerebral haemorrhage, **3**: 710
Cerebral lesion
  breakdown of languages, **3**: 560
Cerebral palsy, **1**: 219, 222, 225, 460
Cerebral responsiveness
  blind children, **3**: 407
  contingent negative variations, **3**: 405
  disturbed children, **3**: 407
  encephalitis, **3**: 411
  epilepsy, **3**: 406

Cerebral responsiveness—*cont.*
  'intention' wave, **3:** 409
  normal children, **3:** 404
  organic disorders, **3:** 410
  'readiness' wave, **3:** 409
  secondary negative component, **3:** 404
  visceral distraction, **3:** 406
Cerebral thrombosis, **3,** 710
Cerebrovascular disease
  memory, **2:** 124
Ceruloplasmin, **2:** 15
Character traits
  child, **3:** 189
Chemical processes (*see also* Biochemistry)
  memory, **2:** 87
Child (*see also* Infant *and* Toddler)
  abstract concepts, **3:** 192-193
  adaptation, **3:** 72
  compulsions, **3:** 195, 381
  'difficult', **3:** 69, 70
  dreams, **3:** 215
  emotional health, **3:** 157
  fantasies, **3:** 194, 210-215
  first year of life, **3:** 162
  identification, **3:** 194
  independence, **3:** 194
  maternal deprivation (q.v.)
  needs (six to twelve years), **3:** 192
  parental guidance, **3:** 195
  psychoanalysis, **3:** 200
  punishment, **3:** 140, 184, 310
  toddler (q.v.)
  unorganized, **3:** 73
Child-birth
  activity and passivity conflicts, **3:** 93
  animal studies, **3:** 90
  intolerance of passivity, **3:** 93
  mother-infant relations, **3:** 80
  mother-infant first interaction, **3:** 88
  mother's reactions to infant, **3:** 90
  repugnance, **3:** 90
  return home after, **3:** 93
  unfamiliarity, **3:** 90
Child care, **3:** 255-258
  collective, **3:** 323
  maternal, **3:** 256
  parenting, **3:** 257
  practices, **3:** 77
  separation (child-parent) q.v.
Child-care institutions, **3:** 764 (*see also* Residential care of children)
  internal life, **3:** 766
  monotony, **3:** 767
  requirements, **3:** 765
  site, **3:** 766
  training of personnel, **3:** 766
Child development, **2:** 456
  abstract operational stage, **1:** 76
  blind children, **3:** 236-238
  concrete operational stage, **1:** 74

conflicts, **3:** 235
delinquency, **1:** 376, 381
deviations, **3:** 161, 187
emotional, **1:** 81, 82
father, **3:** 141
Hampstead Clinic studies, **3:** 230
handicapped children, **1:** 210
interaction with mother, **3:** 115
interference, **3:** 235
intuitive stage, **1:** 71
longitudinal studies, **3:** 66
maternal deprivation (q.v.)
mental functioning, **2:** 456
mothering, **2:** 457
New York Longitudinal Study, **3:** 63, 67
oedipal phases, **3:** 232, 235
parental controls internalization, **2:** 462
perception, **1:** 85
personality development, **2:** 451, 452, 471
Piaget's theory, **1:** 58-84, 87, 88, 90, 94, 95, 98, 188, 213, 214, 376; **3:** 415
precocity, **1:** 199
pre-operational stage, **1:** 67
psychoanalytic studies, **3:** 215-217
in psychosis, **1:** 479
quotient, **1:** 566
scales, **1:** 223
semantic communication, **1:** 212, 336; **2:** 456
sensory-motor stage, **1:** 61
smiling response, **2:** 456
social reinforcement, **1:** 139
tests, **1:** 566
theories, **3:** 61
trauma and, **3:** 249
verbal communication, **1:** 212, 336; **2:** 456
Child guidance, **1:** 252
Child guidance clinics, **3:** 201, 770
  Boston Habit Clinic, **3:** 6
  contribution to child psychiatry, **3:** 6
Child personality
  social class, **3:** 309
Child psychiatric clinics, **1:** 256, 534
  architecture, **1:** 259
  clinical team, **1:** 260
  functions (in-patient units) **1:** 535
  Hampstead Child Therapy Clinic, **2:** 476; **3:** 220-250
  siting of units, **1:** 258, 538
  staff, **1:** 260, 539
Child psychiatric services
  organization, **1:** 251-284
Child psychiatrist, **1:** 261
  functions, **1:** 262
  recruitment, **1:** 261
  training, **1:** 261
Child psychiatry, **3:** 1 (*Capitalized items denote chapter in Vol. 1*)
  Accident Proneness, **1:** 350-369

SUBJECT INDEX

Aetiology of Mental Subnormality, **1**: 496-522
Application of Learning Theory to Child Psychiatry, **1**: 104-169
Child Psychology, **1**: 235-248
Child Therapy: A Case of Anti-Social Behaviour, **1**: 523-533
Children's In-Patient Psychiatric Units, **1**: 534-561
clinical investigation, **3**: 375, 387
comparison by age group method (q.v.)
compensation processes, **3**: 385
contribution of child guidance clinics, **3**: 6
contribution of criminology, **3**: 4
contribution of education, **3**: 4
Contribution of Ethology of Child Psychiatry, **1**: 20-37
contribution of psychiatry, **3**: 2
contribution of psychoanalysis, **3**: 5
Contribution of Psychological Tests to Child Psychiatry, **1**: 562-586
contribution of psychology, **3**: 5
contribution of studies on mental deficiency, **3**: 3
correction of disorders, **3**: 385
Delinquency, **1**: 370-402
Development of Perception, **1**: 85-103
Disorders of Speech in Childhood, **1**: 336-349
Exceptional Children, **1**: 192-209
Freudian, **3**: 61
Genetical Aspects of Child Psychiatry, **1**: 38-57
history, **1**: 251; **3**: 1-15, 375
learning theory, **1**: 104-169; **3**: 62
Neuropsychiatry of Childhood, **1**: 452-472
Normal Child Development and Handicapped Children, **1**: 210-234
Organization of Child Psychiatric Services, **1**: 251-284
paediatrics, **3**: 8
Piaget's Theory, **1**: 58-84
Psychiatric Aspects of Adoption, **1**: 428-451
Psychiatry of Adolescents, **1**: 285-305
Psychoses of Childhood, **1**: 473-495
Psychosomatic Approach in Child Psychiatry, **1**: 306-335
psychotherapy, **3**: 13
Research Methodology and Child Psychiatry, **1**: 3-19
Suicidal Attempts in Childhood and Adolescence, **1**: 403-427
therapy, **3**: 387
Thinking, Remembering and Imagining, **1**: 170-191
trends, **3**: 1
usage of term, **3**: 1

Child psychoanalysis, **3**: 220
Child psychotherapist, **1**: 262, 523
Child rearing
culture and, **3**: 292-317
feeding, **3**: 310
kibbutz, **3**: 321-344
material success, **3**: 312
neo-Freudian influences, **3**: 297-304
overprotection, **3**: 303
personality, **3**: 301
school, **3**: 745
Sioux Indians, **3**: 190, 298
social class, **3**: 309
toilet training, **3**: 310
Ute, **3**: 298
Child training
personality, **3**: 313
Childhood depression, **3**: 247
Childhood psychosis, **1**: 235, 473-495; **2**: 412, 435, 444; **3**: 589, 649-676 (see also Childhood schizophrenia)
acute, organic (see Acute organic psychoses in childhood)
aetiology, **3**: 147, 653
atypical development, **3**: 658
autism, early infantile (q.v.)
autonomic nervous system, **3**: 669
brain damage, **3**: 650
childhood schizophrenia (q.v.)
classification, **3**: 650
definition, **3**: 649
dementia infantilis (q.v.)
dementia praecox (q.v.)
dementia praecocissima (q.v.)
development of speech, **3**: 557
ego psychology, **3**: 660
emotional deprivation, **3**: 659
fantasies, **3**: 214
Hampstead Clinic, **3**: 228, 238
Heller's syndrome (see Dementia infantilis)
historical notes, **3**: 651
mother-infant experiences, **3**: 162
nature of, **3**: 649-676
organic factors, **3**: 661
psychoanalysis, **3**: 660
residential care, **3**: 773
sleep disorders, **3**: 425, 443
symbiotic psychosis, **3**: 653, 658
therapeutic management, **3**: 685-705
Childhood schizophrenia, **1**: 473-485; **2**: 412, 435; **3**: 610, 614, 652, 653 (see also Childhood psychosis)
adaptation, **3**: 666
adaptive deficiencies, **3**: 689
aetiology, **1**: 477, 484; **3**: 653, 691
age of onset, **2**: 7, 397, 398, 414, 434, 435, 439, 444; **3**: 382
arrest in psychological growth, **2**: 396
asynchronous maturation, **1**: 479

SUBJECT INDEX

Childhood schizophrenia—*cont.*
atypical child, **3**: 13
autism, early infantile (q.v.)
biochemical studies, **3**: 670
biological aspects, **1**: 482; **2**: 14, 17, 626, 627
chemotherapy, **3**: 696
chromosomal aberration, **2**: 16, 17, 35, 37, 38, 39
classification, **1**: 474; **2**: 400, 440
clinical description, **1**: 475; **2**: 4
community planning, **3**: 703
comparison-by-age-group method, **3**: 378, 382
convulsion therapy, **1**: 491
corrective socialization, **3**: 688
diagnosis, **3**: 686, 688
double bind, **2**: 396, 399, 404, 406, 407, 409, 466
double communication, **2**: 397
Ego psychology, **3**: 660
emotional deprivation, **2**: 464
environment, **1**: 479; **3**: 691, 692
and epilepsy, **1**: 478
family dynamics, **2**: 464, 465, 466
family psychopathology, **2**: 391-424, 641
family treatment, **3**: 701
father-schizophrenic relationship, **2**: 411
genetic factors, **1**: 481; **2**: 3-19, 444
hysteria, **1**: 484
individual therapy, **3**: 698
insulin therapy, **1**: 492
language, **3**: 671
maternal deprivation, **2**: 457, 458
and mental deficiency, **3**: 13
milieu therapy, **3**: 698
mother-schizophrenic relationship, **2**: 394, 395, 396, 411, 457
neurotic symptoms, **1**: 484
Oedipus complex, **2**: 410
organic factors, **3**: 661
parent-schizophrenic relationship, **2**: 411
pink spot, **2**: 15, 627
professional co-ordination, **3**: 695
pseudo-schizophrenic syndrome, **1**: 483
psychoanalysis, **3**: 655
psychological studies, **3**: 671
psychotherapy, **1**: 492
relationship to adult schizophrenia, **1**: 481
rituals, **1**: 476
services, **3**: 703
and suicide, **1**: 413
syndrome, **1**: 475
treatment, **1**: 491; **3**: 685-705
treatment duration, **3**: 703
treatment objectives, **3**: 692
treatment unit size, **3**: 703
whirling test, **3**: 655
withdrawal, **1**: 476

Children's Apperception Test, **1**: 577
Chlorpromazine, **2**: xxiii, 628
as teratogen, **3**: 52, 53
Chorea, **3**: 711
Chromosomal abnormality, **1**: 47-51, 512; **2**: 16, 17, 20, 33-43; **3**: 47, 51
maternal age and, **1**: 47, 49, 511; **2**: 30
Chromosomes, **1**: 46
autosomal anomalies, **1**: 47
cytological techniques, **1**: 51; **2**: 31
euchromatic, **2**: 22
heterochromatic, **2**: 22, 27
LSD effect on, **2**: 279
mongolism (q.v.)
mosaicism, **2**: 27, 28
nuclear sexing (q.v.)
sex chromatin, **1**: 50, 513; **2**: 21
sex chromosomes anomalies, **1**: 49, 513; **2**: 33-43
Cingulectomy, **2**: 120
Cleft lip
pregnancy stress, **3**: 45, 46, 47, 50
Cleft palate, **3**: 23, 27, 45, 46, 47, 50, 55
Clinical investigation
catamnestic, **3**: 388
epidemiological, **3**: 388
methods, **3**: 387
perspective study, **3**: 387
retrospective, **3**: 388
Clinical psychology
behaviour therapy, **2**: 376
conceptions, **2**: 357
contributions to psychiatry, **2**: 353
courses, **2**: 355
description of patient, **2**: 374
diagnosis, **2**: 365
dynamic approach, **2**: 357
equipment, **2**: 384
experimental approach, **2**: 360
explanation, **2**: 379
growth, **2**: 354
laboratory, **2**: 384
post-graduate education, **2**: 355
psychological tests, **1**: 276, 374, 455, 562; **2**: 358
psychometric approach, **2**: 360
psychotherapy, **2**: 361
research, **2**: 363, 371
teaching, **2**: 382
training, **2**: 354, 384
Clinical services
in schools, **3**: 754
Criminology, **3**: 4
juvenile delinquency, **3**: 4
Cocaine, **2**: 279
Cognitive disorganization
sensory isolation, **2**: 301
sleep deprivation, **2**: 291
Cognitive theory
feedback, **2**: 244

SUBJECT INDEX

programming, 2: 244
sensory deprivation, 2: 243
Colectomy, 3: 507
Colic
  in infants, 3: 171
Collective hypnosis (see Group hypnosis)
Colour
  in child psychiatry clinics, 1: 259
  in psychiatric hospitals, 2: 726
Colour association, 1: 177
Colour blindness, 1: 177; 2: 176, 177
Colour vision test, 1: 582
Coma, 3: 724
  of newborn, 3: 170
Communication
  hospital, 2: 717
  infant, 3: 166
  semantic, 3: 207
Community
  psychiatry (see Community psychiatry)
  therapeutic, 2: 675, 691
Community care
  schizophrenia, 2: 412
Community psychiatry, 2: 675
  definition, 2: 676
  development, 2: 679
  doctor-patient relationship, 2: 687
  family doctor, 2: 686
  future, 2: 682
  hospital treatment, 2: 678
  local authorities, 2: 683
  patient government, 2: 692
  psychiatric social worker, 2: 684, 685
  psychiatrist's role, 2: 686
  staff meeting, 2: 689
  therapeutic community, 2: 691
  therapeutic culture, 2: 693
  training, 2: 688
  transference, 2: 693
  treatment in the community, 2: 679
  ward behaviour, 2: 693
  ward meeting, 2: 689
Comparison-by-age-group method
  neurosis, 3: 379-380
  psychosis, 3: 378-379
  symptoms and syndromes, 3: 380-382
Compensation processes
  mental diseases, 3: 385
Complementarity, 2: 395
Completion techniques, 1: 578
  Rosenzweig picture frustration test, 1: 578
  sentence completion, 1: 578
  story completion, 1: 578
Comprehension, 3: 553
Compulsions
  in adolescents, 3: 381
  in children, 3: 195, 381
Concentration camp
  analysis of young victim, 3: 240

Conception
  extra-marital, 3: 32, 33, 34
  pre-marital, 3: 32, 34
  season of, 3: 27, 32
Concussion, 2: 115
Conditioned reflex, 2: 109, 111, 150, 151, 174, 321, 322, 334, 342, 347 (see also Conditioning)
  conditioned closure, 2: 534, 535
  conditioned response, 2: 535
  environmental conditions, 2: 534
  extinction, 2: 546
  motor skills, 2: 345
  Pavlovian theory, 2: 532
  reinforcement, 1: 139, 141; 2: 535
Conditioning, 1: 104, 108, 555; 2: xxiv, 313, 376, 378, 531 (see also Learning and Learning Theory)
  anorexia nervosa, 2: 569
  asthma, 2: 572
  aversive, 1: 163; 2: 567
  clinical application, 1: 113; 2: 546, 557
  conditioned reflex (q.v.)
  cortical excision, 2: 321
  deconditioning, 1: 110
  delinquency, 2: 570
  diagnostic testing, 2: 378, 379
  drugs, 1: 111
  electrical activity, 2: 537
  enuresis, 1: 116; 2: 569
  epilepsy, 2: 536, 547
  experiments, 2: 539-543
  extinction, 2: 546, 568
  homosexuality, 1: 162; 2: 568
  instrumental (see operant)
  learning therapies, 2: 557
  motor reaction, 2: 535
  negative induction, 2: 546, 547
  operant, 1: 105, 134; 2: 569
  Pavlovian theory, 2: 531-556
  placebo, 2: 603, 607
  schizophrenia, 2: 536, 547, 548, 550, 551, 552, 570
  senile dementia, 2: 547
  skills, 2: 319
  social reinforcement, 1: 139
  spatial inter-relationship, 2: 538
  spatial synchronization, 2: 539, 545, 547, 550, 551, 554
  verbal, 3: 551
Confabulation, 2: 115, 120, 121
Conforming
  kibbutz, 3: 329, 341
Confusional states
  in children, 3: 720
Congenital dislocation of the hip
  maternal emotional stress, 3: 36
Congenital myxoedema, 3: 714
Connections
  inhibitory, 2: 536

SUBJECT INDEX

Connections—*cont.*
  temporary, **2:** 536
Consciousness, **2:** 339-343
  attention, **2:** 346
  awareness, **2:** 344
  coma, **2:** 343; in children, **3:** 724
  diencephalon, **2:** 343, 345
  disorders in children, **3:** 718-725
  memory, **2:** 346
  motor output, **2:** 345
  motor skills, **2:** 345
  neuronal action, **2:** 343, 347
  sensory input, **2:** 344
  sleep, **2:** 343
  stream of, **2:** 339, 343, 346
Constipation (psychosomatic), **1:** 323
Constriction
  in hypnosis, **2:** 150
Contemporary society
  fathering, **3:** 149
Contingent habituation, **2:** 166, 167, 169
  mechanism, **2:** 168
Contingent negative variation (CNV)
  autistic children, **3:** 402, 403
  autonomic variables, **3:** 403
  in children (normal), **3:** 404 (disturbed), **3:** 407
  encephalitis, **3:** 411-413
  evoked responses, **3:** 402
  function, **3:** 401
  origin, **3:** 401
  psychopaths, **3:** 399
Control group, **3:** 789
Conversion hysteria, **2:** 172; **3:** 14; (in adolescents) **1:** 292
  culture, **3:** 314
Convulsion therapy, **1:** 491; **2:** xxiii, 366
  camphor induced, **2:** xxii
  depression, **2:** 633
Coprophagia, **3:** 173
Corporeal awareness, **2:** 130 (*see also* Body image)
  blindness, **1:** 218; **2:** 133
  body-concept, **2:** 136
  body-segments, **2:** 132
  definition, **2:** 131
  in disease-states, **2:** 140
  exteroceptive data, **2:** 132
  face, **2:** 132
  heautoscopy, **2:** 139
  labyrinthine components, **2:** 132
  narcissism, **2:** 141, 142
  ontogeny, **2:** 131
  parietal disease, **2:** 144
  phantom phenomena, **2:** 131, 133-136, 172, 272
  self-portraiture, **2:** 141
  tactile factors, **2:** 132
  terminology, **2:** 131
  visual factors, **2:** 132

Cortegan (*see* Thalidomide)
Cortical excitability, **2:** 50
Cortical mechanisms, **2:** 543
  convulsive discharges, **2:** 544
  cortical-subcortical interaction, **2:** 543
  spatial synchronization, **2:** 543, 547, 550, 551, 554
Cortical neurons
  cytology, **2:** 68
Cousin marriage
  and schizophrenia, **2:** 11
Couvade, **3:** 126, 145, 299, 316
Cranial nerves, **2:** 313
Cretinism, **1:** 507
Culture
  catatonia, **3:** 314
  child rearing, **3:** 292-317
  conversion hysterias, **3:** 314
  definition, **2:** 698
  father, **3:** 293
  illegitimacy, **3:** 308
  Japanese, **3:** 350
  mental disorders, **2:** 700-706; **3:** 294
  psychogenic retardation, **3:** 534-536, 538
  schizophrenia, **3:** 314
  schoolchild, **3:** 748
  social processes, **3:** 309
  stress, **2:** 702
  therapeutic, **2:** 693
  transcultural psychiatry, **2:** 697
  treatment, **2:** 706
Cultural deprivation
  psychogenic retardation, **3:** 534
Cultural values
  changes, **3:** 311
Cybernetics, **2:** 187
Cytochemistry, **2:** 51
  ultramicrotechniques, **2:** 52
  ultrastructural, **2:** 52
Cytogenetics, **1:** 46
  anomalies, **1:** 47-51, 511, 513; **2:** 16, 17, 20, 30, 33-43
  chromosomes (q.v.)
  nuclear sexing (q.v.)
  techniques, **1:** 51; **2:** 31
Cytology, **1:** 46; **2:** 20
  brain cells, **2:** 50
  brain tumours, **2:** 81
  cerebellar cortex, **2:** 69
  cerebral cortex, **2:** 66
  cerebral cortex neurons, **2:** 68
  chromosomes (q.v.)
  cultured nervous tissues, **2:** 50, 77
  diseased nerve tissue, **2:** 81
  neuroglia, **2:** 61
  nuclear sexing (q.v.)

Dasein, **2:** 491-518
Daseinsanalysis (*see* Existential analysis)
Day hospital, **1:** 560; **2:** 683, 713

SUBJECT INDEX

Deafferentation, **2**: 223, 266
Deafness, **1**: 339
  auditory hallucinations, **2**: 272
  hypnotic, **2**: 173-176
  institutional care (children), **3**: 769
  intelligence test, **1**: 572
  speech development, **3**: 554
Death
  concept, **1**: 441
  fear, **2**: 470
  parental, **3**: 283
Decerebrate preparations, **2**: 314, 315
Defectology, **1**: 189
Defence mechanisms, **3**: 216, 294
Dehydrogenase, **2**: 54
Deiters' neurons, **2**: 92, 93
Déjà vu, **1**: 178; **2**: 335
Delinquency, **1**: 242, 370
  in adolescence, **1**: 293, 386
  aetiology, **1**: 377
  aftercare, **3**: 782
  child-parent separation, **3**: 281
  classification, **1**: 372, 395
  conditioning, **2**: 570
  corrective establishments, **1**: 394
  detention departments, **3**: 781
  and development, **1**: 376, 381
  father implication, **3**: 145
  heredity, **1**: 43, 380
  home background, **1**: 375, 397
  homosexuality, **1**: 387
  and illness, **1**: 382
  and intelligence, **1**: 374, 381
  juvenile residential care, **3**: 778
  Klinefelter's syndrome, **2**: 42
  lying, **1**: 179, 525
  neurological damage, **1**: 383
  parental attitude, **1**: 375, 385, 525
  personality, **1**: 382
  predisposing factors, **1**: 385
  psychoanalytic study, **3**: 228
  punishment seeking, **1**: 389
  school homes, **3**: 779
  social factors, **1**: 378
  statistics, **1**: 371
  and suicide, **1**: 413
  treatment, **1**: 390, 523; **2**: 570
  vocational schools, **3**: 780
Delirium
  acute and febrile, in children, **3**: 722
  in children, **3**: 706, 722, 727
  LSD, **2**: 279
Delusion
  in adolescents, **3**: 381
  in children, **3**: 380
  oneiroid, of Cotard, **2**: 431, 436
  schizophrenic, **2**: 430, 433
Dementia, **2**: 114, 120, 425
  memory, **2**: 117
  paralytica, **2**: 114, 120

  praecocissima (q.v.)
  praecox (q.v.)
  senile, **2**: 124, 441; **3**: 533, 563
Dementia infantilis (Heller's syndrome), **3**: 4, 589, 610-616, 646, 662, 675
  dementia praecocissima, **3**: 610
  early symptoms, **3**: 611
  encephalitis lethargica, **3**: 615
  follow-up studies, **3**: 613
  idiotic regression, **3**: 612
  malaria therapy, **3**: 613
  stages, **3**: 613
Dementia praecocissima, **2**: 5, 8; **3**: 589, 590, 593, 594, 597, 599, 611, 646, 651
  and dementia infantilis, **3**: 610
  diagnosis, **3**: 600
Dementia praecox, **2**: 4, 440; **3**: 590-607, 610
  aetiology, **3**: 593
  age of onset, **3**: 593
  comitans, **3**: 594, 595
  diagnosis, **3**: 601
  pathological anatomy, **3**: 606
  premonitory signs, **3**: 605
  prognosis, **3**: 598
  retardata, **3**: 594, 601, 604
  and sexual functions, **3**: 606
  subsequens, **3**: 594, 595
Dementia simplex, **3**: 591
Dendrites, **2**: 59
Dentritic fibres, **2**: 51
Denial syndrome, **2**: 144
Dependence, **3**: 352
  kibbutz, **3**: 329
Depersonalization, **2**: 138, 139
  acute organic psychosis, **3**: 725
  age of onset, **3**; 382
  mescaline, **2**: 280
  schizophrenia, **2**: 306
  sensory deprivation, **2**: 228
  sleep deprivation, **2**: 291
Depression
  in adolescents, **1**: 290
  age of onset, **3**: 382
  anaclitic, **3**: 209, 299, 300, 315
  anti-depressant drugs, **1**: 421; **2**: 622, 623, 631, 632
  childhood, **3**: 247
  clinical picture, **1**: 486
  ECT, **2**: 633
  Harlow's experiments, **3**: 315
  insomnia, **2**: 208
  manic, (in adolescents) **1**: 295 (in children) **1**: 487
  maternal, **3**: 173
  and parental death, **3**: 283
  post-partum, **3**: 81
  in primitive societies, **2**: 701
  reactive (of childhood), **1**: 485, 529
  schizophrenic, **2**: 430, 431, 436

Depression—*cont.*
  suicide, **1**: 410, 412, 421 (*see also* Suicide)
Depressive position, **3**: 175
Deprivation
  cultural, **3**: 534-536, 538
  emotional, **3**: 659
  family, **3**: 535
  maternal (*see* Maternal deprivation)
  of parenting, **3**: 138
  paternal, **2**: 464
  perceptual, **1**: 86
  psychological, **3**: 9
  sensory (*see* Sensory deprivation)
  and separation, **3**: 254-289
  sleep, **2**: 202
Deprived child
  asthma, **3**: 167
Depth psychology, **2**: 505
Desensitization, **1**: 114, 127; **2**: 563-566
Development
  child (*see* Child development)
  electrocerebral, **3**: 413
  personality, **2**: 451, 452
  psychosexual, **2**: 453
  psychosocial, **3**: 413
Developmental differentiation, **3**: 84
Developmental quotient, **1**: 566
Developmental shifts, **3**: 84
Diabetes, **3**: 43
  psychotic symptoms, **3**: 713
Diagnosis
  clinical psychologist, **2**: 365
  treatment choice, **2**: 366, 367, 368
Diencephalon, **2**: 318, 321, 343, 345, 346, 348
Disinhibition phenomena, **2**: 266
Disseminated sclerosis
  corporeal image, **2**: 140
Distaval (*see* Thalidomide)
Divorce, **2**: 640
  emotional, **2**: 394, 396, 413
DMPE (3,4-dimethoxyphenylethylamine), **2**: 15
DNE (deoxyribonucleic acid), **2**: 22, 23, 27, 51, 52, 57, 62, 89, 90, 94, 187
  somatic mutations, **2**: 90
Double bind, **2**: 396, 399, 406, 407, 409, 466
  definition, **2**: 404
Double communication, **2**: 397
Down's disease (*see* Mongolism)
Dreams, **1**: 82, 176, 526, 529; **2**: 193, 270
  brain injury, **2**: 200
  children, **3**: 215
  deprivation, **3**: 418
  electroencephalogram, **2**: 201, 209
  existential interpretation, **2**: 512
  external stimuli and content, **2**: 201
  function of, **3**: 419

  need, **2**: 201
  psychoanalysis, **2**: 449
  REM sleep, **3**: 419
  sexual symbolism, **2**: 202
Drever-Collins Test, **1**: 572
Dromic conduction, **2**: 325
Drowsiness, **2**: 193, 194, 198, 199; **3**: 719
  hypnagogic hallucinations, **2**: 198
Drugs, **1**: 281, 302 (*see also* Psychopharmacology)
  addiction (*see* Drug Addiction)
  anti-depressants, **1**: 421, 491, 546; **2**: 622, 623, 631, 632
  anti-hypnotics, **2**: 622
  behaviour and, **2**: xxiii, 277
  in brain damage, **1**: 459
  butyrophenones, **2**: 629
  conditioning and, **1**: 111
  hallucinogenics, **2**: 622, 623, 636 (*see also* Hallucinogens)
  hypnotics, **2**: 622, 623
  inactive (*see* Placebo)
  inert (*see* Placebo)
  indole alkaloids (q.v.)
  neuroleptics, **2**: 622, 623, 628, 630
  oneirogenic, **2**: 622, 623
  phenothiazines, **2**: 628
  placebo (q.v.)
  psycho-analeptics, **2**: 622, 623
  psychoanalysis and, **2**: 477
  psychodysleptics, **2**: 622, 623
  psycholeptics, **2**: 622, 623
  psychotomimetic, **2**: 301
  psychotropic, classification, **2**: 623
  sedatives, **1**: 547; **2**: 622, 623
  as teratogens, **3**: 50
  tranquillizers, **2**: xxiii, 622, 623; **3**: 502
  withdrawals and nightmares, **2**: 210
Drug addiction, **2**: 282, 634, 635
  avoidance conditioning, **2**: 568
  treatment, **2**: 366
Dualism of body and mind, **2**: 489
Duchenne muscular dystrophy, **2**: 28
Duodenal ulcer in children, **3**: 472
Dynamic approach
  clinical psychology, **2**: 357
Dysarthria, **1**: 337
Dyslalia, **1**: 345
Dyslexia, **1**: 137, 344
  heredity, **1**: 44
  latent learning, **1**: 166
Dysmenorrhea
  hypnosis, **2**: 178
Dysmaturation, **3**: 654
Dysphasia, **3**: 567

Echolalia, **1**: 476; **3**: 555, 556, 646, 656
Ecstasy, **2**: 271

ECT (electroconvulsive therapy), 2: 366
  amnesia, 2: 116, 120
  depression, 2: 633
Eczema
  baby-mother conflicts, 2: 459; 3: 172
  hypnosis, 2: 182
  infantile, 3: 171
Education
  contribution to child psychiatry, 3: 4
  kibbutz, 3: 322, 325, 334-336, 339
  remedial, 1: 134; 3: 4, 387
Educational arrest, 3: 592
Educational attainment tests, 1: 580
EEG (electroencaphalography), 1: 454; 2: xxiv; 3: 391
  abnormalities, 3: 393
  affective function, 3: 393
  alpha range, 3: 392
  autonomic and somatic variables, 3: 392
  delta band, 3: 392
  dreams, 2: 201
  encephalitis, 3: 395
  epilepsy, 1: 463-469; 3: 393
  evoked responses, 3: 396
  feature provenance, 3: 414
  hypnosis, 2: 155
  insomnia, 2: 207, 208
  intrinsic rhythms functions, 3: 395
  intrinsic rhythms interpretation, 3: 392
  IQ, 3: 414
  K-complex, 2: 201
  narcolepsy, 2: 206
  nightmares, 2: 209
  organic disorders, 3: 410
  psychosocial factors, 3: 415
  rocking, 2: 213, 214
  schizophrenia, 2: 550
  sensory deprivation, 2: 233, 237, 300
  sleep, 2: 194, 195, 196, 198, 199, 200, 206, 209, 211, 214, 270; 3: 391, 395
  sleep deprivation, 2: 294
  sleep-walking, 2: 210, 211
  telemetry, 3: 393
  theta band, 3: 392
  young children, 3: 391
Ego
  adaptation, 3: 302, 306
  development, 1: 237
  diffusion, 3: 544
  disorders, 1: 241; 3: 725
  feeling, 3: 543
  identity, 3: 302, 543
  integrity, 2: 470
  loss, 2: 469
  synthesis, 2: 468
  weakness, 1: 245
Egocentricity
  peptic ulcers, 3: 483
Ego psychology
  psychotic children, 3: 660

Eidetic imagery, 1: 179; 2: 268
Elderly
  memory disorders, 2: 124
Electra complex, 2: 156; 3: 293
Electric trauma, 3: 715
Electrocerebral activity
  in children, 3: 391
  conditioning, 2: 537
  evoked potentials, 2: 538
  spatial pattern, 2: 550
  synchronization of brain rhythms, 2: 537
Electrocerebral development
  psychosocial development, 3: 413
Emotion, 1: 214
Emotional adjustment (testing), 1: 226
Emotional changes
  hypnosis, 2: 162
  plasma cortisol levels, 2: 162
  schizophrenia, 2: 432, 433
Emotional deficiency diseases, 3: 174
  anaclitic depression, 3: 174
  hospitalism, 3: 175
Emotional disorders (see Neurosis)
Emotional health
  child, 3: 157
  newborn, 3: 158
Emotional stress
  foetal deaths, 3: 34
  malformations, 3: 29-36
  pregnancy, 3: 27-37
Empathy, 1: 171
Encephalitis, 1: 518; 2: 114, 120, 193; 3: 411
  contingent negative variation, 3: 411-413
  EEG, 3: 395
  herpetic, 3: 711
  infectious diseases, 3: 711, 712
  somnolence, 2: 212
Encephalitis lethargica, 3: 615
Encopresis, 1: 138, 167
Endocrine disorders, 3: 713
Engrams, 2: 266, 267, 273
Enuresis, 1: 245; 2: 212, 213; 3: 450, 451
  aetiology, 1: 44
  conditioning, 1: 113, 116, 163; 2: 212, 569
  kibbutz, 3: 342
  latent learning, 1: 167
Environment
  enriched, 2: 88, 89, 102, 103
  failure and schizophrenia, 2: 457; 3: 691
  manipulation in ulcerative colitis, 3: 521
  personality development, 2: 454
  temperament interaction, 3: 70
Ependymal cells, 2: 62, 64
Epidemiology
  clinical investigation, 3: 388
Epilepsy, 1: 461; 2: 114, 122, 141, 314, 321, 326, 327, 328, 336; 3: 712
  amnesia, 2: 116
  brain functional localization, 2: 323

SUBJECT INDEX

Epilepsy—cont.
  cerebral palsy, 1: 460
  cerebral responsiveness, 3: 406
  classification, 1: 462
  cortical excision, 2: 324
  and delinquency, 1: 384
  EEG, 1: 463; 2: 232; 3: 393
  grand mal, 1: 461; 3: 712
  institutional care (children), 3: 777
  and intelligence, 1: 464
  Klinefelter syndrome, 2: 42
  Korsakoff's syndrome, 2: 120
  myoclonic, 2: 199
  petit mal, 1: 461; 3: 396, 712
  photic activation, 3: 396
  and schizophrenia, 1: 478; 2: xxii, 434, 435
  sleepwalking, 3: 436
  social problems, 1: 470
  television, 3: 396
  toxoplasmosis, 3: 25
Epithelial phenomena
  hypnotic, 2: 179-186
Ethology, 1: 21
  definition, 1: 21
  function in psychiatry, 1: 24
  methods, 1: 21
  mother-infant relations, 3: 82
Evoked responses
  contingent amplification, 3: 399
  contingent attenuation, 3: 399
  contingent negative variation (q.v.)
  detection, 3: 396
  dispersive convergence, 3: 397
  electronic computation, 3: 397
  expectancy wave, 3: 399
  features, 3: 397
  frontal cortex, 3: 396
  habituation, 3: 399
  idiodromic projection, 3: 399
  modality signature, 3: 399
Existential analysis, 2: 488
  acting out, 2: 511, 512
  analysis of dasein, 2: 497
  anxiety, 2: 492, 493
  being-and-having, 2: 296
  being-in-the-world, 2: 498
  body-psyche dichotomy, 2: 501
  communication, 2: 497
  dasein, 2: 491-519
  dreams interpretation, 2: 512
  guilt, 2: 492, 493, 513, 514, 515
  hallucinations, 2: 507
  hysteria, 2: 503
  interpretation of symbols, 2: 509
  neurotic disorders, 2: 504
  pleasure principle, 2: 514
  psychiatry and, 2: 513
  psychoanalysis, 2: 499
  psychosomatics, 2: 502
  psychotherapy, 2: 508
  psychotic disorders, 2: 504
  schizophrenia, 2: 507
  subject-object dichotomy, 2: 495, 496
Existential philosophy, 2: 490
  historical development, 2: 491
Existentialism
  existential analysis (q.v.)
  historical development, 2: 491
  psychiatry and, 2: 513
  schizophrenia, 2: 410
Exogenous psychoses, 2: 441, 442
Exogenous trauma
  schizophrenia, 2: 410
Experimental approach
  clinical psychology, 2: 360
Experimentation
  design, 1: 6
  methods, 1: 9
Exploited child, 3: 579
  definition, 3: 579
  description, 3: 580
  parents, 3: 582
Extinction, 1: 157; 2: 378
  conditioning, 2: 546
  experimental, 2: 568
Eye
  abnormal movements, 1: 219
  movement in sleep, 2: 194, 196, 200, 209, 270

Facilitation, 2: 326, 348
Factor analysis, 1: 106
Family, 3: 125
  of accident-prone children, 1: 361
  aetiological importance (in neurosis), 1: 271
  anniversary reactions, 2: 653
  assessment, 2: 659
  Attitudes Test, 1: 577
  autistic children, 3: 646, 656
  casework, 1: 556
  community interaction, 2: 646
  definitions, 3: 133
  delinquency, 1: 385
  dimensional approach, 2: 644
  doctor, 1: 272; 2: 656, 686 (*see also* General Practitioner)
  dynamics, 2: 652; (in Japan) 3: 356-368
  extended, 3: 134
  genetical counselling, 1: 52-55
  of gifted children, 1: 201
  group diagnosis, 1: 277; 2: 659
  group properties, 2: 645
  group therapy, 1: 281; 2: 397, 641, 642, 663
  groups, 2: 638, 639
  kibbutz, 3: 322, 335
  material circumstances, 2: 645

SUBJECT INDEX

mental retardation, 1: 498, 509; 2: 648, 651
model, 2: 643
motivation, 2: 653
neurosis, 1: 271; 2: 648, 649, 650
nuclear, 3: 133, 134
patriarchy, 3: 137
patrilineal, 3: 137
patrilocal, 3: 137
patrinomal, 3: 137
polygamous, 3: 134, 135
psychiatry (*see* Family psychiatry)
psychogenic retardation, 3: 335, 538
psychosis, 2: 648, 650, 651
Relations Indicator, 1: 577; 2: 660; 3: 147
Relations Test, 1: 579
relationship, 2: 645
scapegoat, 2: 653
schizophrenia, 2: 641, 650, 666; 3: 664, 701
school child, 3: 745
social system, 2: 646
structure (in Japan), 3: 351
and suicide, 1: 422; 2: 653
symptomatology of dysfunctioning, 2: 648
therapy, 1: 279; 2: 661
vulnerability of member, 2: 652
Family doctor, 1: 272; 2: 656, 686 (*see also* General Practitioner)
Family dynamics
in Japan, 3: 356-368
schizophrenia, 2: 464, 465, 466
ulcerative colitis in children, 3: 498
Family psychiatry, 2: 637; 3: 127, 285
advantages, 2: 641
anniversary reactions, 2: 653
attention-giving symptoms, 2: 654
charts of relationships, 2: 660
communicated symptomatology, 2: 653
day hospital, 2: 668
definition, 1: 257; 2: 637
Department of, 1: 257; 2: 647
dyadic therapy, 2: 663
family dynamics, 2: 652
family group diagnosis, 2: 659; 3: 147, 148, 520
family group therapy, 2: 641, 642, 663
family model, 2: 643
family motivation, 2: 653
family psychotherapy, 2: 662
Family Relations Indicator, 1: 577; 2: 660; 3: 147
follow-up, 2: 662
group therapy, 2: 667
home therapy, 2: 668
individual psychotherapy, 2: 663
in-patient observation, 2: 661
Institute of, 2: 647
intake procedure, 2: 656
investigation, 2: 642, 658

manic-depressive psychosis, 2: 651
mental retardation, 2: 648, 651
neurosis, 2: 648, 649
organic psychosis, 2: 651
organization of services, 2: 652
physical methods, 2: 668
play diagnosis, 2: 660
play therapy, 2: 667
practice, 2: 647
presenting family member, 2: 652, 658
psychological procedures, 2: 660
psychopathology, 2: 391-424, 642, 648
psychosis, 2: 391-424, 648
questionnaires, 2: 660
records, 2: 661
referral service, 2: 642, 654
residential care, 2: 668
salutiferous society, 2: 672
selection of cases, 2: 657, 668
scapegoat, 2: 653
schizophrenia, 2: 391-424, 650, 666
symptomatology, 2: 642, 648
theoretical aspects, 2: 638
therapy, 2: 642, 661; 3: 286
vector therapy (q.v.)
vulnerability, 2: 652
Family psychopathology, 2: 642, 648-654
schizophrenia, 2: 391-424
Family Relations Indicator, 1: 577; 2: 660; 3: 147
Family schisms, 2: 402, 413
Family skews, 2: 402, 413
Family stresses
congenital disadvantage, 3: 43, 44
Fantasies
of early childhood, 3: 63
genesis, 3: 212
masturbatory, 3: 211
psychotic children, 3: 214
Father
absence, 3: 140
aetiology of schizophrenia, 3: 146
child development, 3: 141
in clinical practice, 3: 147
definitions, 3: 136
delinquency and, 3: 145
deprivation, 2: 464
dominance, 3: 363
incestuous, 3: 145
kibbutz, 3: 330
newborn child and, 3: 158
participation, 3: 143
peptic ulcers in children, 3: 490
primitive culture, 3: 293
psychosomatic disorders, 3: 145
relationship in schizophrenia, 2: 411
role, 3: 142
separation from, 3: 140, 145, 259-267, 274, 275
treatment and, 3: 146

850 SUBJECT INDEX

Fathering, **3:** 125-156
  Christian religion, **3:** 149
  in contemporary society, **3:** 138, 149
  cultural patterns, **3:** 137
  incidence by social class, **3:** 143
  national practices, **3:** 139
  neglect of (in child psychiatry), **3:** 150
  and psychiatry, **3:** 144
Fear
  in children, **3:** 381
Fecal play
  maternal depression and, **3:** 173
Feeblemindedness
  children, **3:** 611
Feedback, **2:** 242, 244; **3:** 237
Feeding
  anorexia, **1:** 114, 292, 324; **2:** 649; **3:** 713
  pattern in infants, **3:** 94
  problems, **3:** 167
Female sexuality
  psychoanalysis, **2:** 450
Fertility
  and schizophrenia, **2:** 11
Field of forces, **2:** 638, 642, 643
  vector therapy, **2:** 642
First encounter
  mother-infant, **3:** 89
Fixation, **3:** 235, 236
Fixed action pattern, **3:** 82
Flashback
  electrical recall, **2:** 337, 347
  experiential, **2:** 336, 337, 347
Flexibilitas cerea, **2:** 151, 157, 177
Flicker-fusion frequency, **2:** 163, 164
Flight
  confusion of stimuli, **1:** 26
  stimuli, **1:** 25, 26
Foetus
  hazards of, **3:** 19-56
  interaction with mother, **3:** 81
  motility and mother's emotional state, **3:** 83
Folie à deux, **2:** 654
Folklore
  baby's physical condition, **3:** 86
  infant's gender, **3:** 85
Follow-up studies, **3:** 785-803
  adoption, **1:** 443
  biased outcome, **3:** 802
  child psychiatry, **1:** 282, 531, 560; **3:** 785-803
  control group, **3:** 789
  co-operation, **3:** 801
  design, **3:** 787
  evaluation of therapy, **3:** 785
  family therapy, **2:** 662, 666
  Hampstead Clinic studies, **3:** 241
  identifying data, **3:** 793
  inclusion of subjects, **3:** 799
  index cases, **3:** 796
  interviews, **3:** 795
  locating subjects, **3:** 799
  natural history, **3:** 785
  post facto, **3:** 792
  problems, **3:** 797
  prospective, **3:** 792
  psychosomatic disorders, **1:** 331
  records, **3:** 793, 795
  sampling, **3:** 788
  stratification, **3:** 789
  study group, **3:** 787
  study population, **3:** 787
  time intervals, **3:** 797
  uses, **3:** 785
Forced choice techniques, **1:** 578
  Family Relations Test, **1:** 579
  Mooney Problem Check List, **1:** 579
Foster care, **3:** 288, 289
Foster parents, **3:** 129
Frigidity
  hypnosis, **2:** 178
  learning therapy, **2:** 567
Frontal cortex
  evoked responses, **3:** 396
Frontal lobes, **2:** 326
  planned initiative, **2:** 326
Frustration
  infant, **3:** 166
  peptic ulcers, **3:** 482
Fungi
  intoxication, **3:** 714

Galvanic skin response
  sensory deprivation, **2:** 233, 237, 300
  sleep deprivation, **2:** 293
Games (children)
  unconscious content, **3:** 215
Gargoylism, **1:** 507
Gastric mucosa
  peptic ulcer, **3:** 475
Gender
  folklore, **3:** 85
  prediction, **3:** 85
  role, **2:** 38
Gene activity
  and nerve function, **2:** 87, 88, 89
General Practitioner, **1:** 258, 269, 273, 276, 278, 310 (*see also* Family doctor)
Genes
  role in memory, **2:** 91
Genetic mosaicism, **2:** 22, 27, 28, 29
Genetics, **1:** 38
  biochemical, **1:** 45
  chromosomal abnormality (q.v.)
  cytogenetics, **1:** 46
  delinquency, **1:** 43, 380
  genetical counselling, **1:** 52
  history, **1:** 39
  Huntington's chorea, **1:** 53, 511, 514
  Mendelian principles, **1:** 52, 510

mental subnormality (q.v.)
mongolism (q.v.)
neurosis, **1**: 40
nuclear sexing (q.v.)
population studies, **1**: 42
research, **1**: 52
schizophrenia, **1**: 42, 481; **2**: 3-17, 38
special samples, **1**: 43
twin studies, **1**: 39, 380; **2**: 13
Geneva school of genetic psychology
  psychoanalysis, **3**: 176
Genius, **1**: 198
Geriatric psychiatry, **2**: 249
Germ cells, **2**: 30
Gesell's categories of embriological development, **3**: 654
Gesell Developmental Schedules, **1**: 566
Glial cell multiplication, **2**: 88
Gliosomes, **2**: 62
Glucose - 6 - phosphate dehydrogenase (G-6-PD), **2**: 28
Glycolysis, **2**: 54
Glycoprotein neuraminic acid, **2**: 16
Golgi complex, **2**: 53, 56, 60, 64, 66, 68, 69, 70, 72, 77, 78
Gonadal dysgenesis (*see* Turner's syndrome)
Griffiths Mental Development Scale, **1**: 566
Group, **2**: 638
  diagnosis (family), **1**: 277; **2**: 659
  family, **2**: 638, 639 (*see also* Family)
  identification, **3**: 328
  integration, in hospital, **2**: 718
  peer group, **3**: 326, 328
  perceptual relations, **3**: 327
  properties, **2**: 645
  relation, in hospital, **2**: 717
  social bond, **1**: 33
  solidarity, **3**: 329
  structure, **1**: 33
  therapy (q.v.)
Group hypnosis, **2**: 577
  development in USSR, **2**: 577
  group hypnotherapy (q.v.)
  theory, **2**: 579
  therapist's role, **2**: 581
Group hypnotherapy, **2**: 582
  degree of suggestibility, **2**: 586
  gynaecology, **2**: 593
  internal diseases, **2**: 593
  methodology of suggestion, **2**: 584
  neurological disorders, **2**: 593
  neuroses, **2**: 590
  organization in USSR, **2**: 592
  physiological foundation, **2**: 582
  reinforcement of suggestibility, **2**: 587
  shortcomings, **2**: 588
  suggestion and personality, **2**: 587
  symptom substitution, 2: 586
  unities of suggestion, 2: 585

Group therapy, **1**: 281, 540, 550; **2**: 397, 641, 642, 663, 667
  hypnotherapy (*see* Group hypnotherapy)
  psychoanalysis, **2**: 477
  theory, **2**: 579
  ulcerative colitis, **3**: 520
Growth cone
  cytologic features, **2**: 81
Guilt
  catharsis, **2**: 604
  existential analysis, **2**: 492, 493, 513, 514, 515
Gynaecomastia, **2**: 40
Gyrectomy, **2**: 327

Habituation, **2**: 96
Hallucinations, **2**: 265
  auditory, **2**: 272
  autohypnosis, **2**: 271
  autoscopy (*see* heautoscopy)
  chemically induced, **2**: 273
  in children, **3**: 726
  collective, **2**: 273
  cortical changes, **2**: 166, 167
  definitions, **2**: 230, 265
  existential analysis, **2**: 507
  experiential flashbacks, **2**: 336
  hallucinogens (q.v.)
  heautoscopy, **2**: 139, 271
  historical survey, **2**: 265
  hypnagogic, **1**: 178; **2**: 198, 199, 205, 209, 231, 269, 270
  hypnopompic, **1**: 179; **2**: 270
  hypnotic, **2**: 164-170, 271, 272
  mandala, **2**: 271
  monotony, **2**: 272
  negative, **2**: 165
  phantom limb, **2**: 272
  positive, **2**: 165
  related conditions, **2**: 269
  schizophrenic, **1**: 481; **2**: 283, 430, 431
  sensory deprivation, **2**: 228, 229, 230, 245, 271, 280
  sensory input (q.v.)
  sleep deprivation, **2**: 203, 291
  specular, **2**: 139
  theory, **2**: 266
  visual, **2**: 272
  yantra, **2**: 271
Hallucinogens, **2**: 15, 266, 273-283, 622, 623, 626
  adrenochrome, **2**: 281
  amphetamines, **2**: 280
  animal behaviour, **2**: 277
  cannabinols, **2**: 281
  clinical use, **2**: 282
  electrophysiological changes, **2**: 274
  indole alkaloids, **2**: 278
  LSD, **2**: 274, 275, 276, 278, 279, 281, 282
  marihuana, **2**: 274, 281, 282

Hallucinogens—cont.
  mechanism of action, 2: 275, 276
  mescaline, 2: 15, 275, 276, 280
  peyotism, 2: 281
  phenylethylamines, 2: 280
  piperidine derivatives, 2: 279
  psilocybin, 2: 274, 275, 278
  psycho-social aspects, 2: 281
Hallucinosis, 2: 425
  in children, 3: 727
  schizophrenic, 2: 430, 433, 437, 439
Hampstead Child Therapy Clinic, 3: 200-250
  adolescents in treatment, 3: 227
  blind children nursery group, 3: 224
  blind children's development, 3: 227, 236-238
  borderline children, 3: 228, 238
  clinical concept research, 3: 227
  clinical services, 3: 223
  community education, 3: 229
  delinquency, 3: 228
  historical development, 3: 221
  index of case material, 3: 225-227, 245-250
  nursery school, 3: 224
  parents and children simultaneous analysis, 3: 229, 244
  play group for toddlers and mothers, 3: 225
  prevention and education, 3: 224
  profile research, 3: 225
  psychotherapy research, 2: 476
  psychotic children, 3: 228, 238
  publications, 3: 230-250
  referral, 3: 222
  research project and study, 3: 225
  selection of cases, 3: 222
  staff, 3: 223
  support from research foundations, 3: 223
  technical problems, 3: 244
  well-baby clinic, 3: 225, 241
Hand dominance, 2: 328
  protein metabolism, 2: 101
  RNA changes, 2: 92, 93
  speech, 1: 346
Handicapped children
  co-operation, 1: 213
  development, 1: 210
  developmental scales, 1: 224
  emotion, 1: 214
  emotional adjustment, 1: 226
  Hampstead Clinic studies, 3: 239
  institutional care, 3: 768
  intelligence tests, 1: 572
  orthopaedically, 1: 222
  perception, 1: 217
  relationships, 1: 211
  speech and language, 1: 231

  total care, 1: 231
  verbal communication, 1: 212
Handling of infants
  quality, 3: 95
Hartnup disease, 3: 715
Hashish
  intoxication, 3: 715
Hayfever
  hypnosis, 2: 182, 184
Headache, 1: 245
Head banging, 2: 213; 3: 163, 236
Head injury, 2: 321
  amnesia, 2: 115, 116, 120, 125
Health promotion, 1: 282; 2: 672
Hearing
  development of blind child, 3: 237
Heat stroke, 3: 715
Hebephrenia, 2: 425, 432, 439; 3: 592, 594, 652
Heller's syndrome (see Dementia infantilis)
Hemianaesthesia, 2: 135
Hemihypaesthesia, 2: 141
Hemiparesis, 2: 141, 144
Hemiplegia, 1: 217, 340, 341; 2: 144
  corporeal image, 2: 135, 140
Hepatic disorders
  psychotic manifestation, 3: 713
Heredity, 2: 3 (see also Genetics)
Hermaphroditic children, 2: 36
  gender role, 2: 36
Heteropycnosis
  in X chromosomes, 2: 25
Higher nervous activity, 2: 533, 554
  conditioned brain activity, 2: 534
  conditioned reflex, 2: 534
  cortical activity, 2: 534
  inhibition, 2: 533
  subcortical structure, 2: 534
Hippocampal lesions
  amnesia, 2: 118, 127
Histidinaemia, 2: 14
History
  child psychiatry, 1: 251; 3: 1-15, 375
  hypnosis, 2: 147
  social, 1: 263, 276
Homicide
  primitive society, 2: 704
  sleep walking, 2: 211
Homosexuality
  in adolescents, 1: 294; 3: 239
  chromosomes, 1: 51
  conditioning, 1: 162; 2: 568
  cultural aspects, 2: 702
  in delinquency, 1: 387
  role identity, 3: 146
Hospital
  accident records, 1: 353
  admission of adolescents, 1: 300
  child-parent separation, 3: 270
  discharge of adolescents, 1: 303

hospitalization (q.v.)
in-patient units (q.v.)
  psychiatric (see Psychiatric hospital)
  reaction to admission, **1:** 80, 81
  records, **1:** 276
  reports, **1:** 278
  sensory deprivation in, **2:** 248
Hospitalism, **3:** 175, 209, 659
Hospitalization, **1:** 86, 126, 200, 214
  babies, **1:** 220; **3:** 9
  children, **1:** 534
  mental patient, **2:** 715
  sensory deprivation, **2:** 248
Humphrey paradox, **2:** 378
Huntington's chorea, **1:** 511, 514; **2:** 7, 14
  genetics, **1:** 53
Hurler's disease, **1:** 507
Hydantoinate, **3:** 715
Hydrochloric acid, **3:** 475
Hydrocephalus
  toxoplasmosis, **3:** 24
Hydrohypodynamic environment, **2:** 226
Hyperemesis, **3:** 45, 47
Hypertelorism, **3:** 33
Hyperthymic child, **3:** 174
Hypno-analysis, **2:** 165
Hypnosis, **2:** xxi, 146
  in animals, **2:** 147, 148
  athletic training, **2:** 178
  autohypnosis, **2:** 271
  classification of phenomena, **2:** 154-186
  collective (see Group hypnosis)
  definition, **2:** 146, 147, 151
  experimental, **2:** 152
  form of suggestion, **2:** 153
  group (see Group hypnosis)
  history, **2:** 147
  induction, **2:** 149, 152
  learning, **2:** 157
  monotony, **2:** 272
  phylogeny, **2:** 150
  physiological phenomena. **2:** 154, 155, 157, 158, 159, 160, 172-186
  psychoanalysis, **2:** 477
  psychological phenomena, **2:** 154, 155, 156, 157, 161-172
  rapport, **2:** 156
  semantics, **2:** 174
  simultaneous, **2:** 582
  suggestibility, **2:** 585, 586, 587
  symptom substitution, **2:** 586
  trance depth, **2:** 152
Hypnotic drugs, **2:** 215
  memory and, **2:** 109
  prescription statistics, **2:** 207
Hypochondriasis, **2:** 520, 521, 523
Hypothermia
  memory after, **2:** 109
  psychosymptomatology, **3:** 715

Hypotheses
  refutation, **1:** 8
  research, **1:** 8
  selection, **1:** 9
  verification, **1:** 8
Hypoxic encephalopathy, **2:** 114
Hysteresis, **2:** 171
Hysteria, **2:** xxv, 149, 150
  Anna O.'s case, **3:** 293
  conversion symptoms, **2:** 172; **3:** 14; (in adolescents) **1:** 292
  cultural distribution, **2:** 702; **3:** 14
  cultural symptomatology, **2:** 704
  Dora's case, **3:** 293
  existential analysis, **2:** 503
  and psychosis, **1:** 484
  stammer, **1:** 347
  suggestibility test, **2:** 374
  treatment, **2:** 366
Hysterical mutism, **1:** 348

Ideation
  content, **3:** 246
  irrational, **2:** 402
Identification
  sexual, **3:** 303
  social, **3:** 303
Identified patient (see Presenting patient)
Identity
  in schizophrenia, **2:** 398, 402
  sexual, **3:** 315
  social, **3:** 315
Identity concept, **1:** 246
Idioglossia, **1:** 348
Ileostomy, **3:** 507
  clubs, **3:** 520
Illegitimacy
  culture, **3:** 308
  malformations, **3:** 33, 36
  perinatal deaths, **3:** 34, 36
  prematurity, 3, 34
Illusions, **2:** 335, 336
  déjà vu, **1:** 178; **2:** 335
  sleep deprivation, **2:** 203
Imagery, **1:** 172
  body image (q.v.)
  emotive, **2:** 565
  déjà vu, **1:** 178; **2:** 335
  hypnagogic, **1:** 178; **2:** 198, 199, 205, 209, 231, 269, 270
  imaginary companion, **1:** 180
  predominant, **1:** 173
  range, **1:** 174
  strength, **1:** 174
Imagination, **1:** 170
  abstract thinking, **1:** 77
  development, **1:** 68
Immaturity
  schizophrenia, **2:** 394, 413

SUBJECT INDEX

Immigrants
  mental disorders, 2: 703
Immobilization
  sensory deprivation, 2: 248
Impotence
  hypnosis, 2: 178
  learning therapy, 2: 567
Imprinting, 1: 34; 3: 82
  critical period, 3: 82
  gender role, 2: 36
Inborn reflexes, 2: 322
Incestuous preoccupation, 2: 402
Incisures of Schmidt-Lantermann, 2: 58
Indicating patient (*see* Presenting patient)
Individuality
  temperamental, 3: 68
Indole alkaloids, 2: 278
  bufotenine, 2: 278
  harmine, 2: 278
  LSD, 2: 278 (*see also* LSD)
  piperidine derivatives, 2: 279
  psilocin, 2: 278
  tryptamine derivatives, 2: 278
Indole alkylamines, 2: 276
Industry
  psychoanalysis, 2: 477
  vocational guidance, 1: 581
Infant (*see also* Child *and* Toddler)
  ability to love, 3: 168
  abstract intelligence, 3: 168
  anaclitic depression (q.v.)
  anger, 3: 166
  anticipatory excitement, 3: 163
  anxiety, 3: 166
  asthma, 3: 167
  auto-erotic practices, 3: 167
  autonomy, 3: 164
  awareness, 3: 167
  capacity for attention, 3: 167
  coma, 3: 170
  communication, 3: 166
  coprophagia, 3: 173
  dependency, 3: 164
  disturbances of elimination, 3: 167
  eating problems, 3: 167
  eczema, 2: 459; 3: 171, 172
  elimination, 3: 162, 164
  emotional deficiency diseases, 3: 174
  emotional needs, 3: 164
  fears, 3: 166
  fecal play, 3: 173
  finger sucking, 3: 165
  frustration, 3: 166
  functional regression, 3: 163
  growth of trust, 3: 166
  head banging, 3: 163
  hyperthymic, 3: 174
  illegitimacy, 3: 34
  lalling, 3: 166
  maternal stress in pregnancy, 3: 30
  memories, 3: 166
  play with genitals, 3: 165
  premental behaviour, 3: 163
  psyche organizers, 3: 168
  psychotoxic diseases, 3: 170, 171
  retarded in speech, 3: 167
  rocking, 3: 163, 172
  selfishness, 3: 164
  self-reliance, 3: 164
  separation from mother, 3: 174
  smile, 3: 94
  speech, 3: 166
  Spitz's studies, 3: 168
  sucking, 3: 163
  tantrums, 3: 166
  three months colic, 3: 171
  toilet training, 3: 164
  word building, 3: 166
Infant Welfare Clinics, 1: 274
Infantile ill-health
  pregnancy stress, 3: 39-41
Infantile psychoses, 2: 2 (*see also* Childhood psychoses)
  classification, 2: 2
  childhood schizophrenia (q.v.)
  dementia infantilis (q.v.)
  dementia praecocissima (q.v.)
Infections,
  in acute organic psychosis, 3: 711
  encephalitis, 3: 712
  in pregnancy 1: 515, 3: 20-27
Influenza (Asian)
  effect on pregnancy, 3: 21, 22
Information
  genetic, 2: 110
  input, 2: 268
  negative entropy, 2: 187
  retrieval, 2: 50
  storage, 2: 50, 109
  theory, 2: 169
Inhibition
  active, 2: 533
  conditioned, 1: 114; 2: 559
  learning, 2: 97-100
  memory, 2: 97-100
  passive, 2: 533
  protective, 2: 150
  reactive, 2: 295, 296
  reciprocal, 1: 114, 128; 2: 559, 560
Initiation rites, 3: 316
Innate releaser mechanism, 3: 82
In-patient units, 1: 215, 264, 534 (*see also* Hospital *and* Residential care)
  adolescents, 1: 265, 297, 301
  case work with families, 1: 556
  children, 1: 534; 3: 289
  day hospitals, 1: 560
  functions, 1: 535
  group therapy, 1: 550
  house-mothers, 1: 548

SUBJECT INDEX

individual therapy, **1**: 552
psychotic children, **1**: 492, 537
school, **1**: 540, 549, 559, 560
speech defects, **1**: 338
staffing, **1**: 266, 539, 540
therapy, **1**: 539
type and character, **1**: 538
visiting, **1**: 556
ward routine, **1**: 539
Insomnia, **2**: 207
  autonomous melancholia, **2**: 208
  electroencephalogram, **2**: 208
  hallucinations, **2**: 271
  hypnotic drugs, **2**: 207, 214, 215
  hypomania, **2**: 207
  in infancy, **3**: 420-422
  sleep walking, **3**: 430-440
Instinct
  maternal, **3**: 92
Insulin therapy, **1**: 492; **2**: xxii, xxiii
Intellectual stimulation
  lack of, **3**: 532
Intelligence
  alpha rhythm, **3**: 414
  changes, **1**: 216
  childhood thinking, **1**: 184
  creativity, **1**: 186
  delinquency, **1**: 374, 381
  epilepsy, **1**: 464, 470
  family background, **1**: 201, 574
  genius, **1**: 198
  mental health, **1**: 205
  mental subnormality (q.v.)
  Piaget's theory, **1**: 58
  reasoning, **1**: 203
  reliability of assessment, **1**: 196, 571
  school achievement, **3**: 745
  sensory deprivation, **2**: 239
  superior, **1**: 192
  tests, **1**: 185, 193, 562, 565; diagnostic use, **1**: 571
  Turner's syndrome, **2**: 34
  underfunctioning, **1**: 207
Interpersonal Perception Method, **2**: 410
Interview
  structured, **3**: 63
Intracranial tumours, **2**: 114, 120
Intrauterine environment (*see* Prenatal influences)
Introspection, **2**: 340
IQ (*see* Intelligence)
Isolation
  child, **3**: 105
  sensory (*see* Sensory isolation)
  socio-cultural, **2**: 402, 413

Japan
  childbirth tradition, **3**: 93
  contemporary family, **3**: 359
  culture, **3**: 350

eldest son, **3**: 350
family dynamics, **3**: 356-368
family structure, **3**: 351
marriage, **3**: 350
parental attitudes, **3**: 347-368
post-war family, **3**: 365
pre-war family, **3**: 362
roles, **3**: 350
social status, **3**: 350
Westernization, **3**: 351
Josiah Macy Jr. Foundation, **3**: 8
Juvenile courts, **3**: 4

Kalmuck idiocy, **3**: 3
Kandinsky-Clerambault syndrome, **2**: 429, 431, 437, 439, 442
  age of onset, **3**: 382
Karyotype, **1**: 48; **2**: 24
Kernicterus, **1**: 518
Kitsunetsuki, **2**: 705
Kibbutz, **3**: 209
  adolescents, **3**: 336-339
  aggression, **3**: 329, 338
  autoerotic activities, **3**: 329
  child care, **3**: 136
  child and community, **3**: 331
  child and parents, **3**: 330
  child rearing, **3**: 321
  collective child care, **3**: 323
  community, **3**: 321
  conforming, **3**: 329, 341
  criticism, **3**: 338
  dependency, **3**: 329
  differentiation of sexes, **3**: 329
  discontinuous mothering, **3**: 343
  disturbance of behaviour, **3**: 342
  education, **3**: 322, 325, 334-336, 339
  family, **3**: 322, 335
  familistic trends, **3**: 332
  father, **3**: 330
  group identification, **3**: 329
  group living, **3**: 344
  group pressure, **3**: 329
  group solidarity, **3**: 329
  higher education, **3**: 339
  intermittent mothering, **3**: 340
  liberation of women, **3**: 335
  marriage, **3**: 322
  maternal deprivation, **3**: 340
  mental health planning, **3**: 344
  metapelet, **3**: 323-326
  mothers, **3**: 330, 334, 340, 343, 344
  multiple mothering, **3**: 340
  Oedipus complex, **3**: 329, 341, 343, 344
  peer group, **3**: 326
  research, **3**: 339
  sibling rivalry, **3**: 329
  socialization, **3**: 325
  training, **3**: 325

SUBJECT INDEX

Klinefelter's syndrome, **1**: 50, 513; **2**: 17, 27, 39-43
  buccal smear, **2**: 40, 41
  delinquency, **2**: 42
  EEG, **2**: 42
  maternal age, **2**: 30
  mental retardation, **2**: 41, 43
  psychosexuality, **2**: 41, 42
  testicular hystopathology, **2**: 40
  transvestism, **2**: 42
Koro, **2**: 705, 706
Korsakoff's syndrome, **2**: 113, 114, 118, 442
  aetiology, **2**: 120
  clinical features, **2**: 120
  nature, **2**: 121
  pathology, **2**: 120

Labour
  complicated delivery, **3**: 88
  dependence in, **3**: 87
  events during, **3**: 86
  general anaesthesia and paranoid ideation, **3**: 88
  mother's concerns before, **3**: 85
  mother's psychological transformation, **3**: 86
  passivity, **3**: 87
  second stage, **3**: 88
  shift of relationships, **3**: 85
  verbal interchange, **3**: 87
Lactic acid, **2**: 16
Lalling, **1**: 348; **3**: 166, 207
Langdon Down's disease (*see* Mongolism)
Language, **1**: 336 (*see also* Speech)
  development, **1**: 94, 336
  early infantile autism, **3**: 656
  learning, **2**: 329, 334
  psychogenic retardation, **3**: 537
  schizophrenic children, **3**: 671
  stammer, **1**: 114, 136, 343, 345; **2**: 171
  stutter, **1**: 136, 345
  vocabulary, **1**: 204
Latah, **2**: 705
Latency period
  needs of child, **3**: 195
La Verrière, **2**: 714, 719-727
Lead poison, **3**: 714
  brain damage, **1**: 519
Learning, **2**: 108, 376 (*see also* Memory *and* Conditioning)
  conditioned reflex, **2**: 347
  consolidation period, **2**: 380
  difficulties, **1**: 82, 458
  drugs effect, **2**: 93
  educational attainment tests, **1**: 580
  emotional, **2**: 561
  encoding in CNS, **2**: 380
  experiments, **2**: 89
  facilitation, **2**: 326, 348
  hypnotic, **2**: 157
  inhibition, **2**: 97-100
  latent, **1**: 164
  maturation, **1**: 85
  perceptual, **3**: 531
  Piaget's theory, **1**: 59, 80
  placebo, **2**: 603, 607
  protein formation, **2**: 101
  psychogenic retardation, **3**: 537
  role of chemical processes, **2**: 89
  schizophrenics, **2**: 380, 381
  sensory deprivation, **2**: 240
  sleep, **2**: 199
  sleep deprivation, **2**: 291
  studies on, **2**: 92
  theory (*see* Learning theory)
  therapy, **1**: 154, 155; **2**: 557
  uncommitted cortex programming, **2**: 326, 340
  visual, **2**: 111
Learning theorists, **3**: 81
Learning theory, **1**: 104; **2**: 377
  child development, **3**: 62
  clinical application, **1**: 113; **2**: 557
  conditioned inhibition, **1**: 114
  conditioning (q.v.)
  conduct problems, **1**: 106
  desensitisation, **1**: 114
  enuresis, treatment of, **1**: 113, 116, 163: **2**: 212, 569
  generalization of responses, **1**: 142
  intermittent reinforcement, **1**: 141
  modification of conduct, **1**: 378
  negative practice, **1**: 114
  operant conditioning, **1**: 105, 134; **2**: 569
  personality problems, **1**: 106
  phobias, **1**: 118
  reciprocal inhibition, **1**: 128; **2**: 560
  school phobia, **1**: 130
  shaping, **1**: 143
  social reinforcement, **1**: 139
  tics, **1**: 115; **2**: 377
Leucotomy, **2**: xxiii, 327
  dreaming, **2**: 200
Light stimulation, **2**: 89
Limbic system, **2**: 202
Lipochondrodystrophy, **1**: 507
Local Authorities clinics, **1**; 256
Logical Types, **2**: 404
Lying, **1**: 179, 525
Lyon hypothesis, **2**: 22, 25, 27, 38
LSD (lysergic acid diethylamide) **2**: 266, 273, 274, 275, 278
  antidotes, **2**: 279
  body image, **2**: 141
  chromosomal changes, **2**: 279
  clinical use, **2**: 282
  comparison with Sernyl, **2**: 302
  intoxication, **3**: 715
  model psychoses, **2**: 279, 301
  psychopathological reactions, **2**: 279

SUBJECT INDEX

psycho-social aspects, 2: 282
serotonin interaction, 2: 276
Lysergic acid diethylamide (*see* LSD)
Lysosome, 2: 57

Macroglia, 2: 62
Macrosomatognosia, 2: 140
Magnetism, 2: 147, 148
Malaria therapy, 3: 613
Mal de mère, 3: 71
Malformations, 3: 20-45, 52
    illegitimacy, 3: 33
    prenatal influences, 3: 20-46, 51, 52
Mandala, 2: 271
Mania, 2: 425
    chronic, 2: 439
    insomnia, 2: 208
    schizophrenic, 2: 430, 431
Manic-depressive psychosis, 2: 6, 439, 440, 444
    in childhood, 3: 652
    cyclothymia, 2: 439
    family, 2: 651
    personality development, 2: 451
    psychoanalysis, 2: 448
Manifest patient (*see* Presenting patient)
Marihuana, 2: 274, 281
Marriage
    of cousins and schizophrenia, 2: 11
    Japanese culture, 3: 350
    kibbutz, 3: 322
    monogamy, 3: 135
    plural, 3: 135
    polyandry, 3: 135
    polygyny, 3: 135
    trial, 3: 299
Marital schism, 3: 363, 364
Marital skew, 3: 363
Masturbation, 3: 236
    fantasies, 3: 211
    infantile, 3: 429
    sleep disorders, 3: 429, 436, 438
Maternal age
    and chromosomal abnormality, 1: 47, 49, 511; 2: 30; 3: 27
Maternal behaviour, 3: 82
Maternal deprivation, 1: 215, 243, 244; 2: 299; 3: 138, 201, 209
    childhood psychoses, 3: 659
    definition, 3: 254
    Harlow's experiments, 1: 35; 2: 249, 299, 449, 457; 3: 210, 284, 300, 314, 315, 659
    kibbutz, 3: 340
    pica, 3: 465, 468
    psychoanalysis, 2: 450, 456, 457, 458
    psychogenic retardation, 3: 536
    reversibility of effects, 1: 216
    and separation, 3: 254-289
    transmission theory, 1: 243

Maternal dominance, 3: 363
Maternal instinct, 3: 81
Maternal overprotection
    peptic ulcers, 3: 485, 488
Matriarchy
    child rearing, 3: 307
Maximow chamber, 2: 73-76
Maze-learning
    sedatives during pregnancy, 3: 52
Measles
    in pregnancy, 3: 23
Medical progress
    and war, 2: xx
Meiosis, 2: 30
Melancholia, 2: 425
Memory, 2: 87-107, 108-128, 267, 268
    (*see also* Learning)
    amnesia (q.v.)
    amphetamine, 2: 624, 625, 634
    anatomy, 2: 112
    antibody formation, analogy, 2: 90, 91
    autistic children, 3: 640
    brain lesions, 2: 113
    'cannibalism' experiment, 2: 95
    chemical processes, 2: 87
    child, 3: 185
    consciousness, 2: 346
    development, 1: 67
    disorders in the elderly, 2: 124
    electroconvulsive shock, 2: 99, 109
    fundamental nature, 2: 109
    genes' role, 2: 91
    head injury, 2: 115, 116
    immunological, 2: 110
    inhibition, 2: 97-100
    interpretive cortex, 2: 339, 347
    long-term, 2: 89, 98, 99, 101
    meaning of, 2: 108
    molecular basis, 2: 68, 87, 90
    molecular storage, 2: 110
    neurology of, 2: 125
    neuronal record, 2: 346
    short term, 2: 99
    specific defects, 2: 124
    storage, 2: 110, 126, 127
    studies on, 2: 92
    topographical, 2: 124
    transfer by proteins, 2: 96, 97, 103
    transfer by RNA, 2: 94, 95, 96, 103
    Wechsler Memory Scale, 2: 119
Meningiomas, 2: 81, 82, 83
Meningitis, 1: 518; 2: 114
    amnesia, 2: 116
    meningococcal, 3: 711
    tubercular, 3: 711
Menninger Study
    psychoanalytic therapy, 2: 449, 450, 471, 476
Mental deficiency (*see* Mental subnormality)

Mental disease
  cultural epidemiology, 3: 314
  dimensional system of classification, 2: 365
Mental health, 1: 205
Mental hospital (see Psychiatric hospital)
Mental illness (general)
  and culture (see Transcultural psychiatry)
  compensation processes, 3: 385
  correction of disorders, 3: 385
  cultural relativity, 3: 294
  cultural symptomatology, 2: 703
  definition, 2: 698
  development, 3: 386
  endogenous, 2: 7
  methods of investigation, 3: 387
  immigrants, 2: 703
  migration, 2: 703
  polimorphism, 3: 387
  in primitive cultures, 2: 700
  relative frequency, 2: 701
  total frequency, 2: 700
Mental retardation (see Mental subnormality)
Mental set, 2: 272
Mental subnormality, 1: 496; 3: 532
  aetiology, 1: 496, 503
  Alpert's syndrome, 1: 511
  carbon monoxide poison. 1: 519
  and childhood schizophrenia, 3: 13
  chromosomes anomalies, 1: 49, 50, 52, 504, 512; 2: 34, 37, 38, 39, 41, 43
  development of handicapped children, 1: 210
  diagnosis, 1: 224
  direct transmission, 1: 510
  disturbed behaviour, 3: 42
  encephalitis, 1: 518
  environmental factors, 1: 513; 3: 532
  errors of metabolism, 1: 46, 504, 505; 2: 14
  family, 2: 648, 651
  genetical counselling, 1: 52
  historical contributions, 3: 3
  hospital surveys, 1: 501
  Huntington's chorea, 1: 511
  infection during pregnancy, 1: 515
  intra-uterine influences, 1: 514
  kernicterus, 1: 518
  lead poisoning, 1: 519
  lipid metabolism, 1: 507
  maternal pregnancy, 3: 26, 37, 38
  meningitis, 1: 518
  mongolism, 1: 47, 511, 512
  perinatal factors, 1: 516
  phenylketonuria, 1: 505
  Piaget's theory, 1: 82
  prevention, 1: 519
  protophrenia, 3: 532
  pseudo, 2: 651

  residential care (children), 3: 774, 776
  schools, 3: 774, 776
  sensory deprivation, 2: 249
  severe, 3: 532
  social factors, 1: 497
  specific post-natal factors, 1: 517
  speech defects, 1: 338
  speech development, 3: 555
  temperament, 3: 74
  timing of insult, 1: 514
  Turner's syndrome, 2: 34
Meprobamate
  as teratogen, 3: 52
Merrill-Palmer Scale, 1: 567
Mescaline, 2: 15, 275, 276, 280
  body image, 2: 141
  peyotism, 2: 280
Mesencephalon, 2: 318
Metabolism
  disorders of, 3: 713
  glutamic acid, 2: 626
  inborn errors, 1: 45
  mental subnormality, 1: 46, 504, 505
  phenylketonuria (q.v.)
  porphyrins, 2: 626
  schizophrenia, 2: 14, 626, 627
Metachromatic leucodystrophy, 2: 82, 83
Metapelet, 3: 323, 324, 340
  functions, 3: 325
  training, 3: 326
Metapsychology, 3: 233
Methodology of research, 1: 3
  classification, 1: 7
  comparative, 1: 13
  cross-sectional, 1: 12
  evolutionary, 1: 12
  genetic, 1: 12
  longitudinal, 1: 13
  Mill's Canons, 1: 10
  retrospective, 1: 13
  statistical, 1: 14
  validation, 1: 17
Microglia, 2: 62, 64, 65
Migraine, 1: 325; 3: 710
  body image, 2: 141
Migration
  psychological effects, 2: 703
Mill's Canons, 1: 10
Mind (see also Thought)
  brain mechanism, 2: 340
  conditioned reflex (q.v.)
  duality of approach, 2: 341
Ministry of Education, 1: 255
Misoplegia, 2: 144
Mitochondria, 2: 56, 57
Model psychoses, 2: 274, 288
  LSD, 2: 279, 289
  psychotomimetic drugs, 2: 301
  schizophrenia, 2: 288, 289, 301

SUBJECT INDEX

sensory isolation, **2:** 289
Sernyl, **2:** 280, 289, 302, 303, 306
sleep deprivation, **2:** 289
Mongolism (Down's disease), **1:** 47, 511, 512; **2:** 24; **3:** 4, 54
  birth order, **3:** 27
  chromosomal anomalies, **1:** 47; **3:** 47, 51
  genetic counselling, **1:** 54
  maternal age, **1:** 47, 49, 511; **2:** 30; **3:** 27
  maternal factors, **3:** 22, 27
  pregnancy stresses, **3:** 47-50
Monoamine oxidase inhibitors, **2:** 276
Monogamy
  incidence, **3:** 135
Monotony, **2:** 198, 272
  child-care institutions, **3:** 767
Mooney Problem Check List, **1:** 579
Moral insanity, **3:** 597
Morita's theory, **2:** 519
  aetiology of nervosity, **2:** 520
  obsession, **2:** 525
  phobia, **2:** 525
  psychoanalysis, **2:** 522
  symptomatology of nervosity, **2:** 520, 524, 525
  therapy (*see* Morita therapy)
Morita therapy, **2:** 526, 707
  principle, **2:** 526
  results, **2:** 528
  recovery, **2:** 528
  stages, **2:** 526
Mortality
  perinatal and illegitimacy, **3:** 34, 36
  perinatal in zoo mammals, **3:** 90
  ulcerative colitis (in children), **3:** 496, 508
Mosaicism, **2:** 22, 27, 28, 29
Mossy cells, **2:** 62
Mother
  autonomy, **3:** 91
  biological function, **3:** 125
  emotional state of and foetal motility, **3:** 83
  inadequacy, **3:** 94
  interaction with child, **3:** 99-121
  kibbutz, **3:** 330, 334, 340, 343, 344
  narcissistic, **3:** 103
  newborn child and, **3:** 159
  ritual support of, **3:** 93
Mother-child interaction, **3:** 99-121
  at age one, **3:** 106
  areas, **3:** 113
  beginning and end, **3:** 106
  case studies, **3:** 100-106
  content, **3:** 108
  emotional content and child's development, **3:** 115-120
  emotional content of relationship, **3:** 113
  evolution of pattern, **3:** 114
  form, **3:** 107
  frustration, **3:** 105
  intensity and quality of investment, **3:** 113
  maturity level, **3:** 113
  modes, **3:** 108
  mutual pleasure, **3:** 115
  quantity of, **3:** 106
  in relation to closeness/distance, **3:** 112
  in relation to space, **3:** 111
  and relationship, **3:** 111
  tone, **3:** 108
Mother-child relationship, **1:** 35; **2:** 455, 456, 457; **3:** 80-121
  asthma, **3:** 473
  congenital differences, **3:** 95
  conversation with baby, **3:** 91
  emotional content, **3:** 115
  evolution of interaction, **3:** 89
  first interaction after birth, **3:** 88
  hostility, **3:** 171
  improper, **3:** 170
  infant's contribution, **3:** 93
  infantile eczema, **3:** 171
  infantile sleep disturbances, **3:** 423
  insufficient, **3:** 170
  and interaction, **3:** 111
  in Japan, **3:** 352
  maternal deprivation (q.v.)
  newborn coma, **3:** 170
  peptic ulcers, **3:** 473, 478, 481
  quality, **3:** 92
  rejection, **2:** 411; **3:** 170
  schizophrenia, **2:** 394, 395, 411
  somatic reciprocation, **2:** 396
  species-specific structures, **3:** 82
  studies in, **3:** 81
  symbiotic, **2:** 397, 409, 411
  symbiotic psychosis, **3:** 658
  three months colic, **3:** 171
  transactional aspects, **3:** 92
  ulcerative colitis, **3:** 497
Mothering, **3:** 125, 256
  discontinuous, **3:** 343
  Hampstead Clinic studies, **3:** 241
  inadequate, **3:** 299
  intermittent, **3:** 340
  multiple, **3:** 129, 340, 344
Mother surrogate, **1:** 35
Motivation
  animal, **1:** 32
  family, **2:** 653
Motor apparatus, **2:** 315
  cerebral palsied children, **1:** 218, 219, 222, 225, 460
  conscious control, **2:** 321, 345
  motor sequence, **2:** 318
  motor skills, **2:** 345
  primary sensory areas, **2:** 318
  voluntary movement, **2:** 318, 319

Motor disorder
  institutional care, 3: 769
Motor reaction
  conditioning, 2: 535, 539
Mutuality, 2: 398
Myelin formation, 2: 57
Mystification, 2: 410, 413, 466

Narcissism, 2: 141, 142, 464; 3: 204
Narco-analysis, 2: 624
Narcolepsy, 2: 205
  paranoid symptoms, 2: 205
Narcotics (*see also* Hypnotic drugs)
  memory after, 2: 109
National character, 3: 298
National Committee for Mental Hygiene, 3: 6
Nativists, 3: 81
Negative practice, 1: 114; 2: 568
Negativism, 1: 321, 483
Neglected child, 3: 355, 575
  definition, 3: 575
  description, 3: 575
  parents, 3: 577
Neonate's three primary hungers, 3: 161
Neophrenia, 3: 652
Nerve function
  and gene activity, 2: 87, 88, 89
Nervosity, 2: 519 (*see also* Morita's theory)
  aetiology, 2: 520
  differential diagnosis, 2: 523
  symptomatology, 2: 520, 524, 525
Nervous tissue
  protein formation, 2: 100
Nervous tissues in culture
  dynamic studies, 2: 73
  maintaining methods, 2: 73
Neurasthenia, 2: 520; 3: 606
Neuroblasts, 2: 79
Neurocytology, 2: 50
Neurofilaments, 2: 56, 57
Neuroglia, 2: 50
  activity, 2: 80
  contingent negative variations, 3: 401
  cytology, 2: 61
Neuroleptanalgesy, 2: 624
Neurological impairment, 1: 239, 339 (*see also* Brain damage)
  ataxias of articulation, 1: 342
  bilateral athetosis, 1: 342
  congenital cerebral diplegia, 1: 340
  congenital hemiplegia, 1: 341
  congenital suprabulbar paresis, 1: 340
  and delinquency, 1: 383
  double hemiplegia, 1: 341
  hemiplegia, 1: 217, 340, 341; 2: 135, 140, 144
  nuclear affections, 1: 342
  sensory deprivation, 2: 247
Neuro-motor phenomena
  hypnosis, 2: 177-178
Neuronal action, 2: 314
  consciousness, 2: 343
  definition, 2: 347
Neuronal nucleus, 2: 55
Neurons
  electron microscopy, 2: 55
  structure, 2: 53
Neurophysiological theory
  sensory deprivation, 2: 245
Neuropil, 2: 72
Neuropsychiatry
  of childhood, 1: 452-472
Neuro-sensory phenomena,
  hypnosis, 2: 172-177
Neurosis
  accident proneness, 1: 362
  in adolescents, 1: 288; 3: 379
  aetiological importance of family, 1: 271, 289
  anxiety (q.v.)
  behaviour disturbances, 1: 290
  behaviour therapy (q.v.)
  in children (general), 1: 257; 3: 379
  choice of organ, 2: 506
  choice of symptoms, 2: 506, 650
  classification of symptoms, 1: 107, 108; 2: 650
  comparison-by-age group method, 3: 379
  conduct problems, 1: 106, 293
  depression (q.v.)
  emotional learning, 2: 561
  existentialism, 2: 504
  experimental, 1: 127; 2: 558, 569
  family, 1: 271; 2: 648, 649, 650
  family psychiatry (q.v.)
  father importance, 3: 144
  group hypnotherapy, 2: 590
  historical, 2: xxi
  incidence, 2: 648, 650
  infantile, 3: 235
  inherited tendency, 1: 106
  latent learning, 1: 164
  learned behaviour, 1: 105; 2: 558
  learning therapies, 1: 154, 555; 2: 557
  Morita's theory (q.v.)
  Morita's therapy (q.v.)
  Pavlov's definition, 2: 590
  personality problem, 1: 106, 293
  phobias (q.v.)
  psychosis relationship, 1: 484
  psychosomatic disorders (q.v.)
  psychotherapy (q.v.)
  sleep disorders in children, 3: 418-453
  syndromes, 1: 291
  and war, 2: xxi
Neurosyphilis, 2: 114
Newborn
  coma, 3: 170

SUBJECT INDEX

father of, **3**: 158
mother of, **3**: 159, 160
narcissism, **3**: 204
needs of, **3**: 158
relationship with mother, **3**: 80-96
responses, **3**: 203
sex, **3**: 159
smile, **3**: 204
Nightmares, **2**: 209; **3**: 419, 433, 434, 438, 439, 440, 446, 450, 451
   castration fear, **3**: 448
   drugs withdrawal, **2**: 210
   EEG, **2**: 209
   enuresis, **3**: 451
   pavor nocturnus (q.v.)
   repetition compulsion, **3**: 446
Night terrors (*see* Pavor nocturnus)
Nihilism, **2**: 494
Nissl substance, **2**: 51, 53, 55, 56, 57, 59, 68, 69, 73, 79, 100
Nodes of Ranvier, **2**: 57
Nominal dysphasia, **3**: 551
Non-complementarity, **2**: 399
Non-mutuality, **2**: 398
Non-process psychosis, **2**: 391
NREM (non-rapid-eye-movement), **2**: 194
Nuclear complex, **3**: 293
Nuclear rotation, **2**: 79
Nuclear sexing, **1**: 50; **2**: 20-49
   buccal smear, **2**: 31
   clinical conditions in females, **2**: 33
   clinical conditions in males, **2**: 38
   Lyon hypothesis, **2**: 22, 25, 27, 38
   methods, **2**: 21
   sex chromosomes complexes, **2**: 28
   sex chromatin, **2**: 21
   techniques, **2**: 31
Nursing
   children in hospital, **1**: 266, 539-549
   supervision of mental patients, **2**: 723, 724

Obesity
   father implication, **3**: 145
Object relations (in children), **3**: 201
   anxiety, **3**: 206
   non-differentiation, **3**: 202
   pre-objectal stage, **3**: 202
   recognition, **3**: 206
   responses of newborn, **3**: 203
   semantic communication, **3**: 207
   smile, **3**: 204
Obsession
   in adolescents, **1**: 292
   autism, **3**: 646
   avoidance conditioning, **2**: 568
   in children, **3**: 247
   cultural distribution, **2**: 702
   Morita's theory, **2**: 525
   schizophrenic, **2**: 430, 436, 437

Occupational therapist, **1**: 262, 539, 550; **2**: 660, 664, 665, 667
Oedipus complex, **2**: 156; **3**: 144, 212, 213, 244, 293
   child, **3**: 181
   kibbutz, **3**: 329, 341, 343, 344
   resolution, **2**: 467
   schizophrenia, **2**: 410
   stage of development, **2**: 451, 453, 461
Oedipal family, **3**: 294
Oedipal structured society, **3**: 294
Oligodendrocytes, **2**: 58, 62, 64, 65, 77, 78, 79, 82
Oneirism, **3**: 721
   age of onset, **3**: 382
Oneirophrenia, **2**: 438
Oneiroscopy, **2**: 625
Operative thinking, **3**: 214
Organ idiom, **2**: 506
Organic delirium
   sleep deprivation, **2**: 292
Organic disorders
   cerebral responsiveness, **3**: 410
   EEG, **3**: 410
Organic psychoses, **1**: 488-490; **2**: 441, 442
   (*see also* Brain damage *and* Neurological impairment)
   acute, in children (*see* Acute organic psychoses in children)
   aetiology in children, **1**: 488
   clinical picture in children, **1**: 489
   piperidine derivatives, **2**: 279
Overprotection, **3**: 303, 349, 351

Paediatrics and child psychiatry, **3**: 8
Pain
   corporeal image, **2**: 140
   mental, **3**: 247
   precordial, in hypnosis, **2**: 167
   sensory deprivation, **2**: 237
Palsy
   cerebral, **1**: 219, 222, 225, 460
   hypnotic, **2**: 177
Pan-encephalitis of Pette-Doring, **3**: 411
Paralysis
   corporeal image, **2**: 140
   progressive, **2**: 441
   sleep, **2**: 205
Paranoia
   alcoholic, **2**: 442
   general anaesthesia, **3**: 88
   narcolepsy, **2**: 205
   schizophrenic, **2**: 431, 432, 436, 439
Paraphrenia, **3**: 652
Paraplegia, **2**: 136
   sensory deprivation, **2**: 248
Parent role, **3**: 65
Parental attitudes, **3**: 348
   delinquency, **1**: 375, 385, 525
   determinants of, **3**: 350

Parental attitudes—*cont.*
  in Japan, **3:** 347-368
  overprotection, **3:** 303, 349, 351
  pathological, **3:** 349
  perfectionism, **3:** 349, 355
  psychosomatic disorders, **1:** 313-327
  rejection, **3:** 349, 354
  schizophrenia, **2:** 394-412
  suicide, **1:** 415
Parental care, **3:** 256
  animals in laboratory, **3:** 127
  animal studies, **3:** 127
  in anthropoids, **3:** 131
  in a crèche, **3:** 129
  equal care by parents, **3:** 128
  by father, **3:** 130
  fathering (q.v.)
  by female, **3:** 129
  foster parents, **3:** 129
  by group, **3:** 129
  mothering (q.v.)
  multiple mothering, **3:** 129, 340, 344
  no care by parents, **3:** 128
  personality development, **2:** 453
  by servants, **3:** 129
  by siblings, **3:** 130
  switching of roles, **3:** 129
Parental control
  school child, **3:** 746
Parental effectiveness, **3:** 75, 76
Parental guidance
  child's need for, **3:** 195
Parenting, **3:** 128, 136, 257
  in animals, **3:** 148
  dysfunctions of, **3:** 571-584
  importance, **3:** 150
  kibbutz, **3:** 136
Parietal disease
  corporeal awareness, **2:** 144
Parkinson's disease, **2:** 89, 136
Partially sighted children
  intelligence tests, **1:** 572
Passalong (Alexander) test, **1:** 572
Passive transfer, **2:** 182
Patent ductus arteriosus, **3:** 36
  maternal emotional stress, **3:** 36
Paternal deprivation
  schizophrenia, **2:** 464
Pathogenic influences
  selectivity of child responses, **3:** 65
Pavlovian theory
  basic concepts, **2:** 532
  clinical applications, **2:** 546
  cortical mechanisms, **2:** 543
  electrical activity, **2:** 537
  higher nervous activity, **2:** 533
  mental disorders, **2:** 534
  motor reaction conditioning, **2:** 535
  recent development, **2:** 531
  spatial inter-relationship, **2:** 538

  spatial synchronization, **2:** 545, 547
Pavor nocturnus, **3:** 431, 440-453
  fugue states, **3:** 445
  hallucinations, **3:** 445
  hypermotility, **3:** 442, 445
  neurotic, **3:** 442
  over-stimulation, **3:** 442
  psychotic, **3:** 442
  retrograde amnesia, **3:** 442, 445
  sleepwalking, **3:** 445
  traumatic, **3:** 447
Penicillin
  malformation, **3:** 52
Pepsin, **3:** 475
Peptic ulcer
  hypnosis, **2:** 180, 181
Peptic ulcer in children, **1:** 319, 320;
    3: 471-492
  acute phase, **3:** 487
  adaptive immaturity, **3:** 485
  adaptive maturity promotion, **3:** 488
  adjustment problems, **3:** 476
  anxiety, **3:** 471, 487
  clinical observations, **3:** 476
  developmental history, **3:** 478
  diagnosis, **3:** 472
  dynamic formulation, **3:** 481
  egocentricity, **3:** 483
  emotional stress, **3:** 475
  family history, **3:** 477
  fathers, **3:** 490
  frustration, **3:** 482
  gastric function, **3:** 475
  hospitalization, **3:** 487
  impaired self-esteem, **3:** 484
  incidence, **3:** 471
  innate predisposition, **3:** 474
  maternal overprotection, **3:** 485, 488
  mother-child relationship, **3:** 473, 478, 481
  perceptual immaturity, **3:** 483
  personality, **3:** 479
  physiological predisposition, **3:** 474
  presenting problems, **3:** 476
  projective play, **3:** 487
  psychopathology, **3:** 472
  school phobia, **3:** 486
  separation anxiety, **3:** 485, 487
  theoretical models, **3:** 474
  treatment, **3:** 486
  work with child, **3:** 490
  work with parents, **3:** 488
  work with teacher, **3:** 491
Perception
  abnormal, in children, **1:** 217, 241, 476
  auditory, **1:** 94
  body image (q.v.)
  definition, **2:** 163, 340
  development, **1:** 85
  experiential flashbacks, **2:** 336, 337
  hallucinations (q.v.)

SUBJECT INDEX

hypnosis, **2**: 164-170
illusions, **2**: 335, 336
in infants, **1**: 88
interpretive cortex, **2**: 335, 339
interpretive signals, **2**: 336
mental set, **2**: 272
non-verbal, **2**: 341
of objects, **1**: 90
Piaget's theory, **1**: 58
of picture, **1**: 96
psychical responses, **2**: 335
psychoanalysis, **2**: 449
psychogenic retardation, **3**: 531
sensory, **1**: 85
of shape, **1**: 91
of space, **1**: 98, 218
uncommitted cortex, **2**: 338
Perceptual function
  infant, **3**: 205
Perceptual immaturity
  peptic ulcers, **3**: 483
Perceptual isolation, **2**: 296 (*see also* Sensory deprivation)
Perceptual release theory, **2**: 266
Perfectionism
  parental, **3**: 349, 355
Performance
  sensory deprivation, **2**: 239
Perikaryon, **2**: 53, 55, 56, 57, 79
Perinatal death, **3**: 30, 36
Perineuronal satellite cells, **2**: 62
Perivascular satellites, **2**: 64
Permissiveness, **3**: 310
Personality, **1**: 105
  accident-proneness, **1**: 356, 360
  adolescence, **1**: 293; **2**: 468
  adulthood, **2**: 469
  anal stage, **2**: 451, 453, 460
  child care and, **3**: 301
  child training, **3**: 313
  delinquency, **1**: 382
  development, **2**: 451, 452
  environmental factors, **2**: 454, 455
  epigenesis concept, **2**: 452
  extraversion, **1**: 106, 107
  hypochondriacal, **2**: 520, 523
  influence on test performance, **1**: 574
  introversion, **1**: 106, 107
  latency period, **2**: 467
  maternal deprivation, **2**: 457
  mothering, **2**: 457
  oedipal (phallic) stage, **2**: 451, 453, 461
  oral stage, **2**: 451, 453, 454, 464
  parental care, **2**: 453
  problems, in children, **1**: 106
  psychogenic retardation, **3**: 543
  psychosexual concepts, **2**: 455, 471
  psychosexual development, **2**: 453
  psychosocial concepts, **2**: 455, 471
  psychosomatic disorders, **1**: 316

  research, **1**: 108
  schizophrenic, **2**: 432
  school phobic children, **1**: 132
  social class, **3**: 310
  ulcerative colitis, **3**: 497
Peyotism, **2**: 280, 281
Phantasies (*see* Fantasies)
Phantom-body, **2**: 133
Phantom limb, **2**: 131, 133-136, 172, 272
  in leprosy, **2**: 134
  after surgery, **2**: 134, 135
  thalidomide babies, **2**: 135
Phenylpetonuria, **1**: 45, 504, 505, 511; **2**: 14, 626; **3**: 4
  counselling, **1**: 52
Phenylpyruvic oligophrenia (*see* Phenylketonuria)
Phobia, **1**: 113, 118; **2**: 560
  in adolescence, **1**: 291
  aetiology, **1**: 119
  of animals, **3**: 225
  behaviour therapy (q.v.)
  cat, **1**: 158
  confinement, **1**: 121
  extinction, **1**: 158
  imaginal desensitization, **2**: 565
  horse, **3**: 200
  learning theory, applied to children, **1**: 104-151
  little Hans's case, **3**: 200, 293
  Morita's theory, **2**: 525
  school, **1**: 130, 245, 291, 560
  sleep, **3**: 452
  systematic desensitization, **1**: 118; **2**: 563, 569, 571, 572
  treatment in children, **1**: 126, 129
Phocomelia, **3**: 50, 51
Photic activation, **3**: 396
Phrenasthenia, **3**: 594, 598
  progressive, **3**: 592
Piaget's theory, **1**: 58-84, 87, 88, 90, 94, 95, 98, 188, 213, 214, 376; **2**: 243, 448, 452, 726
  criticism of, **1**: 78-79
Pica, **3**: 455-469
  addiction and, **3**: 467
  aetiology, **3**: 455
  constitutional factors, **3**: 462
  definition, **3**: 455
  distribution, **3**: 455
  environmental factors, **3**: 462
  incidence, **3**: 455
  maternal deprivation, **3**: 465, 468
  medical evaluation, **3**: 467
  nutritional factors, **3**: 464
  outpatient treatment, **3**: 467
  preventive measures, **3**: 469
  psychiatric study, **3**: 456
  psychodynamic factors, **3**: 464
  psychopathology, **3**: 465
  research study, **3**: 456

864 SUBJECT INDEX

Pink spot, 2: 15, 627
Pinocytic vesicles, 2: 81
Pinocytosis, 2: 78
Placebo, 2: 596
   active, 2: 611, 612
   age, 2: 602
   anxiety, 2: 603
   attitude towards results, 2: 606
   attitude towards treatment, 2: 606
   catharsis, 2: 604
   clinical applications, 2: 610
   conditioning, 1: 111; 2: 603
   defence mechanisms, 2: 604
   definition, 2: 598
   direct iatroplacebogenesis, 2: 605
   double blind procedure, 2: 612
   effect, 2: 600, 613
   environmental factors, 2: 610
   evaluation of therapy, 2: 611
   faith, 2: 603
   historical, 2: 596
   indications for use, 2: 610
   indirect iatroplacebogenesis, 2: 608
   inert, 2: 611
   intelligence, 2: 602
   learning, 2: 603, 607
   motivation, 2: 603
   negative reactors, 2: 603
   patient-physician relationship, 2: 600, 605
   personality, 2: 601
   precautions, 2: 611
   primitive cultures, 2: 708, 709
   projective tests, 2: 602
   psychiatric diagnosis, 2: 602
   psychological factors, 2: 610
   sex, 2: 602
   single-blind procedures, 2: 611
   situational variables, 2: 609
   staff attitude, 2: 609
   suggestion, 2: 602
   treatment procedure, 2: 609
   triple-blind procedure, 2: 612
Planaria
   memory transfer experiment, 2: 94, 95
Plasma cortisol levels, 2: 162, 163, 186
Play
   diagnosis, 1: 277; 2: 660, 667
   handicapped children, 1: 213
   interpretation, 3: 211, 213
   observation, 3: 215
   practice, 1: 69
   symbolic, 1: 69; 1: 211
   therapy, 1: 280; 2: 667
Pleasure principle, 2: 514
Poliomyelitis
   in pregnancy, 3: 23
Polyandry
   Adelphic, 3: 135
   incidence, 3: 135

Polygyny
   incidence, 3: 135
   sororal, 3: 135
Polysomes, 2: 56
Population mobility, 3: 309
Porphyria, 2: 626; 3: 713
Possession states, 2: 705
Postoperative psychosis
   sensory deprivation, 2: 248
Post-partum depression, 3: 81
Posture, 2: 130
Poverty, 3: 311
Prausnitz-Küstner reaction, 2: 182, 185
Precocity, 1: 199
Preconscious stream, 2: 275
Pregnancy, 3: 159
   antepartum haemorrhage, 3: 43, 53
   anxiety states, 3: 38
   emotional stress, 3: 27-37
   infections, 1: 515; 3: 20-27
   prenatal influences (q.v.)
   psychoanalysis, 3: 83
   psychological climate, 3: 126
   studies in mental stress in, 3: 35
Premature birth
   illegitimacy, 3: 34
   mother-infant relations, 3: 82-83
   social class, 3: 27
Premature ejaculation
   learning therapy, 2: 567
Prenatal influences
   anencephaly, 3 :23, 26 ,27, 30, 31, 32, 33
   animal studies, 3: 20
   behaviour disturbance, 3: 28, 42-45
   birth mark, 3: 19
   cleft lip, 3: 27, 45, 46, 47, 50
   cleft palate, 3: 23, 27, 45, 46, 47, 50, 55
   drugs, 3: 50-53
   emotional stress in pregnancy, 3: 27
   folklore, 3: 19
   infantile ill-health, 3: 39-41
   malformations, 3: 20-45, 51, 52
   mental subnormality, 3: 26, 37, 38
   mongolism, 3: 22, 27, 47-50
   mother-child separation, 3: 20
   research perspectives, 3: 53
   rubella (q.v.)
   social conditions, 3: 27
   virus infection, 3: 20-23
Presbyphrenia, 3: 652
Presenting patient, 2: 652, 658
Primary process, 2: 267
Primitive law, 3: 293
Process psychosis, 2: 391
Professional body of psychiatrists (U.K.), 1: 258
Progressive Matrices, 1: 570, 573
Progressive paralysis, 2: 441
Projection
   schizophrenia, 2: 395

Projective play
  treatment of peptic ulcers, 3: 487
Projective techniques, 1: 575; 2: 357, 369
  'association' techniques, 1: 576
  Children's Apperception Test, 1: 577
  classification, 1: 576
  'completion' techniques, 1: 578
  'constructive' techniques, 1: 577
  definition, 1: 575
  'expressive' techniques, 1: 579
  Family Attitudes Test, 1: 577
  Family Relations Indicator, 1: 577; 2: 660; 3: 147
  'forced choice' techniques, 1: 578
  schizophrenia, 2: 400
  Symonds Picture Story Test, 1: 576
  Two-Houses Technique, 1: 579
Propaganda, 2: 240 (see also Brainwashing)
  sensory deprivation, 2: 240
Propositus (see Presenting patient)
Prosopagnosia, 2: 124
Proteins
  formation in nervous tissue, 2: 100
  learning, 2: 101
  synthesis, 2: 110
  synthesis inhibitors, 2: 98
  transfer of memory, 2: 96
Protophrenia, 3: 532
Psammoma bodies, 2: 82
Pseudo-feeblemindedness, 2: 651
Pseudohermaphroditism, 2: 36
  environmental influences, 2: 36
  gender role, 2: 36
  imprinting, 2: 36
Pseudo-integration, 3: 363
Pseudo-mutuality, 2: 395, 398, 399, 466; 3: 363
Psilocybin, 2: 274, 275
Psoriasis, 2: 171
Psychiatric hospital
  architecture, 2: 719
  colours, 2: 727
  communication, 2: 717
  décor, 2: 726
  doors, 2: 724
  economic consideration, 2: 718
  group relations, 2: 717
  integration of groups, 2: 718
  La Verrière, 2: 714, 719-727
  materials, 2: 727
  medical centre, 2: 721
  principles of construction, 2: 713
  reassuring areas, 2: 720
  reception, 2: 725
  safety, 2: 725
  sensory deprivation, 2: 249
  shapes, 2: 726
  siting, 2: 716
  size, 2: 717
  social centre, 2: 722

  social consideration, 2: 717
  solitude, 2: 718
  supervision, 2: 723, 724
  windows, 2: 724
Psychiatrist
  child, 1: 261, 262
  training in psychoanalytic theory, 3: 233
  training in psychology, 2: 382
Psychiatry
  child (see Child psychiatry)
  clinical psychology contribution, 2: 353
  community: 2: 675
  fathering and, 3: 144
  industrial, 2: 246
  military, 2: 246
  prospects today, 2: xxiv
  retrospect, 2: xix
  social, 2: 676
  transcultural, 2: 697
Psychoanalysis, 2: xxi, 489
  anthropology, 3: 295, 296
  chemical, 2: 625
  child therapy, 1: 523; 2: 476, 479; 3: 200, 220
  childhood schizophrenia, 3: 655
  contribution to child psychiatry, 3: 5
  dreaming, 2: 449
  drug therapy, 2: 477
  ego identity, 2: 468
  ego integrity, 2: 470
  ego loss, 2: 469
  ego synthesis, 2: 468
  ethology, 2: 450
  evaluation, 2: 448-487
  existential analysis, 2: 499
  female sexuality, 2: 450
  free association, 2: 150
  general practitioner, 2: 477
  Geneva school of genetic psychology and, 3: 176
  group therapy, 2: 477
  guilt, 2: 461, 463
  Hampstead Child Therapy Clinic, 2: 476; 3: 220
  infantile sexuality, 2: 467; 3: 5
  laboratory experiments, 2: 477
  labour-management relations, 2: 477
  manic-depressive psychoses, 2: 448
  maternal deprivation, 2: 450
  Menninger Study, 2: 449, 450, 471, 476
  Morita's theory, 2: 522
  patient assessment, 2: 472
  perception, 2: 449
  personality development, 2: 451, 452, 471
  pregnancy, 3: 83
  psychosomatics, 2: 477
  psychotherapy predictions, 2: 475
  research, 2: 471
  schizophrenia, 2: 448, 457, 458, 477
  sensory deprivation, 2: 244, 278

SUBJECT INDEX

Psychoanalysis—*cont.*
  sensory isolation, 2: 449
  simultaneous of mother and child, 3: 423
  social psychiatry, 2: 477, 478
  symbolic realization, 2: 457
  systematization, 2: 449
  Tavistock Clinic, 2: 477
  ulcerative colitis, 3: 511
Psychogenic retardation, 3: 531-545
  cultural deprivation, 3: 534-536, 538
  culture factors, 3: 535
  ego diffusion, 3: 544
  ego feeling, 3: 543
  ego identity, 3: 543
  ego theories, 3: 541
  family deprivation, 3: 535
  family studies, 3: 538
  individual studies, 3: 540
  lack of intellectual stimulation, 3: 532
  language, 3: 537
  learning, 3: 537
  maternal deprivation, 3: 536
  perception, 3: 531
  personality, 3: 543
  social factors, 3: 535
  vulnerability factors, 3: 541
Psycholinguistics, 3: 547
Psychological deprivation (early), 3: 9
Psychologist
  clinical, 1: 262, 539; 2: 353, 390
  educational, 1: 254, 539, 580
  training, 2: 354, 355, 384
Psychology
  and child psychiatry, 1: 562
  clinical, 2: 353-390
  contribution to child psychiatry, 3: 5
  development of perception, 1: 85
  personalist, 2: 490
  Piaget, 1: 58
  reports, 1: 263, 583
  Soviet research, 1: 188
  tests (q.v.)
  unitary-and-structural, 2: 490
Psychometric approach
  in clinical psychology, 2: 360
Psychomotor disorders
  catalepsy in children, 3: 729
Psycho-pharmacology, 2: xxiii, 620-636
  (*see also* Drugs)
  amphetaminic shock, 2: 624
  amphetaminic sub-narcosis, 2: 625
  biochemical psychiatry, 2: 626
  chemical psychoanalysis, 2: 625
  classification, 2: 621
  clinical perspectives, 2: 620
  narco-analysis, 2: 624
  neuroleptanalgesy, 2: 624
  nomenclature, 2: 621
  oneiroscopy, 2: 625
  pharmaco-dynamics, 2: 624

  psychoses, 2: 627, 629
  risks, 2: 633
  weck-analysis, 2: 624
Psychosensory disorders
  in children, 3: 726
Psychoses
  in adolescents, 1: 294
  aetiology, 1: 236, 240, 477, 484, 485, 488
  alcoholic, 2: 442
  asynchronous maturation, 1: 479
  behaviour, 1: 135
  biochemistry, 1: 482; 2: 14, 17, 626
  chemotherapy, 2: 627
  childhood (*see* Childhood psychosis)
  children of psychotics, 1: 43
  classification, 1: 474; 2: 391; 3: 650
  clinical picture, 1: 475, 489
  comparison-by-age group method, 3: 378
  conditioning, 2: 536
  cultural symptomatology, 2: 704
  definition, 1: 490; 3: 649
  depressive, 1: 485, 487; 2: 6, 439, 440, 444, 448, 451, 651
  ECT, 1: 491; 2: 116, 120, 366, 633
  environmental factors, 1: 479; 2: 13, 17
  and epilepsy, 1: 478
  existentialism, 2: 504
  exogenous, 2: 441, 442
  family, 2: 648, 650, 651
  genetics, 1: 42, 481; 2: 3
  incidence, 1: 268; 2: 648, 650
  infantile (*see* Infantile psychosis)
  insulin therapy, 1: 492; 2: xxii, xxiii
  model, 2: 288-312
  neuroleptics, 2: 629
  neurotic symptoms, 1: 484
  organic, 1: 488; 2: 441, 442, 651; 3: 706-731
  parents (of psychotics), 1: 235
  pathogenesis, 1: 240
  pseudo-schizophrenic syndrome, 1: 483
  psychotherapy, 1: 492
  reactive, 1: 296, 485
  schizophrenia (q.v.)
  sensory, 3: 602
  somnolence, 2: 212
  and suicide, 1: 413
  syphilis, 2: 442
  treatment, 1: 491
  treatment in primitive cultures, 2: 707
  units for psychotic adolescents, 1: 265
  units for psychotic children, 1: 265
Psychosexual attitudes, 2: 35, 36
Psychosexual development, 3: 243
Psychosocial development
  electrocerebral development, 3: 413
Psychosocial factors
  EEG patterns, 3: 415
Psychosomatic disorders
  abdominal pain, 1: 324

SUBJECT INDEX

in adolescents, **1:** 296
anorexia nervosa, **1:** 114, 292, 324; **2:** 569, 649
asthma, **1:** 317, 329; **2:** 181, 182, 572
in children (general), **1:** 306
constipation, **1:** 323
cultural distribution, **2:** 702
emotional stress, **1:** 308
existential analysis, **2:** 502
father's implication, **3:** 145
hypnosis, **2:** 178
migraine, **1:** 325
negativism, **1:** 321
obesity, **3:** 145
operative thinking, **3:** 214
parental attitudes, **1:** 313
peptic ulcers, **3:** 471-492
personality, **1:** 316
psychoanalysis, **2:** 477
psychogenesis, **1:** 307
syndrome shift, **1:** 312; **2:** 181, 397, 571, 586
treatment, **1:** 327
ulcerative colitis, **1:** 319; **2:** 180; **3:** 145, 494-525
Psychotherapy, **1:** 152, 311; **2:** xxiii, 489
of brain-damaged children, **1:** 459
child therapy, **1:** 523; **3:** 13
clinical psychologist, **2:** 361
in delinquency, **1:** 392, 396
drawing, **1:** 526
dreams, **1:** 526, 529
existential analysis, **2:** 508
learning, **2:** 557
Morita therapy, **2:** 519
psychoanalysis (q.v.)
in psychosis, **1:** 492
research, **2:** 362
social need, **2:** 361
ulcerative colitis, **3:** 504, 508, 509, 510, 511
Psychotic behaviour
experimentally induced (*see* Model psychoses)
psychotomimetic drugs, **2:** 301
sensory deprivation, **2:** 228
sleep deprivation, **2:** 203, 204
Psychotic parents, **1:** 43; **2:** 6
Psychotogens (*see* Hallucinogens)
Psychotomimetic drugs, **2:** 301
Psychotomimetic states (*see* Model psychoses)
Psychotoxic diseases
of infancy, **3:** 170, 171
Puberty, **1:** 287
Punishment
of child, **3:** 140, 184, 310
Purkinje cells, **2:** 68-73, 75, 77, 78
Pyloric stenosis
mental stress in pregnancy, **3:** 35
Pyramidal cells, **2:** 68

Pyramidal neurons, **2:** 66
Pyruvic acid, **2:** 16

Rabies, **3:** 711
Radiation, **3:** 715
Radio telemetry
EEG, **3:** 393
Reaction formations, **3:** 216
Reactive depression
in children, **1:** 485, 529
treatment, **2:** 366
Reading
dyslexia (q.v.)
neurophysiology, **2:** 334
Reality principle, **2:** 514
Reasoning
in exceptional children, **1:** 203
Recall
inaccuracies of, **3:** 63
Reciprocal inhibition, **1:** 128; **2:** 560 (*see also* Learning theory)
in children, **1:** 114, 128
Redirection, **1:** 29
Referrals
agencies, **2:** 655
children, **1:** 269, 271
family, **2:** 642, 654
Hampstead Clinic, **3:** 222
Reflex action, **2:** 314
mechanisms, **2:** 313
temperature control, **2:** 314
Regression, **2:** 266; **3:** 235, 236
in child, and parental tension, **3:** 188
functional, **3:** 163
pathological (maternal), **3:** 95
sensory deprivation, **2:** 245
toddler, **3:** 187
ulcerative colitis in children, **3:** 509, 516
Reinforcement, **2:** 535, 559
intermittent, **1:** 141
social, **1:** 139
Rejection
maternal, **3:** 170
parental, **3:** 349, 354
Relapse, **1:** 160
Relationship
during labour, **3:** 86-88
family, **2:** 645
mother-child (q.v.)
patient-physician, **2:** 600, 605; **3:** 503
psychodynamic, **1:** 313
in schizophrenia, **2:** 393-424
Relaxation
differential, **2:** 563
responses, **2:** 562
Remedial teaching, **1:** 134; **3:** 4, 387
Replacement therapy, **3:** 516
Reproduction
methods of, **3:** 128
REM (rapid-eye-movement), **2:** 196, 200, 209

Remembering, **1:** 170
Reports, **1:** 276, 278, 282
 psychological, **1:** 263, 583; **2:** 374
Research
 into adoption, **1:** 445
 in child psychiatry, **1:** 267
 clinical psychologist, **2:** 371-374
 in defectology, **1:** 189
 difficulties, **1:** 15
 genetical, **1:** 52
 hypotheses, **1:** 8
 on learning and memory, **2:** 92
 methodology, **1:** 3-19
 model psychoses (q.v.)
 operational, **1:** 5
 Pavlovian theory (q.v.)
 personality, **1:** 108
 Piaget's theory (q.v.)
 play techniques, **1:** 16
 psychotherapy, **2:** 362, 471-478
 schizophrenia (q.v.)
 selection of problem, **1:** 7
 Soviet developmental psychology, **1:** 188
 in transcultural psychiatry, **2:** 709
Reserpine, **2:** xxiii, 629
 as teratogen, **3:** 53
Residential care of children, **3:** 764-783
 (*see also* In-patient units)
 blind, **3:** 769
 character disorders, **3:** 772
 deaf, **3:** 769
 delinquents, **3:** 778
 emotional disorders, **3:** 772
 epileptic children, **3:** 777
 future developments, **3:** 782
 institutions (*see* Child care institutions)
 motor disorders, **3:** 769
 physically handicapped, **3:** 768
 psychiatric indications, **3:** 770
 psychotic children, **3:** 773
 retarded children, **3:** 774
 social indications, **3:** 767
Resistance, **2:** 501
Respiratory changes
 hypnosis, **2:** 158
Resynthesis, **1:** 23
Retardation (*see* Mental subnormality)
Retrospective investigation
 inaccuracies of recall, **3:** 63
 problems, **3:** 62
Ribonuclease, **2:** 95, 97
Ribosomes, **2:** 55, 55, 65, 100
Rituals
 childhood, **3:** 381
 in primitive cultures psychiatry, **2:** 708
 schizophrenic, **2:** 430
 schizophrenic children, **1:** 476
 sleep, **3:** 452, 453
RNA (ribonucleic acid), **2:** 22, 27, 51, 52, 53, 55, 56, 68, 110

 changes, **2:** 100, 102, 103
 inhibitors of synthesis, **2:** 97, 98
 polymerase activity, **2:** 94
 synthesis, **2:** 90
 transfer and memory, **2:** 94, 95, 96
Rocking, **2:** 213; **3:** 163, 172, 236
 EEG, **2:** 213, 214
 institutionalized children, **2:** 213
 mental defectives, **2:** 213
Role
 of anxiety, **3:** 77
 conflict, **2:** 408
 diffusion, **1:** 246
 distortion, **2:** 408
 father, **3:** 142
 homosexuality, **3:** 146
 identity, **3:** 146
 imprinting of gender, **2:** 36
 in Japanese family, **3:** 350
 parent, **3:** 65
 sexual, **2:** 402
 social, **2:** 408
 stereotyped, **2:** 413
 structure, **2:** 399
 subcultural groups, **3:** 311
Roller tube, **2:** 74, 75, 76
Rolling, **3:** 163
Rorschach test, **2:** 368, 369, 370
Rose chamber, **2:** 74, 75, 76
Rosenzweig Picture Frustration Test, **1:** 578
Royal Medico-Psychological Association, **1:** 258
Rubella, **1:** 339, 515; **3:** 26, 36, 38, 54
 statistics of effects on foetus, **3:** 20, 21
 stillbirth, **3:** 45, 46

Samadhi, **2:** 271
Sampling, **3:** 788
Scapegoat
 family, **2:** 653
 primitive culture, **2:** 708, 709
Schematia, **2:** 130
 dysschematia, **2:** 141
 hyper-schematia, **2:** 140
Schizophrenia
 acute toxic delirium, **2:** 414
 adaptation, **3:** 666
 in adolescence, **1:** 295; **2:** 408, 412, 413, 434
 affective psychoses, **2:** 5
 affective syndrome, **2:** 430
 age of onset, **2:** 5, 7, 17, 397, 398, 414, 434, 435, 439, 444; **3:** 378, 382
 anomalies of family functioning, **2:** 393, 413
 arrest in psychological growth, **2:** 396
 asthenic syndrome, **2:** 430, 436, 442
 auto-immune response, **2:** 15
 automatism, **2:** 437

SUBJECT INDEX

biochemical aspects, **1**: 482; **2**: 14, 17, 626, 627; **3**: 383
catatonic, **2**: 425, 431, 433, 435, 438, 439
childhood (*see* Childhood schizophrenia)
chromosomal aberration, **2**: 16, 17, 35, 37, 38, 39
circular, **2**: 439
classification, **2**: 400, 440
clinical description, **2**: 4
clinical forms, **2**: 437
community care, **2**: 412
comparison-by-age group method, **3**: 378, 382
complementarity, **2**: 395
conditioning, **2**: 536, 547, 548, 550, 551, 570
continuous, **2**: 431, 433, 434
continuous-progressive, **2**: 438, 439
cousin marriages, **2**: 11
culture, **2**: 701, 704; **3**: 310
cytogenetic surveys, **2**: 38
definition, **2**: 392
delusion, **2**: 430, 431, 433, 436
dementia, **2**: 414
depression, **2**: 430, 431, 436
diagnostic criteria, **2**: 412
double bind, **2**: 396, 399, 404, 406, 407, 409, 466
double communication, **2**: 397
drug therapy, **2**: 477
EEG, **2**: 550
emotional changes, **2**: 433
emotional deprivation, **2**: 464
emotional divorce, **2**: 394, 397 413
emotional flattening, **2**: 432
emotional fragility, **2**: 432
energy reduction, **2**: 433, 437
environment, **2**: 13, 17
environmental failure, **2**: 457
epidemiological investigation, **2**: 444
epilepsy, **2**: xxii, 434, 435
existential analysis, **2**: 507
existentialism, **2**: 410
exogenous trauma, **2**: 410
family (a case study), **3**: 664
family constellations, **3**: 310
family dynamics, **2**: 464, 465, 466
family group therapy, **2**: 397, 666
family homeostasis, **2**: 404
family psychiatry, **2**: 650
family psychopathology, **2**: 391-424, 641
family schisms, **2**: 402, 413
family skews, **2**: 402, 413
familial concentration, **2**: 10
father-schizophrenic relationship, **2**: 411; **3**: 146
and fertility, **2**: 11
genetics, **1**: 481; **2**: 3-19, 444
hallucinations, **2**: 283, 430, 431, 433, 437, 439

hebephrenic, **2**: 425, 432, 439
historical concepts, **2**: 425-428
hysteria, **1**: 484
immaturity, **2**: 394, 397, 413
incestuous preoccupation, **2**: 402
in infants, **3**: 669
index of alpha-synchronization, **2**: 552
Interpersonal Perception Method, **2**: 410
intra-psychic ataxia, **2**: 426, 437
irrational ideation, **2**: 402
Japanese family study, **3**: 359
Kandinsky-Clerambault syndrome, **2**: 429, 431, 437, 439, 442; **3**: 382
learning, **2**: 380
Logical Types, **2**: 404, 405, 406
mania, **2**: 430, 431, 439
model psychoses, **2**: 288, 301, 306, 414
mother-schizophrenic relationship, **2**: 394, 395, 396, 411, 457
mutuality, **2**: 398
mystification, **2**: 410, 413, 466
neurophysiological alterations and stress, **2**: 465
non-complementarity, **2**: 399
non-mutuality, **2**: 398
non-process, **2**: 393
obsessions, **2**: 430, 436, 437
Oedipus complex, **2**: 410
organic brain lesions, **2**: 414
paranoia, **2**: 431, 432, 436, 439
parent-schizophrenic relationship, **2**: 411
perceptual changes, **2**: 306
periodic, **2**: 431, 437
personal identity, **2**: 398
personality development, **2**: 451
pink spot, **2**: 15, 627
potential, **2**: 399
prediction, **2**: 459
predisposition, **2**: 11
process, **2**: 393
prognosis, **2**: 444; **3**: 379
projection, **2**: 395, 413
projective techniques, **2**: 400
proprioceptive hypothesis, **2**: 305
pseudo-mutuality, **2**: 395, 398, 399, 410
pseudo-neurotic states, **2**: 430
psychic-disturbance, **2**: 429
psychoanalysis, **2**: 448, 457, 458, 477
psychotropic drugs, **2**: 433, 434
recessive hypothesis, **2**: 11, 12, 13, 17
recurrent, **2**: 439, 444
risk, **2**: 10
rituals, **2**: 430
role conflict, **2**: 408
role distortion, **2**: 408
role structure, **2**: 399
schub-type, **2**: 431, 433, 438, 439, 444
sensory isolation, **2**: 300, 301, 303
sex, **2**: 5, 436
sexual identity, **2**: 402

Schizophrenia—cont.
  shadow of insanity, 2: 409
  shift-like, 2: 431, 433, 439
  sleep deprivation, 2: 305
  socially determined characteristics, 2: 436
  socio-cultural isolation, 2: 402, 413
  speech breakdown, 3: 564
  speech intrusion, 2: 410
  stereotypy, 2: 433, 436
  stress, 2: 465
  studies, 2: 394-414
  studies of parents, 3: 146
  symbiotic dependencies, 3: 303
  symptom formation, 2: 395, 397
  symptomatology, 2: 428
  symptomatology shift, 2: 397
  syndrome development, 2: 429
  therapy, 2: xxiii, 308, 366, 397, 433, 434, 448, 457, 458, 477, 666
  transfer phenomena, 2: 410
  transitional, 2: 444
  twins, 2: 13, 17
  urine, 2: 277, 627
  variants, 2: 432
  weight discrimination, 2: 304
Scholastic philosophy, 2: 490
School
  antecedents of distress, 3: 743
  clinical services, 3: 754
  constitution and temperament, 3: 743, 745
  cultural gap, 3: 748
  deviant behaviour incidence, 3: 741
  educational attainment tests, 1: 580
  educational psychologist, 1: 254, 580
  emotional problems identification, 3: 740
  ethnic factors, 3: 746
  exceptional children, 1: 193
  family dynamics, 3: 745
  hospital schools, 1: 471
  in in-patient units, 1: 540, 549, 559, 560
  intellectual resources, 3: 744
  intelligence and achievement, 3: 745
  manifestations of distress, 3: 739
  medical officer, 1: 273, 276, 278
  mental health consultations, 3: 753
  nursery school, 1: 125
  parent education, 3: 749
  parental control, 3: 746
  phobia, 1: 130, 133, 245, 291, 560; 3: 486
  pre-school check-up, 3: 753
  prevention of behaviour problems, 3: 749
  psychology service, 1: 273
  psychosocial context, 3: 733
  referral, 3: 755
  remedial education, 1: 134; 3: 4, 387
  report, 1: 276
  retarded children, 3: 776
  self esteem, 3: 745
  sex roles, 3: 747
  social class mediation, 3: 755
  social structure of classroom, 3: 733, 734, 735
  socio-cultural background, 3: 746
  socio-economic factors, 3: 747
  stress, 3: 736
  syndrome search, 3: 739
  system intervention, 3: 754
  teacher power, 3: 735
  teacher training, 3: 751
  underfunctioning, 1: 207
  vocation instruction, 3: 780
Schwann cell, 2: 58, 59, 62, 76, 80, 81
Secondary negative component (SNC), 3: 404
Sedatives
  prenatal effect, 3: 52, 53
Segregation
  urban industrialization, 3: 308
Self esteem
  peptic ulcers, 3: 484
  schoolchild, 3: 745
Self-identification, 3: 302, 315
Self-portraiture, 2: 142, 143
  Assistinzbild, 2: 143
Seminiferous tubule dysgenesis (see Klinefelter's syndrome)
Senile dementia, 3: 533
  breakdown of language, 3: 563
Senility
  premature, 2: 40
Sensation, 2: 316
  sensory apparatus, 2: 315
  sensory areas, 2: 317
Sensory deprivation, 1: 86; 2: 222-264 (see also Sensory isolation)
  affective changes, 2: 227
  biochemical measures, 2: 235
  brainwashing, 2: 224, 240
  clinical implications, 2: 246
  cognitive effects, 2: 238
  deafferentation, 2: 223
  EEG measures, 2: 233, 237
  exteroceptive stimulation, 2: 223, 224, 248
  family therapy, 2: 479
  geriatrics, 2: 249
  hallucinations, 2: 228, 229, 230
  history, 2: 202
  hospitalization, 2: 248
  hydrohypodynamic environment, 2: 226
  impoverished environment, 2: 224
  industrial psychiatry, 2: 246
  intellectual efficiency, 2: 239
  learning, 2: 240
  McGill studies, 2: 224, 230, 237, 240
  mental hospital, 2: 249
  methodological problems, 2: 224
  military psychiatry, 2: 246
  monotonous conditions, 2: 223

neurological disease, 2: 247
ophthalmology, 2: 248
orthopaedics, 2: 248
perceptual-motor effects, 2: 237
performance, 2: 239
personality variables and reactions, 2: 229, 232
physiological effects, 2: 232
psychoanalysis, 2: 478
psychological states, 2: 237, 247
retardation, 2: 249
sensory threshold, 2: 236
skin potential measures, 2: 233, 237
stimulus-hunger, 2: 241
surgery, 2: 248
theories, 2: 243
therapeutic effects, 2: 249
Sensory input, 2: 268, 269
depatterning, 2: 266, 298
diseases, 2: 272
illusions, 2: 266
overload, 2: 270, 273
Sensory isolation, 2: 88, 298 (see also Sensory deprivation)
clinical applications, 2: 307
cognitive disorders, 2: 301
EEG, 2: 299, 301
galvanic skin response, 2: 300, 301
hallucinations, 2: 271
maternal deprivation, 2: 299
McGill experiments, 2: 298, 299
model psychosis, 2: 299
psychoanalysis, 2: 449
schizophrenia, 2: 300, 301
Sensory loss
hypnotic, 2: 174
Sensory psychosis, 3: 602
Sensory shocks, 2: 198
Sensory stimulations, 2: 88, 89
Sensory threshold
sensory deprivation, 2: 236
Sensuality
child, 3: 179
Sentient statue, 2: 223
Separation (child-parent) 1: 214, 244, 485; 2: 313; 3: 20, 99, 109-111, 140, 145, 174, 175, 254-289, 659
anxiety, 1: 131, 214, 244, 302; 3: 659
animal experiments, 3: 283-284 (see also below Harlow's experiments)
avoidance, 3: 101, 110
backward children, 3: 280
boarding schools, 3: 289
care of child during, 3: 276-278
causes, 3: 273-276
day foster care, 3: 288
complete, 3: 289
death of parent, 3: 283
definition, 3: 254
delinquency, 3: 281

depression, 1: 485, 529; 3: 174
and deprivation, 3: 254-289
direct investigation, 3: 258-279
effects of, 3: 267-271
foster home, 3: 289
Harlow's experiments, 1: 35; 2: 249, 299, 449, 457; 3: 210, 284, 300, 314, 315, 659
hospitalization, 3: 270
hostels, 3: 289
incidence, 3: 258-267
in-patient care, 3: 289
maladjusted children, 3: 281
partial, 3: 288
peptic ulcers, 3: 485, 487
practical consideration, 3: 271-273
psychological individuation, 3: 89
reactions, 3: 102
studies on, 3: 279-289
substitute care, 3: 279
therapeutic clubs, 3: 289
therapeutic uses, 3: 284-289
ulcerative colitis, 3: 506
vector therapy, 2: 671; 3: 286
Sernyl, 2: 280
comparison with LSD, 2: 302
model psychoses, 2: 289, 302, 303, 306
Serotonin
LSD interaction, 2: 276
Sex
anomalies, 1: 49 513; 2: 33-43
of child, 3: 159
chromatin (see Sex chromatin)
determining mechanism, 2: 24
nuclear sexing (q.v.)
role, 2: 402; 3: 146, 747
vulnerability, 2: 653
Sex chromatin, 1: 50, 513; 2: 20-23
abnormality, 1: 49, 513; 2: 20, 33-43
derivation, 2: 21, 23
patterns, 2: 28
properties, 2: 24
Sex chromosomes complexes, 2: 28
Sexual development
testicular feminization, 2: 35
in Turner's syndrome, 2: 34
Sexual dreams, 2: 202
Sexual drives, 2: 453
Sexual identity, 2: 402, 461
adolescence, 2: 468
castration fear, 2: 461, 462
imprinting, 2: 36
incestuous wishes, 2: 461
oedipal conflict, 2: 461
Sexual precocity, 3: 240
Sexual psychopaths, 2: 41, 42
Sexuality
in adolescents, 1: 286
arousal, 1: 34
chromosomes anomalies, 1: 49, 513; 2: 33-43

872

SUBJECT INDEX

Sexuality—*cont.*
  homosexuality (q.v.)
  infantile, **2**: 467; **3**: 5
  psychosexual stages, **1**: 246
  sex chromatin (q.v.)
  taboo, **1**: 182
Shell shock, **2**: xxi
Shintoism, **2**: 705
Sibling rivalry
  kibbutz, **3**: 329
Skills
  conditioning, **2**: 319
  motor, **2**: 345
Sleep, **2**: 193
  cerebral basis, **2**: 193
  deprivation (*see* Sleep deprivation)
  depth, **2**: 196
  disorders (*see* Sleep disorders)
  drugs, **2**: 214
  EEG, **2**: 194, 195, 198, 199, 200, 206, 209, 211, 214, 270; **3**: 391, 395
  hallucinations, **1**: 178, 179; **2**: 198, 199, 205, 209, 231, 269, 270
  learning machines, **2**: 199
  NREM (non-rapid-eye-movement) **2**: 194
  paradoxical phase, **2**: 196
  perceptual release, **2**: 270
  pre-sleep period, **2**: 198
  promotion, **2**: 197
  REM (rapid-eye-movement), **2**: 196, 200, 209, 270
  therapy, **2**: 707
Sleep deprivation, **2**: 202, 289
  affect, **2**: 291
  automatic resting, **2**: 295
  biochemistry, **2**: 204, 293
  catechol amines output, **2**: 294
  cognitive disorganization, **2**: 291
  depersonalization, **2**: 291
  EEG changes, **2**: 294, 295
  galvanic skin response, **2**: 293
  hallucinations, **2**: 203, 204, 271, 280, 291
  illusions, **2**: 203
  lapses, **2**: 295, 296, 297
  learning, **2**: 291
  microsleep, **2**: 290
  narrowing of attention, **2**: 298
  organic delirium, **2**: 292
  peripheral physiology, **2**: 293
  phenomenology, **2**: 290
  psychotic behaviour, **2**: 203, 204
  schizophrenia, **2**: 204, 305
  test, **2**: 296, 297
  waking dreams, **2**: 292
Sleep disorders (in adults), **2**: 205-216
  (in children, *see below*)
  bruxism, **2**: 213
  drugs, **2**: 214, 215, 216
  enuresis (q.v.)

  head-banging, **2**: 213
  idiopathic narcolepsy, **2**: 205, 206
  insomnia (q.v.)
  nightmares, **2**: 209, 210
  rocking, **2**: 213, 214
  sleep talking, **2**: 210
  sleep walking, **2**: 211, 213, 265
  snoring, **2**: 212
  somnolence, **2**: 211
  yawning, **2**: 212
Sleep disorders (in children), **1**: 245, 322; **3**: 418-453
  anal phase of development, **3**: 426
  anxiety, **3**: 418
  castration anxiety, **3**: 429, 436, 448, 452
  emotional disturbance, **3**: 423
  enuresis (q.v.)
  head banging, **2**: 213
  in infancy, **2**: 213; **3**: 420-426
  insomnia, **3**: 420-422
  masturbation, **3**: 429, 436, 438
  mother-child relationship, **3**: 423
  neurotic disturbances, **3**: 419, 420
  nightmares, **3**: 419, 433, 434, 436, 438, 439, 440, 446, 451
  Oedipal phase of development, **3**: 428, 449
  oral phase of development, **3**: 429
  overstimulation, **3**: 426, 429
  pavor nocturnus (q.v.)
  phobias, **3**: 451, 452
  psychosomatic symptoms, **3**: 431, 435, 448, 450
  rocking, **2**: 213, 214
  seduction, **3**: 426, 429
  sleepwalking, **3**: 430-440, 445
  soiling, **3**: 450
  treatment, **3**: 427, 436
Sleep phobia, **3**: 451, 452
Sleeping habits
  faulty, of children, **3**: 427
Smile
  first, **3**: 161
  newborn child, **3**: 204
SNC (*see* Secondary negative component)
Social anthropology
  care of young, **3**: 149
Social casework, **3**: 201
Social character, **3**: 297
Social class
  child rearing, **3**: 309
  personality, **3**: 310
Social history, **1**, 263, 276
Social processes
  cultural factors, **3**: 309
  ethnic factors, **3**: 309
Social psychiatry, **2**: 676
  definition, **2**: 676
  psychoanalysis, **2**: 477
Social stratification, **3**: 309

SUBJECT INDEX

Social status
  in Japan, 3: 350
Social Worker
  and adoption, 1: 447
  community psychiatry, 2: 679, 684, 685
  and employment, 1: 582
  family psychiatry, 2: 656, 659
  psychiatric, 1: 524, 556
  qualifications, 2: 262
  vector therapy, 2: 671
Socialization, 1: 110
  after infancy, 3: 307
  schizophrenic children, 3: 688
Socio-cultural background
  school-child, 3: 746
Socio-economic factors
  schoolchild, 3: 747
Solitude, 2: 718
Somatic reciprocation, 2: 396
Somnambulism, 2: 211, 213, 265
  amnesia, 3: 431, 432, 434, 436
  in children, 3: 430-440, 445
  epilepsy, 3: 436
Space-form blindness, 2: 34
Spastic diplegia, 1: 340
Spatial relationship, 2: 330, 332, 336, 338
  disorientation, 2: 336
Spatial synchronization, 2: 539, 545, 547, 550, 551, 553, 554
Species-specific structures, 3: 82
Specular hallucinations, 2: 139
Speech, 1: 336; 2: 328; 3: 547-568 (*see also* Language)
  acquisition of foreign language, 3: 560
  aphasia (q.v.)
  association, 3: 551
  attention, 2: 334
  autistic children, 3: 640
  blank slate, 2: 329
  brain dominance, 2: 328
  breakdown, 3: 560-568
  cerebral lesions, 3: 560
  comprehension, 3: 553
  cortical areas, 2: 325, 330, 335, 339
  cross-modal association, 3: 553, 557
  deafness, 1: 339; 3: 554
  development, 1: 212, 336; 3: 549
  disorders, 1: 336
  dysphasia, 3: 567
  dysarthria, 1: 337
  dyslalia, 1: 345
  echolalia, 1: 476; 3: 555, 556
  early linguistic utterances, 3: 550
  functional disturbances, 1: 345
  hand dominance, 2: 328
  ideational areas, 2: 333, 338
  idioglossia, 1: 348
  in imbecile children, 1: 231
  imitation, 3: 550
  intrusion, in schizophrenia, 2: 410
  lalling, 1: 348; 3: 166, 207
  mechanical defects, 1: 345
  mental deficiency, 1: 338
  nominal dysphasia, 3: 551
  organic disorders of the nervous system, 1: 339
  pattern potentials, 2: 333, 334
  poor articulation, 3: 556
  pre-linguistic utterances, 3: 549
  psycholinguistics, 3: 547
  psychotic children, 1: 348, 476; 3: 557
  retarded, 3: 167
  schizophrenia, 3: 564
  semantic association, 3: 552
  senile dementia, 3: 563
  small vocabulary, 3: 556
  stammer, 1: 114, 136, 343, 345; 2: 171
  stutter, 1: 136, 345
  syntactic association, 3: 552
  subnormal children, 3: 555
  Thorndike-Lange Word Count, 3: 561
  verbal conditioning, 3: 551
  verbal encoding, 3: 558
  visual encoding, 3: 558
  word accessibility, 3: 561
  word frequency, 3: 561
Spina bifida
  emotional stress in pregnancy, 3: 31
Spinal cord, 2: 314, 316
Spinal ganglia cultures
  morphological patterns, 2: 79
Spinal reflexes, 2: 314
Spongioblasts, 2: 62
Spontaneous remission, 1: 134; 2: 376
Staff (in child psychiatry), 1: 260
  administrative, 1: 264
  child psychiatrist (q.v.)
  child psychotherapist, 1: 262, 523
  clinical psychologist, 1: 262, 539
  co-ordination, 1: 263, 277
  of corrective establishments, 1: 396
  Hampstead clinic, 3: 223
  of in-patient units, 1: 266, 539, 540
  occupational therapist, 1: 262, 539, 550
  recruitment, 1: 261
  social worker, (q.v.)
  training, 1: 261, 267
Stammer, 1: 114, 136, 343, 345; 2: 171
Stanford-Binet Intelligence Scale, 1: 570
Stellate granule cells, 2: 68, 69
Stereotypy, 2: 433, 436; 3: 646
Steroids
  psychotic response to, 3: 502
Stigmata
  hypnotic, 2: 172, 180
Stillbirth, 3: 45, 46
  rubella, 3: 20, 21
  toxoplasmosis, 3: 25, 26
Stimulation
  child learning, 1: 213

Stimulation—*cont.*
  exteroceptive, 2: 223, 232, 244, 248
  handicapped children, 1: 220
  interoceptive, 2: 232
  lack of, 3: 236
  rhythmic, 2: 149, 150, 158, 198
  stimulus-hunger (q.v.)
Stimulus-hunger, 2: 241
  feed-back, 2: 242
  sensation-seeking-scale, 2: 242
Strabismus
  toxoplasmosis, 3: 24, 25
Stress
  mental subnormality, 3: 532
  in pregnancy, 3: 27-37
  at school, 3: 736
  selectivity, 3: 70
  ulcerative colitis, 3: 499
Stuporose state, 3: 723
Sturge-Weber syndrome, 3: 710
Subarachnoid haemorrhage, 2: 114
Subcultural group
  roles, 3: 311
Sublimation, 3: 248, 302
Subnormality (*see* Mental subnormality)
Sucking, 3: 236
  finger and thumb, 3: 163, 165
Suggestibility, 2: 585
  degree of, 2: 586
  placebo, 2: 602
  reinforcement, 2: 587
Suggestion
  hypnotic, 2: 153, 155
Suicide
  anniversary reactions, 2: 653
  in children and adolescents (*see below*)
  cultural distribution, 2: 702
  incidence in U.K., 2: 649
Suicide (in children and adolescents), 1: 403
  aetiology, 1: 408, 424
  attempts, 1: 359, 403
  clinical examination, 1: 414
  death concept, 1: 411
  definition, 1: 403
  and delinquency, 1: 413
  emergency treatment, 1: 420
  family background, 1: 422
  incidence, 1: 404
  incidence in Great Britain, 1: 406
  long-term treatment, 1: 422
  parental attitudes, 1: 415
  prognosis, 1: 424
  prophylaxis, 1: 424
  psychopathology, 1: 408
  and psychosis, 1: 413
  special investigations, 1: 424
  treatment of depression, 1: 421
Sun stroke, 3: 715
Super-ego, 2: 514; 3: 245

Supervision
  in psychiatric hospitals, 2: 723, 724
Surgery
  emotional adjustment to, 3: 509
  phantom phenomena, 2: 134, 135
  sensory deprivation, 2: 248
  in ulcerative colitis, 3: 506-510
Susto, 2: 706
Swaddling, 2: 150, 151
Sydenham's chorea, 1: 342
Symbiosis
  prenatal, 3: 159
Symbiotic activity, 3: 211
Symbiotic contact, 3: 105
Symbiotic psychosis, 3: 653, 658
Symbiotic relationship, 2: 397
Symonds Picture Story Test, 1: 576
Symptom
  definition, 2: 428
  formation, 2: 395, 397
  migration, 2: 181
  substitution, 2: 571, 586
Symptomatology
  shift, 2: 397
Synapse, 2: 50, 60
  cleft, 2: 60
  junctions, 2: 60
  knobs, 2: 109
  transmission, 2: 109
  vesicles, 2: 60
Syndrome
  definition, 2: 428
  shift, 1: 312
Syphilis
  cerebral, 2: 441
  psychosis, 2: 442
Systematic Interview Guides, 3: 44, 55, 56

Taboos, 3: 293
Tabula rasa, 2: 161, 223
Tarantism, 2: 705
Taraxein, 2: 15
TAT (Thematic Appperception Test)
  interpretation, 2: 369, 370
Tavistock Clinic
  psychoanalysis, 2: 477
Team concept (in psychiatry), 1, 254
Telemetry
  EEG, 3: 393
Temperament, 1: 108
  brain-damaged children, 3: 74
  categories, 3: 68
  clusters, 3: 69
  environment interaction, 3: 70
  individuality, 3: 68
  mentally retarded children, 3: 76
Temperature control, 2: 314
Template, 2: 266, 272, 273
Teratogens
  drugs, 3: 50

SUBJECT INDEX

emotional stress, **3:** 27-37
folklore, **3:** 19
infections, **3:** 20-27
Terman-Merrill Test, **1:** 573
Tests (psychological), **1:** 276, 374, 455, 562; **2:** 358, 360, 369
 Alexander Passalong Test, **1:** 572
 and anxiety, **1:** 574
 Children's Apperception Test, **1:** 577
 colour vision, **1:** 582
 'completion' techniques, **1:** 578
 'constructive' techniques, **1:** 577
 and cultural influences, **1:** 574
 description of patient, **2:** 374
 developmental quotient, **1:** 566
 diagnostic use of intelligence test, **1:** 571
 Drever-Collins Test, **1:** 572
 educational attainment, **1:** 580
 'expressive techniques', **1:** 579
 Family Attitudes Test, **1:** 577
 Family Relations Indicator, **1:** 577; **2:** 660; **3:** 147
 Family Relations Test, **1:** 579
 'forced choice' techniques, **1:** 578
 Gesell Developmental Schedules, **1:** 556
 Griffiths Mental Development Scale, **1:** 566
 intelligence, **1:** 185, 193, 565
 Inter Personal Perception Method, **2:** 410
 interpretation, **2:** 369
 Merrill-Palmer Scale, **1:** 567
 Mooney Problem Check List, **1:** 579
 organic involvement, **1:** 582
 and personality, **1:** 574
 for physically handicapped children, **1:** 572
 pre-school children, **1:** 565
 Progressive Matrices, **1:** 570
 projective techniques, **1:** 575
 results, **1:** 573, 583
 Rorschach test, **2:** 368, 369, 370
 school-age children, **1:** 568
 scoring, **1:** 564
 Stanford-Binet Intelligence Scale, **1:** 570
 Symonds Picture Story Test, **1:** 576
 Terman-Merrill Test, **1:** 573
 Thematic Apperception Test, **2:** 369, 370
 Two-Houses Technique, **1:** 579
 vocational guidance, **1:** 581
 Wechsler Adult Intelligence Scale, **1:** 571
 Wechsler Intelligence Scale for Children, **1:** 568
Thalamic nuclei, **2:** 315, 316, 333, 334
Thalamus, **2:** 317, 326
 cortico-thalamic connections, **2:** 332
 sensory input, **2:** 344
Thalidomide, **1:** 222, 515; **2:** 135; **3:** 50, 51
Therapeutic clubs, **3:** 289
Therapy, **1:** 279
 aims, **3:** 14

in accident proneness, **1:** 364
in adolescents, **1:** 296, 298, 300, 302
aversion, **1:** 163; **2:** 567
behaviour, **1:** 154; **2:** 557
in brain damage, **1:** 458
child, **1:** 280, 523, 539
childhood psychosis, **1:** 491
childhood schizophrenia, **3:** 685-705
community psychiatry, **2:** 675
conjoint, **2:** 642
cultural aspects, **2:** 707
in delinquency, **1:** 390; **2:** 570
and diagnosis, **2:** 366, 367, 368
drugs (q.v.)
ECT, **2:** 633
evaluation, **3:** 785
extra-clinic, **1:** 281
family, **2:** 661; **3:** 286
family-group, **1:** 281; **2:** 397, 641
family psychiatry, **2:** 637; **3:** 285
father's resistance, **3:** 146
group (*see* Group therapy)
group hypnosis, **2:** 577
Hampstead Child Therapy Clinic (q.v.)
in-patient (child), **1:** 539
intra-clinic, **1:** 279
learning, **1:** 110; **2:** 557
malaria therapy, **3:** 613
Morita therapy (q.v.)
parent, **1:** 281
parent-child separation, **3:** 284-289
placebos, **2:** 610
play, **1:** 280; **2:** 667
prolonged, **1:** 281
psychoanalytic, **2:** 448, 457, 471, 476, 479, 557, 558
psychopharmacology, **2:** 620
psychoses chemotherapy, **2:** 627
psychosomatic disorders, **1:** 327
psychotherapy (q.v.)
religious, **2:** 708
residential care, **2:** 668
sensory deprivation, **2:** 249
sleep, **2:** 707
social psychiatry, **2:** 676
in suicide, **1:** 420
supportive, **1:** 281
therapeutic community, **2:** 675, 691
therapeutic culture, **2:** 693
ulcerative colitis in children, **3:** 500
vector therapy (q.v.)
Thinking, **1:** 170 (*see also* Thought)
 abstract, **1:** 76
 animistic, **1:** 73
 conceptual, **1:** 68
 conservation, **1:** 72, 75
 egocentric, **1:** 73
 and intelligence, **1:** 184
 intuitive, **1:** 71
 operational, **1:** 74

Thinking—cont.
  operative, 3: 214
  Piaget's theory, 1: 58
  pre-conceptual, 1: 67
  reversible, 1: 74
  schemata, 1: 68
  symbolic, 1: 67
  transduction, 1: 70
Thought (see also Thinking)
  brain mechanisms, 2: 322
  consciousness, 2: 343
  frontal lobes and planned initiative, 2: 326
  inborn reflex action, 2: 314
  mind and brain mechanism, 2: 340
  neurophysiological basis, 2: 313
  perception and interpretive cortex, 2: 335
  physical basis, 2: 332
  sensory and motor apparatus, 2: 315
  speech, 2: 328
Thought disorders
  acute delirium syndrome, 3: 727
Thumbsucking, 3: 179, 187
Tics, 1: 115, 293; 2: 377
Toddler (see also Child and Infant)
  aggressive assertiveness, 3: 182
  autonomy of self-direction, 3: 182
  body image, 3: 185
  conflict, 3: 181
  dependency, 3: 178
  destructiveness, 3: 179
  development of character traits, 3: 189
  deviations in development 3: 187
  discrimination 3: 183
  erotic play 3: 180
  fears of mutilation 3: 181
  hostility 3: 179
  hyperactivity 3: 179
  intellectual learning 3: 184
  interest in feces 3: 180
  jealousy, 3: 182
  learning to love, 3: 191
  memory, 3: 185
  needs, 3: 177
  nightmares, 3: 181
  Oedipal manifestations, 3: 181
  parental permissiveness, 3: 188
  phobias of animals, 3: 181
  play group, 3: 225
  punishment, 3: 184
  regression, 3: 187
  rivalry with parents, 3: 181
  self appraisal, 3: 186
  self assertion, 3: 178
  self feeding, 3: 178
  sense of self, 3: 185
  sensuality, 3: 179
  sexual interests, 3: 179
  skills of self-care, 3: 186
  sleeping difficulties, 3: 179
  symptomatic regressiveness, 3: 184
  tendency to regression, 3: 179
  thumb sucking, 3: 179, 187
  toilet training (q.v.)
  whining, 3: 183
Todd's paralysis, 2: 122
Toilet training, 1: 183; 3: 103, 109, 164, 185, 296, 310, 325
Totems, 3: 293
Toxoplasmosis
  brain damage, 3: 24-25
  congenital, 3: 24, 25
  epilepsy, 3: 24, 25
  hydrocephalus, 3: 24
  stillbirth, 3: 25
  strabismus, 3: 24, 25
Trance, 2: 271
  amnesia, 2: 156
  deep-trance subject, 2: 152
  depth, 2: 152
  form of suggestion, 2: 153
  possession states, 2: 705
  recognition of, 2: 153
Tranquillizers, 2: xxiii, 622, 623
  ulcerative colitis in children, 3: 502
Transcultural psychiatry, 2: 697-712
  Amok, 2: 705
  anxiety states, 2: 704
  clinical issues, 2: 700
  comparative studies, 2: 699
  cultural stresses, 2: 702
  definitions, 2: 697
  depression, 2: 701
  drugs, 2: 707, 708, 709
  homicide, 2: 704
  homosexuality, 2: 702
  hysteria, 2: 702, 704
  Japanese family dynamics, 3: 356-368
  Kitsunetsuki, 2: 705
  Koro, 2: 705, 706
  Latah, 2: 705
  mental disorders frequency, (relative) 2: 701; (total) 2: 700
  mental disorders symptomatology, 2: 703
  methodology, 2: 699
  migration, 2: 703
  Morita therapy (q.v.)
  native healers, 2: 707
  obsession, 2: 702
  possession states, 2: 705
  primitive cultures, 2: 700
  psychosomatic disorders, 2: 702
  psychotic behaviour differences, 2: 704
  religious therapy, 2: 708
  research, 2: 709
  scapegoat, 2: 653, 708, 709
  schizophrenia, 2: 701, 704
  suicide, 2: 702
  Susto, 2: 706
  tarantism, 2: 705

SUBJECT INDEX

trance states, 2: 705
treatment, 2: 706
Windigo, 2: 705
Transference, 2: 501, 600
in children's analysis, 3: 249
therapeutic community, 2: 693
Transvestism, 2: 42
avoidance conditioning, 2: 568
Trial marriage, 3: 299
Trisomy (Triplo-X error), 1: 47-50; 2: 36, 37
Tritiated-thymidine, 2: 23, 24
Tumours
intercranial, 3: 711
Tunnel vision, 2: 154, 159
Turner's syndrome, 1: 50, 513; 2: 17, 33, 34, 35
abortuses, 2: 34
EEG, 2: 35
hearing, 2: 35
intelligence, 2: 34
reading ability, 2: 35
sexual development, 2: 34
space-form blindness, 2: 34
Twilight state, 3: 724
Twins
genetics, 1: 39
schizophrenia, 2: 13
studies, 1: 39, 186, 380; 3: 240
Two-Houses Technique, 1: 579

Ulcerative colitis
in children (*see below*)
hypnosis, 2: 180, 181
Ulcerative colitis in children, 1: 319, 320
aetiology, 3: 499
anaclitic therapy, 3: 516
carcinoma of the bowel, 3: 496, 506, 508
chronic, 3: 496
comprehensive approach to treatment, 3: 521
diet, 3: 503
emotional adjustment after surgery, 3: 509
environmental manipulation, 3: 521
epidemiology, 3: 495
extracolonic manifestation, 3: 496, 507
family functioning, 3: 498
family group therapy, 3: 520
fathers, 3: 145, 498
group therapy, 3: 520
hospitalization, 3: 501
ileostomy clubs, 3: 520
incidence, 3: 495
interpretative play, 3: 517, 518
management, 3: 494-525
mortality, 3: 496
mother-child relationship, 3: 497
operative mortality, 3: 508
parent-child interaction, 3: 501

pathology of bowel, 3: 495
patient-physician relationship, 3: 503
personality, 3: 497
post-operative complications, 3: 508
predisposition, 3: 500
prevention, 3: 524
prognosis, 3: 507
psychoanalysis, 3: 511
psychophysiologic interrelationships, 3: 498
psychosocial factors, 3: 496
psychotherapy, 3: 504, 508, 509, 510
regression, 3: 509, 516
replacement therapy, 3: 516
results of psychotherapy, 3: 511
separation, 3: 506
siblings, 3: 498
somatic clinical picture, 3: 495
spontaneous remission, 3: 514
steroid therapy, 3: 502
stress, 3: 499
surgery, 3: 506-510
theoretical models, 3: 499
therapy, 3: 500
tranquillizers, 3: 502
ward management conference, 3: 522
work with parents, 3: 505, 519
Unconscious (the), 2: 505; 3: 214, 246
Unconscious mind
hypnosis, 2: 156
Underfunctioning, 1: 207
segregation, 3: 308
Uraemia
psychotic disorders, 3: 713
Urban industrialization
Utero
child's hazards in, 3: 19-60

Vagotomy, 3: 507
Value orientation
stress, 2: 703
Vascular lesion, 2: 114
Vector therapy, 2: 642; 3: 586-587
application, 2: 671
definition, 2: 669; 3: 286
facilities, 2: 671
psychotherapy, 2: 670
residential care, 2: 668
separation, 2: 671
Vertigo, 2: 132, 140
Vesania, 2: 440; 3: 593, 598
Vigilance, 2: 111
decline, 2: 198
Vitamin B_1 deficiency, 2: 119, 120
Vocabulary, 1: 204
Vocational guidance, 1: 581
Voice control, 2: 333
Vulnerability
age, 2: 653

Vulnerability—*cont.*
  sex, **2:** 653
  stress, **2:** 652

Waiting list, **1:** 274
Waking dream, **2:** 292
War
  and medical progress, **2:** xx
  and neurosis, **2:** xxi
Warts
  hypnosis, **2:** 181
Weaning, **3:** 190, 296
Wechsler Adult Intelligence Scale, **1:** 571
Wechsler Intelligence Scale for Children, **1:** 568

Weck-analysis, **2:** 624
  hysteria, **2:** 624
  intellectual stimulation, **2:** 624
Wernicke's encephalopathy, **2:** 114, 118, 120
Whorls, **2:** 82
Windigo, **2:** 705
Witch doctors, **2:** 151
Word-blindness, **1:** 137, 344
Writer's cramp, **2:** 509, 510

Xg^a blood group, **2:** 28

Yantra, **2:** 271

CONTENTS OF MODERN PERSPECTIVES IN CHILD PSYCHIATRY

EDITOR'S PREFACE

PART ONE
SCIENTIFIC BASIS OF CHILD PSYCHIATRY

I   RESEARCH METHODOLOGY AND CHILD PSYCHIATRY
    H. GWYNNE JONES

II THE CONTRIBUTION OF ETHOLOGY TO CHILD PSYCHIATRY
    EWAN C. GRANT

III THE GENETICAL ASPECTS OF CHILD PSYCHIATRY   VALERIE COWIE

IV PIAGET'S THEORY   MARY WOODWARD

V   THE DEVELOPMENT OF PERCEPTION   M. D. VERNON

VI THE APPLICATION OF LEARNING THEORY TO CHILD PSYCHIATRY
    H. J. EYSENCK and S. J. RACHMAN

VII THINKING, REMEMBERING AND IMAGINING   PETER MCKELLAR

VIII EXCEPTIONAL CHILDREN   E. M. BARTLETT

IX NORMAL CHILD DEVELOPMENT AND HANDICAPPED CHILDREN
    ELSPETH STEPHEN and JEAN ROBERTSON

X   CHILD PSYCHOPATHOLOGY   FREDERICK H. STONE

PART TWO
CLINICAL ASPECTS OF CHILD PSYCHIATRY

XI   ORGANISATION OF CHILD PSYCHIATRIC SERVICES
     JOHN G. HOWELLS

XII THE PSYCHIATRY OF ADOLESCENTS   WILFRID WARREN

XIII THE PSYCHOSOMATIC APPROACH IN CHILD PSYCHIATRY
     PHILIP PINKERTON

XIV DISORDERS OF SPEECH IN CHILDHOOD   C. WORSTER-DROUGHT

XV   ACCIDENT PRONENESS   GERARD VAUGHAN

XVI DELINQUENCY   P. D. SCOTT

XVII SUICIDAL ATTEMPTS IN CHILDHOOD AND ADOLESCENCE
     P. H. CONNELL

XVIII THE PSYCHIATRIC ASPECTS OF ADOPTION   HILDA LEWIS

XIX THE NEUROPSYCHIATRY OF CHILDHOOD   D. A. POND

XX   THE PSYCHOSES OF CHILDHOOD   GERALD O'GORMAN

XXI THE AETIOLOGY OF MENTAL SUBNORMALITY   BRIAN KIRMAN

XXII CHILD THERAPY: A CASE OF ANTI-SOCIAL BEHAVIOUR
     D. W. WINNICOTT

XXIII CHILDREN'S IN-PATIENT PSYCHIATRIC UNITS
      W. J. BLACHFORD ROGERS

XXIV THE CONTRIBUTION OF PSYCHOLOGICAL TESTS TO CHILD
     PSYCHIATRY   JOHN R. LICKORISH

INDEX

CONTENTS OF MODERN PERSPECTIVES IN WORLD PSYCHIATRY

EDITOR'S PREFACE
INTRODUCTION Lord Adrian, o.m.

PART ONE
Scientific

I A CRITICAL SURVEY OF SCHIZOPHRENIA GENETICS
Professor Lionel Penrose, f.r.s.
II THE SIGNIFICANCE OF NUCLEAR SEXING Professor M. L. Barr
III THE CYTOLOGY OF BRAIN CELLS AND CULTURED NERVOUS TISSUES Dr F. H. Kasten
IV THE CHEMICAL PROCESSES OF MEMORY Dr Bruce S. McEwen
V THE MEANING OF MEMORY Lord Brain, f.r.s.
VI CORPOREAL AWARENESS Dr Macdonald Critchley
VII THE PHENOMENA OF HYPNOSIS Dr Stephen Black
VIII SLEEPING AND DREAMING Dr Ian Oswald
IX SENSORY DEPRIVATION Dr Philip Solomon and Dr A. M. Rossi
X HALLUCINATIONS Dr L. J. West
XI MODEL PSYCHOSES Dr Elliot D. Luby and Dr J. S. Gottlieb
XII THE NEUROPHYSIOLOGICAL BASIS OF THOUGHT
Professor Wilder Penfield, o.m., c.c., f.r.s.

PART TWO
Clinical

XIII THE CONTRIBUTIONS OF CLINICAL PSYCHOLOGY TO PSYCHIATRY
Professor H. J. Eysenck
XIV FAMILY PSYCHOPATHOLOGY AND SCHIZOPHRENIA
Dr John G. Howells
XV THE SYMPTOMATOLOGY, CLINICAL FORMS AND NOSOLOGY OF SCHIZOPHRENIA Professor A. V. Snezhnevsky
XVI PSYCHOANALYSIS—AN EVALUATION Dr R. B. White
XVII EXISTENTIAL ANALYSIS Dr G. Condrau and Professor Medard Boss
XVIII MORITA THERAPY Professor Kazuyoshi Ikeda
XIX PAVLOVIAN THEORY IN PSYCHIATRY Professor K. K. Monakhov
XX LEARNING THERAPIES Dr Joseph Wolpe
XXI THEORY AND PRACTICE OF GROUP HYPNOSIS IN U.S.S.R.
Professor N. V. Ivanov
XXII THE PLACEBO RESPONSE Dr A. K. Shapiro
XXIII CLINICAL PERSPECTIVES IN PSYCHOPHARMACOLOGY
Professor Jean Delay and Professor Pierre Deniker
XXIV FAMILY PSYCHIATRY Dr John G. Howells
XXV COMMUNITY PSYCHIATRY Dr Maxwell Jones
XXVI TRANSCULTURAL PSYCHIATRY Professor E. D. Wittkower
XXVII GENERAL PRINCIPLES OF CONSTRUCTION OF PSYCHIATRIC HOSPITALS Professor Paul Sivadon

AUTHOR INDEX

SUBJECT INDEX